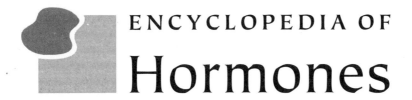

ENCYCLOPEDIA OF
Hormones

VOLUME 3
N–Z, Index

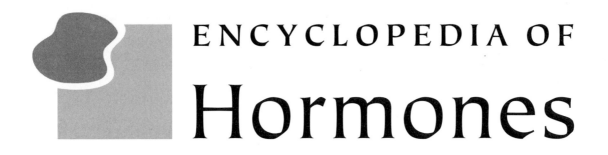

ENCYCLOPEDIA OF
Hormones

EDITORS-IN-CHIEF

HELEN L. HENRY
ANTHONY W. NORMAN
University of California, Riverside

VOLUME 3
N–Z, Index

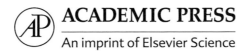

ACADEMIC PRESS
An imprint of Elsevier Science

Amsterdam   Boston   Heidelberg   London   New York   Oxford
Paris   San Diego   San Francisco   Singapore   Sydney   Tokyo

Academic Press
An imprint of Elsevier Inc.
525 B Street, Suite 1900, San Diego, California 92101-4495, USA
http://www.academicpress.com

Elsevier Science Ltd.
The Boulevard, Langford Lane, Kidlington, Oxford OX5 1GB, UK
http://www.elsevier.com

Library of Congress Catalog Card Number: 2003103057

International Standard Book Number: 0-12-341103-3 (set)
International Standard Book Number: 0-12-341104-1 (Volume 1)
International Standard Book Number: 0-12-341105-X (Volume 2)
International Standard Book Number: 0-12-341106-8 (Volume 3)

Printed in the United States of America
03 04 05 06 08 MP 9 8 7 6 5 4 3 2 1

CONTENTS

CONTENTS OF VOLUME 2

CONTENTS BY SUBJECT AREA

FEMALE REPRODUCTION
Evan R. Simpson, Associate Editor

GASTROINTESTINAL HORMONES
George H. Greeley, Jr., Associate Editor

GROWTH FACTORS
Antony W. Burgess, Associate Editor

NEUROENDOCRINOLOGY

Martin J. Kelly and Charles Eugene Roselli, Associate Editors

NUCLEAR SIGNAL TRANSDUCTION

Nancy L. Weigel, Associate Editor

PANCREAS
R. Paul Robertson, Associate Editor

PLANT HORMONES
Paul B. Larsen, Associate Editor

THYROID
Roy E. Weiss, Associate Editor

FOREWORD

The discipline of endocrinology was born with the discovery of hormones, but the concept of endocrinology has been substantially expanded by the more recent discovery of paracrine and autocrine regulators. The field of hormone action was formed to understand the molecular mechanisms by which hormones act in cells, and continues to expand explosively. In the late 1960s, the prevailing view of hormone action ranged from effects on membrane transport of nutrients and precursors for RNA and protein synthesis to effects on the translation of mRNA at the level of ribosomes. Nevertheless, a cadre of voices predicted a possible nuclear action on mRNA synthesis. These voices were correct in that steroid hormones, acting via their receptors, indeed were proved to regulate gene transcription. To the best of my knowledge, the first paper to be presented at the national endocrine meetings in a new field of hormone action was in 1967, and it dealt with hormonal stimulation of oviductal protein synthesis. It was about this time that a small group of scientists interested in hormone effects in cells attended a Gordon Conference in New Hampshire; this was one of the first conferences to focus an entire program on hormone action and mechanisms. The attendees were primarily involved in aspects of steroid hormone and thyroid hormone actions; peptide hormone action was yet to experience its own birth and a similar expansive growth. Only a short time previously, Elwood Jensen had discovered the estrogen-binding protein that eventually became the "estrogen receptor," thus it was logical that the conference dealt mainly with steroid receptors; there were also a few papers presenting data that steroid hormones could induce specific enzyme/protein synthesis in target cells. The mechanisms of these effects were the subject of great debate at this first conference on steroid hormone action, a meeting that persists to this day in New England each summer.

Following the monumental discovery of peptide immunoassays, workers in the peptide field were immersed in the work of measuring hormones, ranging from insulin, to luteinizing hormone, to follicle-stimulating hormone, to thrytropin-releasing hormone, to growth hormone, to name a few. For over a decade, little attention was given to the more difficult task of understanding the functions of their receptors and intracellular signaling pathways. Nevertheless, the advent of this assay methodology, including the ability to synthesize radiolabeled peptide hormones, eventually allowed the identification and quantification of cell surface receptors for peptide and amine-containing hormones. The time of this application was about 1970. Researchers demonstrated that cAMP levels were induced in concert with ligand occupation of certain membrane receptors, and the second messenger cAMP was postulated to initiate intracellular phosphorylation of unknown targets. At this point, the field of peptide hormone action also was born.

The two distinct but related fields, steroid hormone action and peptide hormone action, developed together for much of the next decade. Hormone action conferences invariably contained talks on both types of receptors and progress was rapid and in concert with the development of molecular biology. In the steroid field, progress was more rapid initially, but by the mid 1980s, the peptide field attained equal mechanistic status.

Investigators of steroid hormone action concentrated on first understanding the "pathway of action" for their hormones. Scientists looked for model systems showing large responses to steroids. One approach was to assess changes in enzyme levels in cultured cells. The intact chicken oviduct was another of the more notable systems, in that regard because of the ability of sex steroids (estrogen, progesterone) to induce large increases both in certain egg-white proteins and in their respective mRNAs. Viral proteins also were shown to be induced by glucocorticoids. The finding that purified steroid receptors could bind to DNA directly led to a new understanding of the pathway of steroid, to intracellular receptor, to DNA, to mRNA, to protein, and to function. Still, many complexities remained to be sorted out when the receptor cDNAs were cloned in the 1980s.

Our concept of hormones expanded considerably with the advent of growth factors and cytokines. Arguably, the myriads of growth factors only represent an additional list of peptidelike hormones that often act within the tissue of their origin; they have a strong predilection for growth and cell cycle control. Cytokines have both local and distal actions and are particularly oriented to processes such as smooth muscle function and inflammation and apoptosis.

For a decade, it seems as if the peptide action researchers were unduly fixated on cAMP induction and protein kinase A activation. The complexity of signaling pathways emanating from membrane receptors increased logarithmically with the discovery of the numerous protein kinases that phosphorylated serine and tyrosine, the kinase-kinases, the phosphatases, the calcium and diacylglycerol regulators, and the regulators of all of the phosphorylation intermediates. The types of receptors that proliferated ranged from seven membrane (protein kinase A), growth factors (tyrosine kinase, protein kinase C), cytokine, and eventually even chemokine in nature. The appreciation of G-proteins as upstream targets of the cAMP pathway was key to eventual solutions of the signaling cascade. The discoveries of the ras/raf pathway for mediating the effects of mitogens, and the JAK/Stat pathway as mediator for cytokines and certain peptide hormone effects, were also important milestones in unraveling signal transduction in eukaryotic cells. The realization that CREB and Stat proteins were regulatable transcription factors that eventually acted on DNA united the steroid–peptide fields, in part, at the level of the nucleus. That order was made out of apparent chaos is a striking tribute to the intellectual prowess and perseverance of the workers in this field. Most importantly, the signaling pathways emanating from the membrane have brought new insights to pathologies such as cancer, and have led to an explosive development of new pharmaceutical stimulators and inhibitors, with good promise for therapies of neuropsychiatric disorders, cancer, and other human disorders.

After a consolidation period in the 1970s, the steroid action field heated up again with the cloning of the steroid, thyroid, vitamin D, and retinoic receptors. Certain unpredictable events occurred. Investigators began to clone (by cross-screening) numerous molecules that were similar to steroid receptors, but that were not known to be activated by an existing ligand. The term "orphan receptors" was born and the deduction was made that the steroid receptors were part of a giant superfamily of nuclear receptor transcription factors, numbering 48 in humans. The availability of cloned cDNAs and other reagents allowed mutational analyses of receptors, followed by their reintroduction into cells to monitor effects on synthetic reporter genes; structure–function relationships proved the existence of receptor domains for transcriptional activation, nuclear translocation, and DNA binding. Now at a frenetic pace, information on dimeric DNA binding and heterodimeric partners (retinoic acid X receptor), receptor crosstalk with peptide pathways, ligand-independent receptor activation, and receptor phosphorylation was accumulated. More definitive appreciation of the biology of classical and orphan receptors was accomplished by the emerging transgenic technologies and gene knock-out strategies. The ability to screen for new ligands for orphan receptors extended the range of hormones to lipids (peroxisome proliferator-activated receptors) and other previously unsuspected metabolic regulators. The yearly stream of publications on the physiology of orphan receptors and their novel ligands continued to bring excitement and more expansion to the field. Pharmaceutical companies salivated at the possibilities of new drugs acting at the nuclear level. The tamoxifen paradox (it acts in one tissue as an agonist and in another as an antagonist) provided encouragement for the generation of a successful search for selective receptor modulators that contain tissue- and function-specific profiles.

Still, the field clamored for a greater molecular understanding of how the nuclear receptors worked at the level of DNA. The discovery of receptor-associated regulatory proteins provided this missing link and changed the field of hormone action further. We moved from a situation wherein many believed that intracellular receptors carried out the transcriptional regulation inherent to the actions of steroid/thyroid hormones and vitamins, to an understanding that the receptor-associated "coregulators" are the primary mediators of this genetic response. We now know that the receptor co-activators act as powerful transducers of hormone action, either through inherent enzyme activities or by serving as a scaffold for recruitment of additional co-activator proteins. The coregulators can be divided loosely into two camps: co-activators and co-repressors. Taken together, these molecules mediate the two main tasks of receptors: stimulation and repression of gene expression.

It is perhaps fitting that a burst of recent attention has focused again on the membrane, where both steroids and their receptors have been postulated to have biologically important effects. Actions of nuclear receptors, and also of free hormones binding to traditional membrane receptors or ion channels, are likely to be of increasing future interest to workers investigating hormonal function. In this respect, we have traveled full circle. I have no doubt that the future will see many additional examples of membrane reinforcement of nuclear gene regulation, of important ligand-independent activities of receptors initiated at the membrane, and of pathway crosstalk among the varieties of hormones and their intracellular pathways.

These volumes of the *Encyclopedia of Hormones* represent one of the most ambitious projects completed to date in the field of hormones and their actions. The Editors have assembled articles that address a full spectrum of the biology and cellular physiology of numerous hormones and their actions in many species. This effort allows the reader the opportunity to survey the state of both membrane receptor-initiated signaling and nuclear receptor-initiated signaling from the viewpoints of a wide variety of leading investigators. The history and breadth of this field are evident within the articles of these volumes. The ambitious project will stand as a major reference source for the field, and I predict that readers will have no problem savoring the current rapid progress and heightened excitement that exists in this vast field of molecular endocrinology.

BERT W. O'MALLEY
Thompson Professor and Chair
Department of Molecular and Cellular Biology
Baylor College of Medicine Houston, Texas

PREFACE

The publication of the *Encyclopedia of Hormones* is intended to provide a comprehensive reference work on all known hormones in vertebrate animals, insects, and plants. The list of classical hormones that had been discovered and characterized over the interval from 1914 to 1985 numbered approximately 55; however, as a consequence of the application of modern chemical characterization techniques and molecular biology methodology, this list now exceeds 150 and is still expanding. In fact, during the production interval for the *Encyclopedia,* several new hormones were discovered and new activities for existing hormones were clearly defined. In addition, enormous strides have been made in our understanding of the detailed actions of hormones at the molecular and cellular levels. There have been dramatic applications of this new knowledge in the medical arena with respect to both diagnosis and treatment of diseases; for the plant and insect hormones, new applications have arisen in the realms of agricultural biotechnology and biological control.

Some comment is appropriate concerning the definition of a hormone that has been utilized in compiling entries in the *Encyclopedia.* Of course, the classical definition of a hormone is that it is a chemical messenger in the body: it is secreted by an endocrine gland and is delivered through the circulatory system to target cells that possess receptors specific for the hormone. Occupancy of the receptor by its cognate hormone leads to the initiation of signal transduction processes that result in generation of specific biological responses. But in this post-human-genome era, and with the rich array of technologies used to study and define at the cellular and molecular levels the enormous array of signal transduction pathways employed by cells, the Editors have adopted a broader definition of hormone. Hormones can now be considered to include not only chemical messengers in the classical sense, but also local paracrine and autocrine signals. Thus, the *Encyclopedia* includes articles on many growth factors, interleukins, and intracellular mediators of signal transduction.

The *Encyclopedia of Hormones* is intended to serve as a useful and comprehensive source of information spanning all aspects of the general subject of hormones. It consists of nearly 300 articles that collectively describe hormones from several key perspectives: (1) the cellular and subcellular sites of functioning of the hormone, (2) the major physiological system(s) in which it is operative (e.g., reproductive, immune, neuroendocrine, digestive, and developmental), (3) the nature of the receptor and signal transduction pathway(s) used by the hormone (e.g., nuclear or membrane signal transduction), and (4) for the vertebrate hormones, the important diseases of deficiency or excess or other instances for which there is unusual molecular insight available. We expect that the *Encyclopedia of Hormones* will be as useful to the scientific expert concerned with cutting-edge questions as it will be to students and interested nonscientists.

Given the broad scope of such a major reference work, it was essential to assemble a team of Associate Editors. Each of these 14 individuals has dedicated his or her professional career to researching scholarly endeavors in a specific domain of hormones and, as a consequence of the breadth and depth of achievement in this area, is an acknowledged leader in their field. These interests include the hormone domains of adrenal cortex, calcium-regulating hormones, cytokines, female reproduction, male reproduction, gastrointestinal hormones, growth factors, thyroid, membrane signal transduction, neuroendocrinology, nuclear signal transduction, pancreas, plant hormones, and insect hormones.

The *Encyclopedia* was launched at a two-day meeting of the Editors, Associate Editors, and Elsevier–Academic Press representatives in La Jolla, California, in April, 2001. Here the preliminary list of article titles prepared by the Editors was refined and a list of potential authors created. Each Associate Editor was then responsible for the crucial process of recruiting authors for the individual entries. As the manuscripts were received by Academic Press, they were critically reviewed by the Associate Editors and Editors, as well as by the editorial staff at Academic Press. The final total of 296 articles entered production in only 16 months.

All of the articles are formatted according to the same blueprint and each is intended to be a self-contained presentation. Each article begins with a brief topical content outline that provides the reader with a listing of the major topics presented in the article. The article body begins with an introductory paragraph that defines the topic under discussion and summarizes the content of the article. Following the article are reference citations to provide the reader with access to further in-depth consideration of the topic at hand and a cross-reference to related entries in the *Encyclopedia*. A glossary list defines key terms that may be unfamiliar to the reader and are important to an understanding of the article. A compilation of all glossary terms appearing in the complete multivolume *Encyclopedia* is presented in the final volume as a dictionary of subject matter relevant to hormones.

If the *Encyclopedia* has merit, it is due largely to the contributions of the authors of all the articles, and as well to the dedication of the Associate Editors. Shortcomings are, of course, the responsibility of the Editors and we would appreciate having them brought to our attention. The completion of this large project in the relatively short time, from launch meeting to the actual printing of the *Encyclopedia* (only 23 months), is the result of much hard work and dedication. Certainly the primary credit must go to the some 500 authors who prepared their contributions in a timely fashion. The board of Associate Editors also provided exceptional leadership and service. The Editors thank them all.

Finally, thanks are due to the staff of Elsevier–Academic Press, including Tari Paschall, Judy Meyer, Chris Morris, and Carolan Gladden, who each provided skillful and friendly ongoing management of the project.

HELEN L. HENRY
ANTHONY W. NORMAN

GUIDE TO USING
THE ENCYCLOPEDIA

The *Encyclopedia of Hormones* is a comprehensive description of all known hormones in vertebrate animals, insects, and plants. It includes hormones in the classical sense of the term (chemical messengers) and also in the expanded contemporary sense (local paracrine and autocrine signaling).

This reference work consists of three separate volumes and includes about 300 different articles on various aspects of the subject of hormones. Each entry in the encyclopedia provides a focused description of the given topic, intended to inform a broad spectrum of readers, ranging from research professionals to students to the interested general public.

In order that you, the reader, will derive the greatest possible benefit from your use of the *Encyclopedia of Hormones*, we have provided this guide. It explains how the encyclopedia is organized and how the information within it can be located.

Organization

For the purpose of this encyclopedia, chief editors Dr. Helen Henry and Dr. Anthony Norman, in collaboration with the various associate editors, have defined the study of hormones as consisting of 14 distinct subject areas, as follows:

Adrenal Cortex
Calcium Regulating Hormones
Cytokines
Female Reproduction
Gastrointestinal Hormones
Growth Factors
Insect Hormones
Male Reproduction
Membrane Signal Transduction
Neuroendocrinology
Nuclear Signal Transduction
Pancreas
Plant Hormones
Thyroid

Each of these subject areas was then assigned by the chief editors to an associate editor with particular expertise in that discipline. The editor in question was primarily responsible for the selection of topics and authors in this area, and for the review and approval of manuscripts.

Every article in the encyclopedia is designated as part of a particular one of these 14 subject areas. Please see p. xv of this introductory section for a complete listing of the articles in the encyclopedia according to subject area.

Format

All of the articles in the *Encyclopedia of Hormones* are arranged in a single alphabetical sequence by title. Articles whose titles begin with the letters A to F are in Volume 1, articles with titles from G to M are in Volume 2, and articles from N to Z are in Volume 3, along with the glossary and subject index.

So that they can be easily located, article titles generally begin with the key word or phrase indicating the topic, with any generic terms following. Thus, for example, "Erythropoietin, Biochemistry of" is the article title rather than "Biochemistry of Erythropoietin," and "Spermatogenesis, Hormonal Control of" is the title rather than "Hormonal Control of Spermatogenesis."

Outline

Entries in the encyclopedia begin with a topical outline that indicates the general content of the article. This outline provides a preview of the article, so that the reader can get a sense of what is contained there without having to leaf through the pages. It also serves to highlight important subtopics that are discussed within the article. For example, the article "Insect Endocrine System" includes subtopics such as "The Importance of Insect Hormones," "Insect Body Plan and Degrees of Metamorphosis," and "Neurosecretory System."

The outline is intended as an overview and thus it lists only the major headings of the article. In addition, second-level and third-level headings will be found within the article.

Defining Paragraph

The text of each article begins with a single introductory paragraph that is displayed in boldface and set off from the rest of the article. This introduction defines the topic under discussion and summarizes the content of the article. For example, the entry "Glucocorticoids, Pharmacology of" begins with the following defining paragraph:

> **Normal levels of glucocorticoids are essential for the maintenance of physiologic homeostasis and for an adequate response to stress. Both the lack of glucocorticoids (adrenal insufficiency) and excess glucocorticoids (as seen in Cushing syndrome) lead to life-threatening conditions.**

Glossary

The glossary section appears at the end of the article text. It contains terms that are important to an understanding of the article and that may be unfamiliar to the reader. Each term is defined in the context of the particular article in which it is used. The encyclopedia includes approximately 1,500 glossary terms. For example, the article "Gastrin" includes the following glossary entries (among others):

cholecystokinin A peptide hormone produced in the small intestine and the brain that is homologous to gastrin and contains the same carboxyamidated C-terminus.

transforming growth factor-α (TGF-α) A growth factor closely related to EGF (epidermal growth factor). TGF-α is often expressed in neoplastic tissue together with gastrin, and TGF-α (or EGF) stimulates gastrin gene transcription.

Cross-References

All the articles in the encyclopedia have cross-references to other articles. These appear at the end of the article, following the glossary and preceding the further reading section. The encyclopedia contains a little over 2,000 cross references in all.

The cross-references indicate related articles that can be consulted for further information on the same topic, or for information on a related topic. For example, the article "Oxytocin" provides the following cross-references:

> Corpus Luteum in Primates • Corpus Luteum: Regression and Rescue • Decidualization • Endometrial Remodeling • Oxytocin/Vasopressin Receptor Signaling • Placental Development • Progesterone Action in the Female Reproductive Tract • Sexual Differentiation of the Brain • Vasopressin (AVP)

Further Reading

The further reading section appears as the last element in an article. It lists recent secondary sources to aid the reader in locating more detailed or technical information. Review articles and research papers that are important to an understanding of the topic are also listed. For example, the article "Gastrin" has the following references (among others):

Dockray, G. J., Varro, A., Dimaline, R., and Wang, T. (2001). The gastrins: Their production and biological activities. *Annu. Rev. Physiol.* **63,** 119–139.

Edkins, J. S. (1905). On the chemical mechanism of gastric secretion. *Proc. R. Soc. London Sect. B* **76,** 376.

Rehfeld, J. F. (1998). The new biology of gastrointestinal hormones. *Physiol. Rev.* **78,** 1087–1108.

Walsh, J. H. (1994). Gastrin. *In* "Gut Peptides: Biochemistry and Physiology" (J. H. Walsh and G. J. Dockray, eds.), pp. 75–121. Raven Press, New York.

The further reading references are for the benefit of the reader; they provide the author's recommendations for more information on the given topic. Thus they consist of a limited number of entries. They do not represent a complete listing of all the sources consulted by the author in preparing the paper.

Index

A subject index is located at the end of Volume 3. This index is the most convenient way to locate a desired topic within the encyclopedia and thus it should be the starting point for any reader seeking to find a topic. The entries in the index are listed alphabetically and indicate the volume and page number where information on this topic can be found.

Nerve Growth Factor (NGF)

Michael A. Yarski[*] and Ralph A. Bradshaw[†]

[*]Baker Heart Research Institute, Melbourne, Australia ●
[†]University of California, Irvine

Nerve growth factor is a primarily a paracrine hormone (with a few instances of endocrine and autocrine activity) that services a variety of neuronal and nonneuronal cells, inducing differentiative, survival, and mitotic responses. It utilizes two receptor types that can function both independently and in concert to produce these effects. It is part of a larger family of neurotrophins that function similarly and its activities, particularly in the nervous system, are closely tied to these.

I. OVERVIEW

Nerve growth factor (NGF) was first detected over 50 years ago by Levi-Montalcini and Hamburger as a humoral substance, released by two transplanted mouse tumors, that induced neurite outgrowth from sympathetic and sensory neurons. The subsequent development of a bioassay using 8-day-old chicken dorsal root ganglia and the identification of more suitable sources, in particular the adult male mouse submandibular gland, eventually led to the isolation and characterization of the NGF protein(s). This information provided the realization that NGF was representative of what turned out to be a large class of hormone-like substances, including growth factors and cytokines, that impinge on virtually all cells and stimulate, regulate, or contribute to their basal functions, such as differentiation, division, and survival. These substances all initiate their responses by interacting with receptors (of various types), and NGF was ultimately shown to have two distinct types of cell surface receptors that can function

independently or in concert. A detailed description of the structure and function of NGF (and several homologues) and its receptors, including a substantial elucidation of its mechanisms of action, has now evolved, demonstrating involvement of NGF in regulating a wide variety of activities in neuronal and nonneuronal cells. In this article, the primary focus is on describing the chemical/biological properties of NGF.

II. AMINO ACID SEQUENCE/SUBUNIT STRUCTURE

Following the initial identification of nerve growth-promoting activity in tumors, serendipitous but astute observations revealed that snake venoms and the adult male mouse submandibular gland were far richer sources of NGF. For the next 30 years, and until recombinant material became widely available, most studies were performed with the mouse protein. The biologically active form of NGF (βNGF) in the mouse submandibular gland is associated noncovalently with two copies each of two additional subunits of the kallikrein family (αNGF and γNGF), and this complex is termed 7S NGF. NGF obtained from the homogenous complex (after dissociation) was originally called βNGF to distinguish it from another preparation (2.5S NGF) that was obtained directly from tissue homogenates (in which the 7S complex was dissociated while in an impure state). After sequence analyses showed 2.5S and βNGF to be essentially identical (except for variable amounts of proteolysis at their termini), the β descriptor was generally adopted for all mouse preparations of the active subunit. Various studies demonstrated that the γ-subunit is an active esteropeptidase with a specificity for arginyl peptide bonds; the α-subunit is catalytically inactive, due to the mutation of several key residues that are required for catalysis. Both are synthesized as prepro structures and the γ-subunit is processed normally, similar to other serine proteases. However, due to an altered activation site, αNGF is not processed normally. Both subunits incur additional endo- and exoproteolytic cleavages, producing substantial microheterogeneity, and each has a single N-linked glycosylation site. The full 7S complex also contains two zinc ions that are important for the stability of the complex and is inactive (with respect both to receptor binding and γNGF catalysis) when chemical cross-linking prevents dissociation.

Thus, 7S NGF appears to be a storage form of NGF and is apparently restricted to this tissue (and perhaps some other rodent submandibular glands and snake venoms).

As was first determined with the 2.5S preparation, βNGF is composed of two identical polypeptide chains, associated noncovalently, and thus the 7S complex is a symmetrical heterohexamer. Sequence determination of 2.5S NGF, one of the earliest proteins to be so analyzed, indicated that the longest chain contains 118 amino acids ($M_w = 14259$) and each subunit has three intrachain disulfide bonds, which are paired 1–4, 2–5, and 3–6. Their unique conformational arrangement, subsequently determined from X-ray crystallographic studies, is a hallmark of the NGF super family (see later). These studies also showed that the N-terminal octapeptide is not present in approximately 50% of the chains and that somewhat lesser amounts of each subunit are missing the C-terminal arginine residue. βNGF isolated from purified 7S NGF has considerably less of both modifications. The importance of these regions to receptor binding, and hence activity, has been extensively studied. Basically, the N-terminal region including part of the octapeptide sequence is important for interaction with TrkA (one of the two NGF receptors; see later) but the C-terminal arginine does not contribute to interactions with either receptor. The 7S complex is maximally stable at neutral pH and dissociates above or below pH 7 (primarily due to the dissociation of one or the other of the kallikrein subunits). In contrast, the polypeptides making up the β-subunit are very tightly associated and require denaturing conditions to cause chain separation. Thus, the βNGF ligand always functions as a dimer.

As expected for proteins of this type, NGF is synthesized as a larger precursor molecule, and the sequence of this entity, termed prepro-βNGF, has been determined from the cDNA. Due to the use of an alternative initiation codon, two precursors are formed but both yield the same mature protein. The sequence of the human precursor is shown in Fig. 1, with an indication of the alternative initiation site. Similar sequence information is now available for NGF from a variety of other species, including the mouse, cow, chicken, guinea pig, and cobra. The prepro-βNGF gene is located on human chromosome 1 at p22 and on mouse chromosome 3.

Comparison of the βNGF sequence against the limited database available at the time of initial studies of NGF suggested a distant but significant relationship with proinsulin; this was strongly supported by similarities in functional responses of the respective target cells. This correctly presaged that NGF was a part of what has turned out to be a greatly expanded field of hormones and hormone-like substances that primarily function in autocrine and paracrine fashions. However, eventual structural data disproved the NGF-insulin relationship; rather, NGF is a member of another family of homologous factors collectively termed neurotrophins. In mammals there are three other known members: brain-derived neurotrophic factor (BNDF), neurotrophin 3 (NT3), and neurotrophin 4 (NT4). NT4 is sometimes referred to NT4/5 due to some early confusion about the identity of these two neurotrophins. Two additional neurotrophins, NT6 and NT7, have been identified in lower species but do not have mammalian counterparts. Pairwise comparisons of these sequences (within a single species) show about 50% identity (Fig. 2). There is some variability in length that is manifested at both termini and in short insertions in the BNDF and NT4 sequences. However, the half-cystines are conserved, as is the overall structure of each factor (all four native neurotrophins and two artificial heterodimers have been solved by X-ray crystallographic analysis). Although there are distinct residues involved, the receptor-binding regions are also located in similar places (with the exception of the N-terminal region of NGF).

III. STRUCTURE

Although crystals of βNGF were obtained in 1975, the three-dimensional structure was not obtained until 1991. When it was determined, it described a unique and somewhat unexpected fold (Fig. 3). Each subunit has an elongated structure as opposed to a strictly globular one and there are four extended polypeptide segments that form two pairs of twisted antiparallel β-sheets, giving rise to the extensive, highly hydrophobic interface ($\sim 3000 \text{ Å}^2$) between the two protomers making up the dimer. A "cystine knot" composed of all three intrachain links characterizes one end of this "bundle." Two of these form a circular structure and the third passes through it, providing a quite distinct signature motif. At the opposite end, the β-sheets terminate in three hairpin loops, whereas a fourth, looser loop caps the cystine knot end. The two subunits are oriented in a parallel fashion and a not inaccurate description suggests the overall structure is like a bouquet of flowers.

In addition to the other neurotrophins, which have very similar conformations, there are three other families of hormones/growth factors that share

```
GAG AGC GCT GGG AGC CGG AGG GGA GCG CAG CGA GTT TTG GCC AGT GGT CGT
GCA GTC CAA GGG GCT GGA TGG CAT GCT GGA CCC AAG CTC AGC TCA GCG TCC
GGA CCC AAT AAC AGT TTT ACC AAG GGA GCA GCT TTC TAT CCT GGC CAC ACT
```

```
              -121                                          -110
              M   S   M   L   F   Y   T   L   I   T   A   F
GAG GTG CAT AGC GTA ATG TCC ATG TTG TTC TAC ACT CTG ATC ACA GCT TTT
```

```
                -103        -100
L   I   G   I   Q   A   E   P   H   S   E   S   N   V   P   A   G
CTG ATC GGC ATA CAG GCG GAA CCA CAC TCA GAG AGC AAT GTC CCT GCA GGA
```

```
        -90                                      -80
H   T   I   P   Q   V   H   W   T   K   L   Q   H   S   L   D   T
CAC ACC ATC CCC CAA GTC CAC TGG ACT AAA CTT CAG CAT TCC CTT GAC ACT
```

```
                -70                                      -60
A   L   R   R   A   R   S   A   P   A   A   A   I   A   A   R   V
GCC CTT CGC AGA GCC CGC AGC GCC CCG GCA GCG GCG ATA GCT GCA CGC GTG
```

```
A   G   Q   T   R   N   I   T   V   D   P   R   L   F   K   K   R
                            -50
GCG GGG CAG ACC CGC AAC ATT ACT GTG GAC CCC AGG CTG TTT AAA AAG CGG
```

```
    -40                                  -30
R   L   R   S   P   R   V   L   F   S   T   Q   P   P   R   E   A
CGA CTC CGT TCA CCC CGT GTG CTG TTT AGC ACC CAG CCT CCC CGT GAA GCT
```

```
            -20                                  -10
A   D   T   Q   D   L   D   F   E   V   G   G   A   A   P   F   N
GCA GAC ACT CAG GAT CTG GAC TTC GAG GTC GGT GGT GCT GCC CCC TTC AAC
```

```
                        1                                10
R   T   H   R   S   K   R   S   S   H   P   I   F   H   R   G
AGG ACT CAC AGG AGC AAG CGG TCA TCA TCC CAT CCC ATC TTC CAC AGG GGC
```

```
                            20
E   F   S   V   C   D   S   V   S   V   W   V   G   D   K   T   T
GAA TTC TCG GTG TGT GAC AGT GTC AGC GTG TGG GTT GGG GAT AAG ACC ACC
```

```
    30                                  40
A   T   D   I   K   G   K   E   V   M   V   L   G   E   V   N   I
GCC ACA GAC ATC AAG GGC AAG GAG GTG ATG GTG TTG GGA GAG GTG AAC ATT
```

```
                50                                  60
N   N   S   V   F   K   Q   Y   F   F   E   T   K   C   R   D   P
AAC AAC AGT GTA TTC AAA CAG TAC TTT TTT GAG ACC AAG TGC CGG GAC CCA
```

```
                        70
N   P   V   D   S   G   C   R   G   I   D   S   K   H   W   N   S
AAT CCC GTT GAC AGC GGG TGC CGG GGC ATT GAC TCA AAG CAC TGG AAC TCA
```

```
    80                                  90
Y   C   T   T   T   H   T   F   V   K   A   L   T   M   D   G   K
TAT TGT ACC ACG ACT CAC ACC TTT GTC AAG GCG CTG ACC ATG GAT GGC AAG
```

```
        100                                      110
Q   A   A   W   R   F   I   R   I   D   T   A   C   V   C   V   L
CAG GCT GCC TGG CGG TTT ATC CGG ATA GAT ACG GCC TGT GTG TGT GTG CTC
```

```
                120
S   R   K   A   V   R   R   A   OPA
AGC AGG AAG GCT GTG AGA AGA GCC TGA
CCT GCC GAC ACG CTC CCT CCC CCT GCC CCT TCT ACA CTC TCC TGG GCC CCT CCC TAC CTC
AAC CTG TAA ATT ATT TTA AAT TAT AAG GAC TGC ATG GTA ATT TAT AGT TTA TAC AGT TTT
AAA GAA CTA TTA TTT ATT AAA TTT TTG GAA GC
```

FIGURE 1 The nucleic and amino acid sequences of human prepro-βNGF. The amino acid positions are numbered beginning with the first amino-terminal residue of the mature βNGF molecule. The signal peptide consists of residues −121 to −104 whereas the propeptide is composed of residues −103 to −1. The initiation site is at position −121, with an alternative site at position −119, both of which are indicated by bold text.

the cystine knot/four-strand β-sheet core structure and thus form a superfamily with the neurotrophins. Although each family contains several members, they are represented by platelet-derived growth factor, transforming growth factor-β and chorionic gonadotropin. However, substantial differences, including protomer orientation and the presence of interchain disulfide bonds, distinguish the families. Beyond the conservation of the participating half-cystines, there is no recognizable sequence relatedness between members of the superfamily. This motif has also been found in some other nonhormonal molecules.

The crystal structure of the 7S complex defines the interactions between the kallikrein-like subunits

```
           1         10        20        30        40
NGF   -----SSSHPIFHRG EFSVCDSVSV WVG--DKTTATD IKGKEVMVLG
BDNF  HSDPARRHSDPARRG ELSVCDSISE WVTAADKKTAVD MSGGTVTVLE
NT3   ------YAEHKSHRG EYSVCDSESL WVT--DKSSAID IRGHQVTVLG
NT4   ---GVSETAPASRRG ELAVCDAVSG WVT--DRRTAVD LRGREVEVLG
             *  *  ****** *  **           *    *   *  **
```

```
          50        60        70        80
NGF   EVNI-NNSVFK QYFFETKCRD PNPVDS-------GCRG IDSKHWNSYC
BDNF  KVPV-SKGQLK QYFYETKCNP MGYTKE-------GCRG IDKRHWNSQC
NT3   EIKT-GNSPVK QYFYETRCKE ARPVKN-------GCRG IDDKHWNSQC
NT4   EVPAAGGSPLR QYFFETRCKA DNAEEGGPGAGGGGCRG VDRRHWVSEC
             ***  ** *                    ****  *  ** *
```

```
          90       100       110
NGF   TTTHTFVKAL TMDGKQ-AAWR FIRIDTACVC VLSRKAVRRG
BDNF  RTTQSYVRAL TMDSKKRIGWR FIRIDTSCVC TLTIKRGR--
NT3   KTSQTYVRAL TSENNKLVGWR WIRIDTSCVC ALSRKIGRT-
NT4   KAKQSYVRAL TADAQGRVGWR WIRIDTACVC TLLSRTGRA-
          *  **       **  ***** ***   *
```

FIGURE 2 Alignment of the amino acid sequences (single-letter code) of human nerve growth factor (NGF), brain-derived neurotrophic factor (BDNF), neurotrophin-3 (NT3), and neurotrophin-4 (NT4). Numbers correspond to positions in the NGF sequence. Residues important for p75 receptor binding are indicated by boldface type and residues of NGF known to interact with the TrkA receptor are shaded. Conserved residues are marked with an asterisk. Dashes represent gaps introduced for alignment purposes. Note that, because of differences in the lengths of the N-termini of the different neurotrophins, homologous positions in different molecules do not have equivalent numbering.

and those of βNGF. The αNGF subunits, which show a "locked zymogen" conformation consistent with their unprocessed state, bind to the core pleated sheets and the γNGF molecules interact mainly with the C-terminal region of the βNGF subunit. This latter interaction includes the C-terminal arginine residue of βNGF, which is bound in the active site of the γNGF. These interfaces are in the range of 2000–2500 Å². The two γ-subunits also have a major interaction (~2600 Å²) but there is no contact between the α-subunits. The zinc ions occur at the interface (~1600 Å²) of the α/γ-subunits and each contributes two metal ligands. Although α/β and β/γ dimers are stable in solution under certain conditions, α/γ dimers are not. Both kallikreins are monomeric in solution.

IV. BIOSYNTHESIS/EXPRESSION

The signal peptide of human prepro-βNGF is 18 residues in length and the pro sequence contains 103 residues, yielding a full-length zymogen of ~30 kDa. *In vivo* and *in vitro* labeling experiments had initially detected a 22-kDa precursor that could be converted

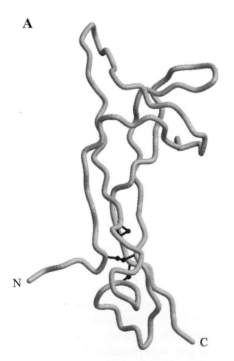 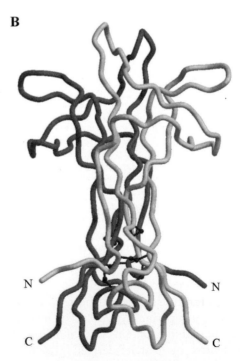

FIGURE 3 Three-dimensional representation of nerve growth factor. (A) The unique tertiary fold for the individual NGF subunit, consisting of the "cystine knot" (indicated by the dark ball-and-stick representation). (B) The NGF dimer with one subunit represented in a darker color for clarity.

by the γ-subunit, among other proteases, to the mature form, and this species was consistent with an intermediate arising from cleavage at a pair of arginine residues. However, the high concentrations required and the lack of specificity argued against γNGF as the pro-βNGF-processing enzyme *in vivo*, and recent studies have identified furin, which is involved in other similar processing events, to be the causative entity. There is also a C-terminal extension, usually of two residues, that is removed in the mouse submandibular protein, probably through the agency of the γ NGF, but this is not apparently the case with the NGF of other species. A possible role for pro-NGF as a preferred ligand for the p75 receptor (see later) has been recently postulated.

NGF is expressed in both glia and neurons in the peripheral and central nervous systems (PNS and CNS), both during development and in the adult, as well as in several nonneuronal tissues. In keeping with the initial identification, NGF is expressed by non-neural target cells of afferent sympathetic and nociceptive sensory neurons and provides support for them via retrograde transport, the basis of the "neurotrophic hypothesis" (see later). The expression of NGF is also up-regulated in some of these tissues in response to injury and inflammation. This is particularly true of Schwann cells, in which, in the adult, it is synthesized only at very low levels, but following injury it is substantially induced by cytokines. In the CNS, the NGF gene is expressed in neurons, the highest levels of mRNA being found in the hippocampus and the cerebral cortex. NGF is also synthesized in astrocytes and microglia and a variety of factors and conditions also affect these levels.

Generally, NGF appears to provide target-derived support for CNS neurons and NGF synthesis by both neurons and support cells is enhanced following injury or other deleterious conditions. However, it should be noted that there have been many identifications of NGF synthesis and expression that are not fully explained. This includes the immune system, in which many types of leukocytes express βNGF, including mast cells, monocytes, T and B lymphocytes, and macrophages. This suggests a major role for NGF in the neural-immune axis, but descriptions of this important physiological system lack detail.

V. RECEPTORS

βNGF interacts with two cell surface receptors: TrkA is a member of the receptor tyrosine kinase (RTK) family and elicits most of the known classical βNGF biological responses; the other receptor, p75NTR, is a pan neurotrophin receptor that binds all of the neurotrophins with similar affinity. The p75NTR induces a largely different set of responses but can also modulate the binding of βNGF to TrkA. TrkA was identified from a chimeric oncogene that contained a portion of tropomyosin fused to the endodomain of an RTK, thus giving rise to the name tropomyosin-related kinase (Trk). The identification of TrkA followed by several years the isolation and characterization of p75NTR and resolved several conflicting reports regarding the signaling entity responsible for the survival and differentiation activities of NGF.

TrkA is a typical single-pass transmembrane RTK. The extracellular part is glycosylated and contains five domains: (1) a cysteine-rich region, (2) three leucine-rich repeats, (3) a second cysteine-rich region, and (4 and 5) two immunoglobulin (Ig)-like domains. NGF binds to the most proximal Ig-domain (domain 5) and a structure of the NGF-domain 5 complex has been determined. Similar structures have also been determined for TrkB and TrkC, the specific receptors for BDNF and NT3. The importance/role of the other domains in TrkA function is less clear. The TrkA-binding site on βNGF has been deduced from several mutagenesis/chemical modification studies and confirmed by the three-dimensional structure. Basically, it is composed of three regions of NGF; the first two have been termed the "specificity patch" and the "conserved patch." The third is less well defined and involves residues in two of the hairpin loops at the end of the molecule opposite the cystine knot. The specificity patch is made up of residues in the N-terminus and the conserved patch is made from residues in the β-sheet core. The residues of TrkA that contact the specificity patch are in a quite hydrophobic pocket that is considerably more hydrophilic in TrkB and absent altogether in TrkC. This interaction is quite consistent with a number of derivatives with various N-terminal modifications that show decreased affinity for TrkA. The conserved patch is made up of several hydrophobic residues and is actually contributed by side chains from both βNGF protomers. There is great deal of similarity in this region in all the neurotrophins and this presumably reflects the commonality of this binding site in all the Trks. The last binding site occurs on the linker segments that connect domain 5 with the transmembrane segment. The βNGF residues involved are less well defined because this interaction has not been observed in the NGF–domain 5 complex.

The p75NTR is also a transmembrane glyco-protein with a single spanning segment. It has a relatively small endodomain containing a "death domain" motif. It also contains a less well-character-ized segment of 29 residues, located near the membrane; this segment has been designated "chop-per" and can induce cell death when incorporated into other proteins or when expressed in a membrane-bound form. The role of either of these domains in p75NTR activity is unclear. The ectodomain contains four cystine-rich sequences (each containing three disulfide bonds) that are similar to those found in the TNF receptor. As a result, a plausible model has been proposed (there are no crystallographic data). All four appear to be required for NGF binding, with the second being of most importance. The p75NTR binding site appears to be composed of two groups of residues—one contributed by loop 3 (near the cystine knot) and one by a group of basic residues in loops 1 and 4 at the opposite end of the molecule. The former seems to represent a common site found in the other neurotrophins as well. The latter is more specific to NGF.

There is substantial indirect evidence that p75NTR and TrkA can interact and it has been suggested that the high-affinity binding observed for NGF results from such a complex. However, physical evidence for the formation of a p75NTR-TrkA complex, with or without NGF, is lacking. Model building suggests that it would be possible for both receptors to bind NGF simultaneously, which would place the cystine knot end of NGF away from the membrane (given the orientation of NGF in complex with the TrkA domain 5). Association of p75NTR with this complex requires an orientation that is inconsistent with domain 2 of p75NTR providing a major binding site. For that to be achieved, the cystine knot must be located toward the membrane. Because both receptors can function in the absence of the other, it is possible that NGF binds to p75NTR in one orientation with the isolated receptor but in the opposite way in a ternary complex.

VI. CELL SIGNALING

Signaling of all receptors is to some degree cell specific. Most of the information available for NGF signaling is derived from studies with PC12 cells, a rat pheochromocytoma line. These cells differentiate into a phenotype quite similar to that of sympathetic neurons on exposure to NGF (among other agents). Although not strictly neuronal cells, they have been extremely valuable in defining the signaling

properties of the NGF receptors. As with other RTKs, the ligand-activated form of TrkA is a dimer. It is stabilized by the phosphorylation of two tyrosine residues in the activation loop and has two additional principal sites for downstream signaling. Tyrosine 490 (Y490), in the endodomain juxtamembrane region, is a docking site for Shc and FRS2, which are scaffolds for assembling signaling complexes, leading to the activation of Ras/ERK1/2 and phos-phatidylinositol 3-kinase (PI3K) among other moi-eties. The former is associated with the differentiative responses whereas the latter is related to survival. Tyrosine 785 (Y785) similarly binds phospholipase C-γ leading to its activation as well. There are additional entities that have also been implicated, such as Src and Abl, but the mechanisms leading to their activation are not well understood.

The p75NTR is activated by NGF to produce ceramide by the activation of sphingomyelinase. The death domain may be responsible for this activity. This receptor also binds and activates tumor necrosis factor receptor-associated factors (TRAFs), leading to the production of nuclear factor κ (NF-κB). Interest-ingly, TrkA also activates this cytoplasmic transcrip-tion factor, but in an Shc-dependent fashion. It has also been suggested that p75NTR may function in a ligand-independent manner to produce cell death based on the overexpression of the intracellular domain. At least some of these effects may be mediated through RhoA and actin cytoskeleton rearrangement.

VII. PHYSIOLOGY

βNGF has a multiplicity of roles in the development and maintenance of the nervous system. It also has less well-defined activities in other tissues. During development, it functions primarily with sympathetic and selected sensory neurons in the PNS and with striatal and cholinergic neurons in the CNS. The PNS activities were the basis for the initial identification by Levi-Montalcini and Hamburger and, indeed, it was the determination that NGF is specifically taken up and retrogradely transported to the perikarya of dependent peripheral neurons the led to the elucida-tion of the neurotrophic hypothesis. However, NGF, as well as other neurotrophic factors, certainly plays some role in maintaining these neurons before synapses are formed.

The availability of βNGF during development is important in determining the phenotypic rate and numbers of βNGF-responsive sensory neurons in the adult. A combination of βNGF antibody-blocking experiments and gene knockout experiments in mice has identified two populations of neurons that are reduced by as much as 80% in the absence of βNGF (the dorsal root ganglion and trigeminal ganglion). The antibody-blocking experiments also suggest that a subset of sensory neurons is βNGF dependent during development, including the nociceptive neurons. A role for βNGF in sensory neuron regeneration is also indicated by its neurite proliferation activity and up-regulation. In adult animals, sensory neurons do not require βNGF for their continued survival. Sympathetic neurons show even a greater dependency on βNGF. In gene knockout mice (both TrkA −/− and βNGF −/− mice), more than 90% of the sympathetic neurons disappear in the cervical ganglion. These data are supported by βNGF-blocking antibody experiments in which the same phenotype is observed. Unlike the sensory neurons, βNGF is required for the continued survival of the sympathetic neurons in the cervical ganglion of adult animals. In the CNS, there are similar observations, particularly in the gene knockout animals for the basal forebrain cholinergic neurons. However, it is also clear that the dependency of neurons on trophic stimulation is complex and even transient. Many neurons depend on more than one factor, and these allegiances can change with time.

There is clearly less neuronal dependency on NGF in adult animals, in which activities are more focused on synaptic function, synaptic plasticity, and repair. As a rule, target-derived support becomes less important although it does not completely disappear. However, other activities of NGF may become more important in the adult animal. One of these is a critical role for endogenous βNGF in inflammation and pain suggested by the increased levels of βNGF in damaged or inflamed tissue. Cytokines, such as interleukin-1β (IL-1β), typically involved in tissue damage and inflammatory processes, increase βNGF levels both *in vitro* and *in vivo*. Administration of antibodies that block βNGF prevents the heat and the mechanical hyperalgesia that normally follow tissue inflammation, without affecting the inflammation. The basis for this action includes an up-regulation of peptide neurotransmitters expressed by neurons concerned with the detection of potentially painful stimuli (nociceptors). TrkA −/− animals do not have nociceptive neurons, supporting these observations.

VIII. PATHOLOGY

The neurotrophic hypothesis that envisioned neurons as dependent on target-derived sources of NGF (and other neurotrophic factors) suggested that any disruption in this flow would lead to neuronal death. Thus, a putative link to neural degenerative diseases was readily forged. However, as it became clear that this dependency was reduced, this hypothesis lost attractiveness, particularly in view of the fact that NGF levels were particularly reduced in patients with Alzheimer's disease. However, further studies have suggested that defects in retrograde transport may be more important. Thus, there maybe a connection with NGF and neurodegeneration that can be eventually exploited. NGF has also been documented to be associated with a variety of autoimmune diseases and inflammatory diseases. Increased levels of βNGF in circulating plasma are found in patients suffering from multiple sclerosis, systemic lupus, and arthritis. The nature of the NGF involvement is unknown.

Early attempts to utilize NGF and other neurotrophins therapeutically were not successful, mainly because of a variety of undesirable side effects. There may well be potential therapeutic targets for PNS and CNS disorders for NGF (or small-molecule antagonists or agonists), but these must first deal with the substantial range of activities of this hormone that underlies the negative responses.

IX. SUMMARY

Nerve growth factor has proved to be a scientific "Rosetta Stone" in that it has provided insights into many groundbreaking areas of endocrinology; over many years, initial insights have been ultimately found to have broad applicability to roles of other hormones and growth factors. It is appropriate, therefore, that the humoral substance first discovered gave rise to the term "growth factor" that is so widely used today.

Glossary

cystine knot proteins Superfamily of proteins, including four growth factor families, all of which contain the distinctive motif made up of a circle of two disulfides (and the intervening peptide chains) through which passes a third disulfide bond.

glial cells Nonneuronal support cells of the nervous system. Schwann cells are found in the peripheral nervous system and astrocytes and oligodendrocytes are found in the central nervous system.

neurotrophic factor Any one of several hormonal substances that provide tropic support for neurons by interacting with cell surface receptors and stimulating the metabolic and transcriptional responses required for maintenance of viability, differentiation, and other activities.

paracrine substances Hormones and growth factors that act in a paracrine fashion are not transported systemically, but rather diffuse from the cell of origin to the target cell. If these are the same type of cell, the mechanism is said to be autocrine. Substances that are transported through the circulation are considered to be endocrine.

prepro structures (zymogens) Precursor forms of proteins that are exported from the cell by removal of the pre sequence (to initiate transfer into the endoplasmic reticulum) and then the pro peptide, to yield the active mature protein. Such structures are common for hormones and hydrolases, for example.

receptor tyrosine kinases A superfamily of plasma-membrane-bound glycoproteins that specifically bind hormones and growth factors, leading to activation of their intracellular tyrosine kinase domains and thus inducing any of several signaling cascades, usually by sequential activation of other kinases.

See Also the Following Articles

Folliculogenesis, Early • Neurotrophins

Further Reading

Angeletti, R. H., and Bradshaw, R. A. (1971). Nerve growth factor from mouse submaxillary gland: amino acid sequence. *Proc. Natl. Acad. Sci. USA* **68**, 2417–2420.

Cohen, S., Levi-Montalcini, R., and Hamburger, V. (1954). A nerve growth-stimulating factor isolated from sarcomas 37 and 180. *Proc. Natl. Acad. Sci. USA* **40**, 1014–1018.

Cowan, W. M. (2001). Viktor Hamburger and Rita Levi-Montalcini: The path to the discovery of nerve growth factor. *Annu. Rev. Neurosci.* **24**, 551–600.

Dechant, G. (2001). Molecular interactions between neurotrophin receptors. *Cell Tissue Res.* **305**, 229–238.

Hamburger, V. (1993). The history of the discovery of the nerve growth factor. *J. Neurobiol.* **24**, 893–897.

Huang, E. J., and Reichardt, L. F. (2001). Neurotrophins: Roles in neuronal development and function. *Annu. Rev. Neurosci.* **24**, 677–736.

Kaplan, D. R., Hempstead, B. L., Martin-Zanca, D., Chao, M. V., and Parada, L. F. (1991). The trk proto-oncogene product: A signal transducing receptor for nerve growth factor. *Science* **252**, 554–558.

Kaplan, D. R., and Miller, F. D. (2000). Neurotrophin signal transduction in the nervous system. *Curr. Opin. Neurobiol.* **10**, 381–391.

Levi-Montalcini, R. (1987). The nerve growth factor 35 years later. *Science* **237**, 1154–1162.

Miller, F. D., and Kaplan, D. R. (2001). Neurotrophin signalling pathways regulating neuronal apoptosis. *Cell. Mol. Life Sci.* **58**, 1045–1053.

Neet, K. E., and Campenot, R. B. (2001). Receptor binding, internalization, and retrograde transport of neurotrophic factors. *Cell. Mol. Life Sci.* **58**, 1021–1035.

Scott, J., Selby, M., Urdea, M., Quiroga, M., Bell, G. I., and Rutter, W. J. (1983). Isolation and nucleotide sequence of a cDNA encoding the precursor of mouse nerve growth factor. *Nature* **302**, 538–540.

Shooter, E. M. (2001). Early days of the nerve growth factor proteins. *Annu. Rev. Neurosci.* **24**, 601–629.

Sofroniew, M. V., Howe, C. L., and Mobley, W. C. (2001). Nerve growth factor signaling, neuroprotection, and neural repair. *Annu. Rev. Neurosci.* **24**, 1217–1281.

Wiesmann, C., Ultsch, M. H., Bass, S. H., and de Vos, A. M. (1999). Crystal structure of nerve growth factor in complex with the ligand-binding domain of the TrkA receptor. *Nature* **401**, 184–188.

Neuroactive Steroids

ANDRE H. LAGRANGE[*] AND MARTIN J. KELLY[†]

[*]*Vanderbilt Medical Center* • [†]*Oregon Health and Sciences University*

I. INTRODUCTION
II. STEROID SYNTHESIS
III. REGULATION OF SYNTHESIS
IV. CELLULAR EFFECTS OF NEUROSTEROIDS/NEUROACTIVE STEROIDS
V. CLINICAL/PHYSIOLOGICAL RELEVANCE
VI. CONCLUSIONS

Many steroids are produced within the central nervous system, allowing for the possibility of local control of hormone synthesis. Other steroids are produced peripherally but affect neural tissues via the bloodstream. Both centrally and peripherally produced neurosteroids have nongenomic effects; they alter a variety of neuronal functions, including those involving ion channels and ionotropic and G-protein-coupled receptors.

I. INTRODUCTION

Steroid hormones are a broad class of lipophilic, polycyclic chemicals that control a wide variety of physiological functions. Despite the diversity of their actions, these hormones have long been thought to have a common mechanism of action. By regulating gene expression, steroid hormones control physiological processes ranging from immune function to metabolism to reproduction. However, there is mounting evidence that these compounds have important functions that are independent of any genomic effects. One of the earliest indications for a nongenomic mechanism of steroid action was the report by Hans Seyle that progesterone and ring A reduced metabolites have very rapid, robust anesthetic actions. In particular, the steroid derivative 3α-hydroxy-5α-pregnane-11,20-dione (also known as alphaxalone) is a potent anesthetic that has been used in human surgery. The anesthetic effect is stereospecific in that the closely related isoform betaxalone (3β-hydroxy-5α-pregnane-1,20-dione) has essentially no anesthetic action.

The powerful actions of synthetic steroid derivatives led researchers to explore the possibility that there are endogenously produced steroids that might influence central nervous system (CNS) function. Various steroids and their derivatives have been detected in the brain; due to their lipophilic nature, brain steroid hormone levels are often higher than serum levels. In some rat models, brain levels have been estimated to be as high as 10–100 nM. Levels of some steroid hormones persist in the CNS even several weeks after peripheral production of hormone is halted by gonadectomy and adrenalectomy. Subsequent work has shown that these hormones are synthesized *de novo* within the CNS, and thus the name 'neurosteroids' was adopted. This article reviews some of the neurosteroid effects in different cellular and whole animal physiologic models.

II. STEROID SYNTHESIS

A. Overview of Steroid Synthesis

All steroid hormones are synthesized from cholesterol precursors (Fig. 1). Cytochrome P450scc is a hydroxylase that is responsible for side chain cleavage of cholesterol, which results in the formation of pregnenolone. From pregnenolone, there are two interdependent pathways, one leading to mineralocorticoid/glucocorticoids and another that produces sex steroids. Although progesterone is a sex steroid, it stands at an important crossroad within this pathway and may be converted to other sex steroids, to glucocorticoids, or to 3α,5α-reduced neurosteroids.

The glucocorticoid pathway starts with 3β-hydroxysteroid dehydrogenase/isomerase (3β-HSD), which converts pregnenolone to progesterone. Progesterone can be converted by P450c21 to 11-deoxycortisone, which is then transformed to corticosterone and aldosterone by P450c11. The sex steroid synthetic pathway starts with P450c17, which converts pregnenolone or progesterone to 17-OH complexes. These compounds are then further converted to sex steroids by the same enzyme. The first

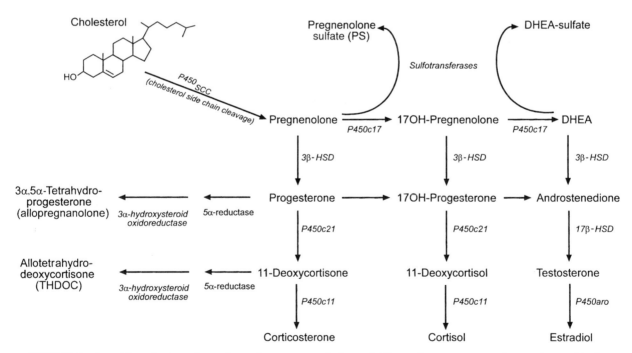

FIGURE 1 Steroid synthetic pathway from the precursor cholesterol. The major enzymes are shown along with the intermediate steroid compounds in the synthetic pathway to the neuroactive steroids [e.g., allopregnanolone, tetrahydrocorticosterone, pregnenolone sulfate, dehydroepiandrosterone sulfate, and 17β-estradiol]. DHEA, Dehydroepiandrosterone; 3β-HSD, 3β-hydroxysteroid dehydrogenase; see text for discussion of the different P450 enzymes.

sex steroid (other than progesterone) is dehydroepiandrostenedione (DHEA), which may be converted by 17β-hydroxysteroid oxidoreductase to androstenedione and then by 3β-HSD to testosterone, and is subsequently aromatized (P450aro) to 17β-estradiol (E2).

B. Neurosteroids and Neuroactive Steroids

The gonads and adrenal glands produce steroid hormones (Fig. 2). They reach the brain, the spinal cord, and the peripheral nerves via the bloodstream. These hormones, which then have specific, nongenomic affects on neural tissue, are often referred to as "neuroactive steroids," to differentiate them from the neurosteroids, which are synthesized within the nervous system. For example, progesterone that is synthesized in the gonads or in glial cells can act as a neurosteroid or can be converted to other neurosteroids. Although the distinction between neuroactive steroid and neurosteroid may be heuristically useful, it is becoming clear that this is an artificial distinction. Steroids and steroid intermediates, including pregnenolone, progesterone, and DHEA, are made both in the CNS and in peripheral tissues. These lipophilic hormones easily cross the blood–brain barrier and so

the physiologic importance of peripherally derived versus CNS-synthesized steroid hormones remains very ambiguous.

Cholesterol can be synthesized *de novo* within the CNS from low-molecular-weight precursors (e.g., mevalonate). The rate-limiting enzyme for steroid hormone synthesis in both the periphery and CNS is P450scc. This enzyme is found in the mitochondria of oligodendrocytes, some astrocytes, and possibly a small number of neurons. Isolated glia are able to produce pregnenolone, which may serve as an intermediate for further steroid synthesis. The next step is the conversion of pregnenolone to progesterone by 3β-HSD. This enzyme is found in both neurons and glia and is widely distributed within the brain, including the cortex, hippocampus, amygdala, and midbrain. As mentioned previously, pregnenolone and progesterone serve as important intermediaries from which glucocorticoids, sex steroids, and 3α,5α-reduced and sulfate derivatives may be formed.

Glucocorticoids can be synthesized from progesterone through the action of P450c21 and P450c11. Although P450c11 enzymatic activity has been demonstrated within the CNS, the same is not true for P450c21. Therefore, it is unclear whether

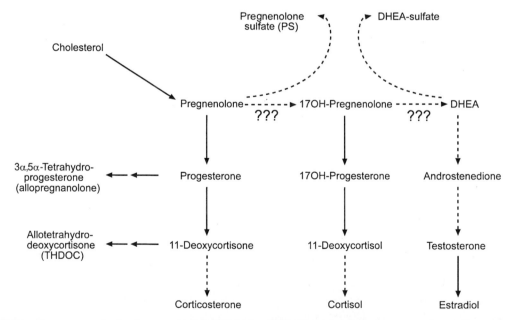

FIGURE 2 *De novo* synthesis of neurosteroids within the CNS. Steps that have been experimentally confirmed are represented by solid lines; steps for which the evidence is incomplete are shown as dashed lines. The enzymes mediating these steps are the same as those in the adrenals/gonads, with the exception of the conversion of progesterone to dehydroepiandrostenedione (DHEA). The P450c17 enzyme that mediates this conversion in the adrenal glands/gonads is not found in the adult CNS. Instead, if *de novo* synthesis of DHEA occurs within the CNS, it is probably mediated by an incompletely characterized Fe^{2+}-dependent enzyme.

there is *de novo* synthesis of glucocorticoids and the important reduced metabolite $3\alpha,5\alpha$-tetrahydro-deoxycorticosterone (THDOC) in the CNS.

Within the sex steroid pathway, DHEA is both an early intermediary and a neurosteroid. Within the adult CNS, there is no P450c17 protein or mRNA. Thus, there should be no *de novo* synthesis of sex steroids through the usual pathway. However, DHEA is found to persist in the brain after gonadectomy/adrenalectomy or with inhibition of P450c17 by an antagonist. Recent work suggests there may be an alternative Fe^{2+}-dependent pathway in oligodendroglia and astrocytes for creating this steroid from progesterone. However, the physiological significance of this pathway remains uncertain, because high (10 mM), probably supraphysiologic, levels of Fe^{2+} are necessary to produce significant quantities of DHEA. DHEA may be converted to androstenedione by 3β-HSD, and then to testosterone by 17β-hydroxysteroid oxidoreductase. However, although the enzymatic machinery for conversion of DHEA to testosterone is present, the physiological importance of this step in the CNS is uncertain. Unlike DHEA, the level of testosterone drops rapidly to undetectable levels after adrenalectomy/gonadectomy. Therefore, testosterone in the CNS is probably derived from peripheral sources. However, aromatase (P450aro) is found within the brain and can convert peripherally derived testosterone to 17β-estradiol.

The addition of sulfate moieties causes some very interesting and potentially important changes in the biological activities of neurosteroids. Pregnenolone sulfate (PS) and DHEA-sulfate (DHEA-S) are the most well-studied examples at this time. *De novo* synthesis of sulfated neurosteroids from isolated CNS cells has not yet been specifically demonstrated, and these compounds are known to be taken up from the blood. However, the brain contains the necessary sulfotransferases and sulfohydrolases to interconvert these compounds, and the levels of PS and DHEA-S in the CNS remain constant after adrenalectomy/ovariectomy, despite undetectable serum levels. It is therefore unclear whether sulfated steroids are synthesized *de novo* within the CNS or are derived from peripheral sources, or both.

Finally, the $3\alpha,5\alpha$-reduced steroids are among the best characterized neurosteroids. Both 5α-reductase and 3α-reductase (3α-hydroxysteroid reductase) are found in neurons and glia in the pituitary, hypothalamus, medulla, thalamus, and cerebellum. These hormones can convert progesterone to $3\alpha,5\alpha$-tetrahydroprogesterone (allopregnanolone) and corticosterone to $3\alpha,5\alpha$-tetrahydrodeoxycorticosterone.

These two neurosteroids have broad, powerful regulatory effects in several systems.

In summary, there is clear evidence for the *de novo* synthesis of neurosteroids in the CNS. The synthesis of progesterone from low-molecular-weight precursors has been established. The conversion of progesterone to allopregnanolone is well established, but synthesis of sex steroids and glucocorticoids is not as well documented. Progesterone is possibly converted to DHEA within the CNS, but testosterone, which is converted to estrogen, appears to be derived from peripheral sources. It remains completely unclear whether glucocorticoids or sulfated steroid derivatives are centrally or peripherally derived.

III. REGULATION OF SYNTHESIS

The physiological regulation of neurosteroid synthesis remains largely unknown. Nonetheless, some early studies have shown that stress can change the levels of CNS steroid hormones. For example, significant elevations of pregnenolone and allopregnanolone have been observed in the frontal cortex following a swim stress in rats. Perhaps even more interesting is the fact that the stress of adrenalectomy/gonadectomy, although abolishing peripheral synthesis of steroid hormones, actually serves to increase brain tissue concentrations of allopregnanolone, PS, DHEA, and THDOC to physiologically active levels. Little else is known concerning the regulation of steroid synthesis in the nervous system. However, there is clear evidence that the levels of these hormones vary in response to diverse stimuli, and this remains a field wide open for further investigation.

IV. CELLULAR EFFECTS OF NEUROSTEROIDS/NEUROACTIVE STEROIDS

A. GABA$_A$

γ-Aminobutyric acid (GABA), an inhibitory neurotransmitter that is distributed widely throughout the brain, activates two broad classes of GABA receptors, ionotropic GABA$_A$ and G-protein-coupled GABA$_B$ receptors. The G-protein-coupled GABA$_B$ receptors modulate a variety of effectors, including activation of K^+ channels and inhibition of Ca^{2+} channels. GABA$_A$ receptors are composed of five subunits with an intrinsic chloride channel (Fig. 3). A vast majority of inhibitory postsynaptic currents in the brain are due to the activation of this conductance. Currently, there are six α, four β, three γ, one δ, one ε, one π,

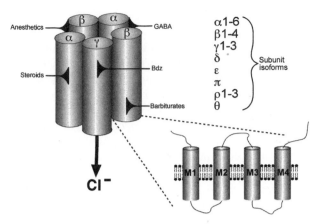

FIGURE 3 γ-Aminobutyric acid type A (GABA$_A$) receptor heteropentameric structure with multiple allosteric modulatory sites. The different subunit isoforms are shown. The inset in the lower right shows the four transmembrane domains of each individual subunit.

three ρ, and one θ known subunit isoforms. Although there are an enormous number of possible subunit arrangements to produce receptors, only a relatively discrete number of actual arrangements have been demonstrated in brain. *In vivo*, these subunits combine to form heteropentamers, likely composed of two α, two β, and either a γ, δ, ε, π, or θ subunit. In addition to a GABA binding site, these proteins contain several other distinct allosteric modulatory sites for agents such as benzodiazepines (sedative-hypnotics), barbiturates (sedative-hypnotic/anesthetic), etomidate (general anesthetic), zinc, and furosemide (diuretic). Although the roles of these modulatory sites in normal physiology remain unknown, they are important targets for clinical manipulation. Examples include the use of phenobarbital in the treatment of epilepsy and propofol as a general anesthetic. As previously mentioned, the anesthetic action of the steroid derivative alphaxalone was one of the earliest indications for a neurosteroid effect. A variety of experimental paradigms have shown that, like several other general anesthetics, alphaxalone is an allosteric modulator of GABA$_A$ currents. Alphaxalone increases both the potency and efficacy for the GABA$_A$ receptor agonist, muscimol. Although alphaxalone does not directly activate GABA$_A$ receptors, it increases both the frequency of opening and the mean open time of the GABA$_A$ channels that have been activated by GABA. This modulation is mediated by a novel independent allosteric modulatory site on the GABA$_A$ receptors. Benzodiazepine antagonists do not inhibit the actions of alphaxalone. Instead of competing at

benzodiazepine or barbiturate binding sites, the addition of alphaxalone actually increases the binding of these agents.

Further studies have shown that physiologically relevant levels of the endogenously synthesized neurosteroids allopregnanolone and THDOC enhance GABA$_A$ channel activity. A similar effect is seen with the compound 3α-OH progesterone (3α-OHP), thus the 3α-OH group appears to be necessary for biologic action. In contrast, betaxalone, corticosterone, hydroxycortisone, pregnenolone, and the biologically inactive 3β-OHP isomer have no effect in this system. Although this effect is mediated by a unique allosteric modulatory site, the exact binding site on the GABA$_A$ receptor remains unknown. However, there is some information that the subunit composition of GABA$_A$ receptors may be important in mediating the neurosteroid response(s). Oocytes injected with the α$_2$β$_1$γ$_2$ combination have a greater neurosteroid modulation than do those expressing α$_1$β$_1$γ$_2$ subunits. Those oocytes with no α-subunits (β$_1$γ$_2$ only) are much less sensitive to neurosteroids. Furthermore, the δ-subunit appears to convey resistance to neurosteroids. This effect of subunit composition is particularly interesting in light of the fact that the GABA$_A$ receptor subunit combinations throughout the brain vary with development and over the reproductive cycle. Furthermore, modulation of GABA$_A$ receptors by allopregnanolone also varies over the reproductive cycle, being most potent at times of high levels of serum estrogens.

In animal studies, allopregnanolone and progesterone enhance the ability of muscimol to impair the righting reflex (the ability to turn over during a fall). Furthermore, inhibition of endogenous allopregnanolone synthesis with a 30-min exposure to a 5α-reductase inhibitor reduces the muscimol sensitivity. This effect was reversed with administration of 5α-dihydroprogesterone, an intermediate compound between 5α-reductase and 3α-reductase. Patch-clamp recording from cortical neurons taken from these animals confirmed that this inhibition of endogenous allopregnanolone synthesis resulted in a smaller muscimol response compared to control. Thus, there is both cellular and behavioral data that neurosteroid modulation of GABA$_A$ responses may be physiologically important.

Interestingly, the sulfated neurosteroids PS and DHEA-S have exactly the opposite effect on GABA$_A$ receptor function. These steroids serve as noncompetitive antagonists that reduce the opening frequency of these channels and increase desensitization to GABA in neurons from multiple preparations, including primary chick spinal cord and rat hippocampal neurons, and in *Xenopus laevis* oocytes expressing $\alpha_1\beta_2\gamma_{2S}$ GABA$_A$ receptors. The switch from a positive to negative allosteric GABA$_A$ receptor modulator seems to depend on the negative charge, because the inhibitory activity is retained when hemisuccinate is substituted for sulfate at the C-3 position. The interaction between steroid negative and positive modulators is not competitive, indicating that steroid negative and positive modulators act through distinct sites.

B. Glycine Receptors

The glycine receptor is a ligand-gated chloride channel that is highly homologous to the GABA$_A$ receptors, so it is not a surprise that these receptors are modulated by neurosteroids as well. Although there is no effect of allopregnanolone or alphaxalone, the maximum response to glycine is enhanced by PS. The mechanism and physiological significance of this effect remains unexplored.

C. Glutamate Receptors

Glutamate is the most widespread excitatory neurotransmitter within the brain. There are three broad classes of glutamate receptor: N-methyl-D-aspartate (NMDA), non-NMDA, and metabotropic receptors. As the name implies, the metabotropic receptor is a G-protein-coupled glutamate receptor, which, among other things, modulates the turnover of intracellular inositol trisphosphate. There are several variations of the non-NMDA receptors, which are activated by various ligands, including kainic acid and 3-amino-3-hydroxy-5-methyl-4-isoxazole propionic acid (AMPA). All of these receptors have an intrinsic mixed sodium/potassium ion channel. Activation of this receptor/ion channel complex is the basis for many of the excitatory postsynaptic potentials within the brain. The NMDA receptors appear to be much more complicated. The receptors require multiple factors for activation. Opening of the intrinsic sodium/potassium/calcium channel requires binding of both NMDA/glutamate and glycine at two separate sites. There are additional sites for allosteric modulators, such as polyamine peptides. Even after binding of glutamate and glycine, the ion channel pore is blocked by Mg^{2+}. The pore can conduct current only if this magnesium blockade is removed by depolarization of the cell. If non-NMDA and NMDA receptors are simultaneously activated, the non-NMDA receptor-induced depolarization may be sufficient to remove the magnesium block of the

NMDA receptors. Activation of NMDA receptors serves to depolarize the postsynaptic cells further. Moreover, some forms of this current are permeable to calcium, which may act as an intracellular messenger, resulting in long-term changes in postsynaptic cell function. The complex interactions among the glutamate receptors appear to play many important physiological functions, ranging from learning to excitotoxicity.

1. NMDA Receptors

Like the GABA$_A$ receptors, there are allosteric modulatory sites on the NMDA receptors. Pregnenolone sulfate acts at the neurosteroid modulatory site to increase the response to glutamate, but does not actually activate the receptor. In contrast, allopregnanolone sulfate (not allopregnanolone) is a negative modulator of NMDA currents. Finally, nanomolar concentrations of estrogen enhance NMDA-mediated excitatory postsynaptic potentials (EPSPs) in hippocampal CA1 pyramidal cells and high doses of this compound are associated with seizure activity in male rats. On the other hand, estrogens attenuate the neuronal damage seen after a variety of insults, including hypoglycemia, hypoxia, and glutamate agonists. It is currently unclear whether these various neurosteroids act by binding the same or different allosteric sites.

2. Non-NMDA Receptors

Estrogen increases the epileptogenicity of systemically administered kainate, more strongly in males than females. Based on *in vitro* intracellular recordings from CA1 pyramidal cells, administration of E2 increased synaptic excitability by enhancing the magnitude, but not the potency, of AMPA and kainate receptor-mediated responses. This effect is stereospecific, rapidly reversible, and does not appear to be due to a direct interaction between 17β-estradiol and the receptor channel. Rather, this effect appears to be mediated by activation of the cAMP/protein kinase A (PKA) pathway (Fig. 4). The actions of E2 are mimicked by PKA activators and blocked by PKA antagonists. The actual estrogen receptor remains unknown but possibly involves a novel binding site. Estrogenic modulation of non-NMDA receptors is seen robustly in a mouse line in which the α isoform of the classical estrogen receptor (ER-α) has been transgenically knocked out. Furthermore, this effect is not blocked by ICI 182,780, which is a potent antagonist at the ER-α and ER-β receptors. These effects may involve a G-protein-coupled receptor in that they are blocked

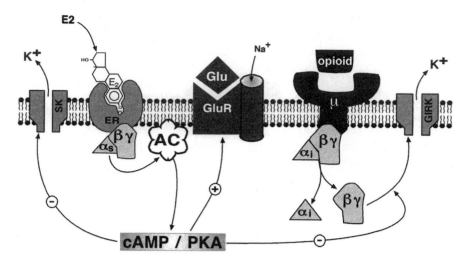

FIGURE 4 Schematic overview of the multiple rapid effects of 17β-estradiol (E2) in CNS neurons. In some cells (e.g., hypothalamic neurons), E2 binds to the estrogen receptor (ER), which stimulates adenylyl cyclase (AC) to produce cyclic adenosine monophosphate (cAMP), possibly via activation of $G_{\alpha s}$. Increased cellular levels of cAMP activate protein kinase A (PKA), which can uncouple μ-opioid (μ) receptors from their effector system (i.e., the inwardly rectifying K^+ channels, or GIRK) through phosphorylation of a protein [e.g., the $G_{\alpha i,o}$ (GIRK) channel]. In other cells (e.g., hippocampal CA1 pyramidal neurons), PKA can phosphorylate Ca^{2+}-dependent K^+ channels (SK), and inhibit their activity (outward K^+ current). Finally, PKA can phosphorylate a glutamate receptor/ionophore to increase its activity (inward cation current) in some neurons (e.g., hippocampal CA1 pyramidal neurons). Although this stylized figure shows the ER in the membrane, the actual subcellular localization of the receptor is not known.

by 5′-O-(2-thiodiphosphate) (GDPβS), which is a nonhydrolyzable GDP analogue that competitively inhibits G-protein activation by guanosine triphosphate (GTP), and they are mimicked by the toxin from *Cholerae vibrio* (cholera toxin), which is known to stimulate $G_{\alpha s}$.

D. Calcium Channels

Neurosteroids also modulate N- and L-type calcium channels. Pregnenolone, THDOC, and PS, but not progesterone, all depress the maximal current up to 60%, as well as slow activation and deactivation of these calcium channels in hippocampal CA1 neurons. This effect may be mediated by an extracellular receptor because intracellular dialysis with PS has no effect. Furthermore, neurosteroids may work through action of G-protein-coupled receptors because pretreatment with toxin from *Bordetella pertussis* (pertussis toxin), an inhibitor of $G_{\alpha i,o}$, or intracellular dialysis with GDPβS blocks the effects of PS. The neurosteroid binding site mediating these effects is pharmacologically distinct from the GABA$_A$ modulatory site. Unlike PS actions at GABA$_A$ receptors, both the neurosteroids and their sulfated derivative have similar effects. The replacement of the sulfated group with acetate abolishes the physiological activity of PS, and progesterone has no effect.

In an independent series of experiments, picomolar concentrations of estrogen were shown to inhibit rapidly (within seconds) L-type calcium channels in acutely dissociated striatal neurons. Unlike estrogenic modulation of glutamate receptors, E2 coupled to bovine serum albumin (E2–BSA) readily mimicked the effect of free E2, suggesting an extracellular binding site. As with the other neurosteroids, the effects of estradiol may involve activation of G-proteins. Those cells that were dialyzed with 5′-O-(3-thiotriphosphate) (GTP-γ), which is a G-protein-activating GTP analogue that is more resistant to hydrolysis than GTP, had an irreversible suppression of Ca^{2+} channels. Interestingly, a similar inhibition of L-type calcium current by estrogen, but not progesterone, has been demonstrated in vascular smooth muscle.

E. Potassium Channels

Estrogen exerts complex control of neuronal potassium channels. Intracellular recordings in hypothalamic neurons have shown that perfusion of 17β-estradiol hyperpolarizes a subset of hypothalamic neurons in an *in vitro* preparation within seconds and that this effect reversed within minutes of washing out estrogen. Similar actions of E2 were demonstrated in hypothalamic ventromedial nucleus and amygdala neurons, even in the presence of protein synthesis inhibitors. The E2-mediated hyperpolarization of hypothalamic and amygdala neurons appears to be the result of the opening of an inwardly rectifying K^+ channel. In another set of hypothalamic neurons, the application of E2 causes a rapid depolarization that is due to the closure of a tonically active potassium conductance. It turns out that both the hyperpolarizing effects of E2 in one group of neurons and the depolarizing actions in another group are enhanced by coperfusion with a phosphodiesterase inhibitor. Interestingly, the hyperpolarizing effects of 17β-estradiol are mimicked by 8-bromoguanosine 3',5'-cyclic monophosphate (8Br-cGMP), a cell-permeable analogue of cGMP, whereas this agent has no effect on that neuron subset that is depolarized by estrogen. Instead, application of 8-bromoadenosine 3',5'-cyclic monophosphate (8Br-cAMP), a cell permeable analogue of cAMP, or stimulation of endogenous adenylyl cyclase with forskolin mimics the effects of estrogen to depolarize a subset of cells.

F. G-Protein-Coupled Receptors

The discussion thus far has been limited to neurosteroid modulation of ionotropic receptors and ion channels. The effects of many neurotransmitters are also mediated by intracellular G-proteins, which subsequently serve to regulate a variety of intracellular processes. Estrogen is probably the most well-studied neurosteroid modulator of these receptors.

1. μ-Opioid

Activation of μ-opioid receptors hyperpolarizes hypothalamic neurons by opening a G-protein-coupled, inwardly rectifying potassium channel (Fig. 4). Perfusion of E2 in vitro results in a fourfold decrease in the potency of μ-opioid agonists to inhibit β-endorphin, but not gonadotropin-releasing hormone (GnRH) neurons. This effect is not mimicked by the inactive isomer 17α-E2, and selective estrogen receptor antagonists block this effect of E2. Estrogenic modulation of hypothalamic μ-opioid potency is mimicked either by stimulation of adenylyl cyclase with forskolin or by direct PKA activation with selective activators. Furthermore, selective PKA antagonists block the effects of E2. The apparent involvement of the cAMP/PKA pathway is highly reminiscent of estrogenic modulation of non-NMDA receptors. Moreover, the potency of the estrogenic effects is similar in both systems (effective concentration $EC_{50} \approx 10$ nM) and is not mimicked by

extracellular BSA–E2, implying that there may be a common receptor and/or intracellular mechanism mediating these estrogenic effects.

In hypothalamic neurons, $GABA_B$ and μ-opioid receptors are coupled to the same K^+ channels. Interestingly, E2 also produces a fourfold increase in the EC_{50} of a $GABA_B$ agonist in the same β-endorphin neurons in which it reduces μ-opioid potency, thus implying that E_2 is modulating signaling pathways shared by both receptors.

2. Catecholamines

Voltage-independent, Ca^{2+}-activated K^+ currents underlie the long-lasting afterhyperpolarizations (AHPs) in a number of CNS neurons, including hippocampal, hypothalamic neurosecretory, midbrain dopamine, vagal motor, and cortical pyramidal neurons. These AHPs limit the firing frequency of neurons and are responsible for spike frequency adaptation in regular-firing cortical neurons and phasically bursting neurosecretory neurons. The slow AHP current is mediated by small-conductance, Ca^{2+}-activated K^+ (SK) channels, and three SK channel genes have recently been cloned. In hippocampal CA1 pyramidal neurons, these currents are regulated by monoamine neurotransmitters, which suppress the slow AHP. The effects of norepinephrine, serotonin, and histamine on the slow AHP are mediated via $β_1$, type 4 5-hydroxytryptamine (5-HT_4), and type 2 histamine (H_2) receptors, respectively. Interestingly, one of the long-term effects of corticosteroid is to increase the slow AHP in CA1 neurons, presumably via a genomic mechanism because protein synthesis inhibitors block these actions of the adrenal steroid. Recently, however, it was found that E2 inhibits the slow AHP current and potentiates the $β_1$-adrenergic receptor-mediated ($G_{αs}$ coupled) inhibition of slow AHP current in CA1 hippocampal neurons (Fig. 4). Because the slow AHP is involved in spike frequency adaptation, these effects of E2 may be critical in increasing the firing frequency of hippocampal pyramidal neurons that are involved in arousal, attention, and memory.

G. Summary

In summary, recent advances in our understanding of the mechanisms mediating neurosteroid action have helped support the idea that steroids may have a rapid, nongenomic effect to regulate neuronal function (Table 1). Although there are almost certainly multiple pathways, the current understanding allows us to differentiate these into two broad categories.

TABLE 1 Summary of the Effects of Neuroactive Steroids[a]

Effect on	Prog	AlloPreg	THDOC	E_2	PS	DHEAS
$GABA_A$-R	±	↑I_{max}, ↑potency	↑I_{max}, ↑potency	—	↓I_{max}	↓I_{max}
Glycine-R	—	∅	—	—	↑I_{max}	—
Non-NMDA-R	—	—	—	±	↓I_{max}	—
NMDA-R	±	∅	—	↑, ±	↑I_{max}	—
I_{Ca}	∅	↓	↓	↓, ±	↓	—
I_K	—	—	—	↓	—	—
μ-Opioid-R	—	—	—	↓ Potency	—	—
$GABA_B$-R	—	—	—	↓ Potency	—	—

[a]Abbreviations: R, receptor; Prog, progesterone; AlloPreg, allopregnanolone (3α, 5α-tetrahydroprogesterone); THDOC, 3α, 5α-tetrahydrodeoxycorticosterone; E2, 17β-estradiol; PS, pregnenolone sulfate; DHEA-S, dihydroepiandrostenedione sulfate; I_{max}, maximum response; potency, potency of agonist binding to receptor; ∅, no measured effect; ±, small or variable effect.

The oldest, most well-established mechanism of action is the modulation of $GABA_A$ and NMDA receptors by progesterone derivatives and sulfated neurosteroids. Although the actual binding site has not yet been identified, these steroids clearly alter neurotransmitter receptors by binding a specific allosteric modulatory site, resulting in well-defined changes in receptor kinetics.

Although the mechanism of estrogenic neuroactive steroid action is less clear, data from multiple systems may be converging on elucidating a single biochemical pathway. Biochemical studies in uterine tissue have shown that estrogen rapidly increases cAMP levels, thereby activating PKA. The ability of estrogen to rapidly uncouple G-protein-coupled receptors, inhibit non-NMDA glutamate receptors, and close potassium channels may all be mediated through cAMP/PKA. It is unknown whether this implies a common mechanism of estrogen action, or simply a single convergent point among multiple complicated pathways. The actual binding site for estrogen remains unknown as well. Several labs have shown a modulation of calcium channels. This may be mediated by a G-protein-coupled membrane estrogen receptor. Whether this is a completely different pathway or another example of the cAMP/PKA family remains undetermined at this point.

V. CLINICAL/PHYSIOLOGICAL RELEVANCE

A. Anesthetic

As previously mentioned, the first hint of neurosteroid existence was the discovery that progesterone and some of its derivatives have potent anesthetic actions. In fact, the drug althesin (mixture of alphaxalone and alphadolone acetate) has been used in human surgery.

B. Regulation of Reproduction

The quintessential role of estrogen in the mammalian CNS is its negative and positive feedback actions on the hypothalamic–pituitary axis to regulate the reproductive cycle. In all mammalian species, the rapid negative feedback actions of estrogen on the hypothalamic GnRH neurons is a critical event for the activation and synchronization of GnRH neurons at the time of ovulation. Synchronous release of GnRH into the portal system produces maximal stimulation of pituitary gonadotrophs to secrete a 'surge' of luteinizing hormone (LH) to cause ovulation. An insight into the mechanism by which estrogen rapidly inhibits GnRH neurons was provided in the 1970s when it was found that E2 could rapidly inhibit hypothalamic neuronal activity. Therefore, the rapid effects of E2 on GnRH neurons may play a role in estrogen's negative feedback on the hypothalamus. In addition, estrogen regulates the reproductive axis through an effect on endogenous opioids. β-Endorphin neurons, originating in the hypothalamic arcuate nucleus, synapse directly on GnRH neurosecretory cells, and these neurons are an integral component of estrogenic negative feedback on the hypothalamic–pituitary axis. The opioid antagonist naloxone blocks the E2 negative feedback and advances the LH surge in women. Activation of μ-opioid receptors mimics E2 negative feedback on GnRH/LH release and has been shown to hyperpolarize directly, and thereby inhibit, GnRH neurons via opening G-protein-activated, inwardly rectifying potassium channels. As previously mentioned, the potency of μ-opioids to hyperpolarize β-endorphin neurons is greatly attenuated by brief application of estrogen (Fig. 4). Because β-endorphin is an endogenous ligand at μ-opioid receptors, these may serve as autoreceptors. By inhibiting β-endorphin autoinhibition, estrogen may cause increased β-endorphin release. Those cells that are impervious to this estrogenic effect (e.g., GnRH neurons) will remain sensitive to μ-opioids in the presence of increased concentrations of extracellular β-endorphin. Therefore, estrogen may serve to inhibit GnRH release through modulation of μ-opioid transynaptic regulation. The interaction between the direct inhibition and modulation of inhibitory input by estrogen has yet to be explored.

Neurosteroid modulation of reproduction may also be mediated by GABA$_A$ receptors. The activity of 3α-hydroxysteroid oxidoreductase is inversely correlated with E2 concentrations. Ovariectomy increases 3α-hydroxysteroid oxidoreductase activity, and this effect is abolished by subsequent administration of E2 (replacement therapy). Interestingly, allopregnanolone concentrations peak between proestrus and estrus in the rat, and the effects of allopregnanolone on the GABA$_A$ receptor vary over the reproductive cycle, being the most potent during the early follicular phase when the levels of serum estrogens are high. Furthermore, in ovariectomized rats, there is a nearly twofold reduction in the potency of allopregnanolone to modulate GABA$_A$ receptor.

C. Striatal Function/Movement Disorders

Clinically, the basal ganglia (also referred to as the corpus striatum) are important target areas for estrogen's actions outside of the hypothalamus. The basal ganglia are actually composed of several nuclei, including the caudate putamen and globus pallidus. This area is important in the regulation of both movement and motivation. Dopaminergic input from the substantia nigra modulates the function of the basal ganglion and its dysregulation is involved in several diseases, including Parkinson's disease and tardive dyskinesia (TD). TD, a disorder that is characterized by involuntary movements, develops after prolonged exposure to dopamine-antagonist antipsychotic drugs (e.g., haloperidol). This disorder has a 2:1 higher incidence in women versus men. There are some other hyperkinetic movement disorders that are associated with estrogen. Women who are pregnant or receiving estrogen supplementation occasionally develop multifocal rapid movements (chorea gravidarum) that resolve when the pregnancy is over or when the estrogen supplementation is discontinued. In contrast, Parkinson's disease is a hypokinetic movement disorder associated with deficient dopamine. There are reports that there is a worsening of symptoms in women during the premenstrual period, when estrogen levels are falling. There is some preliminary evidence that postmenopausal estrogen replacement therapy is associated with a reduced risk of Parkinson's disease in women and a lower disease severity in women with early Parkinson's disease who are not yet taking 1,3,4-dihydroxyphenylalanine (L-DOPA, precursor for dopamine).

Estrogen has multiple short-term effects in the corpus striatum. It potentiates rotational behavior induced by amphetamine in ovariectomized, 6-hydroxydopamine-lesioned (unilateral) rats. This pronounced behavioral effect is recapitulated at the cellular level. Acute administration of E2 also increases dopamine turnover and amphetamine-induced striatal dopamine release within 30 min as measured by *in vivo* microdialysis. A similar effect has been shown in the nucleus accumbens, a target site of ventral tegmental dopamine neurons. Local injection of E2 (but not 17α-estradiol) rapidly (<2 min) potentiates K$^+$-stimulated dopamine release as measured by *in vivo* voltammetry.

In addition to modulating dopamine release, E2 affects the postsynaptic response to this neurotransmitter by uncoupling type 2 dopamine (D$_2$) receptors within the same period. This is consistent with an earlier report that acute E2 treatment reduces the number of caudate neurons that are inhibited by dopamine. Continued exposure to E2 (2 weeks) down-regulates D$_2$ receptor mRNA and attenuates D$_2$ inhibition of adenylyl cyclase in striatal neurons. Interestingly, D$_2$ receptors, like μ-opioid and GABA$_B$ receptors, are G$_{\alpha i,o}$-coupled receptors. In contrast, long-term exposure to E2 potentiates type 1 dopamine receptor (D$_1$)-stimulated adenylyl cyclase activity. Dopamine D$_1$ receptors are coupled to G$_{\alpha s}$, suggesting that the nature of estrogen's effects depends on the intracellular biochemical processes being activated. In fact, some of estrogen's actions may be mediated by alterations in G-proteins. Estrogen enhances the pertussis toxin-catalyzed adenosine diphosphate (ADP)-ribosylation of G$_{\alpha i,o}$, which indicates that E2 modifies the G-protein, possibly through protein kinase A phosphorylation. This is analogous to the rapid effects of E2 in the hypothalamus and hippocampus; therefore, this mechanism of 'uncoupling' G$_{\alpha i,o}$-coupled monoamine receptors may be via a common pathway in the CNS and peripheral tissues.

Although the striatum is a prime target for estrogen modulation of motor activity, there is virtually no ER-α receptor mRNA expression and very little ER-β mRNA expression in this dopamine-rich pathway, suggesting that E2 activates another receptor subtype in this region. Evidence for a membrane receptor for E2 is substantiated by studies showing that membrane-impermeable E2–BSA rapidly stimulates dopamine release from striatal slices. Other studies have shown that femtomolar concentrations of E2 and E2–BSA rapidly inhibit whole-cell L-type calcium currents in medium spiny (GABAergic) caudate putamen neurons.

D. Epilepsy

Given the preponderance of data on neurosteroid modulation of GABA$_A$ and glutamate receptors, it is perhaps no surprise that there is strong evidence that both endogenous and exogenous neurosteroids can affect seizures. Studies in epileptic women have correlated high serum E2 levels with an increased risk of seizures and increased frequency of interictal epileptiform (IED) activity on electroencephalograms (EEGs). Exogenous estrogen administration reduces the latency and increases the severity of kainate-induced seizures in both male and female rats. Inversely, progesterone administration increases the electroshock- or kainate-induced seizure threshold in female rats. In women, high progesterone levels are associated with reduced IEDs. In fact, approximately one-third of epileptic women have a greater than twofold increase in their seizure frequency prior to their menses, when progesterone levels normally drop precipitously (catemenial epilepsy). This is particularly important in epileptic women with inadequate luteal phase syndrome, in which the progesterone levels do not stay sufficiently elevated for the entire luteal phase of the menstrual cycle. This results in irregular menstrual periods, infertility, and a significant increase in seizure frequency before and during menstrual periods. In some studies, it has been shown that administration of progesterone analog reduces seizure frequency by 39% in women with catemenial epilepsy.

At the cellular level, progesterone has a high affinity for intracellular progesterone receptors but has weak actions at GABA$_A$ receptors. However, allopregnanolone is devoid of activity at intracellular progesterone receptors but is a highly effective modulator of GABA$_A$ receptor complexes. There is increasing evidence that the antiseizure effects of progesterone may be mediated by conversion to allopregnanolone. Intravenous or intracerebroventricular administration of allopregnanolone has been shown to suppress seizures in animal models ranging from *in vivo* perforant path stimulation to

injection of picrotoxin or bicuculline. Although both progesterone and allopregnanolone inhibit seizures, the effects of progesterone are greatly inhibited if co-administered with 5α-reductase inhibitors. Allopregnanolone may be an endogenous modulator of seizure threshold as well. Although there is no difference in serum allopregnanolone levels in epileptic and nonepileptic women, there is a significant increase in serum allopregnanolone within 15 min of partial-onset seizures.

VI. CONCLUSIONS

The classic model of steroid hormone action is one in which (neuroactive) steroids are produced in the adrenals/gonads and travel through the bloodstream to the brain, where they alter protein synthesis by genomic actions at nuclear receptors. In contrast, neurosteroids, many of which are produced within the CNS, have nongenomic effects (alteration of a variety of neuronal functions, including those involving ion channels and ionotropic and G-protein-coupled receptors), allowing for the possibility of local control of hormone synthesis. Other steroids (e.g., testosterone) are taken up from the blood and may provide a mechanism for coordinating CNS and peripheral (outside the CNS) physiology. Additionally, there is a wide variety of steroid derivatives and they have an equally wide range of specific physiological actions. Given the broad range of neurosteroid action in various cellular physiological systems, it is not surprising that these compounds may be in involved in multiple arenas of CNS neurophysiology. There is good evidence at systemic and cellular levels for a role of neurosteroids in physiological/pathophysiological processes, ranging from reproduction to epilepsy. We have barely scratched the surface in understanding neurosteroid physiology and the prospect of expanding this field is exciting. In addition to increasing our understanding of normal physiology, steroid derivatives may offer important therapeutic options in the future. The broad range of action of neurosteroids may prove to be valuable ammunition in the arsenal of clinicians.

Glossary

dehydroepiandrostenedione Neurosteroid that is synthesized in the central nervous system.
γ-aminobutyric acid The most prominent inhibitory neurotransmitter in the central nervous system.
G-protein-coupled receptor Membrane receptor that activates intracellular G-proteins.

ionotropic receptor Membrane receptor with an intrinsic ion channel.

N-methyl D-aspartate Selective ligand for one class of glutamate receptors.

P450aro Cytochrome P450 (aromatase); enzyme that converts testosterone to estrogen.

P450c11 Cytochrome P450 (11β-hydroxylase); enzyme that converts 11-deoxycorticosterone to corticosterone, 11-deoxycortisol to cortisol, and 18-hydroxycorticosterone to aldosterone.

P450c17 Cytochrome P450 (17α-hydroxylase/C-17,C-20 lyase); enzyme that converts pregnenolone to 17α-hydroxypregnenolone, then to dehydroepiandrosterone.

P450c21 Cytochrome P450 (21-hydroxylase); enzyme that converts progesterone to 11-deoxycorticosterone.

P450scc Cytochrome P450 (cholesterol side chain cleavage); enzyme that converts cholesterol to pregnenolone.

pregnenolone sulfate Neurosteroid that modulates glutamate channel activity.

17β-estradiol Female gonadal steroid that is a neuroactive steroid in the central nervous system.

testosterone Male gonadal steroid that is converted to 17β-estradiol in the central nervous system.

3α,5α-tetrahydrocorticosterone Neurosteroid that modulates GABA$_A$ channel activity.

3α,5α-tetrahydroprogesterone (allopregnanolone) Neurosteroid that modulates GABA$_A$ channel activity.

See Also the Following Articles

Estrogen Receptor-α Structure and Function • Estrogen Receptor-β Structure and Function • Membrane Steroid Receptors • Progesterone Receptor Structure/Function and Crosstalk with Cellular Signaling Pathways • Steroid Hormone Receptor Family: Mechanisms of Action • Steroidogenic Acute Regulatory (StAR) Protein, Cholesterol, and Control of Steroidogenesis

Further Reading

Balieu, E. E. (1998). Neurosteroids: A novel function of the brain. *Psychoneuroendocrinology* **23**, 963–987.

Barker, J. L., Harrison, N. L., Lange, G. D., and Owen, D. G. (1987). Potentiation of gamma-aminobutyric-acid-activated chloride conductance by a steroid anaesthetic in cultured rat spinal neurones. *J. Physiol.* **386**, 485–490.

Compagnone, N. A., and Mellon, S. H. (2000). Neurosteroids: Biosynthesis and function of these novel neuromodulators. *Front. Neuroendocrinol.* **21**, 1–56.

Ffrench-Mullen, J. M. H., Danks, P., and Spence, K. T. (1994). Neurosteroids modulate calcium currents in hippocampal CA1 neurons via a pertussis toxin-sensitive G-protein-coupled mechanism. *J. Neurosci.* **14**, 1963–1977.

Foy, M. R., Xu, J., Xie, X., Brinton, R. D., Thompson, R. F., and Berger, T. W. (1999). 17β-Estradiol enhances NMDA receptor-mediated EPSPs and long-term potentiation. *J. Neurophysiol.* **81**, 925–929.

Gu, Q., Korach, K. S., and Moss, R. L. (1999). Rapid actions of 17β-estradiol on kainate-induced currents in hippocampal

neurons lacking intracellular estrogen receptors. *Endocrinology* **140**, 660–666.

Herzog, A. G. (1999). Progesterone therapy in women with epilepsy: A 3 year follow up. *Neurology* **52**, 1917–1918.

Lagrange, A. H., Rønnekleiv, O. K., and Kelly, M. J. (1997). Modulation of G protein-coupled receptors by an estrogen receptor that activates protein kinase A. *Mol. Pharmacol.* **51**, 605–612.

Majewska, M. D., Harrison, N. L., Schwartz, R. D., Barker, J. L., and Paul, S. M. (1986). Steroid hormone metabolites are barbiturate-like modulators of the GABA receptor. *Science* **232**, 1004–1007.

Mermelstein, P. G., Becker, J. B., and Surmeier, D. J. (1996). Estradiol reduces calcium currents in rat neostriatal neurons via a membrane receptor. *J. Neurosci.* **16**, 595–604.

Nicoletti, F., Speciale, C., Sortino, M. A., *et al.* (1985). Comparative effects of estradiol benzoate, the antiestrogen clomiphene citrate, and the progestin medroxyprogesterone acetate on kainic acid-induced seizures in male and female rats. *Epilepsia* **26**, 252–257.

Park-Chung, M., Malayev, A., Purdy, R. H., Gibbs, T. T., and Farb, D. H. (1999). Sulfated and unsulfated steroids modulate gamma-aminobutyric acid A receptor function through distinct sites. *Brain Res.* **830**, 72–87.

Pinna, G., Uzunova, V., Matsumoto, K., Puia, G., Mienville, J. M., Costa, E., and Guidotti, A. (2000). Brain allopregnenolone regulates the potency of the GABA(A) receptor agonist muscimol. *Neuropharmacology* **39**, 440–448.

Prince, R. J., and Simmonds, M. A. (1992). Steroid modulation of the strychnine-sensitive glycine receptor. *Neuropharmacology* **31**, 201–205.

Quinn, N. P., and Marsden, C. D. (1986). Menstrual-related fluctuations in Parkinson's disease. *Mov. Disord.* **1**, 85–87.

Seyle, H. (1941). Anaesthetic effects of steroid hormones. *Proc. Soc. Exp. Biol.* **46**, 116–121.

Neuropeptide Regulators of Juvenile Hormone Production

STEPHEN S. TOBE[*] AND BARBARA STAY[†]

*University of Toronto • †University of Iowa

I. INTRODUCTION
II. IS JUVENILE HORMONE PRODUCTION REGULATED?
III. ALLATOTROPINS
IV. ALLATOSTATINS

The juvenile hormone of insects is a primary regulator of growth, metamorphosis, and reproduction in most insect species. As a consequence, it is essential that juvenile hormone production be precisely regulated so that it is present only during appropriate periods necessary for the control of these processes. The presence of juvenile hormone at inappropriate times can result in disruption to metamorphosis and development and, in some cases, to disturbances in female reproduction. For this reason, complex mechanisms that regulate the production of juvenile hormone have evolved and, in many cases, neuropeptides are the primary regulators.

I. INTRODUCTION

In larval insects, the presence of juvenile hormone (JH) directs cells to continue development in a larval direction, whereas its presence in adult females directs specific cells to produce molecules associated with reproduction. In the absence of JH, metamorphosis of larval insects proceeds, either directly to the adult stage, in the hemimetabolous species (e.g., grasshoppers, bugs, cockroaches), or through an intervening pupal stage, in holometabolous species (e.g., beetles, moths and butterflies, flies, bees). The presence or absence of JH therefore determines the direction of development and reproduction in all

insects at all stages of the life cycle. It is for this reason that the regulation of production of JH plays a central role in the life cycle of the insect. This article provides an overview of the neuropeptides that are known to regulate JH production in insects.

II. IS JUVENILE HORMONE PRODUCTION REGULATED?

Is there evidence that JH production in insects is in fact regulated? As a central regulator of both development and physiology of the insect, the importance of JH and precisely controlled changes in its production cannot be overestimated. Figure 1 demonstrates that in both larval and adult stages, the production of JH undergoes dramatic and predictable changes. In the larval stages, these changes are associated with the ecdysis or molt, whereas in the adult, these changes are associated with the reproductive cycle and the production of eggs. In both cases, distinct peaks occur, and these are invariably associated with important physiological events,

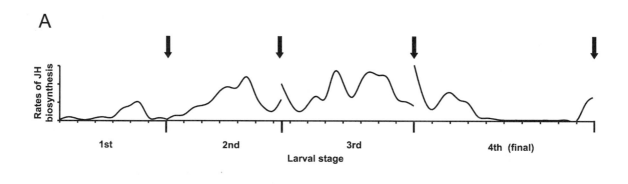

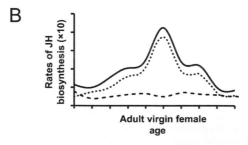

FIGURE 1   Juvenile hormone (JH) biosynthesis as a function of age throughout the larval stage (A) and in the adult virgin female (B) in the cockroach *Diploptera punctata*. Arrows denote the time of molting (A). (B) The results of unilateral cautery of the lateral neurosecretory cell region of the brain of virgin females that do not normally show a cycle of JH biosynthesis. The solid line represents JH biosynthesis by corpora allata on the unoperated side plus the corpora allata from the operated side; the line with long dashes represents JH biosynthesis by the single control unoperated corpus allatum; and the line with short dashes represents JH biosynthesis by the single operated corpus allatum.

including the time of deposition of the next cuticle in larvae and the synthesis of the yolk protein and its uptake by developing oocytes in adult females.

Profiles of JH production have been obtained for only a tiny number of existing insect species but all of these have revealed distinctive and predictable changes in production. In most cases, the periods of maximal production precede the larval molts or are associated with oocyte production in females. Rates of production of JH change dramatically over short periods of time, with changes of 10- to 20-fold being commonplace. In the very few studies that have examined the relationship between JH production and the circulating titer of hormone in the hemolymph, there is a high correlation. Accordingly, JH production mirrors the titer of the hormone.

Assuming that JH production is precisely regulated, how is this process in turn controlled? As with most other endocrine glands, the regulation of hormone production by the corpora allata is effected by neuropeptides and neurohormones. The principal neuropeptide regulators in insects are known as allatotropins (stimulators) and allatostatins (inhibitors) and a range of compounds that show such activity have been isolated. However, it should be noted that most assays for biological activity of these neuropeptides have employed short-term experiments *in vitro*, whereby the compounds in question are incubated with the corpora allata outside of the animal. In very few instances have the neuropeptides been shown to have high activity *in vivo*. Nonetheless, it is now widely believed that neuropeptides were some of the earliest neurotransmitters in the invertebrates and play a major role in the regulation of hormone production in all animals.

III. ALLATOTROPINS

Nomenclature for insect neuropeptides is confusing. Peptides have been named on the basis of the function for which they were originally discovered, which may not be the true function or may be only one of several physiological functions. At present, there are two naming systems, a three-letter prefix, employing the first two letters of the genus and the first letter of the species of the insect in which the peptide was originally discovered, followed by the functional name of the peptide; and a five-letter prefix using the first three letters of the genus and the first two letters of the species (e.g., for *Manduca sexta* allatotropin: Mas-allatotropin or Manse-latotropin).

Neuropeptides known as allatotropins are responsible for the stimulation of JH production.

Such stimulation is important to the insect, to raise the titer of JH in the hemolymph at appropriate times during development or reproduction. The allatotropin appears to exert its stimulatory effect directly on the corpus allatum, the site of biosynthesis and release of the JH. To date, a single type of allatotropin, a 13-amino-acid peptide, has been isolated and identified from the hornworm, *M. sexta*. The amino acid sequence of the Manse-allatotropin is Gly-Phe-Lys-Asn-Val-Glu-Met-Met-Thr-Ala-Arg-Gly-Phe-NH$_2$.

This peptide has been demonstrated to stimulate JH production *in vitro* and structurally related peptides are known to occur in other members of the Lepidoptera, as well as in flies, mosquitoes, locusts, and cockroaches. However, these peptides do not show appreciable allatotropic activity (i.e., the ability to stimulate JH production) in these species, except for the Lepidopteran species. As with many peptides, the allatotropin peptide is not necessarily active at all times of the life cycle and the tissues of the insect show distinct periods of sensitivity. In fact, allatotropin was believed to be active only in adult hornworms, but more recent evidence indicates that it is active at specific times during larval life of some Lepidoptera. In addition, allatotropin exerts effects on tissues other than the corpora allata, including the stimulation of heart/dorsal vessel contraction and inhibition of ion transport across the larval midgut. Such actions are considered pleiotropic and emphasize the multifunctional nature of this peptide as well as of the allatostatins (see below).

Allatotropin is produced by cells in both the brain/central nervous system (CNS) of larvae and adults of *M. sexta* and is prominent in cells of the stomatogastric nervous system (e.g., ganglia and nerves along the foregut) and in the ganglia of the ventral nerve cord. In *Drosophila melanogaster* larvae, immunoreactivity to allatotropin is found in individual cells distributed in the lateral and tritocerebral regions of the brain and in the anterior portion of the ventral ganglion (Fig. 2).

The gene encoding the *Manduca* allatotropin has been cloned and characterized in this species as well as in other Lepidoptera and in *Drosophila*. It is expressed, as predicted from the above discussion, in several tissues, particularly the brain and ventral nerve cord, and at specific times during the life cycle (Fig. 2). The allatotropin peptide can be derived from each of three different precursor proteins and these proteins appear to arise as a result of alternative splicing of the allatotropin gene. The precursors also contain other allatotropin-like peptides that

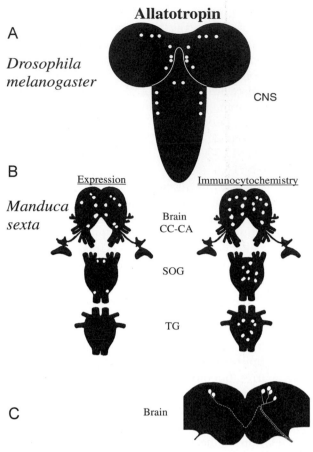

FIGURE 2 Distribution of allatotropin immunoreactivity and expression in larval *Drosophila melanogaster* CNS (A) and in larval (fifth stage) *Manduca sexta* (B). (C) The pathway of cerebral allatotropin-immunoreactive neurons in the larval (fifth stage) *Manduca* brain. (A) *Drosophila* data from P. M. Koladich (2002), Ph.D. thesis, University of Toronto; (B) *Manduca* data from T. R. Bhatt (1998), Ph.D. thesis, University of Nevada, Reno; (C) data from Zitnan *et al.* (1995), modified and redrawn, with permission. CC, corpora cardiaca; CA, corpora allata; CNS, brain + ventral ganglion; SOG, subesophageal ganglion; TG, thoracic ganglion.

show biological activity. Allatotropin is expressed in the brain in larval stages (i.e., mRNA for allatotropin is present), indicating a potential role in the stimulation of JH production, in addition to the midgut function.

Alternative splicing is a common mechanism to increase the capacity and diversity of genes and their protein/peptide products and to regulate gene expression. In addition, the regulation of alternative splicing shows developmental and tissue specificity and may itself be hormonally controlled. It is significant that only a single allatotropin family has been identified to date, and the occurrence of

alternative splicing may permit diversity in the function and developmental profile for the peptide.

IV. ALLATOSTATINS

A. Structure and Action

The two mechanisms that potentially regulate JH production involve either stimulation or inhibition of the biosynthetic process for the hormone within the corpora allata. The stimulation of biosynthesis would appear at first glance to represent the simplest means of regulating hormone production—in the presence of stimulatory factors, JH would be produced, presumably in a dose-dependent fashion, and in the absence of such factors, production would cease. An equally viable means of regulation is the inhibition of hormone production. In many species, this appears to be the primary mode of regulation of JH production; that is, corpora allata are normally inhibited or restrained in a dose-dependent fashion, and in the absence of the inhibitory signal, the glands are released and able to produce JH once again. However, in this instance, an increased dose of inhibitory factors would reduce JH production, and in most species studied to date, JH production cannot be completely inhibited by these factors, nor do corpora allata appear to be completely inhibited in the *in vivo* situation. It is likely that the corpora allata produce JH at a basal level, irrespective of the mode of regulation. That is, glands that operate by way of a stimulatory pathway do produce JH even when the allatotropin is not present, albeit at much lower levels than in the presence of the allatotropin (stimulation appears to be in the range of 4- to 10-fold). Conversely, glands that operate by way of an inhibitory pathway produce JH at low levels, even in the presence of the allatostatin. In both instances, such basal rates of JH biosynthesis are important, since they do indicate that the pathway for the production of JH is extant; the presence of the pathway permits a rapid response of the corpora allata to the neuropeptide signals. Glands that are completely inactive (and hence may lack the enzymes of the biosynthetic pathway for JH) may require a longer interval to respond to neuropeptide signals if biosynthesis of the enzymes is required.

The allatostatins or equivalent inhibitory factors have been hypothesized to exist for more than 50 years. Inhibition of the corpora allata and hence of JH production was inferred by studies on the effect of transection of nerves on the volume of the corpora allata, on production of eggs, or on the nature of the molt in larvae. Similar effects were subsequently obtained following cautery of selected regions of the brain, particularly following destruction of the lateral neurosecretory cells (see Fig. 3). Such operations resulted in the stimulation of JH production (see Fig. 1B) and a stimulation of the physiological

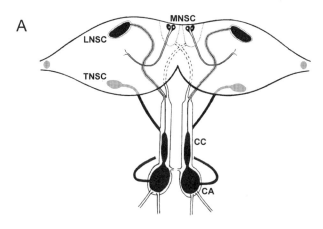

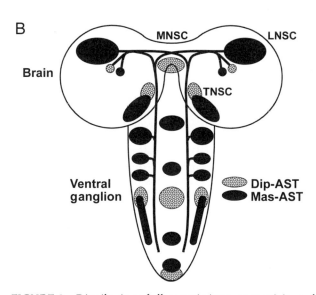

FIGURE 3 Distribution of allatostatin immunoreactivity and expression in the brain and retrocerebral complex of adult female *Diploptera* (A) and CNS of larval *Drosophila* (B), dorsal view. In *Drosophila*, immunoreactivity to both cockroach and *Manduca* allatostatin is shown. In A, lightly shaded regions represent cell groups visible from the ventral perspective. MNSC, medial neurosecretory cells; LNSC, lateral neurosecretory cells; CC, corpora cardiaca; CA, corpora allata. Reprinted from Stephen S. Tobe (1999), Allostatins, *In* "Encyclopedia of Reproduction" (E. Knobil and J.D. Neill, eds). With permission from Elsevier.

processes regulated by JH. Such experiments led workers, including Berta Scharrer, to the conclusion that the corpora allata in cockroaches were normally inhibited by factors from specific neurosecretory cells in the brain.

The allatostatin neuropeptides can be categorized into three families, based on similarities in their amino acid sequences. The largest, most diverse, and most ubiquitous family is the cockroach allatostatins, or the Phe-Gly-Leu-amide family (FGLa) (see Fig. 4). All of these peptides share this common carboxyl-terminus. The five C-terminal amino acids can be generalized as the consensus sequence Tyr/Phe-Xaa-Phe-Gly-Leu-amide, although some minor substitutions do occur in some species (Fig. 4). To date, over 170 FGLa peptides have been either isolated or predicted on the basis of gene sequences and, although commonly called the cockroach allatostatins, actually occur throughout the insects as well as the crustaceans. Similar sequences or immunoreactivity to FGLa-like compounds has also been found in helminth worms, in mollusks, and in platyhelminths.

Figure 4 shows the 14 allatostatin peptides predicted from the coding region of the allatostatin gene of the American cockroach, *Periplaneta americana*, and the precursor polypeptide structure. Studies on other cockroach species have revealed that this family of peptides is remarkably conserved across the order Dictyoptera, suggesting important and ancient functions for the allatostatins. However, this function may not necessarily be the inhibition of JH production, since these peptides appear to be active only in this respect in cockroaches and closely related species such as crickets. In all other insect orders studies, the FGLa peptides are inactive in terms of JH biosynthesis *in vitro* but are potent myomodulators.

Cockroach allatostatins occur in all other orders that have been studied but at present, the identity of these compounds has been established definitively only in crickets and in selected members of the Lepidoptera and Diptera. It is clear that flies, including *Drosophila*, have different compounds capable of inhibiting JH production, but to date, these have not been sequenced. It will be particularly important to isolate and identify the *D. melanogaster* allatostatins in view of the genetic significance of this species and the availability of the genome sequence.

A second group of allatostatins has been isolated and identified from crickets. These peptides are characterized by tryptophan (W) residues at the N-terminal 2 and 9 positions. The generalized structure of these peptides is shown in Table 1 and this group is

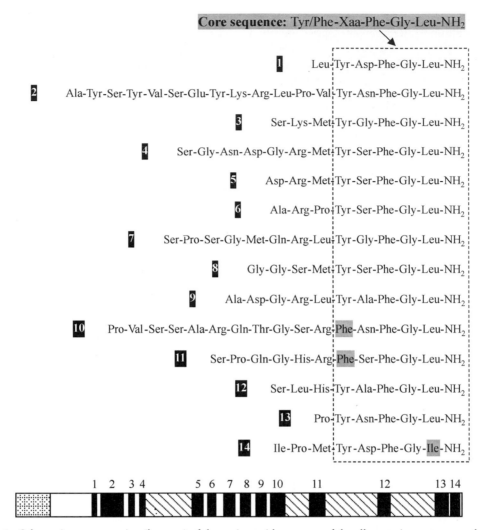

Core sequence: Tyr/Phe-Xaa-Phe-Gly-Leu-NH$_2$

1 Leu-Tyr-Asp-Phe-Gly-Leu-NH$_2$

2 Ala-Tyr-Ser-Tyr-Val-Ser-Glu-Tyr-Lys-Arg-Leu-Pro-Val-Tyr-Asn-Phe-Gly-Leu-NH$_2$

3 Ser-Lys-Met-Tyr-Gly-Phe-Gly-Leu-NH$_2$

4 Ser-Gly-Asn-Asp-Gly-Arg-Met-Tyr-Ser-Phe-Gly-Leu-NH$_2$

5 Asp-Arg-Met-Tyr-Ser-Phe-Gly-Leu-NH$_2$

6 Ala-Arg-Pro-Tyr-Ser-Phe-Gly-Leu-NH$_2$

7 Ser-Pro-Ser-Gly-Met-Gln-Arg-Leu-Tyr-Gly-Phe-Gly-Leu-NH$_2$

8 Gly-Gly-Ser-Met-Tyr-Ser-Phe-Gly-Leu-NH$_2$

9 Ala-Asp-Gly-Arg-Leu-Tyr-Ala-Phe-Gly-Leu-NH$_2$

10 Pro-Val-Ser-Ser-Ala-Arg-Gln-Thr-Gly-Ser-Arg-Phe-Asn-Phe-Gly-Leu-NH$_2$

11 Ser-Pro-Gln-Gly-His-Arg-Phe-Ser-Phe-Gly-Leu-NH$_2$

12 Ser-Leu-His-Tyr-Ala-Phe-Gly-Leu-NH$_2$

13 Pro-Tyr-Asn-Phe-Gly-Leu-NH$_2$

14 Ile-Pro-Met-Tyr-Asp-Phe-Gly-Ile-NH$_2$

FIGURE 4 Schematic representation (bottom) of the amino acid sequence of the allatostatin precursor polypeptide in the cockroach *Periplaneta americana*. The hydrophobic leader sequence (signal sequence) precedes an untranslated region (clear), which is then followed by the allatostatin peptides. Black boxes represent individual allatostatins, which are numbered according to their position relative to the amino-terminus, and the amino acid sequences of each, corresponding to the numbers, are shown at the top. Acidic regions are indicated as diagonally striped areas. Shaded residues in the peptide sequences represent conservative substitutions.

commonly referred to as the W$_2$W$_9$ amide or W$_2$W$_9$a family of allatostatins. To date, these peptides are known to occur in crickets and in stick insects, but they are able to inhibit JH production only in crickets and at concentrations that are an order of magnitude greater than those of the FGLa family. The occurrence of these peptides in stick insects has necessitated a change in name of this family because the peptides are of variable length; hence, the designation W(X)$_6$Wa is more appropriate. The structure of the gene encoding this family of peptides has recently been described in *Drosophila* although the peptides have yet to be isolated in this species.

A third group of peptides capable of inhibiting JH production in Lepidoptera is known as the PISCF family of allatostatins (see Table 1). Currently, only two members have been identified (isolated and sequenced). The *Manduca* peptide is a 15-amino-acid nonamidated, N-terminally blocked peptide originally isolated from *M. sexta* but subsequently found in other Lepidopteran species (Table 1). This peptide is unique, both from the structural perspective, in that it does not occur in any order other than Lepidoptera, and from the functional perspective, since the peptide is capable of inhibiting JH production completely (i.e., 100% inhibition), at least in

TABLE I Allatostatin Amino Acid Sequences

Gryllus bimaculatus W(X)$_6$Wa allatostatins

Gly-Trp-Gln-Asp-Leu-Asn-Gly-Gly-Trp-NH$_2$

Gly-Trp-Arg-Asp-Leu-Asn-Gly-Gly-Trp-NH$_2$

Ala-Trp-Arg-Asp-Leu-Ser-Gly-Gly-Trp-NH$_2$

Ala-Trp-Glu-Arg-Phe-His-Gly-Ser-Trp-NH$_2$

Ala-Trp-Asp-Gln-Leu-Arg-Pro-Gly-Trp-NH$_2$

Manduca sexta PISCF allatostatin

gGlu-Val-Arg-Phe-Arg-Gln-Cys-Tyr-Phe-Asn-Pro-Ile-Ser-Cys-Phe-OH

Drosophila melanogaster PISCF allatostatin/flatline

gGlu-Val-Arg-Tyr-Arg-Gln-Cys-Tyr-Phe-Asn-Pro-Ile-Ser-Cys-Phe-OH

Manduca. No other peptide is capable of reversibly inhibiting JH production to this degree. Furthermore, this peptide has no effect on JH production in non-Lepidopteran species and also appears to affect JH production in larvae and adults of selected Lepidoptera differentially.

A peptide very similar to the Manse-allatostatin (Manse-AST) has been identified in the genome of *D. melanogaster*, with a precursor organization similar to that of the *Manduca* precursor. This peptide is identical to Manse-AST, with the exception of a Tyr substituted for a Phe at N-position 4 of the peptide. This peptide does not inhibit JH production in flies but is a very effective modulator of heart muscle contraction, rapidly and reversibly suppressing contractions at specific developmental stages. For this reason, the peptide and associated gene have been named "*flatline*."

B. Distribution of Allatostatins

Studies on the distribution of the allatostatins provide information not only on sites of release but also on potential target organs. Such information can provide insights into the functions of these peptides, which is particularly important for the allatostatins in light of their very large number, their extensive distribution, and the many different functions that they appear to perform (pleiotropism). Most of the information has been obtained from studies on the FGLa and the PISCF families and principally using immunocytochemistry and to a lesser extent *in situ* hybridization. In view of the role of the allatostatins in the inhibition of JH production, cells innervating the corpora allata can be expected to have immunoreactivity to these peptides. Figures 3 and 5 show diagrammatic representations and micrographs of the innervation of the corpora allata by cells in the brain. Innervation arises principally from the lateral neurosecretory cells although medial neurosecretory cells also appear to be important. The neurons arborize extensively within the corpora allata and there are apparent release sites within the glands. In the case of the *Drosophila* larval CNS, both FGLa immunoreactivity and PISCF immunoreactivity are apparent (Fig. 3B). In *Drosophila* as well, the transection of the nerves innervating the corpora allata, as in the cautery experiments with *Diploptera* noted in Fig. 1B, prevent the release of the peptides in the target tissue, thus releasing the corpora allata from the inhibition of the allatostatins. Not all allatostatins are released from the brain by way of axonal tracts to targets outside the brain. Within the brain, axons from the lateral, medial, and tritocerebral groups all arborize extensively and appear to innervate other neurons and thus can be regarded as interneurons.

Figure 5 also demonstrates extensive innervation of the hindgut of the termite by allatostatin-immunoreactive neurons and reveals the very wide distribution of allatostatin immunoreactivity in most insects. A similar distribution can be found in the midgut, foregut, and hindgut of many species, as well as in the reproductive system, in the optic lobes and antennal lobes, and throughout the CNS. Allatostatins are also found in high concentrations in the hemolymph (blood) serum and some hemocytes of cockroaches. Although it is not possible to define the serum source of the peptides, the extensive release sites observed in and on many tissues including the gut and CNS suggest that these tissues are important contributors.

C. Receptors for Allatostatins

The clear action of the FGLa allatostatins as inhibitors of JH production in cockroaches and in crickets demands the presence of appropriate receptors in the target tissues, including the corpora allata. Since there are multiple allatostatins in these organisms, multiple receptors for the peptides may also exist. In addition, the corpora allata show major differences in sensitivity to the allatostatins at selected developmental times, suggesting that receptor occurrence or expression is regulated. In general, in adult females, the glands show a low level of sensitivity at times of high production of JH, whereas in larvae, although a similar relationship exists early in the stadium, at times of minimal JH production, the corpora allata also appear to be insensitive at later times in the stadium.

The other biological actions of the FGLa allatostatins, particularly the ability to modulate myotropic

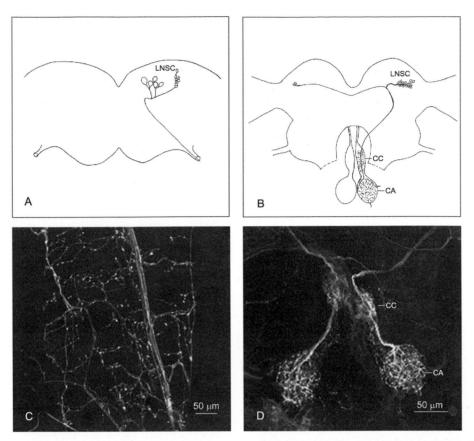

FIGURE 5 Allatostatin immunoreactivity in *Diploptera punctata*, *Manduca sexta*, and *Reticulotermes flavipes*. (A) Diagram of cells in brain of last-stage larva of *Manduca* that innervate the corpora allata and are immunoreactive for Manse-AST (from Zitnan *et al.*, 1995, *Journal of Comparative Neurology* 356, pp. 83–100). (B) Diagram of cells in adult brain of *Diploptera* that innervate the corpora allata and are immunoreactive for Dippu-AST (from Chiang *et al.*, 1999, *Journal of Comparative Neurology* 413, pp. 593–602, Copyright 1999 Wiley. Reprinted by permission of John Wiley & Sons, Inc.). (C) Micrograph of nerves on the muscles of the colon of a termite, *R. flavipes*, that are immunoreactive for Dippu-AST. The varicosities are neuropeptide release sites. Stacked confocal microscope images of twenty-two 2 μm sections. (D) Micrograph of corpora allata and corpora cardiaca of a 45-day embryo of *Diploptera* that are immunoreactive for Dippu-AST. Stacked confocal microscope images of fifteen 2 μm sections. LNSC, lateral neurosecretory cells; CC, corpus cardiacum; CA, corpus allatum.

activity of the midgut and hindgut, also suggest the occurrence of multiple receptors or subtypes for these peptides. These actions are quite distinct from the inhibitory action on the corpora allata and may involve different signaling pathways (see Table 2). To date, two receptor subtypes have been cloned from *Drosophila* and at least one has been cloned from cockroaches. These receptors have been confirmed to be members of the G-protein-coupled superfamily and are structurally related to vertebrate galanin and somatostatin receptors, neither peptide of which is known to occur in insects. These receptors all exhibit seven membrane-spanning domains characteristic of the G-protein-coupled superfamily. The most con-

served regions are the transmembrane domains facing the intracellular side of the membrane known to interact with G-proteins, which appear to be effectors both in the vertebrate system and in the insect system. The greatest difference in the receptors is on the extracellular side of the membrane in the ligand-binding region. This suggests that during evolution, the G-protein-binding domains were conserved, whereas the ligand-binding regions have undergone "rapid" change in response to the variety of ligands available.

As noted earlier, the different allatostatins of the FGLa family show different biological activities, with respect to both their ability to inhibit JH

TABLE 2 Rank Order of Effectiveness of Dippu FGLamide Allatostatins

Peptide designation	Length (amino acid residues)	Muscle contraction	JH Production
Dippu-AST1	6	7	13
Dippu-AST2	18	9	1
Dippu-AST3	8	10	11
Dippu-AST4	9	5	6
Dippu-AST5	8	8	2
Dippu-AST6	8	11	5
Dippu-AST7	13	3	3
Dippu-AST8	9	2	10
Dippu-AST9	10	1	8
Dippu-AST10	16	6	4
Dippu-AST11	11	4	7
Dippu-AST12	6	12	9
Dippu-AST13	8	2	12

production and their ability to modulate myotropic activity (Table 2). With the elucidation of at least two receptors in insect systems, it is likely that these differences in biological activities are attributable to differences in the affinity of the receptors for the different allatostatins. The relative distribution of different receptor subtypes probably permits differences in the responses of target tissues.

The core region responsible for biological activity of the allatostatins is the C-terminal pentapeptide (Fig. 4). This sequence, which is conserved throughout the FGLa family of peptides, interacts with the extracellular surface-binding domain of the receptor(s) and shows full biological activity, albeit at high concentrations. This peptide appears to represent the minimal number of amino acid residues necessary for full potency. This suggestion has now been confirmed using expressed receptor in the frog oocyte expression system.

D. Evolution of Allatostatins

The original function of the FGLa allatostatins is clearly unknown, but in view of the ubiquitous nature of the peptides in insects and other invertebrates, it is likely that they performed a myomodulatory function, as they do in modern species. Nonetheless, the remarkable sequence conservation in the cockroaches does suggest that these peptides are ancient and that their co-opting for the purposes of regulation of JH biosynthesis probably occurred before speciation. Thus, the various cockroach allatostatins can be regarded as orthologues.

The large number of extant peptides of the FGLa allatostatin family (at present, over 170 peptides have been isolated or predicted from gene sequences) might also indicate that specific allatostatins have specific functions, at least in cockroaches and related species. It is possible that at least some of the different allatostatins are not replaceable, effecting only narrowly defined functions. There is some suggestion of this in the different rank order of the allatostatins in terms of the ability to inhibit JH biosynthesis versus modulation of myotropic activity in cockroaches, whereby allatostatins that are the most active in terms of one function often show only very low biological activity in the other function (see Table 2). On the other hand, the great profusion of allatostatins suggests that the allatostatins may be replaceable for a particular function, reflecting some flexibility in the receptor-binding domain. The only region in which amino acid differences are not possible for retention of function is in the core region.

It is likely that the additional functions of allatostatins remain to be defined. At present, it is known that the FGLa family of peptides is able to:

(1) inhibit JH biosynthesis in cockroaches and crickets;
(2) modulate muscle contraction, both spontaneous and proctolin-induced;
(3) modulate neuronal activity in crab CNS;
(4) inhibit vitellogenin production in cockroaches; and
(5) modulate digestive enzyme activity in cockroaches.

The same allatostatin can exert several target-specific effects. The redundancy in the FGLa allatostatin function could allow for the proliferation of the peptides throughout evolution. Immunocyto-chemistry has putatively identified a very large number of different FGLa peptides in the invertebrates. In insects, in any given species in orders more recently evolved than cockroaches, there is a reduction in the number of members of the allatostatin family (based on gene sequences). For example, this number is reduced from 13 or14 in cockroaches to between 5 and 9 in flies and moths. It is significant, however, that there has been a concurrent loss in functionality of the FGLa peptides since they have no effect on JH production in these orders. At this point, it is impossible to determine whether the loss of inhibitory function (and hence a loss of receptor) preceded the reduction in number of the peptides. It is instructive to observe that in the locust, there has been a reduction in the FGLa family to 10 members and a loss in sensitivity to inhibition of JH production. Accordingly, a loss in biological activity may accompany the loss in the peptides expressed in a given species. In crickets, a family in which allatostatins are effective in the inhibition of JH production, there remain 14 putative peptides in the precursor deduced from cDNA sequences.

The neuropeptide regulators of corpus allatum function are important not only with respect to their modulation of JH production but also in their many other functions and in the insight they may provide into the evolution of neuropeptide families.

Glossary

corpora allata Insect endocrine glands associated with and receiving innervation from the central nervous system; the site of production of juvenile hormone.

juvenile hormone Sesquiterpenoid compound, derived from farnesyl biphosphate, that regulates metamorphosis and reproduction in many insect species.

orthologue Peptides from a pair of genes in related species, derived from a single gene in the last common ancestor, which arose as a result of a speciation event; genes of different species that have a common origin. Orthologue assignments do not involve function.

paralogue When a peptide gene is duplicated giving rise to two copies in the genome, the two genes and their products are considered paralogous; involves a duplication and not a speciation event.

pleiotropism The phenomenon whereby one peptide or peptide family exerts multiple physiological effects on target tissues.

preprohormone The entire polypeptide encoded by an mRNA for a peptide hormone or hormones before processing by prohormone convertase enzymes to remove signal sequences and other nonfunctional regions.

prohormone The polypeptide encoded by an mRNA for a peptide hormone following removal of the signal sequence. Cleavage of the prohormone to individual peptides by prohormone convertases results in the release of the final peptide sequences with biological activity.

See Also the Following Articles

Insect Endocrine System ● Juvenile Hormone Action in Insect Development ● Juvenile Hormone Action in Insect Reproduction ● Juvenile Hormone Biosynthesis ● Juvenile Hormones, Chemistry of

Further Reading

Belles, X., Graham, L. A., Bendena, W. G., Ding, Q., Edwards, J. P., Weaver, R. J., and Tobe, S. S. (1999). The molecular evolution of the allatostatin precursor in cockroaches—A guide to methods and applications. *Peptides* 20, 11–22.

Bendena, W. G., Donly, B. C., and Tobe, S. S. (1999). Allatostatins: A growing family of neuropeptides with structural and functional diversity. [Neuropeptides: Structure and Function in Biology and Behavior]. *Ann. N. Y. Acad. Sci.* 897, 311–329.

Hoffmann, K. H., Meyering-Vos, M., and Lorenz, M. W. (1999). Allatostatins and allatotropins: Is the regulation of corpora allata activity their primary function? *Eur. J. Entomol.* 96, 255–266.

Lee, K.-Y., Chamberlin, M. E., and Horodyski, F. (2002). Biological activity of *Manduca sexta* allatotropin-like peptides, predicted products of tissue-specific and developmentally-regulated alternatively spliced mRNAs. *Peptides* 23, 1933–1941.

Meyering-Vos, M., Wu, X., Huang, J., Jindra, M., Hoffmann, K. H., and Sehnal, F. (2001). The allatostatin gene of the cricket *Gryllus bimaculatus*. *Mol. Cell. Endocrinol.* 184, 103–114.

Nichols, R., Bendena, W. G., and Tobe, S. S. (2002). Myotropic peptides in *Drosophila melanogaster* and the genes that encode them. *J. Neurogenet.* 16, 1–28.

Richter, D. (2001). Neuropeptides and their receptors—Evolutionary insights. In "Perspectives in Comparative Endocrinology, Unity and Diversity," (H. J. Th. Goos, R. K. Rastogi, H. Vaudry, and R. Pierantoni, eds.), pp. 455–464. Monduzzi Editore, Bologna, Italy.

Stay, B. (2000). A review of the role of neurosecretion in the control of juvenile hormone synthesis: A tribute to Berta Scharrer. *Insect Biochem. Mol. Biol.* 30, 653–662.

Stay, B., Tobe, S. S., and Bendena, W. G. (1994). Allatostatins: Identification, primary structures, functions and distribution. *Adv. Insect Physiol.* 25, 267–338.

Tobe, S. S., and Bendena, W. G. (1999). The regulation of juvenile hormone production in arthropods: Functional and evolutionary perspectives. [Neuropeptides: Structure and Function in Biology and Behavior] *Ann. N. Y. Acad. Sci.* 897, 300–310.

Tobe, S. S., Zhang, J. R., Bowser, P. R. F., Donly, B. C., and Bendena, W. G. (2000). Biological activities of the allatostatin family of peptides in the cockroach, *Diploptera punctata* and potential interactions with receptors. *J. Insect Physiol.* **46**, 231–242.

Truesdell, P. F., Koladich, P. M., Kataoka, H., Kojima, K., Suzuki, A., McNeil, J. N., Mizoguchi, A., Tobe, S. S., and Bendena, W. G. (2000). The molecular characterization of *Pseudaletia unipuncta* allatotropin. *Insect Biochem. Mol. Biol.* **30**, 691–702.

Neuropeptides and Control of the Anterior Pituitary

MEGHAN M. TAYLOR AND WILLIS K. SAMSON
Saint Louis University School of Medicine

I. INTRODUCTION
II. HYPOTHALAMIC COMMUNICATION WITH THE ANTERIOR PITUITARY: LONG AND SHORT PORTAL VESSELS
III. HORMONE-SECRETING CELLS OF THE ANTERIOR PITUITARY GLAND
IV. REGULATION OF HORMONE SECRETION
V. SUMMARY

Neuropeptides are short chains of amino acids that are produced in neurons throughout the body; when released, they bind to specific receptors on target cells, thereby communicating neural information to other neurons or to nonneural tissues (e.g., hormone-secreting cells of the anterior pituitary gland, vascular smooth muscle, and secretory glands). Neuropeptides access the anterior pituitary via a portal vessel system and set into action complex pathways of neuroendocrine control.

I. INTRODUCTION

Peptides are produced in neurons that have axons terminating at the base of the hypothalamus, in a specialized region named the median eminence; these neuropeptides gain access by diffusion to the unique vascular system that links the brain to the anterior pituitary gland. In this manner, neural signals are communicated to the hormone-secreting cells of the gland and, by controlling the release of those hormones, to the entire body. Each type of anterior pituitary hormone-secreting cell is regulated by a balance of stimulatory and inhibitory neuropeptides released from axon terminals in the median eminence, against a background of information (long loop feedback) received from factors secreted into the general circulation by the cells that are the targets of those anterior lobe hormones. Against that background of information from the periphery, it is the relative balance of releasing and release-inhibiting peptides reaching the gland, and the pattern of the exposure to those factors, that determine hormone production and secretion from the anterior pituitary. That balance defines the field of neuroendocrinology.

II. HYPOTHALAMIC COMMUNICATION WITH THE ANTERIOR PITUITARY: LONG AND SHORT PORTAL VESSELS

The adult human pituitary gland weighs, under normal conditions, approximately 0.5 g, except in pregnancy, when the gland may double in size. Located in a protected cradle within the sphenoid bone, the pituitary measures approximately 1.0–1.5 cm in length and width and 0.5 cm in depth (Fig. 1). It is composed of the posterior lobe, which is neural in origin, and the anterior lobe, which is nonneural in origin. The anterior lobe, which contains the hormone-producing and -secreting cells of the gland, arises from the roof of the oral cavity

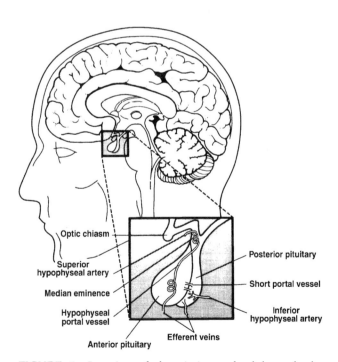

FIGURE 1 Location of the pituitary gland beneath the hypothalamus. The hypothalamo-pituitary portal vessels are idealized for simplicity. Reprinted from "Encyclopedia of Human Biology," Vol. 6 (1991), Academic Press, with permission.

during embryologic differentiation. Between weeks 4 and 6 of gestation, cells destined to become the anterior lobe have budded off of what will become the roof of the mouth, organized into a spherical shape, and migrated upward toward the developing neural tube. This migration is halted by apposition to the base of the forebrain adjacent to the floor of the third cerebroventricle, which is the ventral aspect of the hypothalamus. At the same time, clusters of hypothalamic neurons are extending their axons downward toward the floor of the third ventricle, some stopping near the midline and others protruding out of the neural tube to lie alongside the developing anterior lobe (the. adenohypophysis), as a collection of axons terminating in what will be the posterior lobe (the neurohypophysis). Hypothalamic cells having axons that comprise the posterior lobe deliver two important neuropeptides to the general circulation, vasopressin and oxytocin. These neurons can be considered endocrine cells, because they release their peptides directly into the general circulation.

The cells that project to the floor of the third ventricle deliver neural products (i.e., peptides and biogenic amines) to a region that is invaded during the fifth and sixth weeks of gestation by mesenchymal elements (precursors of blood vessels), organizing into the vascular link between hypothalamus and the hormone-secreting cells of the anterior lobe. Those mesenchymal elements form the superior hypophyseal artery, a branch of the internal carotid artery, and this artery supplies blood to the hypothalamus and, via the portal vessels, the anterior lobe of the pituitary gland. The superior hypophyseal artery terminates in a series of fenestrated capillaries in the midline of the floor the hypothalamus, giving the tissue its characteristic tufted, vascular appearance. This protrusion on the ventral surface of the hypothalamus is called the median eminence and it is here that neuropeptides and biogenic amines access the portal vessel system for delivery to the anterior lobe. These neural factors are not released directly into the circulation, instead diffusing after release in the parenchyma of the median eminence through the fenestration of the capillary endothelial cells of the portal vessels and then out of those long portal vessels into the sinusoids of the adenohypophysis. Because these peptides are produced in neurons, but are delivered to their target tissue (the cells of the adenohypophysis) not via the general circulation but instead via a specialized circulation (the hypophyseal portal vessels), they are true neuroendocrine substances, as opposed to hormones per se. The superior hypophyseal arteries and thus the long portal vessels provide the majority of the

blood flow to the adenohypophysis; the remaining supply comes from superficial, capsular arteries that arise from the inferior hypophyseal artery, which is a major source of flow to the posterior lobe.

Although only a minor component when compared to the contribution of the long portal vessels, a vascular connection between the posterior and the anterior lobes of the pituitary gland has been observed. These short portal vessels, formed from mesenchymal elements that give rise to the inferior hypophyseal artery, are an avenue by which the hormones (vasopressin and oxytocin) released into the general circulation draining the neurohypophysis might gain access to the cells of the adenohypophysis.

III. HORMONE-SECRETING CELLS OF THE ANTERIOR PITUITARY GLAND

There are five major classes of hormone-secreting cells in the anterior pituitary gland. All are encapsulated in a dense collagenous matrix in the gland and are arranged in a sinusoidal fashion adjacent to the thin-walled vascular elements. All five classes exhibit spontaneous (constitutive) secretory activity, but are controlled primarily by tropic factors delivered by the portal vessels (factors originating both in the periphery and in the hypothalamus). In addition, the secretory activity of these endocrine cells can be modulated by locally produced substances acting in a paracrine (after diffusion from neighboring cells) or autocrine (self) fashion. Tropic effects also are exerted by nonendocrine cells of the gland, particularly the folliculostellate cells found among the hormone-secreting cells.

Percentages of cell types in the gland vary with physiologic state, and cell size can similarly vary, dependent on physiologic state. For example, although lactotrophs (prolactin secreting cells) make up approximately 10–15% of the endocrine mass of the tissue under most conditions, during pregnancy and lactation they may contribute as much as 25% of the cell number. Hormone status in general also can affect the size of individual cell types. After menopause, when circulating gonadal steroid levels have fallen and their negative feedback effects are lost, gonadotrophs (cells producing luteinizing and follicle-stimulating hormones) increase in size (volume) by as much as two- to threefold.

In the past, cell types were classified by affinity for basic or acidic dyes; now, using more selective histologic techniques, cell types of the anterior pituitary gland are characterized by their hormone content (Table 1). The endocrine cells of the

TABLE I Hormone-Secreting Cells of the Anterior Pituitary Gland

Cell type	Hormone content	Percentage of total cell number
Somatotroph	Growth hormone	50%
Lactotroph	Prolactin	10–25%
Corticotroph	Pro-opiomelanocortins (adrenocorticotropin, lipotropins, endorphins)	15–20%
Thyrotroph	Thyroid-stimulating hormone	<10%
Gonadotroph	Luteinizing hormone (LH) and follicle-stimulating hormone (FSH)	10–15%

adenohypophysis fall into two classes—those that produce and secrete unmodified protein hormones (prolactin, growth hormone, and adrenocorticotropin) and those that produce and secrete glycosylated proteins (thyroid-stimulating hormone, luteinizing hormone, and follicle-stimulating hormone).

IV. REGULATION OF HORMONE SECRETION

Located beneath the thalamus at the ventral surface of the diencephalon forming the walls of the third cerebroventricle, the hypothalamus is small in size (about 4 g in adults) but is a major crossroad for emotional, autonomic, and endocrine circuitry within the brain. Afferents to the hypothalamus provide extero- and enteroceptive information that is then processed into the neural and hormonal signals responsible for maintenance of normal cardiovascular, renal, visceral, and endocrine function, as well as for the expression of appropriate and conditioned behavioral responses to the environment. Neurons in the hypothalamus are organized into dense clusters of cells called nuclei. These nuclei are integrative centers (microprocessors) that assess neuronal, and in some cases humoral, input and send afferent output (nerve fibers) to relay stations (other nuclei in brain) or to the region where the hypophyseal portal vessels form at the ventral surface of the hypothalamus, just at the point where the infundibular stalk penetrates the diaphragma sella. After diffusion into the portal vessels, these tropic substances control production and release of the anterior lobe hormones. Those tropic substances, which can be either small proteins (i.e., neuropeptides) or neurotransmitters such as dopamine or norepinephrine, can act to either inhibit or stimulate the release/production of hormones in the various anterior pituitary cell types.

A. Growth Hormone

Growth hormone (GH), a protein hormone (191 amino acids) produced in somatotrophs of the adenohypophysis, circulates mainly free (i.e., not bound to carrier proteins) in plasma [plasma half-life $(t_{1/2}) = 20$ min; circulating levels are 2–4 ng/ml in adults (4–8 ng/ml in adolescents)]. Growth hormone acts to decrease blood amino acid levels, decrease blood urea nitrogen (positive nitrogen balance), increase DNA, RNA, and protein synthesis, decrease respiratory quotient due to increased fat oxidation, stimulate somatic growth, stimulate growth and calcification of cartilage, and, at high concentration, cause insulin resistance. Growth hormone secretion can be stimulated by exercise, arginine infusion, insulin-induced hypoglycemia, stress, dopamine, and α-adrenergics. Growth hormone is secreted in a pulsatile fashion, with a major daily secretory event occurring at the onset of sleep during Stages III and IV [non-rapid eye movement (REM) sleep]. Growth hormone secretion is inhibited by REM sleep, GH (autofeedback inhibition), insulin-like growth factors (long loop negative feedback), β-adrenergics, and hyperglycemia.

The hypothalamic component of feedback regulation of GH secretion has two major factors (Fig. 2). Growth hormone-releasing hormone (GHRH) is produced in neurons located in the arcuate nucleus and, above that, in the medial aspects of the ventromedial and dorsomedial hypothalamic nuclei. The predominant form of GHRH in humans is a 44-amino-acid peptide that is the final posttranslational product of a prohormone reported to be either 107 or 108 amino acids in length. GHRH is released into the median eminence in a pulsatile fashion, contributing thus to the pulsatile pattern of GH secretion. It acts by binding to a specific somatotroph receptor that is a member of the superfamily of G-protein-coupled, seven-transmembrane domain receptors. Binding results in activation of adenylyl cyclase, the formation of cyclic adenosine monophosphate (cAMP), an elevation in intracellular calcium levels, and both increased GH gene transcription and GH release. Non-cAMP-dependent signaling pathways may also mediate the effects of GHRH on the somatotroph.

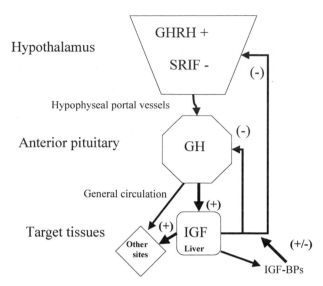

FIGURE 2 Hypothalamic regulation of growth hormone (GH) secretion. The 191-amino-acid hormone has a plasma half-life of 20 min; plasma levels are 2–4 ng/ml in adults and daily surges occur postprandially and at onset of sleep. GHRH, Growth hormone-releasing hormone; SRIF, somatotropin release-inhibiting factor; IGF, insulin-like growth factor; IGF-BPs, IGF-binding proteins.

Growth hormone release also is under inhibitory control, exerted by somatostatin produced in neurons of the anterior hypothalamus, adjacent to the ependymal lining of the third cerebroventricle (the periventricular zone). It, too, is produced by post-translational processing of a larger prohormone form (116 amino acids) and exists in both a 14- and a 28-amino-acid form. Somatostatin, or somatotropin release-inhibiting factor (SRIF), inhibits not only the release of GH, but thyroid-stimulating hormone and prolactin as well. The peptide exerts wide-ranging effects, most inhibitory, in a variety of other tissues. Multiple SRIF receptors have been identified, all being structurally related. In the pituitary gland, SRIF activates inhibitory G-proteins, resulting in decreased cAMP levels and lowered intracellular levels of free calcium. It acts to antagonize the actions of GHRH on adenylyl cyclase and blocks the effects of GHRH downstream of cAMP formation. The action to lower the cytosolic free-calcium levels is thought to be an important mechanism of action, mediated via an effect on voltage-gated calcium channels.

Studies utilizing opioid analogues have revealed the existence of a receptor mechanism, independent of GHRH and SRIF, that controls GH release. The endogenous ligand for that receptor was recently identified to be a novel 28-amino-acid peptide with a unique *n*-octanoyl modification of the serine in position 3 that is necessary for bioactivity. This peptide, called ghrelin, is produced in specialized endocrine cells of the gut, and some production in cells of the hypothalamic arcuate nucleus has also been reported. Thus ghrelin can access the adenohypophysis via the general circulation (from the stomach) or via the hypophyseal portal vessels following release into the median eminence. The ghrelin receptor is a G-protein-coupled, seven-trans-membrane-spanning domain protein with homology to the motilin receptor. Binding of ghrelin results in activation of phospholipase C and the formation of inositol 1,4,5-trisphosphate ($InsP_3$). The physiologic relevance of the GHRH-like actions of ghrelin is still being established and the interactions between GHRH, SRIF, and ghrelin merit further scrutiny.

The nonhypothalamic control of GH release from the somatotroph includes, in addition to gut-derived ghrelin, the long loop negative feedback actions of the insulin-like growth factors (IGFs). Although GH can act directly to stimulate growth and metabolism in a variety of tissues, it is clear that its major actions are to stimulate the production and release of protein hormones that are structurally similar to insulin, hence the term IGFs. These peptide growth factors are produced primarily in liver, but also in bone, brain, prostate, and mammary tissues, where they can exert paracrine or true endocrine actions. In addition, the IGFs act in brain to inhibit GHRH release, and stimulate the release of SRIF, thus exerting long loop negative feedback on the hypothalamic regulation of GH secretion. The IGFs also can act directly in the adenohypophysis to antagonize the action of GHRH.

B. Prolactin

Prolactin (PRL) is a protein hormone (198 amino acids.) produced in lactotrophs of the adenohypophysis; it circulates mainly free in plasma [plasma $t_{1/2} = 20–30$ min; plasma levels are 10 ng/ml in nonpregnant/nonlactating females (slightly lower in males and adolescents), slightly higher in lactating females, and 200–300 ng/ml during nursing]. PRL is cleared from the circulation in liver and kidney. The high catabolic clearance rate indicates very high synthetic capability of the lactotroph (45 ml/min/m²). Pulsatile secretion occurs, with a minor circadian (daily) peak in early morning.

PRL was originally thought to be solely a hormone of reproduction. Indeed, PRL acts to stimulate mammary gland development (ductal and lobuloalveolar growth) and milk production in properly primed breast tissue. Prolactin also has been reported to organize the neural basis of maternal behaviors. In the adrenal cortex and ovary, PRL stimulates cytochrome P450 side chain cleavage enzyme (P450scc), resulting in the precursor for steroid synthesis. However, PRL has recently been recognized to have a broader spectrum of action, including immune modulation and potential actions on bone mineralization, vascular growth, and sodium homeostasis. Prolactin receptors belong both to a class of cell surface, tyrosine-kinase-linked receptors and to a class of intranuclear receptors (such as those for the steroid hormones). Promitogenic actions of PRL are related to both signaling pathways.

Prolactin secretion is stimulated by stress, hypothermia, tactile stimuli (vaginal or nipple stimulation), gonadal steroids (estrogens), and numerous neuropeptides (Fig. 3). The predominant hypothalamic regulation of PRL release is inhibitory in nature. Dopamine (DA), produced in the tubero-infundibular neurons of the arcuate nucleus, is released in a relatively constant fashion into the median eminence, and therefore PRL secretion is tonically inhibited. Dopamine exerts its inhibitory action on the lactotroph via binding to the D_2 subtype of the family of dopamine receptors. The receptor is another one of the G-protein-coupled, seven-transmembrane-spanning domain region proteins. Once activated by DA, the receptor links to a decrease in cellular levels of cAMP and inositol trisphosphates as well as to a decrease in intracellular calcium levels. The major cue for PRL release is the withdrawal of this inhibitory,

dopaminergic tone, although stimulatory effects of some neuropeptides can be expressed even in the presence of physiologic levels of DA.

Stimulatory factors controlling PRL release originate in at least three locations. Estrogens of ovarian origin stimulate both PRL gene transcription and hormone release. Estrogens may also stimulate lactotroph proliferation by releasing a locally produced peptide, galanin, which then acts in a paracrine fashion within the gland. Neuropeptides of hypothalamic origin also can stimulate PRL release following delivery in the hypophyseal portal circulation. The most potent of these is the tripeptide, thyrotropin-releasing hormone (TRH), which is also the major regulator of TSH secretion. TRH stimulates PRL release even in the presence of physiologic, inhibitory levels of DA, a fact that separates it from the other peptidergic PRL-releasing factors (PRFs). TRH is the posttranslational product of a much larger prohormone that is produced in cells in the most medial aspects of the hypothalamic paraventricular nuclei. This is the major site of production that leads to peptide being delivered to the median eminence; however, TRH is produced in a variety of other sites. In the lactotroph, TRH binds to G-protein-coupled, seven-transmembrane-spanning domain receptors on the lactotroph, resulting in activation of phosphoinositide hydrolysis by phospholipase C and the subsequent activation of protein kinase C. The resulting elevation in intracellular free calcium levels certainly underlies the PRL secretory event, and perhaps even the elevation in cAMP levels that occurs concomitantly. Additional neuropeptides can stimulate PRL release from cultured pituitary cells and in some select situations in vivo. Both vasoactive intestinal polypeptide (VIP), a gut peptide also produced in neurons in the paraventricular nuclei, and oxytocin (OT), a neurophyseal hormone more traditionally considered part of the posterior pituitary system, can access the lactotroph following release into the median eminence and delivery by the portal circulation. Results from animal studies clearly demonstrate that both VIP and OT may be physiologically relevant PRFs, but this has not yet been established firmly in humans. OT may access the lactotroph via a second route, delivery by the short portal vessels connecting the posterior (neural) lobe with the adenohypophysis. In addition, there appears to be at least one additional factor (peptide?) of neural lobe origin that accesses the lactotroph via the short portal vessels, but the identity of this PRF has remained elusive.

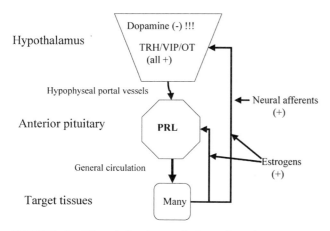

FIGURE 3 Hypothalamic regulation of prolactin (PRL) secretion. The 198-amino-acid hormone has a half-life of 20–30 min; plasma levels are 10 ng/ml, except during pregnancy, laction, and stress. Minor daily surges occur in the morning. TRH, Thyrotropin-releasing hormone; VIP, vasoactive intestinal peptide; OT, oxytocin.

C. Adrenocorticotropic Hormone

Adrenocorticotropic hormone (ACTH; adrenocorticotropin) is derived from a large glycoprotein prohormone, pro-opiomelanocortin (POMC), which is produced in corticotrophs. Corticotrophs in the adenohypophysis produce mainly the 91-amino-acid protein β-lipotropic hormone (LPH; lipotropin) and the 39-amino-acid peptide ACTH. ACTH can be further processed to the 13-amino-acid long α-melanocyte-stimulating hormone (MSH), which stimulates pigment deposition in melanocytes. β-LPH can be further processed to β-endorphin (31 amino acids) and γ-LPH. Corticotrophs derived from the fetal intermediate lobe further process γ-LPH to β-MSH and produce γ-MSH from the N-terminal fragment of POMC.

ACTH circulates free in plasma with a half-life of 20 min and is cleared in kidney and liver. Levels under unstressed conditions are low (about 10 pg/ml) and secretion is pulsatile (20-min intervals); peak levels are present between 2:00 and 8:00 AM. ACTH stimulates activation of cytochrome P450 side chain cleavage enzyme, the rate-limiting step in cholesterol metabolism, and cholesterol esterase activities in the adrenal cortex, resulting in increased levels of glucocorticoids, mineralocorticoids, and adrenal androgens. At high levels, ACTH causes increased skin pigmentation because it also binds to the MSH receptor. ACTH acts via a membrane-bound receptor linked to adenylyl cyclase, increasing cAMP formation in hormone-producing cells of the adrenal cortex. The initial increase in cortisol secretion observed following ACTH infusion is due to increased adrenal blood flow and stimulation of conversion of cholesterol to pregnenolone (P450sccc activation). Prolonged actions of ACTH include stimulation of increased synthesis of the rate-limiting enzymes in adrenal steroidogenesis.

Secretion of ACTH is stimulated by stress, hypothermia, inflammatory substances (pyrogens), hypoglycemia, epinephrine (adrenaline), and several neuropeptides (Fig. 4). Cortisol from the adrenal cortex is the major inhibitory agent controlling ACTH production and release.

Neuroendocrine regulation of ACTH release is primarily stimulatory due to the neuropeptide, corticotropin-releasing hormone (CRH). CRH is a 41-amino-acid peptide produced in the parvocellular elements of the hypothalamic paraventricular nuclei. Actylcholine, serotonin, interleukins, and other cytokines all act to stimulate CRH release into the median

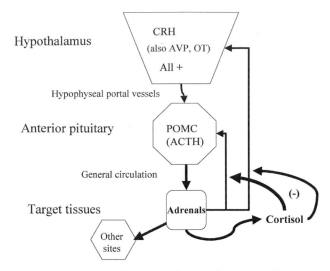

FIGURE 4 Hypothalamic regulation of adrenocorticotropic hormone (ACTH) secretion. The 39-amino-acid hormone has a half-life of 20 min; plasma levels are very low (picograms/milliliter) under nonstressed conditions. Secretion is pulsatile (20 min) and there is a daily surge between 2:00 and 8:00 AM. CRH, Corticotropin-releasing hormone; AVP, vasopressin; OT, oxytocin; POMC, pro-opiomelanocortin.

eminence. At the corticotroph membrane, CRH binds a receptor similar to that for GHRH, resulting in activation, via G-protein coupling, of adenylyl cyclase. CRH also stimulates POMC gene transcription, probably via activation of protein kinase A. Within the hypothalamus, γ-butyric acid (GABA) and cortisol inhibit the activity of the CRH-producing neurons and therefore CRH release. Cortisol also acts directly in the anterior lobe to antagonize the action of CRH, resulting lower secretion and production of POMC-derived peptides. As was the case with PRL, there is credible evidence for the physiologic relevance of the ACTH-releasing actions of vasopressin (AVP) and oxytocin released into the median eminence or delivered via the short portal vessels; however, their role as ACTH secretagogues in humans has not been firmly established.

D. Pituitary Glycoprotein Hormones

The three major pituitary glycoprotein hormones, thyroid-stimulating hormone, luteinizing hormone, and follicle-stimulating hormone, each having a molecular weight of approximately 30,000, are formed from two interconnecting amino acid chains. They all share a common α-chain but their unique β-chains give each hormone an individual, characteristic bioactivity.

1. Thyroid-Stimulating Hormone

Thyroid-stimulating hormone (TSH) circulates mainly free in plasma at levels of 1–4 ng/ml under normal conditions. TSH half-life is 50–60 min and it is cleared (degraded) primarily by the kidneys. Secretion is pulsatile, with a circadian rhythm characterized by highest levels between 9:00 PM and 5:00 AM and lowest levels between 4:00 and 7:00 PM. Physiologic surges occur in response to cold exposure (increases), heat (inhibits), starvation (inhibits), and stress (inhibits).

TSH stimulates thyroid hormone production and secretion by several mechanisms. Iodide transport into the thyroid gland is stimulated by TSH. TSH also stimulates thyroglobulin, iodotyrosine, and iodothyronine formation, and thus increases intracellular stores of thyroid hormones. Finally, TSH stimulates thyroglobulin proteolysis, as well as thyroxine (T4) and triiodothyronine (T3) release.

Hypothalamic control of TSH production and secretion (Fig. 5) is primarily exerted by the tripeptide thyrotropin-releasing hormone. Binding of TRH to its receptor (G-protein coupled) on the thyrotroph results not only in rapid secretion of TSH, but also in increased transcription of the β-subunit of TSH. These effects are thought to be signaled by TRH activation of adenylyl cyclase. There is also substantial evidence that TRH controls the final glycosylation (the addition of sugar moieties to the protein backbone of the hormone) of TSH, a step important for the bioactivity of the secreted product. Factors of hypothalamic origin (somatostatin and dopamine) can inhibit TSH secretion by a direct action in the adenohypophysis; however, by far the most significant negative regulation is exerted by T3 and T4 secreted by the thyroid gland (long loop negative feedback). The active agent in pituitary gland is T3, which either reaches the gland via the general circulation or is produced locally by conversion of T4. Triiodothyronine not only inhibits TSH gene transcription, it also down-regulates the TRH receptor.

2. Gonadotropins: Luteinizing Hormone and Follicle-Stimulating Hormone

The 115-amino-acid-long β-subunits of luteinizing hormone (LH) and follicle-stimulating hormone (FSH) confer unique biological activities to each hormone. The β-chain of LH is similar to that of human chorionic gonadotropin (hCG), thus common biologic activities are shared. Plasma levels of LH and FSH are expressed in terms of International Standard preparations (purified human hormones, as opposed to synthetic forms) and thus they are expressed as International Units (IU)/milliliter of plasma. LH and FSH both are secreted in a pulsatile fashion (circhorial in nature, about every 1–2 h) under the influence of gonadotropin-releasing hormone (GnRH), a 10-amino-acid peptide of hypothalamic origin. With the exception of puberty in males, when nocturnal pulses of GnRH entering the hypophyseal portal vessels cause increasing baseline and spike-like discharges of LH, gonadotropin levels remains fairly constant throughout adult life. Females also experience nocturnal gonadotropin pulses that increase in amplitude and frequency during puberty. During the reproductive years, the secretion of gonadotropins in women is circhorial (hourly) and low (basal LH, 0.8–26 mIU/ml; FSH, 1.4–9.6 mIU/ml). Monthly surges occur just prior to ovulation (LH, 25–57 mIU/ml; FSH, 2.3–21 mIU/ml). After menopause, gonadotropins are secreted in a circhorial pattern (LH, 1.3–13 mIU/ml; FSH, 0.9–15 mIU/ml).

In men, gonadotropin levels are low and fairly constant (LH, 1.3–13 mIU/ml; FSH, 0.9–15 mIU/ml). In women, gonadotropin levels fluctuate depending on stage of the menstrual cycle. After menopause, levels rise noticeably due to the absence of normal ovarian negative feed back (LH, 40–104 mIU/ml; FSH, 34–96 mIU/ml).

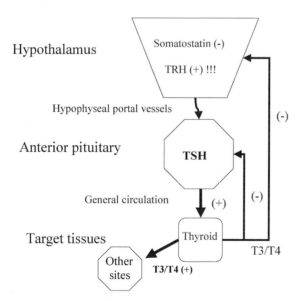

FIGURE 5 Hypothalamic regulation of thyroid-stimulating hormone (TSH) secretion. TSH is a glycoprotein ($M_w = 30,000$) with a half-life of 50–60 min; plasma levels are 1–4 ng/ml. Secretion is circadian, with peaks between 9:00 pm and 5:00 AM and a low between 4:00 and 7:00 PM. TRH, Thyrotropin-releasing hormone; T3, triiodothyronine; T4, thyroxine.

The plasma half-life of FSH is longer than that of LH (about 1 h for LH and 3 h for FSH) and the metabolic clearance rate for FSH (about 10 ml/min/m^2) is slower than that of LH (about 30 ml/min/m^2). These are at least two of the reasons why the midcycle surge of FSH is broader than that of LH. Both gonadotropins are degraded in the liver and kidneys, and some intact hormone is excreted in the urine. In females, LH acts in the ovary to stimulate follicular growth and rupture at ovulation. LH exerts luteotropic effects, stimulating estrogen and progesterone production. FSH also stimulates follicular growth. FSH further stimulates the conversion of androgens to estrogens by activating the enzyme aromatase in granulosa cells, and synergizes with estrogen to induce formation of LH receptors on those cells. In males, LH acts on Leydig cells to stimulate testosterone production. FSH induces LH receptors on those cells, and acts on Sertoli cells to stimulate spermatogenesis. Both LH and FSH signal through unique receptors that are coupled via G-proteins to adenylyl cyclase.

Neuroendocrine regulation of gonadotropin secretion (Figs. 6 and 7) is exerted primarily by the decapeptide hormone gonadotropin-releasing hormone (also called luteinizing hormone-releasing hormone, LHRH). GnRH binds to its cognate receptor (another G-protein-coupled, seven-transmembrane-spanning domain protein) and activates phosphoinositide hydrolysis (phospholipase C activity).

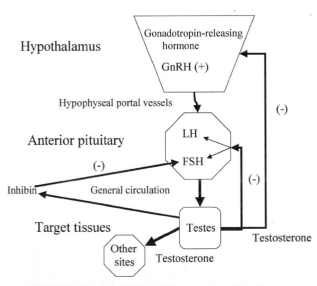

FIGURE 6 Hypothalamic regulation of gonadotropin [luteinizing hormone (LH) and follicle-stimulating hormone (FSH)] secretion in the male. LH half-life, 20–30 min; FSH half-life, 30–40 min; secretion of both hormones is low and constant. GnRH, Gonadotropin-releasing hormone.

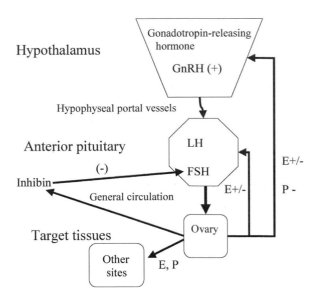

FIGURE 7 Hypothalamic regulation of gonadotropin [luteinizing hormone (LH) and follicle-stimulating hormone (FSH)] secretion in the female. LH half-life, 20–30 min; FSH half-life, 30–40 min; secretion is pulsatile, occurring hourly or monthly. GnRH, Gonadotropin-releasing hormone; E, estrogen; P, progesterone.

The diacylglycerol formed activates protein kinase C and intracellular calcium levels rise, leading to stimulus–secretion coupling and release of LH and FSH. GnRH also stimulates transcription of the GnRH receptor gene and the LH and FSH genes.

Sex steroids exert both positive and negative feedback effects on the hypothalamus and pituitary gland. In females, estrogen at low levels inhibits both LH and FSH secretion, whereas at higher levels the steroid actually stimulates LH β-chain gene transcription and sensitizes the gonadotroph to the actions of GnRH. Progesterone negative feedback is expressed primarily at the level of the GnRH neuron, decreasing pulse frequency of release of the decapeptide into the median eminence. In males, testosterone exerts negative feedback effects in the hypothalamus, similar to those exerted by progesterone in females, and direct inhibitory actions at the pituitary level, similar to those of estrogen in women.

Granulosa cells in the ovary, and Sertoli cells in the testes, also produce a heterodimeric hormone, composed of unique α-and β-subunits, that acts in the gonadotroph to inhibit FSH production and release. The production of this heterodimeric hormone, called inhibin, is in turn stimulated by FSH. It is in all likelihood the loss of inhibin production after menopause that explains the greater rise in plasma FSH levels, compared to LH levels, in the absence of ovarian feedback. Finally, it appears that a homo-dimer of the inhibin β-chain is produced in several tissues, including the pituitary gland. This homo-dimer, called activin, is thought to stimulate FSH production and secretion.

V. SUMMARY

The unique vascular connection between the hypo-thalamus and pituitary gland established by the experiments of Jacobsen and Harris over 50 years ago is the anatomical basis for the science of neuroendocrinology. Peptidergic releasing and inhi-biting factors produced in brain neurons, most localized to the hypothalamus, gain access to their target cells in the anterior lobe of the pituitary gland via this system of portal vessels. The control of peptide release into the median eminence is in turn controlled by neural afferents to the hypothalamus and by blood-borne substances that either cross the blood–brain barrier to act within the hypothalamus or act in the median eminence on the axon terminals containing those peptides, because there is no barrier at this vascularized site. Additional regulation of anterior lobe hormone secretion is determined by direct actions of those circulating hormones (long loop negative and positive feedback) and by intrinsic factors acting in paracrine or autocrine fashion within the adenohypophysis.

Glossary

adenohypophysis The anterior pituitary gland.
autocrine Self-regulation; the release from a cell of a tropic factor that binds to and alters the activity of that same cell.
median eminence Floor of the third cerebroventricle in the hypothalamus; site of the fenestrated endothelium of the capillary loops of the portal vessels.
neuroendocrine Regulation by neural factors reaching the anterior pituitary gland via the portal vessels.
neurohypophyseal Neuronal projections from the supra-optic and paraventricular hypothalamic nuclei to the posterior pituitary gland.
neurohypophysis The posterior pituitary gland.
paracrine Regulation of neighboring cells by a tropic factor that, when released from one cell, diffuses to and acts on another cell.
portal vessels Venous system connecting the capillary loops formed by the superior hypophyseal artery in the median eminence of the hypothalamus with the sinusoids of the anterior pituitary gland.

See Also the Following Articles

Adrenocorticotropic Hormone (ACTH) and Other Proopiomelanocortin (POMC) Peptides ● Amino Acid and Nitric Oxide Control of the Anterior Pituitary ● Cytokines and Anterior Pituitary Function ● Follicle Stimulating Hormone (FSH) ● Ghrelin ● Growth Hormone (GH) ● Growth Hormone-Releasing Hormone (GHRH) ● Luteinizing Hormone (LH) ● Neuropeptide Y (NPY) ● Prolactin (PRL) ● Thyroid Stimulating Hormone (TSH)

Further Reading

Ben-Jonathan, N., and Hnasko, R. (2001). Dopamine as a prolactin (PRL) inhibitor. *Endocr. Rev.* **22**, 724–763.
Buffet, N. C., Djakoure, C., Maitre, S. C., and Bouchard, P. (1998). Regulation of the human menstrual cycle. *Front. Neuroendocrinol.* **19**, 151–186.
Freeman, M. E., Kanyicska, S., Lerant, A., and Nagy, G. (2000). Prolactin: structure, function, and regulation of secretion. *Physiol. Rev.* **80**, 1523–1631.
Muller, E. E., Locatelli, V., and Cocchi, D. (1999). Neuroendocrine control of growth hormone secretion. *Physiol. Rev.* **79**, 511–607.
Ojeda, S. R., and McCann, S. M. (2000). The anterior pituitary and hypothalamus. *In* "Textbook of Endocrine Physiology" (J. E. Griffen and S. R. Ojeda, eds.), pp. 128–162. Oxford, New York.
Reichlin, S. (1998). Neuroendocrinology. *In* "Williams Textbook of Endocrinology," 9th Ed. (J. D. Wilson, D. W. Foster, H. M. Kronenberg, and P. R. Larsen, eds.), pp. 165–248. W. B. Saunders Co., Philadelphia.
Risbridger, G. P., Schmitt, J. F., and Robertson, D. M. (2001). Activins and inhibins in endocrine and other tumors. *Endocr. Rev.* **22**, 836–858.
Rivier, C. (1999). Gender, sex steroids, corticotropin-releasing factor, nitric oxide, and the HPA response to stress. *Pharmacol. Biochem. Behav.* **64**, 739–751.
Taylor, M. M., and Samson, W. K. (2001). The prolactin releasing peptides: RF-amide peptides. *Cell. Mol. Life Sci.* **58**, 1206–1215.
Yen, P. M. (2001). Physiological and molecular basis of thyroid hormone action. *Physiol. Rev.* **81**, 1097–1142.

Neuropeptide Y (NPY)

SATYA P. KALRA AND PUSHPA S. KALRA
University of Florida

I. INTRODUCTION
II. NEUROANATOMY
III. NEUROPEPTIDE Y AND APPETITE
IV. NEUROPEPTIDE Y AND REPRODUCTION
V. NEUROPEPTIDE Y AND NUTRITIONAL INFERTILITY
VI. SUMMARY

The appetitive drive for energy to sustain physiological well-being and to reproduce successfully at the opportune time are two instinctual urges essential for survival of the species against varied evolutionary pressures. Neuropeptide Y is an important neurochemical signal relaying information regarding these instincts.

I. INTRODUCTION

Since the energy cost of reproduction is high and reproductive function is sensitive to nutritional stress and metabolic demands, scarcity and abundance of energy resources must be perceived and relayed continuously to the neural processes governing reproduction. Recent insight into the diversity and interplay of signals in the hypothalamus, a brain structure involved in homeostatic integration, has elevated neuropeptide Y (NPY) to the top of the list of neurochemical signals that relay information bidirectionally between these instinctual drives (Fig. 1). This article collates our understanding of the neurobiology of NPY produced specifically in the arcuate nucleus (ARC) of the hypothalamus. Participation of NPY in neuroendocrine mechanisms that initiate and sustain the drive for energy intake and

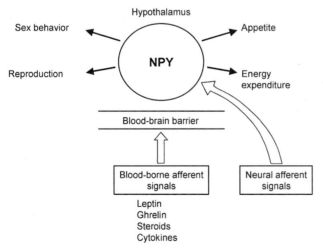

FIGURE 1 Neuropeptide Y (NPY) plays a pivotal role in the hypothalamus in regulating two neuroendocrine functions, reproduction and sex behavior (left) and appetite and energy expenditure to maintain body energy homeostasis (right). In addition to an interconnected circuitry in the hypothalamus (see Figs. 2 and 3), distinct afferent pathways play an important role in regulating NPY release at target sites. Afferent messages from the periphery are relayed by multisynaptic neural pathways through the spinal cord, brainstem, and lateral hypothalamus and then converge onto NPY neurons in the basal hypothalamus. NPY neurons also receive hormonal signals that cross the blood–brain barrier.

expenditure in an orderly manner on the one hand and those that regulate reproduction on the other are described. Subsequently, the ARC NPY links between appetitive and reproductive functions are addressed.

II. NEUROANATOMY

NPY was isolated and chemically sequenced from the brain as a 36-amino-acid peptide closely related to members of the pancreatic polypeptide family. Since NPY is produced exclusively in neural tissue and has tyrosine residues at both the amino- and the carboxy-terminals, it was named neuropeptide tyrosine (Y). The NPY localized in various hypothalamic sites is derived from two main sources. The extrahypothalamic source is a cluster of neurons in the brainstem that co-express a few additional messenger molecules, the most prominent of which are the two catecholamines, norepinephrine (NE) and epinephrine. These NPY and catecholamine neurons are synaptically linked with neurons in the hypothalamus that express various neuroendocrine peptides, neuromodulators, and neurotransmitters. Under certain conditions, co-release of these messenger molecules is important in amplifying or restraining the postsynaptic response of hypothalamic target cells. A denser population of NPY-producing neurons distributed along the ARC and a subpopulation located in the dorsomedial hypothalamus (DMH) are the hypothalamic sources of NPY. NPY-producing neurons in the ARC transsynaptically regulate the synthesis and release of several neurohormones—gonadotropin-releasing hormone (GnRH), growth hormone-releasing hormone, somatostatin, corticotropin-releasing hormone, thyrotropin-releasing hormone, vasopressin, oxytocin, and dopamine. In addition, these ARC NPY neurons innervate other hypothalamic nuclei that regulate appetitive and sexual behaviors and thermogenic energy expenditure.

There is regional heterogeneity in the distribution of NPY neurons in the ARC to selectively regulate various neuroendocrine and behavioral functions. A subpopulation of neurons extensively innervate the median eminence (ME), a neurohumoral junction between the hypothalamus and the anterior pituitary gland. Within the ME, NPY neurons terminate in close proximity of nerve endings of neuroendocrine cells to regulate reproduction. NPY release in the ME evokes the efflux of neuroendocrine messengers into the hypophyseal portal veins for transport to target cells in the anterior pituitary gland. NPY itself is also released into the hypophyseal vessels to potentiate the effects of neuroendocrine hormones on pituitary target cells. ARC NPY neurons that project to the paraventricular nucleus (PVN) secrete NPY in discrete episodes to regulate appetitive behavior. Unlike NPY neurons in the brainstem, the ARC NPY neurons co-express agouti-related peptide (AgrP) and γ-amino butyric acid (GABA); each of these co-transmitters modulates the postsynaptic response of NPY on appetite and reproduction in distinctive ways. Within the ARC itself, NPY neurons are synaptically linked with proopiomelanocortin (POMC)-expressing neurons, an essential component of the neural circuitry involved in the regulation of appetite and reproduction. Since the ARC NPY neurons are strategically positioned inside the weak blood–brain barrier, they receive hormonal afferent messages from peripheral endocrine glands, leptin from adipocytes, ghrelin from stomach, steroids from gonads and adrenal cortex, and cytokines from immune cells (Fig. 1). The ARC NPY neurons also receive messages from ascending neural pathways via the catecholaminergic brainstem neurons and the orexin and melanin-concentrating hormone (MCH)-producing neurons in the lateral hypothalamus (LatH). Thus, the ARC NPY neurons perceive complex afferent messages and propagate command signals for the integration of a spectrum of neuroendocrine and behavioral functions.

Information obtained from investigations across many disciplines to gain insight into the physiology, cellular biology, and molecular biology of this discrete population of ARC NPY neurons in the integration of energy homeostasis and reproduction is summarized below.

III. NEUROPEPTIDE Y AND APPETITE

A. Physiological Orexigen

Among a wide variety of orexigenic neurotransmitters isolated from the hypothalamus, NPY has been found to be the most potent appetite-stimulating signal. Abnormal NPY secretion, as seen in diabetic and genetically altered rodents, produces relentless hyperphagia and increased rate of weight gain, culminating over time in morbid obesity. In laboratory rodents and other mammals, NPY synthesis in the ARC perikarya and storage in nerve terminals in the PVN precede mealtime (Fig. 2). Subsequently, NPY release is triggered by photoperiodically driven neurogenic stimuli from the timing mechanism in the brain. However, in subhuman primates and humans, all these antecedent neurosecretory events are independent of the photoperiodic clock and are entrained to mealtime.

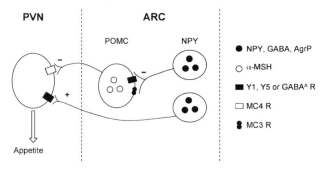

FIGURE 2 A schematic representation of morphological and functional connectivities of neurons that co-express NPY, GABA, and AgrP in the ARC of the hypothalamus (referred to in this and subsequent figures as NPY neurons). These neurotransmitters/neuromodulators are released in the ARC and PVN to evoke appetite. A subpopulation of NPY neurons directly release NPY, AgrP, and GABA in the PVN to stimulate appetite via specific receptors. Another subpopulation of NPY neurons release NPY, AgrP, and GABA in the ARC to transsynaptically curtail the MC4 receptor-mediated restraint on appetite by attenuating the release of α-melanocyte hormone from POMC neurons. This curb on the tonic restraint on appetite is supplemented by AgrP-induced antagonism of MC4 receptors. For details, see text.

NPY release-generating signals evoke the synchronized discharge of high-amplitude episodes at a rapid pace in the PVN. This rhythmic NPY secretion initiates episodic feeding. NPY secretion subsides as animals consume a meal; however, in the absence of readily available food, the episodic NPY discharge persists unabated to sustain the food-seeking drive. This antecedent NPY release is indeed a physiological trigger for appetite as evidenced by findings that prior depletion of the readily releasable NPY stores in the PVN nerve terminals with antisense oligodeoxynucleotides, passive immunoneutralization of the released NPY with NPY antibodies, or blockade of NPY receptors with pharmacologic antagonists suppresses appetite. Although the daily feeding pattern persists in the complete absence of hypothalamic NPY in NPY null mutant mice, these mice do not display increased feeding in response to physiological challenges such as fasting and insulin deficiency, and the hyperphagia and obesity of leptin-deficient ob/ob mice are drastically reduced. Adaptive reorganization during early development within the hypothalamic appetite-regulating network and other hypothalamic orexigenic messengers produced elsewhere in the hypothalamus and co-expressed with NPY in the ARC compensate for NPY deficiency to reinstate the instinctive appetitive drive. Consequently, NPY is a physiologically relevant appetite transducer, and the altered frequency and amplitude of NPY discharge result in the disintegration of the hypothalamic control on energy homeostasis.

B. Mechanism of Action

The orexigenic effects of NPY are mediated by the coordinated participation of three G-protein-coupled receptors, the Y_1, Y_2, and Y_5 receptors, in the ARC–PVN axis (Fig. 2). Y_1 and Y_5 receptor antagonists partially inhibit feeding, whereas germ-line deletions of any of these three receptors elicit varying degrees of altered feeding patterns and hyperphagia, modified response to varied diets, and obesity that manifests at different ages. Normally, a three-pronged interplay under the direction of NPY in the ARC–PVN axis initiates and extinguishes appetitive behavior. First, an increase in NPY and GABA release from the ARC NPY neurons in the PVN generates information to higher brain centers to evoke feeding. Concurrent release of AgrP from the ARC NPY neurons counteracts the tonic restraint exercised by melanocortin 4 (MC4) receptors and amplifies appetite (Fig. 2). Second, at the same time, increased NPY and GABA release within the ARC itself restrains POMC neurons, causing a decreased release of α-melanocyte-stimulating hormone (α-MSH) to diminish the tonic restraint on feeding. This timed and coordinated sequence of dual neurosecretory events, excitation by NPY and GABA and a curb on the tonic restraint on melanocortin signaling in the ARC–PVN axis, stimulates robust and sustained feeding (Fig. 2). Third, a gradual decrease in the release of NPY, GABA, and AgrP in the PVN, evoked by autofeedback through Y_2 receptors on NPY neurons in the ARC, inhibits feeding. Thus, the timely stimulation and termination of NPY release and co-expressed messengers in the hypothalamic ARC–PVN axis constitute an obligatory neurochemical signaling modality to stimulate and inhibit appetite in correlation with the meal pattern on a daily basis.

C. Regulation of Release by Afferent Signals

A complex interplay among diverse neural and hormonal afferent signals under the direction of the central clock precisely times the release of orexigenic signals from NPY neurons in the ARC–PVN axis. The two major hormonal signals from the periphery, leptin from adipose tissues and ghrelin from stomach, restrain and augment, respectively, the ARC NPY efflux (Fig. 1). Neural afferents to the ARC NPY neurons from the ventromedial hypothalamus (VMH) relay inhibitory information generated by circulating leptin. A loss of this relay due to structural

damage in the VMH results in hyperphagia and morbid obesity. Excitatory afferents from the LatH to ARC NPY neurons are relayed independently along the orexin and MCH neural pathways in response to reduced circulating leptin feedback. These neural pathways are strategically located to relay ascending visceral information via the spinal cord and brainstem to ARC NPY neurons for final processing and integration for energy homeostasis.

The most physiologically relevant afferent signals that regulate NPY secretion on a moment to moment basis are transmitted directly by the two functionally opposing afferent hormones, ghrelin and leptin (Fig. 1). Due to widespread action in the PVN, VMH, LatH, and other neighboring sites to produce tonic restraint, leptin is considered a major inhibitory signal. With this new understanding, it is possible to paint a clear picture of the sequential temporal interplay between hormonal afferent signals and hypothalamic effector pathways in governing the daily meal patterning. In anticipation of mealtime, the neural timing device, together with diminished leptin restraint from adipose tissue, stimulates high-frequency and high-amplitude ghrelin pulses from the stomach. This shift from inhibitory to excitatory afferents elicits NPY, GABA, and AgrP secretion from the ARC NPY effector pathway that, as described in the preceding section, propagates expression of hunger and the drive toward an energy source to replenish the depleted energy stores (Fig. 2).

Consumption of a meal reverses this chain of neural and hormonal events. First, there is a steady increase in leptin output, possibly stimulated by a gradual postprandial rise in pancreatic insulin secretion. As the tonic restraint by leptin on ARC NPY effector pathways is reinstated along with a steady decline in excitatory ghrelin generated by ingested food in stomach, appetite subsides. In the case of negative energy balance over long periods, such as that provoked by fasting, malnutrition, scarcity of food, or dieting, leptin secretion is drastically reduced but ghrelin output is markedly augmented. As a result of the concomitant suppression of tonic restraint and elevated stimulatory messages relayed by these functionally opposing hormonal afferents, NPY, GABA, and AgrP are hypersecreted to sustain the appetitive drive. Similarly, the high energy demands of lactation are met by hyperphagia induced by hypersecretion of ARC- and DMH-derived NPY in the PVN.

Afferent hormonal signals from other endocrine systems also employ NPY signaling in the hypothalamus to exert a modulatory effect on energy homeostasis (Fig. 1). Ovarian estrogens inhibit food intake in rodents by both decreasing NPY release in the PVN and increasing leptin secretion from adipocytes. A reduction of appetite and maintenance of reduced weight, consistently observed in response to estrogen therapy in women, are, therefore, likely a result of modified leptin–ARC NPY transmission. On the other hand, since adrenal glucocorticoids stimulate the production and release of hypothalamic NPY, it most likely contributes to hyperphagia and weight gain in patients on glucocorticoid therapy.

D. Eating Disorders: Anorexia and Obesity

During infection, injury in the central nervous system, and other pathological afflictions, anorexia is the predominant condition that results in the loss of body weight and wasting. Under these pathophysiological conditions, the cytokines interleukin 1 and ciliary neurotropic factor are up-regulated. These cytokines efficiently down-regulate NPYergic signaling to produce anorexia and weight loss (Fig. 1). Indeed, NPY replacement therapy has proven beneficial in rodent models as it can counteract cytokine-induced anorexia and weight loss.

The incidence of obesity has increased to epidemic proportions worldwide. A large body of evidence endorses the view that genetic and environmental factors produce an imbalance in the tightly regulated feedback interplay between the peripheral leptin and ghrelin signals and the effector NPY neural pathways. This derangement promotes positive energy balance and enlarged fat tissue to store excess energy fuel. Basically, insufficient leptin restraint along with a rise in the excitatory ghrelin signal to the NPY network contributes to an environmentally induced increase in adiposity and morbid obesity. Recently, gene therapy to circumvent leptin insufficiency and to reinforce the restraint on NPYergic signaling has proven successful. A single injection into the hypothalamus of a nonpathogenic and nonimmunogenic adeno-associated virus vector encoding leptin reinstates the central tonic restraint and suppresses weight gain and adiposity for long periods in rodents consuming a diet rich in calories. This sustained efficacy of leptin gene therapy to suppress weight gain results from a voluntary reduction in food intake and increased energy expenditure. Both of these neural events, in turn, are elicited by a reduced efflux of orexigenic NPY and an increased efflux of anorexigenic α-MSH in the PVN.

IV. NEUROPEPTIDE Y AND REPRODUCTION

A. Anatomical and Functional Links with GnRH

Research spanning nearly two decades documents a crucial regulatory role of NPY in the hypothalamic control of reproduction. NPY is involved in the regulation of GnRH release, a primary brain peptide responsible for the maintenance of reproduction and sexual behavior in both sexes (Fig. 3). GnRH, produced by a network of neurons extending from the rostral septal–medial preoptic area (MPOA) to the ARC–ME caudally in the hypothalamus, stimulates the release of the pituitary gonadotropins luteinizing hormone (LH) and follicle-stimulating hormone (FSH). GnRH is secreted into the hypophyseal portal veins in the ME in a pulsatile manner that represents an optimal mode of communication for pituitary gonadotropins to maintain reproduction in the two sexes (Fig. 3). Two oscillatory patterns of GnRH secretion have been observed in mammals. In general, GnRH is secreted in the form of low-amplitude pulses at more or less regular intervals throughout the 24 h period in males and through various stages of the reproductive cycle in females. These regularly spaced basal GnRH pulses in females are interrupted by an abrupt acceleration in the frequency and amplitude of GnRH discharge, culminating in the preovulatory LH surge release, an event that is essential for induction of ovulation (Fig. 3).

A distinct subpopulation of NPY neurons in the caudal ARC play a critical role in the excitation of pulsatile basal and cyclic GnRH discharge. NPY is also secreted in a pulsatile fashion in the ME with a frequency that coincides with that of GnRH. It acts synergistically with other hypothalamic excitatory signals, such as galanin and NE, to generate the basal GnRH pulses. In addition, NPY is a key excitatory signal for the initiation of the preovulatory secretion of GnRH. The sequential feedback actions of the ovarian steroids estrogen and progesterone on NPY neurons initially activate the synthesis of NPY in ARC perikarya and storage in terminal projections in the ME. This antecedent preparatory event culminates in the clock-driven hypersecretion of NPY, which, by a transsynaptic action on GnRH perikarya and dendrites in the MPOA and nerve terminals in the ME, generates a GnRH surge release into the hypophyseal portal veins (Fig. 3). Along with GnRH, NPY is also discharged into the hypophyseal portal vessels to potentiate the GnRH-induced preovulatory gonadotropin surge. Under certain

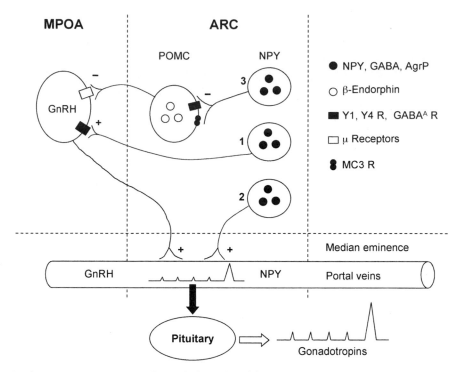

FIGURE 3 A schematic representation of morphological and functional connectivities of NPY-producing neurons in the ARC with the GnRH network in the MPOA and median eminence. NPY acts in three ways to modulate the basal and cyclic release of GnRH into the hypophyseal portal veins for transport to the pituitary gland to stimulate the release of gonadotropins: (1) Pulsatile discharge of NPY in the MPOA and median eminence stimulates GnRH release. (2) NPY is itself released into the hypophyseal portal veins to potentiate GnRH action in releasing pituitary gonadotropins. (3) NPY and GABA act transsynaptically to inhibit opioid release from POMC neurons in the ARC. A decrease in tonic opioid restraint on GnRH secretion facilitates NPY-induced stimulation of GnRH and the preovulatory gonadotropin surge.

environmental insults and physiological challenges, disturbances in NPY pulse patterns inhibit both the basal and the cyclical discharge of GnRH, leading to depressed reproduction and infertility. For example, continuous NPY receptor activation produced by either NPY infusion or excessive endogenous NPY secretion, such as that manifested in genetically obese ob/ob mice and in response to fasting or diet restriction, suppresses reproduction. However, these adverse effects on reproduction correct themselves after normalization of NPY episodic signaling. In the complete absence of endogenous NPY, as in NPY null mutant mice, GnRH–LH surges are only partially attenuated because embryonic neuroendocrine reorganization compensates for the loss.

B. Mechanism of Action

Morphological and experimental investigations have delineated distinct neural pathways mediating the excitatory and inhibitory effects of NPY on GnRH secretion (Fig. 3). NPY stimulates GnRH release on its own by acting through Y_1 receptors located on GnRH cell bodies in the MPOA and nerve terminals in the ME. This direct stimulatory action on GnRH is supplemented indirectly by modulation of the release of β-endorphin from POMC neurons by NPY. Normally, these endogenous opioids exert a tonic restraint on GnRH secretion. This restraint is curtailed by a coordinated interaction of NPY and GABA via Y_1 and $GABA^A$ receptors, respectively, on POMC neurons. Thus, an appropriately timed two-pronged action, the synergistic action of NPY with galanin (GAL), another excitatory neuropeptide produced in the hypothalamus, on GnRH neurons concurrent with a NPY–GABA-induced curb on opioid restraint, promotes GnRH secretion (Fig. 3).

On the other hand, experiments involving germ-line mutations of NPY receptors have identified NPY receptor subtypes that selectively participate in the inhibition of GnRH secretion by continuous NPY secretion. Under these conditions, overstimulation of Y_1 and Y_4 receptors located on POMC neurons in the ARC augments opioid restraint to turn off GnRH secretion. That these dual effects of NPY on GnRH secretion normally operate is endorsed by observations that a dampening of NPY signaling induced either by cytokine therapy or by germ-line deletion of NPY, Y_1, or Y_4 receptors in infertile ob/ob mice restores gonadotropin secretion and fertility.

V. NEUROPEPTIDE Y AND NUTRITIONAL INFERTILITY

It has long been known that nutrition is one of the most important environmental factors to impact human reproduction. Rapid population growth and environmental degradation in the 20th century have severely diminished food resources worldwide. The chronic shortage of food in conjunction with droughts in underdeveloped nations has impacted fertility. Chronic undernourishment and short-term caloric imbalance retard the onset of puberty and diminish fertility in all mammalian species. Limited caloric intake alone or in concert with the energy demands of strenuous exercise adversely impacts reproductive function. Heavy energy demands during lactation are compensated for by hyperphagia and cessation of reproductive cycles. In several genetic models in rodents and humans, hyperphagia and attendant obesity are concomitant with disturbed reproductive cycles and infertility. Is there a commonality in neurochemical signaling that links the neuroendocrine control of energy homeostasis and reproduction and responds appropriately to challenges of varied nutritional environments?

The information in the preceding sections documents a pivotal role of the hypothalamic NPY pathway in governing the neuroendocrine control of energy homeostasis and reproduction. It is obvious that there is spatial and temporal specificity of NPY involvement in these two neuroendocrine functions. The neuroanatomical substrate engaged by the ARC NPY circuitry in regulating reproduction is the GnRH neuronal network resident in the MPOA–ARC–ME axis (Fig. 3). On the other hand, the NPY ARC–PVN pathway represents a final pathway for the synthesis, storage, and release of NPY and other appetite-regulating peptides (Fig. 2). The neural links with neighboring VMH and LatH regions are also important components of the hypothalamic orexigenic network in the daily management of energy

homeostasis. Obviously, the neurochemical link between the circuitries that regulate reproduction and appetitive behavior lies in the commonality of the ARC as the source of NPY and other messenger molecules contacted by NPY neurons, all of which are vulnerable to internal and external environmental challenges of energy supply and hormonal imbalance (Fig. 4).

The intrinsic basal and cyclic patterns of NPY secretion in the MPOA–ARC–ME axis facilitate the secretion of the neurohormone GnRH to sustain reproduction. The rhythmic NPY secretion critical for imparting GnRH pulsatile secretion is modulated by the feedback action of gonadal steroids directly at the level of the ARC NPY subpopulation and the interconnected POMC–GAL pathways. An imbalance of gonadal steroid feedback produced by subnormal or inappropriate patterns of steroid production under nutritional stress disrupts the driving hypothalamic NPY GnRH signals, leading to depressed reproduction. Similarly, deficits in hypothalamic NPY synthesis and release during aging adversely affect GnRH secretion downstream, thereby leading to diminished reproductive and gonadal functions.

Aside from abnormalities in gonadal steroid feedback, deficits in energy fuels are sensed by the NPY network through an imbalance in leptin-ghrelin feedback (Fig. 4). A reduction in leptin feedback relieves the restraint on ARC NPY secretion, which, in concert with heightened stimulation by ghrelin,

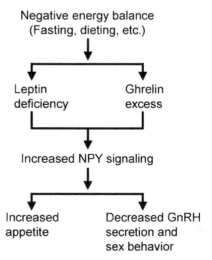

FIGURE 4 Regulatory role of hypothalamic NPY in increasing appetite and concomitantly suppressing reproduction and sex behavior in response to negative energy balance. For details, see text.

up-regulates NPY secretion in both the orexigenic axis of the ARC–PVN and the reproductive MPOA–ARC–ME axis. The overall consequence is robust expression of appetitive behavior to replenish energy fuel through Y_1 and Y_5 receptors at targets both in the ARC and in the PVN. There is concurrent suppression of reproduction and sexual behavior as the inhibitory pathways involving Y_1 and Y_4 receptors on POMC and GnRH neurons and in other sites implicated in regulatory sexual behavior are mobilized. Thus, changes in information flow from the periphery to the NPY network due to severe depletion in energy fuels for short or long periods compromise the intricate communication in the neural network that evokes rhythmic GnRH–gonadotropin secretion. Fortunately, these deleterious effects on reproduction are transient because replenishment of energy fuels reverses these sequelae and reinstates the independent moment to moment control of NPY on energy homeostasis and reproduction. In sum, NPY is an essential messenger molecule in the hypothalamus that serves as a communication bridge between the neuroendocrine processes that regulate reproduction and those that maintain energy homeostasis.

VI. SUMMARY

Information amassed during the past two decades affirms the concept that NPY produced by neurons in the ARC, a discrete subdivision of the hypothalamus, is an obligatory messenger molecule for commanding the two highly regulated innate drives in vertebrates: (1) appetite and the drive toward an energy source and (2) the urge to reproduce. A precise tracking of neural pathways originating in the ARC NPY perikarya has identified two distinct circuitries regulating each of these two hypothalamic regulatory functions. Within these circuitries, ARC NPY neurons, with the aid of intricate interconnections with other neurotransmitter/neuromodulator pathways within the hypothalamus and hormonal and neural afferent information from the periphery, transmit timed signals separately along these two circuitries. Subtle and progressive derangements provoked by environmental, genetic, and hormonal factors propagate molecular events governing the synthesis, release, and signal relay to reciprocally modify NPY transmission along the two circuitries. This commonality of neurochemical signaling has identified vulnerable loci for designing therapies to curb the epidemic of obesity and eating disorders without compromising fertility and, importantly, to alleviate nutritionally based infertility and reproductive disturbances.

Glossary

hypothalamus Area at the base of the brain involved in maintaining body homeostasis and neuroendocrine control of pituitary hormone secretion and appetitive and sex behaviors. Various subdivisions of the hypothalamus, such as the median eminence, arcuate nucleus, ventromedial hypothalamus, lateral hypothalamus, paraventricular nucleus, and medial preoptic area, participate in the regulation of these varied functions.

neurohormones Hormones produced by neurons and released into the hypophyseal portal system in the median eminence of the hypothalamus for transport to the pituitary gland to stimulate or inhibit the release of hormones; for example, gonadotropin-releasing hormone stimulates gonadotropin secretion from pituitary gonadotrophs.

neurotransmitters and neuromodulators Chemicals produced by neurons to transmit messages to other neurons synaptically, for example, neuropeptide Y, γ-aminobutyric acid, agouti-related peptides, norepinephrine, α-melanocyte stimulating hormone, melanin concentrating hormone, and orexins.

orexigen Chemicals produced by cells to stimulate appetite.

pituitary gland An endocrine organ located ventral to the hypothalamus and connected to it neurally and by a specialized vasculature called the hypophyseal portal system.

receptors Proteins in target cells that avidly bind with specific hormones or neurotransmitters/neuromodulators to initiate intracellular signaling responsible for a biological response.

See Also the Following Articles

Appetite Regulation, Neuronal Control ● Eating Disorders ● Growth Hormone-Releasing Hormone (GHRH) ● Leptin Actions on the Reproductive Axis ● Neuropeptides and Control of the Anterior Pituitary ● Peptide YY

Further Reading

Clark, J. T., Kalra, P. S., Crowley, W. R., and Kalra, S. P. (1984). Neuropeptide Y and human pancreatic polypeptide stimulate feeding behavior in rats. *Endocrinology* **115**, 427–429.

Clark, J. T., Kalra, P. S., and Kalra, S. P. (1985). Neuropeptide Y stimulates feeding but inhibits sexual behavior in rats. *Endocrinology* **117**, 2435–2442.

Cowley, M. A., Smart, J. L., Rubinstein, M., Cerdan, M. G., Diano, S., Horvath, T. L., Cone, R. D., and Low, M. J. (2001). Leptin activates anorexigenic POMC neurons through a neural network in the arcuate nucleus. *Nature* **411**, 480–484.

Dhillon, H., Kalra, S. P., and Kalra, P. S. (2001). Dose-dependent effects of central leptin gene therapy on genes that regulate body weight and appetite in the hypothalamus. *Mol. Ther.* **4**, 139–145.

Horvath, T. L., Diano, S., Sotonyi, P., Heiman, M., and Tschop, M. (2001). Minireview: Ghrelin and the regulation of energy balance—A hypothalamic perspective. *Endocrinology* **142**, 4163–4169.

Jain, M. R., Pu, S., Kalra, P. S., and Kalra, S. P. (1999). Evidence that stimulation of two modalities of pituitary luteinizing hormone release in ovarian steroid-primed ovariectomized rats may involve neuropeptide Y Y1 and Y4 receptors. *Endocrinology* **140**, 5171–5177.

Kalra, S. P. (1993). Mandatory neuropeptide–steroid signaling for the preovulatory luteinizing hormone-releasing hormone discharge. *Endocr. Rev.* **14**, 507–538.

Kalra, S. P., and Crowley, W. R. (1992). Neuropeptide Y: A novel neuroendocrine peptide in the control of pituitary hormone secretion, and its relation to luteinizing hormone. *Front. Neuroendocrinol.* **13**, 1–46.

Kalra, S. P., Dube, M. G., Pu, S., Xu, B., Horvath, T. L., and Kalra, P. S. (1999). Interacting appetite-regulating pathways in the hypothalamic regulation of body weight. *Endocr. Rev.* **20**, 68–100.

Kalra, S. P., Dube, M. G., Sahu, A., Phelps, C. P., and Kalra, P. S. (1991). Neuropeptide Y secretion increases in the paraventricular nucleus in association with increased appetite for food. *Proc. Natl. Acad. Sci. USA* **88**, 10931–10935.

Kalra, S. P., and Kalra, P. S. (1996). Nutritional infertility: The role of the interconnected hypothalamic neuropeptide Y–galanin–opioid network. *Front. Neuroendocrinol.* **17**, 371–401.

Kalra, S. P., Pu, S., Horvath, T. L., and Kalra, P. S. (2000). Leptin and NPY regulation of GnRH secretion and energy homeostasis. *In* "The Onset of Puberty in Perspective" (J. P. Bourguignon and T. M. Plant, eds.), pp. 317–327. Elsevier, San Diego, CA.

Larhammar, D., Wraith, A., Berglund, M. M., Holmberg, S. K., and Lundell, I. (2001). Origins of the many NPY-family receptors in mammals. *Peptides* **22**, 295–307.

Sainsbury, A., Schwarzer, C., Couzens, M., Jenkins, A., Oakes, S. R., Ormandy, C. J., and Herzog, H. (2002). Y4 receptor knockout rescues fertility in ob/ob mice. *Genes Dev.* **16**, 1077–1088.

Spiegelman, B. M., and Flier, J. S. (2001). Obesity and the regulation of energy balance. *Cell* **104**, 531–543.

Neurotensin

MICHELE SLOGOFF AND B. MARK EVERS

University of Texas Medical Branch

I. INTRODUCTION
II. THE NEUROTENSIN/NEUROMEDIN N GENE
III. THE NEUROTENSIN/NEUROMEDIN N PEPTIDE
IV. NEUROTENSIN RECEPTORS
V. EFFECTS OF NEUROTENSIN
VI. CONCLUSIONS/FUTURE PERSPECTIVES

Neurotensin, a peptide hormone that is produced in the hypothalamus, plays many important roles in regulatory and activation mechanisms in both the central nervous system and the gastrointestinal tract. Cloning of the neurotensin and closely allied genes and their receptors has provided insights into the physiological roles of these molecules, enhancing the potential for development of clinical/therapeutic applications.

I. INTRODUCTION

During the course of work to isolate the peptide substance P from bovine hypothalamus extracts, Carraway and Leeman discovered a new peptide that produced marked vasodilation of exposed cutaneous areas in rats. Sequencing of this novel peptide revealed a 13-amino-acid peptide that was named neurotensin (NT) because it was found in the brain and exhibited hypotensive activity. Subsequently, NT was isolated from the intestine, where it exhibits endocrine and possibly paracrine effects. In the central nervous system (CNS), NT has a neurotransmitter function and is involved in inhibition of dopaminergic pathways. In the gastrointestinal (GI) tract, NT affects GI motility, pancreatic and biliary secretion, and intestinal mucosal growth. Approximately a decade after the identification of NT, neuromedin N, a structurally related hexapeptide, was isolated from porcine hypothalamus. Neuromedin N has a peripheral distribution similar to that of NT and, in fact, has subsequently been found to be tandemly positioned with NT near the carboxy terminus of the precursor protein. A better understanding of the effects of NT in the CNS and the GI tract has been greatly facilitated by the cloning of the NT/neuromedin N (NT/N) gene, the cloning of the high- and low-affinity NT receptors, and the development of NT receptor antagonists. Moreover, the recent development of NT/N null mice by Dobner and colleagues will provide critical information regarding the precise physiologic role of NT in the CNS and GI tract.

The overview provided here primarily focuses on the most recent findings regarding the NT/N gene (structure, expression patterns, and molecular regulation), the NT/N peptide (structure, localization, and secretion), the NT receptors, and the central and peripheral effects of NT. Additional in-depth reviews on this subject are cited in the bibliography at the end of this article.

II. THE NEUROTENSIN/NEUROMEDIN N GENE

A. Structure

The NT/N gene is highly conserved among species. The cDNA encoding the NT/N gene was first cloned from a canine enteric mucosal library by Dobner and colleagues. Using the canine cDNA probe, the rat NT/N gene was then isolated by screening a rat genomic library. The NT/N gene spans approximately 10.2 kb and is divided into four exons and three introns. The NT and neuromedin N domains are tandemly arrayed on exon 4. Subsequent cloning of the human NT/N gene demonstrated an open reading frame encoding a predicted precursor protein of 170 amino acid residues (Fig. 1). At the nucleotide level, the human NT/N precursor is 92, 91, and 81% identical to canine, bovine, and rat NT/N, respectively; the resulting precursor peptide is similarly conserved (Fig. 2).

B. Expression

NT/N gene expression in the adult is predominantly localized to the small bowel, with increased expression noted in the ileum. In the adult, NT/N gene expression is not detected in the pancreas, stomach, or colon (Fig. 3). Interestingly, unlike the brush border enzymes (e.g., sucrase-isomaltase), the gradient of NT/N expression is not altered by changing the lumenal contents or the transposition of the intestine to other areas along the longitudinal gut axis. These findings suggest an intrinsic program of NT/N gene expression in the gut that is not affected by positional or nutrient alterations.

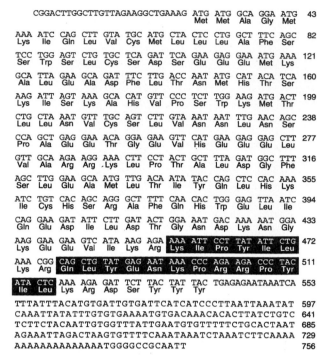

FIGURE 1 Human full-length cDNA clone of NT/N and predicted amino acid sequence of human prepro-NT/N. The neuromedin N and NT coding regions, located in tandem on exon 4, are highlighted in black. Modified from Dong *et al.* (1998), with permission from the *American Journal of Physiology.*

During development, expression of NT/N is noted in a well-defined spatial- and temporal-specific pattern. The earliest NT/N expression in fetal rats, identified by sensitive reverse transcriptase and polymerase chain reaction (RT-PCR) analysis, is

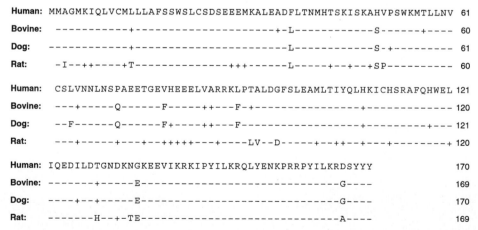

FIGURE 2 Analysis and comparison of the putative amino acid sequence of human NT/N to known sequences of the cow, dog, and rat. −, Identical sequences; +, similar sequences. Modified from Dong *et al.* (1998), with permission from the *American Journal of Physiology.*

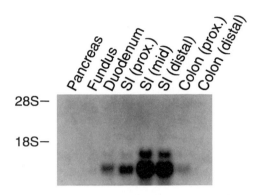

28S—

18S—

FIGURE 3 Localization of NT/N mRNA in the rat. Rat NT/N cRNA was used to probe 10 μg of polyadenylated RNA. Northern blots are from the pancreas, fundus of the stomach, duodenum, three equal segments of small intestine (SI), and two equal segments of colon. Adapted from Evers *et al.* (1991), with permission from *Surgery.*

noted in the primitive foregut at 12 days of gestation. In early fetal development, expression of the NT/N gene is detected in multiple tissues, including colon, pancreas, liver, and stomach; this expression is transient and disappears by the end of the first week of life. In the intestine, NT/N expression is low in both the jejunum and the ileum of fetal rats; steady-state NT/N mRNA levels rise rapidly after postnatal day 1 to assume the adult topographical distribution of increasing NT/N expression along the jejunoileal axis of the small bowel. By postnatal day 28, the pattern of expression is that of an adult, with no expression detected in the pancreas, liver, and stomach, minimal expression in the jejunum, and the majority of NT/N gene expression in the ileum. Developmental expression of NT/N in humans follows a similar pattern; NT/N expression is found in the fetal colon and liver but is not apparent after 24 weeks of gestation. This widespread distribution of NT/N expression in the developing GI tract suggests the presence in the primitive gut of a shared ancestral stem cell that is capable of multidirectional differentiation.

In addition to the fetal colon expression of NT/N during a gestational stage in which the colon resembles the small bowel, expression of NT/N has been detected in human colon cancers. Approximately 25% of freshly resected colon cancers demonstrate NT/N gene expression, although NT/N expression is not apparent in the adjacent normal mucosa. Furthermore, NT/N gene expression has been detected in human colon cancer cell lines. Similar to the expression of sucrase-isomaltase or carcinoembryonic antigen (CEA), the re-expression

of NT/N in certain colorectal cancers further suggests the reversion to a more fetal intestinal pattern. Similarly, NT/N expression has been noted in a variant of hepatocellular cancer (i.e., fibrolamellar cancer) as well as a nonfibrolamellar hepatocellular cancer (Hep3B). Taken together, these findings demonstrate a complex pattern of NT/N expression with well-localized and highly regimented expression in the adult GI tract, a more diffuse expression during fetal development, and re-expression in certain cancers.

C. Molecular Regulation

We have analyzed the molecular factors regulating the constitutive expression of NT/N using the BON endocrine cell line, which was derived from a functioning human carcinoid tumor and established in our laboratory. BON cells, like the terminally differentiated N cells of the small bowel, express high levels of NT/N mRNA, synthesize and secrete NT peptide, and process the NT/N precursor protein in a fashion identical to that of the N cells. Transient transfection assays using the rat NT/N promoter identify the proximal 216 base pairs (bp) of 5′ flanking sequences essential for high-level constitutive NT/N expression. A critical element located in the proximal NT/N promoter binds both activator protein 1 (AP-1) and cAMP-responsive enhancer binding (CREB)/activating transcription factors (ATF) and is critical for NT/N expression in BON cells. Mutation of the cAMP response element (CRE)/AP-1 site almost completely abolishes NT/N expression. This functional "cross talk" between different transcriptional pathways converging on a single binding site within a promoter greatly enhances the combinatorial possibilities of these transcription factors to regulate gene expression. Dobner and colleagues have also shown that elements contained within the proximal 216 bp are important for inducible NT/N gene expression. In contrast to constitutive NT/N expression in BON cells, the elements responsible for NT/N gene induction in the rat pheochromocytoma cell line, PC12, involve the cooperation of multiple elements of the NT/N promoter, including a distal consensus AP-1 site, the proximal CRE/AP-1 site, a near-consensus CRE site, and a near-consensus glucocorticoid response element (GRE) (Fig. 4). Therefore, these results suggest that a different array of regulatory elements is required for the constitutive NT/N expression pattern in the gut, in which NT functions as an endocrine agent, compared with NT/N gene induction in the CNS,

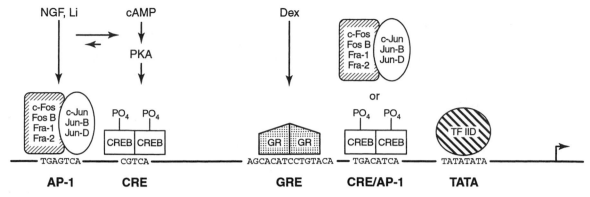

FIGURE 4 Schematic for cooperative regulation of NT/N gene transcription. NGF, Nerve growth factor; AP-1, activator protein 1; cAMP, cyclic adenosine monophosphate; CRE, cAMP response element; CREB, CRE binding protein; GRE, glucocorticoid response element; TF IID, transcription factor IID. Adapted from Dobner *et al.* (1992), with permission from *Ann. N.Y. Acad. Sci.*

in which NT serves as a neurotransmitter or neuromodulator.

The signal transduction pathways resulting in subsequent NT/N expression are also under investigation. In particular, the role of the Ras signaling pathway has been examined. Investigators in our group have shown that Ras (both wild type and activated) enhances expression of the NT/N gene in the Caco-2 human colon cancer cell line, most likely acting through the proximal CRE/AP-1 site. Furthermore, overexpression of Src kinase, another signaling protein in the Ras pathway, is associated with an increase in NT/N promoter activity. Mutation of the proximal promoter element inhibits Ras-mediated NT/N induction. Ras and Src can stimulate the binding activity of AP-1 proteins (e.g., c-Jun); therefore, we speculate that Ras, acting through AP-1 proteins, induces NT/N gene expression.

In addition to transcription factor binding, gene methylation regulates expression of various genes. Methylation appears to play a critical role in the expression of a number of genes during both normal development and malignant transformation. Investigators in our laboratory have shown, by complementary approaches, that DNA methylation plays a role in NT/N gene suppression in certain hepatocellular and colon cancer cell lines. Treatment with a demethylating agent, 5-azacytidine, partially activates the suppressed NT/N gene in the HepG2 hepatocellular cancer. Moreover, our group has shown that DNA methylation plays a role in NT/N gene silencing in the human colon cancer KM20 and that NT/N expression in the KM12C cell line is associated with demethylation of CpG sites in the NT/N promoter. These studies suggest that methy-

lation status may be directly related to NT/N re-expression in certain cancers and may account for gene repression during development. In addition, we speculate that gene methylation may play a role, in combination with transcription factors, in providing the strict tissue-specific regulation of NT/N gene expression noted in various tissues.

III. THE NEUROTENSIN/NEUROMEDIN N PEPTIDE

A. Structure

NT is a peptide composed of 13 amino acids. The amino terminus is a pyrrolidone carboxylic acid and resists proteolytic degradation; the inactive degradation product is NT(1–8). The bioactive core, NT(9–13), resides in the carboxy terminus, which is highly conserved among species. The metabolism of NT(1–13) is rapid; therefore, the majority of circulating NT is in the form of the stable NH_2-terminal fragments, primarily NT(1–8) or, less commonly, NT(1–11). The neuromedin N peptide is structurally related to NT, with conservation of the carboxy terminus. Although distribution of neuromedin N is similar to that of NT, the effects of neuromedin N and NT may be different. NT is not lipophilic and thus does not penetrate the blood–brain barrier.

B. Localization

In the GI tract, the NT peptide is localized to enteroendocrine cells (i.e., N cells), predominantly in the small bowel and proximal colon. Similar to the expression pattern of the NT/N gene, N cells are found in greatest abundance in the distal ileum mucosa. NT immunoreactivity has also been identified in the muscle layers of the gut, mostly in the myenteric plexus. Presumably, in this location, NT functions as a neurotransmitter as it does in the CNS. Within the brain, NT immunoreactivity is primarily located in the substantia nigra, periaqueductal gray matter, amygdala, nucleus accumbens, and some hypothalamic nuclei; lower concentrations are found in the caudate, hippocampus, and globus pallidus.

C. Secretion

The precise signaling mechanisms regulating NT secretion are not entirely known. Fat in the proximal intestine appears to be the most potent stimulus. The initial NT release occurs within 10 min of eating, long before chyme reaches the ileum. Studies have shown that infusion of fat into the jejunum leads to an increase in NT release, whereas infusion of fat into the ileum does not. However, ileal resection abolishes release of NT. Atropine also abolishes this response but truncal vagotomy does not. These findings suggest that NT is released from the ileum via a humoral or neural stimulus from the proximal intestine. Furthermore, the process appears to be cholinergic, but not vagally mediated.

In addition to lipids, *in vitro* experiments using short-term ileal mucosal cell cultures demonstrate that the peptide bombesin directly stimulates NT release that is not abolished by atropine (in contrast to lipid-stimulated release). Catecholamines appear to stimulate NT release via a β-adrenergic receptor. Carbachol stimulates NT release in segments of perfused ileum but has no effect on basal NT release in short-term N cell cultures. In fact, carbachol inhibits β-adrenergic-stimulated NT release; the possible mechanism for these actions has yet to be elucidated. Similarly, substance P stimulates release of NT in neurons and in perfused ileum but not in short-term N cell cultures. Taken together, the data imply that there is more than one pathway affecting NT release (at least one pathway is cholinergically mediated and another is not) and that other mechanisms in the intact organism are required for the activation of release of NT by certain mediators.

IV. NEUROTENSIN RECEPTORS

After secretion, the NT peptide must bind to a receptor in order to produce an effect. Three NT receptors have been identified. The first two receptors, the high-affinity NTS1 and low-affinity nts2, are G-protein-coupled receptors that differ slightly in structure. The recently identified third receptor, nts3, has an altogether different structure compared with NTS1 and nts2.

A. NTS1 Receptor

The high-affinity NTS1 receptor is sensitive to Na^+ ions and guanosine triphosphate (GTP); both substances decrease the affinity of the receptor for NT. This high-affinity receptor is insensitive to levocabastine, an antihistamine-1 that blocks lower affinity binding sites. The NTS1 gene has been sequenced and encodes 424 amino acids (in rats) and 418 amino acids (in humans). The protein has seven transmembrane domains and is considered a G-protein-coupled receptor (Fig. 5). Expression of the NTS1 gene has been identified in the brain and intestine of rats and humans. *In situ* hybridization studies demonstrate high levels of expression in the diagonal band of Broca, medial septal nucleus, nucleus basalis magnocellularis, suprachiasmatic nucleus, supramammillary area, substantia nigra, and ventral segmental area in the brain. In the GI tract, the NTS1 receptor has been identified throughout the small intestine, large intestine, and liver. Following binding with NT, 60–70% of the NTS1 receptor internalizes in a temperature-dependent process; the receptor is not recycled to the cell membrane. After NT binds to this G-protein-coupled receptor, phospholipase C is activated, inducing phosphatidylinositol turnover and mobilization of intracellular calcium. Recent studies have shown that NT binding increases activation of extracellular signal-related kinase (ERK) and c-Jun N-terminal kinase (JNK) (kinases in the Ras pathway). These findings suggest that, like other GI peptides (e.g., cholecystokinin and gastrin), NT activates the Ras pathway via its NTS1 receptor. These observations implicate the Ras pathway in the subsequent downstream effects of NT. Two nonpeptide receptor antagonists synthesized by Gully and colleagues effectively bind NTS1 and prevent many of the actions of NT. SR48692 has been shown to block a number of peripheral and central effects of NT but does not appear to inhibit the hypothermic and analgesic effects of NT. This antagonist binds to a binding site separate from but overlapping that of the NT peptide, thus blocking a portion of the receptor crucial for NT binding. Another antagonist, SR142948A, has been found to have a broader spectrum of activity and also inhibits the

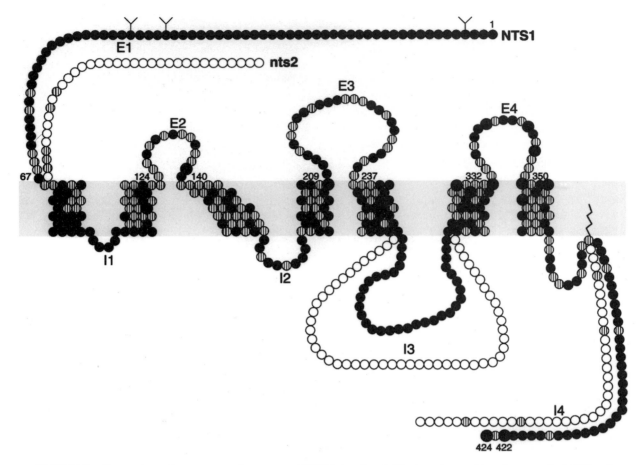

FIGURE 5   Comparison of rat neurotensin receptors NTS1 (•) and nts2. The invariant residues between the NTS1 and nts2 receptors are noted by circles with vertical lines. Regions of the nts2 receptor that vary greatly from NTS1 and are noted by open circles. The N-terminus (1) and C-terminus (424) and the first residues of each extracellular segment of the NTS1 receptor are numbered. Glycosylation sites are highlighted (Y). Residues 422 and 424 are crucial for NTS1 internalization. The third intracellular loop (13) contains a region essential for coupling to phospholipase C. Adapted from Vincent *et al.* (1999), with permission from *Trends Pharmacol. Sci.*

hypothermia and analgesia induced by intracerebroventricular injection of NT.

B. nts2 Receptor

The nts2 receptor is also a G-protein-coupled receptor with seven transmembrane domains. This receptor, in contrast to NTS1, is a low-affinity receptor that can be blocked by levocabastine and is relatively insensitive to Na^+ ions and GTP. The replacement of Asp by Ala or Gly in the second transmembrane domain is believed to be responsible for the decreased affinity of the receptor. This receptor has been localized mostly in the brain. It is specifically expressed in the olfactory system, cerebral and cerebellar cortices, hippocampal formation, and certain hypothalamic nuclei. The nts2 receptor is implicated in NT-induced analgesia. For example, intracerebroventricular injection of antisense oligonucleotides, which specifically block nts2 expression, inhibits NT-induced analgesia. These oligonucleotides have no effect on other receptors. Furthermore, SR48692, which does not block nts2, also does not inhibit NT analgesia.

C. nts3 Receptor

In contrast to the first two receptors, the nts3 receptor is not a G-protein-coupled receptor but has a gp95/sortilin structure (Fig. 6). This receptor has an N-terminal signal peptide, a cleavage site for furin, a long lumenal domain, a single transmembrane domain, and a short cytoplasmic tail; it is stored in vesicles and inserted into the membrane in response to NT. No data are yet available regarding the specific physiologic functions of this newly cloned receptor.

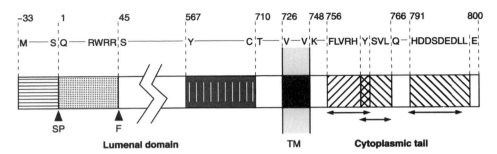

FIGURE 6 The human nts3/gp/sortilin receptor. Numbers indicate the signal peptide (SP) (726–747), the propeptide released by furin (F) cleavage (1–44), the cysteine-rich domain homologous to Vps10p, a yeast receptor for carboxypeptidase Y sorting (567–709), the transmembrane (TM) domain (726–747), and the three internalization/sorting signals in the cytoplasmic tail homologous to the cation-independent mannose 5-phosphate/insulin-like growth factor-II receptor (456–765 and 791–799). Note the partial overlapping between two of these signal sequences. Adapted from Vincent *et al.* (1999), with permission from *Trends Pharmacol. Sci.*

V. EFFECTS OF NEUROTENSIN

NT produces an array of effects in both the CNS and the GI tract. In the CNS, NT functions as a neurotransmitter or a neuromodulator, whereas in the periphery NT can exert its actions via endocrine, paracrine, or neuromodulatory effects.

A. CNS Effects

NT produces significant CNS effects, including hypothermia and a naloxone-insensitive analgesia. NT blocks behaviors associated with activation of dopaminergic pathways, possibly by decreasing the binding efficiency of dopamine to its receptors. Centrally administered NT has been shown to mimic the actions of many antipsychotic drugs. NT, like antipsychotic medications, potentiates the sedation elicited by barbiturates and ethanol, decreases amphetamine-induced locomotor activity, and induces muscle relaxation and hypothermia. Administration of various antipsychotic drugs increases NT concentrations in the caudate nucleus and nucleus accumbens. This effect is preceded by an increase in c-*fos* mRNA levels in the dorsolateral stratum. Typical antipsychotic medications (e.g., haloperidol) induce NT/N expression in the striatum and nucleus accumbens. On the other hand, administration of atypical antipsychotic medications (e.g., clozapine), which are not associated with extrapyramidal side effects (EPSs), results in increased NT/N expression in the nucleus accumbens only. Recent studies using NT/N null mice demonstrate that NT is required for haloperidol-elicited activation of a specific population of striatal neurons; however, the incidence of catalepsy (the model for EPS in mice) was not different in NT/N null mice. These findings indicate that NT mediates the effects of a specific subset of antipsychotic agents but does not contribute to the generation of extrapyramidal side effects.

B. Peripheral Effects

1. Vascular and Hemodynamic Effects

The NT peptide was initially described as a "hypotensive peptide." In reality, the vascular and hemodynamic effects are more complicated than initially described. NT release can lead to either hypotension or hypertension by inducing either histamine release or adrenergic release, respectively. Other hemodynamic effects include decreasing blood flow to adipose tissue and increasing blood flow in the intestine without altering heart rate or blood pressure.

2. Immune Function

Similar to other gut peptides, NT has an effect on immune function. Macrophages demonstrate enhanced phagocytosis in response to NT treatment. Mast cells respond to NT by releasing histamine; the response can be antagonized in rats with diphenhydramine (an antihistamine). In lymphocytes, NT can enhance proliferation, adherence, and chemotaxis. Because the small intestine has a high concentration of immunologically active cells, NT may affect immune function via paracrine effects. In rats, NT has also been shown to be a proinflammatory agent in the colonic inflammation associated with *Clostridium difficile* pseudomembranous colitis. This proinflammatory action is blocked by SR48692.

3. Effects on GI Nutrient Absorption, Motility, and Secretion

Some of the physiologic effects of NT in the GI tract are related to motility. An infusion of NT mimics the consumption of a fat-rich meal (the most potent stimulator of NT release) in the following ways: NT decreases lower esophageal sphincter pressure, slows gastric emptying and intestinal transit while increasing colonic motility, and inhibits the migrating motor complex (MMC).

In addition to effects on GI motility, NT inhibits gastric acid secretion in a vagally dependent manner. Some debate exists regarding whether concentrations of NT that are present physiologically are sufficient to induce this effect. In contrast to gastric acid secretion, NT stimulates pancreatic bicarbonate and protein secretion in a dose-related fashion and has an additive effect in combination with secretin and/or cholecystokinin. NT potently stimulates biliary secretion of water, bicarbonate, and bile salts. Secretin is more effective than NT in stimulating secretion of bicarbonate and bile salts, but NT is more effective in stimulating secretion of bile water. A recent study demonstrates that NT also enhances jejunal absorption of conjugated bile acids and their return to the liver. Additional effects of NT include a net fluid secretion into the postduodenal small intestine and facilitation of lipid absorption from the proximal intestine.

4. Trophic Effects

NT, given exogenously, has trophic effects on normal tissues as well as on certain cancers. Given in high doses, NT can induce growth of the gastric antrum, small intestine, and pancreas. In rats given an elemental diet, intestinal mucosal atrophy ensues; administration of NT can prevent this atrophy in the jejunum but not in other areas of the small bowel. NT can also augment the adaptive hyperplasia of intestinal mucosa associated with small bowel resection. Other studies demonstrate that NT stimulates mucosal growth in defunctionalized, self-emptying jejunoileal loops or isolated loops of small bowel (Thiry–Vella fistulas). Moreover, NT has been shown to restore gut mucosal integrity in rats and to prevent translocation of indigenous bacteria after radiation-induced mucosal injury.

In addition to its effects on normal tissues, NT has been shown to have a trophic effect on pancreatic and colon cancers that possess NT receptors. NT receptors have also been found in non-GI tumors, such as prostate cancer, in which NT has a similar trophic effect. Recent studies utilizing sensitive RT-PCR procedures have identified NT receptor expression in a majority of pancreatic adenocarcinomas. Although not universally expressed in human colon cancer cell lines, NT receptor expression has been identified in a

more metastatic colon cancer cell line (i.e., KM20 cells). *In vitro* and *in vivo* experiments using the human pancreatic cancer line MIA PaCa-2, which possesses high-affinity NT receptors, have demonstrated growth in response to NT. NT treatment of athymic nude mice bearing MIA PaCa-2 xenografts results in increased tumor size, weight, and DNA and protein content. The NT receptor antagonist SR48692 inhibits these trophic effects. NT enhances colon carcinogenesis in rats and stimulates growth of MC-26 (mouse) and LoVo (human) colon cancer cells. These findings suggest a role for NT in the growth of GI cancers with high-affinity NT receptors. Therefore, analogous to current treatment strategies for endocrine-responsive breast and prostate cancers, NT receptor antagonists may play an adjuvant role in the treatment of certain GI and pancreatic cancers.

VI. CONCLUSIONS/FUTURE PERSPECTIVES

Since its initial description almost 30 years ago, much has been learned regarding the regulation and actions of the NT peptide. The cloning of the NT/N gene in multiple species, the identification and cloning of the NT receptor genes, the synthesis of potent NT receptor antagonists, and the development of NT/N knockout mice are recent important developments that have greatly facilitated our understanding of these functions. Collectively, NT has been identified as an important contributory hormone for the maintenance of both gut structure and function. In the GI tract, NT affects intestinal motility, pancreaticobiliary secretion, fat absorption, and growth of normal and neoplastic tissues. In the CNS, an apparent important role for NT appears to be related to the blockade of dopaminergic pathways that have important ramifications in the effects of many psychotropic agents.

Future studies will further extend our current understanding of the effects of NT. Previous studies have identified the NT/N gene as a "model" intestinal gene to further delineate the complex differentiation pathways leading to gut development and maturation, as well as the process of fetal "dedifferentiation" noted in certain colon cancers. Understanding the factors regulating NT/N expression will yield important information on the regulation and attainment of the complete gut phenotype, thus not only providing a better understanding of normal gut development and function, but also providing a model to better understand the cellular events leading to gut neoplasia. The multitude of actions of NT, particularly its trophic and neuroleptic effects, suggest a potential future role for NT as a pharmacologic agent. The fact that NT is secreted in response to a fatty meal and induces delayed gastric emptying and intestinal motility suggests that NT may play a role in satiety and may be useful in the treatment of obesity. The trophic effects of NT on normal intestinal mucosa suggest that NT may be useful in stimulation of intestinal growth during periods of gut disuse, after small bowel resection, or with administration of chemotherapeutic agents. Furthermore, blocking NT receptors using potent receptor antagonists may be useful as adjuvant therapy in the treatment of certain NT receptor-positive colon and pancreatic cancers. Overall, the analysis of NT in the past has yielded important and clinically relevant information regarding its structure, expression pattern, role in development, secretion, and diversity of actions. It is anticipated that future studies, utilizing sophisticated molecular models and more specific receptor antagonists, will provide additional important information regarding the precise role of this novel peptide in GI and CNS functions, as well as exciting new therapies with diverse clinical implications.

Glossary

Gp95/sortilin receptor Type of receptor that contains only one transmembrane domain.

G-protein-coupled receptor Type of receptor that contains seven transmembrane domains.

N cells Enteroendocrine cells localized to the intestine; produce and secrete neurotensin and neurotensin-related peptides; categorized as "open" cells, in which the apical microvilli are in contact with the intestinal lumen.

neuromedin N Hexapeptide that is encoded on the same gene as neurotensin and has a similar distribution pattern.

neurotensin Tridecapeptide that is found in the brain and gastrointestinal tract.

See Also the Following Articles

Gastrointestinal Hormone-Releasing Peptides ● GPCR (G-Protein-Coupled Receptor) Structure ● Motilin

Further Reading

Castagliuolo, I., Wang, C. C., Valenick, L., Pasha, A., Nikulasson, S., Carraway, R. E., and Pothoulakis, C. (1999). Neurotensin is a proinflammatory neuropeptide in colonic inflammation. *J. Clin. Invest.* **103**, 843–849.

Dobner, P. R., Barber, D. L., Villa-Komaroff, L., and McKiernan, C. (1987). Cloning and sequence analysis of cDNA for the canine neurotensin/neuromedin N precursor. *Proc. Natl. Acad. Sci. U.S.A.* **84**, 3516–3520.

Dobner, P. R., Fadel, J., Deitemeyer, N., Carraway, R. E., and Deutch, A. Y. (2001). Neurotensin-deficient mice show altered responses to antipsychotic drugs. *Proc. Natl. Acad. Sci. U.S.A.* **98**, 8048–8053.

Dobner, P. R., Kislauskis, E., and Bullock, B. P. (1992). Cooperative regulation of neurotensin/neuromedin N gene expression in PC12 cells involves AP-1 transcription factors. *Ann. N.Y. Acad. Sci.* **668**, 17–29.

Dong, Z., Wang, X., Zhao, Q., Townsend, C. M., Jr., and Evers, B. M. (1998). DNA methylation contributes to expression of the human neurotensin/neuromedin N gene. *Am. J. Physiol.* **274**, G535–G543.

Ehlers, R. A., Kim, S., Zhang, Y., Hellmich, M. R., Ethridge, R. T., Murillo, C., Hellmich, M. R., Evans, D., Townsend, C. M., Jr., and Evers, B. M. (2000). Gut peptide receptor expression in human pancreatic cancers. *Ann. Surg.* **23**, 838–848.

Evers, B. M. (1999). Expression of the neurotensin/neuromedin N gene in the gut. *In* "Gastrointestinal Endocrinology" (J. G. H. Greeley, ed.), pp. 423–438. Humana Press, Totowa.

Gui, X., and Carraway, R. E. (2001). Enhancement of jejunal absorption of conjugated bile acid by neurotensin in rats. *Gastroenterology* **120**, 151–160.

Iwase, K., Evers, B. M., Hellmich, M. R., Kim, H. J., Higashide, S., Gully, D., Thompson, J. C., and Townsend, C. M., Jr. (1997). Inhibition of neurotensin-induced pancreatic carcinoma growth by a nonpeptide neurotensin receptor antagonist, SR48692. *Cancer* **79**, 1787–1793.

Kislauskis, E., Bullock, B., McNeil, S., and Dobner, P. R. (1988). The rat gene encoding neurotensin and neuromedin N. Structure, tissue-specific expression, and evolution of exon sequences. *J. Biol. Chem.* **263**, 4963–4968.

Le, F., Groshan, K., Zeng, X. P., and Richelson, E. (1997). Characterization of the genomic structure, promoter region, and a tetranucleotide repeat polymorphism of the human neurotensin receptor gene. *J. Biol. Chem.* **272**, 1315–1322.

Merchant, K. M., Dobie, D. J., and Dorsa, D. M. (1992). Expression of the proneurotensin gene in the rat brain and its regulation by antipsychotic drugs. *Ann. N.Y. Acad. Sci.* **668**, 54–69.

Seethalakshmi, L., Mitra, S. P., Dobner, P. R., Menon, M., and Carraway, R. E. (1997). Neurotensin receptor expression in prostate cancer cell line and growth effect of NT at physiological concentrations. *Prostate* **31**, 183–192.

Tanaka, K., Masu, M., and Nakanishi, S. (1990). Structure and functional expression of the cloned rat neurotensin receptor. *Neuron* **4**, 847–854.

Vincent, J. P., Mazella, J., and Kitabgi, P. (1999). Neurotensin and neurotensin receptors. *Trends Pharmacol. Sci.* **20**, 302–309.

Neurotrophins

Y.-A. BARDE

Friedrich-Miescher Institute for Biomedical Research, Switzerland

I. NEUROTROPHIN: BIOCHEMISTRY AND MOLECULAR BIOLOGY
II. NEUROTROPHIN RECEPTORS
III. NEUROTROPHINS AND NEURONAL SURVIVAL
IV. NEUROTROPHINS AND NEURONAL PLASTICITY

The neurotrophins constitute a small family of structurally related proteins. They are primarily known for their ability to affect key aspects of the biology of vertebrate neurons, including neuronal survival and death, dendrite and axonal elongation, and activity-dependent plasticity. The term "neurotrophin" was introduced subsequent to the finding that the sequence of the protein brain-derived neurotrophic factor was related to that of nerve growth factor. In mammals, two additional genes have been identified and they are designated neurotrophin-3 and neurotrophin-4. All four neurotrophins act through two structurally unrelated receptors designated Trk and p75. Neurotrophins can both prevent program cell death and cause it. In addition, they affect the shape of neurons as well as synaptic transmission.

I. NEUROTROPHIN: BIOCHEMISTRY AND MOLECULAR BIOLOGY

A. Biochemistry

All neurotrophins are small (approximately 120 amino acids), basic (pI 9–10) proteins (Fig. 1). They are strongly similar in primary structure and are found in solution as noncovalently, tightly linked homodimers. They are secretory proteins and their cleavable leader sequence is followed by a pro-sequence of variable length [80 aa for the shortest one, human neurotrophin-4 (NT4)]. Cleavage of the pro-sequence occurs at a consensus sequence of the furin type found in all neurotrophins (R-X-K/R-R) to yield the mature and biologically active neurotrophins. However, recent evidence indicates that pro-neurotrophins may also be secreted and that in comparison with mature neurotrophins they have a higher affinity for the neurotrophin receptor p75 and a lower affinity for the Trk receptors. The functional consequence of this characteristic would be a shift toward the death-promoting activity of neurotrophins.

Each mature monomer comprises six cysteine residues involved in the formation of three disulfide bridges. The crystal structure of the neurotrophin dimers has revealed that the disulfide bridges are all grouped at one end of the molecule in the homodimers in an arrangement similar to that found in the transforming growth factor-β superfamily and in the platelet-derived growth factors.

Nucleotide sequences are available for several mammalian species, and approximately 50% of the amino acids are common to all neurotrophins,

including the six cysteine residues. With the exception of NT4, neurotrophins are highly conserved between species. For example, there are no amino acid replacements in the mature sequence of brain-derived neurotrophic factor (BDNF) and neurotrophin-3 (NT3) in most mammals. Additional neurotrophin sequences have been reported in teleost fishes, but no neurotrophin sequence has been detected in the genome of *Caenorhabditis elegans* and *Drosophila melanogaster*. Similarly, these latter two genomes do not contain sequences corresponding to the neurotrophin receptors p75 or Trks.

B. Molecular Biology

In human, *ngf* (nerve growth factor gene) has been localized to chromosome 1q21–q22.1, *bdnf* has been localized to 11q13, *nt3* has been localized to 12q13, and *nt4* has been localized to 19q13.3. The neurotrophin genes are large (at least 40 kb) and contain several small 5′ exons and a larger 3′ exon that contains most of the translated sequence. The neurotrophin genes encode several transcripts from at least four different transcription start sites. Also, they have short or long 3′-untranslated regions. These genes are transcribed as a major transcript of approximately 1.3 to 1.6 kb and often a larger transcript of approximately 4.3 kb. Their relative abundance depends on the tissue in question. In the brain, neurons are the major cellular site of neurotrophin gene expression and there are considerable differences in the degree of expression between different brain areas and developmental stage. Typically, gene expression is regulated by electrical activity. In particular, increased activity leads to rapid increased transcription of the *ngf* and *bdnf* genes, and decreased activity reduces the expression of *bdnf*. Outside of the central nervous system (CNS),

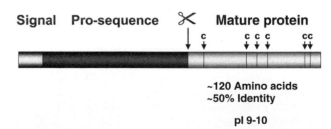

FIGURE 1 Neurotrophins are synthesized as pre-pro proteins. Cleavage occurs following a cluster of basic amino acids. The six cysteine residues indicated in the mature proteins are involved in the formation of three disulfide bridges. Neurotrophins occur in solution as tightly packed homodimers.

numerous cell types express the neurotrophin genes, including Schwann cells, skeletal muscle cells, and smooth muscle cells, as well as cells from heart and lung tissue. Expression has also been detected in cells of the immune system, including lymphocytes.

II. NEUROTROPHIN RECEPTORS

Neurotrophin signaling is quite complex and diverse. There are two different receptor types that bind the neurotrophins, p75, and the Trks (Fig. 2). These receptors can mediate actions as diverse as promoting or preventing the death of neurons. Also, these two receptor types associate in the membrane, and these associations lead to increases in the specificity and affinity of the receptor complex.

A. p75

The neurotrophin receptor p75 was the first member of a large family of receptors, which includes both tumor necrosis factor receptors and CD95, to be molecularly cloned. It was initially designated the nerve growth factor (NGF) receptor. This designation was revisited following the realization that all neurotrophins bind to this receptor and that the Trk receptors also bind neurotrophins (see below). At least two proteins are encoded by *p75*, one of them lacking three of the four cysteine-rich domains that characterize the extracellular domains of all

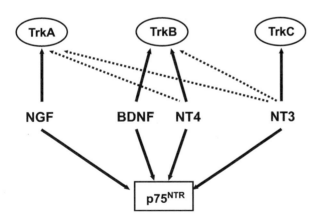

FIGURE 2 Neurotrophins bind two different kinds of receptors. All bind to the receptor p75 with an affinity of at least 10^{-9} M. They also bind to the Trk family of tyrosine kinase receptors. TrkC binds exclusively to NT3, TrkA shows a preference for binding to NGF, and TrkB binds preferentially to BDNF and NT4. NT3 also binds to TrkA and TrkB. All three Trk receptors associate with p75, and this association modulates both the binding specificity and the affinity of the Trk receptors.

members of the p75 family. Like all other members, p75 has no intrinsic catalytic activity and it transduces signals by associating with, or dissociating from, cytoplasmic partners. There are several protein association motifs in the cytoplasmic domain of p75, one being distantly related to the so-called "death domain" of other members of the family. Also of note is a short sequence of the intracellular domain of p75 that is related to the sequence of mastoparan, a 14-mer peptide derived from wasp venom and capable of directly activating G-proteins. The C-terminus forms a consensus sequence found in several other proteins associating with postsynaptic densities, such as postsynaptic density-95. A number of proteins have been shown to associate with the cytoplasmic domain of p75.

All mature neurotrophins tested bind to p75 with an affinity of approximately 10^{-9} M. Recently, pro-NGF was demonstrated to bind to p75 with a 10-fold higher affinity than mature NGF and to bind to the TrkA receptor with a distinctly lower affinity than mature NGF.

B. Trk Receptors

In mammals, three Trk receptors have been identified: TrkA, TrkB, and TrkC. TrkA binds NGF and to a lesser extent NT3, TrkB binds preferentially to BDNF and NT4, though NT3 can also bind to and activate TrkB, especially in the absence of p75 co-expression, and TrkC binds to NT3 exclusively (Fig. 2). As with the neurotrophins, additional Trk receptors have been identified in teleost fishes. Ligand binding leads to receptor-mediated tyrosine phosphorylation. This triggers the activation of pathways leading to some of the best known actions of the neurotrophins, including the prevention of programmed cell death and neuronal differentiation. Three main signaling cascades are activated by the Trk receptors and their substrates: the Ras/Raf/MEK/mitogen-activated protein kinase pathway, phosphatidylinositol 3-kinase, and phospholipase C-γ. At the level of the nerve terminals, the association of neurotrophins with Trk receptors triggers the process of retrograde transport, allowing signals to be transported from the terminals back to the cell body of neurons.

A number of splice variants have been described for the Trk receptors. The most abundant variants are forms of TrkB and TrkC that lack the kinase domain. These truncated TrkB receptors are often expressed in nonneuronal cells in the absence of TrkB.

C. Expression of Neurotrophin Receptors

The expression of both types of neurotrophin receptors is tightly regulated. Typically, only specific subgroups of neurons express one particular Trk receptor. The specificity of the neurotrophins for subgroups of sensory neurons correlates strongly with the selectivity of Trk receptor expression on these neurons. In the peripheral nervous system (PNS), neurotrophins are often expressed in the peripheral targets of those neurons needing neurotrophins for survival in the embryo. In the adult, these target-derived neurotrophins regulate the functional properties of the neurons, including the levels of neurotransmitters and dendritic development. As in the central nervous system, some of the neurotrophin genes are also expressed by neuronal cell bodies, and BDNF in particular is expressed by some sensory neurons and transported in an anterograde manner. It is released by NGF-dependent neurons in the spinal cord, where it affects neurotransmission. p75 is co-expressed with the Trk receptors in many neuronal populations. Its expression profile is highly developmentally regulated. During postnatal development, p75 is down-regulated in most parts of the central nervous system, but it is rapidly induced after nerve lesion or seizure. This receptor is also expressed by many cells, such as neural crest cells, by the time they become postmitotic cells and/or migrate.

III. NEUROTROPHINS AND NEURONAL SURVIVAL

A. Neurotrophins Promote Neuronal Survival

Neurotrophins typically support the survival of embryonic neurons that die in their absence. Thus, antibodies to NGF, like the deletion of the *ngf* or *trkA* gene, lead to the virtually complete destruction of the peripheral sympathetic nervous system as well as to the loss of many neural crest-derived sensory neurons. BDNF, NT3, and NT4 also support the survival of subpopulations of peripheral sensory neurons, including those derived from epidermal placodes, which are not supported by NGF. With the exception of NGF, neurotrophins support the survival of embryonic rat motoneurons *in vitro*, and BDNF prevents their death *in vivo* after axotomy. NGF and to a lesser degree BDNF prevent the loss of cholinergic function seen after axotomy in adult animals. BDNF also supports the survival of dopaminergic neurons dissociated from the rodent mesen-

cephalon as well as of retinal ganglion cells. In the mature nervous system, neurotrophins are involved in the maintenance of neuronal phenotypes; in particular, antibodies to NGF decrease the levels of enzymes synthesizing catecholamines as well as neurotransmitters such as substance P in the peripheral nervous system of adult animals. Neurotrophins also act on some nonneuronal cells, and NT3 in particular contributes to the division and survival of oligodendrocyte precursors. In aged, learning-deficient rats, the intraventricular injection of NGF can reverse the learning deficiencies in simple behavioral tests. Decreased levels of BDNF mRNA have been noted in the hippocampus of patients with Alzheimer's disease.

B. Neurotrophins Cause Programmed Cell Death

Like other receptors belonging to the same family, such as CD95, p75 causes the death of neurons in the developing CNS. This occurs in the developing retina and spinal cord. Also, basal forebrain cholinergic neurons express p75 at high levels, and its complete elimination leads to a long-lasting increase in the number of basal forebrain cholinergic neurons. Cultured oligodendrocytes up-regulate p75 expression and they can be killed by the addition of NGF. NGF is not the only ligand able to activate p75 to cause cell death, and in developing sympathetic ganglia, BDNF also causes cell death through p75.

IV. NEUROTROPHINS AND NEURONAL PLASTICITY

A. Regulation of Process Outgrowth

Beyond their effects on the control of neuronal survival, neurotrophins also have pronounced effects on the size of neurons, on the rate of axonal elongation, and on the growth and branching of dendrites. In adult animals, the administration of NGF causes the length of dendrites of sympathetic neurons to increase. Conversely, antibodies to NGF decrease the length of these dendrites. When such experiments are performed in newborn animals, the increased number of dendrites caused by NGF administration is accompanied by a very large increase in the number of preganglionic axons. In mice carrying a deletion in the pro-apoptotic gene *bax,* the effects of neurotrophins on axonal elongation can be examined in the absence of effects on survival. In such animals, the lack of neurotrophins or of their corresponding Trk receptors causes a dramatic reduction in the number of peripheral axons. Neurotrophins are required for the elongation of peripheral nerves. Indeed, the acute application of a combination of function-blocking monoclonal antibodies causes a marked reduction in the elongation of both sensory and motor nerves. Also, the neurotrophins are able to attract sensory and sympathetic nerves. Similar mechanisms seem to operate in the CNS, as exemplified by work using live tadpoles and slices of the visual cortex. The effects of neurotrophins appear to be complex and different for apical or basal dendrites. The effects are also specific for each neurotrophin tested and the results indicate that each neurotrophin can act to modulate particular patterns of dendritic arborization. The regulation of cortical dendritic growth by neurotrophins requires endogenous electrical activity.

B. Neurotrophins and Synaptic Transmission

Neurotrophins regulate the number of synapses and the efficacy of synaptic transmission. NGF levels modulate both the strength and the number of presynaptic inputs in sympathetic ganglia. In mice overexpressing BDNF in sympathetic neurons, increased numbers of synapses are observed, whereas in *bdnf* − / − animals, a decreased number of synapses are found. Presynaptic alterations and a decreased number of synapses are observed in the absence of TrkB and TrkC receptors.

Neurotrophins rapidly modulate neurotransmission, both in the PNS and in the CNS. Some of these effects occur very rapidly after the application of the neurotrophins. Within milliseconds, BDNF and NT4 cause depolarization and elicit action potentials in pyramidal cells of the hippocampus or cortex and in Purkinje cells of the cerebellum. This depolarization results from an increased conductance for sodium ions, and it is as rapid as that induced by the neurotransmitter glutamate.

BDNF modulates synaptic transmission in the hippocampus, as reflected by its role in long-term potentiation. This has been demonstrated in animals lacking *bdnf*, as well as by the use of specific monoclonal antibodies.

BDNF is not only stored in neurons, it is also released from internal stores by activity-dependent mechanisms. It is present in presynaptic nerve terminals and also in dendrites, where it co-localizes with the postsynaptic markers.

In the visual cortex, neurotrophins are involved in activity-dependent developmental plasticity. Neurotrophins influence the formation of ocular dominance columns in the visual cortex and promote the maturation of cortical inhibition.

C. Neurotrophins and Behavior

Detailed explorations of the heterozygous *trkB* and of conditional mutants reveal that these animals become increasingly impaired over time with regard to their spatial learning behavior, similar to the phenotype in mice with hippocampal lesions. *Bdnf* + / − animals develop an enhanced aggressiveness and hyperphagia, accompanied by weight gain. BDNF is also necessary for canaries to learn new songs. Interestingly, testosterone treatment increases the levels of BDNF in the high vocal center.

Glossary

brain-derived neurotrophic factor Protein purified from pig brain in the 1980s by monitoring its ability to prevent the death of peripheral sensory neurons.

nerve growth factor (NGF) The first neurotrophin to have been identified in the 1950s. It was purified on the basis of its ability to elicit neurite outgrowth from ganglionic explants. The extraordinary and unexplained abundance of NGF in the adult male mouse submandibular gland was a prerequisite for its early characterization.

neurotrophin-3 Identified on the basis of sequence homologies to the previously sequenced proteins nerve growth factor and brain-derived neurotrophic factor.

neurotrophin-4 First identified in *Xenopus laevis* cDNAs and subsequently detected in rodents and humans. Its sequence is more variable between species than the other three neurotrophins. It was initially designated neurotrophin-4 or neurotrophin-5 but it is likely to be the same protein in different species.

p75 A glycoprotein of 75,000 Da that binds all neurotrophins. It was identified in the mid-1980s by expression cloning.

tropomyosin receptor kinases (Trks) A small group of closely related tyrosine kinase membrane receptors that are activated by neurotrophin binding. Trk was first recognized as an oncogene made up of the kinase domain of Trk fused with a portion of *tropomyosin*. The proto-oncogene was later found to be a nerve growth factor receptor.

See Also the Following Articles

Brain-Derived Neurotrophic Factor • **Nerve Growth Factor (NGF)**

Further Reading

Bibel, M., and Barde, Y.-A. (2000). Neurotrophins: Key regulators of cell fate and cell shape in the vertebrate nervous system. *Genes Dev.* 14, 2919–2937.

Bothwell, M. (1995). Functional interactions of neurotrophins and neurotrophin receptors. *Annu. Rev. Neurosci.* 18, 223–253.

Chao, V., and Bothwell, M. (2002). Neurotrophins: To cleave or not to cleave. *Neuron* 33, 9–12.

Davies, A. M. (2000). Neurotrophins: Neurotrophic modulation of neurite growth. *Curr. Biol.* 10, 198–200.

Dobrowsky, R. T., Carter, B. D. p75 neurotrophin receptor signaling: Mechanisms for neurotrophic modulation of cell stress? *J. Neurosci. Res.* 61, 237–243.

Hallböök, F. (1999). Evolution of the vertebrate neurotrophin and Trk receptor gene families. *Curr. Opin. Neurobiol.* 9, 616–621.

Huang, E. J., and Reichardt, L. F. (2001). Neurotrophins: Role in neuronal development and function. *Annu. Rev. Neurosci.* 24, 677–736.

Kaplan, D. R., and Miller, F. D. (2000). Neurotrophin signal transduction in the nervous system. *Curr. Opin. Neurobiol.* 10, 381–391.

McAllister, A. K., Lo, D. C., and Katz, L. C. (2001). Neurotrophins and synaptic plasticity. *Annu. Rev. Neurosci.* 22, 295–318.

Schinder, A. F., and Poo, M. M. (2000). The neurotrophin hypothesis for synaptic plasticity. *Trends Neurosci.* 23, 639–645.

Schuman, E. M. (1999). Neurotrophin regulation of synaptic transmission. *Curr. Opin. Neurobiol.* 9, 105–109.

Sofroniew, M. V., Howe, C. L., and Mobley, W. C. (2001). Nerve growth factor signaling, neuroprotection and neural repair. *Annu. Rev. Neurosci.* 24, 1217–1281.

NGF

See *Nerve Growth Factor*

Nitric Oxide

Derek P. G. Norman[*] and Anthony W. Norman[†]

*Harvard University • †University of California, Riverside

I. INTRODUCTION
II. CHEMISTRY, BIOSYNTHESIS, AND SECRETION
III. BIOLOGICAL ACTIONS OF NO
IV. SUMMARY

Nitric oxide (NO) is one of the body's many hormones. It is unique in that it is the only animal hormone that is a gas. NO, however, is somewhat water soluble and is able to function as a chemical messenger, particularly in cells of the vascular endothelium, immune, and neural systems. Virtually all of the known biological actions of NO on the cardiovascular system are mediated by the activation of a guanylate cyclase, which produces the second messenger cyclic GMP that leads to vasorelaxation (lowered blood pressure).

I. INTRODUCTION

A relatively surprising addition to the family of chemical messengers is nitric oxide (NO). NO is a free radical gas of limited solubility in water. Because NO is noncharged, it can rapidly diffuse across cell membranes and into cells; it has been shown to act as both an intracellular and an intercellular (paracrine) messenger to elicit a wide spectrum of biological responses. A physiological function for NO was first established in the vascular system when the endothelin-derived relaxing factor (EDRF) could be quantitatively explained by the formation of NO. NO is now known to be an integral participant in the signal transduction processes associated with the vascular, immune, and neural systems.

II. CHEMISTRY, BIOSYNTHESIS, AND SECRETION

The formation of NO is an enzyme-mediated reaction (see Fig. 1); the nitrogen donor is the amino acid L-arginine and the oxygen donor is molecular oxygen. The reaction is catalyzed by an NADPH-requiring nitric oxide synthase (NOS). NOS enzymes are structurally related to cytochrome P450 reductase and range in size from 13 to 160 kDa.

NOS exists both as a constitutive enzyme, which is regulated by Ca^{2+} and the calcium-binding protein, calmodulin, and as an inducible enzyme, which is not

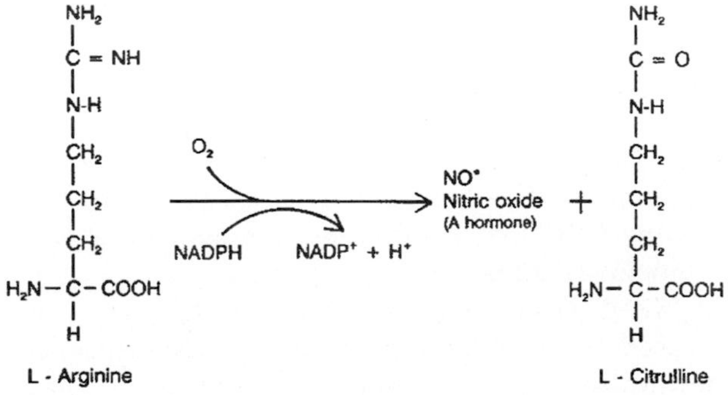

FIGURE 1 Enzymatic reaction catalyzed by nitric oxide synthase (NOS).

regulated by calmodulin. The regulatable forms of NOS are induced by interferon-α (INF-α), tumor necrosis factor-α (TNF-α), interleukin-1β (IL-1β), and estradiol and are inhibited by glucocorticoids. The inducible forms of NOS are associated with components of the host defense immune system.

There is clear evidence that under some physiological circumstances the classical estrogen receptor, when occupied by its cognate hormone, estradiol, can initiate a signal transduction process that activates NOS. One novel aspect of this activation process is that the estrogen receptor for this biological response is localized not in the nucleus but in caveolae found in the cell's plasma membrane. Caveolae and caveolae-related membrane domains are enriched in molecules that play pivotal roles in intracellular signal transduction. In this setting, the steroid hormone estradiol is not working with its receptor to regulate the traditional response of regulation of gene transcription (over hours to days), but is instead generating a rapid response (over seconds to minutes) via a non-nuclear signal transduction process that results in NOS activation. This system of signal transduction has been particularly documented to occur in vascular endothelial cells where estradiol is known to modulate the local cell biology.

III. BIOLOGICAL ACTIONS OF NO

The wide spectrum of biological actions of NO in the cardiovascular, nervous, and host defense systems is summarized in Table 1. Only the actions of NO in the cardiovascular system are discussed in this article.

TABLE I Biological Actions of Nitric Oxide in the Cardiovascular, Nervous and Host Defense Systems

System	Response
Cardiovascular	
Smooth muscle	Initiate vasorelaxation; control of regional blood flow and blood pressure
Platelets	Limitation of aggregation and adhesion
Nervous	
Peripheral	Neurotransmission (penile erection, gastric emptying)
Host defense	
Macrophages	Defense against bacteria, fungi, protozoans, parasites, and viruses
Leukocytes	
Monocytes	

After the generation of NO in the endothelial cell by the NOS enzyme, the NO diffuses to an adjacent smooth muscle where it acts as an agonist to initiate biological responses (see Fig. 2). Virtually all of the known biological actions of NO on the cardiovascular system are mediated by the activation of a soluble guanylate cyclase. The guanylate cyclase has a heme prosthetic group to which NO binds tightly to this moiety. The resulting activation of the guanylate cyclase results in the production of cGMP, which is then postulated to have actions on protein kinases, nucleotide-sensitive phosphodiesterases,

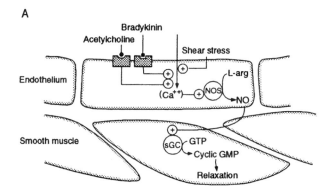

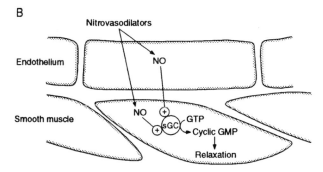

FIGURE 2 Model for the synthesis of NO in endothelial cells and its paracrine actions in smooth muscle cells. In (A), shear stress or receptor activation of vascular endothelium by bradykinin or acetylcholine results in an influx of calcium. The consequent increase in intracellular calcium stimulates the constitutive nitric oxide synthase (NOS). The nitric oxide (NO) formed from L-arginine (L-Arg) by this enzyme diffuses to nearby smooth muscle cells, in which it stimulates the soluble guanylate cyclase (sGC), resulting in enhanced synthesis of cyclic GMP from guanosine triphosphate (GTP). This increase in cyclic GMP in the smooth muscle cells leads to their relaxation. In (B), nitrovasodilators such as sodium nitroprusside and nitroglycerin release NO spontaneously or through an enzymatic reaction. The liberated NO stimulates the soluble guanylate cyclase in the vascular smooth muscle cell, resulting in relaxation. [Adapted from Moncada, C., and Higgs, A. (1993). The L-arginine-nitric oxide pathway, *New Engl. J. Med.* **329**, 2002–2012.]

ion channels, or other unknown cellular proteins that are linked to the generation of the smooth muscle response of vasodilation and also to the inhibition of platelet adhesion and aggregation.

NO is a short-lived agonist in the cellular environment. NO is inactivated either by its chemical linkage to proteins (nitrosylation) or by oxidation to nitrite (NO_2^-) and then nitrate (NO_3^-).

IV. SUMMARY

In the normal physiological state in humans, the distribution, composition, and volume of body fluids are held within relatively narrow limits, despite wide variations in the intake of water and Na^+. Such homeostasis or stability of the internal environment requires a multifactoral collaboration of the hormones and other physiological processes that affect electrolyte and water metabolism. A diverse array of hormones (aldosterone, angiotensin II, rennin, atrial natureatic protein or ANP, NO, endothelin, vasopressin, prostaglandins, and kinins) and signal transduction systems, each responding to different stimuli, is integrated to provide the kidney and cardiovascular system with coherent messages to effect the collective regulation of blood pressure, electrolyte concentration, and water volume.

Glossary

caveolae Sub-domains of the cell's plasma membrane that have a typical flask-like membrane structure where signal transduction molecules may congregate.
endothelium The monolayer of cells lining the inner wall of the vascular system.
estradiol A steroid hormone that belongs to the family of estrogens.
free radical A molecule, usually short-lived and highly reactive, that contains an unpaired electron. All molecules containing an odd number of electrons are free radicals.
nitric oxide A molecule composed of one atom of oxygen and one atom of nitrogen, with the chemical formula NO, which chemically is a free radical. NO is one of the body's many hormones; it is unique in that it is the only animal hormone that is a gas.

See Also the Following Articles

Amino Acid and Nitric Oxide Control of the Anterior Pituitary • Calmodulin • Estrogen Receptor-β Structure and Function

Further Reading

Bogdan, C. (2001). Nitric oxide and the immune response. *Nat. Immunol.* **2**, 907–916.
Chambliss, K. L., Yuhanna, I. S., Anderson, R. G., Mendelsohn, M. E., and Shaul, P. W. (2002). ERb has nongenomic action in caveolae. *Mol. Endocrinol.* **16**, 938–946.
Ignarro, L. J. (1989). Endothelium-derived nitric oxide: Actions and properties. *FASEB J.* **3**, 31–36.
Ignarro, L. J., Buga, G. M., Wood, K. S., Byrns, R. E., and Chaudhuri, G. (1987). Endothelium-derived relaxing factor produced and released from artery and vein is nitric oxide. *Proc. Natl. Acad. Sci. USA* **84**, 9265–9269.
Lala, P. K., and Chakraborty, C. (2001). Role of nitric oxide in carcinogenesis and tumour progression. *Lancet Oncol.* **2**, 149–156.
Liu, L., Hausladen, A., Zeng, M., Que, L., Heitman, J., and Stamler, J. S. (2001). A metabolic enzyme for *S*-nitrosothiol conserved from bacteria to humans. *Nature* **410**, 490–494.
Lowik, C. W., Nibbering, P. H., van de Ruit, M., and Papapoulos, S. E. (1994). Inducible production of nitric oxide in osteoblast-like cells and in fetal mouse bone explants is associated with suppression of osteoclastic bone resorption. *J. Clin. Invest.* **93**, 1465–1472.
Mann, G. E., Yudilevich, D. L., and Sobrevia, L. (2003). Regulation of amino acid and glucose transporters in endothelial and smooth muscle cells. *Physiol. Rev.* **83**, 183–252.
McMahon, T. J., Moon, R. E., Luschinger, B. P., Carraway, M. S., Stone, A. E., Stolp, B. W., Gow, A. J., Pawloski, J. R., Watke, P., Singel, D. J., Piantadosi, C. A., and Stamler, J. S. (2002). Nitric oxide in the human respiratory cycle. *Nat. Med.* **8**, 711–717.
Palmer, R. M., Ferrige, A. G., and Moncada, S. (1987). Nitric oxide release accounts for the biological activity of endothelium-derived relaxing factor. *Nature* **327**, 524–526.
Schini, V. B., Durante, W., Elizondo, E., Scott-Burden, T., Junquero, D. C., Schafer, A. I., and Vanhoutte, P. M. (1992). The induction of nitric oxide synthase activity is inhibited by TGF-beta 1, PDGFAB and PDGFBB in vascular smooth muscle cells. *Eur. J. Pharmacol.* **216**, 379–383.
Stamler, J. S., Lamas, S., and Fang, F. C. (2001). Nitrosylation: The prototypic redox-based signaling mechanism. *Cell* **106**, 675–683.
Stamler, J. S., Singel, D. J., and Loscalzo, J. (1992). Biochemistry of nitric oxide and its redox-activated forms. *Science* **258**, 1898–1902.
Wyckoff, M. H., Chambliss, K. L., Mineo, C., Yuhanna, I. S., Mendelsohn, M. E., Mumby, S. M., and Shaul, P. W. (2001). Plasma membrane estrogen receptors are coupled to endothelial nitric-oxide synthase through Gai. *J. Biol. Chem.* **276**, 27071–27076.

Non-Insulin-Dependent Diabetes Mellitus

See *Diabetes Type 2*

Oncostatin M

MINORU TANAKA AND ATSUSHI MIYAJIMA
University of Tokyo

Oncostatin M (OSM) is a soluble 28 kDa glycoprotein that belongs to the interleukin-6 cytokine family. OSM acts on many types of cells *in vitro* and *in vivo* and functions in diverse biological processes, such as growth regulation, differentiation, gene expression, and cell survival.

I. INTRODUCTION

Cytokines are subdivided into several families based on their biological and structural properties, as well as their receptor components. Oncostatin M (OSM) is a multifunctional cytokine and belongs to the interleukin-6 (IL-6) subfamily that includes IL-6, IL-11, leukemia inhibitory factor (LIF), ciliary neurotropic factor (CNTF), cardiotropin-1, and novel neutrophin-1/B-cell-stimulating factor-3. Among these family members, OSM is the most closely related to LIF structurally, genetically, and functionally. In humans, these two cytokines act on a wide variety of cells and elicit diverse, overlapping biological responses, such as growth regulation, differentiation, gene expression, and cell survival, whereas OSM also exhibits unique activities that are not shared with LIF.

II. BIOCHEMICAL AND GENETIC PROFILE OF OSM

OSM was initially recognized for its ability to inhibit the proliferation of the A375 melanoma cell line as well as numerous other tumor cells. OSM is a secreted 28 kDa glycoprotein originally isolated from phorbol ester-stimulated human histiocytic lymphoma U937 cells. OSM forms a secondary structure with a four-α-helix-bundle motif, characteristic of this cytokine family. OSM is secreted from activated T cells and monocytes. The human OSM (hOSM) gene encodes the precursor polypeptide of 252 amino acid residues, which becomes the mature 196-amino-acid form by removal of the 25-amino-acid N-terminal signal sequence and the 31-amino-acid C-terminal region. On the other hand, mouse OSM (mOSM) was identified as an immediate-early gene induced by IL-2, IL-3, and erythropoietin (EPO) through the Janus kinase/signal transducer and activator of transcription 5 (JAK/STAT5) pathway. OSM mRNA is abundant in hematopoietic tissues, such as bone marrow, thymus, and spleen. The hOSM gene is located on human chromosome 22q12, and the mOSM gene is on mouse chromosome 11. Among the members of the IL-6 cytokine subfamily, not only are OSM and LIF structurally related, their genes are tightly linked in the same chromosomal location, suggesting that the two genes arose by duplication.

III. BIOLOGICAL ACTIVITIES OF OSM (I)

OSM exhibits diverse biological activities on a wide variety of cells *in vitro* and *in vivo*. OSM modulates the growth of tumor and nontumor cells. OSM inhibits the growth of several types of cells, such as solid tissue tumor cells, melanoma cells, and glioma cells. Moreover, OSM induces the differentiation as well as the growth inhibition of several cell types. hOSM is a differentiation factor of the myeloid leukemia cell line M1, and it inhibits the differentiation of mouse embryonic stem cells. mOSM induces the differentiation of fetal hepatocytes in an *in vitro* culture system, e.g., expression of the differentiation marker gene, accumulation of glycogen and lipids, and morphological changes. OSM stimulates the proliferation of fibroblasts, endothelial cells, and plasmacytoma cells and also stimulates DNA synthesis of rabbit vascular smooth muscle cells. In addition, OSM is an autocrine growth factor for acquired immune deficiency syndrome-related Kaposi's sarcoma cells. mOSM stimulates the growth of endothelial-like cells in the primary culture of aorta–gonad–mesonephros cells derived from fetal mouse and stimulates the development of definitive hematopoiesis. OSM is also known to be involved in the modulation of expression of various genes, e.g., up-regulation of the low-density lipoprotein receptor on the cells of the hepatoma cell line HepG2, expression of the plasminogen activator in fibroblasts and endothelial cells, production of endothelin-1 and basic fibroblast growth factor in human umbilical vein endothelial cells, and expression of granulocyte colony-stimulating factor and granulocyte/macrophage colony-stimulating factor in human endothelial cells. On the other hand, OSM has been reported to down-regulate the expression of cytochrome P450 in human hepatocytes.

IV. BIOLOGICAL ACTIVITIES OF OSM (II)

OSM is secreted from activated T cells and monocytes stimulated by cytokines, T-cell activators, and phorbol 12-myristate 13-acetate (PMA) and plays roles in several inflammatory reactions. OSM increases the secretion of acute-phase proteins (APPs), such as haptoglobin, α1-antichymotrypsin, and fibrinogen, in liver cells at the early phase of inflammation. In the inflammatory process, the remodeling of the extracellular matrix is important for healing the damaged tissue induced by inflammatory responses. Matrix metalloproteinases (MMPs) are involved in extracellular matrix breakdown, and tissue inhibitors of metalloproteinases (TIMPs) inhibit the action of MMPs. Therefore, the balance between TIMPs and MMPs is important for the remodeling of the extracellular matrix. OSM induces TIMP-1 expression and inhibits IL-1β-induced TIMP-3 in cultured human synovial-lining cells. OSM induces the expression of MMP-1 and MMP-3 in astrocytes and of MMP-1 and MMP-9 in fibroblasts. Thus, OSM may be involved in wound healing by modulating the balance between TIMPs and MMPs. It is also known that another family member, IL-6, strongly affects inflammatory reactions. In fact, IL-6-deficient mice exhibit the reduced production of APPs and the delayed repair of the liver injury induced by carbon tetrachloride. Since OSM induces the IL-6 receptor in human hepatoma HepG2 cells and stimulates the production of IL-6 in cultured human endothelial cells, OSM affects inflammation not only directly, but also indirectly through the induction of other members of this family.

V. STRUCTURE OF THE OSM RECEPTOR

It is known that different cytokines exhibit similar biological activities on the same cell type (functional redundancy). The functional redundancy among the cytokines of the IL-6 family is now well explained by their receptor structure. Functional receptors for this family of cytokines consist of multiple subunits including the common signal transducing subunit, gp130 (Fig. 1). The receptor complexes for IL-6 and IL-11 consist of a ligand-specific α receptor subunit and gp130. The binding of each cytokine to its specific α-subunit induces the dimerization of gp130. The LIF receptor consists of the low-affinity LIF-binding protein (LIFRβ) and gp130. LIF binding leads to heterodimerization of LIFRβ and gp130. The CNTF receptor is composed of the CNTF-specific α-subunit, LIFRβ, and gp130. Although OSM is a cytokine that binds with low affinity to gp130 directly, it is not enough to transduce its signals. In human, two types of functional OSM receptor are known: the type I OSM receptor is identical to the high-affinity LIF receptor that consists of gp130 and LIFRβ, and the type II OSM receptor consists of gp130 and the OSM-specific receptor β-subunit (OSMRβ). OSMRβ is expressed in a wide variety of cell types, including endothelial cells, hepatic cells, lung cells, skin cells, and many tumor cell lines. Although LIF and OSM share a number of biological functions in common, it is also known that OSM displays some specific biological properties that are not shared by LIF, e.g., growth inhibition of A375 melanoma cells and up-regulation of α1-proteinase inhibitor in lung-derived epithelial cells. Thus, many overlapping biological responses between hOSM and hLIF are mediated by the shared type I receptor, i.e., the LIF receptor, whereas OSM manifests its specific responses through the type II receptor. However, this is not the case for mOSM. Immediately after the isolation of the mOSM cDNA, it was recognized that there are some differences in biological activity between human and murine OSM. For example, it was shown that a more than 30-fold higher concentration of mOSM is required for the growth inhibition of M1 cells compared with hOSM. Likewise, mOSM is much less potent than hOSM in the inhibition of differentiation of mouse embryonic stem (ES) cells. Molecular cloning of mouse OSMRβ cDNA and reconstitution of the high-affinity functional OSM receptor revealed that mOSM transduces signals only through its specific receptor complex composed of gp130 and OSMRβ, but not through the LIF receptor (Fig. 2). Interestingly, hOSM binds to the mouse LIF receptor and transduces signals; however, it fails to transduce signals through the mouse OSM receptor. Thus, the biological functions of hOSM observed in mouse cells are likely to represent mouse LIF functions.

VI. SIGNAL TRANSDUCTION PATHWAY

Cytokines bind to their receptors on the target cells and then initiate various downstream signaling cascades (Fig. 3). The IL-6 family cytokine receptors

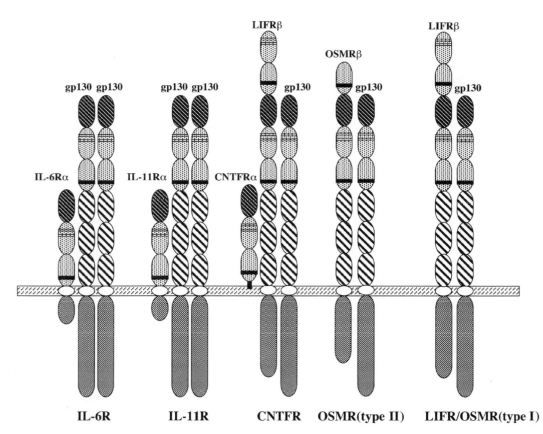

FIGURE 1 Composition of the IL-6 family cytokine receptor complex. IgG-like domains and fibronectin type III-like domains are shown as dark gray and diagonally striped symbols, respectively. The light gray area shows a cytokine-binding module containing the conserved cysteine residues (thin horizontal lines) and WS motifs (thick horizontal lines).

do not possess an intrinsic tyrosine kinase but utilize JAKs/STATs as major mediators of their signals. The first step in receptor activation is the ligand-induced homo- or heterodimerization of signal-transducing receptor subunits. As each signal-transducing receptor subunit binds one JAK (JAK1, JAK2, and Tyk2), dimerization of the subunits leads to the reciprocal phosphorylation and activation of JAKs. The activated JAKs phosphorylate tyrosine residues in the intracellular domain of the receptor, creating docking sites for STATs as well as various signaling molecules with an SRC homology 2 (SH2) domain. These molecules that are recruited to the receptors are then activated by JAKs. Phosphorylated STATs (STAT1, STAT3, and STAT5) then form homo- or hetero-dimers and translocate to the nucleus, where they are involved in gene regulation. A difference in signal transduction between type I and type II OSM receptors has also been reported. STAT5b is pre-dominantly activated by the OSM-specific type II receptor in the A375 cell line. The IL-6-type cytokines stimulate not only the JAK/STAT signaling pathway

but also the Ras/Raf/mitogen-activated protein kinase signaling pathway. It is known that several adapter molecules, such as SHP-2 (SH2 domain-containing protein tyrosine phosphatose 2), Grb2 (growth factor receptor-bound protein 2), and Gab1 (Grb2-associated binder-1), are involved in this pathway. Thus, OSM regulates complex biological responses, such as cell growth, differentiation, and apoptosis, through these signaling pathways.

VII. SUMMARY

OSM is a member of the IL-6 cytokine family. Of all the members of this family, OSM is most closely related to LIF structurally and functionally. In addition, the genes for OSM and LIF are closely linked on the same chromosome. It is also known that the genes for their receptor β-subunits are present in close proximity on mouse chromosome 15. Co-localization of the OSMRβ and LIFRβ genes as well as OSM and LIF genes strongly suggests that they were created by duplication during evolution.

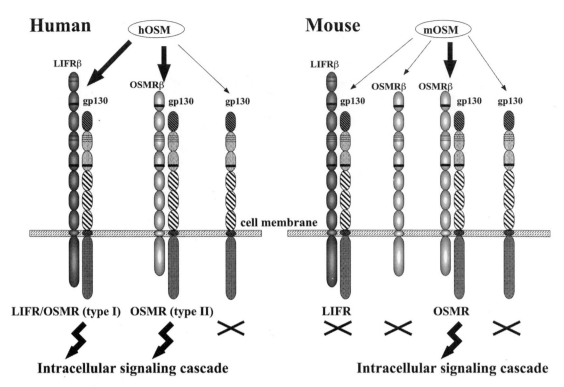

FIGURE 2 Formation of the functional receptor complexes for hOSM and mOSM. Thin arrows show low-affinity binding of OSM to each receptor component and thin arrows indicate high-affinity binding. Broken arrows indicate the relay of the intracellular signaling cascade. X, no signaling.

Since hOSM and hLIF showed various common biological activities, OSM has been thought to be the second LIF. However, hOSM also exhibits unique activities including growth inhibition of A375 melanoma cells, growth stimulation of Kaposi's sarcoma, and induction of TIMP-1 in fibroblasts. Molecular cloning of the hOSM receptor subunit and reconstitution of the functional hOSM receptor indicated that there are two types of functional receptor for hOSM. Although the type I OSM receptor is identical to the high-affinity LIF receptor and shares signaling pathways with LIF, the type II OSM receptor is utilized for OSM-specific signaling. The existence of two functional OSM receptors provides a molecular basis for the biological activities shared in common between LIF and OSM as well as for OSM-specific activities. It should be noted that mOSM uses only the OSM-specific receptor but not the LIF receptor.

Glossary

interleukin-6 A pleiotropic cytokine that acts on a wide variety of cells and exhibits many biological activities, e.g., the induction of B-cell differentiation to antibody-forming plasma cells, differentiation of myeloid leukemic cell lines into macrophages, megakaryocyte matu-

ration, acute-phase protein synthesis in hepatocytes, and development of osteoclasts.

Janus kinases (JAKs) Intracellular tyrosine kinases with molecular masses of 120–140 kDa that bind to cytokine receptors. A typical kinase domain is located at the C-terminus, preceded by a kinase-like domain. Four JAKs (JAK1, JAK2, JAK3, and Tyk2) have been identified.

leukemia inhibitory factor A pleiotropic cytokine that was originally identified as a factor that inhibits leukemic cells and exhibits many biological activities, e.g., induction of monocytic differentiation of the murine leukemic cell line M1, suppression of differentiation of pluripotent embryonic stem cells, and inhibition of adipogenesis.

signal transducers and activators of transcription (STATs) A family of latent cytoplasmic transcription factors with an SH2 domain, members of which are activated by cytokines and translocate to the nucleus to participate in gene expression. Seven mammalian STAT genes (STAT1, 2, 3, 4, 5a, 5b, and 6) have been identified.

tissue inhibitors of metalloproteinases Specific inhibitors of matrix metalloproteinases, a family of enzymes that are responsible for the degradation of collagens, proteoglycans, and glycoproteins of the extracellular matrix.

See Also the Following Articles

Interleukin-6 • Leukemia Inhibitory Factor (LIF)

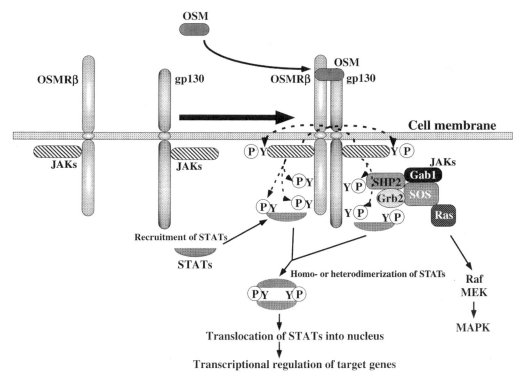

FIGURE 3 Signal transduction pathways of OSM. Binding of OSM to the receptor components induces heterodimerization of the subunits, leading to the reciprocal phosphorylation and activation of JAKs. The activated JAKs phosphorylate the tyrosine residues of the receptor subunits, creating distinct binding sites for STATs and SHP2. The STATs recruited to the receptor are phosphorylated by JAKs, and homo- or heterodimerized STATs are translocated to the nucleus, where they regulate the transcription of target genes. The SHP2 recruitment is required for the mitogen-activated protein kinase (MAPK) pathway. Encircled P, phosphorylation; MEK, MAPK kinase; SOS, son of sevenless; Y, tyrosine residue.

Further Reading

Auguste, P., Guillet, C., Fourcin, M., Olivier, C., Veziers, J., Pouplard-Barthelaix, A., and Gascan, H. (1997). Signaling of type II oncostatin M receptor. *J. Biol. Chem.* **272**, 15760–15764.

Gatsios, P., Haubeck, H. D., Van De Leur, E., Frisch, W., Apte, S. S., Greiling, H., Heinrich, P. C., and Graeve, L. (1996). Oncostatin M differentially regulates tissue inhibitors of metalloproteinases TIMP-1 and TIMP-3 gene expression in human synovial lining cells. *Eur. J. Biochem.* **241**, 56–63.

Gomez-Lechon, M. J. (1999). Oncostatin M: Signal transduction and biological activity. *Life Sci.* **65**, 2019–2030.

Heinrich, P. C., Behrmann, I., Muller-Newen, G., Schaper, F., and Graeve, L. (1998). Interleukin-6-type cytokine signalling through the gp130/Jak/STAT pathway. *Biochem. J.* **334**, 297–314.

Hirano, T., Ishihara, K., and Hibi, M. (2000). Roles of STAT3 in mediating the cell growth, differentiation and survival signals relayed through the IL-6 family of cytokine receptors. *Oncogene* **19**, 2548–2556.

Ichihara, M., Hara, T., Kim, H., Murate, T., and Miyajima, A. (1997). Oncostatin M and leukemia inhibitory factor do not use the same functional receptor in mice. *Blood* **90**, 165–173.

Kortylewski, M., Heinrich, P. C., Mackiewicz, A., Schniertshauer, U., Klingmuller, U., Nakajima, K., Hirano, T., Horn, F., and Behrmann, I. (1999). Interleukin-6 and oncostatin M-induced growth inhibition of human A375 melanoma cells is STAT-dependent and involves upregulation of the cyclin-dependent kinase inhibitor p27/Kip1. *Oncogene* **18**, 3742–3753.

Lindberg, R. A., Juan, T. S., Welcher, A. A., Sun, Y., Cupples, R., Guthrie, B., and Fletcher, F. A. (1998). Cloning and characterization of a specific receptor for mouse oncostatin M. *Mol. Cell. Biol.* **18**, 3357–3367.

Miyajima, A., Kinoshita, T., Tanaka, M., Kamiya, A., Mukouyama, Y., and Hara, T. (2000). Role of oncostatin M in hematopoicsis and liver development. *Cytokine Growth Factor Rev.* **11**, 177–183.

Takahashi-Tezuka, M., Yoshida, Y., Fukada, T., Ohtani, T., Yamanaka, Y., Nishida, K., Nakajima, K., Hibi, M., and Hirano, T. (1998). Gab1 acts as an adapter molecule linking the cytokine receptor gp130 to ERK mitogen-activated protein kinase. *Mol. Cell. Biol.* **18**, 4109–4117.

Tanaka, M., Hara, T., Copeland, N. G., Gilbert, D. J., Jenkins, N. A., and Miyajima, A. (1999). Reconstitution of the functional mouse oncostatin M (OSM) receptor: Molecular cloning of the mouse OSM receptor β subunit. *Blood* **93**, 804–815.

Oocyte Development and Maturation

KATHLEEN H. BURNS AND MARTIN M. MATZUK

Baylor College of Medicine

Female gametogenesis begins in embryonic life, and important events both preceding and following sexual maturity mediate follicular development and the acquisition of oocyte competence. This article will examine aspects of these processes with an emphasis on transgenic mouse models that have shed light on the molecular bases of ovarian function and failure.

I. PRIMORDIAL GERM CELL DIFFERENTIATION AND MIGRATION

Primordial germ cell (PGC) precursors of oocytes are first discernible by alkaline phosphatase staining in the developing female mouse at embryonic day 6.5 (E6.5) when they are located in the extraembryonic mesoderm. From E7.5 to E13.5, these cells migrate along the allantois to the embryonic hindgut and then caudally across the dorsal mesentery to the left and right genital ridges. Throughout their migration, PGCs undergo mitotic divisions to give rise to the full complement of gametes to be allocated over the individual's reproductive lifespan. Mitotic divisions are completed between E12.5 and E13.5 in the mouse, and the germ cells synchronously arrest in the dictyate stage of prophase I of meiosis (Fig. 1). Complex paracrine signaling involving neighboring somatic cells and components of the extracellular matrix is necessary for PGC migration and proliferation, and several mouse models have demonstrated the roles of particular factors in these pathways.

Several growth factors are critical in specifying PGC fate during female reproductive tract development. One of the most well-researched is stem cell factor (kit ligand), which is elaborated by cells along the PGC migration route and binds to KIT, a tyrosine kinase receptor expressed by the germ cells.

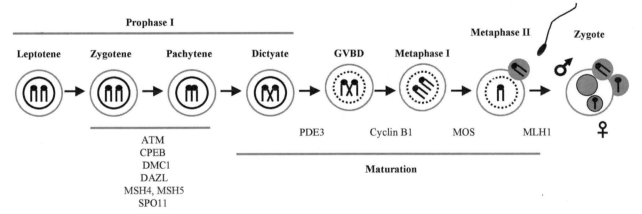

FIGURE 1 Stages of oocyte development and maturation. Oocytes undergo the first stages of prophase I of meiosis during embryonic development. During the leptotene stage, sister chromatids condense and are associated with one another by axial element proteins. Homologous chromosome synapsis and crossover events are mediated during the zygotene and pachytene stages. During the dictyate stage, which is established during the perinatal period, homologous pairs begin to separate, and points of crossover can be appreciated. It is at this stage that oocyte development arrests until ovulation. After the LH surge and immediately prior to cumulus–oocyte complex release, meiosis I proceeds with the dissolution of the nuclear membrane; this is termed germinal vesicle breakdown. The completion of meiosis I is marked by the separation of the first polar body and meiosis is arrested at metaphase II until fertilization. After fertilization, meiosis II is completed, the second polar body is formed, and male and female pronuclei undergo restructuring. Factors that mediate steps in oocyte development and maturation as demonstrated *in vivo* by mouse models are shown.

Mutations affecting the kit ligand (*Kitl*) and *Kit* loci in Steel (*sl*) and white spotting (*w*) mouse models, respectively, cause failures in the proliferation, survival, and migration of the PGCs. Similarly, signaling pathways elicited by members of the transforming growth factor-β (TGF-β) superfamily are necessary for PGC development and have been implicated in PGC migration and in the control of PGC proliferation. Knockout mouse models with mutations in bone morphogenetic protein 4 (*Bmp4*), *Bmp8b*, *Smad1*, or *Smad5* exhibit complete or nearly complete loss of the PGC population. More recently, double-mutant studies generating *Bmp2* $^{+/-}$, *Bmp4* $^{+/-}$ double heterozygotes have revealed co-operative functions of these related proteins in PGC development. Thus, multiple TGF-β superfamily ligands (i.e., BMP-2, BMP-4, and BMP-8B) signaling through the intracellular proteins SMAD1 and SMAD5 play key roles in PGC development.

In addition to soluble growth factors and the intracellular signaling proteins that mediate their response pathways, structural proteins that form contacts between cells and from cells to the extra-cellular matrix are important in PGC development. Knockout mice lacking the gap junction protein connexin 43 demonstrate decreased numbers of PGCs as early as E11.5. In contrast, integrin β1$^{-/-}$ chimeras demonstrate that integrin β1 is dispensable for early PGC differentiation but is essential for their migration to the putative gonad.

Germ cell-deficient (*gcd*) and atrichosis (*at*) mutant models exhibit early embryonic loss of PGCs, though the molecular causes underlying these defects are as yet unknown. Identification of the genes disrupted in *gcd* and *at* mutant mice will further elucidate the proteins required for PGC development and function.

II. PRIMORDIAL FOLLICLE ORGANIZATION AND FOLLICULOGENESIS

Single layers of squamous granulosa cells surround oocytes during the perinatal period, and complex bidirectional communications established at this time between oocytes and these somatic cells function during all stages of follicle development and are crucial for female fertility. It is clear that signals from oocytes participate in the assembly of primordial follicles in the newborn ovary as knockout mice that lack factor in the germ line α (FIGα), an oocyte-specific helix loop helix transcription factor, fail to form primordial follicles and lose their oocytes within the first days of life. This suggests that FIGα regulates one or more factors that are critical for either the recruitment of granulosa cells to the oocyte or the adherence of these granulosa cells to the oocyte.

Recruitment of primordial follicles to initiate folliculogenesis is marked morphologically by oocyte and granulosa cell growth, and stages of subsequent follicular development are characterized by granulosa cell proliferation (see Fig. 2). Factors required for the initial recruitment of primordial follicles to form primary (one-layer) follicles are unknown. Oocyte–granulosa cell interaction is crucial to preantral

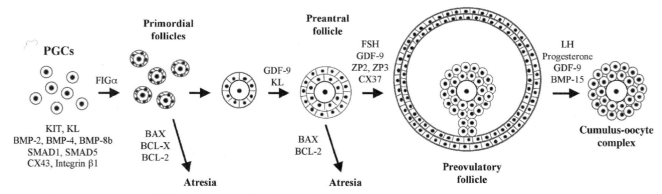

FIGURE 2 Stages of folliculogenesis and its key regulatory proteins. Primordial germ cells proliferate and migrate to the putative gonad during embryonic development and organize granulosa cells to form primordial follicles within a few days after birth in the mouse. Primordial follicles that are not lost to attrition are available to be recruited to the growing pool of follicles, first evidenced by a change in the shape of the granulosa cells from squamous to cuboidal. The mechanisms that regulate the measured recruitment of follicles over a female's reproductive lifespan are as yet unknown. Granulosa cells proliferate during the ensuing stages of folliculogenesis, and large antral preovulatory follicles develop in response to endocrine factors. At ovulation, cumulus–oocyte complexes are released from these dominant follicles, and the remnant cells undergo luteinization. Some of the factors that mediate steps in follicular development as demonstrated by phenotypes of mouse models are shown.

follicle development beyond the primary follicle stage. Growth differentiation factor-9 (GDF-9), a TGF-β superfamily member secreted by oocytes, kit ligand, which is derived from granulosa cells, and kit receptor, expressed on the oocyte surface, are key signaling proteins in these reciprocal interactions. Mice homozygous for a null allele at the *Gdf9* locus or for a hypomorphic *Kitl* allele exhibit female infertility due to blocks in follicular development before the formation of secondary follicles that contain two layers of granulosa cells.

Multilayered follicles become subject to regulation by extraovarian factors, namely, the gonadotropin hormones, and require follicle-stimulating hormone to achieve a crescendo of granulosa cell proliferation and become large antral preovulatory follicles. It is now appreciated that oocyte-derived factors influence granulosa cell proliferation and establish during these later stages of folliculogenesis characteristics unique to the cumulus granulosa cell population (i.e., the granulosa cells closest to the oocyte in the antral follicle as opposed to the mural granulosa cells closest to the follicle wall). For example, GDF-9 has been shown to: (1) stimulate the formation of the cumulus–oocyte complex (COC) by inducing hyaluronan synthase 2 and suppressing urokinase plasminogen activator; (2) promote both the elaboration and the response to prostaglandins in preovulatory granulosa cells, which in turn up-regulate progesterone production during ovulation; and (3) suppress the luteinization of cumulus granulosa cells by inhibiting the production of luteinizing hormone receptor. A related TGF-β superfamily protein, BMP-15, is also expressed in oocytes throughout most stages of follicular development and through ovulation and functions in a cooperative manner with GDF-9 to maintain the integrity of the COC and maximize female fertility in mice. Interestingly, the sheep orthologue of BMP-15, like mouse GDF-9, is crucial for early stages of follicular development and may also affect later events of follicle growth and ovulation. Point mutations occurring in the *BMP15* coding sequence in *Inverdale* (*FecX*[I] mutation) and *Hanna* (*FecX*[H] mutation) sheep cause defects beyond the primary follicle stage and infertility in homozygote ewes, but enhance ovulation in heterozygotes. Thus, the presence of the mutant BMP-15 in heterozygote sheep may interfere with or promote GDF-9 and/or BMP-15 homodimerizations or heterodimerizations or the interactions of these ligands with their receptors.

In addition to growth factors such as GDF-9 and BMP-15, oocytes produce and extrude structural proteins during follicular development that form their encasing zona pellucida matrix. Knockout mice lacking zona pellucida protein 3 (ZP3) or ZP2 demonstrate defects in early antral and preovulatory follicle development, respectively. Disrupted cumulus–oocyte complex formation and decreased ovulation in response to gonadotropins also contribute to both the infertility of the *Zp3* knockout and the subfertility of the *Zp2* knockout. Interestingly, blastocysts derived from *in vitro* maturation and fertilization of eggs from $Zp2^{-/-}$ and $Zp3^{-/-}$ females are not capable of completing development after transfer to pseudo-pregnant recipients. This suggests that zona matrix proteins are important in mediating granulosa cell signals to oocytes that optimize their later developmental potential. Interestingly, *Zp1* knockout females exhibit a more subtle subfertility phenotype, the first discernible compromise being a premature loss of zona integrity that affects early embryogenesis.

III. CONTROL OF EARLY MEIOSIS AND APOPTOSIS IN OOCYTES

Mitotic divisions during PGC migration give rise to a complement of approximately 26,000 germ cells in the female mouse, and the size of this pool and the rate of its depletion are key determinants of the duration of reproductive potential. In addition to interactions with somatic cells during PGC migration and follicular organization, several factors intrinsic to the germ cells have proved critical to germ cell survival, including proteins involved in the control of early meiosis and apoptosis programs.

Several events of meiosis I precede the dictyate-stage block, which persists until ovulation. Replicated sister chromatids connected by axial elements condense and synapse with their homologous chromosomes by the pachytene stage; the maintenance of dictyate germ cells depends on cross-over exchanges that then occur between homologous chromosomes. Several proteins are known to play key roles between the zygotene and pachytene stages (Fig. 1). Chromosome condensation and the formation of synaptonemal complexes are blocked in knockout mice lacking ATM kinase or the DMC1 recombination protein, and in both of these models, female germ cells degenerate during embryogenesis. Translational control of synaptonemal complex proteins and perhaps other participants in early meiosis is exercised at this stage; knockout mice lacking CPEB or DAZL RNA-binding proteins have defects evident at the pachytene stage. Mismatch repair proteins encoded by the *Msh4* and *Msh5* loci are also critical for synapsis, and germ cells in these knockout mice have defects in the zygotene/pachytene stage and are lost within a few days postpartum. Similarly, oocytes in *Spo11* knockout mice, which lack an endonuclease that initiates recombination, die in the perinatal ovary. Thus, meiosis prior to the prophase I block requires the cooperative function of many factors and represents a period in oocyte development that is closely "monitored" to prevent the progression of abnormal gametes.

Functional antagonism between BAX and the anti-apoptotic factors BCL-X and BCL-2 regulates programmed cell death in oocytes. After the completion of PGC mitosis, apoptosis is key in controlling the size of the germ cell reserve during perinatal oocyte attrition and postnatally during follicular atresia in response to gonadotropin deprivation and environmental toxins. *Bax* knockout females have a reduction in postnatal loss of primordial and primary follicles, a threefold increase in the number of primordial follicles at sexual maturity, and an extended lifespan of ovarian function. Although late embryonic and perinatal oocyte loss is not measurably inhibited in the single knockouts, BAX is expressed in embryonic PGCs and has been implicated in the loss of PGCs in BCL-X hypomorphic mouse embryos. Like BCL-X, BCL-2 counters early oocyte apoptotic pathways; *Bcl2* knockout mice establish fewer primordial follicles, and many of these follicles are devoid of oocytes owing to germ cell degeneration. Conversely, oocyte expression of a *Bcl2* transgene increases the number of nonatretic maturing follicles, decreases follicular atresia and spontaneous oocyte loss, and suppresses oocyte apoptosis induced by doxorubicin. Thus, both loss-of-function and gain-of-function transgenic models have illustrated important *in vivo* roles for these apoptotic regulators in controlling the size of the finite oocyte pool after the completion of germ cell mitosis in embryogenesis and throughout the lifespan of ovarian function.

IV. ACQUISITION OF MEIOTIC COMPETENCE AND COMPLETION OF OOCYTE MATURATION

In the periovulatory period, oocytes acquire competence to resume meiosis if separated from their surrounding granulosa cells, which normally control the prophase I block release. Coincident with the rise in serum luteinizing hormone (LH) and ovulation, oocytes from preovulatory follicles complete maturation; they undergo germinal vesicle breakdown, complete the reductional meiotic division, extrude the first polar body, and proceed to an arrest in metaphase of meiosis II.

Signals from the cumulus granulosa cells are critical to this progression. Defects in meiotic maturation are evident in oocytes from *Gja4* knockout mice lacking gap junction protein connexin 37, as well as in oocytes from connexin 43 knockout ovaries grafted into recipient mice to allow for follicular development. It is not clear from these models whether the meiotic phenotype reflects specific functions of these pores in discrete stages of oocyte maturation or whether the defects arise because normal intercellular communications within the follicle are never established. It has been speculated that gap junctions serve as a conduit for granulosa cell-to-oocyte movement of cyclic AMP (cAMP) prior to the LH surge, with oocyte cAMP being important in maintaining meiotic arrest. Consistent with this model, the LH surge induces connexin 43 phosphorylation changes, clearance of connexin 43 protein, and down-regulation of the connexin 43 mRNA. Paralleling these changes, decreases in oocyte cAMP levels, dependent on the activity of oocyte phosphodiesterase PDE3, allow for the resumption of meiosis. In addition to inhibiting oocyte maturation via cAMP, cumulus granulosa cells may provide stimulatory signals that promote meiotic progression. It has been hypothesized that granulosa cell-derived Ca^{2+} and a lipophilic sterol (4,4-dimethyl-5α-cholesta-8,14,24-triene-3β-ol; meiosis-activating sterol) function in promoting meiotic resumption in response to the gonadotropin hormones. Investigating how these and other signals are transmitted to the oocyte and coordinate the regulation of meiosis in response to the hormonal environment *in vivo* represents an exciting field of ongoing research (see Fig. 3).

Oocyte factors are also important regulators in directing the completion of meiosis. Female knockouts lacking the endothelial isoform of nitric oxide synthase, expressed on the surface of oocytes, show compromised ovulation, delayed meiotic progression from metaphase I, and subfertility. The mechanism by which nitric oxide interfaces with the cell cycle machinery directing the metaphase I exit is not known, though mouse models have identified some factors relevant to metaphase transitions during mammalian oogenesis. For example, B-type cyclin proteins have been implicated in directing the commitment to complete both metaphase I and metaphase II as regulatory components of the maturation-promoting

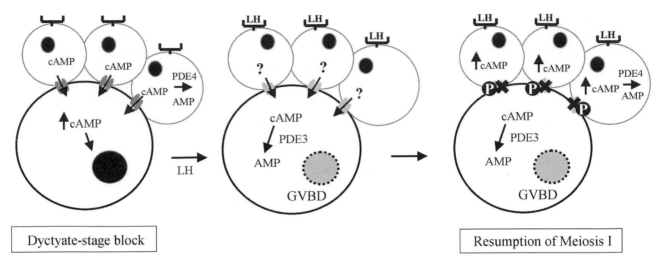

FIGURE 3 A hypothetical model for the resumption of meiosis I. Prior to the preovulatory surge of LH, oocytes are maintained in a prophase I dictyate-stage block, in part by inhibitory signals from the surrounding granulosa cell compartment. It has been proposed that cAMP produced in the granulosa cells is communicated to the oocyte to maintain the dictyate nucleus and prevent germinal vesicle breakdown. The LH surge produces an increase in granulosa cell cAMP, which may affect the phosphorylation, closure, and clearance of gap junction channels by protein kinase cascades. This can be re-created by pharmacologically inhibiting granulosa cell phosphodiesterase (PDE4) activity, which promotes the resumption of meiosis in the absence of LH. It has been postulated that, prior to gap junction closure, a positive effector of meiosis (Ca^{2+} or inositol 1,4,5-trisphosphate) is communicated to the oocyte, where it up-regulates phosphodiesterase enzyme (PDE3) and may mediate other intracellular events that promote oocyte maturation. The gap junction closure effectively isolates the oocyte as a compartment unto itself for the regulation of cAMP metabolism. The subsequent reduction in oocyte cAMP levels is a prerequisite for germinal vesicle breakdown and the release of the dictyate-stage block. Interfering with oocyte PDE3 blocks maturation even in the presence of LH and presumably an intact granulosa cell LHR response. *In vitro* studies have implicated PKA and PKC pathways as downstream mediators of cAMP effects in both the granulosa cells (releasing the meiotic block) and the oocyte (maintaining the meiotic block).

factor complex. B-type cyclin levels increase before each meiotic metaphase, and their ubiquitin-mediated degradation coincides with the metaphase–anaphase transition. Cyclin B1 is expressed in oocytes in this pattern and injection of cyclin B1 antisense mRNA causes defects during the completion of meiosis I and in the onset of metaphase II. Embryonic lethality in cyclin B1 knockout mice has thus far precluded *in vivo* studies of this protein's function in oocytes. Cyclin $B2^{-/-}$ females exhibit a subfertile phenotype, which has not yet been further characterized but may further establish the importance of this cyclin in mouse oogenesis.

The establishment of the block at metaphase II is important biologically to preclude parthenogenic activation of oocytes. This is compromised in *Mos* knockout mice lacking the oocyte-expressed MOS kinase, which is a component of the cytostatic factor complex implicated in maturation-promoting factor stabilization. Female *Mos* knockouts are subfertile and their oocytes have visible abnormalities in chromatin organization after the completion of

meiosis I. A naturally occurring defect intrinsic to oocytes in the LTXBO mouse strain also causes a high incidence of parthenogenic activation, which is associated with delayed entry into anaphase I. Oocytes from these mice have elevated protein kinase C activity in late metaphase I, and inhibition of PKC in these oocytes promotes the timely onset of anaphase I and reduces spontaneous activation. These findings suggest that abnormal regulation of protein kinase C in the oocytes of this strain of mice is causal for their defects. Thus, LTXBO mice provide a valuable model for studying the molecular mechanisms underlying the late stages of oocyte meiosis and the onset of embryonic mitosis.

V. FERTILIZATION AND EARLY EMBRYONIC DEVELOPMENT

Fertilization depends upon sperm–egg fusion molecules expressed by the gametes. Integrin α6β1 dimers and an associated tetraspanin protein, CD9, on the surface of oocytes are thought to be important in interacting with ADAM (a disintegrin and a metallprotease domain) proteins expressed by sperm, facilitating sperm binding and penetration. Corroborating this finding, knockout female mice lacking CD9 have severely compromised fertility owing to defects in the capacity for spermatozoa to bind to CD9 null oocytes.

Mammalian oocytes are normally released from their metaphase II block upon fertilization and this is marked morphologically by the separation of the second polar body. This represents the completion of oocyte maturation and the female gamete may be hereafter referred to as an egg. At least one mismatch repair protein, MLH1, though seemingly dispensable for meiosis I, is critical to the progression through meiosis II. *Mlh1* knockout females are completely sterile. Their oocytes develop, ovulate, and fertilize normally, but postfertilization development is blocked and extrusion of the second polar body is not accomplished. This unique block suggests the presence of a distinct checkpoint in meiosis II governing the completion of oocyte maturation, which involves the detection of aberrant DNA structures and arrests development in gametes with defective heteroduplex repair pathways.

Until sperm DNA decondensation and reorganization of a diploid nucleus are completed, many events of early embryogenesis cannot rely on *de novo* transcription from either parental genome, and factors that are required for embryonic development must be supplied by the oocyte. Disruptions of the maternal genome that cause phenotypes in embryonic development are termed maternal effect mutations and several have been recently characterized in mice using knockout technology. In each case, the gene product is normally accumulated in growing oocytes and persists in the early developing embryo, and the phenotype affects the offspring of homozygote females, regardless of their genotype or gender. Knockout females lacking a PHD-containing protein, ZAR1 (zygote arrest 1), are infertile due to a block in the development of their fertilized eggs to two-cell embryos. Similarly, a maternal effect gene encoding MATER (maternal antigen that embryos require) is necessary for development beyond the 2-cell stage and has been implicated in establishing embryonic genome transcription patterns. A third gene encodes DNMT1o, an oocyte-specific DNA methyltransferase critical for maintaining imprinting patterns established in the embryonic genome and the viability of the developing mouse during the last third of gestation. Transient nuclear localization of the DMTO1o protein during the 8-cell-stage embryo suggests that it normally

functions during the fourth S phase and is required for the transmission of methylation patterns to each daughter cell produced in the 16-cell-stage embryo. Presumably, many other oocyte-derived factors mediate the complexities of early embryogenesis—both the dramatic morphological changes that herald early development and the compositional changes in mRNA and protein of reserves of eggs and zygotes around the time of fertilization.

VI. CONCLUDING REMARKS

Our descriptive understanding of mouse oocyte and early embryo development has enabled us to invent transgenic technologies that hold the promise to reveal the molecular aspects of these biological processes. Future knockout models, multiple mutant studies, and the development of temporal and tissue-specific knockouts will allow us to more thoroughly examine the *in vivo* functions of gene products. The conservation of many genes and their functions across species indicates the potential of such studies in our pursuits to understand and affect the biology of female gameotogenesis in humans.

Acknowledgments

Transgenic mouse research in the Matzuk lab has been supported by Wyeth Research, National Institutes of Health Grants CA60651, HD32067, and HD33438, and the Specialized Cooperative Centers Program in Reproduction Research (HD07495).

Studies of oocyte biology in the Matzuk lab have been supported in part by National Institutes of Health grants and the specialized Cooperative Centers Program in Reproduction Research (HDO 7495). K.H.B. is a student in the Medical Scientist Training Program supported in part by NIH Grant T32GM-07330.

Glossary

folliculogenesis The process by which oocytes and ovarian somatic cells develop to ovulate a fertilizable egg. The first steps in follicle development are directed by intraovarian factors and result in proliferation of granulosa cells surrounding the oocyte and the recruitment of a layer of theca cells. The development of large antral follicles and ovulation depend on the actions of the pituitary gonadotropin hormones, follicle-stimulating hormone and luteinizing hormone. The stages of follicular development are summarized in Fig. 2.

meiosis A specialized cell division program completed during the formation of haploid gametes. In the first stage of meiosis (meiosis I), homologous pairs of replicated chromatids separate into daughter cells, and there is a reduction in both the DNA content and the ploidy. The second stage (meiosis II) involves the separation of paired chromatids. In mammalian female gametogenesis, the completion of each division results in the extrusion of a polar body so that one haploid egg is produced from the two divisions. There are arrests in meiosis at prophase I and metaphase II; these are released upon ovulation and fertilization, respectively. The stages of meiosis are summarized in Fig. 1.

mitosis Cell division that produces daughter cells with the same DNA content as the parental cell. The process begins after DNA replication and involves four phases as follows: (1) prophase, which is subdivided into stages describing chromosome morphology; (2) metaphase, when condensed chromosomes are aligned; (3) anaphase, when chromatids separate to opposite poles; and (4) telophase, which is followed by nuclear and cytoplasmic division.

transgenic mice Mice with heritable, engineered manipulations of the genome. These mice can have genes introduced for ectopic expression or can have endogenous genes or sequences altered. When the expression of an endogenous gene is completely abrogated, mice homozygous for the null allele are called knockout mice.

See Also the Following Articles

Corpus Luteum in Primates ● Extracellular Matrix and Follicle Development ● Fecundity Genes ● Follicle Stimulating Hormone (FSH) ● Folliculogenesis, Early ● Implantation ● *In Vitro* Fertilization ● Ovulation

Further Reading

Ackert, C. L., Gittens, J. E., O'Brien, M. J., Eppig, J. J., and Kidder, G. M. (2001). Intercellular communication via connexin43 gap junctions is required for ovarian folliculogenesis in the mouse. *Dev. Biol.* 233(2), 258–270.

Byskov, A. G., Andersen, C. Y., Leonardsen, L., and Baltsen, M. (1999). Meiosis activating sterols (MAS) and fertility in mammals and man. *J. Exp. Zool.* 285(3), 237–242.

Chang, H., Brown C. W., and Matzuk, M. M. (2002). Genetic analysis of the mammalian TGF-β superfamily. *Endocrine Reviews.* 23(6), 787–823.

Dong, J., Albertini, D. F., Nishimori, K., Kumar, T. R., Lu, N., and Matzuk, M. M. (1996). Growth differentiation factor-9 is required during early ovarian folliculogenesis. *Nature* 383, 531–535.

Donovan, P. J., and de Miguel, M. P. (2001). The role of the c-kit/kit ligand axis in mammalian gametogenesis. *In* "Transgenics in Endocrinology" (M. M. Matzuk, C. W. Brown and T. R. Kumar, eds.), pp. 147–163. Humana Press, Totowa, NJ.

Edelmann, W., Cohen, P. E., Kane, M., Lau, K., Morrow, B., Bennett, S., Umar, A., Kunkel, T., Cattoretti, G., Chaganti, R., Pollard, J. W., Kolodner, R. D., and Kucherlapati, R. (1996). Meiotic pachytene arrest in MLH1-deficient mice. *Cell* 85, 1125–1134.

Galloway, S. M., McNatty, K. P., Cambridge, L. M., Laitinen, M. P., Juengel, J. L., Jokiranta, T. S., McLaren, R. J., Luiro, K., Dodds, K. G., Montgomery, G. W., Beattie, A. E., Davis, G. H., and Ritvos, O. (2000). Mutations in an oocyte-derived growth factor gene (BMP15) cause increased ovulation rate and infertility in a dosage-sensitive manner. *Nat. Genet.* 25(3), 279–283.

Howell, C. Y., Bestor, T. H., Ding, F., Latham, K. E., Mertineit, C., Trasler, J. M., and Chaillet, J. R. (2001). Genomic imprinting disrupted by a maternal effect mutation in the Dnmt1 gene. *Cell* 104(6), 829–838.

Matzuk, M. M., Burns, K. H., Viveiros, M. M., and Eppig, J. J. (2002). Intercellular communication in the mammalian ovary: Oocytes carry the conversation. *Science* 296, 2178–2180.

Matzuk, M. M., and Lamb, D. J. (2002). Genetic dissection of mammalian fertility pathways. *Nat. Med.* 8(S1), S41–S49.

Soyal, S. M., Amleh, A., and Dean, J. (2000). FIG(alpha), a germ cell-specific transcription factor required for ovarian follicle formation. *Development* 127(21), 4645–4654.

Tilly, J. L. (2001). Commuting the death sentence: How oocytes strive to survive. *Nat. Rev. Mol. Cell. Biol.* 2(11), 838–848.

Tong, Z. B., Gold, L., Pfeifer, K. E., Dorward, H., Lee, E., Bondy, C. A., Dean, J., and Nelson, L. M. (2000). Mater, a maternal effect gene required for early embryonic development in mice. *Nat. Genet.* 26(3), 267–268.

Wu, X., Viveiros, M. M., Eppig, J. J., Bai, Y., Fitzpatrick, S. L., and Matzuk, M. M. (2003). Zygote arrest 1 (Zarl) is a novel maternal-effect gene critical for the oocyte-to-embryo transition. *Nat. Genet.* 33(2), 187–191.

Yan, C., Wang, P., DeMayo, J., DeMayo, F. J., Elvin, J. A., Carino, C., Prasad, S. V., Skinner, S. S., Dunbar, B. S., Dube, J. L., Celeste, A. J., and Matzuk, M. M. (2001). Synergistic roles of bone morphogenetic protein 15 and growth differentiation factor 9 in ovarian function. *Mol. Endocrinol.* 15(6), 854–866.

Ying, Y., and Zhao, G. Q. (2001). Cooperation of endoderm-derived BMP2 and extraembryonic ectoderm-derived BMP4 in primordial germ cell generation in the mouse. *Dev. Biol.* 232(2), 484–492.

Orphan Receptors, New Receptors, and New Hormones

DAVID D. MOORE

Baylor College of Medicine

I. INTRODUCTION
II. THE FIRST GENERATION OF THE NUCLEAR RECEPTOR SUPERFAMILY: IDENTIFICATION OF CLASSICAL RECEPTORS AND ORPHANS
III. THE NEXT GENERATION: LIGANDS AND FUNCTIONS FOR THE NEW RECEPTORS
IV. FUTURE GENERATIONS: FUNCTIONS OF THE CURRENT ORPHAN RECEPTORS
V. SUMMARY AND PROSPECTS

There are 48 members of the nuclear hormone receptor superfamily in the human genome. Currently, these proteins can be divided into 23 conventional receptors with known ligands and 25 proteins, called orphan receptors, which do not have known ligands.

I. INTRODUCTION

The nuclear hormone receptor superfamily comprises two groups: the conventional receptors, those with known ligands, and the orphan receptors, those that do not have known ligands. The conventional receptors can be further subdivided into the classical receptors for a series of hormones and signaling molecules that were known to have nuclear receptors before any of the genes encoding these proteins were cloned, and the new receptors for more recently identified compounds. The ligands for the former group consist of estrogens, androgens, progestins, glucocorticoids, mineralocorticoids, vitamin D, thyroid hormone, and retinoic acid. Those for the new receptors include fatty acids, prostaglandins, oxysterols, bile acids, and xenobiotics, as well as an increasing number of synthetic ligands. Several of these synthetic ligands have already been found to be valuable therapeutic agents. This article focuses on the discovery of these new ligands, some of which were not expected to have such direct biologic regulatory functions, and their emerging roles in regulating lipid metabolism. The potential functions of several of the current orphans are also outlined.

II. THE FIRST GENERATION OF THE NUCLEAR RECEPTOR SUPERFAMILY: IDENTIFICATION OF CLASSICAL RECEPTORS AND ORPHANS

The cloning and characterization of the cDNA encoding the glucocorticoid receptor (GR) by the laboratories of Keith Yamamoto and Ron Evans in 1984 and 1985 immediately revealed the existence of at least a small family of nuclear receptor proteins, based on the striking similarity of the GR cDNA sequence to that encoding the cellular proto-oncogene c-erbA. The subsequent isolation of clones encoding additional steroid receptors by the laboratories of Bert O'Malley, Pierre Chambon, and others resulted in the identification of the structurally conserved DNA-binding and ligand-binding domains shared by the family members and the initial characterization of the molecular mechanism of action of these receptors. In this mechanism, the DNA-binding domain functions to recognize specific sequences in appropriate target genes. The binding of the hormone to the structurally separate ligand-binding domain results in an allosteric effect that is now known to allow the binding of a series of different co-regulator proteins. Thus, hormone binding results in the recruitment of these co-regulator proteins to the target genes, where they exert their appropriate transcriptional regulatory effects.

However, the isolation of these additional receptors left open the question of what hormone might activate c-erbA. At the time, the main candidates were a small number of signaling molecules known to have nuclear receptors: thyroid hormone (triiodothyronine, T3), all-*trans*-retinoic acid (t-RA), 1,25-dihydroxyvitamin D_3, and dioxin. It did not take long for the laboratories of Ron Evans and Bjorn Vennstrom to identify T3 as the ligand for both c-erbA, which became the thyroid hormone receptor α isoform, TRα, and the closely related TRβ protein. Thus, these proteins were the first to move from the orphan column to the conventional receptor column.

A similar strategy allowed the identification of a protein originally isolated as the target of hepatitis B virus insertions in hepatoma as the retinoic acid receptor α isoform (RARα), which was joined by the RARβ and RARγ isoforms. The last receptors identified in this initial generation were the retinoid X receptors (RXRα, β, and γ), which were initially identified as RAR relatives that were activated by high concentrations of t-RA, but were unable to bind it directly. The identification of the stereoisomer 9-*cis*-retinoic acid (9-*cis*-RA) as a specific agonist ligand for the RXRs was the first example of the use of what was then an orphan receptor to identify a new signaling molecule. Although the physiological significance of 9-*cis*-RA activation of the RXRs remains unclear more than 10 years after their identification, this exciting finding has led to the identification of specific synthetic RXR agonists that have recently received approval as cancer chemotherapeutic agents.

In 1996, estrogen receptor-β (ERβ) was the last of the classical receptors to be identified. This former orphan was found to be an alternative estrogen receptor on the basis of its sequence similarity to the previously identified ERα. The existence of the β isoform was not anticipated based on classical studies of estrogen function.

As these classical receptors were characterized, the list of the orphans that was initiated with estrogen receptor-related receptor-α (ERRα) and ERRβ quickly began to lengthen. The current status of the family, as revealed in the human genome sequence and summarized in Table 1, is 48 total members, 14 of which are receptors for these classical ligands and 8 of which have more recently identified ligands as described below. The remaining 26 are still orphan receptors.

TABLE 1   Nuclear Hormone Receptor Subgroups

Conventional receptors	
Classical	**New**
Steroid	Fatty acid
ERα, ERβ (3A1, 2), PR (3B3), AR (3B4)	PPARα, PPARδ, PPARγ (1C1–3)
GR (3B1), MR (3B2), VDR (1I1)	
Thyroid	Cholesterol/bile acid
TRα, TRβ (1A1, 2)	LXRα (1H3), LXRβ (1H2), FXR (1H4)
Retinoid	Xenobiotic
RARα, RARβ, RARγ (1B1–3)	PXR (1I2), CAR (1I3)
RXRα, RXRβ, RXRγ (2B1)	

Orphan receptors
ERRα, ERRβ, ERRγ (3B1–3)[a]
COUP-TFI, II (2F1, 2), ear2 (2F6)
HNF-4α (2A1), HNF-4γ (2A2)
SF-1, LRH-1, (NR5A1, 2)
NGF-IB, Nurr1, Nor1 (4A1–3)
RevErbAα, RevErbAβ (1D1, 2)
RORα, RORβ, RORγ (1F1–3)
TR-2, TR-4, (2C1-2)
TLX (2E1), PNR (2E3)
GCNF-1 (6A1)
SHP, DAX-1 (0B1, 2)

Note. Conventional and orphan receptors are grouped based on ligand-binding properties. Many of the nuclear properties have a number of different names and/or different isoforms genereated by alternate splicing or promoter utilization, but only a single commonly used name is included here for each. See http://www.ens-lyon.fr/LBMC/laudet/NucRec/nomenclature_table.html for a more comprehensive list and GenBank accession numbers. In a standardized nomenclature for the nuclear receptors, each is referred to as "NR" followed by a three-character code based on evolutionary relatedness. This code is indicated in parantheses for each family member.

[a]Synthetic inverse agonist ligands have been identified.

In retrospect, it was misleading that the examples provided by these classical receptors clearly predicted that the "hormones" for the remaining orphans would share properties similar to those already described. Thus, it was anticipated that these new hormones would combine potent biologic regulatory effects with quite specific and high-affinity binding to their receptors. A major problem with this prediction was the significant discrepancy between the very limited number of remaining compounds with such properties and the much larger number of orphan receptors. The focus on high-affinity ligands stymied progress in this area for several years.

III. THE NEXT GENERATION: LIGANDS AND FUNCTIONS FOR THE NEW RECEPTORS

A. PPARα, PPARγ, and PPARδ

The next generation in the evolution of the understanding of the nuclear hormone receptors began in 1990 with the identification of a series of compounds previously known to increase numbers of peroxisomes in hepatocytes as ligands for a receptor termed the peroxisome proliferator-activated receptor (PPARα) (Table 2). This linkage was consistent with the prediction that a receptor ligand should have a potent biological effect. However, the fact that some of these ligands were active only at very high concentrations did not fit well with assumptions based on the classic hormones. This issue became even more significant when it was proposed that fatty acids were the endogenous ligands for the three PPAR isoforms. Although it is well known that consumption of different fatty acids can have significant effects on metabolism, it was not thought that such effects were due to a specific receptor for such fatty acids. Moreover, simple considerations of equilibrium binding dictate a basic trade-off between binding affinity and specificity that associates low-affinity interactions with decreased specificity. This argues strongly for quite limited specificity for binding of compounds that occupy a receptor at concentrations more than a million times higher than the picomolar

TABLE 2 Some New Ligands for Nuclear Hormone Receptors

Receptor	Endogenous	Synthetic/exogenous
PPARα	Fatty acids, prostaglandins	Fibrates, other peroxisome proliferators
PPARδ	Fatty acids, prostaglandins	Carbaprostacyclin
PPARγ	Fatty acids, prostaglandins	Thiazolidinediones, new-generation anti-diabetic agents
LXR	Oxysterols	T09031
FXR	Bile acids	GW4064, guggulsterone[a]
CAR	Androstanes[b] (bilirubin)[d]	TCPOBOP[c] (phenobarbital)[d]
PXR	Bile acids	Many drugs, catatoxic steroids and steroid antagonists
ERRs	?	DES and 4-hydroxytamoxifen[b]

[a]Antagonist.
[b]Inverse agonists.
[c]Rodent CAR only.
[d]Indirect activator.

levels associated with the effects of T3 and other high-affinity ligands. Thus, even though the concentrations of fatty acids required for PPAR activation may correspond to their endogenous levels, a signaling mechanism based on such poorly binding ligands must incorporate significant compromises in specificity relative to the conventional hormones. Such considerations predict that the PPARs would be unable to distinguish between various fatty acid species or even to exclude the effects of compounds not closely related to these endogenous ligands.

An elegant series of structural studies with the PPARs provided additional focus to these issues and addressed some of the associated concerns. These studies have revealed that the ligand-binding pocket of the PPARs is unusually capacious relative to more conventional receptors with high-affinity ligands. The ability of fatty acids to occupy this large pocket was directly confirmed by an X-ray crystal structure of eicosapentaenoic acid bound to PPARδ. This structure also confirmed the lack of specificity of such binding, since two quite different conformations of this flexible ligand were observed in the crystals.

Importantly, the crystal structures also explained the ability of additional synthetic ligands to bind these receptors with high affinity. A series of fibrate compounds associated with lipid-lowering effects were among the first compounds identified as activators of PPARα and were subsequently shown to be direct ligands. The initial identification of PPARγ as a factor promoting fat cell differentiation led to the identification of a class of compounds known as thiazolidinediones as relatively high-affinity PPARγ ligands, since such compounds were known to promote adipocyte differentiation. As expected, X-ray crystal structures demonstrate that the thiazolidinediones occupy a much larger fraction of the PPARγ ligand-binding pocket and make a good overall fit.

Based on both knockouts (genetically engineered null mice) and pharmacologic approaches, it is now clear that PPARα functions in the liver to stimulate fatty acid oxidation and PPARγ functions in fat cells to promote adipogenesis and expression of fat-specific genes. PPARγ also functions in macrophages to promote the return of cholesterol to the liver via the reverse transport pathway. The function of the third PPAR isoform, usually called PPARδ, is less clear. It is much more broadly expressed than the other two, and intriguing recent pharmacologic results suggest that PPARδ agonists may be therapeutically useful in treatment of the metabolic problems associated with obesity in syndrome X.

B. Liver X Receptor-α, Liver X Receptor-β, and Farnesoid X Receptor

Three former orphans have been identified as receptors for primary metabolites of cholesterol with roles in cholesterol homeostasis. The first of these was liver X receptor (LXRα), which is activated by hydroxylated cholesterol derivatives called oxysterols. In agreement with the fact that these compounds had previously been identified as potential regulators of the expression of proteins involved in cholesterol homeostasis, and also its expression in the liver, LXRα knockout mice showed a profound defect in hepatic cholesterol metabolism. Normal mice are able to manage even relatively high levels of dietary cholesterol. However, the LXRα knockouts are unable to metabolize and eliminate the excess cholesterol, which accumulates in the liver. The closely related LXRβ isoform is also activated by oxysterols and is expressed in a number of tissues, including the liver, but the phenotype of the LXRα knockout animals demonstrates that LXRβ is unable to fully compensate for the loss of the former isoform. The LXRβ knockout also fails to show the same strong cholesterol accumulation phenotype as the LXRα knockout. However, the double-knockout animals have an even more severe phenotype, indicating some degree of functional overlap.

The phenotype of the LXRα knockout raised the possibility that LXR agonists could be useful in the treatment of hypercholesterolemia. Unfortunately, however, the synthetic agonist T09031 was found to significantly increase triglyceride levels in rodent models. This undesirable side effect is associated with the induction of the transcription factor sterol response element binding protein-1c (SREBP-1c), which promotes fatty acid synthesis.

In addition to their roles in lipid metabolism in the liver, the LXRs also function with PPARγ in the process of reverse cholesterol transport mentioned above. In this pathway, PPARγ activation in macrophages results in induction of LXRα expression, which, in turn, activates target genes responsible for cholesterol efflux, including the ABCA1 active transport pump and apolipoprotein E. Thus, LXR agonists may have beneficial effects in both the liver and the periphery if the triglyceride problem can be circumvented.

Another former orphan that functions in cholesterol homeostasis is farnesoid X receptor (FXR), which is directly activated by bile acids. Bile acids are downstream metabolites of cholesterol. They are produced in large amounts in the liver and are essential for the emulsification and absorption of dietary lipids. Although they are very efficiently reabsorbed in the gut after their release in bile, they represent the primary pathway for elimination of cholesterol from the liver. The potential function of FXR in bile acid and cholesterol homeostasis was supported by results with knockout animals, which show significant defects in these processes, including the inability to appropriately down-regulate bile acid biosynthesis in response to increased bile acid levels.

Like the cholesterol efflux from macrophages, this down-regulation is apparently also a consequence of a nuclear receptor cascade. In this case, activation of FXR by bile acids results in increased expression of an unusual orphan receptor named small heterodimer partner (SHP), which lacks a DNA-binding domain and functions to inhibit transactivation by other nuclear receptors. The orphan receptor liver receptor homologue-1 [LRH-1, also known as fetoprotein transcription factor (FTF)] is particularly sensitive to this repression and its activity is essential for the expression of the rate-limiting enzyme in bile acid biosynthesis, encoded by the Cyp7A1 gene. Thus, the induction of FXR by bile acids results in decreased Cyp7A1 expression via a pathway dependent on both SHP and LRH-1.

Like the LXRs, FXR is also a potential target for the modulation of cholesterol levels. Recently, guggulsterone, a natural product found to lower serum low-density lipoprotein levels in humans, was identified as an antagonist ligand for FXR. Treatment with this plant-derived steroid results in decreased accumulation of cholesterol in the liver of wild-type but not FXR knockout mice challenged with a high-cholesterol diet. Thus, it is possible that this or other, more specific FXR antagonists may be useful in the treatment of hypercholesterolemia.

C. Constitutive Androstane Receptor and Pregnane X Receptor

The former orphans constitutive androstane receptor (CAR) and pregnane X receptor (PXR) are each other's closest relatives within the receptor superfamily. Interestingly, they are in the same branch of the evolutionary tree as LXRα, LXRβ, and FXR. The final receptor in this cluster is the vitamin D receptor (VDR). All six of these receptors are expressed to at least some degree in the liver and all are RXR heterodimer partners. They are also all ligand dependent, with CAR and PXR sharing a rather complex overlapping network of xenobiotic agonists/ activators and also target genes.

The term xenobiotic refers to all the compounds that organisms encounter that are not normal constituents of the body. This category includes an enormous range of agents present in foods, drugs, and environmental contaminants. It is well known that exposure to particular foreign compounds can increase the capacity of the liver to metabolize both the initial xenobiotic stimulus and other compounds. Both genetic and pharmacologic approaches have demonstrated that CAR and PXR mediate two particularly well-known xenobiotic responses.

In the first step of drug metabolism, called Phase I, a series of cytochrome P450 enzymes with a particularly wide range of substrates catalyzes the hydroxylation of xenobiotic compounds. In Phase II, a variety of other enzymes add a number of other functional groups, often to the site of initial hydroxylation. In general, this results in the inactivation and elimination of the xenobiotic substrate. Both CAR and PXR induce coordinate responses of Phase I and Phase II enzymes, as well as multidrug resistance transporters and other components of the drug metabolism pathway. Such responses are the basis for a class of clinically significant drug-drug interactions in which the presence of one drug affects the activity or half-life of another. In such interactions, the first drug is a direct activator of CAR or PXR, whereas the second is a substrate for the drug-metabolizing machinery.

The mouse PXR was first described as a receptor for a series of steroids and steroid antagonists that had previously been known to induce a characteristic xenobiotic response centered on the *Cyp3A* gene. A knockout of the mouse PXR gene confirmed its importance in this response, but also helped resolve a complication associated with the fact that the ligand-binding domain of the human PXR (also called SXR) diverges much more from the mouse PXR ligand-binding domain than is common within the superfamily. This divergent sequence had been shown to result in response to different agonist ligands. For example, the human receptor is potently activated by the antibiotic rifampicin, a well-known inducer of *Cyp3A* expression in human patients, but the mouse protein is completely unresponsive. As predicted from the activity of the isolated receptors, a mouse expressing the human PXR/SXR instead of its own PXR gains the ability to induce *Cyp3A* expression in response to rifampicin.

CAR shares a similar, if somewhat more complex, function. The barbiturate drug phenobarbital, used to treat seizures, also induces a characteristic xenobiotic response that centers on *Cyp2B* enzymes. Again, a knockout mouse model was used to demonstrate that this response is mediated by CAR. The pharmacology of this response is complicated somewhat by the fact that phenobarbital is not a ligand for either the mouse or the human CAR. Instead, it induces a specific translocation of the receptor from the cytoplasm of the hepatocyte to the nucleus. Little is known about this process, but it is thought to contribute to the activation of CAR by many other xenobiotics in addition to phenobarbital. Once in the nucleus, this receptor apparently relies on its ligand-independent or constitutive transcriptional activation function to stimulate the expression of appropriate target genes. Such constitutive activity is not a general characteristic of the ligand-dependent nuclear receptors described above. As described below, however, it is a common feature among the remaining orphan receptors.

The constitutive activity of mouse CAR can be further increased by a compound known as TCPOBOP (1,4-bis-[2-(3,5,-dichloropyridyloxy)] benzene), which is both a direct CAR agonist and a potent inducer of *Cyp2B* expression. It can also be blocked by androstanol and androstenol, which are inverse agonist ligands and can inhibit the activation of *Cyp2B* expression by TCPOBOP. As with PXR, the human and mouse CAR ligand-binding domains are divergent and neither of these murine CAR ligands binds the human receptor.

The functions of the two receptors in the xenobiotic responses overlap to a significant degree. For example, CAR is also able to activate *Cyp3A* expression and PXR can activate *Cyp2B*. They also share some activators, such as the antifungal agent clotrimazole, which can activate both human PXR and mouse CAR (but is a weak inverse agonist for human CAR). This overlap of targets and ligands is certainly not complete, however, and the specific and overlapping functions of these two receptors remain to be defined.

One area where they appear to show more specific activities is in their responses to endogenous compounds. Thus, PXR but not CAR has been associated with a protective response to toxic bile acids that is based on their function as both PXR ligands and substrates for *Cyp3A*. CAR, in contrast, functions to activate the clearance of bilirubin, a toxic breakdown product of heme that is specifically metabolized and eliminated by the liver.

IV. FUTURE GENERATIONS: FUNCTIONS OF THE CURRENT ORPHAN RECEPTORS

In general, much less is known about those members of the nuclear receptor superfamily that remain orphans. In some cases, however, key insights into their roles have come from knockouts or other sources. The potential functions of some of the better characterized orphans will be briefly outlined here.

A. ERRα, ERRβ, and ERRγ

The estrogen receptor-related receptors are closely related to the estrogen receptors and were among the first true orphans to be described. Like several of the other orphans, but not the classical receptors, they are evolutionarily ancient with an apparent homologue in *Drosophila*. The recent identification of the synthetic ER ligands diethylstilbestrol and 4-hydroxy-tamoxifen as inverse agonists strongly suggests that the identification of natural or endogenous ligands will soon relocate these proteins to the conventional receptor category. Although their overall functions remain uncertain, they also share DNA-binding sites, co-regulators, and target genes with the conventional estrogen receptors ERα and ERβ and may function to modulate estrogen signaling pathways.

B. Steroidogenic Factor 1

In contrast to the isolation of many of the orphans using approaches such as low-stringency hybridization, steroidogenic factor 1 (SF-1) was first identified based on its ability to bind a series of related sites in the promoters of steroid hydroxylases. Also, unlike other orphans that bind DNA as homodimers or heterodimers, SF-1 binds as a monomer to an extended consensus element that includes a single copy of the nuclear receptor-binding hexamer. Like many other orphans, however, SF-1 functions as an apparently constitutive transcriptional activator.

The potential role of SF-1 in the regulation of adrenal steroidogenesis was strongly supported by the observation that the loss of SF-1 function in mice resulted in the absence of adrenals, gonads, and the ventromedial hypothalamus, as well as male-to-female sex reversal of internal and external genitalia. Thus, SF-1 is a key regulator of the development of important endocrine tissues. It is also expressed in these tissues in the adult, where its role remains an interesting question.

C. Hepatic Nuclear Factor 4

Hepatic nuclear factor 4α (HNF-4α) is another orphan originally identified based on its ability to recognize specific sites, in this case in various promoters that are active in the liver. It binds these sites as a homodimer. Additional studies revealed that it is also expressed in the kidney, intestine, and pancreas, particularly the insulin-producing beta cells. A wide variety of target genes have been identified, including genes involved in fatty acid and cholesterol metabolism, glucose metabolism, urea biosynthesis, and liver differentiation. HNF-4α null mouse embryos die at a very early stage of development. The heterozygotes do not show an obvious phenotype. In humans, however, heterozygous loss of HNF-4α results in defective pancreatic beta-cell function and a characteristic syndrome called MODY (mature onset diabetes of the young). HNF-4α is MODY1; heterozygous loss of function of several other nonreceptor transcription factors that function in the beta cell results in a similar phenotype.

HNF-4 is another orphan that functions as an apparently constitutive transcriptional activator. Thus, it was a surprise when the recent X-ray crystal structure of HNF-4γ revealed a fatty acid occupying an unusually small putative ligand-binding pocket. This clearly suggests that the function of this important metabolic regulator could be modulated by appropriate synthetic ligands. However, its location in the structure and other lines of evidence suggest that this fatty acid may play a structural role more analogous to the zinc atoms in the DNA-binding domain than the much more dynamic functions of conventional nuclear receptor ligands. Thus, the potential ligand responsiveness of the HNF-4 isoforms remains to be established.

D. Chicken Ovalbumin Upstream Transcription Factor I and II

These two closely related orphans are the mammalian homologues of an ancient orphan with unusually close relatives in Drosophila and a number of other invertebrates. The chicken ovalbumin upstream transcription factors can bind a wide variety of response elements as homodimers. They generally function as transcriptional repressors, but positive effects have been observed in some contexts. Although their activities appear very similar and their patterns of expression overlap significantly, the knockout of either chicken ovalbumin upstream transcription factor I (COUP-TFI) or COUP-TFII is lethal. In the former case, death is perinatal and is caused by multiple defects in development of the central and peripheral nervous system. In the cerebral cortex, for example, layer IV of the cortex is absent, a defect that is apparently secondary to a failure of the appropriate innervation of these neurons and subsequent cell death. In contrast, COUP-TFII null mice die at embryonic day 10 with a variety of heart and vascular defects. Interestingly, some of these defects resemble those observed in mice lacking angiopoeitin 1 or its receptor. The marked decrease in angiopoeitin expression in the knockouts suggests that COUP-TFII is an important upstream regulator of the expression of this important angiogenic factor. Thus, it is possible that modulation of COUP-TFII activity could control angiogenesis in pathologic processes including carcinogenesis.

E. Nur-related Factor 1

Nur-related factor 1 (Nurr1) is one of three related receptors in a group that shows particularly flexible modes of DNA binding. Thus, nerve growth factor inducible B (NGFI-B) was the first orphan shown to bind with high affinity as a monomer, a property shared by the other two family members and also a subset of other orphans. At least in some cases, however, members of this family can also bind specific DNA sites as homodimers or as heterodimers with each other. In addition, Nurr1 and NGFI-B, but not neuron-derived orphan receptor 1 (Nor1), can bind distinct sites as heterodimers with RXR.

Of these three related orphans, the Nurr1 knockout showed the most dramatic phenotype, a complete loss of mesencephalic dopamine neurons. It is an interesting possibility that this orphan may be involved in disease processes that impact such dopaminergic neurons, such as Parkinson's disease and schizophrenia. Some support for this possibility is provided by the identification of Nurr1 gene mutations in a small number of schizophrenic patients.

F. Reverse ErbAα

Reverse ErbAα (RevErbAα) is an orphan with an unusual genomic location: the coding region for its final exon overlaps with that of the final exon of the variant TRα2 isoform. It has a close relative, RevErbAβ, which is also linked to the TRβ locus but does not share a similar overlap. It is interesting that TRα and RevErbAα are also linked to RARα, whereas TRβ and RevErbAβ are linked to RARβ on a different chromosome, suggesting that a single, ancient duplication generated the two sets of isoforms for the three receptors.

A recent clue to the potential function of RevErbAα was provided by the unexpected demonstration that its expression is very strongly regulated by circadian rhythm. Somewhat less marked circadian variations were observed with RevErbAβ and also ROR isoforms, which can bind similar DNA-response elements. In RevErbAα knockout animals, circadian rhythms are significantly altered, but not absent. RevErbAα and RevErbAβ function as apparently constitutive repressors in co-transfection assays, and results with knockout models show that at least RevErbAα functions *in vivo* to represses the expression of Bmal1, a central component of the molecular circadian clock in mammals. Overall, these results confirm both the role of RevErbAα in the regulation of the circadian clock and the existence of redundant mechanisms in this important and complex pathway.

G. SHP and DAX-1

SHP and dosage-sensitive sex reversal-adrenal hypoplasia congenita critical region on the X chromosome 1 (DAX-1) are unique orphans that lack a nuclear receptor DNA-binding domain. SHP directly interacts with a number of other nuclear receptors and inhibits their ability to activate transcription. As described above, results with SHP knockouts supported a specific role proposed for SHP in an FXR-dependent pathway for negative feedback regulation of bile acid biosynthesis. Interestingly, there are apparently also additional, redundant mechanisms for this process, since SHP null mice do show the expected loss of repression in response to a synthetic FXR agonist, but to a large degree maintain the repressive effect of high levels of dietary bile acids.

In contrast to SHP, which consists solely of a ligand-binding domain, DAX-1 includes an additional N-terminal domain. This domain has been associated with various DNA-binding activities, but the significance of this potential function remains uncertain. Loss of function of the human DAX-1 gene causes an X-linked form of adrenal hypoplasia congenita that is associated with hypogonadotropic hypogonadism. Like SHP, DAX-1 functions as a transcriptional repressor and it is thought that the loss of this repression function accounts for this phenotype. The transcriptional targets of DAX-1 remain unknown but several lines of evidence, including direct interaction and similar patterns of expression, suggest that it modulates SF-1 function.

V. SUMMARY AND PROSPECTS

Two broad themes have emerged from studies of orphan receptors over the past 15 years. Starting with the TRs and RARs and continuing through the recent identification of the ERRs as potential targets of selective estrogen receptor modulators, the first is the identification of new ligands for orphan receptors. This has led to important and in some cases quite unexpected advances in several areas. Perhaps the most notable is the identification of the PPARs, LXRs, and FXR as key regulators of lipid metabolism. These and other receptors will continue to be important targets for the identification of new therapeutic approaches to regulate important metabolic pathways.

The potential therapeutic importance of these receptors highlights the significance of an intriguing question: Will ligands eventually be defined for all of the remaining orphans? This question can be further divided into whether such ligands will be endogenous ligands with important regulatory functions or synthetic compounds identified by high-throughput functional tests. In the former case, one might predict that many of the current orphans will remain orphans, since there is not a pool of remaining candidate compounds with the expected regulatory functions. Of course, this may be more reflective of a lack of imagination than a lack of such ligands, and it seems very likely that endogenous ligands will be identified for the ERRs and potentially other orphans. Nonetheless, several evolutionary arguments have suggested that the function of the progenitor of the superfamily may not have been ligand regulated and it is quite possible that other processes, such as phosphorylation, control the function of the remaining orphans.

Even if a significant number of the orphans do not have endogenous ligands, it remains an interesting possibility that synthetic ligands could be identified, for example, by efficient high-throughput screening technologies. The isolation of inhibitory peptides capable of binding to estrogen receptor isoforms with high affinity and specificity suggests a different approach to modulate the activity of orphans. With the continuing definition of the functions of the orphans from knockout studies and other studies, the motivation to identify appropriate ligands will be strong.

A second theme is the emergence of a number of important developmental functions of the orphans. Although the conventional receptor knockouts often show relatively limited phenotypes unless they are appropriately challenged, a number of the orphan receptor knockouts result in very early embryonic lethality or other dramatic developmental phenotypes. It is striking that comparisons of the complete human and *Drosophila* genome sequences reveal that the human nuclear receptors with *Drosophila* relatives are not the classical steroid thyroid and retinoid receptors, but the orphans. Though the existence of multiple isoforms of individual receptor types complicates matters, it is also appears that the knockouts of the mammalian receptors with the closest *Drosophila* relatives, such as the COUP-TFs and HNF-4α, show particularly strong embryonic phenotypes.

Whereas a number of such developmental functions have been identified for the conserved orphans, the apparent role of RevErbAα in circadian rhythm clearly suggests that there will be exceptions. It is a simple prediction that the orphans that remain less well characterized have some interesting surprises in store for us.

See Also the Following Articles

Co-activators and Corepressors for the Nuclear Receptor Superfamily ● Crosstalk of Nuclear Recepors with STAT Factors ● Estrogen Receptor Crosstalk with Cellular Signaling Pathways ● Ligand Modification to Produce Pharmacologic Agents ● Lipoprotein Receptor Signaling ● Peroxisome Proliferator-Activated Receptors (PPARs) ● Steroid Hormone Receptor Family: Mechanism of Action

Further Reading

Chawla, A., Repa, J. J., Evans, R. M., and Mangelsdorf, D. J. (2001). Nuclear receptors and lipid physiology: Opening the X-files. *Science* 294, 1866–1870.

Enmark, E., and Gustafsson, J. A. (2001). Comparing nuclear receptors in worms, flies and humans. *Trends Pharmacol. Sci.* 22, 611–615.

Giguere, V. (1999). Orphan nuclear receptors: From gene to function. *Endocr. Rev.* 20, 689–725.

Giguere, V., Ong, E. S., Segui, P., and Evans, R. M. (1987). Identification of a receptor for the morphogen retinoic acid. *Nature* 330, 624–629.

Kliewer, S. A., Lehmann, J. M., and Willson, T. M. (1999). Orphan nuclear receptors: Shifting endocrinology into reverse. *Science* 284, 757–760.

Lu, T. T., Repa, J. J., and Mangelsdorf, D. J. (2001). Orphan nuclear receptors as eLiXiRs and FiXeRs of sterol metabolism. *J. Biol. Chem.* 276, 37735–37738.

Sap, J., Munoz, A., Damm, K., Goldberg, Y., Ghysdael, J., Leutz, A., Beug, H., and Vennstrom, B. (1986). The c-erb-A protein is a high-affinity receptor for thyroid hormone. *Nature* 324, 635–640.

Weinberger, C., Thompson, C. C., Ong, E. S., Lebo, R., Gruol, D. J., and Evans, R. M. (1986). The c-erbA gene encodes a thyroid hormone receptor. *Nature* 324, 641–646.

Willson, T. M., and Moore, J. T. (2002). Minireview: Genomics versus orphan nuclear receptors—A half-time report. *Mol. Endocrinol.* 16, 1135–1144.

Osteogenic Proteins of the TGF-β Superfamily

U. Ripamonti

Medical Research Council/University of the Witwatersrand, Johannesburg, South Africa

I. INTRODUCTION
II. TRANSFORMING GROWTH FACTOR-β SUPERFAMILY
III. BONE MORPHOGENETIC PROTEINS/OSTEOGENIC PROTEINS
IV. ENDOCHONDRAL BONE INDUCTION BY TGF-β ISOFORMS
V. GEOMETRIC INDUCTION OF BONE FORMATION

The normal repair and regeneration of bone constitute a complex process that is temporally and spatially regulated by soluble and insoluble signals. The bone morphogenetic proteins or osteogenic proteins, members of the transforming growth factor-β supergene family, are morphogens endowed with the striking prerogative to initiate *de novo* bone formation by induction in heterotopic extraskeletal sites of animal models.

I. INTRODUCTION

The three most important requirements for successful tissue engineering of bone are a suitable extracellular matrix substratum, capable responding cells, and soluble osteoinductive signals, which are members of the transforming growth factor-β (TGF-β) supergene family. The reconstitution of bone morphogenetic proteins/osteogenic proteins (BMPs/OPs) (the soluble signals) with biomimetic matrices (the insoluble substratum) provides a bioassay for *bona fide* initiators of bone differentiation as well as delivery systems for therapeutic local osteogenesis. Contrary to all the results obtained in the rodent bioassay, heterotopic implantation of naturally derived or recombinant human (h) TGF-β isoforms induces vigorous endochondral bone induction in the *rectus abdominis* muscle of the adult primate *Papio ursinus*. The binary applications of doses of recombinant hBMPs/OPs with relatively low doses of hTGF-β1 interact synergistically to rapidly induce massive heterotopic and orthotopic ossicles in the rectus abdominis muscle and calvarial defects, respectively.

The discovery that specific surface and geometric characteristics of sintered porous hydroxypatites can induce bone in heterotopic sites of primates in the absence of exogenously applied BMPs/OPs paves the way for the formulation and therapeutic application of smart porous substrata that lead to the formation of predictable tissue types via intrinsic osteoinductivity. The incorporation of specific biological activities into sintered hydroxypatites defined as geometric induction of bone formation elicits therapeutic osteogenesis in clinical contexts. The intrinsic osteoinductivity of porous substrata in primates indicates that the bone induction cascade is initiated by endogenously produced BMPs/OPs bound to the surface of the smart concavities of the substratum, with induction of bone as a secondary response. The concavities of the substratum are geometric regulators of growth endowed with shape memory, recapitulating events that occur in the normal course of embryonic development and appearing to act as gates that give or withhold permission to grow and differentiate. Extensive studies in animal models, particularly nonhuman primates, have made possible the use of both hOP-1 and hBMP-2 for craniofacial and orthopedic applications in clinical contexts.

II. TRANSFORMING GROWTH FACTOR-β SUPERFAMILY

The initiation of bone formation during embryonic development and postnatal morphogenesis and osteogenesis involves a complex cascade of molecular and morphogenetic processes that ultimately lead to the architectural sculpture of precisely organized multicellular structures. Elucidating the nature and interaction of the signaling molecules that direct the generation of tissue-specific patterns during the initiation of endochondral bone formation is a major challenge of contemporary molecular, cellular, developmental, and tissue engineering biology.

Quantum leaps in these rapidly evolving fields have dramatically advanced our understanding of tissue induction and morphogenesis. First, the putative signaling molecules or morphogens, defined as form-generating substances capable of imparting specific different pathways to responding cells initiating the cascade of pattern formation and the attainment of tissue form and function, have been purified and cloned and their *in vivo* functions have been identified.

Nature relies on common yet limited molecular mechanisms tailored to provide the emergence of specialized tissues and organs. The distilled summary of this research effort is surprisingly simple: first, that tissue regeneration in postnatal life recapitulates events that occur in the normal course of embryonic development and morphogenesis and second, that both embryonic development and tissue regeneration are equally regulated by a select few and highly conserved families of morphogens. In addition, these gene products are members of the TGF-β superfamily, and purification and expression cloning yielded an entirely new family of protein initiators, the BMPs/OPs.

III. BONE MORPHOGENETIC PROTEINS/OSTEOGENIC PROTEINS

The BMP/OP family is indeed an elegant example of nature parsimony in programming multiple specialized functions deploying molecular isoforms with minor variations in amino acid motifs within highly conserved carboxy-terminal regions.

Members of the BMP/OP and TGF-β families are pleiotropic morphogens that have potent and diverse effects on cell proliferation, differentiation, motility, and matrix synthesis. They are powerful regulators of cartilage and bone differentiation in embryonic development and in postnatal life and are soluble mediators of tissue morphogenesis and regeneration. They exert their biological activities through heteromeric serine/threonine kinase complexes of type I and II receptors and are predominantly synthesized as glycosylated homodimers with a carboxy-terminal region containing characteristic cysteine motifs. In addition to bone induction in postnatal life, BMPs/OPs are involved in inductive events that control pattern formation during embryonic morphogenesis and organogenesis in such disparate tissues as the kidney, eye, nervous system, lung, teeth, skin, and heart. These strikingly pleiotropic effects of BMPs/OPs spring from minor amino acid sequence variations in the carboxy-terminal region of the proteins, as well as in the transduction of distinct signaling pathways by individual Smad proteins after transmembrane serine/threonine kinase receptor activation.

The three mammalian TGF-β isoforms share limited homology with members of the BMP/OP family. A striking and discriminatory feature of the BMP/OP proteins is their ability to induce *de novo* cartilage and bone formation by induction when implanted in extraskeletal heterotopic sites of mammals as recapitulation of embryonic development. This ability, originally solely assigned to the BMP/OP family, has been extended to other TGF-β supergene family members including decapentaplegic and 60A gene products expressed early in *Drosophila melanogaster* development, demonstrating evolutionary conservation of related proteins from phylogenetically distant species.

IV. ENDOCHONDRAL BONE INDUCTION BY TGF-β ISOFORMS

In the *bona fide* heterotopic assay for bone induction in rodents, the TGF-β isoforms, either purified from natural sources or expressed by recombinant techniques, do not initiate endochondral bone formation. More strikingly and recently, TGF-β isoforms themselves have shown a marked site- and tissue-specific endochondral osteoinductivity yet remarkably this occurs in primates only. Induction of osteogenic differentiation has also been shown, at least in rodents, by growth and differentiation factor-5 and Hedgehog proteins with an activity synergistically regulated and enhanced by recombinant hBMP-2.

The presence of several related but different molecular forms with osteogenic activity poses important questions about the biological significance of this apparent redundancy, additionally indicating multiple interactions during both embryonic development and bone regeneration in postnatal life. The fact that a single hBMP/OP initiates bone formation by induction does not preclude the requirement and interactions of other morphogens deployed synchronously and synergistically during the cascade of bone formation by induction, which may proceed via the combined action of several BMPs/OPs, resident within the natural milieu of the extracellular matrix of bone. Thus, it is likely that the endogenous mechanisms of bone repair and regeneration in postnatal life necessitate the deployment and concerted action of several of the BMPs/OPs resident within the natural milieu of the extracellular matrix. The presence of multiple molecular forms with bone inductive activity also points to synergistic interactions during endochondral bone formation. Indeed, a potent and accelerated synergistic induction of endochondral bone formation was shown with the binary application of recombinant or native TGF-β1 with hOP-1, in both heterotopic and orthotopic sites of primates (Fig. 1). Whether the biological activity of partially purified BMPs as shown in long-term experiments in the adult primate *P. ursinus* is the result of the sum of a plurality of BMP activities or is a truly synergistic interaction among BMP/OP family members deserves appropriate investigation. It is noteworthy, however, that in the identical orthotopic model, the long-term efficacy of single applications of gamma-irradiated hOP-1 delivered by a xenogeneic bovine collagenous matrix in regenerating large defects of membranous bone of the adult primate was demonstrated (Fig. 2). Ultimately, it will be necessary to gain insights into the potential distinct spatial and temporal patterns of expression of other BMPs/OPs during morphogenesis and regeneration elicited by a single application of hOP-1. *In vivo* studies should now design therapeutic approaches based on information about gene regulation by hOP-1.

The TGF-β isoforms are powerful inducers of endochondral bone when implanted in the *rectus abdominis* muscle of the primate *P. ursinus* at doses of 1, 5, and 25 μg per 100 mg of collagenous matrix as carrier, yielding large corticalized ossicles by day 90 (Fig. 3). Endochondral bone induction initiated by TGF-β isoforms expresses mRNA of bone induction markers including BMP-3 and OP-1. An additional and significant striking result is that the bone inductivity of TGF-β isoforms in the primate is site- and tissue-specific, with rather substantial

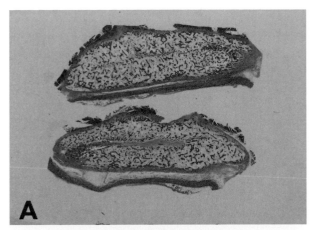

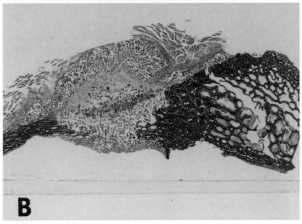

FIGURE 1 Tissue morphogenesis by binary applications of recombinant hOP-1 and TGF-β1. (A) Generation of large ossicles that formed 30 days after implantation of 25 μg hOP-1 and 1.5 μg hTGF-β1 in the *rectus abdominis* of the adult primate *Papio ursinus*. (B) Tissue induction and morphogenesis of bone on day 30 on implantation of 100 μg hOP 1 in combination with 5 μg platelet-derived porcine TGF-β1, culminating in gross displacement of the pericranial tissues. Original magnification: (A) × 3.2 (B) × 2.8.

endochondral bone induction in the *rectus abdominis* muscle but absent osteoinductivity in orthotopic sites on day 30 and limited osteogenesis in orthotopic sites on day 90 (Fig. 4).

V. GEOMETRIC INDUCTION OF BONE FORMATION

Importantly, to induce the cascade of endochondral bone differentiation, the soluble signals must be reconstituted with an insoluble signal or substratum that triggers the bone differentiation cascade. Bone regeneration in clinical contexts requires three key components: an osteoinductive signal, an insoluble substratum that delivers the signal and acts as a scaffold for the induction of new bone formation, and host recipient cells that are capable of differentiation into bone cells in response to the osteoinductive signals. All of the components are amenable to manipulation: the signals to be delivered and the nature of the carrier matrix, which additionally can be loaded with the responding cells and tissues. Although molecular biology has made quantum leaps in the mechanistic understanding of cellular and subcellular activities of soluble signals, less knowledge and fewer mechanistic insights have characterized the quest for optimal delivery systems. Such systems would include insoluble substrata that are inorganic and nonimmunogenic, carvable, and amenable to contouring for optimal adaptation to the various shapes of bone defects and initiating optimal osteogenic activity with relatively low doses of recombinant hBMPs/OPs. They would promote rapid vascular invasion, angiogenesis, and mesenchymal invasion when brought into contact with BMPs/OPs previously absorbed onto the carrier and would be capable of remodeling and resorbing once the regenerative processes are well under way. Finally, they would have optimal surface characteristics and geometric configurations, which are of critical importance in the induction of bone

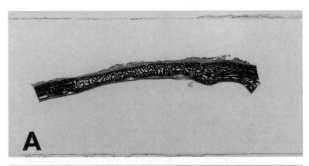

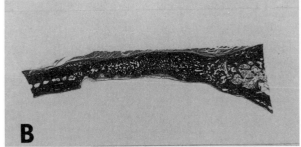

FIGURE 2 Low-power microphotographs of calvarial specimens harvested on days 90 (A) and 365 (B) from the primate *Papio ursinus*. Complete reconstruction and regeneration of the defects after implantation of doses of 0.1 (A) and 0.5 mg (B) of gamma-irradiated hOP-1 delivered by 1 g of gamma-irradiated xenogeneic bovine collagenous matrix. Original magnification: × 2.5.

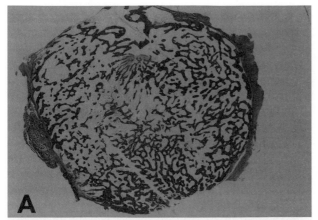

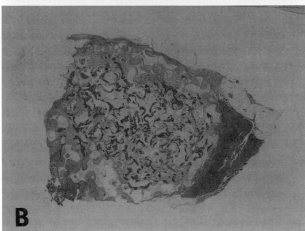

FIGURE 3 Induction of bone formation by hTGF-β2 in the *rectus abdominis* muscle of the primate *Papio ursinus* on implantation of 5 µg hTGF-β2 delivered by the insoluble collagenous matrix as carrier (A) and 1 µg hTGF-β2 delivered by sintered highly crystalline porous hydroxyapatite (B) harvested on day 90. Original magnification: × 3.5.

with and without the exogenous applications of BMPs/OPs. The critical role of the geometry of the carrier substratum in the regulation of bone differentiation has been amply documented using different geometric configurations of collagenous matrix and porous hydroxyapatites, providing evidence that tissue induction and morphogenesis can be greatly altered by the geometry of the carrier.

Since regenerative phenomena recapitulate events that occur in the normal course of embryonic development, the observed multiple patterns of expression of BMPs/OPs in developing tissues and organs may help to devise therapeutic approaches based on recapitulation of embryonic development and ample evidence is accruing regarding the efficacy and safety of two members of the BMP/OP family now available in recombinant form, hOP-1 and hBMP-2, currently the

subject of extensive preclinical and clinical research for orthopedic and craniofacial applications.

The finding that heterotopic bone induction in primates is initiated by naturally derived BMPs/OPs and TGF-βs, recombinant hBMPs/OPs and hTGF-βs, and sintered and highly crystalline hydroxyapatites with a specific geometric configuration indicates that heterotopic ossicles develop as a mosaic structure in which members of the TGF-β superfamily singly, synergistically, and synchronously initiate and maintain the developing morphological structures and play different roles at different time points of the morphogenetic cascade.

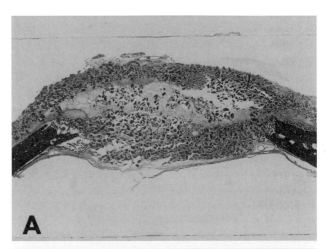

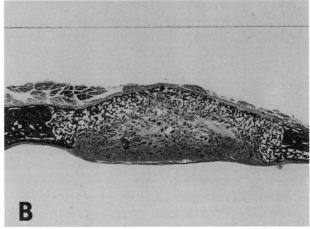

FIGURE 4 Morphology of calvarial regeneration by hTGF-β2 in conjunction with collagenous matrix as carrier. (A) Lack of bone formation on implantation of 100 µg of hTGF-β2 on day 30 with prominent mesenchymal tissue influx and displacement of the collagenous matrix. (B) Limited osteogenesis only pericranially on implantation of 100 µg hTGF-β2. Note the delicate trabeculae of newly formed bone facing scattered remnants of collagenous matrix particles, embedded in a loose but highly vascular connective tissue matrix. Original magnification: × 2.8.

Biomimetic matrices endowed with intrinsic osteoinductive activity, i.e., capable of initiating *de novo* bone formation in heterotopic sites of primates even in the absence of exogenously applied BMPs/OPs, have been developed (Fig. 5). Our findings in nonhuman primates also demonstrate extensive bone formation by hOP-1 adsorbed onto sintered porous hydroxyapatites, indicating that predictable osteogenesis in clinical contexts for the treatment of craniofacial bone defects may be engineered using inorganic, nonimmunogenic, and carvable delivery systems that initiate osteogenesis with relatively low doses of recombinant morphogens, thus mimicking the macro- and microstructures of living bone.

The use of biomimetic matrices capable of initiating bone formation via intrinsic osteoinduction is quickly altering the horizons of therapeutic osteogenesis, leading to a quantum leap in bone tissue engineering. The geometry of the substratum profoundly regulates the expression of the osteogenic phenotype and is defined as geometric induction of bone formation. The intrinsic osteoinductivity regulated by the geometry of the substratum is helping to engineer morphogenetic responses for therapeutic osteogenesis in clinical contexts.

Members of the TGF-β supergene family, BMPs/OPs and TGF-β isoforms endowed with endochondral osteoinductivity in adult primates, are helping to engineer skeletal regeneration and tissue morphogenesis in molecular terms. This prediction is based on a surprisingly simple and fascinating concept: morphogens exploited in embryonic development can be reexploited for the initiation of postnatal morphogenesis and regeneration.

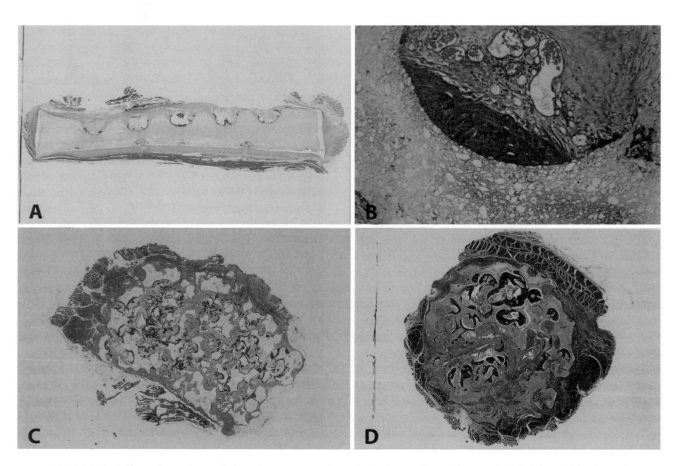

FIGURE 5   Effect of geometry of the substratum on tissue induction and morphogenesis. (A) Monolithic discs of sintered highly crystalline hydroxyapatite with concavities on both planar surfaces were implanted in the *rectus abdominis* muscle of the primate *Papio ursinus* and harvested on day 90 after surgery. Bone forms only within the concavities of the substratum. (B) Note the vascular invasion and angiogenesis close to newly formed and induced bone. (C and D) Low-power photomicrographs of sintered porous hydroxyapatite specimens harvested from the *rectus abdominis* on day 90. Note the intrinsic and spontaneous induction of bone formation within the porous spaces of the hydroxyapatite, essentially initiating in concavities of the substratum. Original magnification: × 8.

Acknowledgments

This work is supported by grants from the South African Medical Research Council, the University of the Witwatersrand, Johannesburg, the National Research Foundation, and the Council for Scientific and Industrial Research, and by *ad hoc* grants of the Bone Research Unit.

The Bone Research Unit and the Medical Research Council acknowledge the CSIR Manufacturing and Materials Technology Unit for the preparation of the sintered hydroxy-apatite implants.

Glossary

bone morphogenetic proteins/osteogenic proteins Pleiotropic glycosylated protein members of the transforming growth factor-β superfamily initiators of bone formation by induction.

intrinsic osteoinductive activity Induction of bone formation by specific geometric configurations of biomimetic matrices in the absence of exogenously applied bone morphogenetic proteins/osteogenic proteins.

transforming growth factor-βs Proteins secreted by transformed cells that can stimulate the growth of normal cells.

See Also the Following Articles

Bone Morphogenetic Proteins • Colony-Stimulating Factor-1 (CSF-1) • Thyroid Hormone Action on the Skeleton and Growth • Vitamin D and Cartilage • Vitamin D: Biological Effects of 1,25(OH)$_2$D$_3$ in Bone

Further Reading

Duneas, N., Crooks, J., and Ripamonti, U. (1998). Transforming growth factors β1: Induction of bone morphogenetic protein gene expression during endochondral bone formation in the baboon, and synergistic interaction with osteogenic protein-1 (BMP-7). *Growth Factors* **15**, 259–277.

Reddi, A. H. (1992). Regulation of cartilage and bone differentiation by bone morphogenetic proteins. *Curr. Opin. Cell. Biol.* **4**, 850–855.

Reddi, A. H. (2000). Morphogenesis and tissue engineering of bone and cartilage: Inductive signals, stem cells, and biomimetic biomaterials. *Tissue Eng.* **6**, 351–359.

Ripamonti, U., and Duneas, N. (1998). Tissue morphogenesis and regeneration by bone morphogenetic proteins. *Plast. Reconstr. Surg.* **101**, 227–239.

Ripamonti, U., and Reddi, A. H. (1997). Tissue engineering, morphogenesis and regeneration of the periodontal tissues by bone morphogenetic proteins. *Crit. Rev. Oral Biol. Med.* **8**, 154–163.

Ripamonti, U., and Vukicevic, S. (1995). Bone morphogenetic proteins: From developmental biology to molecular therapeutics. *S. Afr. J. Sci.* **91**, 277–280.

Ripamonti, U., Crooks, J., and Kirkbride, A. N. (1999). Sintered porous hydroxyapatites with intrinsic osteoinductive activity: Geometric induction of bone formation. *S. Afr. J. Sci.* **95**, 335–343.

Ripamonti, U., Crooks, J., Matsaba, T., and Tasker, J. (2000). Induction of endochondral bone formation by recombinant human transforming growth factor-β2 in the baboon (*Papio ursinus*). *Growth Factors* **17**, 269–285.

Ripamonti, U., Duneas, N., van den Heever, B., Bosch, C., and Crooks, J. (1997). Recombinant transforming growth factor-β1 induces endochondral bone in the baboon and synergizes with recombinant osteogenic protein-1 (bone morphogenetic protein-7) to initiate rapid bone formation. *J. Bone Miner. Res.* **12**, 1584–1595.

Ripamonti, U., Ramoshebi, L. N., Matsaba, T., Tasker, J., Crooks, J., and Teare, J. (2001). Bone induction by BMPs/OPs and related family members in primates. The critical role of delivery systems. *J. Bone Joint Surg. Am.* **83A**, S1116–S1127.

Ripamonti U., Teare J., Matsaba T., Renton L (2001). Site, tissue and organ specificity of endochondral bone induction and morphogenesis by TGF-β isoforms in the primate *Papio ursinus*. Proceedings of the FASEB Summer Conference: The TGF-β superfamily: Signaling and development, Tucson, Arizona, USA, July 7–12.

Ripamonti, U., van den Heever, B., Crooks, J., Tucker, M. M., Sampath, T. K., Rueger, D. C., and Reddi, A. H. (2000). Long-term evaluation of bone formation by osteogenic protein-1 in the baboon and relative efficacy of bone-derived bone morphogenetic proteins delivered by irradiated xenogeneic collagenous matrices. *J. Bone Miner. Res.* **15**, 1798–1809.

Wozney, J. M. (1992). The bone morphogenetic protein family and osteogenesis. *Mol. Reprod. Dev.* **32**, 160–167.

Osteoporosis: Hormonal Treatment

NORMAN H. BELL

Medical University of South Carolina

I. ESTROGEN
II. RALOXIFENE
III. SALMON CALCITONIN
IV. PARATHYROID HORMONE (1–34)
V. SUMMARY

Estrogen, raloxifene, nasal salmon calcitonin, and parathyroid hormone (1–34) are the only hormones or hormonal analogues that have been approved by the Food and Drug Administration (FDA) for the treatment of osteoporosis in the United States.

I. ESTROGEN

It is well established that estrogen deficiency at the time of menopause leads to increases in skeletal remodeling and the rate of bone loss and, in some patients, to osteoporosis and fractures. It is also well established that restoration of estrogen levels via hormone replacement therapy (HRT) reduces skeletal remodeling and not only prevents bone loss but increases bone mineral density (BMD). Whether estrogen prevents fractures, however, is controversial. Analysis of the Study of Osteoporosis Fracture indicated that current estrogen use was associated with a 61% decrease in the incidence of fractures of the wrist and a 34% decrease in nonvertebral fractures. The incidence of hip fractures was significantly reduced in current users by 61% but only when HRT was begun within 5 years of menopause. In an open, randomized, placebo-controlled study from Finland of women treated with HRT beginning shortly after menopause, the incidence of nonvertebral fractures was significantly reduced by 61%. On the other hand, the incidence of fractures was not reduced by HRT in a prospective, double-blind, placebo-controlled study in postmenopausal women less than 90 years of age.

Earlier epidemiological studies indicated that HRT prevents myocardial infarctions and fatal heart attacks in postmenopausal women. However, the recent prospective, randomized, placebo-controlled Heart and Estrogen/Progestin Replacement Study in postmenopausal women with established heart disease found that the incidence of cardiovascular events was not different in HRT- and placebo-treated groups even though there was an 11% reduction in low-density lipoprotein cholesterol and a 10% increase in high-density lipoprotein cholesterol in the HRT-treated group. Previous to these findings, estrogen was considered to be effective with regard to treatment of coronary artery disease. In view of these findings, the use of HRT for prevention of coronary artery disease is no longer recommended. This recommendation has been confirmed. Recently, the Women's Health Initiative, a prospective, randomized clinical trial with conjugated equine estrogen and medroxyprogesterone acetate in 16,608 postmenopausal women, had to be stopped after 5.2 years because it was found that per 10,000 person years there were 7 more events of cardiovascular disease, 8 more strokes, 8 more pulmonary emboli, 8 more invasive breast cancers, 6 fewer colorectal cancers, and 5 fewer hip fractures in the patients than in the controls. Thus, the risks exceed the benefits from use of combined estrogen and progestin treatment in postmenopausal women.

II. RALOXIFENE

Raloxifene is a member of a group of drugs known as selective estrogen receptor modulators (SERMs) that have a more favorable therapeutic profile than estrogen. Raloxifene is an agonist for bone but, unlike estrogen, is an antagonist for breast and uterine tissue. It is therefore safer than HRT. Raloxifene modestly reduces bone turnover and increases BMD and significantly decreased the incidence of fractures of the spine by 30% (at 30 mg/day) and by 50% (at 60 mg/day) in postmenopausal women. In preliminary studies, it reduced the incidence of breast cancer in postmenopausal women. Raloxifene is undergoing a large clinical trial, Study of Raloxifene and Tamoxifen, for comparison with tamoxifen, the current drug of choice, to determine its efficacy in the prevention of breast cancer. Whether raloxifene prevents coronary heart disease is not known. This question is being addressed in another large clinical trial.

III. SALMON CALCITONIN

In the Prevent Recurrence of Osteoporotic Fractures study, nasal salmon calcitonin at 200 IU daily modestly reduced skeletal remodeling and increased BMD of the spine and significantly reduced the incidence of vertebral fractures by 33% in postmenopausal women. Nasal salmon calcitonin was ineffective in this regard at daily doses of 100 and 400 IU. Nevertheless, the drug is approved for treatment of postmenopausal osteoporosis.

IV. PARATHYROID HORMONE (1–34)

Daily injections of parathyroid hormone (1–34) for less than 2 years significantly increased BMD and reduced the incidence of vertebral fractures by more than 60% and of nonvertebral fractures by more than 50% in postmenopausal women with one or more prevalent fractures. Parathyroid hormone (1–34) given by daily injection is anabolic for the skeleton and does not cause bone resorption.

V. SUMMARY

Estrogen, raloxifene (a SERM), salmon calcitonin, and parathyroid hormone (1–34) are four hormones or hormonal analogues that have been approved for the treatment of osteoporosis. Each was shown to decrease skeletal remodeling and increase BMD by inhibiting bone resorption. Whether estrogen prevents fractures as well as coronary artery disease, however, has not been established. These questions may be answered by results of the Women's Health Initiative. Raloxifene was shown to diminish the incidence of vertebral fractures and has the advantage of inhibiting the growth of breast and uterine cancer and uterine tissue. It may prove useful for the treatment of breast cancer. Nasal salmon calcitonin at a dose of 200 IU daily was shown to reduce the incidence of vertebral fractures but doses of 100 and 400 IU daily were ineffective. Parathyroid hormone (1–34), an anabolic peptide, diminished the rate of both vertebral and nonvertebral fractures when given by daily injection.

Glossary

osteoporosis A bone disease in which decreased bone mass and alteration in microarchitecture result in increased skeletal fragility and risk of fracture. It occurs in postmenopausal women as a consequence of estrogen deficiency.

parathyroid hormone (1–34) The N-terminal biologically active portion of parathyroid hormone, which is produced by the parathyroid glands and increases bone resorption and tubular reabsorption of calcium by the kidney.

raloxifene A selective estrogen receptor modulator that is an agonist for bone and, unlike estrogen, is an antagonist for uterine and breast tissue.

salmon calcitonin A hormone produced by the parafollicular C cells of the thyroid gland; it inhibits osteoclastic bone resorption and tubular reabsorption of calcium by the kidney. Salmon calcitonin has a different structure than human calcitonin and is more potent.

selective estrogen receptor modulator A drug that has a profile that is similar to or different than that of estrogen with regard to being an agonist or antagonist for skeletal, uterine, breast and other tissues.

See Also the Following Articles

Aromatase and Estrogen Insufficiency • Calcitonin • Estrogen and Progesterone Receptors in Breast Cancer • Estrogen Receptor Biology and Lessons from Knockout Mice • Osteoporosis: Pathophysiology • Parathyroid Hormone • SERMs (Selective Estrogen Receptor Modulators)

Further Reading

Bryant, H. U. (2001). Mechanism of action and preclinical profile of raloxifene: A selective estrogen receptor modulator. *Rev. Endocrinol. Metab. Dis.* **2**, 129–138.

Cauley, J. A., Black, D. M., Barrett-Connor, E., Harris, F., Shields, K., Applegate, W., and Cummings, S. R. (2001). Effects of hormone replacement therapy on clinical fractures and height loss: The Heart and Estrogen/Progestin Replacement Study (HERS). *Am. J. Med.* **110**, 442–450.

Cauley, J. A., Seeley, D. G., Ensrud, K., Ettinger, B., Black, D., and Cummings, S. R. (1995). Estrogen replacement therapy and fractures in older women. *Ann. Int. Med.* **122**, 9–16.

Chesnut, C. H., III, Silverman, S., Andriano, K., Genant, H., Gimona, A., Harris, S., Kiel, D., Le-Buff, M., Maricic, M., Miller, P., Moniz, C., Peacock, M., Richardson, P., Watts, N., and Baylink, D. (2000). A randomized trail of nasal spray salmon calcitonin in postmenopausal women with established osteoporosis: The prevent recurrence of osteoporotic fractures study. PROOF Study Group. *Am. J. Med.* **109**, 267–276.

Delmas, P. D., Bjarnason, N. H., Mitlak, B. H., Ravoux, A. C., Shah, A. S., Huster, W. J., Draper, M., and Christiansen, C. (1997). Effects of raloxifene on bone mineral density, serum cholesterol concentrations and uterine endometrium in postmenopausal women. *N. Engl. J. Med.* **337**, 1641–1747.

Draper, M. W., Flowers, D. E., Huster, W. J., Neild, J. A., Harper, K. D., and Arnaud, C. (1996). A controlled trial of raloxifene HCl: Impact on bone turnover and serum lipid profile in healthy postmenopausal women. *J. Bone Miner. Res.* **11**, 835–892.

Ettinger, B., Black, D. M., Mitlak, B. H., Knickerbocker, R., Nickelsen, T., Genant, H. K., Christianson, C., Delmas, P. D., Sanchetta, J. R., Stakkestad, J., Gluer, C. C., Krueger, K., Cohen, F. J., Eckert, S., Ensrud, K. E., Avioli, L. V., Lips, P., and Cummings, S. R. (1999). Reduction of vertebral fracture risk in postmenopausal women with osteoporosis treated with raloxifene. *J. Am. Med. Assoc.* **282**, 637–645.

Hully, S., Grady, D., and Bush, T. (1998). Randomized trial of estrogen plus progestin for secondary prevention of coronary heart disease in postmenopausal women. *J. Am. Med. Assoc.* **280**, 605–613.

Journal of the American Medical Association (2002). Risk and benefits of estrogen plus progestin in healthy postmenopausal women: Principal results from the Women's Health Initiative randomized controlled trial. *J. Am. Med. Assoc.* **288**, 321–333.

Komulainen, M., Kröger, H., Tuppurainen, M. T., Heikkinen, A.-M., Alhava, E., Honkanen, R., and Saarikoski, S. (1998). HRT and Vit. D in prevention of non-vertebral fractures in postmenopausal women: A 5 year randomized trial. *Maturitas* **31**, 45–54.

Lufkin, E. G., Wahner, H. W., O'Fallon, W. M., Hodgson, S. F., Kotowitz, M. A., and Lane, A. W. (1998). Treatment of postmenopausal osteoporosis with transdermal estrogen. *Ann. Int. Med.* **44**, 131–136.

Neer, R. M., Arnaud, C. D., Sanchetta, J. R., Prince, R., Gaich, G. A., Reginster, J. V., Hodsman, A. B., Eriksen, E. F., Ish-Shalom, S., Genant, H. K., Wang, O., and Mitlak, B. H. (2001). Effect of parathyroid hormone (1–34) on fractures and bone mineral density in postmenopausal women with osteoporosis. *N. Engl. J. Med.* **344**, 1341–1434.

Reginster, J.-Y., Bruyere, O., Audran, M., Avouac, B., Body, J.-J., Bonvenot, G., Brandi, M. L., Gennari, C., Kaufman, J.-M., Lemmel, E.-M., Vanhaelst, L., Weryha, G. J., and Devogelaer, J. P. (2000). Do estrogens effectively prevent osteoporosis-related fractures? *Calcif. Tissue Int.* **67**, 191–194.

Osteoporosis: Pathophysiology

J. Christopher Gallagher and Prema B. Rapuri

Creighton University

Osteoporosis is a bone disorder characterized by bone fractures, primarily in the elderly, as a result of decreased bone mass density and deteriorated bone tissue microarchitecture. Increased longevity and an ever-enlarging aging population contribute to a growing population of osteoporotic patients. Understanding the mechanism and pathophysiology of osteoporosis is important in the process of developing successful therapeutic interventions.

I. INTRODUCTION

Osteoporosis is now recognized as a major metabolic bone disease affecting elderly subjects, often leading to permanent disability and nursing home admissions. The incidence of osteoporosis is increasing by about 30% each decade, in part because of the increase in the aging population. The classification of osteoporosis is still limited by our lack of knowledge about its pathogencsis, although there have been large strides forward in understanding the bone remodeling process. Though there are currently several effective therapies for osteoporosis, new treatments can be expected to emerge as the bone remodeling process is elucidated. Expectations are strong for therapies that actually build new bone and completely reverse osteoporosis.

II. DEFINITION OF OSTEOPOROSIS

The syndrome of postmenopausal osteoporosis was first described by Albright, and referred to women with vertebral fractures. This traditional description has been retained but refined; osteoporosis is now described as a skeletal disorder characterized by reduced bone mass and deterioration of bone microarchitecture, leading to increased fracture risk. Osteoporotic fractures are most common in the hip, vertebrae, and radius.

Based on the well-documented inverse relationship between bone mineral density (BMD) and fracture risk, new diagnostic criteria for osteoporosis have been proposed by a World Health Organization (WHO) study group. Based on these criteria (Table 1), osteoporosis is defined as a BMD of the spine and/or proximal femur that is more than 2.5 standard deviations (SDs) below normal mean premenopausal peak bone mass. Patients with BMD 1.0–2.5 SDs below the mean peak bone mass of healthy young adults are described as osteopenic. The presence of osteopenia predisposes an individual to increased fracture risk. The term "established osteoporosis" is used to describe a situation in which one or more fragility fractures occur in addition to low BMD. However, these criteria were derived using the mean bone density values of young, adult white women determined by dual-energy X-ray absorptiometry (DXA) of the hip and so are of limited use for men, children, women of other ethnic groups and for BMD measurements at other skeletal sites. Because BMD at any age is related to peak bone mass, the BMD value is expressed as a T score (1 T = 1 SD).

TABLE 1 Definition of Osteoporosis Based on World Health Organization Criteria[a]

Category	Bone mineral density[b]	T score
Normal	≤1 SD below average peak BMD of young adult	
Osteopenia	1.0–2.5 SD below average peak BMD of young adult	−1 to −2.5
Osteoporosis	≥2.5 SD below the mean BMD of young adult	≥ −2.5
Established osteoporosis	≥2.5 SD below the mean BMD of young adult and history of nontraumatic fracture	≥ −2.5

[a]From The WHO study group. Assessment of fracture risk and its application to screening for postmenopausal osteoporosis. Report of a WHO study group. WHO Technical Report Series, No. 8431994. Geneva, World Health Organization (1994).

[b]BMD, Bone mineral density; SD, standard deviation.

III. CLASSIFICATION OF OSTEOPOROSIS

Osteoporosis can be categorized into primary and secondary forms based on the absence or presence of associated medical diseases that predispose to bone loss. Primary osteoporosis is the most common form and is due to age-related loss of bone from the skeleton. Secondary osteoporosis is associated with specific defined clinical disorders that lead to osteoporosis; some of the well-known disorders are given in Table 2.

In 1947, Albright divided osteoporotic patients into postmenopausal and senile groups. He clearly implicated the role of estrogen deficiency in postmenopausal osteoporosis. More recently, based on pathogenic mechanisms, Riggs and Melton used a new terminology: Type I, for postmenopausal osteoporosis, and Type II, for senile osteoporosis. This classification of Riggs and Melton does not include patients with osteoporosis resulting from other diseases and conditions. Appropriately, this latter group of osteoporotics has been classified as Type III. Type I osteoporosis characteristically affects women within 15 to 20 years of menopause, presents principally with vertebral crush fractures and Colle's fractures of distal forearm, and is due mainly to trabecular bone loss as a consequence of estrogen deficiency. Type II (age-related osteoporosis) occurs in both men and women 75 years of age and older and is usually manifested by hip and vertebral fractures. Type II osteoporosis is believed to be mainly due to age-related trabecular and cortical bone loss. Type III osteoporosis, or secondary osteoporosis, occurs in both men and women and is caused by a specific defined clinical disorder or medical treatment. A brief summary of the main features of these three osteoporotic types is shown in Table 3.

IV. PEAK BONE MASS

Peak bone mass can be defined as the maximum level of bone mass attained in an individual as a result of normal growth. It is usually achieved in the first few years of the second decade of life, the early 20s. It is one of the two principal factors that determine lifelong skeletal health, the other being the bone loss. High peak bone mass provides a larger reserve later in life and offers a protective advantage when bone density declines as a result of aging or other causes. Achievement of peak bone mass is mainly determined by genetics, but nutritional, hormonal, and environmental factors and mechanical loading also influence bone mass.

Data from twin studies suggest that BMD at a number of skeletal sites has a strong genetic component and it is estimated that about 60–80% of peak bone mass is determined genetically. Family studies also provide evidence for a genetic impact on BMD; daughters of women with osteoporosis have a lower BMD than do daughters of women with a normal BMD. Another approach to identify specific genes that influence peak bone mass is to use the candidate gene approach. Using this approach, allelic variation in the vitamin D receptor was first shown to be associated with BMD. The association studies have expanded to other candidate genes known to play a role in normal bone physiology. Common allelic variations in the genes of collagen type Iα1, transforming growth factor-β (TGF-β), interleukin-6 (IL-6), and estrogen receptor have also been found to be associated with BMD in diverse populations. However, results of the association studies have been highly inconsistent. Recently, in a single extended pedigree, Johnson *et al.* reported the linkage of a genetic locus (named HBM, for high bone mass) in the human genome to a phenotype of very high spinal bone density. This HBM phenotype was further demonstrated to be due to a mutation in the low-density lipoprotein receptor-related protein 5 gene (LRP5). However, this mutation was not found in osteoporotic patients. There are probably several other major genes involved in the determination of bone mass.

Calcium is an important nutrient for attaining the peak bone mass. Higher calcium intake during skeletal growth period helps in achieving optimal

TABLE 2 Major Causes of Secondary (Type III) Osteoporosis

Drug use	Corticosteriods
	Anticonvulsants
	Radiotherapy
	Heparin
Gastrointestinal	Malabsorption syndromes
	Primary biliary cirrhosis
Blood diseases	Myeloma
	Thalassemia
	Skeletal metastases
Endocrine	Thyrotoxicosis
	Cushing's syndrome
	Turner's/Klinefelter's syndrome
	Primary hyperparathyroidism
Others	Immobilization
	Transplantation
	Alcoholism
	Chronic renal failure
	Osteogenesis imperfecta

TABLE 3   Classification of Osteoporotic Types[a]

Factor	Type I (postmenopausal)	Type II (senile)	Type III (secondary)
Age	55–70	75–90	Any age
Years past menopause	5–15	25–40	Any age
Sex ratio (F:M)	20:1	2:1	1:1
Fracture site	Spine	Hip, spine, pelvis, humerus	Spine, hip, peripheral
Bone loss			
Trabecular	+++	++	+++
Cortical	+	++	+++
Contributing factor			
Menopause	+++	++	++
Age	+	+++	++
Biochemistry			
Parathyroid hormone	↓	↑	↓↑
$1,25(OH)_2 D_3$	↓	↓	↓↑
Calcium absorption	↓	↓	↓
1α-Hydroxylase response to parathyroid hormone	↑	↓	?

[a] Adapted from Gallagher (1992) with permission from W.B. Saunders Company.

peak mass. Endocrine reproductive status affects peak bone mass, because early menarche, pregnancy, and the use of oral contraceptive pills are associated with higher bone mass. Sex steroids, estrogen and testosterone, contribute to sexual dimorphism of the skeleton and lead to increased growth velocity at puberty and cessation of linear growth. Increase in bone mass during adolescence results from increases in bone length, bone diameter, cortical bone width, and cancellous bone density. Smoking and alcohol consumption during adolescence and early adult life may have an adverse effect on peak bone mass. Similarly, exercise also modifies bone mass and bone quality through an effect of mechanical loading on the skeleton. Optimum calcium intake and exercise during the early 20s may increase peak bone mass by about 0.5 standard deviations.

V. MODELING AND REMODELING OF BONE

The adult skeleton is a dynamic tissue that remodels throughout life by a coordinated action of osteoblasts, osteoclasts, and osteocytes. It is composed of 80% cortical (compact) bone and 20% cancellous (trabecular) bone. Bone modeling involves both growth and shaping of bones and occurs during the first 20 years of life in humans. The process of bone modeling involves both bone formation and resorption, the former exceeding the latter. Once the initial modeling and growth of bone are completed, bone is then renewed throughout life by a process known as remodeling. A typical remodeling sequence lasts several months.

It involves an initial state of activation of bone resorption lasting several days, creating a cavity. Once the resorption cavity has been completed, osteoblasts immediately enter the cavity and fill in the space with new bone. This process lasts several weeks and further consolidation occurs over a period of several months. This process of remodeling represents the way that older bone is replaced and renewed with new bone (Fig. 1). It may be that the initial impetus for remodeling of bone is the presence of microfractures, which occur as a result of strain and stress.

The first event during bone remodeling is osteoclast activation followed by osteoclast formation, resorption, and ultimately apoptosis. The major systemic hormones involved in osteoclast activity are parathyroid hormone (PTH), 1,25-dihydroxyvitamin D_3 [$1,25(OH)_2D_3$], sex steroids, and glucocorticoids. None of these hormones appears to act directly on osteoclasts to stimulate resorption, and, in fact, at the present time only calcitonin has been shown to bind directly to receptors on osteoclasts. These hormones do not directly stimulate the osteoclasts but bring about their effects by causing release of a number of other factors generated by osteoblast-like cells. Local hormones may be more important than systemic hormones for the initiation of bone resorption and for normal bone remodeling. Because remodeling occurs in discrete and distinct packets throughout the skeleton, factors generated locally in the microenvironment of bone govern the cellular events. Some of the local cytokines known to be involved in osteoclast activation are tumor

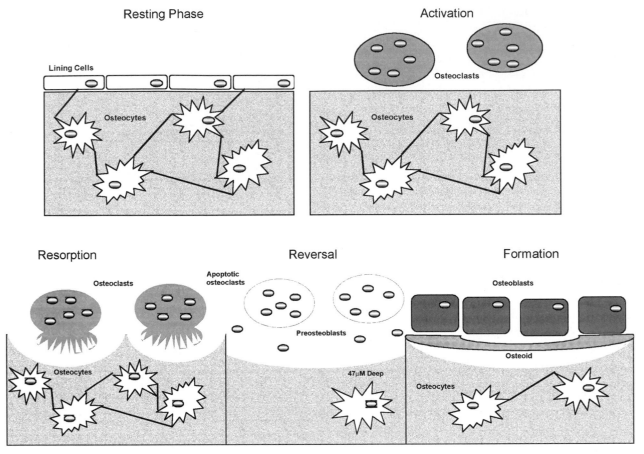

FIGURE 1 Bone remodeling.

necrosis factor (TNF), interleukins (IL-1, IL-6, and IL-18), interferon γ, TGF-β, and colony-stimulating factor (CSF). Some of these factors stimulate osteoclast activity whereas others inhibit the activity. Stimulation of osteoclast activity involves enhancement of proliferation of osteoclast progenitors, differentiation of committed precursors into mature cells, and activation of mature multinucleated cells to resorb bone. Inhibition of osteoclast activity involves blocking proliferation of precursors, inhibiting the differentiation or fusion, and inactivating the mature multinucleated resorbing cells. Current evidence indicates that most factors that stimulate or inhibit osteoclasts act on at least two of these steps. Three new proteins, which are responsible for the interaction between the cells of osteoblastic and osteoclastic lineages and are considered as the final effectors of osteoclast differentiation, have recently been identified. These proteins belong to the family of tumor necrosis factor receptor and have been referred to by different names by different investigators. It has been recommended by a committee that the ligand

(osteoblast-derived paracrine factor) be referred to as receptor activator of nuclear factor κB ligand (RANKL), the receptor on the osteoclast as RANK, and the decoy receptor as osteoprotegerin (OPG). The synonyms for RANK ligand include TNF-related activation-induced cytokine (TRANCE), osteoclast differentiation factor (ODF), and osteoprotegerin ligand (OPGL). The interaction of RANKL and RANK stimulates all aspects of osteoclast function. OPG, produced by cells of osteoblast lineage, acts as a decoy receptor for TRANCE, blocking its interaction with RANK and inhibiting osteoclast formation.

The formation phase of the remodeling sequence involves sequential changes in cells in osteoblast lineage, including osteoblast chemotaxis, proliferation, and differentiation. The formation of mineralized bone follows, and once the new bone is formed, osteoblastic activity ceases. The proliferation and differentiation of osteoblast precursors are also controlled by local osteoblast growth factors. The prominent factors include members of the TGF-β superfamily (TGF-β1 and TGF-β2), platelet-derived growth factor (PDGF), heparin-binding fibroblast growth factor, insulin-like growth factor-I and -II (IGF-I and IGF-II), and bone morphogenetic protein-2 (BMP-2). All of these factors, specifically the TGF-β superfamily members, are important in the coupling that links bone formation to prior bone resorption. The release of local cytokines in the bone remodeling process is another example of autocrine and paracrine control mechanisms.

VI. BONE LOSS

Peak bone mass throughout the skeleton is reached in the late teens, but there is probably a small amount of further consolidation during the next 5 years, which may increase bone density by 3–5%. However, at the radius, a continuous increase is seen in cortical bone mass up to age 40. At the femur and tibia, and to a lesser extent from the trochanter, bone loss starts immediately after peak bone mass has been achieved and proceeds at a rate of 0.5% per year. This loss, however, varies considerably from person to person, starts at different periods of life, and occurs at different rates throughout the skeleton. About 30% of the decrease in BMD of the femoral neck and Ward's triangle in the proximal femur occurs during premenopausal age. At the time of menopause, the bone loss accelerates for a period of 5 to 7 years, and this early postmenopausal phase bone loss is responsible for about one-third of the total lifetime bone loss. Over a 50- to 60-year age span, this steady loss leads to a reduction of about 40% in the bone density of the femoral neck. In contrast, BMD of the spine shows no significant bone loss prior to menopause. At the time of menopause, there is a rapid loss of bone from the vertebral body and about 50% of the lifetime trabecular bone loss occurs within the first 10 years after menopause. Other sites in the body, such as the radius or the humerus, or the total body, also show predominantly menopausal changes in the pattern of bone loss.

Various regions of the skeleton differ in the proportion of cortical and trabecular bone. The variable rates of bone loss that are seen in different regions of the skeleton can be explained by the fact that the trabecular bone has a large surface area for resorption and shows a greater susceptibility to estrogen deficiency at menopause. In cortical bone, resorption occurs primarily at the endosteal surface. In general, the spine is a more hormone-dependent bone than is the femur, while other aging factors are more important in the pathogenesis of bone loss from the proximal femur (neck and trochanter). Thus, up to age 60, 90% of the bone loss in the spine and 40% of bone loss in the femoral neck are due to estrogen deficiency. By the age 85 years, age-related factors cause 75% of femoral neck bone loss and 50% of spine bone loss, whereas estrogen deficiency causes 25% of femoral neck loss and 50% of spine loss.

VII. PATHOGENESIS OF BONE LOSS

Bone loss results as a consequence of an imbalance in the remodeling process whereby the resorption of the bone occurs at a higher rate than the formation, leading to a net decrease in bone density. The age-related bone loss of 0.5% per year occurring before menopause is most likely due to less efficient matrix synthesis by osteoblasts. Immediately following menopause, there is a dramatic increase in bone remodeling process due to estrogen deficiency. The biochemical markers of bone resorption and formation, such as urine cross-links, hydroxyproline, plasma tartrate acid phosphatase, and osteocalcin, are elevated twofold, suggesting an increase in the number of remodeling sites. Usually, bone formation and resorption are coupled efficiently so that bone mass is maintained. However, after menopause, the increase in bone formation is not sufficient to match the increased resorption activity, resulting in a rapid net loss of bone during these years. In bone regions that are primarily trabecular in nature, menopause-induced (estrogen-deficient) bone loss is an important cause of bone loss during the first decade after menopause. Overall, the intensive resorption process after menopause initially leads to thinning of the trabelcula elements, but after several years the trabeculae eventually become completely eroded from continuous resorption, leading to trabecular perforation, loss of continuity of bone structure, and structural damage. During the first phase of trabecular thinning, it is possible to stop resorption and return bone mass to normal, but in the second phase, the antiresorptive agents can only prevent further bone loss.

The mechanism by which estrogen deficiency leads to rapid bone loss is beginning to be clearer. Recent work on the physiology of bone remodeling has further clarified the role of estrogen in maintaining bone health and has provided more evidence for the implication of cytokines in postmenopausal bone loss. Available data suggest that IL-1 and TNF are the main causative agents underlying the bone loss induced by estrogen deficiency, mainly by up-regulating osteoclast formation and activation (Fig. 2). Menopause increases the monocytic production of IL-1 and TNF, which stimulates bone marrow

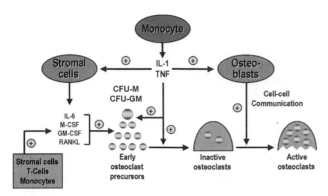

FIGURE 2 Osteoclastic differentiation and activation in estrogen deficiency. IL-1, Interleukin-1; TNF, tumor necrosis factor; CFU-M and CFU-GM, colony-forming units of monocytes, macrophages, and granulocytes; RANKL, receptor activator of nuclear factor κB ligand. Reproduced from *J. Bone Miner. Res.* **11**, 1043–1051 (1996), with permission of the American Society for Bone and Mineral Research.

stromal cells, or their osteoblast progeny, to release factors [IL-6, IL-11, granulocyte/macrophage colony-stimulating factor (GM-CSF), monocyte/macrophage colony-stimulating factor (M-CSF), and RANKL]. These factors in turn stimulate the proliferation of hematopoietic osteoclast precursor cells originating from cells of granulocyte/macrophage colony-forming units (GM-CFUs) and monocyte/macrophage colony-forming units (M-CFUs) lineage. Osteoclast

precursors differentiate into mature inactive osteoclasts in response to IL-1 and TNF. Osteoclast activation is rapidly induced by IL-1, TNF, and RANKL.

Following the initial rapid phase of bone loss after menopause, bone loss continues with age at a slower pace. This late phase of bone loss in women is thought predominantly to be due to age-related factors such as secondary hyperparathyroidism, impaired osteoblast function due to changes in local systemic growth factors or cytokines, and, in some elderly patients, nutrition deficiency of vitamin D. In men, the age-related bone loss is believed to be due to the same age-related factors. Recent evidence suggests that estrogen deficiency is also an important contributor to the late phase of bone loss in both women and men.

VIII. PATHOPHYSIOLOGY IN RELATION TO TYPE OF OSTEOPOROSIS

A. Postmenopausal Osteoporosis (Type I)

Type I osteoporosis (Fig. 3) occurs predominantly in women in the mid-60 age group and is presented primarily as crush fractures of the spine and Colle's fractures. It is associated mainly with the bone loss of trabecular rather than cortical bone, which occurs within 5–15 years of menopause. The spine BMD in these patients is usually more than 2 SDs below the

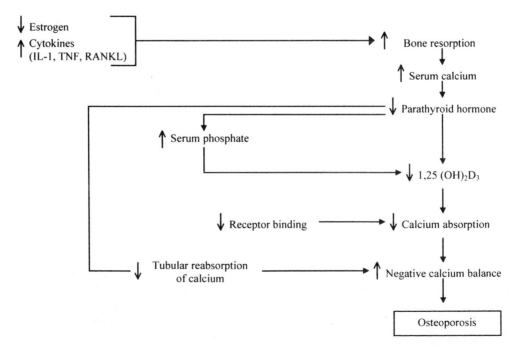

FIGURE 3 Pathogenesis of Type I osteoporosis. IL-1, Interleukin-1; TNF, tumor necrosis factor; RANKL, receptor activator of nuclear factor κB ligand. Adapted from Gallagher (1992) with permission from W.B. Saunders Company.

mean for their age. Histomorphometry of iliac crest biopsies show a reduced bone volume, and about 25% of patients show high bone resorption rates. The rate of bone loss can be anywhere between 1 and 10% per year in the first few years of menopause, and it is likely that women with high rates of bone loss are the ones who develop the fractures due to high-level trabecular bone loss. Another possibility is that these women reach menopause with low peak bone mass, and the menopause-induced bone loss makes them more prone to fractures.

Estrogen deficiency is thought to be the primary factor that underlies Type I osteoporosis. Estrogen deficiency, mediated by changes in cytokines, alleviates bone loss by up-regulating osteoclast formation and activation. The increase in bone resorption is believed to increase serum calcium marginally, which in turn decreases the PTH secretion. The decrease in serum PTH levels down-regulates the production of $1,25(OH)_2 D_3$ and increases renal calcium excretion. A decrease in circulating $1,25(OH)_2 D_3$ also results in impaired calcium absorption, which further increases the bone loss.

B. Senile Osteoporosis (Type II)

Type II (senile) osteoporosis (Fig. 4) occurs both in men and in women who are more than 75 years old. In Type II osteoporosis, there is cortical and trabecular bone loss and the patients present with fractures of the hip, pelvis, humerus, and vertebrae.

Age-related physiological changes contribute to the pathogenesis of Type II osteoporosis. Malabsorption of calcium is quite common in the elderly patient, in part due to low circulating levels of $1,25(OH)_2 D_3$. However, there is evidence for intestinal resistance to endogenous $1,25(OH)_2 D_3$, which results in secondary hyperparathyroidism. Vitamin D deficiency due to inadequate exposure to sunlight or to low dietary intakes of vitamin D and calcium is also common in elderly people who are housebound, and this can contribute to malabsorption of calcium, secondary hyperparathyroidism, and osteomalacia once serum $25OH D_3$ levels fall below 12 ng/ml (30 nmol/liter). The decreased ability of the aging kidney to produce $1,25(OH)_2 D_3$ is another factor responsible for decreased calcium absorption. The decrease in calcium absorption leads to negative calcium balance, which stimulates parathyroid function, which in turn promotes further bone loss.

Recent evidence, however, suggests that low circulating levels of estrogens in the elderly are also important in the pathogenesis of Type II osteoporosis. It has been demonstrated that in women 65 or older with undetectable serum estradiol concentrations (< 5 pg/ml), there is accelerated bone loss and an increased relative risk of 2.5 for subsequent hip or

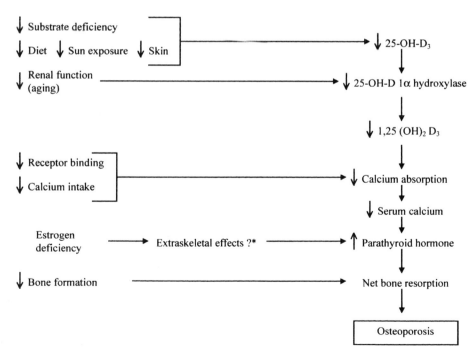

FIGURE 4 Pathogenesis of Type II osteoporosis. The asterisk indicates unitary hypothesis. Adapted from Gallagher (1992) with permission from W.B. Saunders Company.

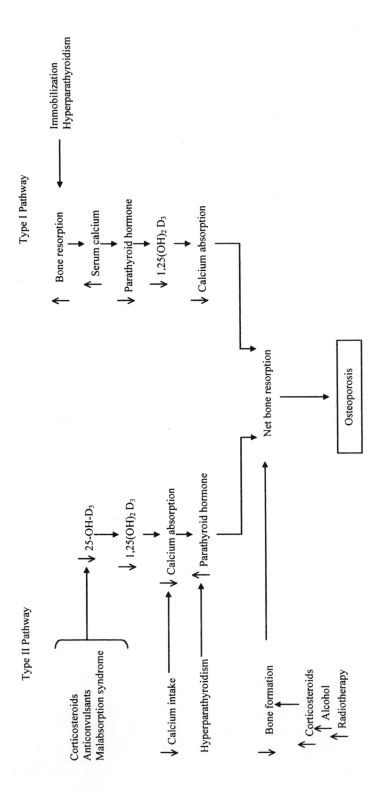

FIGURE 5 Pathogenesis of Type III osteoporosis. Adapted from Gallagher (1992) with permission from W.B. Saunders Company.

vertebral fractures. High serum concentrations of sex hormone-binding globulin, which binds estradiol and decreases its bioavailability, have also been reported to be associated with increased bone loss and increased risk of hip (relative risk of 2.0) and vertebral (relative risk of 2.3) fractures. Further evidence for the role of endogenous estrogens in age-related bone loss is provided by Heshmati *et al.*, who found an increase in bone resorption markers in older postmenopausal women after reducing the already low levels of serum estrogen to near undetectable levels with an aromatase inhibitor, letrozole. Based on this evidence, a unitary model has been proposed, which suggests that estrogen deficiency is the cause for both Type I and Type II osteoporosis. However, this hypothesis needs to be substantiated further.

C. Secondary Osteoporosis (Type III)

Secondary osteoporosis (Fig. 5) is used to describe osteoporosis that can be attributed to specific diseases, surgical procedures, and use of certain drugs. As a result of any of these conditions, Type III patients demonstrate accelerated bone loss, leading to vertebral or hip fracture. Type III osteoporosis can occur equally in men and women and at any age. Vertebral fractures in 20–35% of women and 40–55% men are accounted for by secondary osteoporosis. Some of the common conditions that lead to osteoporosis include hormonal imbalances (Cushing syndrome, thyrotoxicosis, and primary hyperparathyroidism), gastrointestinal disorders (primary biliary cirrhosis and malabsorption syndrome), drug therapy (e.g., corticosteroids, cancer chemotherapy, anticonvulsants, and heparin), neoplasms (multiple myeloma and skeletal metastases), alcoholism, chronic renal failure, immobilization, osteogenesis imperfecta, and transplantation (Table 2). The pathogenesis of the bone loss seen in these conditions could be explained by the mechanisms seen in Type I and Type II osteoporosis. However, in some conditions, the pathogenesis still needs elucidating. In general, patients with secondary causes of osteoporosis present with a hip fracture several years earlier than expected.

IX. THERAPEUTIC CONSIDERATIONS

There are several effective agents for preventing bone loss, and these are grouped together in the category of antiresorptive agents. They include estrogen, selective estrogen receptor modulators (SERMs), bisphospho-nates, calcitonin, calcitriol, and, to a lesser degree, calcium supplements that are used as an adjunctive agent. Newer and more potent antiresorptives in the pipeline include osteoprotegerin and RANKL antagonists. However, antiresorptive agents are limited because they only prevent bone loss. For subjects with severe osteoporosis, agents that increase the formation of new bone are needed. Parathyroid hormone is the first of these systemic agents that increase trabecular thickness and continuity of bone. In addition, BMP proteins, which are osteogenic in vivo, are considered to be therapeutic molecules in the treatment of fractures to induce new bone formation at the site of injury. We can expect more anabolic agents to emerge in the next few years as we explore our understanding of the bone remodeling process.

Glossary

hyperparathyroidism Condition defined by excess parathyroid hormone secretion; leads to accelerated bone turnover.

1,25-dihydroxyvitamin D$_3$ Steroid hormone form of vitamin D; a principal regulator of calcium homeostasis.

osteoblast Cell derived from a pluripotent mesenchymal stem cell; principally involved in bone formation and mineralization of bone.

osteoclast Large multinucleated cell derived from the hematopoietic precursor of monocyte/macrophage cell lineage; involved in resorption of bone.

See Also the Following Articles

Aromatase and Estrogen Insufficiency • Interleukin-1 (IL-1) • Osteoporosis: Hormonal Treatment • Parathyroid Hormone • Parathyroid Hormone-Related Protein (PTHrP) • SERMs (Selective Estrogen Receptor Modulators) • Tumor Necrosis Factor (TNF)

Further Reading

Compston, J. E. (2001). Sex steroids and bone. *Physiol. Rev.* **81**, 419–447.

Cummings, S. R., Browner, W. S., Bauer, D., Stone, K., Ensrud, K., Jamal, S., and Ettinger, B. (1998). Endogenous hormones and the risk of hip and vertebral fractures among older women. Study of Osteoporotic Fractures Research Group. *N. Engl. J. Med.* **339**, 733–738.

Gallagher, J. C. (1992). Pathophysiology of osteoporosis. *Semin. Nephrol.* **12**, 109–115.

Heshmati, H. M., Khosla, S., Robins, S. P., O'Fallon, W. M., Melton, L. J., 3rd, and Riggs, B. L. (2002). Role of low levels of endogenous estrogen in regulation of bone resorption in late postmenopausal women. *J. Bone Miner. Res.* **17**, 172–178.

Johnson, M. L., Gong, G., Kimberling, W., Recker, S. M., Kimmel, D. B., and Recker, R. B. (1997). Linkage of a gene causing high bone mass to human chromosome 11 (11q12–13). *Am. J. Hum. Genet.* **60**, 1326–1332.

Lips, P. (2001). Vitamin D deficiency and secondary hyperpara-thyroidism in the elderly. Consequences for bone loss and fractures and therapeutic implications. *Endocr. Rev.* **22**, 477–501.

Little, R. D., Carulli, J. P., Del Mastro, R. G., Dupuis, J., Osborne, M., Folz, C., Manning, S. P., Swain, P. M., Zhao, S. C., Eustace, B., Lappe, M. M., Spitzer, L., Zweier, S., Braunsch-weiger, K., Benchekroun, Y., Hu, X., Adair, R., Chee, L., FitzGerald, M. G., Tulig, C., Caruso, A., Tzellas, N., Bawa, A., Franklin, B., McGuire, S., Nogues, X., Gong, G., Allen, K. M., Anisowicz, A., Morales, A. J., Lomedico, P. T., Recker, S. M., Van Eerdewegh, P., Recker, R. R., and Johnson, M. L. (2002). A mutation in the LDL receptor-related protein 5 gene results in the autosomal dominant high-bone-mass trait. *Am. J. Hum. Genet.* **70**, 11–19.

Marcus, R., Feldman, D., and Kelsey, J. (1996). "Osteoporosis" (R. Marcus, D. Feldman, and J. Kelsey, eds.), Chaps. 31–38. Academic Press, San Diego.

Pacifici, R. (1996). Estrogen, cytokines, and pathogenesis of postmenopausal osteoporosis. *J. Bone Miner. Res.* **11**, 1043–1051.

Raisz, L. G. (1999). Physiology and pathophysiology of bone remodeling. *Clin. Chem.* **45**, 1353–1358.

Riggs, B. L. (2000). The mechanisms of estrogen regulation of bone resorption. *J. Clin. Invest.* **106**, 1203–1204.

Riggs, B. L., Khosla, S., and Melton, L. J., III (1998). A unitary model for involutional osteoporosis: Estrogen deficiency causes both type I and type II osteoporosis in postmenopausal women and contributes to bone loss in aging men. *J. Bone Miner. Res.* **13**, 763–773.

Sambrook, P. N., Kelly, P. J., White, C. P., Morrison, N. A., and Eisman, J. A. (1996). Genetic determinants of bone mass. *In* "Osteoporosis" (R. Marcus, D. Feldman and J. Kelsey, eds.), pp. 477–482. Academic Press, San Diego.

Stevenson, J. C., and Lindsay, R. (1998). "Osteoporosis" (J. C. Stevenson and R. Lindsay, eds.), Chaps. 2, 3, and 8. Chapman and Hall Medical, London.

Teitelbaum, S. L. (2000). Bone resorption by osteoclasts. *Science* **289**, 1504–1508.

Ovulation

Ariel Hourvitz[*] and Eli Y. Adashi[†]

[*]*Tel Aviv University* ● [†]*University of Utah*

Ovulation, a complex process initiated by the surge of LH, constitutes the ultimate step in the maturation of the ovarian follicle and its contained oocyte. Once initiated, a cascade of events transpires that culminates in the disintegration of the follicular wall and the release of a fertilizable oocyte. This complex series of events inevitably involves specific ovarian cell types and diverse signaling pathways. The individual phases of the normal ovarian life cycle are controlled by a highly synchronized and exquisitely timed cascade of gene expression. Appropriate transition from one phase of the ovarian cycle to the next requires the timely expression of a specific gene(s) to ensure the correct continuation of the process.

I. INTRODUCTION

The teleologic underpinning of ovarian function draws on the fundamental need to preserve the species. Accordingly, the very existence of the ovary, and for that matter the very existence of the reproductive axis as a whole, is designed to subserve a single central objective: the generation of a mature, fertilizable ovum.

The ovary is the master gland in this process, the function of which is made possible by the contribution of the various other components of the reproductive axis. This article will emphasize the cycle of follicular growth and development: recruitment, selection and dominance, ovulation, and corpus luteum formation and demise. In addition, the major operational characteristics of ovulation will be reviewed.

II. FOLLICULAR GROWTH AND DEVELOPMENT: RECRUITMENT, SELECTION, AND DOMINANCE

The primordial follicle consists of an oocyte arrested in the diplotene stage of the first meiotic prophase, surrounded by a single layer of granulosa cells. It is first noted by week 16 of intrauterine life, and it is generally accepted that the formation of follicles ends no later than 6 months postpartum. It is quite certain that this stage of follicular development is entirely gonadotropin-independent.

The preantral growth phase is the phase of follicular development in which the primordial follicles (30 μm in diameter) are converted to mature secondary follicles (120 μm in diameter). Initiated during months 5 to 6 of gestation, the process becomes evident when the granulosa cells undergo proliferation and differentiation combined with theca hypertrophy and the growth and differentiation of the oocyte including the acquisition of the zona pellucida. The resulting mature secondary follicles constitute the pool of preantral follicles from which tonic, likely follicle-stimulating hormone (FSH)-dependent recruitment of follicles takes place.

The term recruitment has been used to indicate that a follicle has entered the so-called growth trajectory, that is, the process wherein the follicle departs from the resting pool to begin a well-characterized pattern of growth and development. Recruitment, although obligatory, does not guarantee ovulation. The recruitment process is a "continuum" process beginning at infancy and stopping when the pool of available oocytes is exhausted. It goes on all times and at all ages, uninterrupted by pregnancy or other periods of non-ovulation. The stimuli for the recruitment of the follicles are unknown but for the process to continue, a specific hormonal environment is needed. The absence of this environment will cause the atresia of most of those follicles. However, the specific hormonal environment present at the beginning of the cycle, mostly the increase in FSH, will enable the formation of a cohort of developing follicles. Following recruitment, the flattened granulosa cells become cuboidal and small gap junctions are formed between the granulosa cells and the oocyte.

The term selection indicates the final winnowing of the maturing follicular cohort (by atresia) down to a size equal to the species-specific ovulatory quota. Accordingly, selection is complete when the number of healthy follicles (i.e., with ovulatory potential) in the cohort equals the ovulatory quota. Like recruitment, selection does not guarantee ovulation. Given its greater temporal proximity to ovulation, however, selection may, with high probability, be expected to be followed by ovulation in a typical cycle.

The leading follicle can be distinguished from other members of the cohort by its sheer size and the high mitotic index of its granulosa cells. Moreover, only the leading follicle at this point in time displays detectable levels of FSH in its follicular fluid. This same follicle also displays significant follicular levels of estradiol. Indeed, it is generally agreed that the capacity to aromatize androgens efficiently is an important determinant of the chosen follicle. Most important, the follicle destined to ovulate displays a granulosa cell mitotic index that is high enough to ensure that smaller, albeit healthy, follicles are unlikely to catch up.

The term dominance refers to the status of the follicle destined to ovulate given its presumed key role in regulating the size of the ovulatory quota. The selected follicle becomes dominant approximately 1 week before ovulation. Consequently, it must maintain its dominance during the week before ovulation. Stated differently, the follicle selected for ovulation is functionally (not merely morphologically) dominant in that it is presumed to inhibit the development of other competing follicles on both ovaries. Inevitably, and for reasons that are not entirely clear, the dominant follicle (i.e., the sole follicle destined to ovulate) continues to thrive in circumstances that it itself has made inhospitable for others. This dominant follicle has produced relatively more estrogen than the other follicles in its cohort. The dominant follicle thus enjoys an orderly sequence of events wherein FSH and estrogen stimulate growth, antrum formation, and the appearance of luteinizing hormone (LH) receptors. The dramatic increase in estrogen production by the dominant follicle, observable during the second half of the follicular phase, is accompanied by falling levels of FSH. As a result, the nondominant follicles fail to thrive. Apparently, the intrafollicular concentrations of gonadotropins and of steroids are central to the self-amplification process.

Experimental findings are consistent with the possibility that the ovary itself may in fact play a zeitgeber role during the menstrual cycle and that this time-keeping function is subserved by the activities of the cyclic structures of the dominant ovary. The 28-day menstrual cycle is thus the result of the intrinsic life span of the cyclic ovarian dominant structures and is not the result of timed changes dictated by the brain or pituitary. The dominant follicle thus determines the length of the follicular phase, with the corpus luteum determining the length of the luteal phase.

These experiments also suggested that the selection of the follicle destined to ovulate had already occurred by day 8 of the cycle. Indeed, it would appear that no other member of the follicular cohort was competent to serve as a surrogate for the follicle to achieve a timely, midcycle ovulation. Thus, it could be suggested that the dominant follicle itself plays a key role in regulating the size of the ovulatory quota by inhibiting the development of any competing follicles in either ovary. A similar function is subserved by the corpus luteum. Thus, the ovulatory follicle, once it is selected during the midfollicular phase, and the corpus luteum are truly dominant ovarian structures. Accordingly, the next round of follicular growth occurs only after the interference by the cyclic structure is removed either artificially, by experimental intervention, or naturally, after the demise of the corpus luteum. Further insight has been gained from studies wherein progesterone-replaced luteectomized primates were evaluated, revealing progesterone to be the principal luteal hormone responsible for the inhibition of luteal follicular growth. It is critical to note that circulating gonadotropin levels were apparently maintained after follicular or luteal ablation and that follicle recruitment occurred without an attendant increment in circulating gonadotropins. Thus, the inhibition of follicular growth by the cyclic structures of the ovary was not due to a decrement in the circulating levels of gonadotropins. Rather, it appeared to be due to local intraovarian influences. The above notwithstanding, careful re-evaluation of these issues may well be warranted in that careful examination of the data suggests at least a slight, albeit transitory, increase in the circulating levels of FSH after ablation.

Further insight has been derived from experiments revealing that the follicle destined to ovulate attains dominance 5 to 7 days after the demise of the corpus luteum. This conclusion was based on the observation that the levels of estradiol in ovarian venous serum were significantly different between ovaries as early as days 5 to 7 of the cycle. This divergence in estrogen secretion between ovaries provides the earliest hormonal index attesting to the emergence of the dominant follicle.

In the late follicular phase, the intrafollicular concentrations of estradiol are maximal at a time when the circulating estradiol levels surge to a peak. With the ovulatory LH surge, the intrafollicular concentrations of estradiol decrease along with parallel decrements in the intrafollicular concentrations of androstenedione. Concurrently, distinct, progressive increments have been noted for the intrafollicular content of both progesterone and 17α-hydroxyprogesterone, reflecting early granulosa cell luteinization.

III. OVULATION

As midcycle approaches, there is a dramatic rise in estrogen and a subsequent LH surge and to a lesser extent an FSH surge that trigger the dominant follicle to ovulate. The LH surge rapidly acts on granulosa cells of the preovulatory follicles to terminate the follicular growth and at the same time induce those genes required for the ovulatory process. Ovulation is characterized by various processes leading to follicle rupture, oocyte maturation, and formation of the corpus luteum.

For reasons that are not well understood, but possibly because of unique microenvironmental circumstances, one (rarely, more than one) follicle ovulates and gives rise to a corpus luteum during each menstrual cycle. In the human, both LH and hCG have been shown to stimulate the rupture of mature follicles. In hypophysectomized rats, however, highly purified FSH can serve as the ovulatory hormone after follicular maturation has been stimulated by the administration of FSH and LH. Interestingly, inhibitors of prostaglandin synthesis (introduced systemically or locally into the antrum) have been shown to inhibit ovulation in rats and rabbits. Because LH has been shown to stimulate prostaglandin biosynthesis by ovarian follicles, increased prostaglandin synthesis might mediate the ovulatory stimulus of LH.

Mechanically, ovulation consists of rapid follicular enlargement with subsequent protrusion of the follicle from the surface of the ovarian cortex. Ultimately, rupture of the follicle results in the extrusion of an oocyte–cumulus complex. In the human ovary, this sequence may well begin 5 to 6 days before the onset of the preovulatory LH surge. It is the latter event, however, that marks the end of the follicular phase of the cycle and precedes actual rupture by as much as 36 h. Fortuitous endoscopic visualization of the ovary around the time of ovulation has revealed that elevation of a conical stigma on the surface of the protruding follicle precedes rupture. Rupture of this stigma is accompanied by gentle, rather than explosive, expulsion of the oocyte and antral fluid, suggesting that the latter is not under high pressure. Indeed, direct measurements have demonstrated that intrafollicular pressure is low in preovulatory follicles.

Several hypotheses have been advanced to account for the rapid increase in size and rupture of the follicle. For one, consideration was given to changes in the composition of the antral fluid during the period of rapid preovulatory follicular enlargement. In addition to changes in the steroid hormone content, an increase in colloid osmotic pressure has been noted. Although the granulosa cell-derived proteoglycans undoubtedly play a critical role in regulating the colloid osmotic pressure, little concrete information regarding the nature of their involvement is in fact available. Thus, a cause and effect relationship between the altered composition of antral fluid and the enlargement and rupture of the follicle remains to be established. Alternatively, stigma formation and rupture may reflect the effects of hydrolytic enzymes acting locally on protein substrates in the basal lamina.

In keeping with this notion, instillation of protease inhibitors into the antral fluid inhibits ovulation. One such proteolytic enzyme, plasminogen activator, has been localized in increasing concentrations in the walls of rat ovarian follicle just before ovulation. Plasminogen activator, a serine protease, stimulates the conversion of plasminogen (a follicular fluid constituent) to the proteolytically active enzyme plasmin. The latter is known to activate collagenase, presumably an obligatory element in the dissolution of the basal membrane and the perifollicular stroma in the course of ovulation. It is thus generally presumed that plasminogen activator-mediated conversion of plasminogen to plasmin may contribute to the proteolytic digestion of the follicular wall, a prerequisite of follicular rupture. Consideration is also being given to the possibility that plasminogen activator may be involved in gap junction disruption and thereby in the delicate communication between the oocyte and the surrounding cumulus cells. Although the ultimate physiologic significance of plasminogen activator remains a matter of study, there is little doubt as to the ability of somatic ovarian cells to produce this protease in measurable amounts in a manner subject to tight hormonal regulation. The FSH-dependent production of plasminogen activators by granulosa cells is particularly well documented.

IV. CORPUS LUTEUM FORMATION AND DEMISE

After ovulation, the dominant follicle reorganizes to become the corpus luteum. Thus, after rupture of the follicle, capillaries and fibroblasts from the surrounding stroma proliferate and penetrate the basal lamina.

Concurrently, the mural granulosa cells undergo morphologic changes collectively referred to as luteinization. These cells, the surrounding theca interstitial cells, and the invading vasculature intermingle to give rise to a corpus luteum.

Clearly, it is this endocrine gland that is the major source of sex steroid hormones secreted by the ovary during the postovulatory phase of the cycle. An important aspect of this phenomenon is the penetration of the follicle basement membrane by blood vessels, thereby providing the granulosa–luteal cells with circulating levels of low-density lipoprotein (LDL). As stated earlier, LDL cholesterol serves as the substrate for corpus luteum progesterone production.

Normally, the functional life span of the corpus luteum is 14 ± 2 days. Thereafter, the corpus luteum

spontaneously regresses, to be replaced (unless pregnancy occurs) at least five cycles later by an avascular scar referred to as the corpus albicans. The mechanisms underlying luteolysis remain unclear. Both estrogens and prostaglandins, however, have been suggested as important factors in the promotion of luteal demise. The above notwithstanding, there is little doubt as to the central role of LH in the maintenance of corpus luteum function. Thus, withdrawal of LH support in various experimental circumstances has virtually invariably resulted in luteal demise.

V. OVARIAN STEROIDOGENESIS

To distinguish steroid hormones secreted by the ovary from those secreted by the adrenal or those produced by peripheral metabolism of precursors, studies have determined and compared the steroid hormone content of ovarian venous effluents and peripheral venous blood. Such studies revealed that the ovaries secrete pregnenolone, progesterone, 17α-hydroxyprogesterone, esterone, dehydroepiandrosterone, androstenedione, testosterone, estrone, and 17β-estradiol. Although such measurements provide significant insight into the steroidogenic pathways under study, they do not identify the specific ovarian cell types involved. In attempts to make these distinctions, steroid hormones have been identified and quantified in medium conditioned by whole (sliced or minced) ovaries, microdissected follicles, or ovarian cell suspensions. It is this combined body of knowledge that underlies our current understanding of adult ovarian steroidogenesis.

Studies using microdissected follicles identified estrone and estradiol as the major products of the follicle. In contrast, progesterone and 17α-hydroxyprocesterone proved to be the major products of the corpus luteum. Studies employing (labeled or unlabeled) C21 and C19 precursors revealed the isolated granulosa cell to be capable of producing mostly progesterone and estrogens along with 17α-hydroxyprogesterone. In contrast, isolated theca cells produced progesterone, 17α-hydroxyprogesterone, and androstenedione.

A. Estrogen Biosynthesis

Granulosa cells are the cellular source of estradiol and progesterone, the two most important ovarian steroids. Although the granulosa cells and their lutein counterparts are capable of producing progesterone independent of other ovarian cell types, the biosynthesis of estrogens requires cooperation between the granulosa cells and their theca neighbors. The participation of these two cell types and of the two gonadotropins (FSH and LH) in ovarian estrogen biosynthesis underlies the two-cell/two-gonadotropin hypothesis, an integrative process required for ovarian estrogen biosynthesis. According to this view, theca-derived, LH-dependent, aromatizable androgens are acted upon by FSH-inducible granulosa cell aromatase activity. Indeed, in virtually all species ovarian estrone and estradiol derive from the androgen precursors androstenedione and testosterone. A broader view of this concept could and probably should allow its extension to include intercellular exchanges of other steroidogenic substrates. Indeed, recent studies strongly suggest that intercellular exchanges of C21 steroids occur at multiple levels of the steroidogenic cascade.

That follicular estrogen biosynthesis requires both granulosa and theca interstitial cells was first discovered by Falck in 1959 through a series of elegant and now classic experiments. The biochemical basis of this two-cell/two-gonadotropin theory was later provided by Ryan and Petro, whose findings revealed the theca interstitial cells to be the producers of C19 androgens, with the granulosa cells being the primary cellular site of aromatization. Moreover, Ryan *et al.* were able to show that the conversion of acetate to estrogen is substantially enhanced by the co-incubation of granulosa and theca cells. This observation, along with a body of related information, was elegantly summarized by Bjersing in 1967: "C19 precursor steroids are elaborated by theca–interstitial cells and are transferred across the basement membrane of the follicle to the granulosa cells where they are aromatized to estrogens." The above notwithstanding, the two-cell/two-gonadotropin hypothesis has been challenged by *in vivo* studies in the subhuman primate.

In keeping with these conclusions, studies of isolated granulosa cells revealed that FSH, but not LH, stimulates estrogen biosynthesis in a manner contingent on the provision of an exogenous aromatizable androgenic substrate. In contrast, isolated theca cells did not produce significant amounts of estrogens in any experimental circumstances. Indeed, aromatase activity of granulosa cells was estimated to be at least 700 times greater than that of theca cells from large preovulatory follicles. As such, these results are consistent with the hypothesis that granulosa cells are the principal site of estrogen biosynthesis in the dominant preovulatory follicle. These observations suggest that androgen (mainly

androstenedione) produced by LH-stimulated theca cells is the main substrate for estrogen biosynthesis by FSH-stimulated granulosa cells. Although estrone may well be the most immediate estrogen produced, it in turn is readily converted to estradiol as a result of the (granulosa cell-based) activity of the steroidogenic enzyme 17β-hydroxysteroid dehydrogenase. The complex aromatization process involves the loss of the angular C19 methyl group and the stereospecific elimination of the 10 and 20 hydrogens of the A ring of the androgen precursor. As such, a total of three hydroxylation reactions are required per mole of estrogen formed.

The hormonal action of both LH and FSH appears to require the intermediacy of the membrane-associated enzyme adenylate cyclase. Indeed, it is generally accepted that gonadotropin-mediated stimulation of adenylate cyclase results in the conversion of intracellular ATP to cyclic AMP. The latter, in turn, is thought to bind to the regulatory subunit of a protein kinase (commonly referred to as A kinase), whereupon the catalytic subunit of the enzyme is activated and dissociated. This in turn phosphorylates key intracellular proteins central to the signal transduction sequence.

B. Progestin Biosynthesis

The granulosa cell, like the theca interstitial cell, is amply endowed to carry out progestin biosynthesis. Central to this process, however, is the availability of abundant supplies of cholesterol, which serves as the starting material for the steroidogenic cascade. Recent studies have shown that cholesterol used for membrane synthesis and steroid hormone production is derived primarily from circulating serum lipoproteins rather than from *de novo* cellular synthesis from acetate. LDL particles are known to bind to specific membrane receptors, with the LDL–receptor complexes entering the cell by receptor-mediated endocytosis. Thereafter, the endocytotic vesicles are known to fuse to lysosomes wherein LDL cholesterol esters are hydrolyzed to yield free cholesterol. The free cholesterol, in turn, is reesterified and stored in the cytoplasm in lipid droplets. Faced with steroidogenic demands, the cholesterol ester is hydrolyzed and the free cholesterol is transported to mitochondria for standard steroidogenic processing.

The importance of LDL cholesterol for ovarian progesterone secretion is demonstrated by the observation that the presence of LDL is required for maximal progesterone secretion by cultured cells.

High-density lipoprotein does not support human ovarian progesterone biosynthesis. Thus, the very availability of LDL to various ovarian compartments could influence steroid hormone production. For example, the relative avascularity of the granulosa cell layer expectedly limits progestin biosynthetic capacity. In keeping with this observation, human follicular fluid contains little or no LDL, thereby limiting the ability of preovulatory granulosa cells to produce progesterone 67. The above notwithstanding, the intrafollicular concentrations of progesterone do rise after the LH surge (before ovulation), suggesting a diminution in the lipoprotein barrier. Moreover, after ovulation occurs, vascularization of the corpus luteum provides the means by which LDL is delivered to the luteinized granulosa cells, thereby allowing progesterone biosynthesis to begin.

Although lipoproteins clearly constitute the most abundant source of cholesterol, endogenously generated cholesterol may also be employed. Cholesterol itself is in turn converted to pregnenolone through the rate-limiting intermediacy of mitochondrial enzyme cholesterol side chain cleavage. The subsequent conversion of pregnenolone to progesterone occurs relatively readily by virtue of the relative abundance of the cytoplasmic enzymes 3β-hydroxysteroid dehydrogenase/Δ5, Δ4-isomerase. Although the human granulosa cell has been reported to contain low levels of 17α-hydroxylase activity and thus has the ability to convert progesterone to 17α-hydroxyprogesterone, the significance of this finding remains uncertain.

C. Androgen Biosynthesis

More recent studies of isolated human theca cells have revealed that the theca layer is the major cellular source of follicular androgen and that LH, rather than FSH, stimulates theca androgen production. In contrast, androgen production by isolated cultured human granulosa cells proved negligible with or without added gonadotropins.

The biosynthesis of C19 androgens is the sole domain of the theca interstitial cell. Accordingly, this cell type is amply endowed with the necessary machinery to generate C21 progestational precursors. More important, however, the theca interstitial cell is amply endowed with 17α-hydroxylase/desmolase (17–20) activity and is capable of converting Δ5 and Δ4 progestational precursors (i.e., pregnenolone and progesterone) to C19 products (dehydroepiandrosterone and androstenedione, respectively). Consequently, the presence of 17α-hydroxylase/desmolase (17–20) activity can be viewed as an exclusive feature of the ovarian theca interstitial cell.

VI. MOLECULAR CHARACTERIZATION OF THE OVULATORY CASCADE

Ovulation, a complex process initiated by the surge of LH, constitutes the ultimate step in the maturation of the ovarian follicle and its enclosed oocyte. Once initiated, a cascade of events transpires, culminating in the disintegration of the follicular wall and the release of a fertilizable oocyte. This complex series of events, inevitably, involves specific ovarian cell types, diverse signaling pathways, and temporally controlled expression of specific genes. To date, a major focus of the research on ovulation has been the analysis of known genes. These studies have led to the establishment of a number of genes as being critical to the murine ovulatory process through the generation of null mutants. Figure 1 depicts those genes

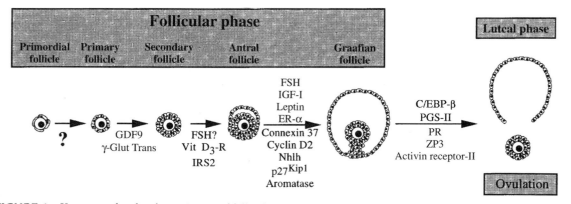

FIGURE 1   Known molecular determinants of folliculogenesis and ovulation. GDF9, growth differentiation factor 9; γ-Glut Trans, γ-glutamyl transferase; Vit D₃-R, vitamin D₃ receptor; ER, estrogen receptor; IRS, insulin receptor substrate; PGS-II, prostaglandin synthase II; PR, progesterone receptor; ZP3, zona pellucida protein 3.

TABLE 1   Gene Mutations Affecting Ovulation and Causing Infertility Due to Ovulation/Fertilization Failure

Disrupted gene	Gene symbol	Ovarian phenotype
Cyclooxygenase type 2	Cox-2 (PGS-2)	Defective ovulatory process; few eggs recovered, none of which were fertilized; the eggs thus recovered proved developmentally abnormal; ovulation failure even when stimulated with gonadotropins
Progesterone receptor	PR	Follicles do not rupture; oocytes become trapped in the ovary
Activin receptor II	ActR-II	Absence of corpora lutea, suggesting ovulatory failure
CCAAT/enhancer-binding protein β	C/EBPβ	Failure to ovulate; absent corpora lutea
Nuclear receptor-interacting protein 1	Nrip 1	Complete failure of oocyte release from mature follicles but luteinization appears normal
Early growth-response protein 1	Egr-1 (Krox-24)	Ovulatory failure due to an inhibition in the expression of the LHβ subunit and LH receptor genes
Ca^{2+}/Calmodulin-dependent protein kinase IV	CaMK-IV	Ovulatory failure with trapped oocytes present in some of the follicles
Cyclin-dependent kinase 4	Cdk4	Abnormal luteinization with disturbed cellularity, trapped oocytes, and a lack of copora lutea; granulosa cells appear normal; increased proestrous and diestrous phases
Cyclin D2	Cd2	Inability of ovarian granulosa cells to proliferate normally in response to FSH; failure to release the oocytes; corpora lutea carrying trapped oocytes
$p27^{Kip1}$	$p27^{Kip1}$	Ovulation is impaired; follicles do not progress to form corpora lutea

identified thus far as obligatory to the ovarian life cycle inclusive of those implicated in ovulation. The genes targeted were mostly those known to be expressed in the ovary and to play a role in follicular growth. Alternatively, a phenotype inclusive of ovulatory failure may be "stumbled upon" in the context of a study of a previously unknown gene or one not previously recognized as being important in ovarian physiology. Tables 1 and 2 display those genes for which the null deletion resulted in ovulation

TABLE 2   Gene Mutations Affecting Ovulation and Causing Reduced Ovulatory Efficiency

Disrupted gene	Gene symbol	Ovarian phenotype
Prostaglandin E2 receptor type 2	EP2	Reduced ovulatory efficiency; cumulus expansion does not occur
Zona pellucida 3	ZP3	Reduced ovulatory efficiency; disorganized cumulus granulosa cells
Colony-stimulating factor-1	CSF-1	Abnormal lengthy estrous cycles; low pregnancy rates; smaller litter sizes
Telomerase RNA	TR	Reduced ovulatory efficiency
Estrogen receptor-β	ER-β	Reduced fertility with altered ovulatory efficiency; increased number of early atretic follicles and sparse presence of corpora lutea, suggestive of arrested folliculogenesis
Nitric oxide synthase	NOS	Reduced fertility with altered ovulatory efficiency; significantly reduced number of ovulated oocytes, longer estrous cycle, and impaired oocyte meiotic maturation
Superoxide dismutase-1	Sod-1	Infertility or reduced fertility with smaller litter size; primary and small antral follicles but few corpora lutea
Urinary trypsin inhibitor	Uti	Severe reduction in fertility; markedly reduced ovulatory efficiency; disorganized corona radiata; large number of retained oocytes
Steroid receptor co-activator-3	Src-3	Decreased ovulation; lower pregnancy rate; small litter size; longer estrous cycling time
c-AMP-specific phosphodiesterase type 4	PDE4D	Reduced number of ovulated oocytes; degeneration of ovulated oocyte; entrapped oocytes

failure (Table 1) or reduced ovulatory efficiency (Table 2) and thus in infertility. Understandably, ovulation failure in the different knockout models is usually associated with additional and often considerable ovarian defects.

In the past few years, the use of advanced molecular biology techniques such as differential display reverse transcription-polymerase chain reaction, subtractive suppression hybridization, DNA array technology, and *in silico* methods has led to the identification of new ovulatory genes. Using these different techniques, researchers were able to identify a multitude of novel ovulatory up-regulated genes. These genes induced by LH include among others, carbonyl reductase, 3α-hydroxysteroid dehydrogenase, regulator of G-protein signaling, tumor necrosis factor-induced gene-6, and early growth regulator-1. The exact role of these genes in the ovulatory process is not clear yet, but their diverse functions and spatial expression in the ovary prove the complexity and global effect of the ovulatory process.

VII. SUMMARY

Recent advances in the human and mouse genome projects, combined with the development of advanced molecular technology such as differential display analysis, subtractive hybridization, and microarray analysis, now provide the opportunity to analyze the expression pattern of thousands of genes. This approach has already led to the identification of new genes that are expressed in the ovary. It will ultimately allow the achievement of a global view of gene expression as it relates to the ovulatory process. Functional studies of these newly discovered genes, based mainly on gene targeting technology, will allow a better understanding of the genetic determinants of the ovulatory cascade and thereby, the endocrine regulation of fertility and its control.

Glossary

dominance The status of the follicle destined to ovulate given its presumed key role in regulating the size of the ovulatory quota.

LH surge Midcycle surge of pituitary luteinization hormone initiating the ovulatory cascade.

luteinization The ovulatory-related process of formation of the corpus luteum from the ovulatory follicle. The corpus luteum comprises luteal and nonluteal cell types. The luteal cells differentiate from the theca and granulosa cells and have the capacity to produce steroids and peptide hormones.

ovulation Release of a fertilizable ovum from the graafian follicle. In its broader sense, the ovulatory response defines the cascade of events following the LH surge and including the resumption of meiosis and oocyte maturation, luteinization, and the rupture of the follicular wall.

ovulatory cascade A highly synchronized and exquisitely timed cascade of specific gene(s) expression to ensure the correct process of ovulation.

recruitment The process wherein the follicle departs from the resting pool to begin a well-characterized pattern of growth and development. Recruitment, although obligatory, does not guarantee ovulation. Stated differently, recruitment is necessary but not sufficient for ovulation to occur.

selection The final winnowing of the maturing follicular cohort by atresia down to a size equal to the species-specific ovulatory quota.

See Also the Following Articles

Corpus Luteum in Primates ● **Corpus Luteum: Regression and Rescue** ● **Decidualization** ● **Endocrine Rhythms: Generation, Regulation, and Integration** ● **Follicle Stimulating Hormone (FSH)** ● **Folliculogenesis** ● **Implantation** ● *In Vitro* **Fertilization** ● **Lipoprotein Receptor Signaling** ● **Luteinizing Hormone (LH)** ● **Oocyte Development and Maturation** ● **Progesterone Action in the Female Reproductive Tract**

Further Reading

Espey, L. L. (1978). Ovarian contractility and its relationship to ovulation: A review. *Biol. Reprod.* **19**(3), 540–551.

Espey, L. L. (1980). Ovulation as an inflammatory reaction—A hypothesis. *Biol. Reprod.* **22**(1), 73–106.

Hizaki, H., Segi, E., Sugimoto, Y., Hirose, M., Saji, T., Ushikubi, F., Matsuoka, T., Noda, Y., Tanaka, T., Yoshida, N., Narumiya, S., and Ichikawa, A. (1999). Abortive expansion of the cumulus and impaired fertility in mice lacking the prostaglandin E receptor subtype EP(2). *Proc. Natl. Acad. Sci. USA* **96**(18), 10501–10506.

Hsu, S. Y., and Hsueh, A. J. (2000). Discovering new hormones, receptors, and signaling mediators in the genomic era. *Mol. Endocrinol.* **14**(5), 594–604.

Leo, C. P., Vitt, U. A., and Hsueh, A. J. (2000). The Ovarian Kaleidoscope database: An online resource for the ovarian research community. *Endocrinology* **141**(9), 3052–3054.

Matzuk, M. M. (2000). Revelations of ovarian follicle biology from gene knockout mice. *Mol. Cell. Endocrinol.* **163**(1/2), 61–66.

Richards, J. S. (1994). Hormonal control of gene expression in the ovary. *Endocr. Rev.* **15**(6), 725–751.

Richards, J. S. (2001). Perspective: The ovarian follicle—A perspective in 2001. *Endocrinology* **142**(6), 2184–2193.

Richards, J. S., Russell, D. L., Ochsner, S., and Espey, L. L. (2002). Ovulation: New dimensions and new regulators of the inflammatory-like response. *Annu. Rev. Physiol.* **64**, 69–92.

Richards, J. S., Russell, D. L., Robker, R. L., Dajee, M., and Alliston, T. N. (1998). Molecular mechanisms of ovulation and luteinization. *Mol. Cell. Endocrinol.* **145**(1/2), 47–54.

Robker, R. L., Russell, D. L., Espey, L. L., Lydon, J. P., O'Malley, B. W., and Richards, J. S. (2000). Progesterone-regulated genes in the ovulation process: ADAMTS-1 and cathepsin L proteases. *Proc. Natl. Acad. Sci. USA* 97(9), 4689–4694.

Robker, R. L., Russell, D. L., Yoshioka, S., Sharma, S. C., Lydon, J. P., O'Malley, B. W., Espey, L. L., and Richards, J. S. (2000). Ovulation: A multi-gene, multi-step process. *Steroids* 65(10/11), 559–570.

Rondell, P. (1970). Biophysical aspects of ovulation. *Biol. Reprod.* 2(Suppl. 2), 64–89.

Sauer, B. (1998). Inducible gene targeting in mice using the Cre/lox system. *Methods* 14(4), 381–392.

Oxyntomodulin

Bo Ahrén

Lund University, Sweden

I. INTRODUCTION
II. OXYNTOMODULIN BIOCHEMISTRY
III. RECEPTORS FOR OXYNTOMODULIN
IV. SIGNALING PATHWAYS OF OXYNTOMODULIN
V. OXYNTOMODULIN PHYSIOLOGY
VI. OXYNTOMODULIN PATHOPHYSIOLOGY

Oxyntomodulin is a gut hormone. This article describes the structure and processing of the hormone, the regulation of its expression and secretion, its effects and mechanisms, as well as possible involvement of the hormone in gastrointestinal disorder.

I. INTRODUCTION

Oxyntomodulin, a 37-amino-acid peptide, is processed from proglucagon in the intestinal L-cells and is released after food intake. Although the physiological role of oxyntomodulin remains to be established, it inhibits gastric acid secretion, gastric emptying, and pancreatic exocrine secretion and stimulates insulin secretion.

The intestinal proglucagon-derived peptide oxyntomodulin works mainly by activating receptors that are more specific for other proglucagon-derived peptides, through actions involving phosphoinositide hydrolysis and formation of cyclic AMP. Physiologically, the peptide may be an enterogastrone and/or an incretin factor; oxyntomodulin may be involved in gastrointestinal disorders, although this has not been established.

II. OXYNTOMODULIN BIOCHEMISTRY

A. Expression of Oxyntomodulin

Oxyntomodulin belongs to the enteroglucagons or the glucagon-like substances in the gut. These substances were initially identified in intestinal mucosa in 1948 by Sutherland and de Duve using bioassay techniques, and in the sixties by Unger and collaborators using radioimmunoassay. Later studies revealed that these substances consist of a variety of several different peptides. All are produced in the gut L-cells, which are of the open type of gut endocrine cells that are located preferentially in the mucosal cell lining of the distal portion of the ileum. All enteroglucagons are encoded by the same glucagon gene, which in humans is located on chromosome 2q36–q37. This gene is also expressed in the pancreatic A-cells and in the brain. It encodes a single proglucagon messenger RNA transcript that is translated into a single 158-amino-acid sequence comprising the proglucagon peptide. Proglucagon, which is identical in all cells expressing the proglucagon gene, is processed through intracellular cleavage, yielding several different peptides (Fig. 1). However, the prohormone processing is different in each cell type expressing proglucagon. In the gut L-cells and in the brain, proglucagon is processed to glicentin, glicentin-related polypeptide (GRPP), oxyntomodulin, glucagon-like peptides (GLP-1 and GLP-2), and intervening peptide-2 (IP-2). In contrast, in the pancreatic A-cells, proglucagon processing gives rise to glucagon, GRPP, major proglucagon factor

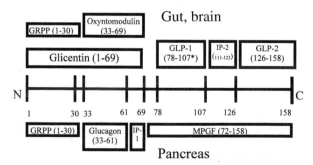

FIGURE 1 Processing of the 158-amino-acid sequence of the proglucagon molecule in the intestinal L-cells and brain (top) versus the pancreatic A-cells (bottom). Numbers denote amino acids. In the gut and brain, proglucagon is processed to glicentin, glicentin-related polypeptide (GRPP), oxyntomodulin, glucagon-like peptide-1 (GLP-1), intervening peptide-2 (IP-2), and GLP-2, whereas in the pancreas, proglucagon is processed to GRPP, glucagon, IP-1 (sequence 64–69), and major proglucagon factor (MPGF). *Indicates oxidation.

(MPGF), and IP-1. The differences in how glucagon is processed in L- and A-cells are explained by tissue-specific differences in expression of the two prohormone convertases (PCs), PC1 and PC2. Thus, oxyntomodulin is formed in cells expressing PC1, as in the L-cells, whereas glucagon is formed in cells expressing PC2, as in the pancreatic A-cells.

B. Formation and Structure of Oxyntomodulin

Formation of oxyntomodulin from proglucagon is a two-step process. First, glicentin is formed through cleavage between amino acids 69 and 70 in the proglucagon sequence. Glicentin is then further processed to form the 30-amino-acid sequence of GRPP and the 37-amino acid sequence of oxyntomodulin through a cleavage of a Lys-Arg dibasic sequence. Oxyntomodulin is equivalent to the C-terminal 37 amino acids of glicentin, corresponding to glicentin(33–69). From a quantitative point of view, approximately 20–40% of the glicentin formed is processed to oxyntomodulin, whereas the majority is released as glicentin. Oxyntomodulin also shows a high degree of structural identity to the other proglucagon-derived peptides, glucagon, GLP-1, and GLP-2 (Fig. 2). In fact, the N-terminal 29-amino-acid sequence of oxyntomodulin, i.e., glicentin(33–61), is identical to pancreatic glucagon. The amino acid sequence of oxyntomodulin is conserved through evolution, as is evident by the identical structure of oxyntomodulin in humans and guinea pigs.

C. Distribution of Oxyntomodulin

Because oxyntomodulin is formed during processing of proglucagon in cells expressing PC1, its cellular distribution is limited to the gut L-cells and certain brain areas. In fact, the rat ileum has a 10-fold higher oxyntomodulin content per gram of tissue, compared to the duodenum, and the content in the colon is approximately double that in the duodenum, which is the same distribution as for L-cells. Studies on oxyntomodulin levels in extracts of various areas of the rat brain show that the most marked expression of oxyntomodulin is in the hypothalamus. Oxyntomodulin is also expressed in the medulla oblongata, although at a 10-fold lower level than in the hypothalamus. In contrast, only trace amounts of oxyntomodulin have been demonstrated in the olfactory bulb, cerebellum, and cortex, and no oxyntomodulin has been detected in the pituitary.

D. Regulation of Expression of Oxyntomodulin

Nutrient ingestion is the primary stimulus for expression of the proglucagon gene in the gut, and therefore for formation of oxyntomodulin. Increased proglucagon gene expression is seen in rats after feeding, whereas fasting is associated with reduced gene expression. Proglucagon gene expression and proglucagon formation are also increased in rats after intestinal injury or intestinal resection. These findings suggest that proglucagon-derived factors are of importance for prandial processes as well as for response to injury.

E. Regulation of Secretion of Oxyntomodulin

After its formation, the mature 37-amino-acid oxyntomodulin is stored in the secretory granules and is secreted extracellularly when L-cells are activated. A rapid secretion of the proglucagon-derived peptides from the L-cells is induced by nutrient ingestion, and both intralumenal carbohydrates and triglycerides have been shown to be of relevance. These nutrients stimulate oxyntomodulin release through activation of L-cells from the gut lumenal side. Nutrient ingestion may, however, stimulate L-cell secretion indirectly through activation of intestinal nerves, as illustrated in rats by a study showing that oxyntomodulin released by intraduodenal administration of oleic acid is inhibited via ganglionic blockade by hexamethonium.

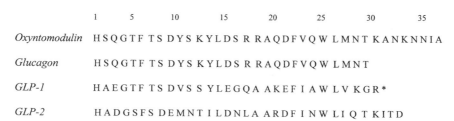

FIGURE 2 Amino acid sequences of oxyntomodulin, glucagon, glucagon-like peptide-1 (GLP-1), and GLP-2. The asterisk indicates amidation.

This is analogous to studies on the potential involvement of nerves in the regulation of GLP-1 secretion, showing that cholinergic nerves and the intestinal neuropeptide gastrin-releasing peptide (GRP) are stimulatory whereas adrenergic nerves are inhibitory.

F. Circulation of Oxyntomodulin

In plasma, circulating fasting levels of oxyntomodulin are approximately 15 pmol/liter in both humans and rats, and these levels are increased approximately twofold following refeeding. The increase in circulating levels is evident within 30 min after meal ingestion. Similarly, a study on the 24-h profile of oxyntomodulin-like immunoreactivity in humans has shown that plasma levels increase after each meal. Pharmacokinetic studies have shown that oxyntomodulin is rapidly eliminated through a two-phase elimination mechanism. In the pig, a rapid first phase has a half-life of 7 min and a slow second phase has a half-life of 20 min. In humans, the plasma half-life of oxyntomodulin has been estimated to 12 min. However, the metabolic pathways responsible for degradation of oxyntomodulin in plasma are not known. The fate of oxyntomodulin differs from the metabolic fates of the two other hormones from the L-cells, GLP-1 and GLP-2, which are both degraded by removal of the two N-terminal amino acids (His-Ala) by the enzyme dipeptidyl peptidase IV, because this enzyme requires for action either alanine or proline in position 2 of the substrate, which is not the case for oxyntomodulin.

G. Effects of Oxyntomodulin

The first described effect of oxyntomodulin was a stimulatory action on the formation of cyclic AMP in the acid-secreting fundic portion of rat stomach, which in fact was the basis for Bataille and collaborators to name the peptide oxyntomodulin. They found that oxyntomodulin was approximately 20 times more potent than glucagon in augmenting cAMP in this system, in contrast to having only 10% of the potency of glucagon in stimulating cAMP formation in membranes from the rat liver. This difference was later reproduced in studies using a preparation of highly enriched rat gastric parietal cells, and it was also shown that oxyntomodulin stimulates acid secretion through a cAMP-dependent mechanism.

However, in several other systems, oxyntomodulin has been shown to inhibit gastric acid secretion. Oxyntomodulin inhibits histamine- and pentagastrin-induced gastric acid secretion in rats *in vivo*

without affecting basal gastric acid secretion; in humans, oxyntomodulin inhibits pentagastrin-stimulated gastric acid secretion. This inhibitory action on gastric acid secretion *in vivo* is explained by a stimulatory action of oxyntomodulin on somatostatin secretion from D-cells; somatostatin in turn inhibits gastric acid secretion. Oxyntomodulin has also been shown to stimulate smooth muscle contraction in the stomach, as demonstrated by a reduced mean length of isolated rat gastric smooth muscle cells, and the peptide also inhibits ion and water transport through the rat small intestine. Moreover, oxyntomodulin inhibits pancreatic exocrine secretion in rats, both in terms of the volume of juice as well as the bicarbonate and protein output, which has been shown to be an indirect action through activation of the vagal nerves. In humans, oxyntomodulin also delays gastric emptying, inhibits postprandial duodenal motility and exocrine pancreatic enzyme secretion, and inhibits pentagastrin-stimulated gastric acid secretion. Therefore, at least under *in vivo* conditions, oxyntomodulin seems to act as a general inhibitory agent on proximal gastro-entero-pancreatic postprandial events, suggesting that it is involved in the small intestinal inhibitory control of these functions.

Oxyntomodulin also affects processes of relevance for carbohydrate metabolism. Infusion of oxyntomodulin in rats increases glucose absorption in the jejunum and promotes glucose release from isolated hepatocytes. Furthermore, oxyntomodulin stimulates insulin and somatostatin secretion from the pig pancreas and augments insulin secretion in the presence of glucose in the perfused rat pancreas. Infusion of oxyntomodulin increases plasma insulin and C-peptide concentrations in humans. Thus, oxyntomodulin has the ability to increase glucose levels through actions on the gut and liver, but also to reduce glucose levels through its stimulation of insulin secretion.

III. RECEPTORS FOR OXYNTOMODULIN

In spite of the various effects induced following exogenous administration of oxyntomodulin, no specific oxyntomodulin receptor has been identified or cloned. Instead, oxyntomodulin has been suggested to act through activation of receptors that are more specific for the other proglucagon-derived peptides. For example, oxyntomodulin increases cAMP formation in a cell line transfected with the GLP-1 receptor, and the peptide displaces radiolabeled GLP-1 bound to these cells, although the potency of oxyntomodulin is lower than that of GLP-1. Similarly, oxyntomodulin stimulates the release of somatostatin from a cell line by activating a GLP-1-selective receptor type and displaces radiolabeled GLP-1 from rat parietal cells. This suggests that oxyntomodulin acts at least partially through the GLP-1 receptors. However, oxyntomodulin has also been shown to bind to pig liver glucagon receptors, although with an affinity of only 2% of that of glucagon, suggesting a low-grade cross-reaction with these receptors. In addition, in isolated smooth muscle cells, oxyntomodulin seems to act through a glicentin/oxyntomodulin receptor type that shows high affinity for glicentin and low affinity for oxyntomodulin. Hence, several different receptor subtypes may transduce actions of oxyntomodulin. In a variety of experimental systems, there has been a general finding that the active site of oxyntomodulin resides in its C-terminal portion, because a C-terminal fragment, oxyntomodulin(19–37), is equipotent with the entire peptide.

IV. SIGNALING PATHWAYS OF OXYNTOMODULIN

Because oxyntomodulin may work through activation of GLP-1 and glucagon receptors, cyclic AMP is a likely second messenger for transducing the effects. This has been confirmed in a few studies of the signaling underlying the effects of oxyntomodulin. It has also been shown, however, that oxyntomodulin may activate other signaling pathways. For example, stimulation by oxyntomodulin of gastric smooth muscle cells is mediated by phosphoinositide hydrolysis, resulting in formation of inositol 1,4,5-trisphosphate ($InsP_3$) and liberation of Ca^{2+} from intracellular stores; this is accompanied by reduced formation of cAMP in a pertussis-toxin-sensitive manner. Oxyntomodulin may therefore activate G-protein-coupled receptors, which are linked to phospholipase C and/or adenylate cyclase.

V. OXYNTOMODULIN PHYSIOLOGY

The physiological role of oxyntomodulin remains to be established. Release of oxyntomodulin after ingestion of a meal suggests that the hormone is involved in regulation of postprandial nutritional or metabolic events. Its main function, to inhibit gastric acid secretion and pancreatic exocrine secretion, suggests that oxyntomodulin is an enterogastrone candidate. Enterogastrones are prandially released gut-derived factors that inhibit proximal events such as gastric acid

secretion, gastric emptying, and pancreatic exocrine secretion, perhaps to prevent excessive acid or exocrine pancreatic secretion. Evidence that oxyntomodulin is an enterogastrone factor includes that it is released after ingestion of each meal and that it inhibits gastric acid secretion and pancreatic exocrine secretion when exogenously administered at dose levels that are equivalent to circulating levels under physiological conditions. Furthermore, one study has shown a negative correlation between circulating levels of oxyntomodulin and gastric acid secretion in humans. On the other hand, the potency of oxyntomodulin to inhibit gastric acid secretion, as demonstrated in dogs, is much lower than the potency of other enterogastrone candidates, such as peptide YY, secretin, and cholecystokinin. Therefore, the role of oxyntomodulin as an enterogastrone remains to be established.

Because oxyntomodulin also stimulates insulin secretion, it may also be an incretin factor. Incretin factors are gut hormones released after meal intake and they stimulate insulin secretion. Again, the evidence that oxyntomodulin may be an incretin factor resides in its release after food intake and its ability to stimulate insulin secretion. However, in comparison with the potency of the two main incretin candidates, GLP-1 and gastric inhibitory polypeptide (GIP), the potency of oxyntomodulin is low. Therefore, although oxyntomodulin is a potential incretin, it remains to be established that such an effect is indeed of physiological relevance.

Although oxyntomodulin is expressed in the brain, particularly in the hypothalamus, no studies so far have shown any effects of the peptide in the central nervous system. For example, oxyntomodulin infused for 7 days in rats has no effect on body weight or food intake. So far, there is no evidence of any role of oxyntomodulin in the regulation of the central nervous system.

VI. OXYNTOMODULIN PATHOPHYSIOLOGY

The potential involvement of oxyntomodulin in various gastrointestinal disorders has been the matter of a few studies. One study in subjects with duodenal ulcer has shown that circulating oxyntomodulin levels do not differ from those in controls. Another study has shown that children with celiac disease display high circulating levels of oxyntomodulin and that oxyntomodulin levels correlate to markers of malabsorption. Although this may suggest that oxyntomodulin is involved in the development of malabsorption, a more likely explanation is that the peptide is involved in an adaptive mechanism. Expression of the proglucagon gene is known to be stimulated by intestinal injury and after intestinal resection, thus oxyntomodulin levels will increase under such conditions. Whether, however, oxyntomodulin has any role in this adaptation, as has been suggested for GLP-2, is not known. Therefore, the role of oxyntomodulin under pathological conditions is far from established.

Glossary

enterogastrones Hormones from the gut that are released after meal ingestion; inhibit gastric acid secretion and gastric emptying.

enteroglucagons Hormones produced in the intestinal glucagon cells (L-cells) through processing of the proglucagon molecule.

glicentin Intermediary 69-amino-acid peptide processed from proglucagon and cleaved to form glicentin-related polypeptide and oxyntomodulin.

glicentin-related polypeptide A peptide that is processed from the N-terminal end of glicentin in the intestinal L-cells.

incretins Hormones from the gut that are released after meal ingestion; stimulate insulin secretion.

oxyntomodulin A 37-amino-acid peptide that is processed from proglucagon in the intestinal L-cells and in the brain, but not in the pancreatic A-cells.

See Also the Following Articles

Glucagon Action • Glucagon-like Peptides: GLP-1 and GLP-2 • Glucagon Processing • Glucose-Dependent Insulinotropic Polypeptide (GIP)

Further Reading

Anini, Y., Jarrousse, C., Chariot, J., Nagain, C., Yanaihara, N., Sasaki, K., Bernard, N., Le Nguyen, D., Bataille, D., and Roze, C. (2000). Oxyntomodulin inhibits pancreatic secretion through the nervous system in rats. *Pancreas* 20, 348–360.

Baldissera, F. G., Holst, J. J., Knuhtsen, S., Hilsted, L., and Nielsen, O. V. (1988). Oxyntomodulin (glicentin-(33–69)): Pharmacokinetics, binding to liver cell membranes, effects on isolated perfused pig pancreas, and secretion from isolated perfused lower small intestine of pigs. *Regul. Pept.* 21, 151–166.

Beales, I. L., and Calam, J. (1996). Truncated glucagon-like peptide-1 and oxyntomodulin stimulate somatostatin release from rabbit fundic D-cells in primary culture. *Exp. Physiol.* 8, 1039–1041.

Fehmann, H. C., Jiang, J., Schweinfurth, J., Wheeler, M. B., Boyd, 3rd, A. E., and Göke, B. (1994). Stable expression of the rat GLP-1 receptor in CHO-cells: Activator and binding characteristics utilizing GLP-1(7–36)-amide, oxyntomodulin, exendin-4, and exendin(9–39). *Peptides* 15, 453–456.

Gros, L., Thorens, B., Bataille, D., and Kervran, A. (1993). Glucagon-like peptide-1-(7–36) amide, oxyntomodulin, and

glucagon interact with a common receptor in a somatostatin-secreting cell line. *Endocrinology* 133, 631–638.

Holst, J. J. (1983). Gut glucagon, enteroglucagon, gut glucagonlike immunoreactivity, glicentin—Current status. *Gastroenterology* 84, 1602–1613.

Jarrousse, C., Batailler, D., and Jeanrenaud, B. (1984). A pure enteroglucagon, oxyntomodulin (glucagon 37), stimulates insulin release in perfused rat pancreas. *Endocrinology* 115, 102–105.

Kervran, A., Blache, P., and Bataille, D. (1987). Distribution of oxyntomodulin and glucagon in the gastrointestinal tract and the plasma of the rat. *Endocrinology* 121, 704–713.

Le Quellec, A., Kervran, A., Blache, P., Ciurana, A. J., and Bataille, D. (1992). Oxyntomodulin-like immunoreactivity: Diurnal profile of a new potential enterogastrone. *J. Clin. Endocrinol. Metab.* 74, 1405–1409.

Le Quellec, A., Kervran, A., Blache, P., Ciurana, A. J., and Bataille, D. (1993). Diurnal profile of oxyntomodulin-like immunoreactivity in duodenal ulcer patients. *Scand. J. Gastroenterol.* 28, 816–820.

Lloyd, K. C., Amirmoazzami, S., Friedik, F., Heynio, A., Solomon, T. E., and Walsh, J. H. (1997). Candidate canine enterogastrones: Acid inhibition before and after vagotomy. *Am. J. Physiol.* 272, G1236–G1242.

Rodier, G., Magous, R., Mochizuki, T., Le Nguyen, D., Martinez, J., Bali, J. P., Bataille, D., Jarrousse, C., and Genevieve, R. (1999). Glicentin and oxyntomodulin modulate both the phosphoinositide and cyclic adenosine monophosphate signaling pathways in gastric myocytes. *Endocrinology* 140, 22–28.

Schepp, W., Dehne, K., Riedel, T., Schmidtler, J., Schaffer, K., and Classen, M. (1996). Oxyntomodulin: A cAMP-dependent stimulus of rat parietal cell function via the receptor for glucagon-like peptide-1 (7–36)NH2. *Digestion* 57, 398–405.

Schjoldager, B. T., Baldissera, F. G., Mortensen, P. E., Holst, J. J., and Christiansen, J. (1988). Oxyntomodulin: A potential hormone from the distal gut. Pharmacokinetics and effects on gastric acid and insulin secretion in man. *Eur. J. Clin. Invest.* 18, 499–503.

Veyrac, M., Ribard, D., Daures, J. P., Mion, H., Lequellec, A., Martinez, J., Bataille, D., and Michel, H. (1989). Inhibitory effect of the C-terminal octapeptide of oxyntomodulin on pentagastrin-stimulated gastric acid secretion in man. *Scand. J. Gastroenterol.* 24, 1238–1242.

Oxytocin

JOHN A. RUSSELL AND ALISON J. DOUGLAS
University of Edinburgh, United Kingdom

I. INTRODUCTION
II. SOURCES OF OXYTOCIN IN THE BODY
III. REGULATION OF OXYTOCIN GENE EXPRESSION
IV. CONTROL OF OXYTOCIN SECRETION
V. OXYTOCIN RECEPTOR
VI. OXYTOCIN IN PARTURITION

Oxytocin is a nonapeptide (Cys^1-Tyr^2-Ileu^3-Gln^4-Asn^5-Cys^6-Pro^7-Leu^8-Gly^9-NH$_2$) that is produced only in mammals. Synthesis occurs in groups of nerve cells (neurons) and (variably, according to species) in reproductive tissues. Circulating oxytocin is entirely from the posterior pituitary gland. Oxytocin in the brain or cerebrospinal fluid is produced in the brain. Parturition, maternal behavior, and lactation are stimulated by oxytocin release.

I. INTRODUCTION

Oxytocin was one of the first hormones to be discovered. At the beginning of the past century, extracts of the posterior pituitary gland were shown to stimulate the contractile activity of the pregnant uterus. This led to the idea that oxytocin had a role in stimulating uterine contractions in parturition, and its name [Gk.: swift (*oxys*) birth (*tokos*)] derives from this action. It was later discovered that posterior pituitary extract is the most effective stimulant of milk let-down or milk ejection in lactating mammals. The other hormonal activity in the posterior pituitary is due to antidiuretic hormone (vasopressin), although it was not until Du Vigneaud characterized and synthesized the vasopressin and oxytocin peptides in the 1950s (for which work a Nobel Prize was awarded) that it was clear these are distinct molecules.

Oxytocin is a nine-amino-acid peptide, comprising a six-member ring formed by sulfide bridges between the two cysteines, and a short tail (~ 1 kDa). Vasopressin differs from oxytocin by having Phe at position 3 and Arg at position 8. Oxytocin is essentially a mammalian hormone (among other vertebrates it has been found only in the ratfish), and its close chemical similarity to vasopressin indicates that it arose in evolution first, by a duplication of the vasopressin gene (or its forebear), and then by mutations. It is clear, in particular from studies on mice with targeted disruption of the oxytocin gene, that oxytocin is indispensable for milk transfer during suckling; consequently, oxytocin is to be regarded as the hormone without which mammalian reproduction would not be possible. The oxytocin and vasopressin genes remain in close proximity to each other (in humans, on chromosome 20), and in opposite orientation, so that they are transcribed left to right and vice versa. Like other peptide hormones, the RNA transcribed from the oxytocin gene includes transcripts from several (three) exons separated by introns, and this heterogeneous nuclear RNA is processed to an mRNA that codes for the oxytocin peptide and for a much larger (~ 10 kDa) protein called oxytocin-neurophysin. This acts as a carrier for oxytocin in the cells in which it is produced, and they are secreted together, but as separate molecules; neurophysin has no known hormonal function, but its measurement in the circulation can be used as an indicator of oxytocin secretion. Among the marsupials, the oxytocin hormone produced is either oxytocin or the similar mesotocin (Ile is substituted for Leu at position 8), or both in some species.

Soon after its synthesis in the laboratory was achieved, industrial production began in the mid-1950s so that oxytocin could be used to promote labor in women, replacing use of the relatively impure posterior pituitary extract that had previously been used. Since its introduction into obstetric practice, millions of human births have been aided by the infusion, usually intravenously, of oxytocin. Also, on delivery of the infant, routine intramuscular injection of oxytocin (together with an ergot) to induce strong uterine contractions is a frontline measure to ensure occlusion of spiral arterioles, which are ruptured when the placenta separates, and thus to prevent post-partum hemorrhage. Conversely, the likely involvement of oxytocin in preterm birth has led to the development of oxytocin receptor antagonists to try to prevent this important cause of neonatal morbidity and mortality.

It became clear in the 1950s that oxytocin is also present in neurons projecting within the brain, where it acts as a neurotransmitter or modulator, with stimulatory roles in neural circuits concerned with affiliative and reproductive behaviors (actions that, together with peripheral effects, have earned oxytocin the title "love hormone"). To date, there is no known naturally occurring oxytocin deficiency state, and no known mutations, although both oxytocin peptide and oxytocin receptor "knockout" mice have been generated.

II. SOURCES OF OXYTOCIN IN THE BODY

A. The Posterior Pituitary Gland

The posterior pituitary gland contains the greatest amount of oxytocin in the body. About three times more oxytocin is stored in the posterior pituitary at the end of pregnancy than is needed to drive the birth process. However, oxytocin stored in the posterior pituitary is not synthesized there: storage occurs in the many thousands of axon terminals of nerve cells that have their cell bodies in the hypothalamus, where oxytocin is continuously synthesized. These nerve cells are concentrated in two paired groups of neurons, or nuclei, in the hypothalamus: the supra-optic and paraventricular nuclei. The oxytocin nerve cell bodies have the general characteristics of neurons. These include dendritic processes, which, like the cell bodies, have many synapses that mediate inputs from many brain areas, using a wide range of excitatory and inhibitory neurotransmitters. Because the neuronal cell bodies produce relatively large amounts of peptide hormone, to achieve effective concentrations in the systemic circulation, they have abundant mRNA for oxytocin (oxytocin mRNA is the most abundant peptide mRNA species in the hypothalamus) and prominent protein synthetic machinery. This includes the Golgi apparatus, where the oxytocin-neurophysin preprohormone is processed and packaged into membrane-bound ves-icles. The cell bodies of the oxytocin neurons are thus larger than other hypothalamic neurons and are visible in histological sections as closely packed "magnocellular" neurons. The similarity between oxytocin and vasopressin has been mentioned already, and this extends to the similarity between the oxytocin neurons and those producing and storing vasopressin. Importantly, magnocellular hypothalamic neurons make either oxytocin or vasopressin, but not both (except for a small percentage of vasopressin neurons that may also express oxytocin when there is a large demand, as in lactation), even though both types of neuron are adjacent to one another in both the supraoptic and the paraventricular nuclei. They can be distinguished from each other with an immunocytochemical technique, using antibodies for oxytocin or vasopres-sin. These neurons differ in other respects that allow them to respond in the most appropriate ways to the different stimuli that activate them and to generate optimal patterns of hormone secretion (see later). What determines whether a magnocellular neuron develops as an oxytocin or a vasopressin neuron is presently not understood; the intergenomic region that links the oxytocin and vasopressin genes evidently contains important sequences that regulate which gene is expressed.

The vesicles containing oxytocin and neurophysin are actively transported within the axon of each neuron, leaving the cell body and arriving several hours later a few millimeters away in the branching terminals in the posterior pituitary. The stalk of the posterior pituitary gland that connects the gland to the hypothalamus mainly comprises these axons, which are packed with the vesicles containing oxytocin (and its neurophysin). Some of the vesicles containing oxytocin are transported from the cell bodies into the dendrites of the neurons, thus remaining in the brain, in the hypothalamus. The secretion of oxytocin by the nerve terminals in the posterior pituitary gland occurs only when the terminals are depolarized by the arrival of action potentials, conducted along the axons from the cell bodies, at $\sim 1\,\mathrm{m\,s^{-1}}$. These action potentials are generated in the cell bodies of the magnocellular oxytocin neurons in the hypothalamus when they are excited by their synaptic input, or are otherwise depolarized. This mechanism can be simulated by electrical stimulation of the pituitary stalk to study the relationship between the frequency and pattern of action potentials and oxytocin secretion, and the signaling mechanisms in the nerve terminals that couple depolarization to the release of oxytocin.

The key event following arrival of action poten-tials is the opening of the membrane channels that allow entry of calcium ions; the increase in cyto-plasmic calcium ion concentration then triggers the intracellular machinery that moves the oxytocin secretory vesicles to the plasma membrane of the nerve terminal, with which they fuse and release their contents into the extracellular space in the process of exocytosis. The peptide released by this neuro-secretory mechanism then passes through the fenestrations in the walls of the adjacent capillaries, to be carried in the systemic circulation to target tissues.

There are two particularly important points about the coupling of the stimulation of the cell bodies of the oxytocin neurons to the secretion of oxytocin from their terminals. The first is that more oxytocin is secreted per action potential if the action potentials are close together (in a "burst"); this is "frequency facilitation" of release. The second is that if all of the oxytocin neurons have a burst of activity at the same time, then the result will be the secretion of a "pulse" of oxytocin into the circulation, achieving a high concentration for a short time. (The importance of this pattern of secretion is explained later.) Once oxytocin is secreted into the circulation it has a half-life of only 2 min or so, being cleared by the tissues on which it acts and by excretion from the kidneys.

B. Oxytocin Within the Brain

Very little, less than 1%, of the circulating oxytocin is able to enter the brain because the blood–brain barrier prevents entry of this peptide, as for most other peptide hormones. However, oxytocin has well-established functions in the central nervous system, the blood–brain barrier effectively allowing the brain and posterior pituitary oxytocin systems to function independently. There are two sources of oxytocin in the brain, the first being the magnocellular neurons of the paraventricular and supraoptic nuclei that secrete oxytocin from their axon terminals in the posterior pituitary, because they also secrete oxytocin from their dendrites, in a way similar to the mechanism operating in the posterior pituitary. Oxytocin from these dendrites has local and probably more distant actions. Second, in the paraventricular nucleus, there are the separate populations of oxytocin neurons that project their axons only centrally, to other brain or spinal cord regions.

C. Peripheral Sources of Oxytocin

The hypothalamic magnocellular neuron-posterior pituitary and the central neuron sources of oxytocin are common to all mammals. There are also peripheral sources of oxytocin that show species or class specificity.

1. Uterus

In pregnancy in humans and in rats, but not in the mouse, cow, or sheep, the oxytocin gene is expressed in the lining of the uterus, placenta, and amnion. Because the adjacent late-pregnant myometrium is a target tissue for oxytocin action, it is possible that oxytocin produced locally acts in this way. However, oxytocin is released not from the side of the cells adjacent to the myometrium, but from the lumenal surface of the uterine epithelium, where there are also oxytocin receptors. It seems unlikely that this source of oxytocin can directly stimulate the myometrium. Instead, this oxytocin is more likely to act by stimulating prostaglandin production by the epithelium or endometrial decidual cells, or in humans by the amnion; in the rat, the amnion lacks the oxytocin receptor.

2. Corpus Luteum

In ruminants (cattle, deer, and sheep), the corpus luteum, formed in the ovary from the follicle after ovulation, produces oxytocin. This acts, together with oxytocin secreted by the neurohypophysis, on the nonpregnant endometrium and stimulates pros-

taglandin F2α secretion, provided oxytocin receptors are expressed; estrogen stimulates the expression of the oxytocin receptors in the endometrium. This prostaglandin F2α is then carried back to the corpus luteum in a local countercurrent circulation to stimulate further oxytocin secretion and to initiate luteolysis. The consequent decrease in progesterone secretion permits gonadotropin stimulation of ovarian follicular development and hence ovulation. This mechanism thus brings forward a further opportunity for conception if the previous ovulation fails to result in pregnancy. Obviously, if pregnancy is to be established, then this mechanism must be prevented. This is achieved by suppression of endometrial oxytocin receptor expression as a result of action of interferon τ produced by the conceptus. This mechanism is thus the key factor in the maternal recognition of pregnancy in these species.

In some other species (e.g., pigs) there is a low level of oxytocin expression in the granulosa cells, which may play a role in luteinization. Studies in pregnant mice show that here low levels of circulating oxytocin maintain the corpora lutea, preventing progesterone withdrawal and paradoxically delaying parturition. Consequently, parturition in mice requires loss of luteal oxytocin receptors as well as up-regulation of myometrial receptors.

3. Heart

In the rat, oxytocin has a natriuretic action. This is consistent with the stimulation of the secretion of both oxytocin and vasopressin by an increase in osmolarity of extracellular fluid in this species. This is usually a result of sodium ion accumulation following food intake or water deprivation; oxytocin promotes sodium excretion, helping to restore normal osmolarity, acting along with vasopressin, which retains water by its actions on the kidney. While oxytocin may act directly on the renal tubules to cause sodium excretion, it now seems that oxytocin also acts on the atria of the heart to stimulate the secretion of atrial natriuretic peptide, which then acts on the kidney to stimulate sodium excretion. It also seems that oxytocin secretion is stimulated by increased blood volume and is important in mediating the subsequent stimulation of atrial natriuretic peptide secretion, which counteracts the volume expansion. Furthermore, the atria evidently produce oxytocin and, if released with atrial distension, as in blood volume expansion, could act locally to stimulate atrial natriuretic peptide secretion in a paracrine fashion.

4. *Immune System*

Oxytocin is synthesized in the thymus gland, particularly in epithelial and nurse cells, although it is not secreted. Nonetheless, oxytocin produced by thymic epithelial cells has been proposed to signal to the differentiating T lymphocytes with which the epithelial cells are in intimate contact. This neuropeptide signaling may be important in the development of immune self-tolerance.

III. REGULATION OF OXYTOCIN GENE EXPRESSION

Regulation of the massive increase in expression of the oxytocin gene in bovine ovarian follicle granulosa cells at ovulation, as they luteinize, has been extensively studied. As yet the factors regulating gene expression in this system remain unclear.

The store of oxytocin in the posterior pituitary increases by about 50% to the end of pregnancy. This may result from reduced release rather than from increased oxytocin gene expression, in as much as the amount of oxytocin mRNA in the magnocellular neurons has not been consistently reported to increase. The upstream region of the oxytocin gene has variations on the AGGTCA motif, a consensus sequence for nuclear hormone receptor binding, but it is not clear what transcription factors regulate the gene. In view of its reproductive functions, regulation of the production of oxytocin by sex steroids has been investigated by many researchers, but the effects are weak and not consistent. Gene expression is increased at parturition, as a consequence of excitation of the neurons during birth, involving withdrawal of inhibitory actions of progesterone in the presence of estrogen. Oxytocin neurons lack progesterone receptors, but there is a strong inhibitory action of progesterone through its metabolite allopregnanolone (a neurosteroid), which is an allosteric modifier at the inhibitory γ-aminobutyric acid ($GABA_A$) receptors on the neurons. Withdrawal of progesterone at the end of pregnancy thus facilitates oxytocin neuron excitation. Although estrogen is reputed to have stimulatory actions on oxytocin gene expression, the mechanism is not known. However, inhibitory effects of estrogen on stimulated oxytocin release, and on oxytocin mRNA expression, have also been described. In the rat, oxytocin neurons express estrogen receptor-β (and not estrogen receptor-α, which the neurons express in some species), but any role in mediating estrogen actions on oxytocin expression is not clear. Estrogen may act on estrogen receptors on the cell surface rather than through intracellular receptors.

In the paraventricular nucleus, which contains centrally projecting neurons, oxytocin gene expression in rats is increased by estrogen. Interestingly, this action of estrogen is interfered with by thyroid hormone, raising the issue of the importance of thyroid status in the functioning of oxytocin neurons. In pregnant sheep, oxytocin mRNA expression is increased in these neurons in pregnancy, but sex steroid actions may not be responsible.

In lactation, the store of oxytocin becomes greatly reduced as it is secreted to drive milk ejections. After a week of lactation, there is marked up-regulation of oxytocin mRNA expression in the magnocellular neurons, leading to increased oxytocin synthesis. This increase has been attributed in part to the decline at this time in progesterone secretion, which is increased for several days after the postpartum estrus. Other factors, such as consequences of continual stimulation of the neurons by suckling, are also involved.

IV. CONTROL OF OXYTOCIN SECRETION

Oxytocin neurons are like other neurons in that they have many synaptic boutons contacting their dendrites and cell bodies. These mediate control of the oxytocin neuron discharge activity by other brain regions and by sensory inputs from the body. These synaptic inputs comprise a rich variety of types of chemical transmitters, such that it is difficult to find a neurotransmitter or neuropeptide that does not act on oxytocin neurons. Thus, there are excitatory amino acid, eicosanoid, monoamine, purine, and peptide actions (e.g., glutamate, noradrenaline, prostaglandin, adenosine, and cholecystokinin), and similarly actions of a range of inhibitory transmitters (e.g., GABA, opioid peptides, and the gas nitric oxide). The effects of these transmitters on oxytocin neurons are, as in other neurons, the result of their depolarizing or hyperpolarizing actions. Again, as for other types of neurons, local modulation of the activity of the synaptic boutons by other transmitters is important in determining the intensity of excitatory or inhibitory barrage. Oxytocin has such a presynaptic action, as do nitric oxide and opioid peptides produced by the oxytocin neurons.

For magnocellular oxytocin neurons, the major inputs in terms of function are those mediating afferent stimuli from the birth canal during parturition and from the mammary glands during suckling (Fig. 1). In the rat, there is an important input from

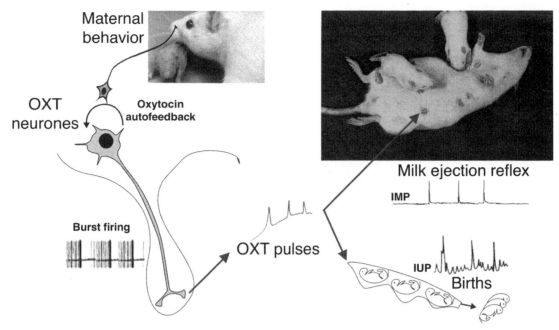

FIGURE 1 Summary of the peripheral and central effects of oxytocin (OXT) in parturition, maternal behavior, and lactation in rats. During the passage of each fetus through the uterine cervix and vagina, afferent nervous impulses from these structures, as they are stretched, are relayed, via the spinal cord and brain pathways, to oxytocin neurons in the hypothalamus. The hypothalamic neurons are excited and send bursts of action potentials to the posterior pituitary, where oxytocin is released into the circulation. Because all of the neurons send bursts at the same time, the result is secretion of a pulse of oxytocin. This stimulates further uterine contractions, increasing intrauterine pressure (IUP) and expelling the fetus. Oxytocin released in the brain at the same time both further excites the oxytocin neurons and evokes maternal behavior. In lactation, the suckling stimulus has similar effects on oxytocin secretion, and now each pulse of oxytocin causes a milk ejection, seen as a sharp increase in intramammary pressure (IMP).

rostral osmosensitive brain structures involved in regulating oxytocin neurones in the context of natriuretic action. Regulation by all of these inputs involves a balance between local GABA and glutamate inputs. These are modulated by actions of oxytocin and nitric oxide released by the dendrites and perikarya of the oxytocin neurons when they are stimulated. Nitric oxide has a local negative feedback effect. In contrast, oxytocin has a local positive feedback effect, provided there is also stimulation by input from the distended birth canal or suckled mammary glands. The neurochemical signature of these inputs is not certain. Noradrenergic neurons projecting from the brain stem, receiving input from the birth canal, are stimulated during parturition, but they are not alone. Similarly, noradrenaline is one of several candidate transmitters mediating excitation of oxytocin neurons by suckling. It seems that there is redundancy in these essential pathways for mammalian reproduction.

In rats, circulating cholecystokinin stimulates oxytocin secretion. As cholecystokinin is secreted by the small intestine during digestion, the consequent secretion of oxytocin helps excrete ingested salt through its natriuretic action. In contrast with the pathways from the birth canal and mammary glands, the pathway for the action of cholecystokinin is clear. It is mediated by vagus nerve afferents and the area postrema and by noradrenergic neurons in the brain stem (nucleus tractus solitarius) that project to oxytocin neurons.

A. Terminal Modulation

The principal determinant of oxytocin release from the posterior pituitary is the frequency of action potentials arriving from the cell bodies in the hypothalamus. However, there is an opportunity for preterminal modulation at this level. First, if the action potentials are clustered, then there is a greater rise in $[Ca^{2+}]$ in the terminals, and hence greater oxytocin release (a mechanism to increase the amount of oxytocin in a pulse). Second, this is a site of inhibition by κ-opioid peptides, which oxytocin neurons also secrete. This mechanism probably reduces basal secretion and in pregnancy helps to build up a store of oxytocin. At the end of pregnancy, this mechanism is down-regulated, facilitating oxytocin secretion during parturition.

B. Suspending Oxytocin Secretion and Parturition

Several species slow or stop the progress of parturition in adverse environmental conditions. In the rat and pig, this seems to be primarily a result of inhibition of oxytocin secretion by activation of central mu opioid peptide receptors on oxytocin neurons. This central opioid mechanism emerges during pregnancy and may also function to prevent premature oxytocin secretion. In mice, stopping parturition in response to stress does not involve opioids, but instead β-adrenergic mechanisms are used.

V. OXYTOCIN RECEPTOR

The actions of oxytocin on target tissues are determined by the level of expression of receptors, their affinity and stability, and their coupling to postreceptor signaling pathways. Both the expression, i.e., the density of oxytocin receptors, and the affinity of the receptors are regulated by steroids. The oxytocin receptor mediates the contractile effects of oxytocin on the myometrial cells of the uterus and the myoepithelial cells of the mammary gland milk-producing alveoli. In marsupials that produce mesotocin rather than oxytocin, the mesotocin receptor seems identical to the oxytocin receptor in other mammals. In the brain, oxytocin receptors mediate the effects of oxytocin on the release of transmitters from nerve terminals and the postsynaptic actions on the electrical activity of neurons.

Like the neurohypophyseal nonapeptides, the oxytocin and vasopressin receptors are also closely related. However, whereas there are three different vasopressin receptors [V1a, V1b (also called V1 and V3, respectively), and V2], each the product of a different gene, there is only one oxytocin receptor gene. The human oxytocin receptor gene is on chromosome 3 and contains four exons and three introns. The oxytocin receptor is a seven-transmembrane domain, class I G-protein-coupled receptor. The second and third extracellular loops and the transmembrane domains of the receptor show remarkable conservation in their amino acid sequences among species, indicating involvement in oxytocin binding. Site-directed mutagenesis studies in expression systems have identified the amino acid residues in the receptor responsible for selectivity. The eighth amino acid (Leu) in oxytocin interacts with several residues in the first and second extracellular loops and Cys-1 then bonds to a Glu residue in the third extracellular loop. The oxytocin ring is then docked in a pocket formed by the transmembrane domains; the interactions between each residue in the oxytocin molecule and residues in the receptor have been derived from computer modeling. The changed configuration of the receptor leads to binding of G-protein to the intracellular domains. Antagonists and oxytocin probably bind to different domains.

The high-affinity state of the receptor in the myometrium has been known for a long time to require Mg^{2+}, and more recently cholesterol and progesterone have been identified as allosteric modulators. Progesterone has been found to interfere with the binding of oxytocin to its receptor in rat (but not in human) myometrium, reducing its affinity. Clearly, this action could explain some of the inhibitory actions of progesterone on oxytocin stimulation of the uterus and the need for progesterone to be withdrawn in many species (although not in the guinea pig) before parturition can be initiated. Another modulatory influence on oxytocin receptor function is the requirement for a cholesterol content of ~60% in the membranes in which the receptor is embedded for high-affinity binding. The receptor has a binding site for cholesterol as well as for oxytocin and cholesterol stabilizes the receptor in the high-affinity state. *In situ*, oxytocin receptors are localized in cholesterol-rich caveoli at the surface of myometrial cells, and in this location internalization is delayed following oxytocin exposure. The involvement of oxytocin and its receptor in positive feedback mechanisms (e.g., luteolysis, parturition, and milk ejection) implies that oxytocin-induced down-regulation or desensitization would cause these loops to fail; the pulsatile secretion of oxytocin may help prevent this.

One of the striking features of the oxytocin receptor is the very large change that is seen in the number of receptors in the uterus as pregnancy advances. Early in pregnancy the uterus is rather insensitive to oxytocin, but the myometrium becomes exquisitely sensitive just before parturition. This correlates with a dramatic increase in oxytocin receptor expression and an increase in affinity. In the rat, the increase in expression occurs on the last day of pregnancy. Hence, increasing stimulation of uterine contractions by oxytocin near the end of pregnancy need not rely on increased oxytocin secretion. In contrast, prolonged exposure to oxytocin, as during labor or oxytocin infusion, causes homologous receptor desensitization with marked decreases in receptor binding, and in oxytocin receptor mRNA expression.

Although the expression of the oxytocin receptor in the myometrium is regulated by the sex steroid changes in pregnancy, and, in particular, expression is inhibited by progesterone and up-regulated by estrogen, this does not seem to be by direct actions on the receptor gene. The regulatory elements of the gene lack the palindromic estrogen response element, although there are half-palindromic motifs. The implication is that estrogen acts through other genes, presumably for specific transcription factors, which then regulate the receptor gene. Of particular interest, in view of the proposed role of infection in preterm labor, is the presence of binding sequences for nucleofactor interleukin-6 in the $5'$ upstream region. Other regulatory signals may be generated by stretching of the myometrium.

In the brain, even in closely related species there are differences in the distribution of oxytocin receptors. These differences are more striking than changes with reproductive state within a species, except that oxytocin receptor expression in the ventromedial hypothalamic nucleus is exquisitely sensitive to regulation by sex steroids (see later).

A. Postreceptor Signaling

The intracellular signaling mechanisms mediating actions of oxytocin are similar among the various target tissues. The oxytocin receptor in the myometrium is predominantly coupled via G_I and $G_{\alpha q/11}$ proteins to phospholipase C-β. This pathway leads to liberation of Ca^{2+} from intracellular stores, and there is also entry of Ca^{2+} from outside, including via L-type Ca^{2+} channels. The increased intracellular $[Ca^{2+}]$ forms complexes with calmodulin, and this then activates myosin light chain kinase (MLCK); phosphorylated myosin then interacts with actin, and the shortening actomyosin contracts the cell. The jointly contracting myometrial cells, which are united by strong junctions, generate the expulsive force required for fetal expulsion. The automatic activation of intracellular Ca^{2+} sequestering mechanisms, and active expulsion of Ca^{2+} from the cells, lead to relaxation. Relaxants such as adrenaline activate adenylyl cyclase via $G_{\alpha s}$ and hence a protein kinase A (PKA) pathway. PKA phosphorylates and inactivates phospholipase C-β and MLCK. The amount of $G_{\alpha s}$ increases in pregnancy but is decreased at term. In pregnancy, there is a change in the proportions of the types of adenylyl cyclase isoforms, which have different properties, expressed in myometrial cells. These changes may contribute to the shift from uterine relaxation in pregnancy to greater responsiveness to oxytocin at term.

A similar mechanism involving increased intracellular $[Ca^{2+}]$ mediates oxytocin stimulation of mammary gland myoepithelial cell contractions, which cause milk ejection. An additional signaling pathway, studied in the amnion (of humans and rabbits), activates cytosolic phospholipase A_2 and hence releases arachidonic acid for prostaglandin synthesis. Here, the oxytocin receptor couples to G_q; the resulting increase in intracellular $[Ca^{2+}]$ contributes to cytosolic phospholipase A_2 activation, which is phosphorylated by extracellular signal-regulated kinase (ERK). Prostaglandin E2 synthesis is then stimulated. In the endometrium of ruminants, oxytocin stimulates prostaglandin F2α production via mobilization of intracellular Ca^{2+}, which activates a protein kinase C-dependent pathway. As described previously, this mechanism produces a luteolytic signal in the absence of conception. A similar stimulation of prostaglandin F2α production by decidual cells reinforces oxytocin actions on the myometrium in parturition.

The actions of oxytocin on neurons bearing oxytocin receptors involve mechanisms similar to those in other tissues. Hypothalamic magnocellular oxytocin neurons (the source of posterior pituitary oxytocin) are stimulated by oxytocin. Oxytocin induces a rapid and long-lasting increase in intracellular $[Ca^{2+}]$, and most of this is released from intracellular stores. This response has a key role in the driving of oxytocin neuron activity during parturition and lactation.

VI. OXYTOCIN IN PARTURITION

As mentioned already, no naturally occurring oxytocin deficiency state is known. The phenotype of this state is partly known from studies in transgenic mice with deletion or inactivation of the oxytocin peptide gene; and more recently from studies of mice with inactivation of the oxytocin receptor gene. Such mice get pregnant and deliver their young, evidently at the appropriate time. However, their young do not survive for long because they cannot obtain milk. The young are rescued if the mothers are given injections of oxytocin. The conclusions from these studies are that oxytocin, and its receptor are not essential for ovarian function, reproductive behavior, or parturition. However, they are essential for milk transfer. The conclusion regarding the essential role of oxytocin in milk transfer is clear enough.

It is not appropriate, however, to conclude that oxytocin has no role in, for example, normal parturition. Rather, the performance of parturition in the absence of oxytocin illustrates how other mechanisms, in particular the uterine production of prostaglandins, and possibly vasopressin, can stimulate uterine contractions. This argues for redundancy in the mechanisms that bring about parturition, which might be expected given the crucial importance for the survival of both mother and offspring of the successful completion of this process. If so, then there should be activation of oxytocin secretory mechanisms, and enhanced oxytocin action, at parturition in mice and other species. The large increase in oxytocin receptor expression in the uterus at term and the changes in intracellular signaling mechanisms so that excitatory pathways predominate (see Section V) are strong circumstantial evidence that oxytocin has a role in parturition.

It does seem clear from studies on several species (humans, rats, and guinea pigs) that although parturition can be initiated at term by systemic infusion with oxytocin, the natural initiation of labor is not a result of increased maternal oxytocin secretion. The role of oxytocin in parturition is to promote the strong uterine contractions in the second stage, leading to the passage of the fetus through the dilated uterine cervix and vagina. Oxytocin then stimulates further uterine contractions that cause placental separation and, in polytocous species, the birth of the next fetus. In human deliveries, these further contractions ensure closure of the ruptured spiral arterioles, preventing a potentially fatal postpartum hemorrhage.

The evidence for increased secretion of oxytocin from the maternal posterior pituitary in parturition is manifold. Oxytocin concentration in the circulation increases in the second stage of labor. In marsupials that produce mesotocin, which has actions identical to those of oxytocin, the concentration of mesotocin in the circulation increases at the birth of the fetus. In humans, measurement of oxytocin in the circulation is difficult because the placenta secretes an aminopeptidase that rapidly destroys oxytocin, and secretion is expected to be pulsatile, so occasional blood samples are unlikely to catch a pulse. Nonetheless, increases in circulating oxytocin have been measured in the second stage. Oxytocin antagonist administration is effective in treating preterm labor in humans and delays births in guinea pigs and slows established parturition in rats. The content of oxytocin in the posterior pituitary gland is decreased by ~30% during parturition. Furthermore, oxytocin is released by the dendrites of the magnocellular neurons during parturition, and local oxytocin antagonist disrupts parturition (probably because it interferes with burst firing). Last, magnocellular oxytocin neurons increase their firing rate, express the immediate-early gene product Fos (a sign of activation of the neurons), and increase expression of the oxytocin gene. Most persuasively, in rats, the oxytocin neurons burst-fire as each pup is born and, furthermore, each burst is followed by a pulse of oxytocin that can be measured in the circulation.

So, what stimulates the secretion of oxytocin in parturition? In the 1940s, Ferguson concluded that oxytocin secretion is stimulated by the distension of the birth canal as the fetus is moved through it and stimulates afferent nerve endings. This is a positive feedback mechanism, which, like all such loops, can only end in an explosion—in this case, the birth of the fetus. Subsequent studies have shown that the pathway for this reflex from the birth canal to the oxytocin neurons is via brain stem nucleus tractus solitarius neurons, including noradrenergic neurons, that project directly to the magnocellular oxytocin neurons. There is an increase in noradrenaline release from the terminals of these neurons in the supraoptic nucleus during parturition, and other evidence suggests a role for this input in driving oxytocin neurons.

VII. OXYTOCIN IN LACTATION

Feeding offspring with milk transferred by suckling is a distinctive feature of mammalian reproduction and is new in evolution, contrasting with parturition that has a long evolutionary connection with egg laying. The production of milk requires stimulation of mammary gland development by sex steroids and the subsequent stimulation by prolactin of milk synthesis and secretion by the epithelial cells of the alveoli. The milk is stored in alveoli (e.g., in rats), in sinuses, which are enlargements of the milk ducts beneath the nipple (e.g., in humans), or in a cistern into which the ducts empty, located beneath the nipple (the udder in cattle and sheep). Oxytocin acts on contractile myoepithelial cells around the alveoli, and the combined action of these cells around the thousands of alveoli causes the movement of milk through the ducts. In species with substantial storage capacity in the sinuses or cistern, this movement comprises milk "let-down." The suckling young then obtain the milk by the milking action as they suck on the nipple and the subjacent storage sites. Milk ejection from the nipple resulting from the action of oxytocin occurs if more milk is let down than can be stored.

It was shown in electrophysiological studies on lactating rats in the early 1970s that a continual suckling stimulus applied to the nipples is converted to intermittent high-frequency action potential discharge of neurons in the supraoptic and paraventricular nuclei. These bursts were found in about half of the neurons recorded and occurred about 7 min apart during suckling. Each burst preceded a sharp increase in intramammary pressure by the time that it takes oxytocin to travel in the circulation from the posterior pituitary to the mammary gland. Later, paired recordings showed that neurons in the supraoptic or paraventricular nuclei burst-fire almost synchronously. Thus, each episode of synchronized bursting leads to the secretion of a pulse of oxytocin, each of which causes a milk ejection and each comprising about 1 pmol (0.5 mU) of oxytocin.

The suckling stimulus applied to the nipples is carried in afferent nerve fibers to the brain stem, and then, via a multisynaptic pathway that is not fully characterized, to the oxytocin neurons. The synapses on oxytocin neurons contain a multitude of neurotransmitter types, but it is not clear which transmitter is of key importance in signaling the suckling stimulus.

VIII. IMPORTANCE OF OXYTOCIN IN THE BRAIN

Oxytocin released within the brain has several actions. There are two broad types of oxytocin action. First, oxytocin has local positive feedback actions on the magnocellular neurons that produce it. In this case, the oxytocin is released from the dendrites of the neurons and it acts back on the oxytocin neurons and their local synaptic inputs to excite the neurons during parturition and suckling. These actions are important in generating the pulsatile pattern of oxytocin secretion at these times. Second, oxytocin is released from the axon terminals of centrally projecting neurons (mainly those with cell bodies in the paraventricular nucleus) at several discrete sites in the brain that are important in organizing reproductive behaviors and associated emotion, or autonomic, outputs.

A. Oxytocin in the Generation of Bursting Activity of Oxytocin Neurons

It is clear that the oxytocin released by dendrites of the oxytocin neurons during the quiet initial period of suckling, before the bursts start, plays an essential role in driving bursts. Oxytocin release in the magnocellular nuclei can be detected by sampling extracellular fluid with a microdialysis probe; bursting is stopped by administration of an oxytocin antagonist into a magnocellular nucleus, and centrally injected oxytocin facilitates bursting.

In addition to actions on the oxytocin neurons, oxytocin also acts presynaptically to suppress excitatory glutamatergic input and to inhibit GABA-ergic input. These actions may lead to periodic increases in local excitatory input. The synchronization of bursting behavior among the oxytocin neurons, without which a pulse of oxytocin could not be secreted, could also follow periodic activation of a local network. Also involved are morphological changes within the magnocellular nuclei due to retractions of glial processes that bring adjacent neurons into more intimate contact, and to the increased density of GABA and glutamate synapses in lactation. Oxytocin release in the bed nucleus of the stria terminalis (a limbic brain region) contributes to facilitation of the bursting activity of magnocellular oxytocin neurons during suckling, and here estrogen has a positive influence. This is one brain area in which oxytocin receptor expression increases in late pregnancy.

B. Oxytocin and Behavior

Oxytocin in the brain has actions on behavior that are congruent with its peripheral reproductive functions.

1. Maternal Behavior

The first observation, in 1979, was that oxytocin injected into the brain in estrogen-treated virgin rats induced the rapid onset of maternal behavior toward foster pups. Without such oxytocin treatment, virgin rats seem fearful of pups. Conversely, oxytocin antagonist infusion into the medial preoptic area or ventral tegmental area, regions known from other studies to be important in maternal behavior, blocked the initiation of maternal behavior postpartum. Part of the action of oxytocin on maternal behavior involves reducing anxiety.

In sheep, oxytocin is released in the brain in response to vagino-cervical stimulation during birth. Bonding of the ewe with its lamb depends on olfactory memory, and this involves oxytocin action in the olfactory bulb. The paraventricular nucleus contains the important population of centrally projecting oxytocin neurons that promote maternal behavior. Oxytocin release from terminals in the brain regions where maternal behavior is organized modulates release of other transmitters that in turn elicit maternal behavior. Once this task is performed immediately postpartum, continued action of oxytocin does not seem to be required to maintain maternal behavior. In contrast, transgenic mice with inactivation of the oxytocin gene show normal maternal behavior, but mice are peculiar in that females show maternal behavior without having been pregnant. Thus, mice do not need the drive provided by oxytocin released in the brain during parturition. Indeed, they lack oxytocin receptors in the forebrain area where oxytocin acts in other species to promote maternal behavior.

2. Female Reproductive Behavior

In the rat and hamster, oxytocin from paraventricular nucleus neurons acts in the hypothalamic ventromedial nucleus and medial preoptic area to facilitate female reproductive (lordosis) behavior. The effectiveness of oxytocin depends on estrogen, which induces oxytocin receptors in the ventromedial nucleus, and receptor distribution is expanded by progesterone. This leads to enhanced electrophysiological responses of the neurons to oxytocin. However, estrogen inhibits oxytocin receptor expression in the mouse, and as a corollary the oxytocin knockout female mouse does not show defects in sexual receptivity.

Marked differences in the affiliative behavior of species of voles have been used to uncover roles of brain oxytocin in bonding between sexual partners. Prairie voles are monogamous and live in social groups, but montane voles are not monogamous and live in isolation. Bond formation between a female prairie vole and the male with which she first mates depends on oxytocin released in the brain during mating. In contrast, montane voles do not form bonds after mating, not even if oxytocin is injected into the brain: indeed, they have very low levels of oxytocin receptor expression in brain areas associated with reward, in contrast with prairie voles. These different patterns of receptor expression reflect differences in the upstream region of the gene that confers tissue-specific expression.

A role for oxytocin in the brain in promoting social interaction is supported by finding defects in transgenic mice with inactivation of the oxytocin gene. Unlike normal mice, these transgenic mice fail to learn to recognize conspecifics with which they have become familiar by repeated social exposure. This is attributable to loss of an essential action of oxytocin in the medial amygdala, part of the limbic, emotional, brain.

3. Ingestive Behavior

Consonant with its natriuretic action in the rat, oxytocin acts within the brain to inhibit salt ingestion when this is inappropriate. It is also one of several peptides that act in the brain to reduce food intake; though this may reflect a primary role to inhibit intake of the salt in food. Through projections to the dorsal vagal complex in the brain stem, oxytocin neurons inhibit gastric motility, an appropriate accompaniment to inhibition of intake.

IX. OTHER ACTIONS OF OXYTOCIN/ANTAGONISTS

A. Oxytocin Actions on the Anterior Pituitary

Oxytocin is present in hypothalamo-hypophyseal portal blood at greater concentrations than in peripheral blood. This oxytocin is secreted from magnocellular neuron axon swellings in the median eminence. Oxytocin acts on V1b receptors on corticotrophs [cells secreting adrenocorticotropic hormone (ACTH), which do not have oxytocin receptors] in the anterior pituitary to augment the action of corticotropin-releasing hormone on ACTH secretion in rats; however, in humans, oxytocin is inhibitory.

The main action of oxytocin on the anterior pituitary is to stimulate prolactin secretion in lactation. This is promoted by a large increase in oxytocin receptor expression in lactotrophs (cells secreting prolactin) at the end of pregnancy, but depends on withdrawal of inhibition by dopamine. However, other factors increase prolactin secretion in lactation. Oxytocin can advance the ovulatory luteinizing hormone surge, though the importance of this is not clear.

B. Oxytocin in Males

The importance of oxytocin is primarily in the context of female reproduction. In males, oxytocin secretion is increased by sexual intercourse and stimulates seminiferous tubule contractions, so it may aid the transport of sperm from the testis. Produced by Leydig cells in the testis, oxytocin locally influences steroidogenesis; oxytocin produced in the prostate affects prostate androgen metabolism. In the brain, oxytocin acts in the paraventricular nucleus to induce penile erection; this probably activates, through a mechanism involving nitric oxide, oxytocin neurons projecting to autonomic outflow neurons in the brain stem and spinal cord. Transgenic male mice without oxytocin show reduced aggressiveness toward intruder males.

C. Oxytocin Receptor Antagonists

Several oxytocin receptor antagonists have been synthesized. Most are peptides based on the non-apeptide prototype. One such peptide, Atosiban, is licensed in Europe for use in the management of imminent preterm birth. Nonpeptide antagonists are not in clinical use. The advantage of targeting the oxytocin receptor for tocolysis (uterine relaxation) over other approaches, such as the use of β_2-adrenergic agonists, is that oxytocin receptors are largely restricted to the pregnant uterus and the mammary gland. Consequently, unwanted actions of selective oxytocin receptor antagonists on other tissues should not be a problem. However, there may be the possibility of actions in the heart, but the main issue is that the antagonists developed so far are also antagonists at V1a receptors. Although this may reinforce tocolytic actions because of the possible involvement of V1a receptors in the stimulation of uterine contractions in parturition, vasopressin stimulation of blood vessel contraction through these receptors will be inhibited. This is a potential problem in the context of defense of blood pressure during hemorrhage. Peptide antagonists are unlikely to enter the brain significantly or to cross the placenta. Atosiban is effective in alleviating the symptoms of dysmenorrhea (pain prior to menstruation), because in this condition vasopressin acting through V1a receptors is responsible for the stimulation of painful uterine contractions.

Glossary

amnion Sac in which the embryo and fetus develop.
axons Thin processes of neurons contacting a target (here, either other neurons or blood vessels in the posterior pituitary); rapidly conduct action potentials (waves of depolarization) from the cell body to the terminals; slowly transport peptide to be secreted from the terminals.
burst Brief, high-frequency cluster of action potentials generated in a neuron; the basis for secretion of a pulse of oxytocin.

corpus luteum Endocrine tissue formed from the ovarian follicle after it ovulates; produces progesterone. Luteolysis is the death of the corpus luteum.
decidua Endometrial lining shed at the end of pregnancy.
dendrites Thick nerve cell processes that receive synapses (contacts) from other nerve cells; also capable of secreting.
endometrium Lining of the human uterus.
hypothalamus Brain region concerned with automatic regulation of many body functions, including controlling secretion of hormones from the pituitary gland.
myoepithelial cells Contractile cells surrounding the milk-secreting glands in the lactating mammary gland.
myometrium Contractile, muscular tissue of the uterus.
natriuresis Stimulated sodium excretion by the kidney.
paraventricular and supraoptic nuclei Areas in the hypothalamus where most of the nerve cells (neurons) in the brain producing oxytocin are located.
posterior pituitary gland Developmentally, a downgrowth from the hypothalamus of the brain. Contains terminals of hypothalamic neurons with stored oxytocin.
preterm birth Emergence of the fetus before it is fully prepared for extrauterine life.

See Also the Following Articles

Corpus Luteum in Primates • Corpus Luteum: Regression and Rescue • Decidualization • Endometrial Remodeling • Oxytocin/Vasopressin Receptor Signaling • Placental Development • Progesterone Action in the Female Reproductive Tract • Sexual Differentiation of the Brain • Vasopressin (AVP)

Further Reading

Dellovade, T. L., Zhu, Y.-S., and Pfaff, D. W. (1999). Thyroid hormones and estrogen affect oxytocin gene expression in hypothalamic neurons. *J. Neuroendocrinol.* 11, 1–10.
Douglas A. J., Leng G., and Ludwig M., Russell J. A. (eds.) (2000). Oxytocin and vasopressin—From molecules to function. Exp. Physiol. 85S, 1–272.
Geenen, V., Kecha, O., and Martens, H. (1998). Thymic expression of neuroendocrine self-peptide precursors: Role in T cell survival and self-tolerance. *J. Neuroendocrinol.* 10, 811–822.
Gimpl, G., and Fahrenholz, F. (2001). The oxytocin receptor system: Structure, function, and regulation. *Physiol. Rev.* 81, 629–668.
Imamura, T., Luedke, C. E., Vogt, S. K., and Muglia, L. J. (2000). Oxytocin modulates the onset of murine parturition by competing ovarian and uterine effects. *Am. J. Physiol.* 279, R1061–R1067.
Ivell, R. (1999). The physiology of ovarian oxytocin. *Reprod. Med. Rev.* 7, 11–25.
Jankowski, M., Hajjar, F., Al Kawas, S., Mukaddam-Daher, S., Hoffman, G., McCann, S. M., and Gutkowska, J. (1998). Rat heart: A site of oxytocin production and action. *Proc. Natl. Acad. Sci. U.S.A.* 95, 14558–14563.

McCracken, J. A., Custer, E. E., and Lamsa, J. C. (1999). Luteolysis: A neuroendocrine-mediated event. *Physiol. Rev.* **79**, 263–323.

Parry, L. J., and Bathgate, R. A. D. (2000). The role of oxytocin and regulation of uterine oxytocin receptors in pregnant marsupials. *Exp. Physiol.* **85S**, 91S–99S.

Pedersen, C. A., Caldwell, J. D., Walker, C., Ayers, G., and Mason, G. A. (1994). Oxytocin activates the postpartum onset of rat maternal behavior in the ventral tegmental and medial preoptic areas. *Behav. Neurosci.* **108**, 1163–1171.

Russell, J. A., and Leng, G. (1998). Sex, parturition and motherhood without oxytocin? *J. Endocrinol.* **157**, 343–359.

Russell J. A., Douglas A. J., Windle R. J., and Ingram C. D. (eds.) (2001). The maternal brain. Neurobiological and neuroendocrine adaptations and disorders in pregnancy and post partum. Prog. Brain. *Res.* **133**, 1–365.

Russell, J. A., Leng, G., and Douglas, A. J. (2003). The magnocellular oxytocin system, the fount of maternity: Adaptations in pregnancy. *Front. Neuroendocrinol.* [in press].

Young, L. J., Lim, M. M., Gingrich, B., and Insel, T. R. (2001). Cellular mechanisms of social attachment. *Horm. Behav.* **40**, 133–138.

Zingg, H. H., Bourque C. W., and Bichet D. G. (eds.) (1998). Vasopressin and oxytocin. Molecular, cellular, and clinical advances. *Adv. Exp. Med. Biol.* **449**, 1–483.

Oxytocin/Vasopressin Receptor Signaling

MELVYN S. SOLOFF AND YOW-JIUN JENG

University of Texas Medical Branch, Galveston

The neurohypophyseal hormones oxytocin and arginine vasopressin are structurally related and signal through a family of G-protein-coupled receptors. The oxytocin receptor is unique and there are three distinct vasopressin receptors: V_1, V_2, **and** V_3. **Oxytocin and vasopressin** V_1 **and** V_3 **receptors are coupled to** $G_{q/11}$ **and** $G_{i/o}$ **heterotrimeric G-proteins, whereas** V_2 **vasopressin receptors act through** G_s.

I. INTRODUCTION

The signal pathways mediating the actions of oxytocin and arginine vasopressin on specific target cells through their unique receptors are highlighted in this article. Although generalizations have been made, some pathways vary with different cell types or species. Even within the same cell type, there may be differences in signaling at different stages of the cell cycle or during development. Exceptions will be noted whenever possible.

II. OXYTOCIN AND VASOPRESSIN

Oxytocin (OT) and arginine vasopressin (AVP) are produced primarily by the supraoptic and paraventricular nuclei of the hypothalamus; they are transported along axons to cell termini in the posterior pituitary, where they are stored in the form of membrane-bound neurosecretory granules. The two neuropeptides are structurally related to each other and to vasotocin, which occurs in fish, reptiles, amphibians, and birds (Fig. 1). These peptides share a disulfide-linked ring structure of six residues that restricts conformational flexibility, and a flexible three-residue amino-terminal tail. The carboxyl-terminal glycine is amidated in all three peptides. Oxytocin and vasopressin differ only at position 3 of the cyclic peptide portion and position 8 of the C-terminal tripeptide amide region. Duplication of a common ancestral gene likely gave rise to the OT and AVP genes. Both genes reside on the same chromosome and, in humans and mice, are only 12 and 3 kb apart, respectively. Both peptides are synthesized in larger precursor forms and are

```
                      1   2   3   4   5   6
Oxytocin      H₂N-Cys-Tyr-Ile-Gln-Asn-Cys-Pro-Leu-Gly-NH₂
                  |_____|


Vasopressin   H₂N-Cys-Tyr-Phe-Gln-Asn-Cys-Pro-Arg-Gly-NH₂
                  |_____|


Vasotocin     H₂N-Cys-Tyr-Ile-Gln-Asn-Cys-Pro-Arg-Gly-NH₂
                  |_____|
```

FIGURE 1   Structures of OT, AVP, and vasotocin. In lysine vasopressin, which is found in pigs, a Lys replaces Arg in position 8.

processed to mature hormones in neurosecretory cells. When the nerve cell membrane is depolarized, OT and AVP are released and pass through endothelial cells to enter the circulation. Oxytocin release is caused by vaginal stretch, by suckling, and, in some species, by osmotic stimuli. Higher centers in the brain are also involved. Vasopressin release occurs in response to stimuli that alter the state of fluids in the body, such as increased plasma osmotic pressure and reduced blood volume and/or blood pressure. Oxytocin stimulates mammary myoepithelial cell contraction and is essential for milk ejection in most mammalian species. Oxytocin also elicits contraction of uterine smooth muscle and probably plays a role in labor initiation. Oxytocin targets in the brain elicit responses associated with social, sexual, and maternal behavior. Vasopressin, or antidiuretic hormone (ADH), is a vasoconstrictor, and it also reduces urinary water excretion by increasing the water permeability of the renal collecting duct. Vasopressin is also a costimulator with corticotropin-releasing hormone (CRH) of adrenocorticotropic hormone (ACTH) release from the anterior pituitary.

The similar structures of the neurohypophyseal peptides account for the overlap in agonist activities. Oxytocin has about 1% of the potency of AVP in increasing rat blood pressure or eliciting antidiuresis. Vasopressin has about 15% of the potency of OT in both rat uterus and rabbit mammary gland assays. Generally, these differences are the reflection of reduced affinities for receptor binding sites; but vasopressin has about twice the apparent K_d for OTRs, compared to OT, yet only 15% of the agonist activity. This paradox may be explained by AVP being a partial OT agonist/antagonist that binds to the OTR to a greater extent than is reflected by signal transduction. The selective binding of OT and AVP to their respective receptors is largely determined by the residue at position 8. In vasopressin, a basic residue fills this position; in OT and OT analogues, the residue is neutral and usually aliphatic.

As might be expected from the common ancestry of OT and AVP, the receptors for the neurohypophyseal hormones, which are G-protein-coupled receptors (GPCRs), are more closely related to each other than to any other GPCR family member. The neurohypophyseal hormone receptors comprise a group of four related proteins expressed by separate genes. The OT receptor (OTR) is largely associated with target cells involved in reproductive processes. The V_2 receptor is expressed predominantly in the

kidney and accounts for the antidiuretic effects of vasopressin. The V_1 and V_3 receptors can be distinguished by their selectivity for AVP analogues, but the primary difference is in their cellular distribution. Vasopressin V_1 receptors are expressed in vascular smooth muscle and other tissues, whereas V_3 receptors are largely restricted to the central nervous system. The two extremes in the family, the V_2R and OTR, are identical in 40% of their sequences, with the highest similarity in the transmembrane and extracellular domains.

III. OXYTOCIN SIGNALING

OTRs are expressed in the lactating mammary gland, uterine smooth muscle (myometrium), uterine epithelium (endometrium or decidua), and the amnion, among other target sites. There have been extensive studies on neural targets for OT, but less information on signaling mechanisms is available. In general, OTRs are highly regulated. In virtually all species studied, the concentration of OTRs in the myometrium is maximal at the time of parturition, rising several 100-fold in women between the beginning and end of pregnancy. The coupling to G-proteins in the rat myometrium is also up-regulated at the end of pregnancy, as determined by gel filtration analysis of solubilized OTR–G-protein complexes. The concentration of OTRs in the endometrium (or decidua) and amnion is also maximal at the end of gestation. Conversely, OTR concentrations in the mammary gland are maximal during lactation, when the concentration of OT in the blood is elevated; the uterine OTRs are down-regulated at this time, so that only mammary myoepithelial cells are stimulated by OT. Although the AVP receptor subtypes are regulated, the magnitude of change is small compared with OTRs.

A. G-Protein and Effector Coupling to the Oxytocin Receptor

The OTR is functionally coupled to both $G_{q/11}$ and $G_{i/o}$, as demonstrated in several target cell types (Fig. 2). Both classes of G-proteins stimulate phospholipase C-β (PLC-β), which leads to the generation inositol 1,4,5-trisphosphate (InsP$_3$) and 1,2-diacylglycerol (DAG). Inositol trisphosphate triggers Ca^{2+} release from intracellular stores, whereas DAG, acting in conjunction with Ca^{2+}, stimulates protein kinase C (PKC). Activation of mitogen-activated protein (MAP) kinase (MEK) in the MAP kinase cascade occurs downstream of PKC phosphorylation.

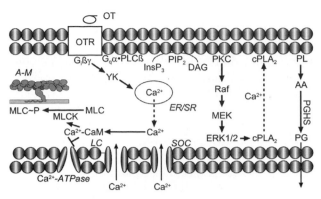

FIGURE 2 Pathways involved in OT signaling result in an increase in myosin light chain (MLC) phosphorylation and contractile activity and/or the stimulation of prostaglandin (PG) synthesis. Both processes are mediated by an increase in $[Ca^{2+}]_i$ from the endoplasmic/sarcoplasmic reticulum (ER/SR) through $G_{q/11}$/phospholipase C (PLC) and $G_{i/o}$/tyrosine kinase activation. The resultant increase in $[Ca^{2+}]_i$ allows the influx of extracellular Ca^{2+} through store-operated channels (SOCs) and L-type voltage regulated channels (LCs). An increase in the binding of Ca^{2+} to calmodulin (CaM) results in inhibition of a sarcolemmal calcium pump (Ca^{2+}-ATPase), resulting in elevated Ca^{2+} levels over a longer time. The Ca^{2+}–CaM complex activates MLC kinase (MLCK) to phosphorylate the myosin light chain 20 of myosin II, which promotes the interaction of actin and myosin (A–M) and the contraction of smooth muscle. The increase in $[Ca^{2+}]_i$ also allows translocation of cytosolic phospholipase A_2 ($cPLA_2$) to internal membranes. Increased protein kinase C (PKC) activity resulting from $G_{q/11}$ activation also leads to successive extracellular signal-related kinase (ERK2/1) and $cPLA_2$ phosphorylations. The activated $cPLA_2$ catalyzes increases in arachidonic acid (AA) levels from membrane phospholipids (PLs) and greater PG synthesis through prostaglandin H synthase (PGHS) activity. OTR, Oxytocin receptor; $InsP_3$, inositol 1,4,5-trisphosphate; PIP_2, phosphatidylinositol 4,5-bisphosphate.

A role for $G_{i/o}$ was initially determined by pertussis toxin (PTX) sensitivity of OT-stimulated signaling pathways (Fig. 2). However, caution is advised in the use of PTX treatment because it elevates intracellular cyclic adenosine monophosphate (cAMP), which inhibits responses to OT that are independent of OTR activation. For example, cAMP-stimulated protein kinase A (PKA) catalyzes the phosphorylation of PLC, resulting in inhibition of OT-stimulated $InsP_3$ production. The inhibition could be reversed by treatment with a selective PKA inhibitor. Thus, at least part of the effects of PTX can be attributed to $G_{i/o}$ that is not coupled to the OTR. Other work, however, has shown that the OTR is associated with $G_{i/o}$; using both coprecipitation with antibody, and assays showing it has been shown that OT

stimulation of GTPase activity in intact myometrial membranes is inhibited by PTX. In addition, OT treatment decreases PTX-stimulated ADP-ribosylation of $G_{\alpha i}$ in myometrial membranes. This decrease is consistent with OT activating heterotrimeric G_i by dissociating $G_{\alpha i}$, because ribosylation of the α-subunit occurs only in the heterotrimer. Inhibition of PLC activity by PKA phosphorylation may partially explain the ability of agents that elevate intracellular cAMP to oppose the actions of OT and to maintain uterine smooth muscle in a quiescent state.

Removal of 51 residues from the C-terminus of the rat OTR expressed in stably transfected Chinese hamster ovary (CHO) cells causes the loss of coupling to $G_{q/11}$. PTX-sensitive increases in intracellular Ca^{2+} concentration ($[Ca^{2+}]_i$), however, are unaffected by receptor truncation. Surprisingly, this signaling is independent of PLC activity; the $G_{i/o}$ pathways leading to increased $[Ca^{2+}]_i$ are yet undefined. Activation of $G_{i/o}$ involves the $G_{\beta\gamma}$ subunits, because transient transfection of the cells expressing truncated OTR with the $G_{\beta\gamma}$ sequestrant βARKct blocks OT-stimulated intracellular Ca^{2+} transients. A generic tyrosine kinase inhibitor also inhibits the effects of OT, suggesting that $G_{\beta\gamma}$ subunits transactivate signaling via tyrosine kinase pathways, as has been shown for other GPCRs. Oxytocin signaling in a mutant lacking 39 residues of the C-terminal tail is indistinguishable from that of the wild-type OTR. Therefore, the region between 39 and 51 residues from the carboxyl terminus appears to be critical for coupling of the OTR to $G_{q/11}$.

B. Many Effects of Oxytocin are Mediated by Increased Intracellular Ca^{2+} Concentrations

The initial rise in $[Ca^{2+}]_i$ following OT treatment of isolated myometrial cells is due mainly to the $InsP_3$-mediated release of Ca^{2+} from intracellular stores in the endoplasmic or sarcoplasmic reticulum, but Ca^{2+} influx from extracellular sources also occurs (Fig. 2). Studies have indicated that the increased influx of Ca^{2+} is regulated by store-operated or capacitative channels, following the rise in $[Ca^{2+}]_i$ from intracellular sites. Other studies indicate that extracellular Ca^{2+} influx occurs through L-type voltage channels. The large difference in Ca^{2+} concentration between the outside and inside of cells is maintained in part by the unidirectional export of Ca^{2+} by a high-affinity Ca^{2+} extrusion pump in the cell membrane. This process, involving Ca^{2+},Mg^{2+}-dependent ATPase activity, occurs in a number of cell types. OT inhibits this ATPase in sarcolemmal (plasma) membranes from the uterine smooth muscle of rabbits, rats, and humans. This process contributes to maintaining elevated $[Ca^{2+}]_i$ in myometrial cells following the increase in Ca^{2+} from intracellular and extracellular sources. The effects of OT are blocked by calmodulin (CaM) inhibition, but the signal pathways require further elaboration.

In uterine smooth muscle cells and mammary myoepithelial cells, which are smooth muscle-like but are derived from ectoderm instead of mesoderm, the rise in $[Ca^{2+}]_i$ leads to Ca^{2+}–CaM stimulation of myosin light chain kinase (MLCK) activity. The phosphorylation of myosin light chain (MLC) 20 allows myosin heads to form cross-bridges with actin filaments, leading to contraction. Yet to be elucidated are the molecular actions of OT on neural targets involved in many behavioral patterns, as well as in memory and learning. It seems likely that OT-stimulated rises in $[Ca^{2+}]_i$ control cellular excitability and modulate firing patterns. These processes almost certainly involve stimulation of gene transcription and protein synthesis.

C. Oxytocin Stimulation of Prostaglandin Synthesis

A second major activity of OT in uterine and other tissues is the stimulation of prostaglandin synthesis. This occurs in endometrial and amnion cells and CHO cells stably transfected with the rat OTR by stimulation of arachidonic acid formation from membrane glycerophospholipids, and the incorporation of arachidonic acid into prostaglandins. OT-induced increases in $[Ca^{2+}]_i$ (described in the preceding paragraph) lead to Ca^{2+} binding to the C-2 domain of cytosolic phospholipase A_2 (cPLA$_2$) and its translocation to the nuclear envelope and endoplasmic reticulum, wherein lie glycerophospholipid substrates for cPLA$_2$-catalyzed arachidonic acid formation. The phospholipase is activated by serine phosphorylation by extracellular signal-regulated protein kinases (ERK1/2), which in turn are activated by OT stimulation of the PKC/MEK pathway. Arachidonic acid is converted to prostaglandins (PGs) through the actions of prostaglandin endoperoxide H synthase (PGHS), also referred to as cyclooxygenase (COX). This bifunctional enzyme catalyzes both the oxidation of arachidonic acid to the prostaglandin endoperoxide, PGG$_2$, and its subsequent reduction to PGH$_2$, the precursor for all prostanoids. There are two PGHS isoforms, each expressed by a separate gene. PGHS-1 is constitutively expressed in most cell types, whereas PGHS-2 mRNA is rapidly and transiently induced. Normally, PGHS-2 is undetectable but is induced in the fashion of an immediate-early gene by a variety of agents, including OT, in the endometrium, myometrium, and amnion. Generally, utilization of PGHS-1 is associated with the early phase of prostaglandin synthesis, occurring within several minutes of stimulation, whereas prostaglandin synthesis occurring over several hours coincides with the induction of PGHS-2 expression.

Depending on the cell type and stimulus, PGHS-2 synthesis can be a rate-limiting step with respect to PG synthesis, or it can enhance production of the relatively low levels of PGs synthesized through PGHS-1. The induction of PGHS-2 is necessary for OT-stimulated PGF$_{2\alpha}$ synthesis in bovine uterine endometrium and prostacyclin production by human myometrial cells. In contrast, the levels of PGHS-1 activity in rabbit amnion are constitutively high and the induction of PGHS-2 does not contribute to increased PGE$_2$ production. The role of PGHS-2 in these cells is presently unknown, as are the pathways involved in OT-induction of PGHS-2 expression. In cultured human myometrial cells, this induction is PTX sensitive, as is activation of the MAP kinase pathway.

D. Down-regulation of Oxytocin Receptors by Endocytosis

Radioligand binding data using intact human myometrial cells have shown that OTR numbers on the cell membrane remain stable for a number of hours after addition of OT. This observation is consistent with physiological observations, because the uterus remains sensitive to OT for a period of time during labor. Human OTRs expressed in human embryonic kidney (HEK) or CHO cell lines, however, are rapidly internalized in response to OT treatment. Internalization is mediated by phosphorylation of two serine clusters in the C-terminal domain of the receptor by PKC, followed by the binding of β-arrestin-2 and uncoupling of the receptor from its G-protein partners. This process results in the termination of OTR signaling. β-Arrestin acts as an adapter protein that links the receptor to components of the endocytic machinery and targets the desensitized receptor to clathrin-coated pits for endocytosis. Like other GPCRs, the internalized OTRs are dephosphorylated in endosomes and recycled back to the cell surface fully resensitized.

It remains to be established whether OTRs in natural target cells, other than myometrial cells, are rapidly internalized. Apart from internalization, the association of receptors with β-arrestin may be involved in initiating and/or regulating signaling pathways. For example, Src recruitment to the β_2-adrenergic receptor is mediated by β-arrestin, which functions as an adapter protein, binding both c-Src and the agonist-occupied receptor. β-Arrestin also appears to function as a molecular scaffold that organizes and recruits components of the MAPK cascade.

E. Atypical Oxytocin Target Cells

Functional OTRs have been described in several tissues and a variety of cell types not typically considered targets for OT. Generally, the signal pathways involved in OT action have only been examined in a perfunctory manner. In most cases the cell types were not in primary cultures but were established cell lines; therefore, signaling by OT is not necessarily representative of OT action in untransformed cells.

Oxytocin has insulin-like activity in stimulating glucose oxidation and lipogenesis in rat adipocytes. These effects occur independently of insulin action and are mediated by OTRs, which have been characterized by ligand binding. Unlike insulin, the effects of OT on glucose oxidation in fat cells are not mediated by increased glucose transport. Instead, OT stimulates polyphosphoinositide breakdown and elevated $[Ca^{2+}]_i$ in adipocytes. The molar concentration of OT-stimulating glucose oxidation is about five times greater than that of insulin, and the maximal effect is only about 20% that of insulin. Oxytocin is also less effective than insulin in stimulating lipogenesis; therefore, it is not certain whether there is a physiological role for OT in fat cell metabolism.

Oxytocin receptors are expressed in both undifferentiated and differentiated human trabecular bone cells with osteogenic capacity in primary culture. The addition of OT rapidly increases $[Ca^{2+}]_i$ and stimulates prostaglandin synthesis. Oxytocin receptors have been demonstrated in the aorta, vena cava, and pulmonary vein by reverse transcription polymerase chain reaction (RT-PCR) and ligand binding analyses. Because OT is also expressed in these same tissues, these blood vessels appear to contain an intrinsic OT system, which may be involved in the regulation of vascular tone as well as vascular regrowth and remodeling. It is likely that OTRs are confined to the endothelium of these vessels. Occupancy of these receptor sites mobilizes intracellular

Ca^{2+} and causes the release of nitric oxide, which is prevented by chelation of extracellular and intracellular Ca^{2+}. Nitric oxide production is associated with vasorelaxation, and presumably OT has a vasodilatory effect on certain blood vessels.

Oxytocin receptors in both atrial and ventricular chambers of the rat heart mediate the OT-stimulated release of atrial natriuretic peptide. This peptide slows the heart and reduces its force of contraction to produce a rapid reduction in circulating blood volume. Oxytocin receptors are found in human breast tumors of epithelial origin, as measured by immunological techniques. There are, however, no clear indications as to whether these receptors are functional. Several breast tumor cell lines have been shown to express OTRs, but the functional role of OT is not clear. Oxytocin receptors have been found in thymocytes, ovarian cells, Leydig cells, and prostate cells, but information regarding signaling pathways in these cell types is still rudimentary.

IV. LACK OF DISEASES ASSOCIATED WITH IMPROPER EXPRESSION OF OXYTOCIN RECEPTORS

No natural mutations in the OTR gene have been described. Oxytocin-null mice fail to lactate, illustrating the importance of OT for survival of the species. There are no changes in the timing of parturition in these mice, but this process is likely dictated by the marked up-regulation of OTRs before labor. It is possible that AVP may replace OT in stimulating uterine contractions when OTRs are up-regulated.

V. DIFFERENTIAL BINDING SITES FOR NEUROHYPOPHYSEAL HORMONE AGONISTS AND ANTAGONISTS

Target size estimation, using radiation inactivation analysis, shows that an OT antagonist binds to a site about half the size of the agonist binding site. These findings suggest that the binding sites for agonists and antagonists are distinct. Indeed, by transfer of domains from the OT receptor into the V_2 vasopressin receptor, chimeric gain-of-function V_2/OT receptors are produced that bind OT agonists with structural requirements distinct from those of antagonists. For agonist binding and selectivity, the first three extracellular receptor domains are the most important. Conversely, the binding site for the OT antagonist d(CH$_2$)$_5$ [Try(Me)^2,Thr^4,Orn^8,Tyr^9-NH$_2$]vasotocin is formed by transmembrane helices 1, 2, and 7, with the upper part of helix 7 contributing to binding affinity. Thus, the antagonist displaces OT by interacting with a distinct binding site, yet behaves as a competitive inhibitor.

VI. VASOPRESSIN SIGNALING THROUGH THE V$_1$ VASOPRESSIN RECEPTOR

The V$_1$ vasopressin receptor (V$_1$R) mediates a range of physiological processes, such as contraction of vascular smooth muscle cells and cell proliferation. Vasopressin also stimulates hepatic glycogenolysis in the rat but in no other species, and is one of several agonists that stimulate platelets to aggregate and secrete their granular contents. Platelet activation is partly mediated by InsP$_3$ production.

Occupancy of the V$_1$R leads to activation of G$_{q/11}$–PLC-β production of InsP$_3$ and the subsequent transient increase in [Ca^{2+}]$_i$ in most of the cell lines studied (Fig. 3). Part of the [Ca^{2+}]$_i$ arises from the influx of extracellular Ca^{2+}. In rat glomerulosa cells, the influx of extracellular Ca^{2+} occurs through L-type channels in a PTX-sensitive manner. Voltage-operated channels, however, do not mediate the influx of Ca^{2+} by vascular smooth muscle cells. Like OT signaling, increases in [Ca^{2+}]$_i$ lead to Ca^{2+}–CaM activation of MLCK and the phosphorylation of MLC. V$_1$ receptor occupancy also results in the release of arachidonic acid by vascular smooth muscle cells and glomerular mesangial cells via activation of PLA$_2$. Arachidonic acid release in rat glomerular mesangial cells is PTX sensitive. Thus, V$_1$ receptors are coupled to both G$_{q/11}$ and G$_{i/o}$ heterotrimeric G proteins, each of which regulates separate pathways.

A. Phospholipase D

A number of studies have implicated phospholipase D (PLD) in AVP action, but the mechanisms have not been thoroughly characterized. Activating PLD converts phosphatidylcholine to choline and phosphatidic acid, which helps regulate specific cellular functions (Fig. 3). Most agonists that activate PLD also induce phosphatidylinositol 4,5-bisphosphate (PIP$_2$) hydrolysis through the stimulation of PLC. The resulting generation of InsP$_3$ and DAG activates Ca^{2+}-sensitive PKC isoenzymes that stimulate PLD. The activation of PLD, however, is not mediated by PKC in all cell types, and it has been suggested that small GTPases of the Rho and ADP ribosylation

factor families also activate PLD. In other cases, βγ- and α-subunits of heterotrimeric G-proteins may stimulate PLD upstream from PKC signaling. Although the regulation of PLD by AVP is still poorly characterized, there is evidence that this pathway may be more relevant that PLC-mediated pathways in mediating smooth muscle contraction. For example,

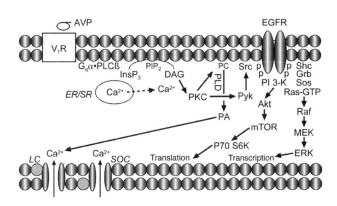

FIGURE 3 Transactivation of the epidermal growth factor receptor by arginine vasopressin (AVP) signaling through the vasopressin V$_1$ receptor. In addition to signaling by pathways that lead to vascular smooth muscle contraction, as outlined for oxytocin stimulation of myosin light chain phosphorylation in Fig. 2, AVP also stimulates cell proliferation by signaling transcriptional and translational events. These processes are thought to involve transactivation of the epidermal growth factor receptor (EGFR), which serves as a scaffold for signaling proteins. The phosphorylation of a Ca^{2+}-dependent tyrosine kinase, Pyk2, by protein kinase C (PKC) creates a ligand for another nonreceptor tyrosine kinase, Src, which is phosphorylated. Src, thus activated, phosphorylates the EGFR, which has phosphotyrosines that interact with proteins containing SH2 domains. Among them, the regulatory subunit of phosphatidylinositol 3-kinase (PI3K) is activated to catalyze the formation of phosphatidylinositol 3,4,5-trisphosphate, which serves as an attachment site for the Akt plekstrin homology domain. Phosphatidylinositol 3,4,5-trisphosphate also activates phosphoinositide-dependent kinase, which catalyzes the phosphorylation of Ser and Thr residues on Akt, resulting in activation of Akt. Akt stimulates mTOR, which in turn activates p70 S6 kinase and phosphorylation of the S6 protein of the 40S ribosomal subunit that is involved in translational control of 5′-oligopyrimidine tract mRNAs. Phosphorylation of the EGF receptor also creates docking sites for Shc, which serves a scaffolding function in signaling for a variety of receptor tyrosine kinases. Grb2/Sos binds to phosphorylated Shc, activating the Ras/Raf/MAPK pathway. The end product ERK phosphorylates transcription factors, leading to an increase in transcriptional activity of target genes. Protein kinase activation of phospholipase D (PLD) causes the release of phosphatidic acid, which signals the influx of extracellular Ca^{2+} and Ca^{2+}-dependent action potentials, leading to smooth muscle contraction (other abbreviations as in Fig. 2).

in A7r5 vascular smooth muscle cells, 10–500 pM AVP stimulates excitation by increasing Ca^{2+} oscillations and Ca^{2+}-dependent action potentials via a PLD-mediated pathway. The PLC pathway is activated only at higher concentrations of hormone.

B. Switching of G-Protein-V₁ Vasopressin Receptor Coupling

The coupling of recombinant V_1Rs to G-proteins has been examined in transfected CHO cells. When expressed at relatively low levels, V_1Rs were coupled solely to G_q. At higher expression levels, however, G_i and G_s were associated with V_1Rs, reflecting the promiscuity in G-protein coupling under contrived conditions. Changes in G-protein coupling, however, also occur naturally during the cell cycle. In proliferating Swiss 3T3 fibroblasts, AVP-induced increases in $[Ca^{2+}]_i$ are mediated by G-proteins of the G_q family. In quiescent cells (G_0/G_1 phase), however, the AVP-induced increase in $[Ca^{2+}]_i$ is partially PTX sensitive, suggesting G_i-protein involvement. The blocking effect of PTX pretreatment in G_0/G_1 cells was mimicked by microinjection of antisense oligonucleotides, suppressing the expression of the $G_{\alpha i3}$ or $G_{\beta\gamma}$ subunits. The significance of both $G_{q/11}$ and G_{i3} coupling is not clear, because both pathways appear to involve activation of phospholipase C-β. Class-switching mechanisms do not appear to be related to any changes in receptor number or type, or to changes in the relative expression of the G-proteins, but may relate to changes in expression level of proteins that are regulators of G-protein signaling (RGS) during the cell cycle.

C. Vasopressin Transactivation of Epidermal Growth Factor Receptors

Kidney mesangial cells, important for maintaining the microcirculation of the glomerulus, contract in response to AVP treatment. Vasopressin is also one of several growth factors that stimulate mesangial cells to proliferate in culture. The growth-promoting effects of AVP are mediated by Ras mitogen-activated protein kinase and the phosphatidylinositol 3-kinase (PI3K) signaling pathways. Treatment with rapamycin, an inhibitor of the p70 S6 kinase activator mTOR, inhibits AVP action downstream from PI3K activation. These activities follow AVP transactivation of the epidermal growth factor (EGF) receptor via tyrosine phosphorylation of the Ca^{2+}/PKC-dependent nonreceptor tyrosine

kinase, Pyk2, leading to Pyk2/c-Src interaction and c-Src activation (Fig. 3). Association of c-Src with EGF receptor results in EGF receptor phosphorylation and creation of docking sites for PI3K and Ras. Thus, like other GPCRs, which transactivate EGF receptor through tyrosine phosphorylation of adapter proteins, the V_1R is able to stimulate cell proliferation. Phosphatidylinositol 3-kinase also mediates the growth-promoting effects of AVP on rat fibroblasts.

Vasopressin also stimulates mitogenesis in vascular smooth muscle cells, 3T3 cells, rat hepatocytes, and adrenal glomerulosa cells. All three MAP kinase pathways, ERK1/2, c-Jun N-terminal kinase (JNK), and p38, are phosphorylated after AVP stimulation of vascular smooth muscle cells. JNK or p38 is involved in AVP-stimulated smooth muscle actin transcription.

VII. VASOPRESSIN V₂ RECEPTOR SIGNALING

The V_2R is expressed in the kidney medulla and mediates the antidiuretic effects of AVP, which involve water transport across the epithelium of the renal collecting duct. Occupancy of receptor sites on the basolateral plasma membrane of ductal cells leads to activation of adenylyl cyclase type IV via G_s coupling.

A. Aquaporin-2 Water Channels

Generation of cAMP and activation of PKA cause translocation of intracellular vesicles containing aquaporin-2 (AQP2) water channels to the apical cell surface (Fig. 4). Phosphorylation of AQP2 by PKA occurs on serine residue 256 in the cytoplasmic carboxyl terminus. This step, which is essential for the translocation of AQP2, requires the anchoring of PKA to intracellular vesicles by PKA anchoring proteins. A variety of vesicular-trafficking processes involve localized increases in intracellular Ca^{2+}. In renal cells, an increase in $[Ca^{2+}]_i$ results from the AVP-stimulated rise in intracellular cAMP. This process occurs in the absence of activation of the phosphoinositide signaling pathway and involves ryanodine-sensitive Ca^{2+} stores in the endoplasmic reticulum and the type 1 ryanodine receptor. Calmodulin also plays a role in the AVP-stimulated redistribution of AQP2. Introduction of a synthetic peptide corresponding to the C-terminus of the $G_{\alpha i3}$ subunit into permeabilized cells, derived from rabbit cortical collecting duct and stably transfected with rat

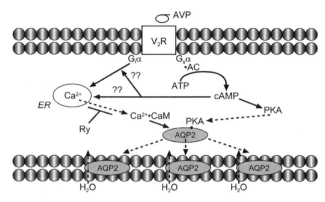

FIGURE 4 Signaling by occupancy of arginine vasopressin (AVP) V_2 receptors (V_2R) involves the generation of cyclic adenosine monophosphate (cAMP), which stimulates the phosphorylation of aquaporin-2 (AQP2) via protein kinase A (PKA) and an increase in Ca^{2+}-calmodulin (CaM). Both events are involved in the targeting of aquaporin-containing intracellular vesicles to the cell surface. Cyclic AMP stimulates Ca^{2+} release from ryanodine-sensitive (Ry) stores in the endoplasmic reticulum (ER) by mechanisms that may involve $G_{\alpha i}$. Translocation events are indicated by broken arrows.

AQP2 cDNA, inhibits cAMP-induced AQP2 translocation. Thus, a member of the G_i family, most likely G_{i3}, is also involved in the cAMP-triggered targeting of AQP2-bearing vesicles to the apical membrane of kidney epithelial cells. The rapid response to AVP involves translocation of AQP2 to the apical cell surface, but longer exposure of cells to AVP (24 h or more) causes an increased abundance of water channels, presumably from increased transcription of the *AQP2* gene.

B. Vasopressin and Urea Transport

Urea transport in the renal medullary loop of Henle and collecting duct is vital for urine concentration and regulation of renal water excretion. Like water channels, there are distinct transporters that regulate the movement of urea across cell membranes. The urea transporter found in portions of the thin descending limb of the loop of Henle is designated as UT-A, to distinguish it from the UT-B transporter expressed in erythrocytes and endothelial cells. AVP increases the expression of the UT-A2 variant of the UT-A gene (UT-A1 is transcribed from a separate promoter). Chronic treatment of rats with AVP almost doubles the level of expression of a Na–K–2Cl cotransporter in the thick ascending limb of the loop of Henle. Increased cAMP levels presumably mediate AVP-stimulated expression of both the UT-

A2 and Na–K–2Cl cotransporter, but the signaling mechanisms are not yet characterized.

C. Desensitized Response to Vasopressin

The V_2R recruits β-arrestin to the plasma membrane after AVP occupancy and is internalized in a β-arrestin- and clathrin-dependent manner into endosomes. This process is mediated by the persistent phosphorylation of a specific cluster of serine residues in the carboxyl-terminal tail of the internalized V_2R, which inhibits recycling of receptors to the plasma membrane and causes a prolonged state of receptor desensitization.

D. Vasopressin Mutations and Diabetes Insipidus

Diabetes insipidus is a disease characterized by a severe disturbance of antidiuresis caused by a lack of AVP. Patients produce large amounts of dilute urine and must drink large amounts of fluid to replace what is lost. This disease occurs most often as a result of damage to the hypothalamus from trauma or metastatic disease, or it occurs as a primary idiopathic disorder. In rare instances, the disorder is hereditary and generally is transmitted in an autosomal-dominant manner. In these cases, mutations have been identified in the coding sequence of the preprovasopressin–neurophysin II gene. The AVP precursor protein consists of four regions that are cleaved proteolytically during processing. Starting from the amino terminus, they include a 19-amino-acid signal sequence for targeting to the endoplasmic reticulum; the nonapeptide sequence of vasopressin; neurophysin II (NPII), a 93-residue carrier for AVP that is involved in the proper targeting, packaging, and storage of AVP; and a 39-amino-acid glycopeptide of unknown function. The signal sequence is cleaved by signal peptidases on translocation of the precursor into the lumen of the endoplasmic reticulum. After folding and disulfide bond formation, pro-AVP passes through the Golgi apparatus into secretory granules, where mature AVP is formed by proteolytic cleavage. Mutations identified in different kindred are located in the sequences encoding the NPII portion, the signal peptide, and in one case the AVP sequence. Diabetes insipidus usually develops gradually over a period of months or years after birth. Postmortem examination usually indicates degeneration of the hypothalamic magnocellular neurons in which the AVP precursor is synthesized.

Thus, impaired transport and/or processing of the mutant precursor may result in its intracellular accumulation, eventually leading to degeneration of the vasopressinergic neurons and the gradual manifestation of clinical symptoms.

E. V_2 Vasopressin Receptor Mutations and Nephrogenic Diabetes Insipidus

Patients with nephrogenic diabetes insipidus (NDI) are unable to produce concentrated urine despite normal or elevated plasma levels of AVP. The AVP receptor 2 gene is located on the X chromosome (Xq28), and about 90% of patients with congenital NDI are males with the X-linked recessive form of the disease. Over 155 mutations within the gene have been characterized. Mutations have also been identified in the *AQP2* gene on chromosome region 12q13. When expressed in transfected cells, most NDI mutations result in receptors that are trapped intracellularly and are unable to reach the plasma membrane. AQP2 mutant proteins have also been found to be misrouted and cannot be expressed at the apical surface. A few types of mutant V_2 vasopressin receptors reach the cell surface but are unable to bind AVP or to properly induce cAMP production. One type of mutation results in perpetual down-regulation of V_2R because of constitutive arrestin-mediated internalization.

F. Rescue of Misrouted V_2 Vasopressin Receptors

Modifying the amino acid sequence of the C-terminus of transfected V_2Rs causes an accumulation of these receptors in the endoplasmic reticulum. Considerable functional activity can be regained, however, by coexpression of the mutant with a C-terminal V_2R peptide (130 amino acid residues) spanning the sequence containing the mutations. In many cases, restoration of receptor activity by the coexpressed receptor peptide is accompanied by a significant increase in receptor numbers on the plasma membrane. In other cases, coexpression allows an increased number of AVP binding sites and stimulation of adenylyl cyclase activity without an increase in surface receptor expression. The mechanisms of this rescue phenomenon are unclear. A physical association between the mutant V_2R proteins and the V_2-tail polypeptide has been demonstrated by coimmunoprecipitation, suggesting that functional rescue involves receptor–polypeptide dimerization.

Certain V_2R mutants have been rescued pharmacologically by incubating transfected cells expressing NDI alleles with membrane-permeant receptor antagonists. Of the 15 mutants evaluated, 8 were rescued to the surface and manifested AVP-stimulated cAMP accumulation. A nonpermeant V_2R antagonist was ineffective in receptor rescue, indicating that the effects of the permeant antagonists occur intracellularly, perhaps by inducing a receptor conformation that allows targeting to the cell surface. The expression of partial receptor peptides, by adenovirus-mediated delivery or the use of permeant AVP antagonists that act as pharmacological chaperones, offers an exciting potential treatment modality for NDI.

VIII. DOMAIN SWAPPING OF V_2 VASOPRESSIN AND OXYTOCIN RECEPTORS TO ELUCIDATE LIGAND BINDING AND G-PROTEIN INTERACTIVE DOMAINS

The neurohypophyseal hormone receptor family is ideal for examining the effects of domain swapping, because only the V_2R is coupled to cAMP production. Expression of the V_1/V_2 hybrid receptors in COS-7 cells shows that proteins containing the V_1R sequence in the second intracellular loop activate the phosphatidylinositol pathway with high efficiency. Only hybrid receptors containing the V_2 receptor sequence in the third intracellular loop are capable of efficiently stimulating cAMP production. These findings indicate that specific, single intracellular receptor domains differentiate between G-proteins.

Chimeric vasopressin OT/V_2 receptors have been used to identify receptor regions involved in ligand binding as well as G-protein coupling. A hybrid containing OTR sequences from the N-terminus to the middle of transmembrane region three had high-affinity OT binding sites that were coupled to activation of adenylyl cyclase. In contrast, a hybrid containing OTR sequences extending from transmembrane helix five to the C-terminus preferentially bound AVP but was not coupled to the V_2-selective $G_{\alpha s}$. Thus, OT binding requires the N-terminal third of the OTR. Use of OT/V_2 receptor chimeras and hybrid hormones (e.g. vasotocin) allows for a detailed analysis of the structural motifs involved in binding. The first two extracellular domains of the OTR are involved in binding to the C-terminal tripeptide of OT. The third extracellular domain of the receptor contacts the cyclic part of OT; the fourth and final outer domain does not appear to be involved in ligand binding.

IX. V$_3$ VASOPRESSIN RECEPTOR SIGNALING

The V$_3$R (or V$_{1b}$R) was initially described in corticotroph cells of the anterior pituitary, where AVP potentiates the release of ACTH. Subsequent cloning of the receptor showed that it was a third member of the AVP receptor family. Although studies on the AVP pituitary receptor revealed a different pharmacological profile compared to those of the V$_1$R and the V$_2$R subtypes, there are no specific AVP analogues that allow V$_3$R signaling to be completely distinguished from V$_1$R signaling. Vasopressin V$_3$R transcripts have been detected throughout the rat brain by reverse transcription polymerase chain reaction and by *in situ* hybridization. These receptors have also been localized immunohistochemically in fiber networks concentrated mainly in the hypothalamus, amygdala, and cerebellum (particularly in those areas with a leaky blood–brain barrier or close to the circumventricular organs). In peripheral tissues, V$_3$R transcripts are expressed in the kidney, pancreas, and adrenal medulla. Because of the difficulty in discriminating V$_3$ from V$_1$ receptor activation, most of what is known about V$_3$R signaling comes from studies in which the receptor has been stably expressed in CHO cells that do not otherwise express AVP receptors. AVP stimulates PLC activity in V$_3$R transfected cells. In clones expressing high levels of receptors, a portion of PLC stimulation is PTX sensitive, and AVP stimulates cAMP synthesis. These results suggest that the V$_3$R has a preferential affinity for G$_{q/11}$ but that at higher concentrations of receptor, it can also interact with G$_{i/o}$ and G$_s$, presumably by promiscuous interactions.

Vasopressin occupancy of V$_3$Rs also stimulates arachidonic acid release by a PTX-sensitive process. Activation of MAP kinases by AVP is dependent on activation of PLC and PKC; both the level and duration of activation are a function of the receptor density. Vasopressin stimulates DNA synthesis in clones expressing medium levels of V$_3$R.

Acknowledgments

We would like to thank Jennifer Desormeaux for secretarial assistance. For editorial and graphic assistance, we thank Ob/Gyn Publications director and staff: R. G. McConnell, Kristi Barrett, John Helms, Traci Morris, and Pam Necessary.

Glossary

amnion Tough fibrous membrane that surrounds the fetus; has a simple (usually low-cuboidal with microvilli) epithelium facing inward.

aquaporin-2 Water channel that is expressed in the renal collecting duct; is translocated from intracellular vesicles to the apical membrane in response to an intracellular signaling cascade that is initiated by binding of vasopressin to its receptor.

endometrium Comprises the mucosal and glandular-containing submucosal lining of the uterus.

mesangial cell Contractile cell of the glomerular mesangium, which is a thin membrane that helps support the capillary loops in a renal glomerulus. Vasopressin stimulates contraction of these cells and stimulates their growth in cell culture.

myometrium Uterine smooth muscle.

pertussis toxin *Bordetella pertussis* protein that catalyzes the ADP-ribosylation of G-protein α-subunits of the G$_i$ family; this modification blocks the receptor-G-protein interaction.

ryanodine receptors/calcium release channels Ca^{2+} is released from the endoplasmic and sarcoplasmic reticulum in a wide range of tissues by specialized types of calcium channels, i.e. ryanodine receptors, by the process of Ca^{2+}-induced Ca^{2+} release.

See Also the Following Articles

Oxytocin • Vasopressin (AVP)

Further Reading

Birnbaumer, M. (2000). Vasopressin receptors. *Trends Endocrinol. Metab.* 11, 406–410.

Chou, C. L., Yip, K. P., Michea, L., Kador, K., Ferraris, J. D., Wade, J. B., and Knepper, M. A. (2000). Regulation of aquaporin-2 trafficking by vasopressin in the renal collecting duct—Roles of ryanodine-sensitive Ca^{2+} stores and calmodulin. *J. Biol. Chem.* 275, 36839–36846.

Gimpl, G., and Fahrenholz, F. (2001). The oxytocin receptor system: Structure, function, and regulation. *Physiol. Rev.* 81, 629–683.

Ghosh, P. M., Mikhailova, M., Bedolla, R., and Kreisberg, J. I. (2001). Arginine vasopressin stimulates mesangial cell proliferation by activating the epidermal growth factor receptor. *Am. J. Physiol.* 280, F972–F979.

Li, Y., Shiels, A. J., Maszak, G., and Byron, K. L. (2001). Vasopressin-stimulated Ca^{2+} spiking in vascular smooth muscle cells involves phospholipase D. *Am. J. Physiol.* 280, H2658–H2664.

Morello, J. P., and Bichet, D. G. (2001). Nephrogenic diabetes insipidus. *Annu. Rev. Physiol.* 63, 607–630.

Soloff, M. S., Jeng, Y.-J., Copland, J. A., Strakova, Z., and Hoare, S. (2000). Signal pathways in oxytocin-stimulated prostaglandin synthesis. *Exp. Physiol.* 85S, 51S–58S.

Thibonnier, M., Coles, P., Thibonnier, A., and Shoham, M. (2001). The basic and clinical pharmacology of nonpeptide vasopressin receptor antagonists. *Annu. Rev. Pharmacol. Toxicol.* 41, 175–202.

Yue, C. P., Kus, C. Y., Liu, M. Y., Simon, M. I., and Sanborn, B. M. (2000). Molecular mechanisms of the inhibition of phospholipase Cβ$_3$ by protein kinase C. *J. Biol. Chem.* 275, 30220–30225.

Pancreastatin

Víctor Sánchez-Margalet[*] and Suad Efendic[†]

[*]*Virgen Macarena University Hospital, Spain* •
[†]*Karolinska Institutet, Sweden*

Pancreastatin (PST), which was first isolated from the porcine pancreas, is a chromogranin A-derived peptide that occurs throughout the neuroendocrine and gastrointestinal systems. Although the physiological role of PST has not yet been established, it is known to have a number of effects in the modulation of secretion of different glands and in the regulation of metabolism. This article describes the synthesis and secretion of PST as well as its biological activities in a number of tissues.

I. INTRODUCTION

Pancreastatin (PST) is a chromogranin A (CGA)-derived peptide that was first isolated from the porcine pancreas. However, PST has subsequently been shown to be present throughout the neuroendocrine and gastrointestinal systems. In fact, PST was the first known biologically active peptide to be derived from CGA, a prohormone for a variety of different peptides.

During the past decade, much evidence indicating that PST is a regulatory peptide has been obtained. Even though the physiological role of PST has not yet been unraveled, many different effects regarding the modulation of endocrine and exocrine secretion from different glands and the regulation of glucose, lipid, and protein metabolism have been described. Autocrine, paracrine, and endocrine activities have been observed in a variety of systems, but the molecular mechanisms underlying most of these still await investigation.

The present article summarizes the synthesis, tissue processing, and secretion of PST. More extensively, the different actions described for PST in a variety of tissues are examined, giving more detail to those effects that have been more thoroughly studied, such as metabolic regulation by PST in the liver and adipose tissue.

II. PANCREASTATIN STRUCTURE

A. Primary Structure

PST was first isolated from porcine pancreas as a 49-amino-acid peptide (5103 Da). The sequence showed no significant homology with any known family of peptides. The only relevant details were the polyglutamate sequence shared with gastrin and the C-terminal Arg-Gly-NH_2 shared with vasopressin. The amidated C-terminus is feature common to many neuropeptides and gastrointestinal hormones.

Variations in the PST sequence among the following species have been described: porcine, bovine, rat, mouse, and human. The homologies are variable, depending on the species being compared. Thus, rat and mouse share 88% of their sequences, whereas the homologies between bovine and mouse and between rat and human are only 45 and 55%, respectively. The human PST sequence shares 71% homology with that of porcine. These homologies are higher when the C-terminal fragment containing the biological activity of the peptide is considered (i.e., 76% between the human and porcine PST sequences).

B. Molecular Forms

Since PST is derived from the proteolysis of the precursor chromogranin A, different molecular forms that represent processing intermediates have been described. All of these conserve the biologically active C-terminal part of the molecule, however.

Thus, peptides of 29 aa (residues 273–301 of hCGA), 48 aa (residues 254–301 of hCGA), 92 aa (residues 210–301 of hCGA), and 186 aa (residues 116–301 of hCGA) have been found in human tumors. Similarly, in the rat, different forms that represent various N-terminal truncations but that conserve the active C-terminal part of the molecule have been described. PST-52 and a larger species of 15–20 kDa have been shown to be the major molecular forms in human plasma.

Different phosphorylated forms of PST have been reported, depending on the localization of the peptide. In fact, there seems to be a correlation between the extent of phosphorylation of the precursor, CGA, and its processing in different tissues. Thus, CGA and PST are highly phosphorylated in the pancreas, from which mature PST is secreted, whereas CGA is poorly phosphorylated in the ileum, from which there is no processing to PST.

III. PANCREASTATIN SYNTHESIS AND SECRETION

Proteolysis of CGA occurs both inside and outside the cell to yield peptides with biological activity. This function of CGA as a precursor of active peptides was first suggested after the isolation of PST, which turned out to have the sequence of a central part of the CGA molecule. This hypothesis was then supported by the observation of pairs of dibasic residues in the sequence of CGA, which usually represent targets for protease cleavage.

Intact CGA is the major component of secretory granules of the adrenal medulla and hypothalamus. Nevertheless, it is generally accepted that degradation products of CGA do exist in chromaffin cells. In the rat pheochromocytoma cell line PC12, intact CGA is present and is processed only at its N-terminus, although mature PST is rare. Chromaffin cells may be the major source of circulating CGA, and they could therefore be the major indirect source of PST in plasma.

The intracellular processing of PST has been fully described for bovine CGA and partially described for rat CGA. The mechanism involves proteases such as prohormone convertase-2 (PC-2) and carboxypeptidase H.

The extracellular processing of CGA may occur as a result of the activities of proteases co-secreted by the chromaffin granule or may be due to exoproteases localized on the extracellular side of the cell plasma membrane. In addition, fragmentation of bovine CGA by plasma kalikrein has also been shown.

The processing of CGA is tissue- and species-specific. Thus, CGA is more fully processed in the stomach, especially in the endocrine cells of the antrum, and in the endocrine pancreas, of which PST is a major product. PST production is higher in insulinoma cells than in primary human islets. In this tissue, PST expression has been found in the beta-, delta-, and alpha-cell populations. The somatostatin-secreting delta-cell line (QGP-1N) also releases PST.

Enterochromaffin-like (ECL) cells, originating from the gastric antrum, represent the best characterized physiological system of PST secretion. These cells respond to gastrin stimulation by increasing both PST secretion and CGA mRNA levels. In the rat *in vivo*, an increase in gastrin levels, either by infusion or by indirect means, leads to the suppression of acid secretion and an increase in PST levels. Conversely, a decrease in gastrin levels by fasting or antrectomy is followed by a decrease in PST levels. Moreover, gastrin receptor antagonists produce a decrease in PST levels. Finally, patients with gastrinomas have increased plasma PST levels, due to an excess of gastrin secreted by the tumor.

Plasma porcine PST-like immunoreactivity levels have been shown to increase 50% (from 100 to 150 pM) in response to a meal. In perfused porcine pancreas, PST-like immunoreactivity is released in parallel with insulin in response to insulinotropic stimuli.

Elevated PST levels have been found in response to a glucose load in type 2 diabetes, in hypertension, and in pregnant women with gestational diabetes, correlating with plasma catecholamine levels.

IV. BIOLOGICAL EFFECTS OF PANCREASTATIN

Many different biological effects of PST in a variety of tissues have been described. PST may act as an autocrine, paracrine, and/or endocrine peptide in many target cells.

A. Endocrine Secretion

There is accumulated evidence for the ability of PST to modulate endocrine secretion in a variety of systems.

1. The Endocrine Pancreas
The first described effect of PST was the inhibition of glucose-stimulated insulin secretion, and especially first-phase insulin secretion, in isolated rat pancreas. PST also potentiates the inhibition of insulin secretion caused by a physiological decrease in glucose concentration. On the other hand, PST has also been shown to prime glucose-stimulated insulin secretion after a second glucose pulse. PST can also inhibit the stimulatory action of other agents, whether these are physiological (arginine), hormonal (GIP, VIP, CCK, glucagon), or even pharmacological (IBMX, sulfonylurea). The inhibitory effect of PST on insulin release has been confirmed *in vivo* in the rat.

On the other hand, other groups have reported no such effect in dogs and pigs, suggesting different effects depending on the species. In general, PST seems to negatively modulate insulin secretion in an autocrine, paracrine, and endocrine manner. Other effects of PST that relate to endocrine pancreatic secretion are the stimulation of glucagon release and the inhibition of pancreatic polypeptide secretion.

However, PST has been shown *in vitro* to be able to modulate the formation of insoluble fibers of amyloid polypeptide. Actually, the formation of amyloid fibers seems to be mediated by an inappropriate balance between the amyloid peptide, insulin, C-peptide, and PST.

2. Parathyroid Secretion

PST has an inhibitory effect on parathyroid hormone (PTH) secretion. This effect has been observed in porcine and bovine parathyroid cells on stimulation with low (but physiological) concentrations of either calcium or phorbol ester (a nonphysiological agent). This effect was confirmed by the demonstration that PTH secretion increases if parathyroid cells are incubated with anti-PST antibodies. Moreover, PST inhibits not only PTH secretion but also transcription of the PTH and CGA genes; the stabilities of these mRNAs are also decreased. The mechanism by which PST exerts these effects is not known, however.

The parathyroid gland is very rich in CGA, but complete processing of this protein to PST is very rare, due to the lack of prohormone convertases PC2 and PC1/3. Therefore, it cannot be concluded that PST has an autocrine role in parathyroid secretion. Nevertheless, processed PST is present in calcitonin-producing C cells, and in this way PST may be involved in the regulation of the thyroid–parathyroid axis.

3. Adrenal Medulla Secretion

The inhibition of secretion from the adrenal medulla by CGA-derived peptides (obtained by tryptic proteolysis) suggested that these peptides (including PST) may have some inhibitory action in chromaffin tissue. Consistent with this hypothesis, PST administration in the rat decreases catecholamine levels during surgical stress. It is not yet known whether this is a direct or an indirect effect of PST, however.

4. Atrial Secretion

PST can also regulate endocrine secretion from the heart. Atrial myocardial cells store and secrete atrial natriuretic peptide. Thus, PST has been shown to stimulate atrial cell secretion by 90%. This result suggests that the PST precursor, CGA, which has been identified in atrial secretory granules, may play an autoregulatory role in atrial secretion.

B. Exocrine Secretion

1. Exocrine Pancreatic Secretion

Evidence showing an inhibitory effect of PST on exocrine pancreatic secretion has been accumulating. *In vivo* studies employing physiological stimuli (a meal), CCK-8, and central vagal nerve stimulation have provided convincing data supporting an inhibitory effect of PST on pancreatic exocrine secretion. These effects seem to be mediated by the presynaptic modulation of acetylcholine release from the vagal system. Therefore, PST has been proposed as a new mediator in the islet–acinar axis.

2. Gastric Secretion

Contradictory *in vitro* versus *in vivo* results regarding the effects of PST on gastric secretion have been reported. Thus, PST inhibits gastric secretion in isolated parietal cells, but *in vivo* seems to enhance gastric acid secretion stimulated by different nutrients.

ECL cells from the gastric antrum are an important source of PST. Therefore, PST may play a role in the paracrine regulation of gastric acid secretion.

C. Hepatic Glycogen Metabolism

PST activates glycogenolysis in the rat liver. Thus, PST increases glucose release from the liver, resulting in a hyperglycemic effect. This effect can be observed *in vivo*, without even a modification of glucagon or insulin levels, suggesting a direct effect on liver metabolism. This observation was confirmed by studies in isolated hepatocytes, in which PST had a glycogenolytic effect similar to that of glucagon in potency, but was independent of cyclic AMP production and dependent on calcium. In fact, this glycogenolytic effect correlates with the dose-dependent increase in intracellular free calcium produced by a PST challenge.

In addition to its glycogenolytic effect, PST inhibits insulin-stimulated glycogen synthesis, but unlike glucagon it does not affect the rate of insulin-stimulated glycolysis. In this way, even though the glycogenolytic effect of PST is comparable to that of glucagon, the latter produces higher levels of hyperglycemia. Conversely, PST inhibits glucagon-stimulated insulin release and thus enhances the hyperglycemic effect of glucagon.

D. Metabolic Effects in the Adipocyte

Another target cell for metabolic regulation by PST is the adipocyte. Here, PST has been shown to modulate glucose, lipid, and protein metabolism in isolated adipocytes. PST also inhibits basal and insulin-stimulated glucose transport, lactate production, glycogen synthesis, and lipogenesis in a dose-dependent manner. It therefore opposes the main metabolic action of insulin in adipose tissue. These effects can be observed at a wide range of insulin concentrations, leading to a shift to the right in the dose–response curve. Maximal effects are obtained at 10 nM PST, with an ED_{50} of 0.1 nM. These counterregulatory effects on insulin action suggest that PST may have a role in insulin resistance. Moreover, PST has a dose-dependent lipolytic effect in isolated adipocytes ($ED_{50} = 0.1$ nM). However, this effect is inhibited by 10 nM insulin. On the other hand, PST has a stimulatory effect on protein synthesis and enhances insulin-stimulated protein synthesis in isolated adipocytes.

E. Insulin Receptor Inhibition

PST signal transduction has been shown to cross-talk with insulin receptor signaling. Thus, PST inhibits insulin receptor tyrosine kinase activity by promoting serine phosphorylation of the insulin receptor β-subunit. Lower tyrosine phosphorylation levels of insulin receptor substrates lead to decreased interactions with the regulatory enzyme phosphatidyl inositol-3 kinase. This is a key enzyme that mediates glucose transport and metabolism in the adipocyte and glycogen synthesis in the hepatocyte. These inhibitory effects of PST on insulin receptor signaling partly mediate the metabolic counterregulatory action of PST and further suggest that PST may have a role in insulin resistance.

Meanwhile, PST stimulates the mitogen-activated protein kinase (MAPK) signaling cascade, potentiating this insulin receptor signaling pathway. In fact, this dual effect on insulin receptor signaling may explain PST's ability to simultaneously inhibit glucose and lipid metabolism and promote protein synthesis in adipocytes.

F. PST Regulation of Cell Growth

PST has been found to have an inhibitory effect on cell growth in a variety of cell lines (pancreatic and hepatic cells). This inhibitory effect of PST has also been observed *in vivo* in islets transplanted into nude mice. Moreover, PST inhibits basal and CCK-stimulated pancreas growth in mice. Consistent with this finding, PST can also inhibit DNA synthesis in rat fetal islets.

Even though PST stimulates MAPK signaling in HTC (hepatoma cells), it has been found that PST inhibits protein and DNA synthesis. The PST-induced inhibition of cell growth observed in HTC hepatoma cells is mediated by nitric oxide (NO) production. If NO production is blocked, PST stimulates cell growth. This stimulatory effect is mediated by activation of the MAPK pathway. In this way, the final effect of PST on hepatocyte growth may depend on NO availability.

G. Effects of PST on Central Nervous System

Peripheral administration of PST has been shown to enhance memory retention in mice. In addition, PST can revert the amnesia produced by the cholinergic antagonist scopolamine. This activity in memory retention seems to be a peripheral rather than a central effect, since intraventricular administration produces only a modest relief. Therefore, these effects may be a consequence of the PST-mediated hyperglycemia previously demonstrated in mice, since hyperglycemia is known to increase memory retention. Moreover, intracranial administration of PST elevates blood glucose and free fatty acids in the rat. This action is opposite to that of insulin, further supporting the counterregulatory effects of PST.

PST may also play a role in the formation of senile plaques in Alzheimer's disease, in which a long 13.5 kDa form of PST seems to be present. The physiological or pathophysiological role of PST in Alzheimer's disease is unknown, however.

H. Immunomodulatory Effect of PST

PST seems to have an immunomodulatory effect. It is able to enhance the mitogenic response of peripheral blood T lymphocytes when they are stimulated by noncognate stimuli (lectins). Therefore, a role for PST as an immunomodulator has been proposed.

V. PUTATIVE PHYSIOLOGICAL ROLE OF PANCREASTATIN

Although the physiological role of PST has yet to be fully established, a multitude of effects have been ascribed, implicating PST in the modulation of secretion and the control of metabolism.

The variety of PST's effects on the modulation of secretion in glands where this peptide is synthesized and processed has led to the hypothesis that PST may have a role as an autocrine and paracrine regulatory peptide of exocrine and endocrine secretion. Nevertheless, further studies to identify the molecular mechanisms underlying these effects are needed to establish a physiological role in the regulation of secretion.

The metabolic actions of PST have been more thoroughly studied and some of the molecular mechanisms by which PST modulates glucose, lipid, and protein metabolism, with effects that are generally counterregulatory to those of insulin, are already known.

Our current hypothesis is that PST plays a role in the physiology of stress, by regulating the supply of energy to the body (especially the muscle and brain). In fact, PST levels may be increased under stressful conditions, during which CGA is co-secreted with catecholamines. Therefore one would expect that the endocrine actions of PST may actually take place under stressful conditions, when circulating PST levels are high enough to interact with specific receptors in target cells. Consistent with this proposal, specific PST receptors and PST-induced signal transduction have been characterized in liver and adipose tissue, providing a basis for the molecular mechanisms of the metabolic effects of PST.

Moreover, PST can modify the insulin/glucagon ratio by modulating secretion to further increase metabolic anti-insulin effects. In this context, PST could also play a role not only in the physiology of stress, but also in pathophysiological conditions such as insulin-resistant states. In support of this concept, increased levels of PST, which correlate with those of catecholamines, have been found in type 2 diabetes, gestational diabetes, and essential hypertension.

These effects of PST may also be considered complementary to those described for other CGA-derived peptides, which have been found to exert different actions, such as the control of catecholamine secretion, vasodilation, and infection.

In conclusion, PST is a regulatory peptide derived from CGA and, therefore, may be regarded as part of the functional axis controlled by this protein, for which the description of a physiological role has been elusive for so long.

Glossary

chromaffin Tissue of neuroectodermic origin with the specialized function of synthesizing and secreting catecholamines.
chromogranin A A glycoprotein that is very abundant in the secretory granules of chromaffin and other neuroendocrine cells.
insulin resistance A pathophysiological condition in which the action of insulin is impaired, so that a higher insulin concentration is needed to result in the same effect.

pancreastatin A chromogranin A-derived peptide that inhibits secretion and impairs insulin action.
regulatory peptide A peptide that is released in response to a stimulus and that exerts specific biological actions. It may function as an autocrine, paracrine, or endocrine agonist or antagonist.

See Also the Following Articles

Insulin Actions ● Insulin Processing ● Insulin Secretion ● Pancreatic Polypeptide ● Parathyroid Hormone ● Stress

Further Reading

Ahren, B., Lindskog, S., Tatemoto, K., and Efendic, S. (1988). Pancreastatin inhibits insulin secretion and stimulates glucagon secretion in mice. *Diabetes* **37**, 281–285.
Efendic, S., Tatemoto, K., Mutt, V., Quan, C., Chang, D., and Ostenson, C. G. (1987). Pancreastatin and islet hormone release. *Proc. Natl. Acad. Sci. USA* **84**, 7257–7260.
Funakoshi, A., Miyasaka, K., Nakamura, R., Kitani, K., and Tatemoto, K. (1989). Inhibitory effect of pancreastatin on pancreatic exocrine secretion in the conscious rat. *Regul. Pept.* **25**, 157–166.
Östenson, G. C., Efendic, S., and Holst, J. J. (1989). Pancreastatin-like immunoreactivity and insulin are released in parallel from the perfused porcine pancreas. *Endocrinology* **124**, 2986–2990.
Ravazzola, M., Efendic, S., Östenson, C. G., Tatemoto, K., Hutton, J. C., and Orci, L. (1988). Localization of pancreastatin immunoreactivity in porcine endocrine cells. *Endocrinology* **123**, 227–229.
Sánchez, V., Lucas, M., Calvo, J. R., and Goberna, R. (1992). Glycogenolytic effect of pancreastatin in isolated rat hepatocytes is mediated by a cyclic-AMP-independent Ca^{2+}-dependent mechanism. *Biochem. J.* **284**, 659–662.
Sánchez-Margalet, V., and Goberna, R. (1994). Pancreastatin inhibits insulin-stimulated glycogen synthesis but not glycolysis in rat hepatocytes. *Regul. Pept.* **51**, 215–220.
Sánchez-Margalet, V., and González-Yanes, C. (1998). Pancreastatin inhibits insulin action in rat adipocytes. *Am. J. Physiol.* **275**, E1055–E1060.
Sánchez-Margalet, V., Gonzalez-Yanes, C., and Najib, S. (2001). Pancreastatin, a chromogranin A-derived peptide, inhibits DNA and protein synthesis by producing nitric oxide in HTC rat hepatoma cells. *J. Hepatol.* **35**, 80–85.
Sánchez-Margalet, V., Lobon, J. A., González, A., Escobar-Jimenez, F., and Goberna, R. (1998). Increased pancreastatin-like levels in gestational diabetes subjects. Correlation with catecholamine levels. *Diabetes Care* **21**, 1951–1954.
Sánchez-Margalet, V., Lucas, M., and Goberna, R. (1996). Pancreastatin: Further evidence for its consideration as a regulatory peptide. *J. Mol. Endocrinol.* **16**, 1–8.
Sánchez-Margalet, V., Santos-Alvarez, J., Gonzalez-Yanes, C., and Najib, S. (2000). Pancreastatin: Biological effects and mechanisms of action. *Adv. Exp. Med. Biol.* **482**, 247–262.
Sánchez-Margalet, V., Valle, M., Lobon, J. A., Maldonado, A., Escobar, F., Olivan, J., Perez-Cano, R., and Goberna, R. (1995). Increased pancreastatin-like immunoreactivity in levels in non-obese patients with essential hypertension. *J. Hypertension* **13**, 251–258.

Sjoholm, A., Funakoshi, A., Efendic, S., Östenson, C. G., and Hellerstrom, C. (1991). Long term inhibitory effect of pancreastatin and diacepan binding inhibitor on pancreatic beta cell deoxyribonucleic acid replication, polyamine content, and insulin secretion. *Endocrinology* **128**, 3277–3282.

Tatemoto, K., Efendic, S., Mutt, V., Makk, G., Feistner, G. J., and Barchas, J. D. (1986). Pancreastatin, a novel pancreatic peptide that inhibits insulin secretion. *Nature* **324**, 476–478.

Pancreastatin Receptor Signaling

VÍCTOR SÁNCHEZ-MARGALET

Virgen Macarena University Hospital, Spain

I. PANCREASTATIN RECEPTOR
II. G-PROTEINS COUPLED TO PANCREASTATIN RECEPTOR
III. EFFECTORS FOR PANCREASTATIN RECEPTOR SIGNALING
IV. CROSSTALK OF PANCREASTATIN RECEPTOR WITH INSULIN RECEPTOR SIGNALING
V. CONCLUSIONS

Pancreastatin (PST) receptor signaling has been thoroughly studied in the rat liver and adipose tissue during the past decade, and it is still an active area of research. PST receptor signaling is a paradigmatic example of the signal transduction of a calcium-mobilizing hormone receptor. Even though the PST receptor has not yet been cloned, the signaling triggered in response to PST has the typical pattern of a seven-trans-membrane-spanning receptor coupled to heter-trimeric G-proteins in the plasma membrane to exert the metabolic actions observed in the liver and adipose tissue. This article describes the different signaling pathways that have been shown to be activated in response to PST and the possible molecular mechanisms underlying the modulation of the metabolic action exerted by PST in the liver and adipose tissue, as well as the counterregulatory effects on insulin action.

I. PANCREASTATIN RECEPTOR

One of the hallmarks confirming the endocrine nature of a peptide is the presence of specific receptors in the plasma membrane. Thus, pancreastatin (PST)-binding sites have been characterized in rat liver, adipose, and heart membranes. Binding data obtained using radioiodinated rat PST in rat liver membranes suggested the presence of specific high-affinity receptors for PST. The PST binding fulfills all the criteria for membrane receptors: it is temperature-, time-, and pH-dependent, and it is saturable and reversible. In addition, the binding of the ligand is very sensitive to the PST sequence, further suggesting the specificity of the receptor. Thus, PSTs from species that share a low level of sequence homology with rat PST, such as human or porcine PST, showed a low level of binding affinity in the studies of radioligand displacement. Analysis of binding data under equilibrium conditions showed similar affinity values in rat liver, HTC rat hepatoma, rat adipose, and heart membranes, indicating the presence of a single site with a K_d ranging from 0.2 to 1 nM. This range of K_d values correlates well with the ED_{50} obtained for the effects of PST in hepatocytes and adipocytes and is in accordance with PST levels found in pig and human plasma. In addition, these values are comparable to those obtained for most peptidic hormone receptors. Therefore, the affinity of the putative PST receptor is consistent with a possible physiological and pathophysiological role for this regulatory peptide.

On the other hand, different concentrations of binding sites have been found depending on the target tissue, from 5 fmol/mg of protein in adipose tissue to 34 fmol/mg of protein in heart membranes, with an intermediate B_{max} of 15 fmol/mg of protein in rat liver membranes. These binding data give an estimate of 1000–5000 binding sites per cell.

Active PST receptors have been solubilized and characterized from rat liver membranes. Molecular analysis of the solubilized receptor by covalent cross-linking and further identification on sodium dodecyl sulfate–polyacrylamide gel electrophoresis indicated a single band of 85 kDa. Gel filtration studies of the solubilized receptors confirmed the 80 kDa molecular mass of the PST receptor. In addition, the solubilized receptor is a glycoprotein that can specifically bind to the wheat-germ agglutinin (WGA) lectin.

Taking advantage of the glycoprotein nature of the receptor, a two-step procedure has been employed as a purification strategy. Thus, WGA semipurification followed by affinity purification using a biotinylated PST analogue has led to the purification of PST receptors in homogeneity. The PST receptor can be purified as an 80 kDa monomeric glycoprotein physically associated with a $G_{\alpha q/11}$ protein. The scale-up of the purification process may yield sufficient amounts of receptor proteins to undertake microsequencing in the near future.

II. G-PROTEINS COUPLED TO PANCREASTATIN RECEPTOR

Heterotrimeric (α, β, γ) GTP-binding (G) proteins are one of the most important transducers of the signaling from receptors in the plasma membrane to the interior of the cell, coupling the activation of the receptor with the triggering of different effector systems. The coupling of the PST receptor with GTP-binding proteins has been demonstrated by different approaches in rat liver, adipocyte, and heart membranes.

The first evidence for the coupling of the PST receptor with G-proteins was revealed by the sensitivity of PST binding to the presence of guanine nucleotides, especially nonhydrolyzable analogues. These results were then confirmed with direct evidence of physical and functional coupling. Thus, GTPase activity, GTP-binding studies, and photolabeling, in combination with pertussis toxin (PT) pretreatment and blocking antibodies against different α-subunits, demonstrated the double coupling of the PST receptor, mainly with a G-protein of the $\alpha_{q/11}$

family and to a lesser extent with a G-protein of the $\alpha_{i1,2}$ family (PT sensitive). Moreover, a physical association was demonstrated by binding studies with radiolabeled PST in anti-$G_{\alpha q/11}$ immunoprecipitates. These results were confirmed by the opposite approach. Thus, $G_{\alpha q/11}$ proteins could be observed along with semipurified and purified PST receptor.

In general, a double system of G-proteins seems to be engaged in PST signaling, a pertussis toxin-sensitive G-protein belonging to the $G_{\alpha i1,2}$ family and a pertussis toxin-insensitive G-protein belonging to the $G_{\alpha q/11}$ family (see Fig. 1). The specific G-protein coupled to the PST receptor has been assessed in rat liver membranes, where $G_{\alpha 11}$ rather than $G_{\alpha q}$ seems to functionally couple to the PST receptor. On the other hand, $G_{\alpha 16}$ (another G-protein of the $\alpha_{q/11}$ family) is the G-protein that couples to the PST receptor in the heart. Since $G_{\alpha 16}$ is not present in liver or adipose tissues, but is present in the heart, the coupling of PST receptor with $G_{\alpha q/11}$ in hepatocytes and adipocytes is compatible with the preferential coupling with $G_{\alpha 16}$ rather than $G_{\alpha q/11}$ in heart membranes.

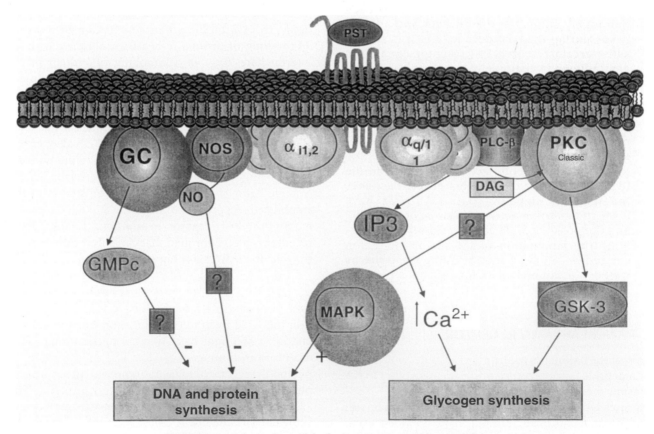

FIGURE I   Schematic model of pancreastatin receptor signaling.

III. EFFECTORS FOR PANCREASTATIN RECEPTOR SIGNALING

A. Phospholipase C Activity

The polyphosphoinositide-specific phospholipase C (PLC) that is activated by seven-transmembrane receptors by coupling heterotrimeric G-proteins is the membrane-associated PLC-β. PST has been shown to stimulate membrane-associated PLC-β activity in rat liver membranes. Four different PLC-β isoforms (β1–4) have been described, although the expression of PLC-β4 is more limited and cannot be found in hepatic, adipose, or heart tissues. The PLC-β3 isoform seems to be the specific isoform activated by PST receptors in rat liver and adipose membranes, although PLC-β1 is also activated in HTC rat hepatoma cells. The activation of PLC by PST is mediated mainly by $G_{\alpha q/11}$ in liver and adipose membranes, but some activation may be accounted for by βγ released by $\alpha_{i1,2}$ or $\alpha_{q/11}$ activation.

On the other hand, PLC-β2 is the isoform preferentially activated in rat heart membranes by PST, although it can also stimulate some activation of β1 and β3 isoforms. This is not striking when it is taken into account that PST preferentially activates $G_{\alpha 16}$ in heart membranes, and this G_α protein preferentially activates PLC-β2, although it can activate β1 and β3 to a lesser extent.

B. Calcium

The role of calcium in PST action has been studied in the hepatocyte. Thus, PST stimulation of isolated hepatocytes induces a rapid increase in intracellular calcium concentration. Consistent with these results, the glycogenolytic effect of PST was found to be cyclic AMP-independent but very dependent on both extracellular and intracellular calcium. In fact, the dose-dependent glycogenolytic effect of PST correlates with the progressive increase in intracellular calcium concentration. Moreover, PST has been found to increase intracellular free calcium concentration by releasing intracellular stores and increasing the influx of extracellular calcium. These effects are mediated by the production of inositol 1,4,5-triphosphate (IP$_3$) resulting from the activation of PLC-β by $G_{\alpha q/11}$.

C. Protein Kinase C

The activation of PLC-β activity in the plasma membrane by PST stimulation leads to the production of IP$_3$ as discussed in the previous section, but also produces diacylglycerol (DAG). DAG in addition to calcium is responsible for the activation of protein kinase C (PKC), more precisely, the classical isoforms of PKC. Thus, PST has been found to activate classical isoforms of PKC (α, βI, and βII) by promoting translocation from the cytoplasm to the plasma membrane in HTC hepatoma cells and rat adipocytes. Moreover, the glycogenolytic effect of PST in the hepatocyte and the inhibition of glucose transport in the adipocyte can be prevented by blocking the activation of PKC. Taken together, these results suggest that PKC activity is a very important effector of PST receptor signaling.

D. Mitogen-Activated Protein Kinase

G-protein-coupled receptors are known to signal to the mitogen-activated protein kinase (MAPK) pathway by two different but complementary mechanisms. Thus, the βγ dimer of heterotrimeric G-proteins can activate the Ras–Raf pathway, whereas the $\alpha_{q/11}$ protein connects with MAPK by activating PKC. Therefore, the reported effect of PST-activating MAPK in hepatoma cells and adipocytes can be explained by this dual mechanism. Thus, PST induces the Ser/Thr phosphorylation of MAPK by activation of MAPK kinase. In fact, this pathway mediates the effect of PST-stimulating protein synthesis in rat adipocytes.

E. Glycogen Synthase Kinase-3 Activity

PST stimulation is able to activate glycogen synthase kinase-3 (GSK-3) activity in rat adipocytes. The phosphorylation level of GSK-3 is negatively correlated with the activity. Thus, PST inhibited basal phosphorylation of GSK-3. The PST stimulation of GSK-3 activity seems to be mediated by PKC since it can be prevented by a specific PKC inhibitor. This effect of PST on GSK-3 activity results in the inhibition of both basal and insulin-stimulated glycogen synthesis in rat adipocytes. This effect of PST can also be prevented by using a PKC inhibitor. Therefore, PKC activation by PST mediates the activation of GSK-3, which is one of the final effectors of PST receptor signaling to regulate glucose metabolism.

F. Nitric Oxide and Cyclic GMP

PST was found to increase the production of the second messenger cyclic GMP (cGMP) in rat hepatocytes by a PT-sensitive mechanism, probably involving $G_{\alpha i1,2}$ activation, although this mechanism still needs experimental confirmation to finally define this signaling pathway. In any case, this effect has been proved to be mediated by nitric oxide (NO) production in hepatoma cells. The production of cGMP may eventually lead to down-regulation of the $G_{\alpha q/11}$–PLC-β signaling by activating protein kinase G (PKG), as observed in other systems for other G-protein-coupled receptors. The role of cGMP/PKG in the counterregulation of PST signaling still needs further investigation, however.

On the other hand, NO and cGMP have been shown to inhibit DNA and protein synthesis in hepatoma cells. Therefore, these effectors seem to mediate the antiproliferative effect of PST in HTC rat hepatoma cells. The antiproliferative effect of the NO–cGMP pathway has been found in other systems. In fact, when NO synthase activity is blocked by pharmacological inhibitors, the effect of PST changes to the stimulation of growth and proliferation, due to the activation of the MAPK pathway. Therefore, the final effect of PST on cellular growth and proliferation may depend on the balance between these two signaling pathways, especially the availability of NO.

IV. CROSSTALK OF PANCREASTATIN RECEPTOR WITH INSULIN RECEPTOR SIGNALING

Crosstalk of the PST receptor with insulin receptor signaling has been studied in hepatoma cells and adipocytes. Similar results have been observed in both systems (Fig. 2).

PST inhibits insulin-mediated autophosphorylation of the insulin receptor β-subunit in a dose-dependent manner. In addition, PST blunts tyrosine phosphorylation of insulin receptor substrate-1 (IRS-1), IRS-2, and p60-70, preventing their association with p85, the regulatory subunit of phosphatidyl inositol 3-kinase (PI3K). This effect results in the inhibition of PI3K activity. Moreover, the insulin activation of the downstream protein kinase B and S6 kinase is also blocked by PST.

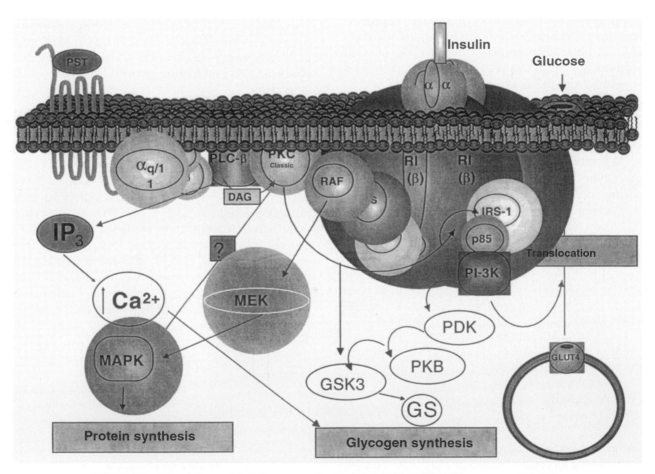

FIGURE 2 Schematic model of the cross talk of pancreastatin with insulin receptor signaling.

These effects of PST in preventing insulin receptor signaling can be fully reversed by blocking protein kinase C activity, strongly suggesting that the PST-induced activation accounts for the crosstalk of both receptors. In fact, PST induces the serine/threonine phosphorylation of insulin receptor β-subunit and IRS-1, which is a well-known mechanism of inhibition of insulin receptor tyrosine kinase activity by counterregulatory hormones. Moreover, the PST-mediated Ser/Thr phosphorylation of the insulin receptor and IRS-1 seems to be caused by the activation of PKC, since this effect can also be prevented by blocking PKC activity. In fact, the PST-mediated activation of PKC has been observed in both the hepatocyte and the adipocyte. PST-inhibited, insulin-stimulated PI3K activity can also be reversed by blocking PKC. In parallel with the signaling results, the PST inhibition of the physiological actions of insulin can also be reversed by preventing PKC activation. Thus, the inhibitory effects of PST on insulin-stimulated glucose transport in adipocytes and glycogen synthesis in hepatocytes are also abrogated by blocking PKC activation.

These findings suggest that PST may exert its anti-insulin effect on the insulin receptor by cross talk with the early signaling events, as a result of PKC-mediated Ser/Thr phosphorylation that inhibits tyrosine phosphorylation in insulin receptor signaling.

V. CONCLUSIONS

Data from PST signaling studies in hepatocytes and adipocytes point to the presence of a specific receptor of high binding affinity and specificity in the plasma membrane. Signal transduction of the PST receptor engages the activation of a double system of G-proteins. On the one hand, a PT-sensitive $G_{\alpha i1,2}$ pathway may mediate the activation of NO and cGMP production, which then may have a role inhibiting the signaling and mediating the inhibitory effect of PST on cell proliferation. On the other hand, a PT-insensitive $G_{\alpha q/11}$ is activated by the PST receptor and certainly mediates the activation of the PLC-β–PKC–MAPK pathway. The activation of classical isoforms of PKC is a central mediator of the metabolic effects of PST and its crosstalk with the insulin receptor, whose signaling and action are subsequently impaired. The balance of both limbs of signal transduction is also important for the final effect of PST on cell growth and proliferation.

Glossary

chromogranin A A glycoprotein that is very abundant in chromaffin and neuroendocrine secretory granules. This protein may function as a prohormone precursor of biologically active peptides.

cyclic GMP Cyclic nucleotide synthesized by guanylate cyclase, an enzyme activated by nitric oxide.

G-protein Heterotrimeric protein (α, β, γ) whose α-subunit has GTPase activity. G-proteins couple seven-trans-membrane-spanning receptors with different effectors.

nitric oxide synthase (NOS) There are three isoforms: inducible, neuronal, and endothelial. The activities of neuronal and endothelial NOS are regulated by extracellular signals and the inducible NOS is regulated at the transcriptional level.

pancreastatin Chromogranin A-derived peptide with autocrine, paracrine, and endocrine effects regulating secretion and metabolism.

phospholipase C Polyphosphoinositide-specific phospholipase, typically producing inositol 1,4,5-triphosphate and diacylglycerol. The phospholipase C β isoform is located in the plasma membrane.

protein kinase C Serine/threonine protein kinase whose activity is dependent on calcium and/or phospholipids.

See Also the Following Articles

Calcium Signaling ● Heterotrimeric G-Proteins ● Insulin Receptor Signaling ● Pancreastatin

Further Reading

González-Yanes, C., and Sánchez-Margalet, V. (2000). Pancreastatin modulates insulin signaling in rat adipocytes. *Diabetes* **49**, 1288–1294.

González-Yanes, C., Santos-Alvarez, J., and Sánchez-Margalet, V. (1999). Characterization of pancreastatin receptors and signaling in adipocyte membranes. *Biochim. Biophys. Acta* **1451**, 153–162.

Gonzalez-Yanes, C., Santos-Alvarez, J., and Sanchez-Margalet, V. (2001). Pancreastatin, a chromogranin A-derived peptide, activates $G_\alpha(16)$ and phospholipase C-β(2) by interacting with specific receptors in rat heart membranes. *Cell Signal.* **13**, 43–49.

Sánchez-Margalet, V. (1999). Modulation of insulin receptor signalling by pancreastatin in HTC hepatoma cells. *Diabetologia* **42**, 317–325.

Sánchez-Margalet, V., and Goberna, R. (1994). Pancreastatin activates pertussis toxin-sensitive guanylate cyclase and pertussis toxin-insensitive phospholipase C in rat liver membranes. *J. Cell. Biochem.* **55**, 173–181.

Sánchez-Margalet, V., González-Yanes, C., and Najib, S. (2001). Pancreastatin, a chromogranin A-derived peptide, inhibits DNA and protein synthesis by producing nitric oxide in HTC rat hepatoma cells. *J. Hepatol.* **35**, 80–85.

Sanchez-Margalet, V., Gonzalez-Yanes, C., Santos-Alvarez, J., and Najib, S. (2000). Characterization of pancreastatin receptor and signaling in rat HTC hepatoma cells. *Eur. J. Pharmacol.* **397**, 229–235.

Sánchez-Margalet, V., Lucas, M., and Goberna, R. (1993). Pancreastatin increases free cytosolic Ca^{2+} in rat hepatocytes involving both pertussis toxin-sensitive and -insensitive mechanisms. *Biochem. J.* **294**, 439–442.

Sánchez-Margalet, V., Lucas, M., and Goberna, R. (1994). Pancreastatin activates protein kinase C by stimulating the formation of 1,2-diacylglycerol in rat hepatocytes. *Biochem. J.* **303**, 51–54.

Sánchez-Margalet, V., Santos-Alvarez, J., Gonzalez-Yanes, C., and Najib, S. (2000). Pancreastatin: Biological effects and mechanisms of action. *Adv. Exp. Med. Biol.* **482**, 247–262.

Sánchez-Margalet, V., Valle, M., and Goberna, R. (1994). Receptors for pancreastatin in rat liver membranes: Molecular identification and characterization by covalent cross-linking. *Mol. Pharmacol.* **46**, 24–29.

Santos-Alvarez, J., González-Yanes, C., and Sánchez-Margalet, V. (1998). Pancreastatin receptor is coupled to a guanosine triphosphate-binding protein of the $G_{\alpha q/11}$ family in rat liver membranes. *Hepatology* **27**, 608–614.

Santos-Alvarez, J., and Sánchez-Margalet, V. (1998). Pancreastatin activates β3 isoform of phospholipase C via $G_{\alpha 11}$ protein stimulation in rat liver membranes. *Mol. Cell. Endocrinol.* **143**, 101–106.

Santos-Alvarez, J., and Sánchez-Margalet, V. (1999). G protein Gaq/11 and Gai1,2 are activated by pancreastatin by pancreastatin receptors in rat liver. Studies with GTP-γ-^{35}S and azido-GTPγ-^{32}P. *J. Cell. Biochem.* **73**, 469–477.

Santos-Alvarez, J., and Sanchez-Margalet, V. (2000). Affinity purification of pancreastatin receptor–Gq/11 protein complex from rat liver membranes. *Arch. Biochem. Biophys.* **378**, 151–156.

Pancreatic Polypeptide

RONALD E. CHANCE

Eli Lilly and Company, Indiana

I. INTRODUCTION
II. CHEMISTRY
III. BIOLOGY

Pancreatic polypeptide is a 36-residue peptide hormone with an amidated carboxyl group at the C-terminus. The hormone was discovered fortuitously in 1968 by scientists at Kansas University during research to purify chicken insulin.

I. INTRODUCTION

Discoverers Joseph Kimmel, Gail Pollock, and Robert Hazelwood named the persistent contaminant avian pancreatic polypeptide (APP; more recently aPP), fully expecting to rename it later once function was established. Because aPP was indistinguishable from glucagon by polyacrylamide disc gel electrophoresis, the peptide was assayed for glucagon bioactivity by William Bromer (Eli Lilly). Even though no hyperglycemic activity was found by the U.S. Pharmacopeia rabbit assay, continued work revealed that aPP was probably a hormone based primarily on a key structural feature. The C-terminal amino acid was amidated (i.e. tyrosinamide). This prompted the author's laboratory at Eli Lilly to further examine some side fractions that the staff had isolated during studies on the characterization of minor components in crystalline insulins (one of these components was already known to be proinsulin). The bovine, human, ovine, and porcine counterparts of aPP were discovered; furthermore, like aPP, all were 36 amino acids in length and all terminated with tyrosinamide.

Antisera against the avian and mammalian pancreatic polypeptides (PPs) along with the respective hormones were widely distributed to investigators by both laboratories in an effort to better understand the physiological role of this newly recognized pancreatic hormone. Immunohistochemistry studies revealed that PP is the product of a fourth type of islet cell, sometimes referred to in earlier literature as the F cell and now known as the PP cell. In mammals, in particular, the PP cell is located on the periphery of the islet; PP-rich islets are often regionally located in the duodenal portion of the pancreas, as shown in Fig. 1. The so-called uncinate process in the canine pancreas is an especially good source of PP cells. Early findings showed that blood levels of PP rose sharply following meals, especially after protein-rich meals. Insulin-induced hypoglycemia was also found to cause a dramatic rise in PP levels. Further investigations revealed that secretion of PP from the pancreas is mediated by vagal, cholinergic mechanisms, and, for this reason, PP responses have sometimes been used in clinical settings to assess vagal function.

Although PP is found primarily in the pancreas, the hormone is often included in discussions on gut hormones. Indeed, an intestinal peptide that is identical to porcine pancreatic polypeptide has been isolated from pig intestinal extracts. Early studies by Tsung-Min Lin (Eli Lilly) showed that bovine pancreatic polypeptide (bPP) administered to dogs did not affect blood glucose like insulin or glucagon but rather was a potent inhibitor of exocrine pancreatic secretion. Similar results in other laboratories led to speculation about using PP to treat pancreatitis. Meanwhile, aPP was studied extensively in chickens by researchers at the University of Kansas

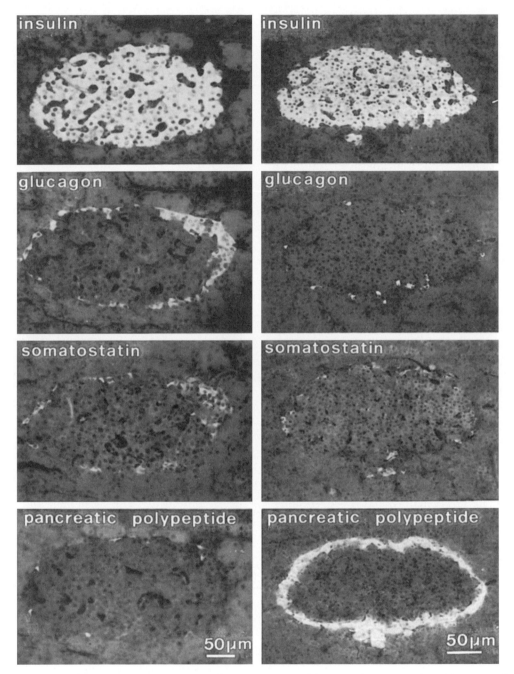

FIGURE 1 Series of four consecutive sections of a rat pancreatic islet stained, respectively, with anti-insulin, anti-glucagon, anti-somatostatin, and anti-pancreatic polypeptide antisera. The pattern shown in the panels on the left-hand side is characteristic of islets situated in the body and tail of the pancreas (the splenic region). The pattern shown in the panels on the right-hand side is characteristic of islets situated in the lower part of the head of the pancreas. The figure is courtesy of Lelio Orci. Reprinted from Hazelwood (1981), with permission.

in collaboration with Robert Hazelwood at the University of Houston. The avian hormone was found to be a powerful gastric stimulant in chickens.

Because PP was a recognized contaminant in therapeutic insulin preparations prior to the advent of highly purified animal insulins, the PP radioimmuno-assay was utilized as a quality control assay on post-1980 purified bovine and porcine insulins. Prior to this, persons with diabetes who received the older traditional and nonchromatographed insulins were sometimes found to have detectable PP antibodies. The assay has also been used in the diagnosis of pancreatic tumors.

II. CHEMISTRY

The primary structures of aPP and several of the mammalian PPs (bovine, human, porcine, ovine, and canine) were reported in the 1970s. This was followed by the discovery and characterization of two peptide hormones that shared considerable homology with the PPs, yet were distinctly different. Using a more elegant and systematic approach to new hormone discovery, Kazuhiko Tatemoto and Viktor Mutt examined intestinal and brain extracts for peptides possessing amidated carboxyl groups and discovered peptide YY (PYY) and neuropeptide Y (NPY) (see comparison of primary structures in Table 1). Based on X-ray crystal studies of aPP, the hairpin-like fold appears applicable to most if not all members of the so-called PP family, which is now referred to as the PP-fold family.

All of the PP-fold peptides are the result of a precursor–product relationship that has been clarified through the use of molecular biology techniques. Whereas the gene for human NPY is on chromosome 7, the genes for PYY and PP are in close proximity on chromosome 17q21.1, and it is thought that gene duplication of the human peptide YY gene (PYY) generated the pancreatic polypeptide gene (gene symbol PPY). The PPY gene product is a 95-residue protein in which hPP is flanked by a 29-residue signal peptide at the N-terminus and a 30-residue C-terminal extension as shown (hPP sequence in boldface type):

Human Prepropancreatic Polypeptide

[1]MAAARLCLSLLLLSTCVALLLQPLLGAQGly↓
APLEPVYPGDNATPEQMAQYA
ADLRRYINMLTRPRYGly↓ Lys↓ Arg↓ HKED-
TLAFSEWGSPHAAVPArg↓ ELSPLDL[95]

Single-letter notation is used for all amino acids except those at the processing sites, which are denoted by 3-letter abbreviations and underlined. Prepropancreatic hPP is matured to hPP through the action of several enzymatic steps. After biosynthesis, the preprohormone is translocated from the endoplasmic reticulum to the *trans*-Golgi network with the removal of the signal peptide by signal peptidase. The prohormone is sorted to a regulated transport site and a proprotein convertase cleaves at the COOH-terminus of the Lys-Arg sequence. Arginine and lysine are removed though the action of carboxypeptidase E. Finally, the remaining Gly becomes a substrate for peptidyl glycine α-amidating monooxygenase, resulting in the carboxyamidation of tyrosine at hPP position 36. An icosapeptide and a heptapeptide result from a trypsin-like cleavage at the single arginine residue in the C-terminal extension peptide.

The primary structures of more than 40 PPs have been reported. A partial list is shown in Table 1. Essentially, all are obvious homologues despite species diversity. X-ray crystal structure studies have been limited to aPP (chicken and turkey have identical sequences), although bPP crystals suitable for X-ray analysis have been grown. A solution

TABLE 1   Primary Structures of Some Members of the PP-Fold Family[a]

	1	2	3	4	5	6	7	8	9	10	11	12	13	14	15	16	17	18	19	20	21	22	23	24	25	26	27	28	29	30	31	32	33	34	35	36
Human PP	A	P	L	E	P	V	Y	P	G	D	N	A	T	P	E	Q	M	A	Q	Y	A	A	D	L	R	R	Y	I	N	M	L	T	R	P	R	Y
Cat PP	-	-	-	-	-	-	-	-	-	-	-	-	-	-	-	-	-	-	-	-	-	-	E	-	-	-	-	-	-	-	-	-	-	-	-	-
Dog PP	-	-	-	-	-	-	-	-	-	-	D	-	-	-	-	-	-	-	-	-	-	-	E	-	-	-	-	-	-	-	-	-	-	-	-	-
Pig PP	-	-	-	-	-	-	-	-	-	-	D	-	-	-	-	-	-	-	-	-	-	-	E	-	-	-	-	-	-	-	-	-	-	-	-	-
Horse PP	-	-	M	-	-	-	-	-	-	-	D	-	-	-	-	-	-	-	-	-	-	-	E	-	-	-	-	-	-	-	-	-	-	-	-	-
Cow PP	-	-	-	-	-	E	-	-	-	-	-	-	-	-	-	-	-	-	-	-	-	-	E	-	-	-	-	-	-	-	-	-	-	-	-	-
Sheep PP	-	S	-	-	-	E	-	-	-	-	-	-	-	-	-	-	-	-	-	-	-	-	E	-	-	-	-	-	-	-	-	-	-	-	-	-
Guinea pig PP	-	-	-	-	-	-	-	-	-	-	D	-	-	-	Q	-	-	-	-	-	-	-	E	M	-	-	-	-	-	-	-	-	-	-	-	-
Rabbit PP	-	-	P	-	-	-	-	-	-	-	D	-	-	-	-	E	-	V	-	-	-	-	-	-	-	-	-	-	-	-	-	-	-	-	-	-
Mouse PP	-	-	-	-	-	M	-	-	-	-	Y	-	-	-	-	-	-	-	-	E	T	Q	-	-	-	-	-	T	-	-	-	-	-	-	-	-
Rat PP	-	-	-	-	-	M	-	-	-	-	Y	-	-	H	-	-	R	-	-	E	T	Q	-	-	-	-	-	T	-	-	-	-	-	-	-	-
Chicken PP	G	-	S	Q	-	T	-	-	-	-	D	-	P	V	-	D	L	I	R	F	Y	N	-	-	Q	Q	-	L	-	V	V	-	-	H	-	-
Human NPY	Y	-	S	K	-	D	N	-	-	E	D	-	P	A	-	D	L	-	R	-	Y	S	A	-	-	H	-	-	-	L	I	-	-	Q	-	-
Human PYY	Y	-	I	K	-	E	A	-	-	E	D	-	S	-	-	E	L	N	R	-	Y	-	S	-	-	H	-	L	-	L	V	-	-	Q	-	-
Homologous positions		P			P			P	G			A															Y		N			T	R		R	Y

[a]Positions differing from the human PP sequence are indicated. Excluding the sheep PP, there are 11 homologous positions. All tyrosines at position 36 are amidated.

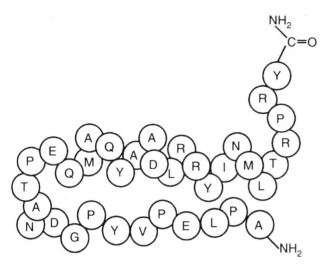

FIGURE 2 Primary structure of human pancreatic polypeptide (hPP) depicted in the PP-fold configuration. The 36-residue peptide begins with an NH₂-terminal alanine and terminates with an amidated tyrosine. See Table 1 for primary structures of several members of the PP-fold family. The computer graphic is courtesy of Don Gehlert (Eli Lilly).

structure of bPP showed a fold remarkably similar to that of aPP. The other PP-family members are considered to fit the so-called PP-fold model, as depicted in Fig. 2. In this model, there is a polyproline type II helix involving residues 2-8, a β-turn, and an α-helical region from residues from ~15 to 32. It is interesting that the prolines at positions 2, 5, and 8 are part of a polyproline-type conformation and interdigitate with the hydrophobic side chains of the helix to form a stable fold.

III. BIOLOGY

The physiologic function(s) of PP is unknown. The hormone does not have readily apparent actions like the other islet hormones. In both birds and mammals, PP seems to mainly involve regulation of various gastrointestinal activities. For instance, aPP is a powerful gastric stimulant in chickens, and bPP has been found to have a wide spectrum of gastrointestinal actions in dogs, the most notable being the relaxation of the gall bladder and the inhibition of pancreatic exocrine secretion. Results from a few small-scale studies conducted in humans are generally in agreement with the results from the research on dogs. In other studies, PP was administered to 11 patients with chronic pancreatitis with a PP deficiency, as shown by lack of response to a test meal. Results indicated some improvement in abnormal glucose metabolism.

A recurring question concerns the role of PP in satiety. Most animal studies have been inconclusive on this matter. When PP was administered to children with the hyperphagia and obesity of the Prader-Willi syndrome (also shown to have a poor PP response to a protein meal), food intake was reduced slightly. In a 2002 review, Katsuura et al. cite recent animal studies showing that peripherally administered PP suppresses food intake and gastric emptying, whereas central administration of PP elicits food intake and gastric emptying. Some of the discrepancies in the literature on this subject may be the result of species specificity for PP. Today, virtually any species of PP can be prepared synthetically with relative ease, whereas older studies were conducted mainly with bovine or porcine PP administered to mice and rats (see Table 1 for PP structural differences). Also, recent transgenic technology is useful in addressing such questions. For example, PP transgenic mice that had overproduction of PP exhibited both decreased food intake and decreased gastric emptying.

The reason that central administration of PP stimulates feeding in several different species of experimental animals may be revealed in the future as PP receptors become better understood. Binding sites for PP have been found in several regions of the rat brain, including sites corresponding to brain regions regulating digestion and autonomic function. Binding sites for PP have been also found in the basolateral membranes of canine small intestinal mucosa as well as the ductus choledochus, duodenum, ileum, adrenal gland, and liver in the rat. In chickens, aPP binding was demonstrated in the spleen, liver, pancreas, gastrointestinal tract, and cerebellum.

Structure–activity studies with PP (bPP) using the canine intestinal mucosa model revealed the importance of the C-terminal tyrosinamide at position 36 for full receptor binding. Removal of this residue abolished receptor binding. Similarly, conversion of the native tyrosinamide to tyrosine also abolished receptor binding. When the carboxyl group was converted to a carboxymethyl form, the receptor binding was restored to 60% receptor recognition. Similar studies confirmed this work using a cloned hPP-preferring receptor, now known as the Y4 receptor, a G-protein-coupled receptor. These studies also demonstrated the importance of the N-terminal portion of PP for full receptor binding.

Future research on the PP-fold family of peptides, and on PP in particular, may reveal the true function of PP.

Glossary

neuropeptide Y A 36-residue neuropeptide hormone with considerable homology to pancreatic polypeptide.

pancreatic polypeptide A 36-residue peptide hormone found predominantly in the pancreas.

peptideYY A 36-residue peptide hormone found predominantly in the gut; it shows homology to both neuropeptide Y and pancreatic polypeptide.

PP cell One of four endocrine cell types in pancreatic islets where pancreatic polypeptide is located. Also known as the F cell.

PP-fold Refers to the U-shaped structural fold assumed by members of the pancreatic polypeptide (PP) family (PP, peptide YY, and neuropeptide Y).

See Also the Following Articles

Appetite Regulation • Pancreastatin • Pancreastatin Receptor Signaling

Further Reading

Berntson, G. G., Zipf, W. B., O'Dorisio, T. M., Hoffmann, J. A., and Chance, R. E. (1993). Pancreatic polypeptide infusions reduce food intake in Prader-Willi syndrome. *Peptides* **14**, 497–503.

Boel, E., Schwartz, T. W., Norris, K. E., and Fill, N. P. (1984). A cDNA encoding a small common precursor for human pancreatic polypeptide and pancreatic icosapeptide. *EMBO J.* **3**, 909–912.

Bordi, C., Azzoni, C., D'Adda, T., and Pizzi, S. (2002). Pancreatic polypeptide-related tumors. *Peptides* **23**, 339–348.

Brunicardi, F. C., Chaiken, R. L., Ryan, A. S., Seymour, N. E., Hoffmann, J. A., Lebovitz, H. E., Chance, R. E., Gingerich, R. L., Andersen, D. K., and Elahi, D. (1996). Pancreatic polypeptide administration improves abnormal glucose metabolism in patients with chronic pancreatitis. *J. Clin. Endocrinol. Metab.* **81**, 3566–3572.

Chance, R. E., Johnson, M. G., Hoffmann, J. A., and Lin, T.-M. (1979). Pancreatic polypeptide: A newly recognized hormone. *In* "Proinsulin, Insulin, C-peptide" (S. Baba, T. Kaneko, and N. Yanaihara, eds.), pp. 419–425. Excerpta Media, Amsterdam-Oxford.

Chen, Z.-W., Bergman, T., Östenson, C.-G., Höög, A., Näslund, J., Norberg, A., Carlquist, M., Efendic, S., Mutt, V., and Jörnvall, J. (1994). A porcine gut pancreatic polypeptide identical to the pancreatic hormone PP (pancreatic polypeptide). *FEBS Lett.* **341**, 239–243.

Conlon, J. M. (2002). The origin and evolution of peptide YY (PYY) and pancreatic polypeptide (PP). *Peptides* **23**, 263–267.

Gehlert, D. R. (1998). Multiple receptors for the pancreatic (PP-fold) family: Physiological implications. *P.S.E.B.M.* **218**, 7–22.

Gehlert, D. R., Schober, D. A., Beavers, L., Gadski, R., Hoffmann, J. A., Smiley, D. L., Chance, R. E., Lundell, I., and Larhammar, D. (1996). Characterization of the peptide binding requirements for the cloned human pancreatic polypeptide-preferring receptor. *Mol. Pharmacol.* **50**, 112–118.

Gingerich, R. L., Akpan, J. O., Gilbert, W. R., Leith, K. A., Hoffmann, J. A., and Chance, R. E. (1991). Structural requirements of pancreatic polypeptide receptor binding. *Am. J. Physiol.* **261**, E319–E324. Endocrinol. Metab. **24**.

Glover, I., Haneef, I., Pitts, J., Wood, S., Moss, D., Tickle, I., and Blundell, T. (1983). Conformational flexibility in a small globular hormone: X-ray analysis of avian pancreatic polypeptide at 0.98-Å resolution. *Biopolymers* **22**, 293–304.

Hazelwood, R. L. (1981). Synthesis, storage, secretion, and significance of pancreatic polypeptide in vertebrates. *In* "The Islets of Langerhans" (S. J. Cooperstein and D. Watson, eds.), pp. 275–318. Academic Press, New York.

Hennig, R., Keksis, P. B., Friess, H., Adrian, T. E., and Büchler, M. W. (2002). Pancreatic polypeptide in pancreatitis. *Peptides* **23**, 331–338.

Katsuura, G., Asakawa, A., and Inui, A. (2002). Roles of pancreatic polypeptide in regulation of food intake. *Peptides* **23**, 323–329.

Kimmel, J. R., Pollock, H. G., and Hazelwood, R. L. (1968). Isolation and characterization of chicken insulin. *Endocrinology* **83**, 1323–1330.

Larsson, L.-I., Sundler, F., and Håkanson, R. (1976). Pancreatic polypeptide—A postulated new hormone: Identification of its cellular storage site by light and electron microscopic immunocytochemistry. *Diabetologia* **12**, 211–226.

Li, X., Sutcliffe, M. J., Schwartz, T. W., and Dobson, C. M. (1992). Sequence-specific ^{1}H NMR assignments and solution structure of bovine pancreatic polypeptide. *Biochemistry* **31**, 1245–1253.

Orci, L. (1982). Banting Lecture 1981. Macro- and micro-domains in the endocrine pancreas. *Diabetes* **31**, 538–565.

Schwartz, T. W. (1983). Pancreatic polypeptide: A hormone under vagal control. *Gastroenterology* **85**, 1411–1425.

Whitcomb, D. C., Puccio, A. M., Vigna, S. R., Taylor, I. L., and Hoffman, G. E. (1997). Distribution of pancreatic polypeptide receptors in the rat brain. *Brain Res.* **760**, 137–149.

Parathyroid Hormone

ROBERT A. NISSENSON

University of California, San Francisco and Veterans' Affairs Medical Center, San Francisco

I. INTRODUCTION
II. BIOSYNTHESIS, SECRETION, AND CHEMISTRY OF PTH
III. PHYSIOLOGICAL ACTIONS OF PTH IN BONE
IV. PHYSIOLOGICAL ACTIONS OF PTH IN KIDNEY
V. MECHANISM OF ACTION OF PTH
VI. DISEASE STATES

Parathyroid hormone (PTH) is a polypeptide hormone that serves as a major regulator of plasma calcium. Increased circulating levels of PTH result in a compensating increase in ionized calcium in the blood by mobilizing calcium form the body's enormous calcium reserves in bone, by reducing renal calcium loss, and by (indirectly) increasing the efficiency of absorption of dietary calcium by the intestine.

I. INTRODUCTION

Parathyroid hormone (PTH) is produced by tiny organs in the region adjacent to the thyroid glands in the neck. Humans generally have four functional parathyroid glands. In evolution, parathyroid glands first appear in terrestrial vertebrates, and their existence is closely linked to the need to maintain adequate levels of ionized calcium in blood. Ionized calcium in the extracellular fluid serves to support a range of essential physiological processes including proper neuromuscular function, exocrine and endocrine secretion, mineralization of bone, and cell growth and differentiation. With the evolution of amphibians, vertebrate life needed to adapt from seawater, which has a very high ambient level of calcium, to land, where calcium must be obtained from dietary sources. A complex endocrine homeostatic system evolved in terrestrial vertebrates in order to ensure maintenance of adequate levels of plasma calcium even under conditions of limited dietary calcium intake. The parathyroid glands play a pivotal role in this homeostatic system, since they are able to detect even small decreases in the level of ionized calcium in the blood and to respond by secreting PTH. This article presents an overview of the current understanding of the biochemistry, physiology, and mechanism of action of PTH as well as a discussion of the clinical diseases associated with abnormalities in this hormonal system.

II. BIOSYNTHESIS, SECRETION, AND CHEMISTRY OF PTH

As mentioned above, the maintenance of adequate levels of plasma ionized calcium ($1.0–1.3$ mM) is required for normal neuromuscular function, bone mineralization, and many other physiological processes. The parathyroid gland secretes PTH in response to very small decrements in ionized calcium in the blood in order to maintain the normocalcemic state. PTH accomplishes this by promoting bone resorption and releasing calcium from the skeletal reservoir, by inducing renal conservation of calcium and excretion of phosphate, and by indirectly enhancing intestinal calcium absorption by increasing the renal production of the active vitamin D metabolite $1,25(OH)_2$ vitamin D. The parathyroid

gland functions in essence as a "calciostat," sensing the prevailing ionized calcium level in the blood and adjusting the secretion of PTH accordingly (Fig. 1). The relationship between ionized calcium and PTH secretion is a sigmoidal one, allowing significant changes in PTH secretion in response to very small changes in plasma ionized calcium.

In addition to providing acute regulation of PTH secretion, ionized calcium is a primary factor controlling chronic secretion of the hormone. Thus, sustained hypocalcemia promotes increased expression of the PTH gene and results in parathyroid hyperplasia. A common example of the latter is the marked parathyroid hyperplasia (secondary hyperparathyroidism) that frequently accompanies chronic renal failure. $1,25(OH)_2$ Vitamin D also serves as a negative regulator of PTH gene expression and parathyroid cell hyperplasia. In chronic renal failure, both hypocalcemia and reduced circulating levels of $1,25(OH)_2$ vitamin D presumably contribute to the progression of secondary hyperparathyroidism.

The plasma membrane of parathyroid cells contains high levels of a calcium-sensing receptor (CaR). Unlike intracellular calcium-binding proteins, which have an affinity for free calcium in the nanomolar range (consistent with intracellular levels of free calcium), the CaR binds calcium in the millimolar range. The receptor is a member of the G-protein-coupled receptor superfamily. It contains calcium-binding elements in its extracellular domain and signaling determinants in its cytoplasmic regions.

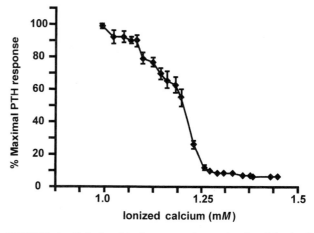

FIGURE 1 Relationship between plasma levels of ionized calcium and the release of PTH(1–84) in normal humans. Variations in plasma ionized calcium were achieved by the infusion of calcium or EDTA. Note the sigmoidal relationship, ensuring significant changes in PTH secretion with small variations in ionized calcium.

Calcium binding to the receptor triggers activation of G-proteins that are able to suppress the synthesis and secretion of PTH. When ionized calcium in the blood falls, there is less signaling by the CaRs on the parathyroid cell and PTH secretion consequently increases. The essential role of the CaR can best be seen in humans bearing loss-of-function mutations in the CaR gene. In the heterozygous state, such mutations result in familial hypocalciuric hypercalcemia, characterized by inappropriately high levels of PTH secretion in the face of hypercalcemia. These individuals are quantitatively resistant to the suppressive effect of calcium on PTH secretion due to the reduced number of parathyroid CaRs. In the homozygous state, patients display a severe increase in PTH secretion with life-threatening hypercalcemia (neonatal severe primary hyperparathyroidism).

The initial translation product of the PTH gene is prepro-PTH. The N-terminal pre-sequence (signal peptide) of the protein facilitates transport across the membrane of endoplasmic reticulum and into the initial biosynthetic pathway where the pre-sequence is proteolytically removed. The amino-terminal pro-sequence is also required for the proper transport of the protein during biosynthesis, and this 6-amino-acid peptide is cleaved in the Golgi by a furin-like peptidase. The resulting product is the mature, 84-amino-acid secretory product of the parathyroid gland, PTH.

Although the biologically active, mature form of PTH is an 84-amino-acid molecule, the major actions of PTH on bone and kidney can be reproduced with synthetic peptides containing as few as the 34 amino acids of the amino-terminus of the protein. The functional importance of the midregion and carboxyl-terminal region of PTH remains unclear. Truncation of merely a single amino acid from the amino-terminus of PTH results in a dramatic loss of biological activity. Thus, the amino-terminus of the peptide appears to have a central role in the ability of PTH to activate its receptor on target cells in kidney and bone. The 1–34 sequence of PTH has been highly conserved throughout the evolution of terrestrial vertebrates, consistent with the important biological function of this region of the molecule. Interestingly, there is a second gene product that shares sequence similarity with the 1–34 region of PTH and is thus able to activate the PTH receptor. The factor is termed PTH-related protein (PTHrP), and its physiological role is to exert local control over the development and function of a number of tissues. For reasons that are unclear, PTHrP is expressed at very high levels by several types of cancers.

With some cancers, circulating levels of PTHrP become high enough to cause excessive bone resorption and increased blood calcium due to the actions of circulating PTHrP on PTH receptors.

Early studies demonstrated that PTH circulates in multiple forms that can be distinguished by radioimmunoassays specific for different regions of the PTH molecule. PTH(1–84) is subject to metabolism within the parathyroid gland, resulting in the secretion of PTH fragments as well as the intact molecule. In addition, PTH(1–84) is metabolized in peripheral tissues. Midregion and carboxyl-terminal fragments of PTH have a much longer half-life in the circulation than does PTH(1–84). As a result, midregion and carboxyl-terminal fragments of PTH circulate at much higher concentrations than does intact PTH(1–84). Rapid plasma clearance of PTH is due primarily to hepatic metabolism, with a lesser contribution by the kidneys. Peripheral metabolism generates midregion and carboxyl-terminal fragments of PTH that resemble those secreted by the parathyroid gland. Midregion and carboxyl-terminal PTH fragments are cleared by renal excretion, and thus circulating levels of these fragments are highly dependent on renal function. Extremely high levels of PTH detected with antibodies against the midregion and carboxyl-terminal region of the hormone in many patients with end-stage renal disease thus reflect a combination of secondary hyperparathyroidism and reduced renal clearance of PTH fragments.

Midregion and carboxyl-terminal PTH fragments lack the amino-terminal 1–34 sequence of the hormone required for binding to PTH/PTHrP receptors and producing the classical effects of PTH on kidney and bone. Metabolism of PTH could produce biologically active, amino-terminal fragments of PTH, but there is little evidence for the presence of significant levels of amino-terminal PTH fragments in the circulation or for significant secretion of such fragments by the parathyroid gland. Presumably, both the parathyroid gland and the peripheral organs contain enzymes that degrade amino-terminal fragments of PTH. This ensures that circulating levels of biologically active PTH are derived exclusively from glandular secretion of PTH(1–84). A few studies have demonstrated potential biological effects of midregion or carboxyl-terminal fragments of PTH, and there is also evidence for the existence of membrane receptors for these fragments. However, the biological role of PTH fragments remains unclear.

III. PHYSIOLOGICAL ACTIONS OF PTH IN BONE

The major physiological role of PTH is to mobilize calcium from bone in order to maintain an adequate level of plasma ionized calcium. In times of dietary calcium deficiency, blood levels of calcium fall slightly and this serves to increase the secretion of PTH by the parathyroid gland. PTH acts directly on bone to increase the number and activity of osteoclasts—the cells that promote bone resorption. During osteoclastic bone resorption, calcium-rich hydroxyapatite bone mineral is converted to soluble calcium, which is transported into the general extracellular space to support the level of blood calcium. PTH also increases the efficiency of transport of calcium from bone to blood.

PTH receptors have been localized to bone-forming osteoblasts and their precursors, but it is not clear whether osteoclasts possess PTH receptors. Indeed, PTH is not able to activate isolated osteoclasts *in vitro* unless osteoblast-like cells are also present. These findings suggest that PTH may produce its actions on osteoclasts indirectly, perhaps through direct interaction with cells of the osteoblast lineage. Indeed, PTH induces an increase in the expression of a molecule termed RANK ligand (RANKL) on the surface of osteoblasts (Fig. 2). Osteoclasts and their precursors (myeloid lineage cells) express the receptor for RANKL, a molecule termed RANK. When PTH-stimulated osteoblasts come into contact with osteoclasts or their precursors, RANKL interacts with RANK, resulting in signaling events that produce increased formation and activity of osteoclasts. Osteoblasts also produce an inhibitor of RANKL (termed osteoprotogerin or

OPG). PTH inhibits the production of OPG, an effect that also promotes increased osteoclast formation and activity.

Although stimulation of bone resorption is the major physiological response of the skeleton to PTH, pharmacological experiments have shown that PTH is also capable of increasing bone formation. Thus, administration of PTH intermittently to animals or humans results in a marked anabolic response of the skeleton. High levels of PTH are known to produce an increase in the number of osteoblasts, which results in part from the coupling between increased osteoclastic resorption and new bone formation. However, intermittent treatment with low doses of PTH produces a direct positive effect on bone formation that is independent of preceding bone resorption. The cellular basis for this action of PTH is not fully understood but could result from an action of PTH to increase the number and/or functional activity of bone-forming osteoblasts. There is currently great interest in exploiting this action of PTH for the purpose of treating individuals with low-bone-mass diseases such as osteoporosis.

IV. PHYSIOLOGICAL ACTIONS OF PTH IN KIDNEY

PTH produces a series of renal actions that help to ensure that calcium mobilized from bone contributes optimally for the maintenance of plasma ionized calcium levels. The renal actions of PTH include inhibition of renal phosphate reabsorption, stimulation of renal calcium reabsorption, and increased production of $1,25(OH)_2$ vitamin D. The ability of PTH to inhibit renal phosphate reabsorption has been known for many years, providing the basis for

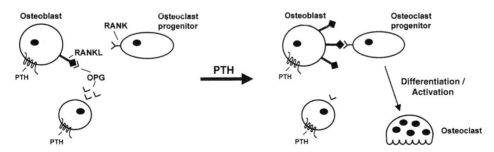

FIGURE 2 Regulation of osteoclast differentiation and activation by PTH. Binding of PTH by receptors on osteoblasts results in increased expression of osteoprotegerin ligand (RANKL) on the cell surface. Activation of PTH receptor can also reduce the secretion of the RANKL inhibitor osteoprotegerin (OPG), which is produced by cells in the bone microenvironment. These effects of PTH promote the action of RANKL on its receptor (RANK) on the surface of osteoclast precursors and mature osteoclasts. RANK signaling, together with the action of macrophage colony-stimulating factor, stimulates the differentiation of osteoclast precursors and promotes the activation of mature osteoclasts.

a clinical test of renal responsiveness to the hormone. Patients with primary hyperparathyroidism display hypophosphatemia and decreased renal tubular reabsorption of phosphate, whereas hypoparathyroid patients are hyperphosphatemic and have increased phosphate reabsorption. Phosphate forms a complex with free calcium in blood. Thus, for a given level of serum calcium, ionized calcium will be reduced as serum phosphate increases. Under conditions of relative hypocalcemia (e.g., during chronic dietary calcium deficiency), PTH secretion is increased, resulting in increased bone resorption. Both calcium and phosphate are released from hydroxyapatite during the process of bone resorption. By promoting renal excretion of phosphate, PTH facilitates a rise in ionized and total plasma calcium. Recently, the molecular basis for PTH-induced inhibition of renal phosphate reabsorption was clarified. PTH inhibits the expression of a specific (type IIa) sodium–phosphate co-transporter in the brush border of proximal renal tubular cells. This results in a reduced V_{max} for phosphate transport and therefore lower efficiency of proximal phosphate reabsorption.

PTH also acts to increase renal calcium reabsorption, thus ensuring that only small amounts of calcium released during PTH-induced bone resorption are lost via renal excretion. The major sites for this effect of PTH are in the distal convoluted tubule and the thick ascending limb of Henle's loop. Recent evidence indicates that distal renal tubular calcium reabsorption is an active process that requires calcium influx through dihydropyridine-sensitive calcium channels located in the apical plasma membrane. Drugs that inhibit these channels are effective in blocking PTH-induced renal calcium reabsorption. Unlike voltage-sensitive calcium channels in excitable tissues, PTH-responsive calcium channels in the distal nephron are activated by membrane hyperpolarization. PTH appears to open calcium channels by inducing hyperpolarization of the apical plasma membrane. Calcium entering the distal renal tubular cell in this manner is transported into the extracellular compartment via a sodium–calcium exchanger present on the basolateral plasma membrane.

PTH promotes intestinal calcium reabsorption indirectly, through an action to increase circulating levels of 1,25(OH)$_2$ vitamin D. This vitamin D metabolite acts directly on intestinal epithelial cells to increase the efficiency of calcium (and phosphate) absorption. Primary hyperparathyroidism is commonly associated with increased circulating levels of 1,25(OH)$_2$ vitamin D, whereas reduced levels of this

metabolite are present in hypoparathyroidism. PTH produces this effect by increasing the rate of production of 1,25(OH)$_2$ vitamin D through activation of the 25(OH) vitamin D-1-hydroxylase enzyme located in the proximal renal tubule. Studies *in vivo* as well as in cultured renal cell lines indicate that PTH increases the expression of the 25(OH) vitamin D-1-hydroxylase gene through a transcriptional mechanism.

The actions of PTH to promote increased bone resorption, reduced calcium excretion, and (indirectly) increased intestinal calcium absorption all help to maintain adequate levels of plasma calcium even under conditions of dietary calcium deficiency.

V. MECHANISM OF ACTION OF PTH

PTH action is initiated by the binding of the hormone to a G-protein-coupled receptor on the surface of target cells in kidney and bone (Fig. 3). The major G-protein activated by the PTH receptor is G_s, the G-protein coupled to activation of adenylyl cyclase and production of cyclic AMP. Indeed, shortly after the discovery of the cyclic AMP signaling pathway, it was found that PTH is capable of increasing the levels of cyclic AMP in target cells through activation of the adenylyl cyclase. Cyclic AMP is a second messenger in the cellular action of a wide variety of hormones and other extracellular regulatory molecules. It activates cyclic AMP-dependent protein kinase A (PKA), which in turns phosphorylates and thereby regulates key proteins that participate in physiological responses. Very little is known about the identity of substrates of PKA that are phosphorylated in response to PTH receptor activation. These presumably include transcription factors, ion channels, transporters, and enzymes involved in cellular metabolism.

The important role of the cyclic AMP pathway in mediating PTH action is underscored by the ability of cyclic AMP analogues (or drugs that directly activate adenylyl cyclase such as forskolin) to reproduce many of the biological effects of PTH. For example, cyclic AMP analogues and forskolin are capable of reducing the expression of the renal type IIa sodium–phosphate co-transporter. The also promote an increase in the expression of RANKL in osteoblasts. Furthermore, genetic deficiency in the α-subunit of G_s (as seen in the human disease pseudohypoparathyrodism type Ia) results in renal and skeletal resistance to PTH action.

PTH receptors also couple to the G-protein G_q, which activates phospholipase C, an enzyme that

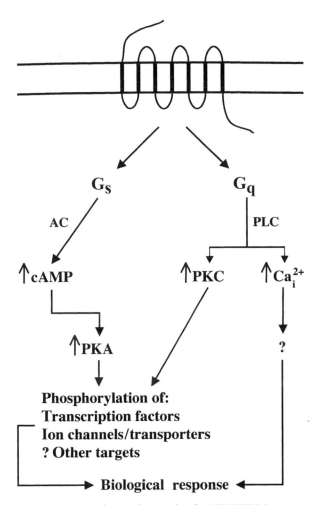

FIGURE 3 Signal transduction by the PTH/PTHrP receptor. PTH and PTHrP bind to determinants in the extracellular domain and in the body of the receptor. This leads to conformational changes in the transmembrane helices and consequent structural changes in the cytoplasmic domain. The latter permit productive interactions between the receptor and the G-proteins G_s and G_q, activating the adenylyl cyclase (AC) and phospholipase C (PLC) signaling pathways, respectively. These pathways are thought to cooperate in determining the cellular response to the receptor activation. Most available evidence supports a primary role of the cyclic AMP/protein kinase A (PKA) pathway in mediating the biological effects of PTH/PTHrP receptor activation, with the PLC pathway playing a modulatory role. PKC, protein kinase C.

hydrolyzes the plasma membrane phospholipid phosphatidylinositol 4,5-bisphosphate to produce diacylglycerol (DAG) and soluble inositol 1,4,5-trisphosphate (IP_3). DAG and IP_3 function as second messengers—the former by activating protein kinase C and the latter by binding to and opening calcium channels on the membrane of the endoplasmic reticulum, thereby increasing cytosolic free calcium.

There is currently great interest in understanding how this pathway contributes to the physiological effects of PTH in bone and kidney.

There has been great interest in understanding how the structure of the PTH receptor contributes to ligand binding and signal transduction. The PTH receptor is a member of the large superfamily of G-protein-coupled receptors. All members are intrinsic plasma membrane proteins with seven membrane-spanning segments that line a central cavity. Ligands (PTH and PTHrP) bind to the large N-terminal extracellular domain of the receptor as well as to the extracellular loops. This facilitates the interaction of the ligand with the transmembrane cavity of the receptor, producing a conformational change in the receptor. In the ligand-bound state, the receptor interacts with and activates its cognate G-proteins on the cytoplasmic surface of the plasma membrane. Many features of this activation mechanism are shared by other (so-called class II) G-protein-coupled receptors that are related to the PTH receptor (e.g., receptors for glucagon, calcitonin, and secretin).

As with most G-protein-coupled receptors, signal transduction by the PTH receptor is under strict regulatory control. After an initial burst of signaling, agonist-occupied PTH receptors lose their signaling capacity. This desensitization results from the phosphorylation of the active PTH receptor by a G-protein-coupled receptor kinase. This phosphorylation event promotes the interaction of the receptor with a cytoplasmic protein called arrestin. When arrestin binds to the PTH receptor, interaction with G-proteins is sterically inhibited and thus signaling is prevented. The desensitized PTH receptor is internalized via clathrin-coated pits and is recycled back to the plasma membrane. It is likely that dephosphorylation of the PTH receptor occurs within endocytic vesicles, allowing resensitization of the receptor prior to its reinsertion in the plasma membrane.

VI. DISEASE STATES

The most common diseases of the PTH endocrine system result from excessive production of ligands for the PTH receptor. Primary hyperparathyroidism most commonly results from a benign tumor affecting one of the four parathyroid glands. Occasionally, all four glands are enlarged. Parathyroid cancer can also occur but is extremely rare. Excessive secretion of PTH results in increased bone resorption, increased renal reabsorption of calcium, and increased production of 1,25(OH)$_2$ vitamin D (and thus increased intestinal calcium absorption). These combined actions result in hypercalcemia and (over time) bone loss due to hyperresorption. A similar syndrome occurs in patients with malignant (nonparathyroid) tumors that secrete large amounts of PTHrP. Optimal treatment for these disorders is the removal of the parathyroid tumor or malignancy responsible for producing excessive PTH or PTHrP, respectively. When surgical treatment is not possible, the hypercalcemia can be treated by the administration of drugs that inhibit bone resorption such as bisphosphonate compounds.

Secondary hyperparathyroidism can occur as a result of conditions that produce chronic hypocalcemia such as chronic renal failure. Hypocalcemia has both a direct stimulatory effect on PTH secretion and an indirect effect by promoting the increased proliferation of parathyroid cells. Over time, chronic hypocalcemia produces a massive increase in the size of the parathyroid glands due to hyperplasia. This results in very high circulating levels of PTH and excessive bone resorption, often resulting in bone pain and fragility. Treatment of this disorder is targeted toward restoring the plasma calcium level and thereby removing the stimulus for further proliferation of parathyroid cells. 1,25(OH)$_2$ vitamin D is often used therapeutically, since it promotes an increase in intestinal absorption of calcium and thus helps to suppress PTH secretion and parathyroid cell growth.

Although much less common, genetic mutations in components of the PTH receptor signaling pathway are also known to be associated with human diseases. Certain mutations in the PTH receptor are known to result in constitutive (i.e., hormone-independent) receptor signaling. Individuals harboring such a mutation display evidence of PTH receptor hyperfunction, including hypercalcemia and increased bone resorption. They also display premature cartilage differentiation reflecting an exaggeration in the normal physiological action of PTHrP (acting through the PTH receptor) on chondrogenesis. This disorder is known as Jansen's metaphyseal chondrodysplasia. Complete loss of the PTH receptor results in Blomstrand's lethal chondrodysplasia due to the generalized failure in the proper development of endochondral bones. Finally, partial loss of the function of the G-protein (G$_s$) that couples receptors to adenylyl cyclase results in a disorder known as pseudohypoparathyroidism type Ia. These individuals show partial resistance to a number of hormones that utilize the G$_s$/adenylyl cyclase signaling pathway. Resistance to PTH action is often particularly severe

due to genetic imprinting of the G$_{s\alpha}$ gene in PTH-responsive tissue. These individuals also have a developmental phenotype (Albright's hereditary osteodystrophy) as a consequence of a deficiency in G$_s$ signaling during embryogenesis and early development.

Glossary

adenylyl cyclase The enzyme responsible for converting ATP to the intracellular second messenger cyclic AMP.
bone mineralization The process by which calcium and phosphate are deposited onto the extracellular matrix of bone, resulting in the formation of hydroxyapatite.
G-proteins A family of peripheral membrane proteins that couple membrane receptors to specific effector molecules such as adenylyl cyclase.
hyperplasia Increase in the size of an organ due to excessive proliferation of the constituent cells.
osteoblasts Cells responsible for promoting bone formation by secreting bone matrix proteins and by facilitating bone mineralization.
osteoclasts Multinucleated cells that attach to the mineralized surface of bone and secrete acid and proteases, resulting in the breakdown of bone (bone resorption).
osteoporosis A disorder of bone characterized by decreased bone mass and decreased bone strength.

See Also the Following Articles

Calcium Signaling • GPCR (G-Protein-Coupled Receptor) Structure • Humoral Hypercalcemia of Malignancy • Osteoporosis: Hormonal Treatment • Osteoporosis: Pathophysiology • Parathyroid Hormone-Related Protein (PTHrP) • Vitamin D: Biological Effects of 1,25(OH)$_2$D$_3$ in Bone

Further Reading

Bastepe, M., and Juppner, H. (2000). Pseudohypoparathyroidism: New insights into an old disease. *Endocrinol. Metab. Clin. N. Am.* 29, 569–589.
Brown, E. M. (2000). Calcium receptor and regulation of parathyroid hormone secretion. *Rev. Endocr. Metab. Disord.* 1, 307–315.
Calvi, L. M., and Schipani, E. (2000). The PTH/PTHrP receptor in Jansen's metaphyseal chondrodysplasia. *J. Endocrinol. Invest.* 23, 545–554.
D'Amour, P. (2002). Effects of acute and chronic hypercalcemia on parathyroid function and circulating parathyroid hormone molecular forms. *Eur. J. Endocrinol.* 146, 407–410.
Friedman, P. A. (2000). Mechanisms of renal calcium transport. *Exp. Nephrol.* 8, 343–350.
Gardella, T. J., and Juppner, H. (2000). Interaction of PTH and PTHrP with their receptors. *Rev. Endocr. Metab. Disord.* 1, 317–329.
Goltzman, D., and White, J. H. (2000). Developmental and tissue-specific regulation of parathyroid hormone (PTH)/PTH-related

peptide receptor gene expression. *Crit. Rev. Eukaryot. Gene Expr.* **10**, 135–149.

Karaplis, A. C., and Goltzman, D. (2000). PTH and PTHrP effects on the skeleton. *Rev. Endocr. Metab. Disord.* **1**, 331–341.

Kronenberg, H. M., Lanske, B., Kovacs, C. S., Chung, U. I., Lee, K., Segre, G. V., Schipani, E., and Juppner, H. (1998). Functional analysis of the PTH/PTHrP network of ligands and receptors. *Rec. Prog. Horm. Res.* **53**, 283–301.

Nissenson, R. A. (2002). Target tissue actions, metabolism, and assay of parathyroid hormone. *In* "Disorders of Bone and Mineral Metabolism" (F. L. Coe and M. J. Favus, eds.), pp. 102–128. Lippincott Williams & Wilkins, Philadelphia.

Nissenson, R. A. (2001). Parathyroid hormone and parathyroid hormone-related protein. *In* "Osteoporosis" (R. Marcus, D. Feldman and J. Kelsey, eds.), pp. 221–246. Academic Press, San Diego.

Seeman, E., and Delmas, P. D. (2001). Reconstructing the skeleton with intermittent parathyroid hormone. *Trends Endocrinol Metab.* **12**, 281–283.

Silver, J., Kilav, R., and Naveh-Many, T. (2002). Mechanisms of secondary hyperparathyroidism. *Am. J. Physiol. Renal Physiol.* **283**, F367–F376.

Spiegel, A. M. (2000). G protein defects in signal transduction. *Horm. Res.* **53**(Suppl. 3), 17–22.

Swarthout, J. T., D'Alonzo, R. C., Selvamurugan, N., and Partridge, N. C. (2002). Parathyroid hormone-dependent signaling pathways regulating genes in bone cells. *Gene* **282**, 1–17.

Parathyroid Hormone-Related Protein (PTHrP)

JOSHUA N. VAN HOUTEN AND JOHN J. WYSOLMERSKI

Yale University School of Medicine

Parathyroid hormone-related protein (PTHrP) is a peptide with the ability to act as a systemic hormone or a local growth factor. It is involved in a wide variety of seemingly disparate functions in development and physiology and it is a key contributor to the pathophysiology of human cancer. In this article, the structures of PTHrP and its gene are characterized and the roles that PTHrP plays in cancer, embryonic development, and reproduction are examined.

I. INTRODUCTION

The isolation of parathyroid hormone-related protein (PTHrP) was the fruit of over 30 years of efforts aimed at understanding the mechanisms underlying the humoral form of hypercalcemia in patients with malignancy. In the 1940s, Fuller Albright predicted that the cause of hypercalcemia in these patients would be a tumor-derived factor related to the calciotropic peptide, parathyroid hormone (PTH). This prediction proved correct when, in the 1980s, PTHrP was isolated concurrently in three laboratories. By the 1990s, the human, mouse, rat, and chicken PTHrP genes had been cloned, and since then the PTHrP gene has also been isolated from a teleost (*Fugu rubripes*) and the sea bream, *Sparus aurata*. Over the past decade, our understanding of the biology of PTHrP has exploded through the study of a variety of transgenic and knockout mouse models. This article will first summarize key aspects of the structure of PTHrP and its gene. Then PTHrP's role in cancer will be discussed. Finally, our new understanding of the biology and comparative physiology of this remarkably versatile protein will be examined.

II. THE PTHrP GENE

As its name suggests, PTHrP is related to parathyroid hormone. The modern versions of these two genes arose from a common ancestor as the result of a tetraploidization event some 200 to 300 million years ago. Several lines of evidence now suggest that, in fact, the PTH gene was derived from an ancestral PTHrP gene, perhaps in response to the new demands of calcium metabolism related to the development of a bony skeleton in fish or to the adaptation of amphibians to a terrestrial environment. Although the two genes have diverged considerably, they share common locations on paired chromosomes, a common genomic organization, and amino-terminal sequence homology, all of which point to their common ancestry. For practical purposes, the last feature is the most important shared trait, for the similar amino-termini of both peptides allows them to bind to and signal through a shared PTH/PTHrP receptor. This unusual arrangement is responsible for the clinical syndrome that led to the discovery of PTHrP (see below).

The human PTHrP gene is located on the short arm of chromosome 12 and is flanked by the genes for lactate dehydrogenase B and the K-ras proto-oncogene. It spans more than 15 kilobases and contains eight exons. It has three different promoters, one that is GC-rich and two that contain typical TATA sequences. There are four noncoding exons at the 5′-end of the gene (Fig. 1) and there is considerable alternative splicing to generate a series of mRNAs with different 5′-ends. In addition, there is alternative splicing at the 3′-end of the gene that gives rise to three distinct classes of transcripts

encoding peptides of different lengths [139, 141, or 173 amino acids (aa)]. Thus, there are a variety of different mRNAs for PTHrP that differ in both their 5′- and 3′-ends. However, the physiological significance of these different mRNA species remains obscure. This complexity is a relatively recent event in the evolution of the gene, as the rodent genes are much simpler and contain only one promoter and use only one 3′-terminus. Transcriptional control of the PTHrP gene will not be discussed in this article. Interested readers are referred to recent comprehensive reviews.

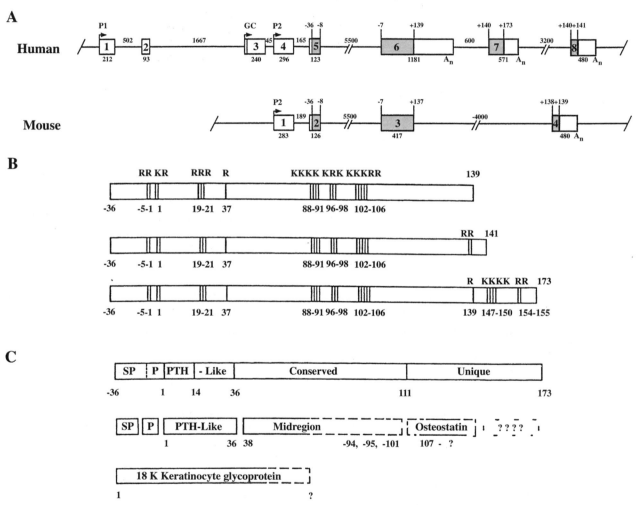

FIGURE 1 Schematic of the human and mouse PTHrP genes. (A) Numbered boxes represent exons, with distances indicated in base pairs. Arrows denote promoters, and amino acid residues are numbered relative to the start of the mature peptide. Polyadenylation sites are marked A_n. Potential multibasic cleavage sites in the three human PTHrP isoforms. (B) Arginine (R) and lysine (K) residues are marked. Functional domains and sequence homologies in PTHrP. (C) Intracellular posttranslational processing removes the signal peptide (SP) and the propeptide (P). The first 36 amino acids constitute the N-terminal PTH-like peptide, reflecting the strong sequence similarity in amino acids 1–13 between PTH and PTHrP. The region between residues 36 and 111 is evolutionarily conserved, whereas the least conserved region of the peptide is the C-terminus (amino acids 111 to 139 or 141). The extreme C-terminus, residues beyond 141, has been found only in humans. Secreted products of PTHrP include the amino-terminal PTH-like fragment (1–36), the glycosylated amino-terminal fragment found in keratinocytes, and midregion peptides. C-terminal species remain ill-defined.

III. PTHrP STRUCTURE AND POSTTRANSLATIONAL PROCESSING

The primary transcript of PTHrP represents a polyprotein analogous to the primary transcript of the proopiomelanocortin gene. Therefore, most cells expressing the PTHrP gene actually secrete several different PTHrP peptides. The primary transcript has a typical prepro sequence encompassing amino acid residues -36 to -1, which confers the ability for secretion from the cell. The mature peptide is very well conserved across species with residues 1–111 being 98% homologous in chickens compared with humans. This area has several stretches of basic amino acids that allow proteolyic cleavage of the primary transcript by prohormone convertases within the Golgi and secretory granules to generate a series of peptides encompassing the amino-terminus, the midregion, and the carboxy-terminus of PTHrP.

The amino-terminus of PTHrP is the portion that is homologous to PTH. Of the first 13 aa of the two proteins, 8 are identical and 3 represent conservative changes. Furthermore, there is considerable similarity in the predicted conformation of the two peptides through residue 34. There are several species containing this amino-terminal region that appear to be secreted by various cells. Most cells produce PTHrP 1–36, which is equipotent with PTH 1–34 at binding and activating the type I PTH/PTHrP receptor (PTH1R). In addition, an "intact" PTHrP molecule that includes at least the first 74 aa circulates in patients with HHM. Finally, keratinocytes have been reported to make a glyco sylated amino-terminal version of PTHrP with a molecular weight of 18 kDa.

Various cells have also been shown to produce midregion peptides that begin at Ala-38 and stretch to amino acids 94, 95, or 101. These peptides have been shown to circulate and their secretion appears to be regulated. This portion of PTHrP appears to function to facilitate placental calcium transport from mother to fetus. However, the receptor for this portion of PTHrP has not been identified. The midregion of the molecule also contains nuclear localization sequences (NLSs) and there is a growing body of literature that suggests that nuclear-targeted PTHrP may have effects on cellular proliferation, differentiation, and apoptosis. At this point, it is unclear whether the midregion portions that are secreted versus targeted to the nucleus are the same or represent distinct peptides, as there are potential processing sites between Ala-38 and the NLS between amino acids 87 and 106. Interestingly, in this regard, recent data have suggested that initiation of PTHrP translation may occur downstream of the signal peptide to generate a nonsecreted form of PTHrP. Other evidence suggests that longer peptides containing both the amino-terminal and the NLS sequences may be imported to the nucleus after binding to cell surface PTH1R. Obviously, there is much information concerning this portion of the molecule that remains to be elucidated.

Finally, carboxy-terminal portions of PTHrP also appear to circulate and have been detected in the urine of normal patients and in the serum of patients with renal failure. Peptides encompassing residues 107–111 and 107–139 have been shown to inhibit bone resorption *in vitro* and this portion of the molecule has been dubbed "osteostatin." However, not all groups have demonstrated this effect and the biological significance of carboxy-terminal PTHrP remains undefined.

IV. PTHrP RECEPTORS

As noted previously, the amino-terminal portion of PTHrP can use the type I PTH/PTHrP receptor (PTH1R) for signal transduction. This receptor does not discriminate between PTHrP and PTH, and both peptides are equipotent at binding and activating signaling. The PTH1R is a seven-transmembrane-spanning, G-protein-coupled receptor that signals via the cyclic AMP (cAMP)/protein kinase A and protein kinase C/calcium transient pathways. The ability of PTH and PTHrP to use the same receptor is the reason that patients with cancers that secrete PTHrP into the circulation develop hypercalcemia. Under physiologic conditions, PTHrP is excluded from the circulation and does not interact with PTH1Rs in bone and kidney meant for PTH. PTHrP target tissues appear to have a lower receptor density and rely on high local concentrations of PTHrP for activation of signaling. The exceptions to this rule may be in the setting of tooth eruption and during lactation. In these cases, PTHrP appears to be involved in the physiologic regulation of bone resorption and thus its action mimics that of PTH. These functions may represent the evolutionary pressure that has preserved the ability of both peptides to use the same receptor. With the exception of placental calcium transport, all the currently well-defined biological effects of PTHrP are mediated through the PTH1R. There are undoubtedly other receptors for the non-amino-terminal portions of PTHrP. However, they have not yet been characterized.

V. PTHrP IN CANCER

A. Humoral Hypercalcemia of Malignancy

Humoral hypercalcemia of malignancy (HHM) is a paraneoplastic syndrome defined by elevated calcium levels in patients with malignancy, but no bone metastases. It is the most common metabolic complication of cancer and results from increased bone resorption and decreased calcium excretion by the kidneys. As noted above, PTHrP was isolated from tumors causing this syndrome and several lines of evidence have established that tumor-derived PTHrP is the cause of the perturbations in calcium metabolism in this syndrome. For example, removal of the tumor or administration of neutralizing antibodies against PTHrP have been shown to reverse the syndrome, whereas infusion of PTHrP into rodents or humans reproduces the syndrome. Since PTH and PTHrP share a common receptor, this syndrome is the result of tumor-derived PTHrP acting on the population of PTH1R in bone and kidney normally reserved for the actions of PTH. Therefore, in HHM the physiological autocrine/paracrine signaling molecule, PTHrP, becomes an endocrine hormone and mimics the pathologic effects of PTH as seen in hyperparathyroidism. Although many types of solid tumors and hematologic malignancies are associated with HHM, squamous cell carcinomas and urothelial malignancies are the most frequent cause.

B. Bone Metastasis

In addition to its role in HHM, PTHrP appears to be important in the development of bone metastases in breast cancer. Several studies have found that, in breast cancer patients, PTHrP is expressed more frequently in bone metastases than in metastases to other sites. Initially, it was thought that PTHrP might be involved in targeting cancer cells to bone and, therefore, that PTHrP expression by a primary tumor might predict the occurrence of bone metastases. However, a recent study of transgenic overexpression of PTHrP in a rodent model of breast cancer did not support this idea. Furthermore, in the only large prospective study performed to date, PTHrP expression within the primary breast tumor did not correlate with the presence of bone metastases. However, there is ample experimental evidence demonstrating that manipulation of PTHrP expression within breast cancer cells can alter the development of osteolytic bone lesions. Currently, it is thought that although PTHrP production in the primary tumor may not predict bone metastases, the ability of breast cancer cells to up-regulate PTHrP production in the bone microenvironment is critical. Guise and colleagues have suggested that tumor-derived PTHrP production stimulates bone resorption, which liberates growth factors from the bone matrix that stimulate tumor cell proliferation, further PTHrP production, and increase bone resorption. It appears that bone matrix-derived transforming growth factor-β (TGF-β) is particularly important in up-regulating PTHrP production by breast cancer cells in bone. If this construct proves to be correct, the TGF-β/PTHrP/PTH1R loop may become an attractive therapeutic target for the treatment or prevention of bone metastases in breast cancer.

C. Proliferation

Another proposed role for PTHrP in tumorigenesis is the regulation of proliferation. PTHrP has been reported to have variable effects on the proliferation and/or differentiation of a variety of cultured cell lines. These effects have generally been modest and there is no existing evidence to suggest that PTHrP has a dominant role in regulating the proliferation of cancer cells. However, it was recently found that transgenic overexpression of PTHrP in the mammary gland resulted in a shorter latency to tumor development and a higher overall incidence of mammary tumor development in mice exposed to a chemical carcinogen. Interestingly, recent experiments have also suggested that the intracellular trafficking of PTHrP may determine whether it regulates the growth of breast cancer cells negatively or positively. For example, overexpression of PTHrP in the MCF-7 breast cancer cell line was reported to be mitogenic, whereas adding PTHrP to the extracellular medium inhibited growth. Another group of investigators has reported that neutralization of the endogenous PTHrP produced by MCF-7 cells led to an acceleration of their growth rate in culture. More data, especially from experiments *in vivo*, will be needed to determine whether PTHrP participates in the regulation of breast tumor growth in a meaningful manner.

VI. PTHrP IN EMBRYONIC DEVELOPMENT

PTHrP is expressed early in development in all three embryonic cell lineages as well as the amnion and the trophoblast. In fact, it has been reported that PTHrP and the PTH1R are the earliest hormone/receptor pair to appear, being first detectable at the morula stage. During the later stages of development, the distribution of PTHrP expression is even broader than in the adult, suggesting its importance as a developmental regulatory molecule. Functionally, in early development, PTHrP appears to participate in the regulation of the differentiation of parietal endoderm from primitive endoderm. During organogenesis, paracrine signaling between PTHrP and the PTH1R appears to be involved in inductive tissue interactions in several organs. The role that PTHrP plays in skeletal development and mammary gland development is discussed below because these systems have been well characterized. However, PTHrP is also necessary for tooth eruption and may be important in the development of the skin, the lung, the heart, and other organs.

A. Skeletal Development

Genetic ablation of PTHrP in mice causes perinatal lethality and short-limbed dwarfism. Upon histological examination, PTHrP null mice exhibit a form of chondrodysplasia in which chondrocytes within the growth plates of endochondral bones differentiate prematurely, leading to early mineralization of endochondral bones and premature loss of linear growth capacity. In contrast, PTHrP overexpression targeted to chondrocytes with a collagen II promoter slows chondrocyte differentiation and inhibits apoptosis of hypertrophic chondrocytes, leading to a delay in the formation of "mature" bone. Thus, the overall effect of PTHrP on endochondral bone formation is to inhibit the program of chondrocyte differentiation and to preserve the proliferative (growth) capacity of the growth plate. These effects are mediated through the PTH1R, since PPR1 null mice phenocopy PTHrP null mice. In humans, Blomstrand's chondrodysplasia, a short-limbed dwarfism similar to that seen in PTHrP and PTH1R null mice, is caused by loss-of-function mutations in the PTH1R gene. Another human disorder, Jansen's metaphyseal chondrodysplasia, results from activating mutations in the PTH1R gene and is similar to the phenotype observed in the collagen II–PTHrP transgenic mice.

The regulation of chondrocyte proliferation and differentiation within the growth plate is complicated and relies on the concerted actions of several families of growth factors and their receptors. It is now known that PTHrP acts together with at least one other of these growth factors, Indian hedgehog (IHH), in a feedback loop to regulate the differentiation of chondrocytes (Fig. 2). PTHrP is expressed in the periarticular region, and the PTH1R is expressed in prehypertrophic chondrocytes. IHH is expressed in the transition zone where proliferating chondrocytes

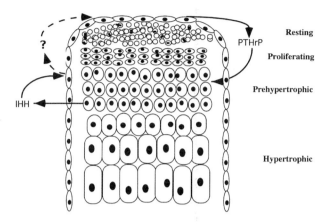

FIGURE 2 Schematic representation of the proposed interactions of PTHrP and Indian hedgehog (IHH) during chondrocyte differentiation in a growth plate. IHH produced by prehypertrophic chondrocytes in the lower zone acts on the adjacent perichondrium to communicate with the PTHrP-producing cells. PTHrP, in turn, acts on PTHR1-expressing prehypertrophic chondrocytes to impair their further differentiation by up-regulating Bcl-2 expression.

become prehypertrophic chondrocytes. Like PTHrP, IHH activity slows the differentiation of chondrocytes in bone explants from wild-type mice, but not in explants from PTH1R null mice. Therefore, IHH from prehypertrophic chondrocytes is thought to act on the perichondrium (possibly through smoothened, patched, and/or hedgehog-interacting protein), to stimulate PTHrP production in the periarticular region, which, in turn, inhibits further procession of the chondrocytes down the differentiation pathway toward hypertrophy and apoptosis.

B. Mammary Gland Development

PTHrP signaling is necessary for the formation of the mammary gland in mouse and human embryos. PTHrP and PTH1R knockout mice, as well as human fetuses with Blomstrand's chondrodysplasia, lack mammary glands and nipples. The first step in the formation of embryonic mammary glands is the formation of an epithelial bud, which is surrounded by a specialized stroma or mesenchyme. During the development of the mammary buds in mice and humans, PTHrP is produced by epithelial cells within the mammary bud, and the PTH1R is expressed by the surrounding mesenchymal cells. Like many developing organs, the mammary glands rely on a constant conversation between epithelial and mesenchymal cells to coordinate proper morphogenesis.

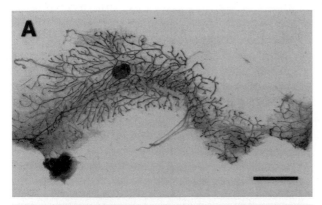

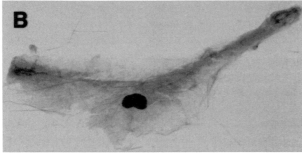

FIGURE 3 Whole-mount analysis of mammary glands from PTHrP null mice rescued from perinatal lethality by targeted expression of PTHrP in chondrocytes (col II-PTHrP/PTHrP null mice) and normal littermates. The normal gland (A) is characterized by a fully branched epithelial duct system surrounding the central lymph node. In contrast, the col II-PTHrP/PTHrP null gland (B) is devoid of epithelial structures; only the lymph node and vasculature are present within the fat pad. These results show that PTHrP is required for the development of mammary epithelium. Scale bar represents 5 mm.

PTHrP participates in this conversation by acting as a message from the mammary epithelial cells that triggers mammary-specific differentiation of the mesenchymal cells. If this message is not received, as in the PTHrP or PTH1R knockout mice, the mesenchyme becomes dermis instead of mammary stroma, the mammary epithelial cells regress, and no further breast development occurs (Fig. 3).

VII. PTHrP IN REPRODUCTION

A. Uterus

In the rat uterus, myometrial PTHrP mRNA levels rise during pregnancy from very low levels in virgin rats to a peak right around the time of birth. Levels then decrease significantly within 4 h after parturition, and by 4 days postpartum, PTHrP mRNA levels have returned to baseline virgin levels. It appears that this profile of expression is related to stretching of the myometrium and not to hormonal changes of pregnancy, as it can be reproduced in virgin rats using mechanical stimuli. However, it has also been reported that uterine PTHrP mRNA expression is also up-regulated by estrogen. Functionally, PTHrP and PTH have been shown to induce uterine smooth muscle relaxation, indicating that this effect is mediated by PPR1 signaling. Therefore, PTHrP expression induced and maintained by some combination of mechanical stretch and estrogen during gestation could serve to prevent premature parturition by inducing uterine relaxation or by antagonizing contractions, allowing the uterus to expand and accommodate the growing fetus. Similar observations in the bladder, stomach, and egg-laying gland of the chicken have suggested that PTHrP might play a more general role in regulating the expansion of hollow, muscular organs.

B. Placenta

There is an uphill gradient of calcium from mother (approximately 9.5 mg/dl) to fetus (approximately 13 mg/dl) that is maintained through the actions of a placental calcium ATPase. Recent data have demonstrated that PTHrP acts to facilitate the placental transport of calcium from mother to fetus. Interestingly, this function of PTHrP appears to be mediated by the midregion portion of the peptide and not by the N-terminal region. In a fetal parathyroidectomized lamb model, midregion PTHrP, but not amino-terminal PTHrP or PTH, was shown to facilitate placental calcium transport. In mice, the maternal–fetal calcium gradient depends upon an intact PTHrP gene, and midregion PTHrP stimulates placental calcium transfer. Thus, there is a considerable body of evidence that now supports a role for midregion PTHrP in regulating placental calcium transport from mother to fetus. However, the nature of the receptor for this portion of PTHrP and the mechanisms by which it stimulates calcium transport remain obscure.

C. Mammary Gland—Lactation

Not long after PTHrP was discovered, several laboratories found it to be expressed in lactating mammary tissue and secreted into milk in large quantities. In fact, milk is the most abundant source of PTHrP in nature. The expression of the PTHrP gene is up-regulated at the beginning of lactation, and PTHrP mRNA is localized to the epithelial cells of the lobuloalveolar units. Expression levels during lactation have been shown to be modulated by systemic prolactin and local signals initiated by suckling.

Great quantities of calcium are secreted in milk each day and large increases in bone resorption and decreases in bone mass occur during lactation, presumably to mobilize calcium from the maternal skeleton to meet the demands for milk production. Given PTHrP's ability to mimic the actions of PTH on calcium metabolism, it has been suggested that PTHrP might participate in this mobilization of skeletal calcium stores. In order for this to be the case, PTHrP from the breast would need to enter the systemic circulation and act on the maternal skeleton. Although not all studies have concurred, the weight of evidence suggests that circulating PTHrP levels are elevated during lactation. Furthermore, it has been reported that circulating PTHrP levels during lactation correlate with increases in rates of bone turnover and decreases in bone density. Case reports suggest that elevated PTHrP may compensate for the lack of PTH in lactating women with hypoparathyroidism. In addition, studies in rats and cows have correlated the suckling-induced increase in mammary PTHrP with a rise in cAMP and phosphate in urine, possibly indicating systemic effects of PTHrP produced in the mammary gland. However, in the only study that attempted to manipulate PTHrP levels during lactation, passive immunization with anti-PTHrP antibodies did not alter calcium metabolism in lactating mice. Thus, although there is considerable evidence to support an endocrine role for mammary gland-derived PTHrP in lactation, the data are not conclusive. Alternative roles for PTHrP produced by the lactating mammary gland include the regulation of blood flow to the mammary gland or the regulation of gut development or calcium homeostasis in neonates.

VIII. OTHER ACTIONS OF PTHrP

A. Pancreas

PTHrP is expressed in all pancreatic islet cell types and in pancreatic ductular epithelium, but not in adult exocrine cells. Although the PTH1R has not been demonstrated on beta cells, N-terminal PTHrP (or PTH) acts on cultured beta cells to increase intracellular free calcium. This might indicate an alternative PTH/PTHrP receptor. The precise role of PTHrP in the pancreas is not well understood; however, data from transgenic mice expressing PTHrP under control of the rat insulin II promoter (RIP–PTHrP mice) suggest that PTHrP might

regulate beta-cell mass. The RIP–PTHrP mice demonstrate islet hyperplasia, due to both an increase in the number of islets and their size. As a result, these mice are hyperinsulinemic and hypoglycemic, conditions that become acutely symptomatic upon fasting. Interestingly, RIP–PTHrP mice are also resistant to the beta-cell-toxic effect of streptozotocin. How these findings relate to the physiologic role of PTHrP in the pancreas is unknown.

B. Cardiovascular System

As mentioned previously, PTHrP may have a general function in the regulation of smooth muscle cell contractility. In tissues such as the uterus, the urinary bladder, and the hen oviduct, PTHrP expression in smooth muscle cells is induced by stretch, with the level of induction proportional to the degree of stretch (or filling). Furthermore, PTHrP acts on smooth muscle cells to cause relaxation. In addition to the organs mentioned above, PTHrP is expressed in the muscularis layer of most vascular beds. In vascular smooth muscle cells, vasoconstrictors, such as angiotensin II, serotonin, endothelin, norepinephrine, bradykinin, and thrombin, induce a potent, but transient, up-regulation of PTHrP expression. As before, mechanical stimulation (stretch) also induces PTHrP expression in vascular smooth muscle cells, but probably through a different pathway than vasoconstrictors. N-terminal PTHrP is a vasorelaxant in many vascular beds, including those of the mammary gland, the placenta, the aorta, the portal vein, the renal artery, and the coronary artery. The ability of PTHrP to relax smooth muscle cells appears to be mediated by a decrease in intracellular free calcium caused by the inhibition of the activity of L-type voltage-sensitive calcium channels (L-VSCC). In addition to its effects on contractility, PTHrP has been reported to modulate vascular smooth muscle cell proliferation. When added exogenously, PTHrP inhibits smooth muscle cell proliferation by inducing the cyclin-dependent kinase inhibitor p27^{kip1}. However, when PTHrP is overexpressed in the A10 smooth muscle cell line, proliferation was increased. This occurred only when the cells expressed PTHrP with an intact nuclear localization signal, suggesting that this was an intracrine effect of PTHrP. These effects are identical to the aforementioned studies with MCF-7 cells, again demonstrating that PTHrP can have opposing effects on the same cells, depending on the trafficking of the protein. Finally, exogenous PTHrP also inhibits migration of vascular smooth muscle cells in response to platelet-derived growth factor. The effects of PTHrP on vascular smooth muscle cell contractility, proliferation, and migration have all generated interest in the potential role of this peptide in atherosclerosis.

In addition to blood vessels, PTHrP has direct effects on the heart. N-terminal PTHrP has been shown to exert positive chronotropic and ionotropic effects in *ex vivo* perfused hearts. It also increases the rate of cardiac myocyte contraction *in vitro*. Although some of the tachycardia caused by systemic infusion of PTHrP is likely related to its ability to cause vasodilation and reduce blood pressure, these experiments also suggest that it may have direct effects on pacemaker function.

C. Skin

The first nonmalignant cell type that was shown to produce PTHrP was the keratinocyte. During development, PTHrP participates in the epithelial–mesenchymal interactions necessary for proper skin appendage formation. In addition, PTHrP may also play a role in the epithelial mesenchymal interactions in the skin of adult animals. Keratinocytes express PTHrP but not the PTH1R, and dermal fibroblasts express the PTH1R but not PTHrP. One likely function of PTHrP in the skin is to regulate the hair growth cycle. Systemic antagonists of the PTH1R have been shown to shorten telogen, lengthen anagen, and inhibit catagen. This suggests that PTHrP may promote the resting or catagen/telogen stage of the hair cycle, thereby causing reduced hair follicle growth. However, somewhat paradoxically, mice expressing no PTHrP in their skin undergo coat thinning over time, rather than the expected increase in hair growth. In addition to any effects on the hair cycle, evidence from mice expressing no PTHrP in their skin and mice overexpressing PTHrP in their skin suggests that PTHrP may also modulate keratinocyte differentiation. It remains unknown whether the effects of PTHrP on keratinocyte differentiation and hair follicle growth result from paracrine signaling to dermal fibroblasts or from autocrine or intracrine pathways. However, current data support the notion that PTHrP participates in the regulation of these processes.

D. Central Nervous System

Both PTHrP and the PTH1R are expressed within the brain. Interestingly, recent studies have demonstrated that other members of the PTH receptor family as well as other potential ligands for these receptors are expressed within the CNS. Therefore, PTH1R signaling is likely to have important yet complex functions in the nervous system. As with vascular smooth muscle cells, PTHrP, acting via this receptor, has been shown to affect the function of L-VSCC in neurons. In response to depolarization-induced L-VSCC calcium influx, PTHrP expression is up-regulated in cerebellar granule cells in culture. In turn, it appears that PTHrP can inhibit calcium entry through L-VSCC. Since calcium entry through these channels can be toxic to neurons (a phenomenon known as excitotoxicity), it has been suggested that PTHrP might participate in a putative neuroprotective short-feedback loop. However, in contrast to its effects on granule cells, PTHrP has been shown to increase L-VSCC activity in PC-12 cells, an effect that leads to an increase in dopamine secretion.

IX. COMPARATIVE BIOLOGY OF PTHrP

A. PTHrP, a Calciotropic Factor in Fish

Fish face a different set of problems than terrestrial mammals in achieving mineral homeostasis. The main challenges to marine fishes are to eliminate excess salts and prevent dehydration. The PTHrP sequence is most similar between fishes and tetrapods at the N-terminus, suggesting that regulation of calcium metabolism could be a conserved function. In support of this hypothesis, PTHrP expression co-localizes with the main sites of active calcium transport in fish (gills, skin, intestine, and opercular epithelium). Furthermore, in sea bream larvae, PTHrP increases the uptake of calcium and decreases total calcium efflux. PTHrP may be a classical endocrine hormone in fish, where it is secreted from the pituitary gland. In elasmobranchs, circulating PTHrP levels correlate positively with potassium and calcium and negatively with sodium, chloride, and urea, suggesting that PTHrP regulates ion transport and/or osmolality.

B. PTHrP in the Avian Oviduct

In the hen, PTHrP is expressed in the immature oviduct of growing animals, but is not highly expressed in the nulliparous adult oviduct. During the egg-laying cycle, expression of PTHrP is greatly up-regulated in the oviduct. The localization of PTHrP mRNA changes with the position of the egg as it descends. When the egg moves through the magnum, PTHrP is expressed most highly in the isthmus, and when the egg moves through the isthmus, PTHrP expression is up-regulated in the shell gland. Finally, when the egg passes out of the shell gland, PTHrP message is rapidly down-regulated. This sequence of events is strikingly similar to what happens in the mammalian uterus, where PTHrP expression is up-regulated until the time of birth and then declines. One possibility is that PTHrP regulates the passage of the egg through the oviduct by relaxing the smooth muscle "ahead" of the egg so that the contracted muscle "behind" the egg will push it forward. PTHrP can, in fact, relax strips of oviduct smooth muscle *in vitro*. Another possibility is that PTHrP regulates calcium transfer from the hen to the egg for shell formation. Interesting parallels can be raised between a function in egg shell formation and the putative roles of PTHrP in regulating placental calcium transfer and calcium transfer to the milk during lactation. Finally, PTHrP could regulate blood flow to the oviduct through its actions on vascular smooth muscle.

Acknowledgments

J. V. H. is supported by Grant 5 F32 DK59719-02 from the National Institutes of Health (NIH). J. W. is supported by NIH Grants CA 94175 and DK 55501 and by ACS Grant RP6-00-037-01-CNE.

Glossary

endochondral bone formation Bone development that occurs at growth plates by mineralization of a cartilaginous framework.

humoral hypercalcemia of malignancy A syndrome characterized by elevated calcium levels in cancer patients without metastases.

intracrine A mechanism of signaling in which a hormone produced by a cell is rapidly transported to the nucleus of that same cell where it exerts its effects.

parathyroid hormone/parathyroid hormone-related protein receptor type 1 A seven-membrane-spanning receptor that can be activated by parathyroid hormone or N-terminal parathyroid hormone-related protein peptides.

polyprotein prohormone A hormone precursor that is posttranslationally processed into multiple active peptide hormones.

See Also the Following Articles

Calcium Signaling • Humoral Hypercalcemia of Malignancy • Parathyroid Hormone

Further Reading

Bilezikian, J. P., Marcus, R., and Levine, M. A. (2001). "The Parathyroids: Basic and Clinical Concepts." Academic Press, New York.

Broadus, A. E., Mangin, M., Ikeda, K., Insogna, K. L., Weir, E. C., Burtis, W. J., and Stewart, A. F. (1988). Humoral hypercalce-

mia of cancer: Identification of a novel parathyroid hormone-like peptide. *N. Engl. J. Med.* **319**, 556–563.

Dunbar, M. E., and Wysolmerski, J. J. (1999). Parathyroid hormone-related protein: A developmental regulatory molecule necessary for mammary gland development. *J. Mamm. Gland Biol. Neoplasia* **4**, 21–34.

Juppner, H. (2000). Role of parathyroid hormone-related peptide and Indian hedgehog in skeletal development. *Pediatr. Nephrol.* **14**, 606–611.

Mannstadt, M., Juppner, H., and Gardella, T. J. (1999). Receptors for PTH and PTHrP: Their biological importance and functional properties. *Am. J. Physiol.* **277**, F665–F675.

Massfelder, T., Fiaschi-Taesch, N., Stewart, A. F., and Helwig, J. J. (1998). Parathyroid hormone-related peptide—A smooth muscle tone and proliferation regulatory protein. *Curr. Opin. Nephrol. Hypertens.* **7**, 27–32.

Philbrick, W. M., Wysolmerski, J. J., Galbraith, S., Holt, E., Orloff, J. J., Yang, K. H., Vasavada, R. C., Weir, E. C., Broadus, A. E., and Stewart, A. F. (1996). Defining the roles of parathyroid hormone-related protein in normal physiology. *Physiol. Rev.* **76**, 127–173.

Strewler, G. J. (2000). The physiology of parathyroid hormone-related protein. *N. Engl. J. Med.* **342**, 177–185.

Vasavada, R. C., Garcia-Ocana, A., Massfelder, T., Dann, P., and Stewart, A. F. (1998). Parathyroid hormone-related protein in the pancreatic islet and the cardiovascular system. *Rec. Prog. Horm. Res.* **53**, 305–338.

Wysolmerski, J. J., and Stewart, A. F. (1998). The physiology of parathyroid hormone-related protein: An emerging role as a developmental factor. *Annu. Rev. Physiol.* **60**, 431–460.

PCOS

See *Polycystic Ovary Syndrome*

PDGF

See *Platelet-Derived Growth Factor (PDGF)*

Peptide YY

Thomas E. Adrian
Northwestern University Medical School

I. CHEMISTRY AND MOLECULAR BIOLOGY OF PYY
II. TISSUE DISTRIBUTION AND ONTOGENY
III. PYY SECRETION AND RELEASE MECHANISM
IV. PYY RECEPTORS AND SECOND-MESSENGER SYSTEM
V. BIOLOGICAL EFFECTS OF PYY

Peptide YY, a hormonal peptide produced by endocrine cells in the intestinal mucosa, was first isolated from porcine small intestine using a novel chemical assay to detect peptides with a carboxy-terminal amide group, a structural feature shared by many regulatory peptides. PYY inhibits cholecystokinin- and secretin-stimulated pancreatic secretions, suggesting a hormonal role. In this article, the biological effects of PYY in the gastrointestinal tract are described and the clinical ramifications of these effects are explored.

I. CHEMISTRY AND MOLECULAR BIOLOGY OF PYY

Peptide YY is a straight-chained 36-amino-acid polypeptide that is structurally related to pancreatic polypeptide (PP) and neuropeptide Y (NPY). All three of these biologically active peptides have both C-terminal and N-amino-terminal tyrosine residues, which is the source of the name assigned to PYY (in the single-letter-code peptide nomenclature, Y represents tyrosine). Human PYY differs from porcine peptide at three residues, whereas the sequences of rat, dog, and pig PYY are identical. The amino acid sequences of the human peptide family are shown in Table 1. Truncated forms of human and canine PYY with 34 residues (PYY 3–36) have been isolated from colonic mucosa. The differences in the biological effects of the truncated and full-length forms of PYY relate to the PYY receptor subtypes (see later). Another posttranslational modification of PYY is phosphorylation of the serine residue in position 13 of the peptide. This phosphorylated form retains biological activity but is slightly less potent than the nonphosphorylated form.

The human and rat PYY genes have been cloned and sequenced. In both cases, the gene is composed of four exons and three introns spanning approximately 1.2 kbp. The human gene resides on chromosome 17q21.1 in a cluster with the PP gene. Two mRNA species are derived from the PYY gene by alternative splicing. The PYY precursor is a 98-amino-acid protein residue in which the PYY sequence is preceded by a signal peptide and followed by the cleavage and amidation sequence of Gly-Lys-Arg, which is followed by a cryptic peptide of another 31 amino acids. Thus, the precursor is similar in structure to that of pancreatic polypeptide and neuropeptide Y, and all are derived from a common ancestor by gene duplication. Indeed, the most recent gene duplication event has led to production on the 17q21 chromosome of a second cluster called the PYY2–PPY2 gene cluster, which has been detected in the cow, baboon, and human genomes. Despite the 92% sequence identity of the two gene clusters, a few specific mutations have resulted in significantly altered peptide sequences. These structural alterations have led to acquisition of new functions. The cow PYY2 gene codes for seminal plasmin, which is involved in reproductive function rather than gastrointestinal physiology.

A peptide with strong sequence identity with PYY has been isolated from the skin of the South American arboreal frog, *Phyllomedusa bicolor*. This peptide, called skin peptide tyrosine-tyrosine (SPYY), inhibits melanotropin release from frog neurointermediate lobes in a manner similar to that of NPY.

II. TISSUE DISTRIBUTION AND ONTOGENY

Cells containing PYY are found in the mucosa throughout the small and large bowel in humans. PYY concentrations increase distally through the gut, reaching peak concentration in the rectal mucosa. Similar gut distributions have been reported in the rat, mouse, dog, and monkey, with concentrations in the colon generally 100- to 200-fold higher than in the duodenum. PYY is colocalized with the glucagon gene products in the intestinal L cells. Interestingly, this

---

TABLE 1   Amino Acid Sequences of Mammalian PYY, NPY, and PP

Peptide[a]	Sequence
PYY (porcine[b])	YPAKPEAPGEDASPEELSRYYASLRHYLNLVTRQRY-NH$_2$
PYY (human)	YPIKPEAPGEDASPEELNRYYASLRHYLNLVTRQRY-NH$_2$
NPY (human)	YPSKPDNPGEDAPAEDMARYYSALRHYINLITRQRY-NH$_2$
PP (human)	APLEPVYPGDNATPEQMAQYAADLRRYINMLTRPRY-NH$_2$

[a]PYY, Peptide YY; NPY, neuropeptide Y; PP, pancreatic polypeptide.
[b]Rat and canine PYY sequences are identical to the porcine sequence.

colocalization is also seen in the glucagon-producing pancreatic islet alpha cells in mice, rats, guinea pigs, cats, dogs, pigs, and cows. These cells expressing glucagon and PYY are the earliest islet cells identified in the fetus and presumably represent the islet stem cells that have differentiated from the pancreatic endoderm. At this early stage, the products of the glucagon gene represent those expressed in the adult intestine (glicentin and the glucagon-related peptides, rather than glucagon), and because of this difference in posttranslational processing, the metabolic hormone glucagon is not made. In the developing mouse pancreas, PYY is transiently co-expressed with insulin, PP, and somatostatin, when the cell types expressing these peptides first appear. PYY expression may thus serve as a marker for islet differentiation. Production of PYY peaks just before term and ceases in the human pancreas shortly after parturition, although PYY continues to be co-expressed with glucagon in the rodent pancreas. In the mouse pancreas, the immunoreactive PYY is mostly confined to a major subpopulation of alpha cells in the splenic lobe. The PYY-expressing cells are also the earliest endocrine cells to appear in the fetal intestine. Once again, co-expression of PYY with other hormones such as secretin, cholecystokinin, neurotensin, gastrin, and somatostatin is seen when these hormones are first expressed. These findings suggest that PYY plays an important role in endocrine cell differentiation in the gut and the pancreas and support the existence of a common endocrine cell progenitor in these tissues.

Peptide YY is found not only in endocrine cells of the gut but also in nerve fibers in the myenteric plexus in several species, including rats, cats, ferrets, pigs, and dogs. In the rat, these are restricted to the stomach, but in cats, ferrets, and dogs, numerous fibers are also found in the upper small intestine. In the pig, only a few fibers are seen in these myenteric plexus locations and no fibers are seen in human gastrointestinal smooth muscle tissues.

III. PYY SECRETION AND RELEASE MECHANISM

As would be expected with a gastrointestinal hormone, circulating concentrations of PYY in humans change with food ingestion. Circulating concentrations rise in response to food intake and the magnitude of the increase reflects the total caloric load ingested. It should be emphasized that the increase in response to a small meal in healthy subjects is small. Ingested fat and protein, in particular, elicit a PYY response in humans. Similar increases in circulating PYY in response to feeding have been noted in a number of species, including rats, pigs, and dogs. In dogs, fat, rather than proteins and carbohydrates, appears to be responsible for PYY release.

The observed rapid PYY response to feeding led to early speculation that the foregut played a role in release of the peptide. It was seen that intraduodenal oleic acid releases PYY into the circulation even when the flow of chyme is prevented, whereas ileocolectomy abolishes PYY release in response to duodenal oleate. Infusion of the upper intestinal hormone, cholecystokinin (CCK), causes concentration-dependent release of PYY into the circulation. Other studies in the dog have shown that response to a fatty meal as well as to CCK infusion is abolished by a specific CCK-A-type receptor antagonist, underlining the importance of CCK-stimulated PYY release in this species. Concentrations of PYY in cord blood are substantially greater than those in normal fasting adults, and the response to feeding in neonates is massive, suggesting a role for the peptide in early adaptations to extrauterine life. Concentrations in neonatal animals, such as the pig, are also high.

Secretion has also been investigated in isolated intestinal endocrine cells cultured *in vitro*. Sodium oleate concentration dependently stimulates PYY release, as does bombesin, epinephrine, and forskolin, but not carbamyl choline. Studies in isolated perfused rabbit left colon have revealed that bile salts, rather than fatty acids per se, are responsible for release of the peptide following colonic stimulation. In contrast, high concentrations of amino acids are more effective at releasing PYY from the dog colon than is fat, glucose, or protein. Bile salts selectively and potently released PYY from the human colon. Although added oleic acid does not increase the PYY response to deoxycholate, this fatty acid causes a concentration-dependent increase in release of glucagon gene products. Because both peptides appear to be secreted from the same cell type, either there must be a difference in the hormone content of granules within the responding endocrine cells or a subpopulation of enteroglucagon secreting cells must be stimulated. Short-chain fatty acids also release PYY from the rabbit colon, a mechanism that could be highly significant in this species, which largely relies on short-chain fatty acids from colonic fermentation for its caloric intake.

Secretion studies in rats show a different spectrum of PYY release in response to nutrients, compared to the other mammalian species just mentioned.

Intraduodenal isocaloric amounts of glucose and amino acids release as much PYY as does a meal; oleic acid in place of a meal is less effective. This is likely to reflect the high tonicity of these solutions, because hyperosmolar saline also releases PYY but isotonic solutions have little effect. Studies in the vascularly perfused isolated rat colon show relatively weak stimulation of PYY by CCK and secretin, but a marked increase in PYY secretion in response to glucose-dependent insulinotropic peptide (GIP). Similarly, blockade of CCK and bombesin receptors is without effect on PYY release in anesthetized rats. With regard to intralumenal stimulation of PYY release in isolated perfused rat intestine, only supraphysiologic concentrations of glucose and amino acids are able to elicit a response. In contrast, some fibers, including pectin and gum arabic, but not cellulose, stimulate marked PYY secretion. The β-adrenergic agonist isoproteranol, the cholinergic agonist bethanechol, and calcitonin gene-related peptide all increase PYY secretion in this model. The effects of these agents are not affected by tetrodotoxin, suggesting direct effects on the PYY cells rather than mediation through the enteric nervous system.

There is some controversy regarding the extrinsic neural release of PYY. Several groups have shown a PYY response to two peptide transmitters, vasoactive intestinal polypeptide (VIP) and gastrin-releasing peptide (GRP), or to the amphibian analogue to GRP, bombesin. Studies in the pig reveal that electrical stimulation of the vagus supplying the pig distal intestine results in PYY release, whereas splanchnic stimulation has no effect. In keeping with this observation, atropine and hexamethonium significantly inhibit the PYY response to food. In contrast, total extrinsic jejunoileal denervation results in an increased PYY response to intralumenal fat stimulation in the dog. Interestingly, the CCK responses to fat are abolished in this denervation model, indicating that the increased PYY responses to fat are not mediated by CCK. Similarly, the PYY responses to food are enhanced by truncal vagotomy. Taken together, these findings suggest that food-induced PYY release is influenced by both an atropine-blockable postganglionic, parasympathetic pathway and a tonic inhibition, probably through a vagal cholinergic pathway.

A variety of other hormones and growth factors can influence the production and secretion of PYY. Pharmacologic inhibition of gastric acid secretion elevates circulating gastrin levels and concomitantly reduces both transcription and secretion of PYY. This inhibition is prevented by the gastrin receptor antagonist LY365,260. This control mechanism may relate to enterogastrone effects of PYY (see later). Insulin-like growth factor stimulates both expression of PYY mRNA and the peptide as well as its secretion into the circulation. A similar effect on tissue and plasma PYY levels, but not its mRNA content, is seen in transgenic mice overexpressing transforming growth factor-α. Somatostatin has been shown to inhibit PYY release in all species studied. This effect is mediated via type 5 somatostatin receptors in the rat and type 2 somatostatin receptors in humans.

IV. PYY RECEPTORS AND SECOND-MESSENGER SYSTEM

The PYY peptide family shares several different receptor (Y receptor) subtypes. There are currently six recognized members of this family, although only five of these (excluding Y3) have been cloned, i.e., Y1, Y2, Y4, Y5, and y6 (it should be noted that the y6 receptor is a pseudo-receptor in humans and pigs, hence the designation y6). The y6 receptor is absent in the rat but is apparently functional in the rabbit and mouse. All of the Y receptors are members of the G-protein-coupled seven-transmembrane-domain "serpentine" superfamily of receptors, which are coupled to inhibition of adenylate cyclase. The G-proteins involved are members of the G_o and G_i family and the effect of receptor activation is generally pertussis-toxin-sensitive, although exceptions in presynaptic receptors have been reported. This is, however, likely to arise from the inability of pertussis toxin to penetrate and activate the G-proteins rather than from a distinct signaling mechanism.

Structure–affinity and structure–activity studies with peptide analogues, together with studies based on site-directed mutagenesis and antireceptor antibodies, have given insight into the individual characterization of each receptor subtype relative to its interaction with ligand, as well as to its biological function. The characteristics of the different Y receptor subtypes, including binding characteristics and examples of locations, functions, and selective agonists and antagonists are summarized in Table 2. This summary is simplified because there are species differences as well as differences in reported activities from different laboratories. PYY binds to all the active subtypes, although it is less potent than NPY on Y1 receptors and much less potent than PP on Y4 receptors. Y2 receptors strongly bind PYY 3–36, a naturally occurring product of PYY produced in the small intestine.

TABLE 2 Subtypes of Receptors for PYY and Other Family Members

Subtype	Binding characteristics	Example locations	Example functions	Selective agonists	Selective antagonists
Y1	NPY > PYY ≫ PP	Gut, brain, heart, kidney	Vasoconstriction, anxiolysis; antisecretory in intestine	[Pro34]PYY, [Pro34]NYY	BIBP 3226, GR231118[a]
Y2	PYY = NPY ≫ PP strongly binds PYY 3-36-NH$_3$	Brain, low levels in peripheral tissues	Presynaptic inhibition of neurotransmitter release	PYY 3-36, PYY 13-36	BIIE0246
Y3[b]	NPY ≫ PYY	Nucleus tractus solitarius, colon, and adrenal	Regulation visceral afferents	None available	None available
Y4	PP > PYY = NPY[c]	Small intestine, colon, prostate, and CNS	Inhibition of pancreatic secretion	PP	GR231118
Y5	PYY = NPY = PP	Brain areas involved in food intake	Increased food intake	Ala-31-Aib$_{32}$ NPY and PP/NPY chimera, [Dtrp32]NPY	None available
Y6	Pseudogene in human and pig brain, absent in rat, functional in rabbit and mouse	Small intestine and adrenal (mouse)	Not known	None available	None available

[a]Putative receptor, not yet cloned.
[b]GR31118 has high affinity for Y1 and Y4 receptors; selectivity toward Y5 is not established.
[c]PYY activates the human but not the rat Y4 receptor.

V. BIOLOGICAL EFFECTS OF PYY

With the considerable overlap between the PP-fold peptides for the various receptor subtypes, it is not surprising that the biological effects of the PYY family overlap, particularly the effects of PYY and NPY. This does not mean that all of these biological effects are important physiological functions of the respective peptides. It is necessary to deliver the appropriate concentration of peptide to receptor, which, in the case of PYY, is via the circulation, with, perhaps, some local effects in the intestine. For NPY, the delivery is made to synaptic receptors in the peripheral and central nervous systems.

The broad range of biological effects of PYY includes gastrointestinal effects, such as slowing of gastric emptying and intestinal transit and inhibition of gastric pancreatic and small intestinal secretions. In peripheral tissues, PYY is also a vasoconstrictor and cardiac stimulant. PYY can reach some brain receptors via the circulation. The central effects of PYY include simulation of food intake as well as effects on circadian rhythm, anxiety, and memory.

Interestingly, PYY 3-36 has been shown to inhibit food intake and to reduce weight gain through the NPY Y2 receptor. PYY 3-36 is released from the intestine postprandially directly in proportion to the amount of calories consumed. The motor and secretory effects on the gastrointestinal tract are seen at circulating concentrations that are within the range seen after physiological stimuli, and are, therefore, undoubtedly physiologically relevant. The physiological importance of the other biological effects of PYY is uncertain.

VI. PHYSIOLOGICAL EFFECTS OF PYY

A. Motor Effects of PYY in the Gastrointestinal Tract

Early investigations of PYY showed inhibitory effects on jejunal and colonic motility together with intestinal vasoconstriction. Infusion studies in humans revealed marked inhibitory effects on gastric emptying and intestinal transit. It is now clear from the work of several groups that, in humans and experimental animals, PYY is responsible for the upper gut inhibitory motor effects that are seen in response to ileal infusion of lipids, known as the "ileal brake." Ileal or colonic infusion of lipid lengthens the interval between migrating complexes and also slows gastric emptying through the stimulation of PYY secretion. These motor effects of PYY appear to be mediated through vagovagal pathways.

There are apparently paradoxical effects of PYY in the stomach. Several studies show that PYY inhibits the ileal brake through the dorsal vagal center. However, under some circumstances, PYY can stimulate gastric motility. Y2 agonists inhibit thyrotropin-releasing hormone (TRH)-stimulated motility, mimicking the suppressive effect of PYY, but have no effect on basal acid secretion. In contrast, Y1 agonists stimulate motor function under basal conditions. This difference is probably due to the localization of Y1 and Y2 receptors in the dorsal vagal complex and the rapid conversion of PYY to a Y2 agonist by the ubiquitous dipeptidyl aminopeptidase.

The role of PYY in gallbladder function is controversial. One group has reported marked relaxation and increased filling of the prairie dog gallbladder in response to modest increases in PYY concentrations. In contrast, studies in the dog have revealed no effect of PYY on gallbladder function.

B. Role of PYY in Gastric Secretion

There is a consensus that PYY is a physiological enterogastrone in several species, including dogs and humans. PYY inhibits gastric acid and pepsin secretion stimulated by pentagastrin, cholinergic agonists, vagal activity, and histamine. The point that is somewhat controversial is the site of action. Most evidence points to inhibitory effects on vagal neurons. However, one group has provided evidence in support of a vagally independent mechanism. It is possible that, in view of the high concentrations of gastrin that are seen in newborns, the very high concentrations of PYY in neonates are important for inhibiting gastric acid secretion, i.e., allowing the tropic effects of gastrin to occur in the gastric mucosa without hyperstimulation of acid secretion.

C. Effects of PYY on Pancreatic Secretion

Multiple studies in dogs and rats have demonstrated that PYY inhibits pancreatic secretion stimulated by CCK, secretin, food, and intraduodenal amino acids, or vagal stimulation by infusion of 2-deoxyglucose. In contrast, a single study in humans showed no effect on CCK- and secretin-stimulated pancreatic secretion.

Although there is complete agreement with regard to the effect of PYY in dogs and rodents, the site of action appears to be different in these two species. In dogs, the inhibitory effect of PYY on pancreatic secretion is independent of the vagus, and PYY inhibits secretion from the denervated canine pancreas even in the presence of atropine. Results from another study on dogs suggest that PYY acts on the intrapancreatic cholinergic nerves rather than on extrinsic pathways. Other explanations from groups working with dogs are that PYY acts, at least partially, by blocking CCK release and reducing blood flow.

In one rat study, PYY predominantly inhibited neurally stimulated secretion and this inhibition was blocked by coinfusion of a cholinergic agonist. Results from a more recent study lead to the conclusion that the effect of PYY in the rat is predominantly mediated through the CCK pathway at a site proximal to convergence with the neural pathway. Immunoneutralization studies in the rat have confirmed that PYY is a physiologically important regulator of food-stimulated pancreatic secretion.

D. Effects of PYY on Small Intestinal and Colonic Secretion

Early studies using Ussing chambers demonstrated that PYY has antisecretory effects in the small intestine and colon. PYY reduces basal and VIP-stimulated increases in short-circuit current as well as VIP-stimulated increases in cAMP production and chloride secretion. PYY also abolished the secretory responses to cholera toxin and forskolin but not to 8-bromo-cAMP, indicating that the effect is mediated through inhibition of receptor-coupled adenylate cyclase.

In vivo, secretion and absorption occur simultaneously and all regions beyond the duodenum normally show net absorption. When infused at concentrations that mimic the postprandial response, PYY causes a substantial increase in net water and electrolyte absorption in Thiry–Vella fistula dogs. Other studies have revealed that infusion of PYY can augment the increase in net absorption that occurs postprandially, and that immunoneutralization with a monoclonal PYY antibody blocks the meal-induced increase in absorption. Whether the proabsorptive effect acts directly on the enterocyte or is mediated indirectly is not clear. One study has shown that the effects on short-circuit current and chloride secretion are blocked by hexamethonium, suggesting neural mediation, whereas another study has concluded that the effects are independent of neural blockade.

E. Growth and Differentiation-Inducing Effects of PYY in the Gut

Some studies in rats and mice have shown that administration of PYY can increase the weight and DNA content of the duodenum, ileum, and colon. However, other infusion studies in the rat have shown no effect on mucosal weight or crypt cell production rate, a very sensitive indicator of intestinal hyperplasia. In Caco-2 intestinal epithelial cells, PYY induces expression of the brush border enzyme alkaline phosphatase and decreases the specific activity of dipeptidyl dipeptidase. These findings suggest that PYY promotes differentiation of Caco-2 cells to a more colonocyte phenotype.

The effects of PYY on preventing the gut hypoplasia that accompanies total parenteral nutrition (TPN) have been assessed after 7 days of TPN in tumor-bearing rats. PYY was coinfused with clenbuterol, an anabolic β-adrenergic agonist. The combination resulted in significant savings in small intestinal weight and protein content, but had no effect in sparing the colon. Histologic analysis of the ileal tissues suggested that the effects of PYY were mostly mucosal, whereas clenbuterol mainly influenced the muscle. The combination treatment also resulted in a significant saving of protein content in the gastrocnemius muscle, suggesting a reduction in the cachectic response. Studies in breast (MCF7 and ZR-75) and pancreatic cancer (MIA PaCa-2) cells have shown significant growth-inhibitory effects of high concentrations of PYY.

F. Other Effects of PYY on the Gastrointestinal Tract and Metabolism

As already mentioned, PYY has vasoconstrictor effects on several vascular beds and, in particular, it reduces intestinal blood flow. Infusion of PYY in humans is accompanied by a small but significant increase in both systolic and diastolic blood pressure. Indeed, it is quite possible that inhibitory effects on secretion and motor activity may be mediated, at least in part, through effects on the splanchnic vasculature.

PYY increases expression of intestinal fatty acid-binding protein, suggesting that PYY plays a role in the trafficking of free fatty acids in the enterocyte. Similarly, physiologically relevant concentrations of PYY increase production of apolipoprotein AIV in the intestinal mucosa. PYY has also been shown to stimulate mucin secretion in the rat colon. PYY has been shown to inhibit the secretion of several gastrointestinal hormones, including motilin and pancreatic polypeptide in humans and cholecystokinin in rats and dogs. In contrast, PYY has no effect on circulating concentrations of glucagon, gastrin, glucose-dependent insulinotropic peptide, neurotensin, or enteroglucagon. A study in dogs has shown that PYY inhibits the insulinotropic effects of GIP, suggesting a role for the peptide in the negative feedback regulation of insulin secretion. Studies in humans show no effect on basal or glucose-stimulated insulin secretion or on the glucose elimination rate after intravenous glucose. Furthermore, PYY has no significant effect on circulating concentrations of glucose, lactate, glycerol, or free fatty acids. It remains to be seen whether PYY influences the enteroinsular axis in humans.

PYY infused at concentrations similar to those seen after a meal had significant effects on renal function in a group of male subjects. The effects included a decrease in glomerular filtration rate, plasma renin activity, and aldosterone levels. Infusion of PYY at a higher dose, which reproduced plasma levels seen in diarrheal illness, resulted in similar changes in function but also reduced renal plasma flow. These findings suggest that PYY may be an important mediator of the postprandial natriuretic response.

G. Orexigenic Effects of PYY

Lateral ventricular injections of PYY and NPY in hamsters induces a dose-dependent increase in food intake but causes a marked reduction in lordosis duration. In rats, injection of these peptides into the paraventricular nucleus causes a dramatic dose-dependent increase in food intake as well as a small increase in water intake. When the animals are able to select from different macronutrient diets, they overwhelmingly select carbohydrate over diets rich in either fat or protein. A recent study showed that infusion of PYY 3-36-NH$_2$ at physiological concentrations has marked inhibitory effects on food intake in humans.

VII. PATHOPHYSIOLOGY OF PYY

In endocrinology, a lot can be learned about the physiological role of a hormone by studying syndromes associated with excessive hormonal secretion and lack of hormonal production. This is the case with PYY, which appears to play an adaptive role in several intestinal disorders and after small bowel resection.

A. PYY in Gastrointestinal Diseases

Circulating basal and postprandial PYY concentrations are grossly elevated in patients with celiac sprue and in patients with postinfective tropical malabsorption (tropical sprue). Patients with these disorders have severe malabsorption resulting from small intestinal mucosal atrophy; in celiac patients this is due to sensitivity to the gliadin fraction of wheat flour and in tropical sprue it is caused by an unknown infective agent. In both conditions, PYY levels normalize with successful treatment with a gluten-free diet or antibiotics, respectively. The increased secretion of PYY is entirely appropriate in these conditions, given the inhibitory roles of PYY on gastrointestinal secretion and motility. PYY is presumably released in response to unabsorbed nutrients that reach the PYY-containing cells in the distal ileum and colon. This contrasts with the normal situation in which nutrients are almost totally absorbed in the proximal small bowel. High concentrations will reduce secretions and therefore the intralumenal volume in the gut and will also slow gastric emptying and intestinal transit. All of these physiological changes tend to enhance absorption by increasing the contact time with the small intestinal mucosa and by increasing local nutrient concentrations.

Smaller elevations of PYY are seen in patients with inflammatory bowel diseases (Crohn's disease and ulcerative colitis) and chronic pancreatitis and in patients recovering from a severe, acute, infective diarrhea. These conditions are associated with a degree of malabsorption, although direct effects of intestinal inflammation may also play a role in enhancing secretion of the hormone in inflammatory bowel disease and diarrhea. Once again, the elevation in diarrhea is appropriate, because PYY will slow nutrient transit and enhance intestinal absorption.

PYY concentrations are normal in meal studies performed in patients with other gastrointestinal disorders, including peptic ulcer, diverticular disease, and irritable bowel syndrome.

B. PYY Abnormalities Following Alimentary Surgery

Peptide YY secretion changes in response to a variety of surgical procedures, which, once again, could be considered to be appropriate adaptive changes. First, a proportion of patients who undergo gastric resection will suffer from "dumping" syndrome. In these patients, rapid emptying of hypertonic chyme into the upper small intestine causes water to pass from the vascular space into the intestinal lumen. This results in a shortness of breath, rapid heart rate, pain, bloating, nausea, vomiting, and even diarrhea. Furthermore, rapid absorption of glucose results in an exaggerated insulin response that can cause a reactive hypoglycemia, with symptoms including weakness, cold sweating, confusion, and headache. PYY levels are markedly increased following oral glucose ingestion in patients with dumping syndrome.

The pattern of secretion after massive small bowel resection is similar to that seen in sprue. This is not surprising, because unabsorbed nutrients rapidly reach the distal bowel, triggering release of the peptide YY. Generally, the more small intestine that is resected, the greater the elevation of PYY levels. Similar increases of PYY secretion are seen in dogs and rats after small bowel resection. In dogs and humans, infusion of PYY at concentrations that raise circulating levels to those seen after resection markedly slows intestinal nutrient transit, inhibits gastrointestinal secretions, and enhances net water and electrolyte absorption throughout the small intestine. As previously mentioned, PYY does not seem to be responsible for the ileal resection-induced adaptive mucosal hyperplasia and hypertrophy that are seen in the remaining bowel in continuity. Indeed, it is now clear that glucagon-like peptide-2 (GLP-2), a product of the same cell but not of the PYY gene, is responsible for the adaptive intestinotropic response to bowel resection. Studies on the expression of the GLP-2 and PYY genes have revealed that their respective mRNA contents are already markedly increased within 6 h after enterectomy, even before the animals are fed. Plasma PYY concentrations are also increased within 24 h. One can only speculate on this early endocrine response to small bowel resection. In the absence of food, it is possible that biliopancreatic secretions reaching the distal intestine are responsible. A modest increase in PYY response accompanies orthotopic jejunoileal autotransplantation in the dog. This is nothing like the magnitude of the increase seen after small bowel resection and is likely to be the result of motor changes in the denervated gut.

In contrast to the effect of massive small bowel resection, colonic resection is associated with low PYY levels. Here the postprandial response reflects the postsurgical anatomy. Levels are very low in patients with an ileostomy; this is not surprising because all of the PYY-containing colonic mucosa is out of the intestinal stream. Responses are a little greater in patients with an ileoanal anastomosis, but there is no difference between straight ileoanal anastomosis and patients who have a J-pouch fecal reservoir. Interestingly, in patients with ileoanal pouches, fecal retention time is related to the plasma PYY response as well as to mouth-to-pouch transit time. This finding suggests that it would be advantageous to maintain PYY responses in patients who have undergone colonic resection. A recent report of a new pouch procedure, the 9-pouch with a recycle segment, reveals that this more physiological approach, with attention to the effects of ileal peristalsis, results in PYY responses that are not different from those of healthy controls and offers a marked improvement in the functional outcome in these patients. The time-course of changes in PYY function has been carefully studied in the dog and rat after colonic resection and ileoanal anastomosis. Both the number of PYY positively stained cells and the PYY content of the ileal J-pouch mucosa are greater than is seen in control ileum and mucosa from straight ileoanal anastomoses. Furthermore, PYY responses increase with time after resection, suggesting that these changes represent an adaptive response that is improving the functional outcome.

PYY levels are modestly increased after total pancreatectomy. This pattern of response is very similar to that in chronic pancreatitis with exocrine deficiency, undoubtedly reflecting the malabsorption.

C. PYY and Tumors of the Intestine

Peptide YY, glucagon gene products, and PP are all common constituents of rectal carcinoid tumors, but PYY is not generally seen in endocrine tumors from other regions of the gut, such as the pancreas. An interesting report of a patient with an ovarian carcinoid revealed that excessive PYY production was associated with severe constipation that resolved after tumor resection. Low concentrations of PYY are seen in colonic cancer tissues and adenomatous polyps, compared with normal mucosa. Extremely low concentrations appear to reflect the malignant potential of these lesions, but this is probably related to the differentiation of the tumors, because concentrations are highest in tubular polyps, lower in villus polyps, and lowest in carcinomas. This is consistent with epithelial dysplasia and incomplete formation of mucosal endocrine cells.

D. PYY in Eating Disorders

A recent report on the measurement of PYY in the cerebrospinal fluid (CSF) in patients with eating disorders showed a dramatic increase in CSF PYY levels in bulimics who had abstained from bingeing for 30 days, compared with controls or their own levels when actively bingeing. No differences were seen in anorexia nervosa patients. It is possible that bulimic behavior corrects a central nervous system abnormality in PYY. Because PYY can profoundly increase food intake, these results are very interesting and worthy of further investigation.

VIII. THERAPEUTIC POTENTIAL

The spectrum of actions of PYY, including slowing of gastrointestinal nutrient transit and inhibition of secretions, make this peptide an ideal candidate for treating a number of different conditions, including acute or chronic diarrheal diseases and patients who have undergone colonic resection. In addition, PYY alleviates experimental pancreatitis, presumably because of its inhibitory effects on pancreatic secretion, so it also has potential for treating this condition.

Problems with the therapeutic use of PYY, however, are that the peptide has a short half-life (about 10 min) in the circulation and is large, making synthesis expensive. It is possible that there will be further development of long-acting analogues of PYY or some of the small-molecule agonists that target the PYY receptors that are responsible for PYY secretory and motor functions. Such compounds would have widespread clinical use. Because of the profound inhibitory effects of PYY on intestinal motor function, it is possible that a PYY antagonist could be useful in the treatment of postoperative ileus.

Glossary

enterogastrone Putative inhibitory hormone from the small intestinal mucosa; inhibits gastric acid secretion.

enteroinsular axis Stimulation of insulin secretion by hormonal signals from the gut; triggered by ingested sugars and amino acids.

ileal brake Inhibitory effects on upper gastrointestinal motor activity; triggered by a distal intestinal hormone that is released in response to intralumenal fat.

ileoanal anastomosis Surgical end-to-end connection between the terminal ileum and distal rectum after total colonic resection.

ileostomy Terminal ileum exteriorized through the abdominal wall; allows intestinal waste to be collected in a bag.

Thiry–Vella fistula Loop of intestine with ends exteriorized through the abdominal wall; allows easy access to intestinal contents. The loop retains its blood and neural supply through intact mesentery.

Ussing chamber Small glass chamber in two halves that sandwich a small piece of bowel or mucosa; used to study ion fluxes. A voltage clamp across the tissue allows measurement of short-circuit currents.

vagovagal reflex Signal transmitted through afferent vagal fibers to the dorsal vagal complex and then back to an abdominal target through efferent vagal fibers.

See Also the Following Articles

Bombesin-like Peptides ● Cholecystokinin (CCK) ● Gastrin ● Gastrointestinal Hormone-Releasing Peptides ● Neuropeptide Y (NPY) ● Secretin ● Somatostatin ● Vagal Regulation of Gastric Functions by Brain Neuropeptides ● Vasoactive Intestinal Peptide (VIP)

Further Reading

Adrian, T. E., Ferri, G. L., Bacarese-Hamilton, A. J., Fuessl, H. S., Polak, J. M., and Bloom, S. R. (1985). Human distribution and release of putative new gut hormone, peptide YY. *Gastroenterology* 5, 1070–1077.

Adrian, T. E., Savage, A. P., Bacarese-Hamilton, A. J., Wolfe, K., Besterman, H. S., and Bloom, S. R. (1986). Peptide YY abnormalities in gastrointestinal diseases. *Gastroenterology* 2, 379–384.

Adrian, T. E., Savage, A. P., Fuessl, H. S., Wolfe, K., Besterman, H. S., and Bloom, S. R. (1987). Release of peptide YY (PYY) after resection of small bowel, colon, or pancreas in man. *Surgery* 6, 715–719.

Batterham, R. L., Cowley, M. A., Small, C. J., Herzog, H., Cohen, M. A., Dakin, C. L., Wren, A. M., Brynes, A. E., Low, M. J., Ghatei, M. A., Cone, R. D., and Bloom, S. R. (2002). Gut hormone PYY_{3-36} physiologically inhibits food intake. *Nature* 418, 650–652.

Bilchik, A. J., Hines, O. J., Adrian, T. E., McFadden, D. W., Berger, J. J., Zinner, M., and Ashley, S. W. (1993). Peptide YY is a physiological regulator of water and electrolyte absorption in the canine small bowel *in vivo*. *Gastroenterology* 3, 1441–1448.

Gomez, G., Zhang, T., Rajaraman, S., Thakore, K. N., Yanaihara, N., Townsen, C. M., Jr., Thompson, J. C., and Greeley, G. H. (1995). Intestinal peptide YY: Ontogeny of gene expression in rat bowel and trophic actions on rat and mouse bowel. *Am. J. Physiol.* 268, G71–G81.

Greeley, G. H., Jr., Jeng, Y. J., Gomez, G., Hashimoto, T., Hill, F. L., Kern, K., Kurosky, T., Chuo, H. F., and Thompson, J. C. (1989). Evidence for regulation of peptide-YY release by the proximal gut. *Endocrinology* 3, 1438–1443.

Guo, Y. S., Fujimura, M., Lluis, F., Tsong, Y., Greeley, G. H., Jr., and Thompson, J. C. (1987). Inhibitory action of peptide YY on gastric acid secretion. *Am. J. Physiol.* 253, G298–G302.

Kohri, K., Nata, K., Yonekura, H., Nagai, A., Konno, K., and Okamoto, H. (1993). Cloning and structural determination of human peptide YY cDNA and gene. *Biochim. Biophys. Acta* 3, 345–349.

Lluis, F., Gomez, G., Fujimura, M., Greeley, G. H., Jr., and Thompson, J. C. (1988). Peptide YY inhibits pancreatic secretion by inhibiting cholecystokinin release in the dog. *Gastroenterology* 1, 137–144.

Michel, M. C., Beck-Sickinger, A., Cox, H., Doods, H. N., Herzog, H., Larhammar, D., Quirion, R., Schwartz, T., and Westfall, T. (1998). XVI International Union of Pharmacology recommendations for the nomenclature of neuropeptide Y, peptide YY, and pancreatic polypeptide receptors. *Pharmacol. Rev.* 1, 143–150.

Savage, A. P., Adrian, T. E., Carolan, G., Chatterjee, V. K., and Bloom, S. R. (1987). Effects of peptide YY (PYY) on mouth to caecum intestinal transit time and on the rate of gastric emptying in healthy volunteers. *Gut* 2, 166–170.

Tatemoto, K. (1982). Isolation and characterization of peptide YY (PYY), a candidate gut hormone that inhibits pancreatic exocrine secretion. *Proc. Natl. Acad. Sci. U.S.A.* 8, 2514–2518.

Upchurch, B. H., Fung, B. P., Rindi, G., Ronco, A., and Leiter, A. B. (1996). Peptide YY expression is an early event in colonic endocrine cell differentiation: Evidence from normal and transgenic mice. *Development* 4, 1157–1163.

Wen, J., Phillips, S. F., Sarr, M. G., Kost, L. J., and Holst, J. J. (1995). PYY and GLP-1 contribute to feedback inhibition from the canine ileum and colon. *Am. J. Physiol.* 269, G945–G952.

Peptidomimetics

MARK T. GOULET AND RALPH T. MOSLEY

Merck & Company, Inc., New Jersey

I. INTRODUCTION
II. "NATURAL" PEPTIDOMIMETICS
III. STRATEGIES FOR PEPTIDOMIMETIC DISCOVERY AND DESIGN
IV. SUMMARY

Many G-protein-coupled receptors can utilize peptides or proteins as their natural ligands for effecting signal transduction. Nonpeptide ligands, or peptidomimetics, that can either reproduce the activity of a peptide agonist or act as an antagonist of that system have been discovered for many of these receptors. Rational peptidomimetic designs rely on structural information derived from the ligand in either the receptor-bound or the solution state. Peptidomimetic ligands can serve as useful tools for the study of receptor signaling pathways and as important pharmacological agents for the treatment of disease.

I. INTRODUCTION

Approximately 60% of known G-protein-coupled receptors (GPCRs) utilize peptides or proteins as their natural ligand for effecting signal transduction. For many of these receptors, non-peptide ligands, or peptidomimetics, have been discovered that can either reproduce the activity of a peptide agonist or act as an antagonist of that system. Natural products derived from the secondary metabolism of lower organism occasionally function as peptidomimetic ligands for GPCRs, but a majority of peptidomimetic ligands are the outcome of a premeditated design as a means of obtaining biologically active receptor modulators with properties distinct from those of peptides. This effort is driven primarily by research in the pharmaceutical industry, because nonpeptides have demonstrated improvements over peptides with respect to oral bioavailability, metabolic stability, and tissue distribution. Many modern drugs are peptidomimetic ligands for receptors that either cause or ameliorate disease. Along with the discovery of peptidomimetics has come an increased understanding of the principles for their design and the nature of the nonpeptide–protein interaction.

For the purposes of classification, three types of peptidomimetics have been described, based primarily on the nature of their interaction with macromolecules. A type I mimetic incorporates an amide bond surrogate, or "isostere," that is intended to mimic the local topography about an amide bond. Often type I mimetics are designed as atom-for-atom replacements of the amide bond and are utilized predominantly in the construction of enzyme (e.g., protease) inhibitors. Type II mimetics are functionally analogous to a given peptide agonist or antagonist, but their mode of binding to the receptor is distinct from that of the original ligand. Thus, type II mimetics do not necessarily mimic the structure of the parent hormone. The type III mimetics possess the necessary groups, arrayed about a nonpeptide core, to mimic the parent ligand topographically. Often these structures bear no obvious resemblance to the original hormone, but because their mode of binding is predicted to be the same as the parent they have been termed "ideal" peptidomimetics. Representatives of the three types of peptidomimetics are shown in Table 1.

II. "NATURAL" PEPTIDOMIMETICS

Evaluation of the biological activity of natural products, isolated primarily from plants and

TABLE 1   Classification of Peptidomimetics

Type	Structure	Peptide	Receptor
Type I	Saquinavir	{-L NF· PI-} (gag-pol)	HIV protease (enzyme)
Type II	CP-96345	R P K P Q Q F F G L M-NH₂ (Substance P)	Neurokinin-1 receptor
Type III		A G C K N F W K T F T S C-OH (Somatostatin)	Somatostatin receptors 1–5

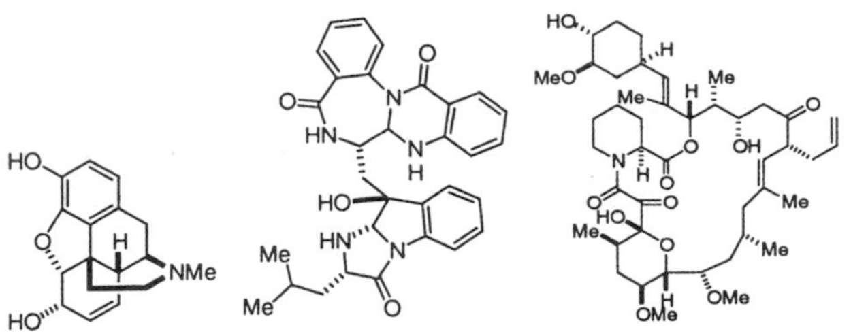

FIGURE 1   Natural product peptidomimetics.

microorganisms, has revealed a number of compounds fitting the description of peptidomimetics. Some representative "natural" peptidomimetics are shown in Fig. 1. Perhaps the most well-known example is the plant-derived alkaloid morphine. Morphine and related structures are agonists of the opioid receptor family and act by mimicking the N-terminal Tyr-Gly-Gly-Phe of the endorphin neuropeptides. Morphine, as well as its synthetic and semisynthetic analogues, has been used extensively for the study of receptor–ligand interactions and subsequent GPCR signaling. Asperlicin is a natural product that acts as an antagonist of the neurotransmitter peptide cholecystokinin (CCK). Although only weakly active as a CCK antagonist ($IC_{50} = 1 \ \mu M$), asperlicin has served as the structural basis for the design of potent and subtype-selective CCKA and CCKB receptor antagonists. The macrocyclic bacterial metabolite FK-506 (Tacrolimus) is an interesting peptidomimetic of clinical relevance to the field of immunosuppression. Through studies relating to the pharmacological mechanism of action, it was discovered that the amidopyranose portion of FK-506 functions as a peptidomimetic ligand for the peptidyl-prolyl isomerase FKBP-12. This complex, in turn, binds and inhibits the serine/threonine phosphatase PP2B (calcineurin) to block signal transduction in activated T cells. It is thought that portions of the polyketide-derived backbone act as a peptidomimetic ligand for PP2B during this second binding event.

III. STRATEGIES FOR PEPTIDOMIMETIC DISCOVERY AND DESIGN

A. Privileged Structures

Certain nonpeptide units that exhibit a propensity for binding to GPCRs and other macromolecules have been termed "privileged structures." In general, these

are hydrophobic assemblages that often contain aromatic rings and are constructed in a manner so as to maintain a defined shape even in an aqueous environment, thereby avoiding what is known as hydrophobic collapse. Several common privileged structures are depicted in Fig. 2. A successful strategy for discovering peptidomimetics is to identify a privileged structure or derivative thereof that exhibits affinity for the desired receptor, then modify this structure by addition of appropriate groups to optimize potency and selectivity for that receptor. At times, the same privileged structure can be used to produce potent peptidomimetics for a variety of receptor types. For example, the biphenyltetrazole privileged structure is found in the angiotensin II antagonist prodrug losartan and in the Merck growth hormone secretagogue (Fig. 3). Preparation of chemical libraries based on a privileged structure has proved to be a successful method for both generation and optimization of pharmacologically active peptidomimetics.

B. Benign Scaffolds

Privileged structures within a peptidomimetic both bind to the macromolecule and provide a site(s) for additional chemical modification. Another strategy for peptidomimetic design is the use of a rigid template, onto which groups that can interact with a receptor are appended. These "benign scaffolds" are not intended to participate directly in the binding event but rather to connect and display the pharmacophore elements in a manner appropriate for binding. One example of a benign scaffold is the sugar core of the type III peptidomimetic shown in Fig. 1. Another is the thyrotropin-releasing hormone (TRH) agonist RO 24-9975, wherein elements of the three amino acid side chains present in TRH are displayed about a 1,3,5-trisubstituted cyclohexane ring (Fig. 4). Computer algorithms that utilize

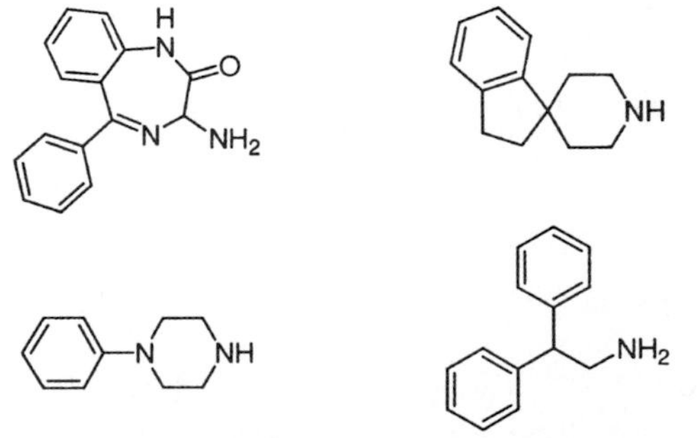

FIGURE 2   Some common privileged structures.

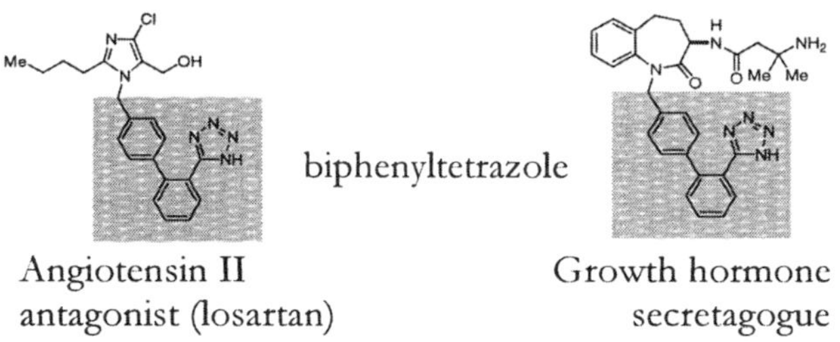

FIGURE 3 An angiotensin II antagonist and growth hormone secretagogue that share a common privileged structure (shaded area).

knowledge of the bound conformation to predict useful benign scaffolds have enhanced the success of this approach to peptidomimetic design.

C. Using Structural Information

The regular nature of α-amino acid amide linkages has facilitated study through biophysical and theoretical methods such that it is possible to predict secondary structure from primary sequence and, in limited cases, to propose reasonable tertiary structures. This amount and type of information also permits the discovery of materials that can mimic large structural motifs, such as entire β-strands and α-helices (which are beyond the scope of further discussion here), as well as smaller structural features, particularly β and γ turns. And, although it can be shown that widely dispersed residues of a peptide hormone make contributive interactions with a receptor for binding and function, it is often the case that small regions of the hormone, comprising three to four amino acids, critical to receptor activation can be identified. This is typically accomplished through amino acid scans (sequential replacement of each residue in the polypeptide strand by an unobtrusive amino acid, typically alanine) and

peptide truncation. Oftentimes, these critical residues are found within a turn region of the peptide. Analysis in this manner results in the development of a conceptual pharmacophore and begins the peptidomimetic design process. Having identified the requisite residues for activity, additional analytical and computational tools, such as X-ray crystallography, nuclear magnetic resonance (NMR), and molecular modeling, are often applied to further refine the structural requirements for peptidomimetic design and optimization.

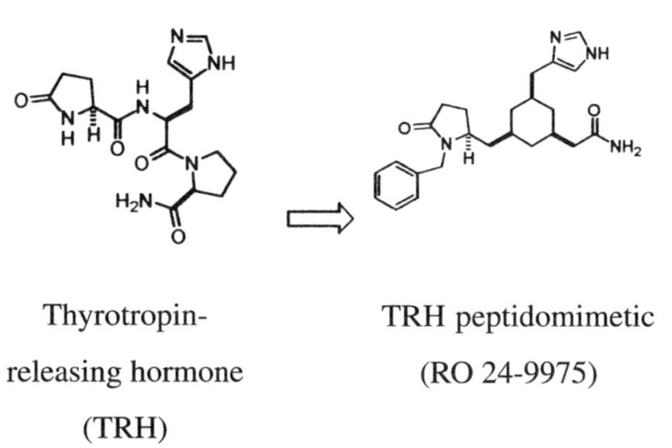

The conformation of the receptor-bound peptide hormone and, by extension, the placement of the peptide side chain moieties would be the most useful information for peptidomimetic design. At present, this information is largely gathered by inference from peptide structure–activity relationships (SARs), receptor mutagenesis, and studies with related peptidomimetics. Alternatively, it might be assumed that the conformation that can be confirmed in the solution phase is relevant, because it is that conformation that is initially "sensed" by the receptor and from which the bound conformation is derived.

The clearest pieces of structural data from solution-state NMR studies include strong nuclear Overhauser effects (NOEs), which typically indicate stable and close proximity (2–2.5 Å) between two protons, small temperature coefficients for amide protons (indicating lack of solvent accessibility and, by extension, involvement in an internal hydrogen bond), up-field chemical shifts of proton resonances (indicating a deshielding environment typically that is found near an aromatic ring system), and coupling constants between vicinal protons (indicating torsion angles between them). These types of information can be used in conjunction with molecular modeling techniques to generate energy-minimized conformations that meet the conditions stipulated by the NMR experiments. The two most prevalent ways to generate conformations are via distance geometry followed by energy minimization or by molecular dynamics (MD) simulations. The NMR-generated data can be used to restrain the calculation, usually the case during MD, or as a postprocessing filter. The resultant peptide conformations can be clustered on the basis of the backbone conformation and energetics to propose the prevalent bioactive conformation.

If NMR information is unavailable, small peptides can be modeled as just described and the resultant low-energy conformers can be examined for any proclivity toward a particular turn type as determined by the Φ–Ψ angles of the main-chain

FIGURE 4 Thyrotropin-releasing hormone mimetic derived from a benign, cyclohexane scaffold.

TABLE 2   Commonly Mimicked Reverse Turns

Turn structure	Turn type	Φ_{i+1}	Ψ_{i+1}	Φ_{i+2}	Ψ_{i+2}	Amino acid turn inducers
	γ classical	70 to 85	−60 to −70	—		—
	γ inverse	−70 to −85	60 to 70	—		—
	βI	−60	−30	−90	0	*i*: D, N, S, C *i* + 1: P *i* + 2: no P *i* + 3: G
	βI'	60	30	90	0	*i* + 1: G *i* + 2: G
	βII	−60	120	80	0	*i* + 1: P *i* + 2: G, N
	βII'	60	−120	−80	0	*i* + 1: G

atoms. Identification of a turn type can be further advanced by examination of the peptide SAR (e.g., increases in potency by use of amino acids known to induce reverse turns in the suspected loop region). Table 2 contains the typical Φ–Ψ angles for the most common reverse turns, as well as some of the amino acids known to contribute to their stabilization.

D. Design Strategies

With this data, there are now several approaches that can be followed to maintain the shape of the peptide while removing much of the peptide character. Which approach is taken depends on the derived SAR. A constrained amino acid via Cα–Cβ cyclization, Cα or Cβ substitution, or N-side chain cyclization can fix the conformation of the side chain (usually measured as the χ angle: N-Cα–Cβ–Cγ) and sometimes the entire turn region. If maintaining the β-strand motif and main-chain atoms is important, the side chains of

residues at the $i + 1$ and $i + 2$ positions in a β-turn can be replaced with a cyclic structure to maintain the β-strand structural motif, a so-called "external scaffold." Finally, if the side chains provide the important contacts, the main chain of these residues can be replaced with some cyclic system, or an "internal scaffold." These different routes of structure stabilization are schematically depicted in Fig. 5.

Choosing to internally cyclize the γ or β reverse turn is equivalent to replacing the hydrogen bond to create a 7-membered or 10-membered ring, respectively. In the latter case, this typically takes the form of a fused bicyclic system. At this point, modeling of the proposed peptidomimetic is typically conducted to ensure that the three-dimensional realization of the design is in agreement with the target. Modeling studies of some turn mimetics have indicated that there can be several conformational families present or that the turn mimetic even fails to meet the desired conformation.

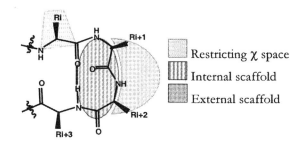

FIGURE 5   Schematic of a β-turn depicting various peptido-mimetic approaches.

Several conclusions from work in the peptidomi-metic field can be proposed:

1. The more sequentially posited the amino acids to be mimicked, the greater the probability for success.
2. Determining the conformation of both the peptide backbone and side chain, particularly for the critical residues, is important and becomes more so as the critical amino acids become less contiguous in the sequence.
3. Identification of a nonpeptide lead through screen-ing approaches (e.g., binding assays), which can then be further developed as a peptidomimetic, rather than *de novo* design based on peptide sequence, is another frequently used method of discovery.

Ultimately, the goal is to imitate or antagonize the function of the peptide ligand, and mimicking the conformation of the peptide is merely one potential means to that end.

E. Database Search Approaches

Rather than design the scaffold, various searching methods can be used to identify scaffolds to replace the main-chain atoms. One approach is to use three-dimensional substructure searches in which the Cα–Cβ bond vectors of the modeled peptide hormone are used as the probe to identify scaffolds that contain similar bond vectors, such as is done in the program

CAVEAT. Or, one might use three-dimensional similarity searches to identify replacements for the main chain directly.

Designing and synthesizing a scaffold or identify-ing one through a database search still requires that care then be taken to incorporate the relevant side chains into the design process. Rather than take this intermediary step, a number of tools exist that can be used to search for replacements of the requisite amino acid side chains directly, either in the form of three-dimensional substructure or three-dimensional simi-larity searches. An example of this is discussed in the following case study for the somatostatin peptidomi-metics. Finally, database searching technologies exist that allow one to forgo the use of three-dimensional information entirely. Markush queries can be readily constructed for two-dimensional substructure searches to identify molecules that contain the side chain moieties of interest. Topological similarity searches are more problematic in that a peptide probe tends to identify other peptides; the recurrence of the peptide bond creates a "signal" that overwhelms that of the side chains. Even here, methods have been developed that circumvent this to identify peptidomi-metics successfully.

F. Case Study: Somatostatin Peptidomimetics

Somatostatin is a neuropeptide known to modulate the secretion of growth hormone, insulin, and glucagon, among others; somatostatin agonist drugs could lead to treatments for diabetes, cancer, and acromegaly. Somatostatin occurs in both a 28- and 14-residue peptide form and binds to five distinct somatostatin receptor (SSTR) subtypes (1-5), which are members of the G-protein-coupled receptor family A (rhodopsin-like). Early SARs showed the importance of Trp-8 and Lys-9 to activity; peptides cyclized via a Cys–Cys disulfide linkage, e.g., the octapeptide Sandostatin, or via regular peptide bonds, e.g., the hexapeptide seglitide (MK-678), are highly potent compounds (Fig. 6). NMR-derived data such as NOEs, vicinal proton coupling constants,

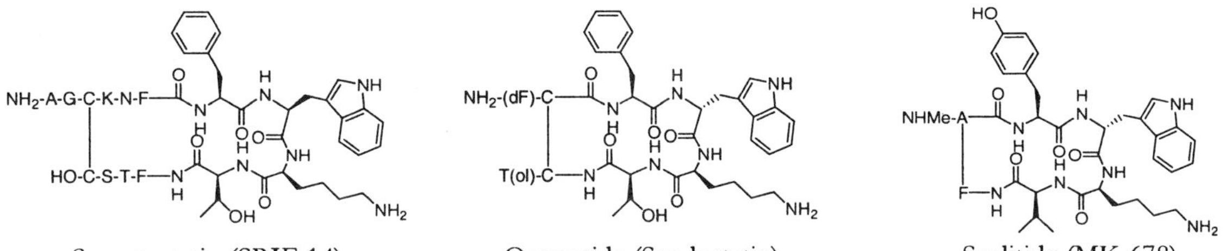

Somatostatin (SRIF-14)   Octreotide (Sandostatin)   Seglitide (MK-678)

FIGURE 6   Somatostatin and related constrained peptide analogues.

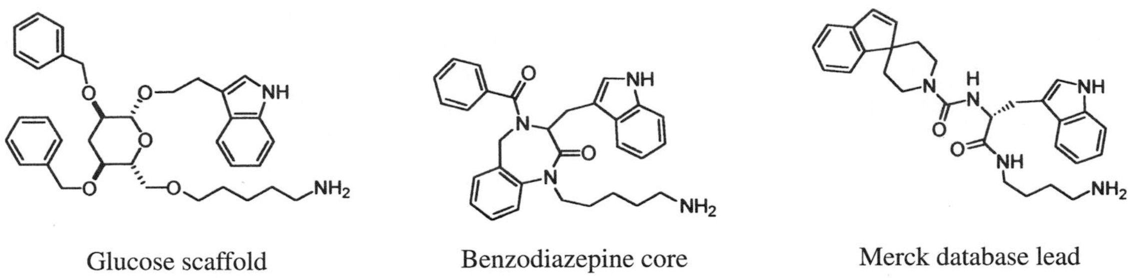

Glucose scaffold   Benzodiazepine core   Merck database lead

FIGURE 7   Somatostatin peptidomimetics.

and small-temperature coefficients indicate the occurrence of a βII′-turn at the DTrp-8–Lys9 of these peptides. Upfield chemical shifts in the NMR spectrum of methylene protons in the Lys side chain indicate proximity to an aromatic system, presumably the indole of DTrp8. Additionally, it is known that the backbone atoms of the peptide are unnecessary for SSTR activation.

As an alternative to the backbone cyclization strategy just described, several attempts have been made to mimic the side chain positions by supporting their equivalents from a central scaffold, such as a sugar or benzodiazepine core (Fig. 7). Typically, this has resulted in compounds with modest agonist activity. A different approach is to use the three-dimensional structure derived from NMR and SAR results to query a database containing three-dimensional models of molecules and thereby identify new leads without predilection for a particular scaffold or other structural constraint to be used as a synthetic starting point. Using a three-dimensional model of one of the cyclic peptides, the probe can be constructed to replicate the SAR using only side chain atoms for

Phe-7–DTrp-8–Lys 9 in which the side chains of DTrp-8 and Lys-9 are near each other. Interestingly, the most potent compounds identified using this search method at Merck Research Laboratories do not contain a central scaffold, but rather mimic the basic amine of the Lys and the aromatics of the Trp and Phe in a linear manner, presumably while maintaining the three-dimensional relationship of the pharmacophoric elements. This is accomplished, in part, by the incorporation of a "privileged structure" unit (Fig. 7).

The Merck database lead was amenable to optimization by both traditional medicinal chemistry and combinatorial chemistry and became the basis for the design and synthesis of analogues with a 10,000-fold increase in binding potency and 1000-fold increase in selectivity for the various receptor subtypes compared to the original lead. The Merck database lead is composed of three units, a diamine to mimic Lys, an amino acid to mimic Trp, and a "privileged structure" amine to mimic Phe. These units are combined in sequence by forming amide and urea bonds between the fragments. In order to facilitate biological screening of what could potentially be a

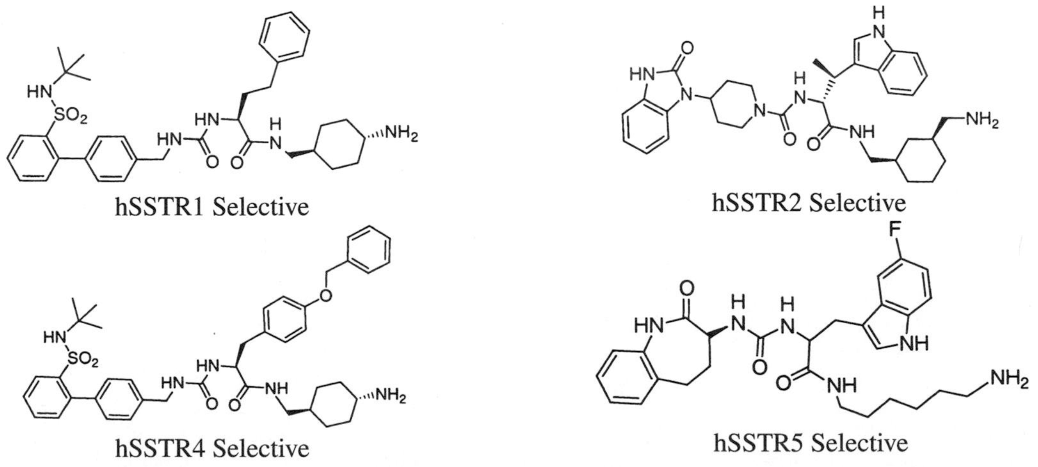

hSSTR1 Selective   hSSTR2 Selective

hSSTR4 Selective   hSSTR5 Selective

FIGURE 8   Selective somatostatin peptidomimetics from a combinatorial approach.

very large chemical library, it was decided to synthesize mixtures of compounds, which could then be quickly and selectively deconvoluted if a particular mixture showed activity in the assay. The library is synthesized by first coupling the diamine to a resin. A protected amino acid is then added to create the amide bond, the amine protecting group is removed, and the urea link to the terminal amine is formed. The products are then cleaved from the resin. Some of the resin is archived after each addition of a subunit to facilitate later deconvolution and identification of active components. Theoretically, 131,670 compounds were prepared in this library of 79 mixtures, when stereo- and regioisomers for the 20 diamines, 20 amino acids, and 79 amines are taken into account.

The design process for peptidomimetics was used in the selection of the library components. The most important consideration was to ensure that the pharmacophoric elements identified for somatostatin were present in the selected starting materials. Most of the amino acids used contained an aromatic group, as did the final amine fragment. Conformational restraints in the form of rings and branching groups were used in all components to further restrict flexibility, with the "privileged structure" amine biased toward piperidines and piperazines to further mimic the database lead. Biological screening followed by iterative deconvolution of components in the active mixtures led to the identification of compounds that were individually selective as agonists for somatostatin receptor subtypes 1, 2, 4, and 5 (Fig. 8).

IV. SUMMARY

Peptidomimetic ligands can serve as useful tools for the study of receptor signaling pathways and as important pharmacological agents for the treatment of disease. One method for their discovery involves activity screening of natural products and other compound collections. Use of "benign scaffolds" and chemical modification of "privileged structures" are two tactics for further refinement of the potency and selectivity of a peptidomimetic lead structure. Principles for rational design have also been put forth that rely on structural information derived from the ligand in either the receptor-bound or the solution state. Application of computational methods has greatly assisted this design process.

Glossary

chemical library A group of chemical compounds generally related by structure and method of preparation.

isostere A chemical equivalence in which an undesired chemical moiety is replaced by an atom or groups of atoms that retain the desired properties of the moiety being replaced.

Markush query Chemical database search tool in which substituents on the core structure do not need to be precisely enumerated.

peptidomimetic Nonpeptidic compound that, when bound to a receptor, can either imitate or block the action of a peptide ligand at the receptor level.

pharmacophore A conceptualization of features, both steric and electronic, minimally required in a molecule in order to elicit some desired biological response.

privileged structure Fragment or group often used in peptidomimetic design; contains elements of both pharmacophore (typically hydrophobic/aromatic) and scaffold.

topography Representation or "mapping" out of three-dimensional features in two-dimensional space.

See Also the Following Articles

Angiotensins • GPCR (G-Protein-Coupled Receptor) Structure • Heterotrimeric G-Proteins • Ligand Modification to Produce Pharmacologic Agents • Multiple G-Protein Coupling Systems • Somatostatin • Thyrotropin-Releasing Hormone Receptor Signaling

Further Reading

Berk, S. C., Rohrer, S. P., Degrado, S. J., Birzin, E. T., Mosley, R. T., Hutchins, S. M., Pasternak, A., Schaeffer, J. M., Underwood, D. J., and Chapman, K. T. (1999). A combinatorial approach toward the discovery of non-peptide, subtype-selective somatostatin receptor ligands. *J. Comb. Chem.* **1**, 388–396.

Freidinger, R. M. (1999). Nonpeptidic ligands for peptide and protein receptors. *Curr. Opin. Chem. Biol.* **3**, 395–406.

Hoffman, R. W. (1992). Flexible molecules with defined shape-conformational design. *Angew. Chem. Int. Ed. Engl.* **31**, 1124–1134.

Hruby, V. J. (2001). Design in topographical space of peptide and peptidomimetic ligands that affect behavior. A chemist's glimpse at the mind–body problem. *Acc. Chem. Res.* **34**, 389–397.

Marshall, G. R. (1993). A hierarchical approach to peptidomimetic design. *Tetrahedron* **49**, 3547–3558.

Müller, G., Hessler, G., and Decornez, H. Y. (2000). Are β-turn mimetics mimics of β-turns? *Angew. Chem. Int. Ed. Engl.* **39**, 894–896.

Olsen, G. L., Cheung, H.-C., Chiang, E., Madison, V. S., Sepinwall, J., Vincent, G. P., Winokur, A., and Gary, K. A. (1995). Peptide mimetics of thyrotropin-releasing hormone based on a cyclohexane framework: Design, synthesis, and cognition-enhancing properties. *J. Med. Chem.* **38**, 2866–2879.

Patchett, A. A., and Nargund, R. P. (2000). Privileged structures—An update. *In* "Annual reports in Medicinal Chemistry," **Vol. 35**, (A. M. Doherty, ed.),. pp. 289–298. Academic Press, San Diego.

Rohrer, S. P., Birzin, E. T., Mosley, R. T., Berk, S. C., Hutchins, S. M., Shen, D.-M., Xiong, Y., Hayes, E. C., Parmar, R. M.,

Foor, F., Mitra, S. W., Degrado, S. J., Shu, M., Klopp, J. M., Cai, S.-J., Blake, A., Chan, W. W. S., Pasternak, A., Yang, L., Patchett, A. A., Smith, R. G., Chapman, K. T., and Schaeffer, J. M. (1998). Rapid identification of subtype-selective agonists of the somatostatin receptor through combinatorial chemistry. *Science* **282**, 737–740.

Sheridan, R. P., Singh, S. B., Fluder, E. M., and Kearsley, S. K. (2001). Protocols for bridging the peptide to nonpeptide gap in topological similarity searches. *J. Chem. Inf. Comput. Sci.* **41**, 1395–1406.

Stigers, K. D., Soth, M. J., and Nowick, J. S. (1999). Designed molecules that fold to mimic protein secondary structures. *Curr. Opin. Chem. Biol.* **3**, 714–723.

Wiley, R. A., and Rich, D. H. (1993). Peptidomimetics derived from natural products. *Med. Res. Rev.* **13**, 327–384.

Peroxisome Proliferator-Activated Receptors

KAREN L. MACNAUL AND DAVID E. MOLLER

Merck Research Laboratories, New Jersey

I. INTRODUCTION
II. STRUCTURE OF PPARs
III. PPAR-α AND DISEASE TARGETS
IV. PPAR-γ AND DISEASE TARGETS
V. PPAR-δ AND DISEASE TARGETS
VI. SUMMARY

Peroxisome proliferator-activated receptors regulate key genes involved in glucose and lipid metabolism. In addition, these receptors are involved in many diverse biological functions, including development of the central nervous system, inflammation, cancer, and fertility. Development of specific, potent ligands for these receptors offers the potential for therapeutic intervention in many debilitating diseases.

I. INTRODUCTION

Peroxisome proliferator-activated receptors (PPARs) are members of a large superfamily of ligand-activated nuclear receptors. Three human isoforms, encoded by separate genes, have been identified in the past decade: PPAR-α [NR1C1], PPAR-δ [NR1C2], and PPAR-γ [NR1C3]. The subtypes share many structural similarities typical of nuclear receptors. Physiologically, PPARs are known to regulate key genes involved in both glucose and lipid metabolism. Synthetic PPAR agonists have been found to be efficacious in decreasing serum glucose, insulin, and lipids. By lowering these parameters in humans, metabolic disorders such as type 2 diabetes and dyslipidemia are improved. With the prevalence of type 2 diabetes and related metabolic disorders such as dyslipidemia and atherosclerosis reaching epidemic proportions in countries consuming a high-fat Western diet, the need for effective, safe therapies is critical.

II. STRUCTURE OF PPARs

PPARs have been identified and cloned from numerous species, including *Xenopus*, rodents, and humans. Like other nuclear receptors, they share characteristic functional domains. The amino-terminal region contains a variable "A/B" domain, which is poorly conserved between the three isoforms and contains a ligand-independent activation function (AF-1) domain. The highly conserved central "C" region contains the DNA-binding domain. This region contains two zinc finger structures that bind to PPAR responsive elements (PPREs) in target genes. Comparing the human isoforms, there is greater than 80% amino acid identity in this region. A flexible hinge region, "D," separates the DNA-binding domain (DBD) from the ligand-binding domain (LBD). The LBD "E" region is also highly conserved, with greater than 60% amino acid identity between human isoforms. The carboxy terminus of the LBD contains a ligand-dependent activation function domain, AF-2 (Fig. 1). The crystal structures of all three PPAR LBDs have been solved, both as apoproteins and co-crystalized with ligands. PPARs are ligand-dependent transcription factors that switch from an inactive form to an active form on binding agonist. The LBDs contain 13 α-helices and a small four-stranded β-sheets (Fig. 2). This structure contains a relatively large hydrophobic ligand-binding pocket in comparison to other nuclear receptors.

As with many nuclear receptors, all three PPAR subtypes are known to heterodimerize with the 9-*cis*-retinoid X receptors (RXRs) (Fig. 3). PPAR:RXR heterodimers are "permissive" in that they can be activated by either PPAR- or RXR-selective agonists. These heterodimers bind to direct repeats (DR-1) of a hexameric nucleotide sequence with the consensus sequence AGGTCA separated by one nucleotide. PPREs are located in the promoter of PPAR target genes. After agonists are bound, the LBD undergoes conformational changes, co-activators are recruited, and transcriptional activation is initiated.

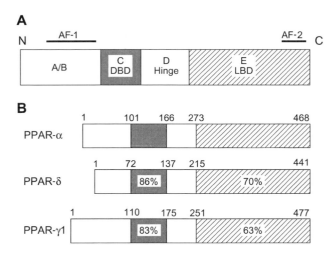

FIGURE 1 Functional domains of the PPARs. (A) The N-terminal A/B domain contains the ligand-independent activation function domain (AF-1). Domain C contains the DNA-binding domain (DBD), connected by hinge region "D" to the "E" region containing the ligand-binding domain (LBD). The C-terminus of the LBD contains a ligand-dependent activation function domain, AF-2. (B) The amino acid identities of DBD and LBD regions of the three human subtypes are compared; the percent identity relative to PPAR-α is indicated within the domains. The numbers above the individual receptors indicate the number of amino acid residues from the N-terminus for the regions.

PPARs can complex with a number of co-activator or corepressor proteins to regulate transcriptional activation or repression, respectively, of PPAR target genes. Binding of co-activators usually occurs at the AF-2 region, which has been located on helix 12 of the LBD. Several PPAR co-activators have been identified to date and can be grouped into three general categories based on their mode of regulation of transcriptional activation. Two prototypes are steroid receptor co-activator-1 (SRC-1) and cyclic adenosine monophosphate response element binding (CREB) protein p300 (CBP/p300); both have histone acetylase activity that is involved in the remodeling of chromatin structure to allow transcription factors access to DNA binding sites. Another class of co-activators that includes members of the vitamin D-interacting protein/thyroid hormone receptor-associated protein (DRIP/TRAP) complex augments basal transcriptional activity by interacting with the basal transcriptional complex. Several additional co-activators, including the PPAR-γ co-activator (PGC-1), receptor-interacting protein-140 (RIP140), and androgen receptor 70-kDa co-activator (ARA70), have been implicated as regulators of PPAR action, although their mechanisms of action are not well understood.

III. PPAR-α AND DISEASE TARGETS

A. Characterization and Ligands

PPAR-α was the first isoform to be identified and cloned from a murine liver cDNA library in 1990. PPAR-α has since been cloned from several other rodent species, *Xenopus*, and humans. The human PPAR-α gene has been mapped to chromosome 22q12–q13. PPAR-α is expressed at highest levels in tissues involved in fatty acid catabolism, such as liver, kidney, heart, skeletal muscle, and cells of the arterial wall. In these tissues, PPAR-α plays a key role in lipid metabolism by regulating genes involved in the β-oxidation of long-chain fatty acids, including acyl-CoA oxidase, enoyl-CoA hydratase/dehydrogenase multifunctional enzyme, keto-acyl-CoA thiolase, CYP4A cytochrome P450 enzymes, and fatty acid binding protein. Fatty acid transport protein (FATP) and fatty acid translocase (FAT, also known as CD36), which are involved in transport of fatty acids across the cell membrane, are up-regulated by

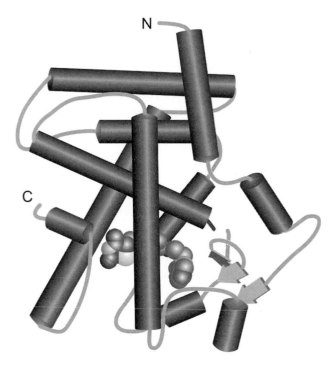

FIGURE 2 Overall structure of the human PPAR-γ ligand-binding domain complexed with rosiglitazone. The α-helices are represented by tubes and the small, four-stranded β-sheet is denoted by arrows. Within the large binding pocket is the thiazolidinedione rosiglitazone, represented by the ball structure, which binds in a U-shaped conformation and occupies only ~40% of the pocket. The AF-2 domain located on the C-terminal α-helix is important for cofactor binding and transcriptional activation.

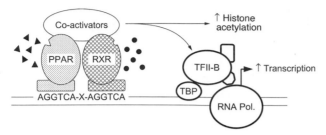

FIGURE 3 The peroxisome proliferator-activated receptor: retinoic acid X receptor (PPAR:RXR) transcriptional complex. PPARs heterodimerize with RXR and bind to specific DNA response elements in the regulatory regions of target genes. PPAR agonists (▲) and RXR agonists (●) bind their respective receptors and undergo conformational changes and recruitment of co-activator proteins. This illustration depicts binding of a co-activator with histone acetylase activity that is involved in remodeling the chromatin structure to allow interaction with basal transcriptional factors (such as TFII-B, TBP, and RNA polymerase).

PPAR-α activation; apoproteins A-I and A-II (apoA-I and apoA-II), the major constituents in high-density lipoproteins, are up-regulated by PPAR-α as well.

Natural ligands for PPAR-α present in human serum are composed of many saturated and unsaturated fatty acids, including palmitic acid, oleic acid, linoleic acid, and arachidonic acid (Fig. 4). These fatty acids bind to PPAR-α with micromolar affinities. However, it is not known if all of these ligands are present in sufficiently high concentrations to be physiologically relevant. Higher affinity naturally occurring PPAR-α activators have been identified, including the lipoxygenase 8(S)-hydroxyeicosatetraenoic acid [8(S)-HETE] and leukotriene B4 (LTB4). However, these ligands also may not be present at sufficient levels in relevant tissues to be considered key endogenous ligands.

PPAR-α can be activated by a diverse range of synthetic compounds, including industrial plasticizers, pesticides, and the fibrate class of drugs prescribed for hypertriglyceridemia. Among the fibrates are clofibrate, gemfibrozil, and fenofibrate. These compounds are relatively weak agonists (30–50 μM) and require large doses clinically in humans for efficacy in hyperlipidemia. In rodents, PPAR-α agonists cause an increase in the size and number of liver peroxisomes, subcellular organelles containing enzymes involved in long-chain fatty acid oxidation. Peroxisome proliferation in rodents progresses to hepatomegaly and hepatocarcinoma. In humans, however, significant hepatic peroxisome proliferation has not been observed on exposure to PPAR-α activators, as evidenced by the long-term clinical

experience with fibrates. Hence, the name "peroxisome proliferator-activated receptors" is a misnomer for this class of human nuclear receptors. It is therefore currently believed that activation of PPAR-α in humans does not warrant concerns for hepatotoxicity. The reason for this species-to-species difference may be because there is 10-fold lower expression of hepatic PPAR-α mRNA in humans, compare to mice. In addition, 30–50% of the PPAR-α expressed in human liver is a truncated splice variant lacking exon 6, which encodes for the ligand-binding domain. This further reduces the amount of functional receptor compared to mice.

B. Dyslipidemia and Atherosclerosis

The increased prevalence of a high-fat Western diet in many societies, coupled with increasingly sedentary lifestyles, has resulted in an increased incidence of metabolic disorders, including type 2 diabetes. Common comorbid conditions are dyslipidemia and progression to atherosclerosis, the leading cause of death among patients with type 2 diabetes. Dyslipidemia, an inappropriate alteration in lipid chemistry, is generally characterized by elevations in serum triglycerides (TGs) and very low-density lipoproteins (VLDLs) and a decrease in high-density lipoproteins (HDLs). PPAR-α activation by fibrates results in the up-regulation of lipoprotein lipase, which enhances

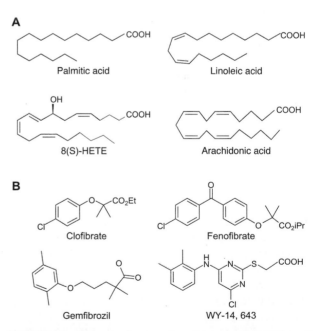

FIGURE 4 The structures of various natural (A) and synthetic (B) PPAR-α ligands. 8(S)-HETE, 8(S)-Hydroxyeicosatetraenoic acid.

the lipolytic activity of triglyceride-rich VLDL particles, and the suppression of hepatic apoC-III gene expression, which increases VLDL clearance. Fibrates, prescribed since the 1960s, have been investigated in humans in several large clinical trials; they have been found to be efficacious in lowering serum TGs and produce a modest increase in HDL levels. Moreover, fibrates have the proved benefit of reducing the risk of atherosclerosis.

PPAR-α null mice have been generated and exhibit a phenotype of significantly higher levels of total serum cholesterol, HDL cholesterol, and apoA-I mRNA. After 6 months of age, these mice exhibit a phenotype of increased body fat and increased hepatic fatty acids, visualized as lipid vesicles in the parenchyma. Unlike wild-type mice, the PPAR-α null animals do not respond to fibrate challenge with an induction of enzymes responsible for fatty acid oxidation. Neither is there a reduction in serum TGs or total serum cholesterol, further illustrating the role of PPAR-α in lipid homeostasis.

The formation of atherosclerotic lesions involves the recruitment of monocytes and their activation to macrophages, followed by their incorporation into the arterial wall via the vascular cell adhesion molecule 1 (VCAM-1). As the lesion progresses, macrophages become laden with cholesterol esters (foam cells) and a fibrous cap is formed from vascular cells and cell debris. Concurrent with this process is a local inflammatory response involving plasma cytokines such as interleukin-1β (IL-1β), interleukin-6 (IL-6), and tumor necrosis factor α (TNFα), as well as the proinflammatory eicosanoid LTB4. As atherosclerotic plaques mature, they protrude into the arterial lumen, restricting circulation. Rupture of these plaques results in thrombosis, which can cause myocardial infarctions and/or stroke.

PPAR-α is expressed in human monocytes, macrophages, endothelial cells, and vascular smooth muscle cells of atherosclerotic lesions. PPAR-α agonists can improve the outcome of atherosclerosis in a number of ways. One mechanism is the down-regulation VCAM-1 expression in human vascular endothelial cells, thus reducing the formation of lesions. Numerous in vitro studies have also shown that PPAR-α activators can inhibit the expression of the inflammatory cytokines IL-6 and IL-1β in a PPAR-α-dependent manner. In addition, arachidonic acid-induced ear-swelling in mice shows that the inflammatory response is prolonged in PPAR-α null mice compared to wild-type mice. However, the most relevant data for humans come from clinical trials in which coronary artery disease (CAD) patients treated

with fibrates for several years show reduced prevalence of recurrent myocardial infarction.

IV. PPAR-γ AND DISEASE TARGETS

A. Characterization and Ligands

PPAR-γ, the most extensively studied PPAR isoform, has been cloned from a wide variety of species, including Xenopus, mice, hamsters, rhesus monkeys, and humans. The level of amino acid conservation across species is highest (95% identity between murine and human receptors) for this isoform. The human PPAR-γ gene has been mapped to chromosome 3p25. PPAR-γ is expressed at high levels in adipose tissue and is a key regulator of fatty acid metabolism and adipocyte differentiation. Recently, PPAR-γ was found to be expressed in foam cells of atherosclerotic plaques, implying a role for this receptor in cardiovascular disease. The three PPAR-γ mRNA isoforms that have been identified in humans, γ1, γ2, and γ3, differ by alternate promoter usage and splice variants. PPAR-γ1 and PPAR-γ3 encode the same protein whereas PPAR-γ2, a splice variant of PPAR-γ1, has an additional 30 amino-terminal amino acids encoded by one exon. The expression pattern of these three isoforms is regulated in a tissue-specific manner. PPAR-γ1 is expressed in a wide range of tissues, including skeletal muscle, heart, colon, intestines, kidney, pancreas, and spleen. PPAR-γ2 is expressed primarily in adipose tissue, where it is the predominant isoform. PPAR-γ3 expression has been detected only in adipose tissue, macrophages, and colon epithelia. Presently, the functional significance of the two protein isoforms and their differential tissue expression is unclear.

PPAR-γ can be activated at micromolar affinity by a range of natural ligands (Fig. 5), including the fatty acids linoleic acid, arachidonic acid, and eicosapentaenoic acid; the 9- and 13-hydroxyoctadecadienoic acids (9-HODE and 13-HODE) that are generated from the conversion of linoleate by 15-lipoxygenase are micromolar PPAR-γ agonists. Additionally, the prostaglandin (PG) derivatives, most notably 15-deoxy-δ^{12,14}-PGJ2, PGH1, and PGH2, have activation affinities of $<10 \mu M$ on the PPAR-γ receptor. The affinities of these natural ligands are within the range of levels normally seen in human serum. However, the physiological level, chemical form, or specificity of these ligands in target cells is not known. Recently, the most potent natural ligand for PPAR-γ, the oxidized alkyl phospholipid, hexadecyl azelaoyl phosphatidylcholine (azPC), was identified and

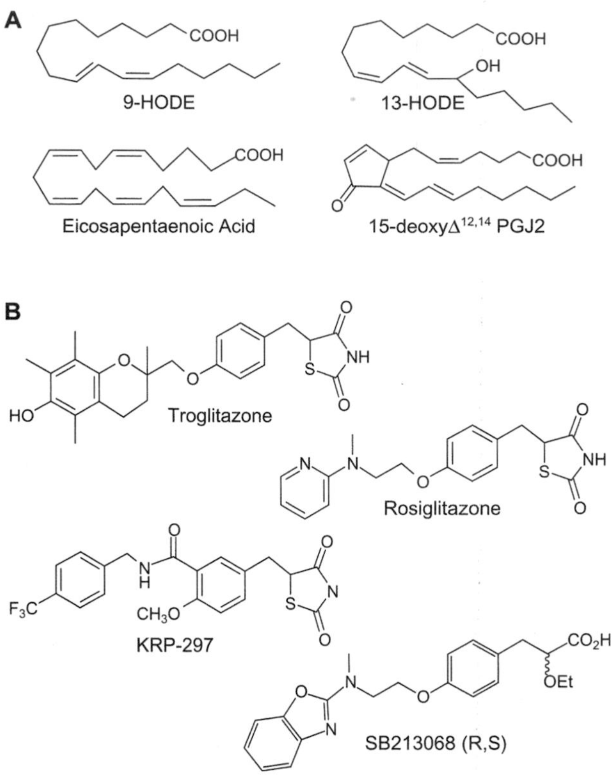

FIGURE 5 The structures of various natural (A) and synthetic (B) PPAR-γ ligands. 9- and 13-HODE, 9- and 13-Hydroxyoctadecadienoic acids; 15-deoxy-$\Delta^{12,14}$-PGJ2, 15-deoxy-$\Delta^{12,14}$-prostaglandin J2.

characterized as a $\sim$40 nM activator. Hexadecyl azPC is formed by oxidation of low-density lipoprotein (LDL) phospholipid particles, which are believed to initiate and maintain vascular inflammation during atherogenesis, linking the expression of PPAR-γ in this disease process to a relevant ligand.

Numerous potent synthetic ligands spanning a range of structural classes have been identified as PPAR-γ agonists. The thiazolidinediones (TZDs), also termed "glitazones," were the first class reported. TZDs were identified through empirical compound screening in insulin-resistant, diabetic rodents and have since been developed as insulin-sensitizing agents in humans. Compounds included in this class are troglitazone, pioglitazone, and rosiglitazone, which have affinities ranging from 20 to 100 nM for the human and murine receptors. These TZDs are relatively selective for PPAR-γ, but a newer TZD, KRP-297, binds potently to both PPAR-γ and PPAR-α. Recently, another compound class has been identified, the α-alkoxy-β-phenylpropionates, represented by SB 236636 and SB 213068, which are potent PPAR-γ agonists with significant PPAR-α

activity. Several nonsteroidal anti-inflammatory drugs (NSAIDs) such as indomethacin and fenoprofen have also been found to activate PPAR-γ and PPAR-α at micromolar concentrations and are able to induce adipocytic differentiation *in vitro*.

B. Type 2 Diabetes

The most extensive use for PPAR-γ agonists is in the treatment of type 2 diabetes in humans. The synthetic TZDs were the first class of compounds shown to have a direct correlation between their *in vitro* potency and their efficacy as insulin sensitizers in diabetic animal models and humans. TZDs increase the sensitivity of target tissues (adipose tissue, liver, and muscle) to the action of insulin. Thus, they improve glucose disposal and inhibit hepatic glucose production, thereby reducing plasma glucose levels. Since 1995, several TZDs have been approved for treatment of patients with type 2 diabetes (troglitazone, rosiglitazone, and pioglitazone), resulting in a major therapeutic advancement in treatment for a metabolic disorder that affects approximately 28 million people worldwide. In March 2000, troglitazone was removed from the market due to idiosyncratic hepatotoxicity, severe enough in some patients to require liver transplants or to cause death. These severe adverse effects have not been seen with rosiglitazone or pioglitazone.

PPAR-γ is expressed at highest levels in adipose tissue, where it has been studied extensively. However, very few PPAR-γ target genes have been identified to explain adequately a mechanism for insulin-sensitizing effects of TZDs. In isolated human adipocytes, rosiglitazone increases expression of p85-α phosphatidylinositol 3-kinase (p85-α PI3K) mRNA, a component of the insulin signaling pathway. Insulin receptor substrate-2 (IRS-2), a key intracellular substrate in the insulin signaling pathway, has also been demonstrated to be increased in cultured adipocytes and human adipose tissue treated with PPAR-γ agonists.

In adipose tissue, PPAR-γ regulates the transcription of several PPAR-responsive genes encoding lipogenic proteins and proteins involved in the differentiation of adipocytes. These genes include the adipocyte fatty acid-binding protein (aP2), phosphoenolpyruvate carboxykinase (PEPCK), lipoprotein lipase (LPL), and the fatty acid transporters FATP and CD36. Currently, it is speculated that altering the expression of fat cell genes may, through a secondary mechanism, result in insulin sensitization of muscle and liver. Confirming this hypothesis, an insulin-resistant, hyperglycemic transgenic mouse model in which adipose tissue has been ablated fails to show significant glucose lowering when treated with a TZD.

PAR-γ null mice have been generated. However, they demonstrate an embryonic lethal phenotype at approximately day 10 of gestation due to severe defects in placental development and myocardial thinning. Studies performed using PPAR-γ-deficient stem cells to generate chimeric mice have shown that PPAR-γ is required for differentiation of adipose tissue. Surprisingly, PPAR-γ heterozygous mice fed a high-fat diet show decreased fat mass, smaller adipocytes, and improved insulin sensitivity relative to wild-type mice. In humans, three individuals with severe insulin resistance have been found to have two different heterozygous loss-of-function (and dominant-negative) mutations in helix 12 of the PPAR-γ ligand-binding domain (P467L and V290M). These mutations also result in the development of type 2 diabetes at an early age.

C. Atherosclerosis

Monocytes and macrophages are key cell types involved in the immune response. They act by releasing inflammatory cytokines such as IL-1β, IL-6, and TNF α, along with inducible nitric oxide synthase (iNOS), an enzyme responsible for the production of a potent oxidant, nitric oxide (NO). These cell types are also important early mediators in the pathogenesis of atherosclerosis. PPAR-γ has been shown to be significantly up-regulated during the differentiation of monocytes into macrophages, and has been found to be expressed in cholesterol-laden, macrophage-derived foam cells within atherosclerotic lesions. Current evidence shows that PPAR-γ agonists may exert both pro- and anti-atherogenic effects via the expression of macrophage genes involved in atherosclerosis. Treatment of macrophages with TZDs and an RXR agonist *in vitro* increases the expression of the class B scavenger receptors, CD36 and SR-B1, involved in the transport of oxidized LDL (Ox-LDL) cholesterol particles into foam cells. In addition, the Ox-LDL-derived products 9- and 13-HODE are PPAR-γ activators, suggesting a positive feedback loop for a pro-atherogenic effect. On the other hand, TZDs have variably been reported to down-regulate the expression of potentially pro-atherogenic proteins, including matrix metalloproteinase-9 (MMP-9; also named gelatinase B, an enzyme implicated in atherosclerotic plaque destabilization) and scavenger

receptor class A (SR-A), along with vascular cell adhesion molecule-1(in vascular cells. Patients treated with troglitazone show a reduction in plasminogen activator inhibitor type 1 (PAI-1), a serine protease inhibitor that promotes thrombosis. These data suggest an anti-atherogenic effect of PPAR-γ agonists. Given that the net effects of PPAR-γ agonist treatment in mouse models of atherosclerosis are to reduce lesion formation, it is hoped that chronic treatment of humans will produce similar effects. However, current clinical data have not yet substantiated this hypothesis.

D. Cancer

PPAR-γ is expressed in a variety of human tumors, including lung carcinoma, breast adenocarcinoma, prostate carcinoma, liposarcoma, renal cell carcinoma, and colorectal carcinomas, in addition to a wide range of human cancer cell lines. PPAR-γ activators have been shown to inhibit the proliferation of fibroblasts *in vitro* during differentiation into normal preadipocytes, leading to the hypothesis that PPAR-γ agonists play a role in inhibiting the growth of adipose tissue-derived carcinoma. This has been demonstrated in metastatic human liposarcoma, a soft tissue malignancy that responds poorly to conventional therapies. Terminal differentiation of this malignant growth cell type has been achieved *in vitro* by treatment with the PPAR-γ activator pioglitazone and an RXRα-specific agonist. In addition, clinical troglitazone treatment of patients suffering from advanced liposarcomas results in inhibition of cell proliferation and terminal differentiation of the solid tumor.

PPAR-γ activators have also been shown to inhibit proliferation of human prostate cells *in vitro*, and patients with advanced prostate cancer treated with troglitazone have a decrease in prostate-specific antigen, a marker for prostate cancer. In human mammary adenocarcinomas, PPAR-γ is also expressed at significant levels and agonists have been reported to inhibit growth and induce terminal differentiation of malignant breast epithelial cells. Although PPAR-γ is expressed in human colonic polyps, primary colon tumors, and colon cancer cell lines, conflicting data as to the benefits vs proneoplastic effects of agonism have been generated from various animal and cellular models of this disease. Further investigation is needed to elucidate the role PPAR-γ may have in cancer and the mechanism by which TZDs exert their antiproliferative effects.

V. PPAR-δ AND DISEASE TARGETS

A. Characterization and Ligands

PPAR-δ, first cloned in 1992 from *Xenopus*, was initially given the name PPAR-β. Subsequently, in various labs it was cloned from humans and mice and was named NUC1 and PPAR-δ, FAAR, or NUC1, respectively. The current accepted nomenclature for all species is now PPAR-δ. The amino acid homology between human and rodent PPAR homologues is 90% in the LBD. The human PPAR-δ gene has been mapped to chromosome 6p21.1–p21.2. PPAR-δ is ubiquitously expressed in adult rat tissues. It has been reported to be expressed in human liver, intestine, kidney, skeletal muscle, brain, abdominal adipose, and skin. Presently, no specific target genes for PPAR-δ have been identified and studies to elucidate its physiological role have just recently begun to emerge.

PPAR-δ binds naturally occurring saturated and unsaturated fatty acids, as well as to their metabolites, including dihomo-γ-linolenic acid, eicosapentaenoic acid, and arachidonic acid, with affinities in the low micromolar range (Fig. 6). Synthetic ligands include L-165041, a compound with 10- to 30-fold selectivity for human PPAR-δ vs PPAR-γ. Recently, GW501516 has been identified as a potent PPAR-δ agonist. This compound is selective for the human, rhesus monkey, and mouse PPAR-δ subtypes vs other nuclear receptors.

B. Dyslipidemia

In *db/db* mice, which serve as a model of type 2 diabetes (increased serum TGs, glucose, and insulin),

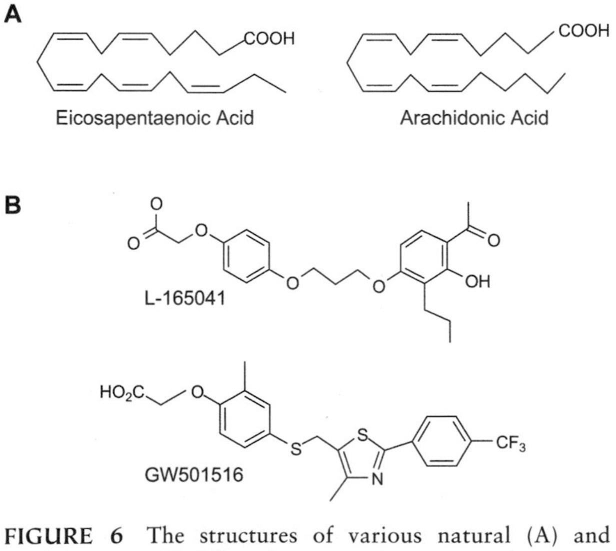

FIGURE 6 The structures of various natural (A) and synthetic (B) PPAR-δ ligands.

L-165041 causes a modest increase in HDL at a dose that does not cause TG or glucose lowering. GW501516 has been studied in a population of obese rhesus monkeys with metabolic parameters similar to those in humans with metabolic syndrome (dyslipidemia, insulin resistance, hyperinsulinemia, and hypertension). In this model, GW501516 induces a significant increase in HDL-cholesterol levels along with a reduction in TG. Elevated levels of plasma insulin are also suppressed by GW501516 treatment, whereas serum glucose levels are unaffected. These results suggest that PPAR-δ agonists may prove useful in the treatment of dyslipidemia, but it is important to note that this was a limited study with respect to species and compounds. The role of PPAR-δ in dyslipidemia requires further investigation.

C. Fertility

In mice, PPAR-δ is the only PPAR subtype expressed at the site of blastocyst implantation. Expression is induced in the stromal layer surrounding the implanting blastocyst and in the decidual layer following implantation. The same expression pattern is seen for cyclooxygenase 2 (COX-2). COX-2 is the rate-limiting enzyme involved in the synthesis of prostaglandins. Several prostaglandins generated from the COX-2 biosynthetic pathway, such as prostacyclin, are PPAR-δ ligands. COX-2 null mice have defects resulting in reduced implantation and decidualization. Treatment of COX-2 null mice with a natural PPAR-δ agonist, carbaprostacyclin, or the synthetic PPAR-δ agonist L-165041, restores implantation to normal in these animals. When PPAR-δ heterozygous null mice are bred, fewer than expected null offspring are produced, indicating that although PPAR-δ may play a role in implantation and fertility, it is not essential.

D. Cancer

PPAR-δ has been recently identified as a downstream target in a pathway involved in colorectal carcinogenesis. PPAR-δ mRNA expression is up-regulated in many human and rodent colon carcinomas. During the development of colorectal carcinoma, an inactivation mutation in the adenomatous polyposis coli (APC) gene occurs. This mutation causes an increase in β-catenin, a cytoplasmic protein involved in cellular adhesion and development. β-Catenin forms complexes with a protein called T-cell factor 4 (TCF-4), which binds DNA and induces genes involved in cellular proliferation. β-Catenin/TCF-4 complexes can bind and activate the PPAR-δ promoter and have been shown to up-regulate the expression of PPAR-δ in colon carcinoma cells. A human colorectal cancer cell line, HCT116, in which the PPAR-δ gene is deleted, was established and injected as xenografts into nude mice. In this model, the PPAR-δ null cells result in fewer tumors with slower progression compared to xenografts of wild-type HCT116 cells. Taken together, these data suggest that inhibition of PPAR-δ expression or function by antagonists may result in colon tumor suppression.

E. Central Nervous System

The expression of PPARs during rat embryonic development, assessed by *in situ* hybridization, shows that PPAR-δ is expressed ubiquitously and earlier in development than PPAR-α or PPAR-γ. Interestingly, PPAR-δ is expressed in embryonic tissues at much higher levels compared to the other isoforms, in sharp contrast to expression levels in adult tissues. Peak expression of PPAR-δ occurs at embryonic day 13.5 (E13.5) in tissues of the developing nervous system, suggesting an important role for this subtype in differentiation of cells within the CNS. *In vitro*, PPAR-δ mRNA is expressed in immature murine oligodendrocytes. These are the major lipid-producing cells in the CNS that differentiate into cells with myelin sheets. Treatment of neonatal primary glial cell cultures, which contain immature oligodendrocytes, with the PPAR-δ selective agonist L-165041 results in accelerated differentiation of oligodendrocytes, increased processes, and the formation of membrane sheets. *In vivo*, PPAR-δ null mice have alterations in the extent of myelination in the corpus collosum compared to wild-type controls. This subregion normally expresses high levels of PPAR-δ.

VI. SUMMARY

Data have emerged over the past decade showing the involvement of the three PPAR isoforms as sensors for fatty acids and lipid metabolites in metabolically active tissues. In these tissues, PPARs transcriptionally regulate target genes that play critical roles in lipid metabolism. Therapeutic use of the fibrates in humans has validated the efficacy of PPAR-α agonists in improving hypertriglyceridemia and reducing the risk for atherosclerosis and subsequent myocardial

infarctions. Both the TZD and the more recently identified non-TZD PPAR-γ agonists have been shown to improve insulin sensitivity and lower serum glucose in patients with type 2 diabetes, a metabolic disorder of epidemic proportions in westernized cultures. In addition, PPAR-γ agonists have demonstrated provocative effects in animal models, implying that there is great potential for their use in treating or preventing atherosclerosis in humans. The role of PPAR-γ in cancer is just emerging. Further investigation is needed to elucidate the mechanisms of action by which this receptor positively impacts on these disease states. PPAR-δ, the isoform for which only limited data have emerged, may have therapeutic utilities in such diverse disorders as dyslipidemia, fertility, cancer, and demyelinating CNS diseases. Specific, potent ligands are being identified that will allow a deeper understanding of the pleiotropic effects of the PPARs.

Glossary

adipocytes Cells that store energy in the form of triglycerides and release energy as free fatty acids during periods of nutritional deprivation.

atherosclerosis Condition caused by progressive thickening and hardening of the walls of medium-sized and large arteries as a result of extensive fat and cellular deposits on their inner lining, ultimately leading to arterial occlusion.

fatty acid Long-chain aliphatic carboxylic acid found in fats, oils, membrane phospholipids, and glycolipids.

hormone receptor Protein in or on the surface of target cells; functions as a sensor for the hormone by binding the hormone and initiating a cellular response.

ligand Small molecule that binds specifically to a larger one; for example, a hormone is the ligand for its specific protein receptor.

metabolic syndrome Condition defined by insulin resistance, hyperinsulinemia, and dyslipidemia (generally elevated serum triglycerides and decreased high-density lipoprotein cholesterol).

peroxisome Subcellular organelles in the cytoplasm of eukaryotic cells; involved in the β-oxidation of long-chain fatty acids.

type 2 diabetes One of the two major types of diabetes, in which the beta cells of the pancreas produce insulin but the body is unable to use it effectively because the target cells have become resistant to the action of insulin.

See Also the Following Articles

Diabetes Type 2 • Ligand Modification to Produce Pharmacologic Agents • Lipoprotein Receptor Signaling

Further Reading

Barak, Y., Nelson, M. C., Ong, E. S., Jones, Y. Z., Ruiz-Lozano, P., Chien, K. R., Koder, A., and Evans, R. M. (1999). PPARγ is required for placental, cardiac, and adipose tissue development. *Mol. Cell* **4**, 585–595.

Barroso, I., Gurnell, M., Crowley, V. E. F., Agostini, M., Schwabe, J. W., Soos, M. A., Maslen, G., Williams, T. D. M., Lewis, H., Schafer, A. J., Chatterjee, V. K. K., and O'Rahilly, S. (1999). Dominant negative mutations in human PPARγ associated with severe insulin resistance, diabetes mellitus, and hypertension. *Nature* **402**, 880–883.

Chao, L., Marcus-Samuels, B., Mason, M. M., Moitra, J., Vinson, C., Arioglu, E., Oksana Gavrilova, O., and Reitman, M. L. (2000). Adipose tissue is required for the antidiabetic, but not for the hypolipidemic, effect of thiazolidinediones. *J. Clin. Invest.* **106**, 1221–1228.

Delerive, P., Fruchart, J.-C., and Staels, B. (2001). Peroxisome proliferator-activated receptors in inflammation control. *J. Endocrinol.* **169**, 453–459.

Kliewer, S. A., Xu, H. E., Lambert, M. H., and Willson, T. M. (2001). Peroxisome proliferator-activated receptors: From genes to physiology. *Recent Prog. Horm. Res.* **56**, 239–263.

Kubota, N., Terauchi, Y., Hiroshi, M., Tamemoto, H., Yamauchi, T., Komeda, K., Satoh, S., Nakano, R., Ishii, C., Sugiyama, T., Eto, K., Tsubamoto, Y., Okuno, A., Murakami, K., Sekihara, H., Hasegawa, G., Naito, M., Toyoshima, Y., Tanaka, S., Shiota, K., Kitamura, T., Fujita, T., Ezaki, O., Aizawa, S., Nagai, R., Tobe, K., Kimura, S., and Kadowaki, T. (1999). PPAR mediates high-fat diet—Induced adipocyte hypertrophy and insulin resistance. *Mol. Cell* **4**, 597–609.

Moller, D. E., and Greene, D. A. (2001). Peroxisome proliferator-activated receptor (PPAR)γ agonists for diabetes. *Adv. Protein Chem.* **56**, 181–212.

Oliver, W. R., Shenk, J. L., Snaith, M. R., Russell, C. S., Plunket, K. D., Bodkin, N. L., Lewis, M. C., Winegar, D. A., Sznaidman, M. L., Lambert, M. L., Xu, H. E., Sternbach, D. D., Kliewer, S. A., Hansen, B. C., and Willson, T. M. (2001). A selective peroxisome proliferator-activated receptor δ agonist promotes reverse cholesterol transport. *Proc. Natl. Acad. Sci. U.S.A.* **98**(9), 5306–5311.

Palmer, C. N. A., Hsu, M., Griffin, K. J., Raucy, J. L., and Johnson, E. F. (1997). Peroxisome proliferator-activated receptor-α expression in human liver. *Mol. Pharmacol.* **53**, 14–22.

Park, B. H., Vogelstein, B. K., and Kinzler, W. (2001). Genetic disruption of PPARδ decreases the tumorigenicity of human colon cancer cells. *Proc. Natl. Acad. Sci. U.S.A.* **98**(5), 2598–2603.

Saltiel, A. R. (2001). New perspectives into the molecular pathogenesis and treatment of type 2 diabetes. *Cell* **104**, 517–529.

Torchia, J., Glass, C., and Rosenfeld, M. G. (1998). Co-activators and co-repressors in the integration of transcriptional responses. *Curr. Opin. Cell. Biol.* **10**, 373–383.

Torra, I. P., Gervois, P., and Staels, B. (1998). Peroxisome proliferator-activated receptor α in metabolic disease, inflammation, atherosclerosis and aging. *Curr. Opin. Lipidol.* **10**, 151–159.

Willson, T. M., Brown, P. J., Sternbach, D. D., and Henke, B. R. (2000). The PPARs: From orphan receptors to drug discovery. *J. Med. Chem.* **43**(4), 527–550.

Willson, T. M., Cobb, J. E., Cowan, D. J., Wiethe, R. W., Correa, I. D., Prakash, S. R., Beck, K. D., Moore, L. B., Kliewer, S. A.,

and Lehmann, J. M. (1996). The structure–activity relationship between peroxisome proliferator-activated receptor gamma agonism and the antihyperglycemic activity of the thiazolidinediones. *J. Med. Chem. Lett.* **6**, 2121–2126.

Pheromone Production in Insects

GARY J. BLOMQUIST
University of Nevada

I. INTRODUCTION
II. PBAN REGULATION IN LEPIDOPTERA
III. JUVENILE HORMONE REGULATION IN COLEOPTERA
IV. JUVENILE HORMONE REGULATION IN BLATTODEA
V. ECDYSTEROID REGULATION IN DIPTERA
VI. CONCLUDING REMARKS

The production of pheromones can be regulated by hormones from the brain, ovary, and corpora allata. In insects, at least three different hormones have been shown to regulate pheromone production: pheromone biosynthesis-activating neuropeptide, juvenile hormone, and ecdysteroids. This article discusses several model insect systems of endocrine regulation of pheromone biosynthesis.

I. INTRODUCTION

The observation that females of certain species have repeated reproductive cycles and that mating occurs only during defined periods of each cycle led to the proposal that pheromone production might be under hormonal control. Studies on a limited number of species demonstrate that pheromone production can be under the regulation of products of the brain, ovary, and corpora allata (CA). At least three distinct hormones have been shown to regulate pheromone production in insects. In many female moths (Lepidoptera), pheromone biosynthesis is regulated by a 33- or 34-amino-acid pheromone biosynthesis-activating neuropeptide (PBAN) (Fig. 1). PBAN alters enzyme activity at one or more steps during or subsequent to fatty acid synthesis during pheromone production. In some species of Coleoptera, Blattodea, and Lepidoptera, juvenile hormone (JH) (Fig. 1) induces pheromone production. In the female housefly, ovarian produced ecdysteroids (Fig. 1) regulate

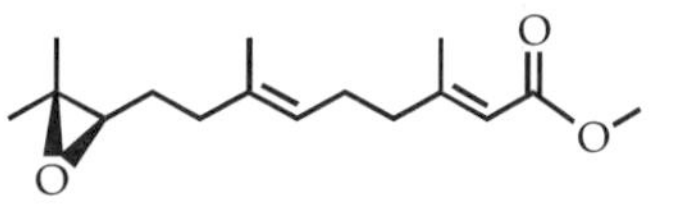

Juvenile hormone III

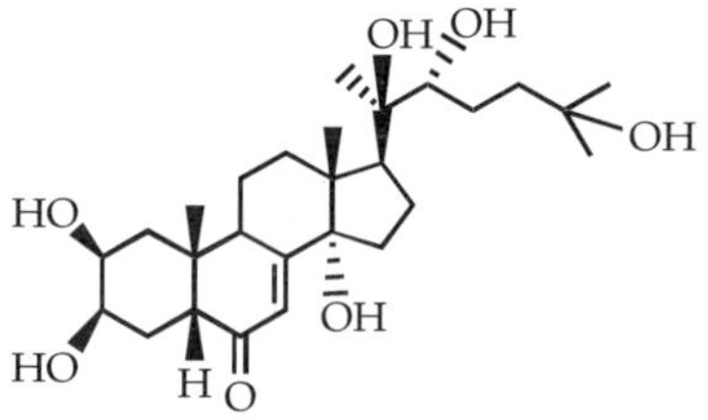

20-Hydroxyecdysone

```
            1              5            10             15
Hez-PBAN  Leu-Ser- Asp-Asp-Met-Pro-Ala-Thr-Pro-Ala-Asp-Gln-Glu-Met-Tyr-Arg-Gln-
Bom-PBAN  Leu- Ser- Glu-Asp-Met-Pro-Ala-Thr-Pro-Ala-Asp-Gln-Glu-Met-Tyr-Gln-Pro-
Lyd-PBAN  Leu-Ala-Asp-Asp-Met-Pro-Ala-Thr-Met-Ala-Asp-Gln-Glu-Val-Try-Arg-Pro-
```

```
                 20            25            30
PBAN     Asp-Pro-Glu-Gln- Ile- Asp-Ser-Arg-Thr-Lys-Tyr-Phe-Ser-Pro-Arg-Leu-NH₂
         Asp-Pro-Glu-Glu-Met-Glu-Ser-Arg-Thr-Arg-Tyr-Phe-Ser-Pro-Arg-Leu-NH₂
         Glu-Pro-Glu-Gln- Ile- Asp-Ser-Arg-Asn-Lys-Tyr-Phe-Ser-Pro-Arg-Leu-NH₂
```

**Amidated C-terminal
pentapeptide**

FIGURE 1   Structures of juvenile hormone, 20-hydroxyecdysone, and PBAN.

the chain length of cuticular alkenes so that the pheromone component (Z)-9-tricosene (muscalure) becomes a major product. It appears that JH induces key regulatory enzymes, whereas ecdysteroids repress specific enzymes to result in pheromone production. Discussed below is work from a limited number of model insect systems in which endocrine regulation of pheromone production has been most extensively studied. It is not by any means an exhaustive list, and excellent work in other insects has been done. Studies on the endocrine regulation of pheromone production to date have utilized relatively few species, and large gaps in our knowledge are readily apparent.

II. PBAN REGULATION IN LEPIDOPTERA

A pheromone biosynthesis-activating neuropeptide was first purified and sequenced from *Heliothis zea* in 1989 by Ashok Raina and co-workers. PBANs from other lepidopterans, including *Bombyx mori*, *Lymantria dispar*, *Agrotis ipsilon*, and *Helicoverpa assulta*, have subsequently been isolated and identified. All of the PBANs examined to date are 33- or 34-amino-acid peptides that share approximately 80% homology and an amidated C-terminus. The minimum sequence necessary for biological activity is the C-terminal pentapeptide (Phe-Ser-Pro-Arg-Leu-NH₂), although the activity of this pentapeptide is an order of magnitude or so lower than that of the intact peptide.

It is becoming clear that in most moths PBAN is released into the hemolymph and acts directly on the pheromone gland to stimulate pheromone biosynthesis. There is evidence, however, that in some species PBAN undergoes neural transport. Regardless, PBAN is produced in the subesophageal ganglia and transported to the corpora cardiaca (CC). In most species, PBAN is then released from the CC (a neurohemal organ) and transported through the hemolymph to the pheromone gland.

The proposed direct mechanism of PBAN involves the binding of PBAN to a specific pheromone gland receptor (Fig. 2). This triggers second messengers, including Ca^{2+} and cyclic AMP, and may involve phosphatidyl inositol. The steps in pheromone biosynthesis that are regulated by PBAN have been examined, and in some species it appears that PBAN increases acetyl coenzyme A (acetyl CoA) carboxylase activity and in others it may affect the reduction of fatty acyl groups to aldehydes and alcohols or other steps in pheromone biosynthesis.

Although PBAN and PBAN-like peptides have been found in all Lepidoptera examined to date as

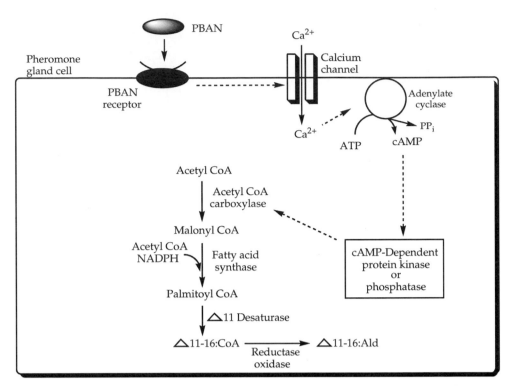

FIGURE 2   Proposed mode of action of PBAN on pheromone production in *Helicoverpa zea.*

well as insects from other orders, in some species they do not appear to regulate pheromone production. For example, in *Trichoplusia ni*, the pheromone gland becomes competent to produce pheromone at adult eclosion and pheromone production continues unregulated for the duration of the life of the female. In some Lepidoptera, JH and ecdysteroids are involved in regulating pheromone production, in some cases apparently regulating PBAN release.

III. JUVENILE HORMONE REGULATION IN COLEOPTERA

Coleoptera (beetles) produce and/or emit pheromones in response to various environmental or physiological factors, with JH often being involved. In many insect species, JH induces vitellogenin production and coordinates other reproductive events, so it is not unexpected that it can also affect pheromone production. A key question for certain species, especially bark beetles, is whether JH stimulates the conversion of host precursors to pheromone or whether it stimulates *de novo* pheromone synthesis. Recent findings, primarily with the pine engraver, *Ips pini*, have demonstrated that JH III can directly induce *de novo* pheromone production.

Perhaps the most complete picture of JH regulation of pheromone production occurs in *I. pini*. Radiotracer studies with male *I. pini* monitoring *in vivo* incorporation of radiolabeled acetate into ipsdienol showed that incorporation increased with increasing topical JH III dose. The *in vivo* incorporation of radiolabeled mevalonolactone into ipsdienol by male *I. pini* was not affected by increasing JH III dose, indicating that the JH regulation of isoprenoid pheromone production occurred at steps between acetyl CoA and mevalonate (Fig. 3). Subsequent studies showed that feeding or topical application of JH III induces the mRNA transcript for 3-hydroxy-3-methylglutaryl CoA reductase (HMG-R) 20- to 30-fold. The emerging picture for this insect is that feeding stimulates JH III production, which in turn induces HMG-R transcript and enzyme activity, resulting in a large increase in pheromone production (Fig. 3). HMG CoA synthase transcript was increased only several fold by JH III, indicating that the main regulatory step is HMG CoA reductase.

Using a mRNA probe to HMG-R, *in situ* hybridization on exposed whole mounts of JH-stimulated male *I. pini* demonstrated that the site of pheromone synthesis is midgut tissue. Furthermore,

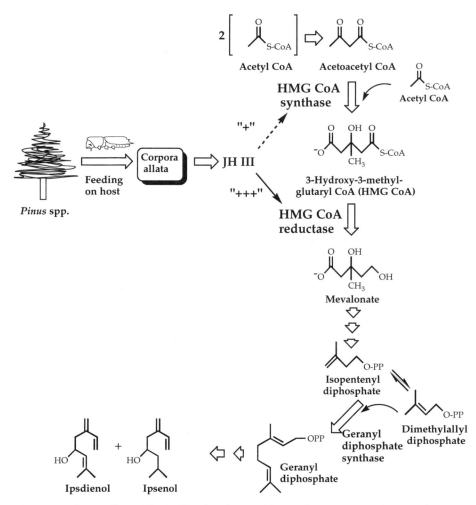

FIGURE 3 Current understanding of the ipsdienol and ipsenol biosynthesis in *I. pini* showing the proposed mode of action of JH III. The major regulatory step induced by JH III is HMG CoA reductase.

isolated midgut tissue incorporated labeled acetate into ipsdienol.

The molecular details of how JH affects transcription and ultimately, coleopteran pheromone biosynthesis, remain to be elucidated. Following release from the CA, lipophilic JH binds to a specific protein (the JH-binding protein) for transport through the aqueous hemolymph and protection from degradative enzymes. Once at the target tissue for pheromone biosynthesis, it would most likely cross the cell membrane and bind to intracellular receptors, although JH has been shown to act at the membrane level in some systems. The isolation and identification of an intracellular receptor for JH remain elusive and controversial. Although it is tempting to extend the intracellular molecular mode of action for steroidal hormones to JH, the diverse physiological phenomena regulated by JH may suggest a more complex

interplay involving an ensemble of regulatory proteins or transcription factors with the putative JH receptor. The large induction of HMG-R transcript by JH apparently acting alone (without the involvement of ecdysteroids as occurs during development) makes the *I. pini* system an attractive model for elucidating the mode of action of JH.

IV. JUVENILE HORMONE REGULATION IN BLATTODEA

By far the best studied and most understood example of JH regulation of pheromone production in the Blattodea was done by Schal and collaborators in female German cockroaches, *Blattella germanica*. *In vivo* synthesis of the contact sex pheromone, 3,11-dimethylnonacosan-2-one (3,11-DMN:Ke) and its accumulation on the cuticle are correlated with the *in vitro* synthesis of JH III by the CA and oocyte development, suggesting common JH regulation of sex pheromone production as well as other reproductive events. Comparison of the patterns of pheromone and hydrocarbon production in starved, allatectomized, and head-ligated females, as well as in females rescued with hormone replacement therapy, suggests two mechanisms of regulation of sex pheromone production: (1) hormonal, a JH-induced conversion of the hydrocarbon precursor to the oxygenated sex pheromone that is related to the CA cycle and oocyte development, and (2) nonhormonal, a JH-independent process, probably related to feeding, that supplies precursors for hydrocarbon (pheromone) biosynthesis.

Dependence of pheromone synthesis on JH levels in female *B. germanica* is supported by the following findings: (1) the pattern of accumulation of 3,11-DMN:Ke and 3,11-dimethylheptacosan-2-one (minor pheromone component) on the cuticle correlates with the pattern of JH synthesis through two gonotropic cycles; (2) the rates of synthesis of methyl ketones, using labeled propionate, correspond to rates of JH synthesis; and (3) pheromone production declines in allatectomized females or females with experimentally inhibited CA (e.g., starved, protein-deprived, ootheca implanted), whereas juvenile hormone analogue (JHA) treatment restores pheromone production in these females.

Whereas pheromone production is completely suppressed in individuals of other allatectomized cockroach species, allatectomized female *B. germanica* produce a small quantity of pheromone. Because JHAs are also less effective inducers of pheromone production in unfed female *B. germanica*, it was hypothesized that feeding might indirectly influence pheromone production by influencing the availability of pheromone precursor (hydrocarbon), and results from recent studies support this hypothesis.

V. ECDYSTEROID REGULATION IN DIPTERA

In several species of Diptera, ecdysteroids have been shown to regulate the female reproductive process of vitellogenesis. Ecdysteroids also regulate sex pheromone production in the female housefly, *Musca domestica*. Pheromone biosynthesis normally begins approximately 2 days after emergence to adult in female *M. domestica*. However, ovariectomy of newly emerged females prevents pheromone biosynthesis. Pheromone production can be restored in ovariectomized females by implantation of ovaries or injection of 20-hydroxyecdysone (20-HE). These and

other studies have led to the conclusion that sex pheromone production in female *M. domestica* is regulated by ecdysteroids.

Male houseflies normally do not produce significant amounts of (Z)-9-tricosene or its oxygenated products. However, implantation of ovaries or treatment with 20-HE induces the production of the female sex pheromone. Immature females and males of all ages normally produce cuticular alkenes of 27 carbons or more. Since 20-HE appears to be a product of the mature ovary in adult houseflies, adult males normally are not exposed to 20-HE. Treatment with 20-HE induces pheromone synthesis, indicating that the male has the biosynthetic machinery to produce pheromone.

An in-depth study of the biochemistry of pheromone production in the housefly led to an understanding of the enzyme activity affected by 20-HE. The endocrine-mediated induction of sex pheromone biosynthesis in the housefly involves a change in the fate of tetracosenoyl CoA (Z15-24:CoA) from one of elongation to one of reduction to the aldehyde and then decarboxylation to the main sex pheromone component, (Z)-9-tricosene (Z9-23:Hy) (Fig. 4). The two most likely regulatory points where 20-HE could exert its effect were (1) the fatty acyl CoA elongation step(s) and/or (2) the reductive conversion of fatty acyl CoA to hydrocarbon formation step(s). *In vitro* enzyme assays demonstrate that ecdysone predominantly affects the elongation enzyme(s) rather than the enzymes functioning in the conversion of Z15-24:CoA to Z9-23:Hy (Fig. 4). It appears that 20-HE exerts its effect primarily if not exclusively by repressing the fatty acyl CoA elongase that converts 24:1-CoA to longer chain fatty acids, resulting in the build up of 24:1-CoA, which is then reduced to the aldehyde and decarboxylated to (Z)-9-tricosene (muscalure). A portion of the (Z)-9-tricosene is then converted to epoxide and ketone, both of which function in the female sex pheromone (Fig. 4).

As is the case with JH III and coleopteran pheromone biosynthesis, the molecular details of how 20-HE influences the enzymatic reactions in dipteran pheromone biosynthesis remain to be elucidated. By analogy to steroidal hormones in other systems, it is reasonable to hypothesize that gene expression would be regulated for key biosynthetic enzymes, in this case repression of a specific fatty acyl CoA elongase. In general, steroid hormones such as 20-HE are thought to diffuse freely through the cell membrane into the cytoplasm and/or nucleus to bind specific intracellular hormone receptors. A dimerized

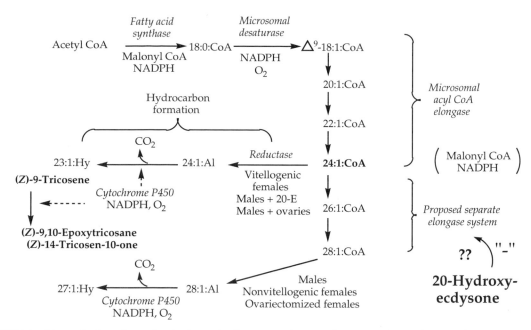

FIGURE 4 Biosynthetic pathway for the housefly pheromone showing the proposed site of action of 20-HE. Reprinted from Tillman *et al.* (1999), with permission from Elsevier Science.

form of the receptor–ligand complex then binds to specific DNA sequences called hormone-responsive elements to affect gene expression. Although the motivation for their study has been insect morphogenesis, ecdysteroid receptors have been isolated from species of Diptera, Lepidoptera, and Coleoptera. These receptors occur in a surprising variety of isoforms and this may have implications for the regulation of pheromone biosynthesis in the Diptera.

VI. CONCLUDING REMARKS

In no model pheromone biosynthetic system are the molecular mechanisms of hormonal regulation completely understood, and studies to address these obvious gaps in our understanding are being pursued in representative species. It is now clear that ecdysone and JH regulate pheromone production by inducing or repressing specific enzymes, but the molecular basis for these changes is not understood. A better understanding of the PBAN receptor and the biochemical steps regulated in pheromone production is needed. In no system are the exact enzymatic steps affected by the pheromone biosynthesis-regulating hormone known with certainty and completeness. Ultimately, just as behavioral chemicals themselves have been extended to pest management, research on pheromone biosynthesis and its hormonal regulation

may be directed toward application and ultimately used in insect control.

Glossary

corpora allata Paired ganglia-like bodies often located just posterior to the corpora cardiaca. They synthesize and secrete juvenile hormone.

corpora cardiaca Paired neurohemal organs located behind the brain and often near the corpora allata. They release neurosecretory material from the brain, including pheromone biosynthesis-activating neuropeptide.

ecdysteroids Polyhydroxy steroids that induce molting during development in insects and that are also involved in reproductive processes in some adult insects, including Diptera.

juvenile hormones Sesquiterpenoids with epoxide and methyl ester functional groups produced by the corpora allata. They serve to keep the insect in the immature state during development and to coordinate reproductive events in many adult insects.

pheromone A chemical (or blend of chemicals) that is released by an organism and causes specific behavioral or physiological reaction(s) a in one or more conspecific individuals.

pheromone biosynthesis-activating neuropeptide A 33- or 34-amino-acid peptide produced in the brain that triggers pheromone production in many species of Lepidoptera.

subesophageal ganglion A large nerve center consisting of the fused ganglia of the original mandibular, maxillary, and labial segments, situated in the head, beneath the esophagus.

See Also the Following Articles

Ecdysteroid Action in Insect Reproduction • Ecdysteroids, Overview • Insect Endocrine System • Juvenile Hormone Action in Insect Development • Juvenile Hormone Action in Insect Reproduction • Juvenile Hormone Biosynthesis • Juvenile Hormones, Chemistry of • Neuropeptides: Roles in Regulation of Juvenile Hormone Production

Further Reading

Adams, T. S., Dillwith, J. W., and Blomquist, G. J. (1984). The role of 20-hydroxyecdysone in housefly sex pheromone biosynthesis. *J. Insect Physiol.* **30,** 287–294.

Chase, J., Touhara, K., Prestwich, G. D., Schal, C., and Blomquist, G. J. (1992). Biosynthesis and endocrine control of the production of the German cockroach sex pheromone, 3,11-dimethylnonacosan-2-one. *Proc. Natl. Acad. Sci. USA* **89,** 6050–6054.

Hall, G. M., Tittiger, C., Andrews, G., Mastick, G., Kuenzli, M., Luo, X., Seybold, S. J., and Blomquist, G. J. (2002). Male pine engraver beetles, *Ips pini*, synthesize the monoterpenoid pheromone ipsdienol *de novo* in midgut tissue. *Naturwissenschaften* **89,** 79–83.

Jurenka, R. A., Jacquin, E., and Roelofs, W. L. (1991). Stimulation of sex pheromone biosynthesis in the moth *Helicoverpa zea*: Action of a brain hormone on pheromone glands involves Ca^{2+} and cAMP as second messengers. *Proc. Natl. Acad. Sci. USA* **88,** 8621–8625.

Jurenka, R. A., and Roelofs, W. L. (1993). Biosynthesis and endocrine regulation of fatty acid derived pheromones in moths. *In* "Insect Lipids: Chemistry, Biochemistry and Biology" (D. W. Stanley-Samuelson and D. R. Nelson, eds.), pp. 353–388. University of Nebraska Press, Lincoln.

Ma, P. W. K., Knipple, D. C., and Roelofs, W. L. (1994). Structural organization of the *Helicoverpa zea* gene encoding the precursor protein for pheromone biosynthesis-activating neuropeptide and other neuropeptides. *Proc. Natl. Acad. Sci. USA* **91,** 6506–6510.

Rafaeli, A., Soroker, V., Kamensky, B., Gileadi, C., and Zisman, U. (1997). Physiological and cellular mode of action of pheromone biosynthesis activating neuropeptide (PBAN) in the control of pheromoneotropic activity of female moths. *In* "Insect Pheromone Research: New Directions" (R. T. Cardé and A. K. Minks, eds.), pp. 74–82. Chapman and Hall, New York.

Raina, A. K. (1993). Neuroendocrine control of sex pheromone biosynthesis in Lepidoptera. *Annu. Rev. Entomol.* **38,** 329–349.

Schal, C., Burns, E. L., Gadot, M., Chase, J., and Blomquist, G. J. (1991). Biochemistry and regulation of pheromone production in *Blattella germanica* (L.). (Dictyoptera: Blattellidae). *Insect Biochem.* **21,** 73–79.

Schal, C., Liang, D., and Blomquist, G. J. (1997). Neural and endocrine control of pheromone production and release in cockroaches. *In* "Insect Pheromone Research: New Directions" (R. T. Cardé and A. K. Minks, eds.), pp. 3–20. Chapman and Hall, New York.

Soroker, V., and Rafaeli, A. (1995). Multi-signal transduction of the pheromonotropic response by pheromone gland incubations of *Helicoverpa armigera*. *Insect Biochem. Mol. Biol.* **25,** 1–9.

Tang, J. D., Charlton, R. E., Jurenka, R. A., Wolf, W. A., Phelan, P. L., Streng, L., and Roelofs, W. L. (1989). Regulation of pheromone biosynthesis by a brain hormone in two moth species. *Proc. Natl. Acad. Sci. USA* **89,** 1806–1810.

Tillman, J. A., Holbrook, G. L., Dallara, P. L., Schal, C., Wood, D. L., Blomquist, G. J., and Seybold, S. J. (1998). Endocrine regulation of *de novo* aggregation pheromone biosynthesis in the pine engraver, *Ips pini* (Say) (Coleoptera: Scolytidae). *Insect Biochem. Mol. Biol.* **28,** 705–715.

Tillman, J. A., Seybold, S. J., Jurenka, R. A., and Blomquist, G. J. (1999). Insect pheromones—An overview of biosynthesis and endocrine regulation. *Insect Biochem. Mol. Biol.* **29,** 481–514.

Tillman-Wall, J. A., Vanderwel, D., Kuenzli, M. E., Reitz, R. C., and Blomquist, G. J. (1992). Regulation of sex pheromone biosynthesis in the housefly, *Musca domestica*: Relative contribution of the elongation and reductive step. *Arch. Biochem. Biophys.* **299,** 92–99.

Phytoestrogens

ALICE L. MURKIES[*] AND MARK FRYDENBERG[†]

*Jean Hailes Centre for Women, Australia • †Monash University, Monash Medical Centre, Australia

I. INTRODUCTION
II. CLASSIFICATION AND METABOLISM
III. FOOD SOURCES AND SAFETY
IV. POTENCY AND BIOLOGICAL ACTIVITY
V. EFFECTS IN HUMANS
VI. PHYTOESTROGENS IN SPECIFIC DISEASES
VII. SUMMARY

Phytoestrogens are plant compounds with binding affinity for the estrogen receptor and consequently have estrogen-like biological activity. Phytoestrogens have physiological effects in humans that vary depending on the phytoestrogens and tissue end-points examined. The most supportive data of the beneficial effects of phytoestrogens in humans are from the effect of soy protein on lipids, lipid profiles, and blood pressure. The active moiety appears to be present in whole foods, which have a greater physiological effect than subfractions or supplements. This article examines the classification and metabolism of phytoestrogens and discusses their biological activities in humans.

I. INTRODUCTION

Historically, estrogenic activity in plants has been referred to in folk medicine. The pomegranate is associated with fertility, and hops were used by German clergy in the Middle Ages to lower fertility.

In 1923, the Allen Doisy bioassay for estrogens was published, and in 1926, plant extracts were reported to exhibit estrogenic activity. By 1975, several hundred plants were reported to have estrogenic activity on bioassay or to contain estrogenically active compounds. Phytoestrogens gained importance in the 1940s due to infertility in sheep grazing on pastures rich in subterranean clover in Western Australia later known as "clover disease."

Setchell reported measurement of urinary phytoestrogens in nonhuman primates in 1979 and in humans in 1982. Based on epidemiological studies, Adlercreutz has suggested that a diet rich in phytoestrogens as consumed by individuals in Asiatic and Mediterranean nations is associated with reduced risk of the so-called Western diseases such as breast and prostate cancer and cardiovascular disease.

Estrogenic activity has been reported in compounds produced by animals, plants, and microorganisms. Industrially manufactured chemicals, including plastics, household products, food packaging, and pesticides, such as DDT, contain weak estrogen-like compounds and are classified as xenoestrogens. These include organochlorine pesticides, polychlorinated biphenyls (PCBs), phenolic compounds, and phthlate esters. Deleterious effects of xenoestrogens have been hypothesized but not substantiated. Of concern are the long-half-life of these compounds and the persistence in fat tissue for many years. Adverse effects have been documented in wildlife but no direct evidence to show a cause and effect relationship has been reported in humans. The estrogenic potency of industrially derived estrogenic compounds is very limited, but the estrogenic potency of phytoestrogens is significant and the classification, metabolism, and biological effects in men and women and disease states will be the essence of this article.

II. CLASSIFICATION AND METABOLISM

There are three main classes of phytoestrogens found in plants or their seeds. Isoflavones and coumestans, also known as isoflavonoids, are synthesized within the plant itself. One plant can contain more than one category of phytoestrogen. The soybean contains predominantly isoflavones and the soy sprout is a rich source of coumestrol, the major coumestan. Lignans are formed from the action of gut microflora on the lignan precursors found in the plant wall. The resorcyclic acid lactones exhibit estrogenic

activity and the active metabolites, zearalenone and zearalenol, are produced by molds that contaminate cereal crops and are better described as mycoestrogens (Fig. 1).

The major isoflavones, genistein and daidzein, exist as inactive glucosides genistin and daidzin. They are also derived from their respective methyl ethers biochanin A and formononetin and after breakdown by intestinal glucosidases are converted to genistein and daidzein. Daidzein can be further metabolized to equol and O-desmethylangiolensin (O-DMA).

The estrogenically active lignans enterodiol and enterolactone are derived from secoisolariciresinol and matairesinol plant precursors found in the aleuronic layer of the grain close to the fiber layer. Enterodiol can be oxidized to enterolactone.

In humans, after consumption of plant isoflavones and lignans, complex enzymatic metabolic conversions occur in the gastrointestinal tract by the microflora, resulting in the formation of heterocyclic polyphenols similar in structure to estrogen (Fig. 2). The absorbed phytoestrogen metabolites undergo enterohepatic circulation and may be excreted in the bile, deconjugated by intestinal flora, reabsorbed, reconjugated by the liver, and excreted in the urine.

Phytoestrogen metabolites have been measured predominantly in urine, in trace amounts in feces, and also in semen, bile, saliva, and breast milk. Measurement of urinary phytoestrogen excretion is considered a reliable indication of dietary phytoestrogen intake. Concentrations of metabolites can vary within individuals even in a controlled setting of isoflavone and lignan supplements. This is attributed to the variation in metabolism determined by gastrointestinal flora, antibiotic use, bowel disease, and concomitant dietary intake of fiber, fruit, and vegetables. Similarly, dietary fat, fiber, protein, alcohol, and micronutrients may affect endogenous estrogen metabolism.

Little is known about the metabolism of coumestans in humans.

III. FOOD SOURCES AND SAFETY

The isoflavones that exhibit estrogenic activity occur almost exclusively in legumes and beans, predominantly the soybean, and in derivative products that contain most or all of the bean.

Second-generation soy foods are produced by adding soy to other manufactured foods and thereby reducing the original isoflavone content, for example, soy yogurt and soy noodles. Lignans are widely

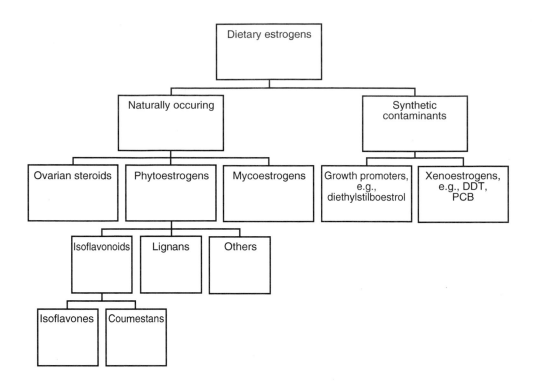

FIGURE 1 Sources and classification of dietary estrogens. Reprinted from Murkies, A.L., Wilcox, G., and Davis, S.R. Clinical review 92: Phytoestrogens. *J. Clin. Endocrinol. Metab.* **83**, 297–303, 1998, with permission. Copyright The Endocrine Society.

distributed in cereals, fruit, vegetables, and seeds, with the highest concentration in flaxseed.

Coumestans occur predominantly with germination, for example, in sprouting beans and fodder crops.

Resorcyclic acid lactone metabolites are produced by *Fusarium* species of mold found growing on crops stored under damp conditions. The compounds are concentrated in the seed hull and are predominantly removed in food processing.

Variation in phytoestrogen content in food can occur due to seasonal variation, genetic differences in plants, infection with fungal diseases, processing, and as part of the plant's defense mechanism.

Promotion of foodstuffs reported to contain a fixed phytoestrogen concentration cannot be substantiated because isoflavone content varies widely between strains in different soybean varieties and between locations of grown soybeans. Soy-enriched breads display a wide range of isoflavone content, from two- to threefold, within and between breads. Due to the natural variation of phytoestrogen concentration, it is probably not prudent for consumption of these foods to be based on isoflavone content alone in the belief that these are constant doses. Products

derived from the whole bean such as soy flour, tofu, and soy milk have the highest concentration of isoflavones.

Phytoestrogens are considered beneficial rather than harmful to humans despite evidence from a number of animal species that phytoestrogen consumption can interfere with reproductive development and function. Observations of Asian societies that have consumed a phytoestrogen-rich diet for centuries and appear not to have any deleterious effects have led to a presumption that phytoestrogens may be safe. Consideration of the safety of phytoestrogens introduced into the adult diet is not unreasonable as up to 60% of processed foods may contain soy derivatives.

Macrobiotics and other vegetarians have the highest excretion values of lignans. Asian populations ares estimated to consume 20–150 mg/day of isoflavones, with a mean of 40 mg from tofu and miso. This can be achieved in Western diets with consumption of modest quantities of soy foods. Consumption of isoflavones in the United States has been estimated at < 1 mg/day. It has been shown that 50 mg isoflavone consumption is sufficient to have endocrine effects in females and it appears that the dose,

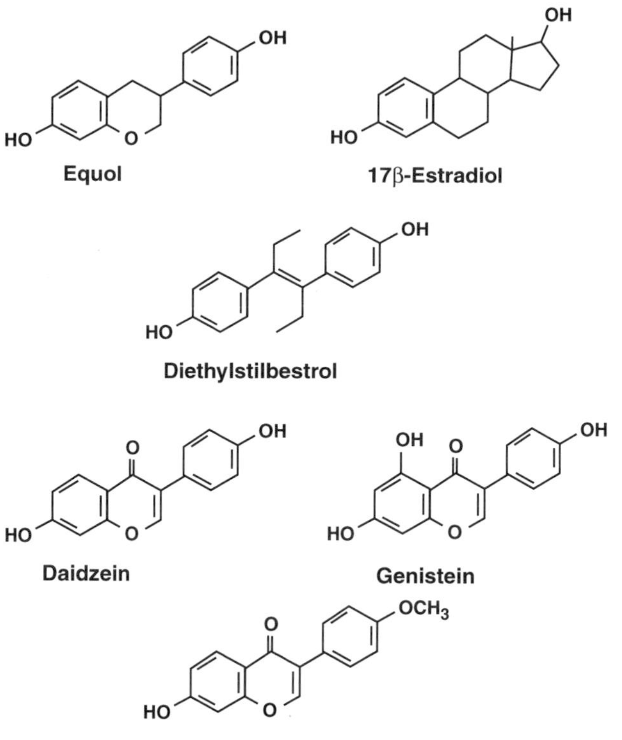

FIGURE 2 A comparison of the chemical structure of the phytoestrogen equol, genistein and daidzein, which are formed in the gastrointestinal tract of humans and animals, 17β-estradiol, and diethylstilbestrol. Reprinted from Setchell, K. D. *et al.* (1984). Non-steroidal estrogens of dietary origin: Possible roles in hormone dependent disease. *Am. J. Clin. Nutr.* 40, 569–578, Reproduced with permission by the *American Journal of Clinical Nutrition* © Am. J. Clin. Nutr. American Society for Clinical Nutrition.

duration, and timing of exposure of intake will influence clinical and biological outcomes.

IV. POTENCY AND BIOLOGICAL ACTIVITY

The biological potencies of phytoestrogens vary greatly. The majority of the compounds are nonsteroidal in structure and vastly less potent than synthetic estrogens (10^{-2} to 10^{-5}). The potency determined by human cell culture bioassays varies with species, routes of administration, and tissue end-points used. With estradiol arbitrarily given the value of 100, the relative potencies of estrogenic isoflavonoids are as follows: coumestrol 0.202; genistein 0.084; equol 0.061; daidzein 0.013; and formononetin 0.0006.

More recently, the relative binding affinity of phytoestrogens to estrogen receptor-α (ER-α) and ER-β has been determined with the relative binding affinity of estradiol arbitrarily assigned at 100.

Observations are comparable with the human cell culture bioassays, with coumestrol being the most potent. Relative binding affinities to ER-α and ER-β, respectively, are as follows: coumestrol 94 and 185; genistein 5 and 36, with a stronger binding affinity of phytoestrogens to ER-β.

A. Estrogenic Activity, Anti-estrogenic Activity, and Other Biological Properties

Varying physiological effects of individual phytoestrogens highlight the complexity of response of the estrogen receptor. Ligands for ER-α and ER-β can act as estrogen agonists, as antagonists, or as partial or selective agonists/antagonists, depending on the tissue receptors, co-regulators, and the interaction on estrogen-regulated genes. Knowledge of the effects of individual phytoestrogens is limited. Genistein is reported to bind in a manner similar to that observed for 17β-estradiol within the three-dimensional structure of the estrogen receptor-β ligand-binding domain. However, the ER-β–genistein complex induces a distinct orientation in the transactivation helix that is not agonist but partial agonist so that the transcriptional response to certain ligands is attenuated. A diagrammatic representation of the receptor sites for ER-α and ER-β in the human body is seen in Fig. 3.

Adverse estrogenic effects have been observed in animals. Reproductive disturbances observed in sheep in 1946 were attributed to the estrogenic effect of the fodder crop. In some but not all studies, estrogenic effects are seen in laboratory animals, with isoflavones stimulating uterine growth. In contrast, genistein administered with estradiol functions as an anti-estrogen, decreasing uterine estradiol uptake in animal models.

Genistein *in vitro* has been shown to exert both proliferative (estrogenic) and anti-proliferative (anti-estrogenic) effects in human cell lines. In the human ER$^+$ MCF-7 breast cancer cell line, the effects are biphasic with stimulation at low concentrations of genistein (10^{-5} to 10^{-8} M) and inhibition at higher concentrations (10^{-4} to 10^{-5} M), the latter probably not mediated via the estrogen receptor. At low concentrations, genistein competes with estradiol for binding to the ER with a 50% inhibition concentration of 5×10^{-7} M, and it stimulates the expression of pS2mRNA, a specific marker of ER-mediated estrogen-like activity. Similar stimulatory effects have been shown with daidzein, equol, and enterolactone.

Most studies to date indicate induction of DNA synthesis in tumor cell lines at concentrations close to

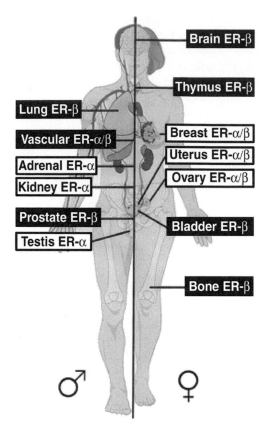

FIGURE 3 Simplified diagram illustrating the anatomical distribution of the newly described estrogen receptor ER-β to sites that are specific targets where classical estrogen replacement is beneficial. Reprinted from Setchell, K.D.R., and Cassidy, A. (1999). Dietary isoflavones: Biological effects and relevance to human health. *J. Nutr.* **129**, S758–S767, with permission from the American Society for Nutritional Sciences.

probable plasma levels in humans, achieved when consuming a high isoflavone intake, and inhibition only at very high concentrations, not achievable by diet.

Isoflavones exhibit anti-carcinogenic activity *in vivo*. Laboratory animals fed soy-fortified diets have less breast tumor proliferation after stimulation with direct and indirect tumor-inducing agents, N-methyl-N-nitrosurea and dimethylbenz(a)anthracene, respectively.

Anti-proliferative effects are demonstrated *in vitro* and appear to be independent of the estrogen receptor. Genistein and possibly other phytoestrogens interfere with the tyrosine kinase activity of activated growth factor receptors and cytoplasmic tyrosine kinases that are essential for transduction of mitogenic signals and hence inhibit tumor growth. Genistein inhibits

epidermal growth factor-receptor (EGF-R) tyrosine autophosphorylation or alternatively exerts inhibitory effects downstream from EGF-R tyrosine autophosphorylation by some other mechanism.

Genistein has been reported to inhibit topoisomerase II, an essential nuclear enzyme involved in DNA replication, and this may result in cell cycle arrest.

Isoflavones exhibit other biological properties *in vitro* and inhibit angiogenesis, cell cycle progression, and aromatase enzyme activity, stimulate sex hormone-binding globulin (SHBG) synthesis, may decrease bioavailable endogenous estrogen, and have antioxidant properties and digitalis-like activity.

V. EFFECTS IN HUMANS

A. Infants

Soy infant formulas contain significantly high levels of daidzein and genistein. Large quantities of phytoestrogens were identified in the plasma and urine in human neonates, raising concerns about possible effects on neuroendocrine developmental processes. This probably arises as neonates have reduced intestinal degradation of the ingested isoflavones and frequent feeds. Cows' milk has been shown to contain isoflavones at low concentrations. A retrospective cohort study examining the association between infant exposure and health in adult life has found that exposure to soy does not appear to lead to different general or reproductive outcomes than cows' milk. This is reassuring about the safety of infant soy formulas.

B. Premenopausal Women

A cyclic pattern of lignan excretion was observed in the menstrual cycle of the vervet monkey and also in humans. Controlled intervention studies with dietary phytoestrogens have shown endocrine-modulating effects with increased cycle length in premenopausal women. Sixty grams of soy protein daily has been reported to increase follicular phase length and to suppress the midcycle follicle-stimulating hormone (FSH) and luteinizing hormone (LH) surges. Thirty-six ounces (1000 ml) of soy milk daily has been reported to decrease serum 17β-estradiol and luteal-phase serum progesterone in young ovulating women. Daily intake of flaxseed at 10 g per day increases luteal-phase length with no difference in follicular phase in normally cycling women. SHBG was not increased in these studies. Supplementation with 60 g soy/day increases breast epithelium proliferation in premenopausal women.

C. Postmenopausal Women

Epidemiological studies comparing Asian and Western populations have suggested that consuming a phytoestrogen-rich diet may ameliorate the symptoms of estrogen deficiency, such as hot flashes at menopause. However, intervention studies have shown no benefit from phytoestrogens as an alternative to hormone therapy in postmenopausal women.

In 1990, mild estrogenic effects in the vaginal-cell maturation index of postmenopausal women were first reported after supplementation with 45 g soy flour for 6 weeks. Subsequent studies have failed to demonstrate a correlation between vaginal-cell estrogenic response and vasomotor symptoms. Also, a strong placebo effect has been noted. Some studies have reported a reduction in hot flashes upon supplementation with soy versus placebo but the effects have not been dramatic. A controlled trial of wheat versus soy unexpectedly found that wheat-supplemented women showed a significant reduction in hot flashes after 3 months and had low urinary isoflavones. These studies highlight the difficulties in treating hot flashes over time due to their natural resolution. The differences in response could be attributed to varying soy products used, study design, and individual variability in response. Specific dosages and formulations cannot be recommended.

Data on the effect of phytoestrogens on serum estradiol FSH, and LH concentrations are also variable. Isoflavone supplements have no benefit beyond placebo for reduction in hot flashes and no effect on plasma hormones including SHBG and FSH.

Phytoestrogens have no effect on the other symptoms of menopause, such as arthralgia, myalgia, headaches, and anxiety, which comprise part of the Kupperman index.

D. Men

Exposure to compounds with estrogenic activity has been postulated to be responsible for adverse changes in male reproductive health, including declining sperm counts, increase in testicular cancer, and testicular genital malformations although currently there are no definitive studies. Data are limited; however, intervention studies in males fed textured vegetable protein or soy protein isolate report no change in serum testosterone.

VI. PHYTOESTROGENS IN SPECIFIC DISEASES

A. Cardiovascular Disease

Vegetarians and individuals in Asian countries have a reduced risk of cardiovascular disease compared with individuals in Western nations, and Adlercreutz suggested that this may be partly attributable to phytoestrogen consumption. Dietary intake of vegetable protein, particularly soy, is associated with decreased cardiovascular disease risk.

1. Lipid Profiles

Intervention studies with soy-supplemented diets indicate that cardiovascular disease benefits may result from improved lipoprotein profiles. It is not known whether the effects are derived from the soy protein isoflavone or other nonphytoestrogen components of soy such as saponins, from fiber, or from a combination of the two. Limited data suggest that soy subfractions are not as effective at decreasing cardiovascular disease risk factors.

Soy in which substantial portions of the isoflavones and saponins are extracted by alcohol is described as isoflavone deplete (soy −) and has been used in primate models and compared with soy protein with isoflavones intact (soy +), to help identify the active moiety in soy protein. Studies in primates and humans overall report a beneficial effect in lipid profile of soy + supplementation comparable with studies of estrogen. Since 1977, soy has been reported as a treatment for hypercholesterolemia. A meta-analysis of 38 published controlled clinical trials of soy protein consumption in humans that averaged 47 g/day and serum lipoprotein concentrations found that soy protein consumption was significantly associated with mean reductions in total cholesterol [9.3% (− 0.6 mmol/liter) decrease, 95% CI 0.35–0.85 mmol/liter], LDL cholesterol [12.9% (− 0.5 mmol/liter) decrease, 95% CI 0.30–0.82 mmol/liter], and triglycerides [10.5% (− 0.15 mmol/liter) decrease, 95% CI 0.003–0.29 mmol/liter], with little change in HDL concentration. The degree of cholesterol reduction is similar to that observed with dietary intervention of plant-based foods such as oat bran and garlic. The hypocholesterolemic effect is more profound in men and women with elevated cholesterol, with only marginal benefit for those with a normal baseline lipid profile.

For example, a soybean protein diet in subjects with type II hyperlipoproteinemia may lower cholesterol on average by 20%. Ingestion of 60 g/day of soy protein isolate by normocholesterolemic men resulted in no change in plasma lipids. Ingestion of 40 g soy supplementation in normocholesterolemic men and women resulted in decreases in triglycerides and an increase in lipoprotein Lp(a) by 15%.

Although results from individual studies are variable and dependent on the original serum cholesterol levels, the Food and Drug Administration approval for labeling of soy foods states "included in the daily diet, they may reduce heart disease."

2. Blood Pressure

Soy supplementation is reported to lower blood pressure in normotensive individuals. In a study of normotensive men and postmenopausal women, 3 months of 40 g daily soy supplementation significantly reduced systolic (2.4 mm Hg lower), diastolic (3.9 mm Hg lower), and mean blood pressure (BP) (4.2 mm Hg lower) compared with the casein-fed placebo group. These changes are greater than reported with dietary intervention alone. Soy supplementation in nonhypercholesterolemic, nonhypertensive, perimenopausal women resulted in a significant decline in diastolic BP (5 mm Hg lower) in the 20 g twice daily soy diet compared with the placebo diet. In contrast, concentrated phytoestrogen supplements did not alter BP in normotensive subjects. This highlights the discrepancy of phytoestrogen doses, the consumption of soy protein in preference to extracts, and the possibility of the hypotensive effect being mediated by nonestrogenic mechanisms.

3. Vascular Compliance and Endothelial Function

ER-β has been shown to be the primary estrogen receptor in the vessel wall and is up-regulated in response to vascular injury. Interest has focused on whether soy has vascular effects similar to those of estrogen. Studies of rhesus monkeys support a reduction in atheromatous plaque with isoflavone-intact soy supplementation and enhanced dilator responses of atherosclerotic coronary arteries to acetylcholine in female monkeys, improving blood vessel dilation and consequent blood flow.

However, a large study of both men and women consuming soy protein reported no beneficial effect on arterial compliance. Two small studies in peri- and postmenopausal women, with no male subjects included, have reported improved systemic arterial compliance of 26% in concentrated phytoestrogen supplements.

Brachial flow-mediated vasodilation (FMD) is a strong predictor of coronary endothelial dysfunction. In the larger previous study, soy supplementation had no effect on FMD in healthy postmenopausal women and unexpectedly reduced FMD in males. In comparison, estrogen administration does not improve FMD in healthy adult males or improve endothelial-dependent vasodilation in the male monkey model.

A small study of postmenopausal women supplemented with an 80 mg phytoestrogen tablet similarly reported no improvement of FMD.

Cross-sectional data from postmenopausal women indicated that women with high genistein intake had a significantly lower body mass index (P-trend = 0.05), waist circumference (P-trend = 0.05), and fasting insulin level (P-trend = 0.07) than those with no daily genistein consumption. Similarly, a population-based cohort of midlife women found that women with a high intake of isoflavones, >40 mg/day, derived from diet were more likely to exercise, were less likely to smoke, had a lower mean body mass index, and observed lifestyle factors that were associated with reduced cardiovascular disease risk.

Dietary soy phytoestrogens may provide cardio-protection via direct lipid effects; however, the response pattern does not follow that of estrogen with respect to BP responses, lipoprotein changes, and vascular function effects and not all effects are beneficial, in particular, elevated lipoprotein Lp(a) and reduced FMD in males. The mechanisms of action are still uncertain. Isoflavones, especially genistein, in vitro are reported to have anti-atherogenic properties and inhibit the process of coagulation, a key promoter of plaque formation, by inhibition of growth factors such as platelet-derived growth factor and inhibition of tyrosine kinase activity, an enzyme central to thrombin formation and inflammation in general. Genistein is the most potent antioxidant of the isoflavones in soy protein.

In summary, phytoestrogens have beneficial effects for cardiovascular disease risk via lipid reduction, particularly in hypercholesterolemic men and women, and reduction in blood pressure in normotensive men and women with no overall beneficial effect on arterial compliance or endothelial function in adult males. Individuals that consume phytoestrogens have healthy lifestyle factors that are preventative of cardiovascular disease.

B. Cancer

The incidence of hormone-dependent cancers is lower among vegetarians and in Asia and Eastern Europe than in Western countries. Breast, ovarian, prostate, and colon cancers show a negative correlation with cereal and phytoestrogen intake when cancer mortality rates and food availability data between countries are compared.

1. Breast Cancer

Some epidemiological studies have suggested an association between high phytoestrogen intake and reduced breast cancer risk. Studies of urinary phytoestrogen excretion in women immediately after diagnosis of breast cancer have shown lower equol, enterolactone, and daidzein excretion in women with breast cancer than in controls, despite similar dietary patterns.

Japanese immigrants to North America have a higher incidence of breast cancer than their counterparts in Japan, with a higher incidence of cancer the younger the age of migration. Such findings support the role of environmental factors in the etiology of breast cancer.

Studies have shown conflicting results. A significant graded inverse association in Japanese women has been reported between risk of breast cancer and consumption of miso (soybean paste soup). A diet high in soy products conferred a low risk of breast cancer in premenopausal women in Singapore, with no effect observed in postmenopausal women. A Chinese study reported no association between soy and breast cancer but did find an inverse correlation between fiber and other nutrient intake and breast cancer rates. Similarly, a progressive reduction in relative risk of breast cancer with each quintile of increasing fiber intake for women has been reported in Australian women. Lower levels of ER-α^+ cells have been shown in normal breast tissue in Japanese women, 9% compared with white Australian women ($>17\%$ for those over 50 years and 12% for those <50 years), and this may contribute to ethnic differences in breast cancer rates.

Isoflavones have been reported to have protective effects in animal models of experimentally induced breast cancer, measured by tumor number, incidence, metastasis, and latency. It may be that prepubertal exposure may confer greater protection by precocious maturation of breast terminal end buds. Breast cancer cell line studies have shown that at low concentrations (equivalent to levels measured in humans consuming a 40 mg isoflavone supplement) genistein stimulates ER$^+$ cells with no effect on ER$^-$ cells. Consistent with these findings, soy supplementation stimulates breast epithelium proliferation in premenopausal women. Genistein at high concentrations, beyond that achieved by diet, inhibits the growth of ER$^+$ and ER$^-$ cell lines. Genistein in cell studies has

been shown to antagonize the anti-estrogenic effect of tamoxifen, and caution is advised regarding supplements in women with breast cancer.

Phytoestrogens have estrogenic effects on the breast and larger long-term studies are needed before concentrated supplements can be safely recommended.

2. Prostate Cancer

Men in Asia were found to have a higher concentration of isoflavones, equol, and daidzein in plasma and prostatic fluid than their counterparts in Europe. This led to the speculation that phytoestrogens may be protective of prostate cancer. Epidemiological studies have reported an association between consumption of lentils, peas, tomatoes, and dried fruits and decreased prostate cancer in 14,000 Seventh Day Adventist men. A study of Japanese immigrants to North America has shown an increased incidence in prostate cancer, the younger the age at migration, supporting the hypothesis of environmental factors, including diet, having an impact on cancer risk.

In the rodent model, an isoflavone-rich diet reduced the incidence of prostate-related cancer and prolonged the disease-free interval by 27%. The effects were observed only when the rodents were fed soy prior to the exposure of cancer, indicating that early exposure to soy supplementation may protect against prostate cancer in later life.

It is plausible that the effects of genistein are mediated via ER-β, in view of the greater affinity of genistein to ER-β versus ER-α and the high levels of ER-β found in the prostate. In human prostate cancer cell lines, high concentrations of genistein and biochanin A inhibit the growth of androgen-dependent cells. In vitro high levels of genistein inhibit 5α-reductase and 17β-hydroxysteroid dehydrogenase in genital skin fibroblasts and prostatic tissue. These two enzymes are involved in androgen and estrogen synthesis. Genistein inhibits the growth of prostatic cells from benign prostatic hypertrophy and prostate cancer cells in histoculture in a dose-dependent manner. In addition, genistein inhibits tyrosine kinase and topoisomerase, which are crucial to cellular proliferation.

Phytoestrogen supplementation with a 160 mg (4 × 40 mg) isoflavone equivalent, made from red clover, was taken for 7 days prior to surgery for an infiltrating low-grade adenocarcinoma of the prostate in one subject. At surgery, the prostatectomy specimen showed a moderately high-grade adenocarcinoma with patchy microvacuolation and prominent apoptosis typical of a response to prior estrogen therapy. Decreased serum testosterone, decreased serum prostate-specific antigen, and altered sexual behavior have been demonstrated in men who were administered an herbal remedy containing phytoestrogens used as treatment for prostate cancer. Further intervention studies are currently being conducted.

C. Osteoporosis

Osteoporosis is related to a number of factors including genetics, aging, hormone deficiency, and diet. Epidemiological studies have shown reduced rates of osteoporosis in Asian women compared with Western women and phytoestrogens have been postulated as a protective factor although many other factors could account for these findings. *In vitro* cell culture has shown that phytoestrogens inhibit osteoclasts and may stimulate osteoblasts. *In vivo* animal studies suggest that in high enough doses, dietary soybean prevents bone loss in ovariectomized rats.

ER-β has been identified in bone and its ligand specificity toward phytoestrogens has been reported. Isoflavones appear to have an effect on osteoblasts via the ER, whereas the effects on osteoclast appear to be non-ER-mediated, such as growth factor activity and cytokine activity. There are limited human studies. Postmenopausal women supplemented with casein, soy protein, or soy protein fortified with isoflavores for 6 months demonstrated increased bone mineral content and density in the spine in the soy fortified group alone compared with controls. Forty-five grams of soy-enriched bread improved bone mineral content in postmenopausal women compared with controls. Long-term data on the efficacy and safety of ipriflavone for prevention of postmenopausal bone loss have been conflicting. Ipriflavone (7-isopropoxy-isoflavone), a synthetic flavonoid, inhibits osteoclast function and 600 mg/day has been reported to prevent bone loss at the distal radius in postmenopausal women. More recently, a 4-year study of 474 postmenopausal women randomly assigned ipriflavone at 200 mg three times per day or placebo found no difference in bone loss prevention and in biochemical markers of bone metabolism. Long-term studies are needed before the role of phytoestrogens in the prevention of osteoporosis can be supported.

VII. SUMMARY

Cancer research is still in its infancy. The epidemiological and animal data suggest that phytoestrogens may play a beneficial role in breast and prostate cancer. It may be that prepubertal exposure is of importance and ingestion needs to be lifelong. Extrapolations from cell line and animal studies need to be viewed with caution. It is probably naive to attribute many health outcomes to one food, and other lifestyle factors, such as exercise, substance abuse, and the diet as a whole, may be relevant.

In contrast to animal studies in which deleterious effects were observed with consumption of a phytoestrogen diet, in humans few adverse effects are observed. In humans, a genetic tolerance may have evolved in nations with a high-soy-intake diet or the varied human diet may be protective of one food group alone dominating and causing adverse effects. The limited studies to date have confirmed that diet can have significant hormonal effects and these may be of benefit in preventing some of the common diseases. Global nutrition is an increasing problem and further knowledge from scientific studies of plant-based foods is warranted.

Glossary

coumestans A potent subgroup of phytoestrogens found in fodder crops.
daidzein An isoflavone metabolite derived from daidzin by gastrointestinal bacteria.
enterodiol A lignan metabolite derived by gastrointestinal bacteria.
enterolactone A lignan metabolite derived by gastrointestinal bacteria.
genistein An isoflavone metabolite derived by gastrointestinal bacteria from genistin.
isoflavones A subgroup of phytoestrogens derived from legumes, e.g., soybean.
lignans A subgroup of phytoestrogens found in vegetables, fruits, nuts, and seeds.
phytoestrogen A plant compound with binding affinity for the estrogen receptor.

See Also the Following Articles

Estrogen and Progesterone Receptors in Breast Cancer
• Estrogen in the Male • Estrogen Receptor Actions through Other Transcription Factor Sites • Estrogen Receptor-α Structure and Function • Estrogen Receptor-β Structure and Function • Follicle Stimulating Hormone (FSH)
• Lipoprotein Receptor Signaling • Luteinizing Hormone (LH) • Sex Hormone-Binding Globulin (SHBG)

Further Reading

Adlercreutz, H. (1990). Western diet and Western diseases: Some hormonal and biochemical mechanisms and associations. *Scand. J. Clin. Lab. Invest.* 50(Suppl.), 2103–2123.
Alexandersen, P., Toussaint, A., Christiansen, C., Devogelaer, J. P., Roux, C., Fechtenbaum, J., Gennari, C., and Reginster, J. Y. (2001). Ipriflavone in the treatment of postmenopausal

osteoporosis: A randomized controlled trial. *J. Am. Med. Assoc.* **285**(11), 1482–1488.

Clarkson, T. B., Antony, M. S., and Hughes, C. L. (1995). Estrogenic soybean isoflavones and chronic disease risk and benefits. *Trends Endocrinol. Metab.* **6**, 11–16.

Consensus Opinion (2000). The role of isoflavones in menopausal health: Consensus opinion of the North American Menopause Society. *Menopause* **7**, 215–229.

Davis, S. R., Dalais, F. S., Simpson, E. R., and Murkies, A. L. (1999). Phytoestrogens in health and disease. *Rec. Prog. Horm. Res.* **54**, 185–210.

Di Paola, R. S., Zhang, H., Lambert, G. H., Meeker, R., Licitra, E., Rafi, M. M., Zhu, B. T., Spaulding, H., Goodin, S., Toledano, M. B., Hait, W. N., and Gallo, M. A. (1998). Clinical and biologic activity of an estrogenic herbal combination (PC-SPES) in prostate cancer. *N. Engl. J. Med.* **339**, 785–791.

Guthrie, J. R., Ball, M., Murkies, A., and Dennerstein, L. (2000). Dietary phytoestrogen intake in mid-life Australian-born women: Relationship to health variables. *Climacteric* **3**, 254–261.

Kuiper, G. G. J. M., Lemmen, J. G., Carlsson, B., Corton, J. C., Safe, S. H., van der Saag, P. T., van der Burg, B., and Gustafsson, J. (1998). Interaction of estrogenic chemicals and phytoestrogens with estrogen receptor B. *Endocrinology* **139**, 4252–4263.

Lawson, J. S., Field, A. S., Champion, S., Tran, D., Ishikura, H., and Trichopoulos, D. (1999). Low oestrogen receptor alpha expression in normal breast tissue underlies low breast cancer incidence in Japan. *Lancet* **354**, 1787–1788.

Murkies, A. L., Wilcox, G., and Davis, S. R. (1998). Clinical review 92: Phytoestrogens. *J. Clin. Endocrinol. Metab.* **83**, 297–303.

Pike, A. C., Brzozowski, A. M., Hubbard, R. E., Bonn, T., Thorsell, A. G., Engstrom, O., Ljunggren, J., Gustaffson, J. A., and Carlquist, M. (1999). Structure of the ligand-binding domain of oestrogen receptor beta in the presence of a partial agonist and a full antagonist. *EMBO J.* **18** (17), 4608–4618.

Schwartz, J. A., Liu, G., and Brooks, S. C. (1998). Genistein-mediated attenuation of tamoxifen-induced antagonism from estrogen receptor-regulated genes. *Biochem. Biophys. Res. Commun.* **253**, 38–43.

Setchell, K. D. R., and Cassidy, A. (1999). Dietary isoflavones: Biological effects and relevance to human health. *J. Nutr.* **129**, S758–S767.

Stephens, F. O. (1997). Phytoestrogens and prostate cancer: Possible preventive role. *Med. J. Aust.* **167**, 138–140.

Strom, B. L., Schinnar, R., Ziegler, E. E., Barnhart, K. T., Sammel, M. D., Macones, G. A., Stallings, V. A., Drulis, J. A., Nelson, S. E., and Hanson, S. A. (2001). Exposure to soy-based formula in infancy and endocrinological and reproductive outcomes in young adulthood. *J. Am. Med. Assoc.* **286**, 807–814.

Teede, H. J., Dalais, F. S., Kotsopoulos, D., Liang, Y., Davis, S. R., and McGrath, B. P. (2001). Dietary soy has both beneficial and potentially adverse cardiovascular effect: A placebo-controlled study in men and postmenopausal women. *J. Clin. Endocrinol. Metab.* **86**, 3053–3060.

Pilosebaceous Unit (PSU)

Dianne Deplewski

University of Chicago

I. INTRODUCTION
II. POSTNATAL GROWTH AND DEVELOPMENT OF THE PSU
III. ANDROGEN ACTION IN THE PSU
IV. ROLE OF NONANDROGENIC HORMONES IN THE PSU
V. DISORDERS OF THE PSU: HIRSUTISM, PATTERN ALOPECIA, AND ACNE VULGARIS

The pilosebaceous unit (PSU) consists of a piliary component and a sebaceous component. Each PSU has the capacity to differentiate into either a terminal hair follicle (in which a large medullated hair becomes the prominent structure) or a sebaceous follicle (in which the sebaceous gland becomes prominent and the hair remains vellus). This article provides an introduction to the role of androgens and other hormones in normal PSU development and in PSU disorders.

I. INTRODUCTION

Androgens play a key role in the development of the pilosebaceous (PSU) in most areas of the body. In androgen-sensitive areas before puberty, the hair is vellus and the sebaceous glands are small. In response to increasing levels of androgens, PSUs become large terminal hair follicles (sexual hairs) in sexual hair areas or they become sebaceous follicles (sebaceous glands) in sebaceous areas. Androgens play a role in PSU disorders, namely, hirsutism, pattern alopecia, and acne vulgaris. However, it is clear that the pathogenesis of these disorders involves more than androgen.

II. POSTNATAL GROWTH AND DEVELOPMENT OF THE PSU

A. Hair Follicle

Hair follicles vary considerably in size and shape depending on their localization in the body. Approximately 5 million hair follicles cover the human body, and this number is established before birth. New follicles are not formed after birth; however, the size of the follicles and hairs can change with time, primarily under the control of androgen. The difference in the apparent density of sexual hair between men and women is due to a different density of terminal hairs rather than a difference in the number of PSUs. Racial differences also affect various features of hair, such as shape and medullation.

Normal development and cycling of the hair follicle depend on the interaction of the follicular epithelium with the dermal papilla, which consists of specialized fibroblasts located at the base of the hair follicle. Hair grows cyclically by reverting from the anagen (growth) phase, through the catagen (shortening) phase, to the telogen (resting) phase (Fig. 1). The dynamics of the hair growth cycle vary between species, between different body sites in the same species, and between different follicle types at the same body site. It is likely that hair follicles have an intrinsic rhythmic behavior that is modulated by multiple growth factors. The duration of the anagen stage is the major determinant of the length to which a hair grows, and it varies with the location of the hair follicle. For example, scalp hairs are in anagen for a

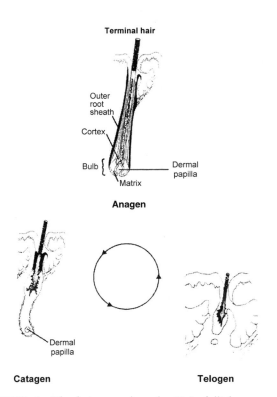

FIGURE 1 The hair growth cycle. Hair follicles progress through repetitive cycles of growth, from anagen (active phase of growth), through catagen (shortening of the hair follicle), to telogen (resting phase of the hair cycle), after which the club hair is shed, and the follicle begins a new hair cycle again. Modified from D. Deplewski and R. L. Rosenfield, Role of hormones in pilosebaceous unit development. *Endocr. Rev.* **21,** 363–392, 2000, with permission. Copyright 2000, The Endocrine Society.

long time (between 2 and 8 years) and produce long hairs, whereas mustache hairs stay in the anagen stage for only 4 months and thus produce short hairs. Other factors influencing hair growth in various areas of the body include the linear growth rate of the hair fiber, as well as the diameter and density of the terminal hairs. During the catagen phase, hair follicles go through a highly controlled process of regression and involution, caused by apoptosis (programmed cell death). This is the shortest phase of the hair growth cycle and lasts from 2 to 3 weeks. During the telogen phase, a club hair develops and is eventually shed from the follicle to make room for new hair growth. This phase lasts for 3 to 4 months. Whereas shaving does not induce hair growth, plucking a resting (telogen) hair causes an advancement in the onset of anagen and thus induces hair regrowth.

B. Sebaceous Gland

The life cycle of sebaceous cells (sebocytes) begins at the periphery of the gland in the highly mitotic basal layer. As sebaceous cells differentiate, they accumulate increasing amounts of lipid and migrate toward the central duct. Eventually, the most mature sebocytes burst and their lipid is extruded into the ducts of the sebaceous gland as the holocrine secretion sebum. The cells of sebaceous glands turn over more rapidly than those of hairs, as they are normally completely renewed every month.

III. ANDROGEN ACTION IN THE PSU

Before puberty, the androgen-dependent PSU consists of a prepubertal vellus follicle, which consists of a virtually invisible hair and a tiny sebaceous gland component (Fig. 2). Under the influence of androgens produced at adrenarche and then puberty, these PSUs differentiate in a distinctive pattern that depends on their location. In the sexual hair areas, a terminal hair follicle develops and the sebaceous gland develops only moderately. In acne-prone areas, androgen causes the prepubertal vellus follicle to develop into a sebaceous follicle in which the hair remains vellus and the sebaceous gland enlarges tremendously. In the balding-prone area of the scalp, PSUs respond to androgen in yet a different manner in individuals predisposed to pattern alopecia. Terminal hair follicles that previously grew without androgen gradually change with each growth cycle to an intermediate kind of follicle in which the hair component reverts to the vellus state, leaving an adult vellus follicle. Hair follicles are still present and cycling, even in

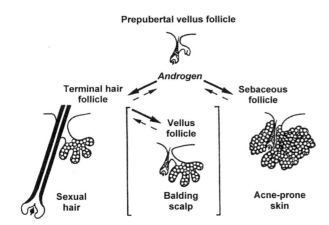

Prepubertal vellus follicle

Androgen

Terminal hair follicle

Sebaceous follicle

Vellus follicle

Sexual hair

Balding scalp

Acne-prone skin

FIGURE 2 Role of androgen in the development of the pilosebaceous unit. Solid lines indicate the effects of androgen; dashed lines indicate the effects of anti-androgens. Hairs are depicted only in the anagen (growing) phase of the growth cycle. In balding scalp (bracketed area) terminal hairs not previously dependent on androgen regress to vellus hairs under the influence of androgen. Reprinted from *Am. J. Med.* **98**, R. L. Rosenfield and D. Deplewski, Role of androgens in the developmental biology of the pilosebaceous unit. pp. 80S–88S. Copyright 1995, with permission from Excerpta Medica Inc.

bald scalp. These phenomena are reversed by anti-androgens: both types of androgen-dependent PSUs revert toward the prepubertal state. The fact that individual PSUs can respond differently to the same circulating hormones illustrates the complexity of the response of the PSU to androgen.

The most direct evidence that androgens are the principal hormones controlling sexual hair growth is that androgens stimulate hair growth in eunuchs and castration reduces hair growth. The latter classic observation illustrates the pliable nature of the PSU response to androgens, i.e., the reversion from terminal to vellus follicles. The sensitivity of PSUs to androgen is determined by their pattern of distribution and generally wanes from pubis to head (Fig. 3). Thus, rising androgen levels recruit an increasing proportion of PSUs in a given area to initiate the growth of terminal hair follicles, each in accordance with its preset genetic sensitivity to androgen. The apparent dose–response curve to androgen is fairly steep, with a mustache typically appearing at plasma testosterone levels just slightly above the upper limits of normal for women and the beard requiring 10-fold higher levels for full growth. There is considerable individual variability. Androgens are thought to control hair growth by influencing the synthesis and release of growth factors from dermal papilla cells that act in a paracrine fashion on the other cells of the hair follicle.

The sensitivity of sebaceous glands to androgens seems to follow a different dose–response curve than the hair follicle, with most sebaceous glands being highly and similarly sensitive to testosterone. Sebum production is at its nadir at approximately 4 years of age and begins to increase between 8 and 11 years of age. Microcomedones (1 mm or less in diameter), which form when desquamated cornified cells of the upper canal of the sebaceous follicle become abnormally adherent and form a plug in the follicular canal, make their appearance in approximately 40% of 8- to 10-year-olds. Thus, sebaceous gland function begins approximately coincident with adrenarche, before true puberty, at levels of androgen below those ordinarily required for the initiation of pubic hair growth (Fig. 4). Seventy-five percent of the normal male amount of sebaceous gland function is achieved at androgen levels normal for women. There is considerable individual variability in the degree of sebum production to a given level of androgen.

It is not yet clear what controls the nature of the response of a PSU to androgen; however, the variability in PSU responsiveness may be related in part to variations in androgen metabolism. Enzymes important in androgen metabolism in skin are shown in Fig. 5. Two forms of 5α-reductase, which are differentially expressed in various tissues, exist. The type 2 isozyme is important for most androgen actions in sexual organs; however, the type 1 isozyme is the major form of 5α-reductase in skin. The activity of 5α-reductase has been found to be higher in

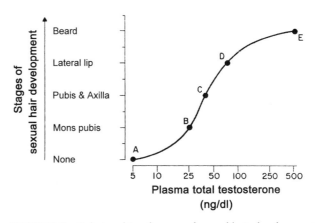

FIGURE 3 Relationship of stages of sexual hair development to testosterone as a representative plasma androgen. Note logarithmic scale for testosterone. (A) Prepubertal; (B) stage 3 pubic hair: (C) stage 5 pubic hair: (D) moderate hirsutism; (E) adult male. Reprinted from Rosenfield, R. L. (1986). Pilosebaceous physiology in relation to hirsutism and acne. *Clin. Endocrinol. Metab.* **15**, 341–362, with permission.

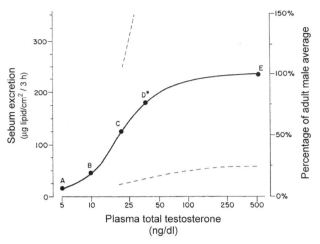

FIGURE 4 Relationship between sebum output and testosterone as a representative plasma androgen. Note the logarithmic scale for testosterone. Dashed lines show the normal range of sebum excretion. (A) 4-year-old children; (B) 7- to 11-year-old prepubertal children; (C) castrated man; (D) 20- to 40-year-old normal adult women; (E) 20- to 40-year-old normal adult men. *Average sebum level of normal 15- to 19-year-old boys and girls. Reprinted from Rosenfield, R. L. (1986). Pilosebaceous physiology in relation to hirsutism and acne. *Clin. Endocrinol. Metab.* 15, 341–362, with permission.

sebaceous glands of the scalp and facial skin (acne-prone skin) than in other skin areas. However, no obvious difference in type 1 isozyme expression has been found between balding and nonbalding areas of adult scalp. In contrast, greater 3β-hydroxysteroid dehydrogenase activity has been found in sebaceous glands from balding scalp than in those from nonbalding scalp. Table 1 depicts the characteristic pattern of androgen metabolism in skin. A summary of the localization of the mediators of androgen signal transduction in the PSU is provided in Table 2.

IV. ROLE OF NONANDROGENIC HORMONES IN THE PSU

In addition to androgen, other hormones including estrogen, growth hormone, insulin-like growth

$$\mathbf{DHEA} \xrightarrow{\mathbf{3\beta\text{-}HSD}} \mathbf{AD} \xleftrightarrow{\mathbf{17\beta\text{-}HSD}} \mathbf{T} \xrightarrow{\mathbf{5\alpha\text{-}R}} \mathbf{DHT}$$

FIGURE 5 Androgen metabolism in skin. The weak androgen dehydroepiandrosterone (DHEA) is metabolized to the more potent androgen dihydrotestosterone (DHT) by specific enzymes as depicted. AD, Androstenedione; T, testosterone; 3β-HSD, 3β-hydroxysteroid dehydrogenase; 17β-HSD, 17β-hydroxysteroid dehydrogenase; 5α-R, 5α-reductase.

factor-I, insulin, glucocorticoids, prolactin, thyroid hormone, retinoids, and others are well recognized to play roles in PSU growth and development, and these are summarized in Table 3.

V. DISORDERS OF THE PSU: HIRSUTISM, PATTERN ALOPECIA, AND ACNE VULGARIS

A. Hirsutism

Hirsutism is typically defined as excessive male-pattern hair growth in women. This definition distinguishes hirsutism from hypertrichosis, which is the term reserved to describe the androgen-independent growth of body hair that is vellus, prominent in nonsexual areas, and most commonly familial or caused by metabolic disorders (e.g., thyroid disturbances, anorexia nervosa, or porphyria) or medications (e.g., phenytoin, minoxidil, or cyclosporine).

B. Pattern Alopecia

Pattern alopecia is the androgen-dependent thinning of hair that occurs progressively with advancing age in genetically susceptible men and women. However, it can begin as soon as the early teenage years. The process is mainly the result of miniaturization of terminal to vellus hair follicles (Fig. 2). The androgen-dependency of pattern alopecia was initially deduced on the basis of eunuchs not suffering from male pattern hair loss unless they are given replacement testosterone. Pattern alopecia is generally thought to be distinct from the diffuse thinning of scalp hair associated with aging. However, it remains possible that pattern alopecia may partially be due to an accentuation of the normal process of hair loss associated with aging. In men, pattern alopecia typically presents as temporo-occipital pattern (male-pattern) balding. In female-pattern alopecia, the thinning typically begins with involvement of the crown of the scalp (rather than the vertex and bifrontal areas as in men) and may become fairly diffuse. Pattern alopecia can be psychologically devastating in both sexes. The genetic predisposition to pattern alopecia is still poorly understood. However, the pattern of inheritance is considered to be polygenic with variable penetrance. It is likely that the penetrance is greatly determined by the height of the plasma androgen level.

Minoxidil and finasteride are hormonal treatments for pattern alopecia. Minoxidil induces and prolongs the anagen stage and converts vellus follicles to terminal follicles. Finasteride inhibits type 2 5α-reductase, which converts testosterone to DHT.

TABLE 1   Pattern of Androgen Metabolism within Skin Organelles of Axilla and Scalp

	Relative enzyme activity (percentage of total)		
	5α-Reductase ($n = 8-10$)	17β-HSD ($n = 6-16$)	3β-HSD ($n = 2$)
Sebaceous gland	17	21	⎫
Hair follicle	8	15	⎬ 50
Sweat gland	60	47	40
Dermis	9	6	8
Epidermis	6	11	2
Total	100	100	100

Note. Regional differences in enzyme activity between axilla and scalp may exist. 17β-HSD, 17β-hydroxysteroid dehydrogenase; 3β-HSD, 3β-hydroxysteroid dehydrogenase. Reprinted from D. Deplewski and R. L. Rosenfield, Role of hormones in pilosebaceous unit development, *Endocr. Rev.* 21, 363–392, 2000, with permission. Copyright 2000, The Endocrine Society.

Finasteride inhibits miniaturization of hairs, converts vellus follicles to terminal follicles, and prolongs the anagen stage in androgen-dependent scalp follicles. Typically, 9 to 12 months of treatment is needed to judge the efficacy of a given treatment on hair growth, because of the long duration of the hair growth cycle. Unfortunately, simply removing androgens does not usually cause a significant conversion of miniaturized vellus follicles to terminal follicles; thus, current treatments for pattern alopecia are less than optimal.

C. Acne Vulgaris

Sebum, the holocrine secretion of sebaceous glands, plays a central role in the pathogencsis of acne vulgaris. Acne occurs at the onset of puberty when plasma androgen levels rise, peaks at midpuberty, and usually resolves by the mid-20s. Virtually all adolescents have at least a few open and closed comedones, which are noninflammatory enlarged sebaceous follicular ducts known as blackheads and whiteheads, respectively. Androgens are an incitant of acne vulgaris since they are necessary for the growth and differentiation of sebaceous glands.

Dehydroepiandrosterone sulfate (DHEAS) plays a role in acne through its conversion to more potent androgens that stimulate sebum production. Plasma DHEAS is likely the most important androgen for the initiation of comedonal acne in early puberty, as it rises first. Excessive DHT formation in skin has also been implicated in the pathogenesis of acne vulgaris, suggesting that the activity of 5α-reductase may also play an important role.

There is more to acne than sebaceous gland growth and sebum production: abnormal sebaceous duct keratinization, bacterial colonization with *Propionibacterium acnes*, and host immune response factors are also important. The pathogenesis of acne is thought by most to commence with plugging of the outlet of the sebaceous gland with desquamated cornified cells of the upper canal of the follicle. The more severe stages of acne are the consequences of obstruction and impaction, with bacterial secondary infection of static sebum occurring in an anaerobic environment. A closed comedone takes 2 months to form from its precursor lesion, the microcomedone. Inflammatory acne, consisting of papules, pustules, nodules, and cysts, is a later phenomenon that develops from comedonal acne.

TABLE 2   Androgen Mechanism of Action in the Pilosebaceous Unit

Parameter	Sebaceous gland		Sexual hair	
	Stroma	Sebocytes	Dermal papilla	Hair epithelium
3β-HSD	?	+++	?	±
17β-HSD	?	+++	Type 3	Type 2
5α-Reductase	?	Type 1	Type 2	Type 1
Androgen receptor	+	++++	++++	±

Note. 3β-HSD, 3β-hydroxysteroid dehydrogenase; 17β-HSD, 17β-hydroxysteroid dehydrogenase. Reprinted from D. Deplewski and R. L. Rosenfield, Role of hormones in pilosebaceous unit development, *Endocr. Rev.* 21, 363–392, 2000, with permission. Copyright 2000, The Endocrine Society.

TABLE 3 Hormone Action on the Pilosebaceous Unit

Hormone	Action on PSU
Androgen	• Has diverse effects on hair follicles depending on their location in body; for example, sexual hairs grow only in certain areas of the body, whereas hair on the scalp undergo regression from a terminal to a vellus type in genetically susceptible individuals • Induces sebaceous gland development in acne-prone areas
Estrogen	• Prolongs the anagen phase of hair growth • Rapid growth postpartum causes telogen effluvium (loss of a large number of hairs due to simultaneous advancement into telogen) • Directly suppresses sebaceous gland function
Insulin	• Hair growth retarded in diabetes mellitus and accelerated with insulin treatment • Essential for hair follicle growth and sebaceous cell growth *in vitro* • May act as an IGF-I surrogate
Growth hormone	• Augments androgen effects on hair growth and sebocyte differentiation • Important for sebocyte growth and development • GH excess of acromegaly is associated with excess output of sebum from the sebaceous gland (seborrhea) • GH receptor found in hair follicles and sebaceous gland
Insulin-like growth factor	• Prevents hair follicles from entering catagen stage • May mediate some of the androgen effects on PSUs—induces the up-regulation of 5α-reductase by DHT in genital skin fibroblasts • Found in both hair follicles and sebaceous glands
Glucocorticoids	• Hypertrichosis (diffuse excessive hair growth) is present in Cushing's syndrome • Glucocorticoid therapy aggravates acne
Prolactin	• Hyperprolactinemia can cause hirsutism and seborrhea • Receptors localized in dermal papilla and sebaceous glands
Thyroid hormone	• Low or high levels can cause telogen effluvium • Low level cause scalp hair to become dull or brittle • Can stimulate sebum production • Receptors found in PSUs
PPARs	• Likely important in sebaceous gland development
Retinoids	• Important in hair follicle formation and patterning • Prolong anagen stage and decrease telogen stage of hair growth cycle • Trace amounts promote sebocyte growth and differentiation; larger doses cause atrophy of sebaceous glands and a decrease in sebum production
Catecholamines	• May be involved in the aggravation of acne by stress
Vitamin D receptor	• Mutations associated with alopecia in humans
Melanocortin-5 receptor	• Targeted disruption in mice causes a decrease in sebaceous lipid production
Parathyroid hormone	• Inhibits hair growth

Note. DHT, dihydrotestosterone; GH, growth hormone; IGF-I, insulin-like growth factor-I; PPARs, peroxisome proliferator-activated receptors; PSU, pilosebaceous unit.

Topical agents and retinoids play an important role in the treatment of acne, and 2 to 3 months may be needed to see the full effect of treatment on acne. Whereas trace amounts of retinoids promote sebocyte growth and differentiation, larger doses cause atrophy of sebaceous glands and a decrease in sebum secretion in both animals and humans. Retinoids have been postulated to inhibit lipid synthesis in sebocytes either directly, through an inhibition of lipogenic enzymes, or indirectly, by decreased cell proliferation. Retinoids have been used for the treatment of acne vulgaris for a long time although the precise mechanism for their efficacy has not been completely elucidated.

Glossary

acne vulgaris A disorder of the sebaceous gland; characteristic lesions include open (blackhead) and closed (whitehead) comedones, papules, pustules, and nodules.

hirsutism Excessive male-pattern hair growth in women.

pattern alopecia The androgen-dependent thinning of hair that occurs progressively with advancing age in genetically susceptible men and women; the process is mainly the result of miniaturization of terminal to vellus hair follicles.

pilosebaceous unit A skin appendage consisting of a hair follicle, a hair shaft, and a sebaceous gland.

sebaceous gland A small sacculated organ within the dermis; composed of acini, which are attached to a common excretory duct that is continuous with the wall of the piliary canal and, indirectly, with the surface of the epidermis.

terminal hair Thick, long, pigmented hair on scalp and body.

vellus hair Thin, short, usually nonpigmented hair.

See Also the Following Articles

Androgen Effects in Mammals • Androgen Receptor-Related Pathology • Androgens: Pharmacological Use and Abuse • Dihydrotestosterone, Active Androgen Metabolites and Related Pathology

Further Reading

Brown, S. K., and Shalita, A. R. (1998). Acne vulgaris. *Lancet* 351, 1871–1876.

Deplewski, D., and Rosenfield, R. L. (2000). Role of hormones in pilosebaceous unit development. *Endocr. Rev.* 21, 363–392.

Hoffmann, R., and Happle, R. (2000). Current understanding of androgenetic alopecia. Part I. Etiopathogenesis. *Eur. J. Dermatol.* 10, 319–327.

Kealey, T., Philpott, M., and Guy, R. (1997). The regulatory biology of the human pilosebaceous unit. *Bailliere Clin. Obstet. Gynecol.* 11, 205–227.

Paus, R., and Cotsarelis, G. (1999). The biology of hair follicles. *N. Engl. J. Med.* 341, 491–497.

Randall, V. A., Hibberts, N. A., Thornton, M. J., Hamada, K., Merrick, A. E., Kato, S., Jenner, T. J., De Oliveira, I., and Messenger, A. G. (2000). The hair follicle: A paradoxical androgen target organ. *Horm. Res.* 54, 243–250.

Rosenfield, R. L., Deplewski, D., Kentsis, A., and Ciletti, N. (1998). Mechanisms of androgen induction of sebocyte differentiation. *Dermatology* 196, 43–46.

Stenn, K. S., and Paus, R. (2001). Controls of hair follicle cycling. *Physiol. Rev.* 81, 449–494.

Whiting, D. A. (1998). Male pattern hair loss: Current understanding. *Int. J. Dermatol.* 37, 561–566.

Zouboulis, C. C. (2000). Human skin: An independent peripheral endocrine organ. *Horm. Res.* 54, 230–242.

Pituitary Adenylate Cyclase-Activating Polypeptide (PACAP) and Its Receptor

JOSEPH R. PISEGNA

VA Greater Los Angeles Healthcare System and UCLA School of Medicine

I. INTRODUCTION
II. PACAP HORMONE
III. THE PAC1 RECEPTOR
IV. PHYSIOLOGY OF PACAP AND ITS RECEPTOR, PAC1
V. CONCLUSIONS

This article provides an overview of the neuropeptide pituitary adenylate cyclase-activating polypeptide (PACAP) and its receptor, PAC1, which were discovered more than a decade ago. The current understanding of the structure and function of the PACAP hormone and an in-depth understanding of the structure and physiology of the PAC1 receptor are presented. The important roles that the PACAP hormone and receptor play in the regulation of physiological actions in the body are examined. Since the receptor and hormone are localized in both the central nervous system and the periphery, their important effects in both systems are described.

I. INTRODUCTION

Pituitary adenylate cyclase-activating polypeptide (PACAP) is the most recently discovered neuropeptide in the vasoactive intestinal polypeptide (VIP), secretin, and glucagon family of peptide hormones. It was designated PACAP because it stimulated adenylyl cyclase in rat anterior pituitary cells in culture and was a polypeptide of 38 amino acids. Since their discovery, PACAP hormone and its receptor, PAC1, have been identified in numerous tissues by immunohistochemistry and radioimmunoassay. Although the exact role of PACAP in the brain has not been determined, its broad distribution and presence during development suggest that it acts as a neurotransmitter or neuromodulatory peptide. Therefore, PACAP appears to play an important role in the growth and development of the brain. Its role as a neuromodulatory hormone will be discussed in more detail below. PACAP is also present in a number of peripheral tissues, including

TABLE 1   Alignment of the Amino Acid Sequences for PACAP and Related Hormones

PACAP-38	**HSDGIFTDSYSRYRKQMAVKKLAAVLG**KRYKQRVKNK-NH$_2$
PACAP-27	**HSDGIFTDSYSRYRKQMAVKKLAAVLG**-NH$_2$
VIP	**HSD**A**V**F**TD**N**Y**T**R**L**RKQMAVKKL**NSILNK-NH$_2$
Secretin	**HSDG**TF**T**SE**L**S**RL**RE**G**A**RL**Q**RLL**Q**G**L**V**G-NH$_2$
Helodermin	**HSD**AIF**T**YSK**LL**ARLA**L**QKYLASILGSRTSPPP-NH$_2$
Glucagon	**HS**QG**T**F**TSDYSK**Y**L**DS**R**RA**QD**FV**Q**WLMNT-NH$_2$
GRF	YAD**A**IF**T**NSYSKV**L**G**QL**SARK**LL**QDIMSRQQGESNQERGARARL-NH$_2$

Note. Boldface type indicate amino acids with complete identity at those positions of the PACAP-38 hormone.

the gastrointestinal tract, adrenal gland, and testis. Another important action of PACAP is its ability to stimulate cellular growth and differentiation. PACAP appears to regulate the growth of a number of tumors and may have important actions in cancer biology.

II. PACAP HORMONE

A. Discovery

Arimura and colleagues isolated fractions of ovine hypothalamic extracts that stimulated adenylyl cyclase activity in anterior pituitary cells. The hormone pituitary adenylate cyclase-activating polypeptide was so named for this activity. The hormone PACAP was shown to contain 38 amino acids, and later a 27-amino-acid form was identified. Since both a 27-amino-acid form and a 38-amino-acid form are biologically active, they are designated PACAP-27 and PACAP-38, respectively. There is significant interspecies conservation of the amino acid structure of the PACAP hormone.

B. Structure

The primary sequence of the PACAP hormone is 68% identical to its closest hormone relative, VIP. These hormones belong to a broader category of hormones including PACAP, VIP, secretin, glucagon, and GRF. As demonstrated in Table 1, there is significant homology of these peptides. The peptides most closely related to PACAP are grouped closest to PACAP at the top of Table 1. The three-dimensional structures of the hormones in this family show close similarity. Minor differences in the α-helix conformation may account for receptor specificity of PACAP and VIP.

C. PACAP Hormone Gene

The PACAP hormone gene has been cloned in mice and humans. The human gene is composed of five exons with a structure that is similar to other members of this family of peptides. This close similarity suggests that all of the members of this family of peptides may originate from a similar ancestral gene through duplication.

D. PACAP Hormone Distribution

The greatest concentration of PACAP is detected in the central nervous system of mammals. The site of greatest activity in the rat is the paraventricular and supraoptic nuclei in the hypothalamus. It is thought that the hormone is transported to the pituitary gland, where the hormone has activity in the anterior pituitary. PACAP-38 immunoreactivity is also present in extrahypothalamic sites, such as the substantia nigra, cerebellum, pons, and the paraventricular nuclei of the thalamus. The spinal cord also contains PACAP that is localized mainly in the dorsal root ganglia and dorsal horn. PACAP has been identified in the gastrointestinal enteric neural plexus, where it is an important mediator of gastric acid secretion and intestinal motility. In the adrenal gland, PACAP is present in the adrenal medulla, where it appears to be a potent stimulator of catecholamine release.

III. THE PAC1 RECEPTOR

A. Cloning and Pharmacological Characterization

There are three receptors with high affinity for PACAP hormone that have been identified and cloned. The first of these receptors to be cloned was the classical VIP receptor (VPAC1). Subsequently, a receptor with affinity for only PACAP was cloned, the type I PACAP receptor (PAC1). The last receptor to be cloned in this family was the VIP2 receptor (VPAC1). These receptors can be differentiated pharmacologically based on their relative affinities for the ligands, as shown in Table 2. PAC1 has affinity for only PACAP-38 and PACAP-27, whereas the

TABLE 2   Relative Affinities of the Three PACAP and VIP Receptors for the Ligands PACAP-27, PACAP-38, VIP, and Helodermin

IUPHAR nomenclature	Relative affinities
PAC1	PACAP-27 = PACAP-38 ≫ VIP > Helodermin
VPAC1	PACAP-27 = PACAP-38 = VIP ≫ Helodermin
VPAC2	Helodermin > PACAP-27 = PACAP-38 = VIP

Note. Classification of the receptors in the PACAP superfamily based on relative affinities to the related peptides. Adapted from Harmar *et al.* (1998), with permission.

VPAC receptors have nearly identical affinities for the ligands PACAP and VIP.

Cloning of the rat PAC1 cDNA identified it as a member of the VIP and secretin family of peptide receptors. The receptor cDNA encoded a putative protein of approximately 50 kDa and 495 amino acids. Similar to the VIP and secretin receptors, the PAC1 receptor contained seven hydrophobic domains, conserved cysteines in the extracellular domains, and several N-linked glycosylation sites. Cloning of the PAC1 gene indicated that the receptor could exist as four major splice variants, which were subsequently identified. As shown in Fig. 1, the four potential splice variants differed in the length of the third intracellular domain and were identified by Spengler and colleagues as hip, hop, hip-hop, and null. More importantly, these investigators identified variations in signal transduction coupling to phospholipase C and differences in the tissue distribution of the splice variants. The PAC1 cDNA was also cloned in a number of other species such as rat, mouse, and bovine. Subsequently, all of the human PAC1 receptor cDNA splice variants were cloned. The cloning of human PAC1 revealed a high level of homology with the rat and mouse receptor and a similar gene organization. However, unlike the rat splice variants, differences in signal transduction coupling were not observed in humans. Instead, a higher efficacy for the hop variant, an intermediate coupling for the hip-hop splice variant, and a lower level of coupling for the hip splice variant for coupling to phospholipase C were observed. Similar to the human receptor gene, the rat PAC1 receptor gene has been shown to be large (~50 kb); however, unlike the human gene, which is localized to chromosome 7, the rat gene is localized to chromosome 4.

B. Signal Transduction Characteristics

The PAC1 receptor is coupled to a dual signal transduction pathway. This was first demonstrated in PC12 cells. With the cloning of the PAC1 receptor, the specificity of PACAP-38 and PACAP-27 was shown. A fourth transmembrane splice variant was shown not to couple to either adenylyl cyclase or phospholipase C, yet it does couple to an L-type Ca^{2+} channel. The region of PAC1 shown to be responsible for signal transduction coupling is the COOH-terminus. Two critical amino acids in this region of the receptor, Ser and Arg, were shown by mutagenesis studies to be coupled to signal transduction intermediates.

C. Localization of PAC1 Receptors

The greatest density of receptors occurs in the hypothalamus, for instance, in the supraoptic nucleus, periventricular nucleus, and lateral hypothalamus. Other areas include the olfactory bulb and regions of the thalamus and cerebellum. In the rat brain, the predominant splice variant is the null variant. PAC1 has been detected by immunohistochemistry as well as electron microscopy in the retina, where it appears to be distributed in the inner plexiform layer.

In peripheral tissues, PAC1 receptors have now been identified in a large number of organs. The greatest density has been identified in the adrenal medulla where the predominant receptor splice variant appears to be of the hop type. Similarly, PAC1 receptors are expressed at high levels in the anterior pituitary gland, where, again, the predominant splice

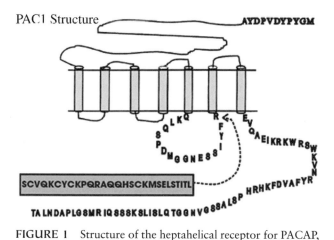

FIGURE 1   Structure of the heptahelical receptor for PACAP, PAC1. The receptor has seven transmembrane domains indicated by the cylinders and a long third intracellular loop. Splice variants are indicated in the shaded rectangle.

variant is the hop type and to a lesser extent the null variant. The human prostate gland also contains PAC1 receptors that are present in conditions such as benign prostatic hyperplasia. PAC1 receptors are also present on germ cells and spermatogonia as well as Sertoli and Leydig cells. The respiratory system contains predominantly VPAC1 receptors with little to no PAC1 receptor expressed, whereas the cardio-vascular system contains all three receptor types. The PAC1 and VPAC 1 receptors have been identified in the gastrointestinal tract with the PAC1 receptor expressed on the gastric enterochromaffin-like (ECL) cells and the VPAC1 expressed on the somatostatin-containing D cells and chief cells of the stomach. The liver appears to contain predominantly VPAC1 receptors, although careful studies examining PAC1 receptor expression in this organ have not been performed. The smooth muscles of the gastrointesti-nal tract contain VPAC1 and PAC1 receptors with the PAC1 receptor well described in the rat taenia coli. Another system that has received much scrutiny recently is the immune system. The PAC1 receptor has been described in macrophages, whereas other PACAP receptor types have been described in a number of tumor cell lines. The cloning of rat PAC1 from the rat pancreatic acinar carcinoma cell line AR42J underscores this observation. PAC1 receptor expression has been described in human lung and breast cancer cell lines. Differences in the expression of splice variants of PAC1 receptors in pituitary tumors have also been shown previously. The rat pheochromocytoma cell line PC12 was one of the classical cell systems in which the signal transduc-tion cascade for PAC1 receptors was reported.

IV. PHYSIOLOGY OF PACAP AND ITS RECEPTOR, PAC1

A. Central Nervous System

PACAP appears to exert a multitude of effects within the CNS. Exogenously administered PACAP increases the activity level as well as amount of vasopressin released. The predominant signal transduction path-way involved in the stimulus and release is the protein kinase A pathway. Intracisternal administration of PACAP has been shown to regulate the release of a number of hormones such as gonadotropin-releasing hormone (GnRH), luteinizing hormone (LH), pro-lactin, somatostatin, and the dopamine analogue DOPAC. PAC1 receptors have been shown to be expressed at relatively high levels within the pineal gland and appear to stimulate melatonin secretion.

Intracerebral injection of PACAP increases rapid eye movement sleep in sleep-deprived rats. Another potential action of PACAP is in the control of appetite as suggested by its distribution in key areas of the hypothalamus. In cultured cell systems, PACAP has been shown to activate the c-fos, c-Jun, and mitogen-activated protein kinase signaling system, indicating its role in regulating the.proliferation of cells. PACAP has been shown to reduce the cytopathic effects of the human immunodeficiency virus envelope protein gp120 in cultured neuroblasts, again supporting a role for this hormone as a neuroprotective factor. In cerebellar granule cells, PACAP appears to reduce apoptosis.

B. Endocrine Organs

PACAP stimulates gonadotropes, somatotropes, lac-totropes, and thyrotropes. Somatotropic cells that release growth hormone are stimulated by PACAP and appear to be additive to the effects of GRF. PACAP activates both adenylyl cyclase and phospho-lipase C in cultured pituitary cells. PACAP appears to be a major regulator of anterior pituitary function by stimulating the release of growth hormone, LH, follicle-stimulating hormone (FSH), prolactin, and the adrenocorticotropic hormone (ACTH). PACAP may act in a synergistic manner with GnRH to stimulate the release of LH and FSH. In cultured lactotropes, PACAP appears to directly stimulate the release of intracellular Ca^{2+}. Unlike the somato-tropes, gonadotropes, and lactotropes, the effect of PACAP on corticotropes appears to be indirect, by stimulating corticotropin-releasing factor, the major stimulus for ACTH release. Similarly, no direct effect of PACAP on the thyrotroic cells of the pituitary has been shown.

The second major endocrine site of physiological activity is in the male and female reproductive tract. PACAP has been localized to the smooth muscles of the female reproductive tract, where it may be involved in muscle relaxation. PACAP has also been localized in the placenta. VPAC2 receptors have also been identified in placental tissue, which is the site of initial cloning of the VPAC2 receptor. The ovary also contains PACAP in the granulosa zone. PACAP appears to stimulate an increase in progesterone production in the preovulatory phase. As described earlier, PACAP and PAC1 receptors have been localized to the male gonadal germ cells. PACAP has been shown to stimulate testosterone release. PACAP has been localized to the epididymis and may be an important trigger for sperm release. A reduction in PACAP may be an important mechanism in penile erection and thus may have a clinical role in male impotence. The adrenal gland contains the highest concentration of PACAP outside of the CNS. It has been shown that PACAP is the most potent stimulator of catecholamine release from the adrenal gland.

C. Respiratory Organs

The major effect of PACAP in the respiratory tree is bronchodilation, an effect that is mediated primarily through the VPAC1 receptor and the activation of cyclic AMP (cAMP). With the discovery that PACAP and VIP may also activate smooth muscle nitric oxide synthesis, this may represent another important action of these hormones. Given the potent actions of PACAP on bronchodilation in humans, the development of potent agonists may be clinically useful.

D. Gastrointestinal Tract

PACAP-containing enteric nerve fibers have been described in the stomach and co-localized with PAC1 receptors on the surface of enterochromaffin-like cells. In the stomach, PACAP appears to be the major neural pathway involved in gastric acid secretion and may account for the observed nocturnal increase in gastric acid secretion. Through its activity on the VPAC1 receptor expressed on the surface of the D cell, PACAP not only activates gastric acid secretion but also, along with galanin, inhibits acid secretion through the release of somatostatin from the gastric D cell (Fig. 2). Another important effect of PACAP is in the regulation of intestinal motility. The action of PACAP is mainly that of relaxation, being mediated through the VPAC1 receptor, but in rat colon, PACAP appears to stimulate apamin-sensitive K^+ channels. The major colonic peristaltic reflex is mediated through VIP, whereas the descending relaxation phase of intestinal peristalsis appears to be regulated by PACAP through its actions on the VPAC1 receptor. Another novel mechanism that has been discovered is the interplay between the hormones VIP and PACAP in nitric oxide synthesis.

E. Cardiovascular System

As shown in both the respiratory and the digestive systems, the primary effect of PACAP is the relaxation of smooth muscles through the activation of cAMP and protein kinase A. Similarly, in the cardiovascular system, PACAP relaxes the smooth muscle in vessels, resulting in an overall reduction in blood pressure. In whole animal studies, intravenous administration of

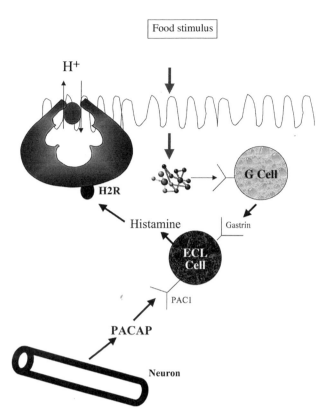

FIGURE 2 Model for the regulation of gastric acid secretion by the hormone PACAP. Released by neurons of the gastrointestinal enteric neural plexus, PACAP binds to the PAC1 receptors of nearby enterochromaffin-like (ECL) cells. PACAP stimulation of ECL cells triggers the release of histamine. Liberated histamine then binds to histamine-2 receptors (H2R) located on the surface of stomach parietal cells, thereby regulating gastric acid secretion.

PACAP results in a biphasic effect with initial vasodilation and a subsequent catecholamine release reflex causing an increase in blood pressure. In cardiac myocytes, PACAP produces a positive inotropic and chronotropic effect and a later reduction in ionotropic effect that appears to be mediated by the resulting vagally released acetylcholine.

F. Immune System

PACAP and VIP have effects on a wide range of immune cells. The role of PACAP in the regulation of cell-mediated immunity has not been thoroughly investigated. In the mouse, PACAP has been shown to activate murine macrophages that would then be able to stimulate T-cell proliferation through specific VPAC1 receptors with a consequent release of interleukin-10 (IL-10) and inhibition of IL-6 and IL-12 production. VIP and PACAP have been shown

TABLE 3　Nomenclature for PACAP and Related VIP Receptors

Receptor type IUPHAR nomenclature	Selective Agonists		Selective antagonists	Fluorescent agonists	Selective antagonist
		Previous nomenclature			
PAC1	PACAP type I	PACAP-38	PACAP 6–38	Fluor-PACAP	PACAP(6–38)
	PVR1	PACAP-27	PACAP 6–27		
		Maxadilan?			
VPAC1	VIP	[Arg^{16}] chicken secretin	Ro-	Fluor-VIP	[Ac-His^1, D-Phe^2, Lys^{15}, Arg^{16}]
	VIP1	[Lys^{15}Arg^{16}Leu^{27}]VIP (1–7)GRF(8–27)-NH$_2$			VIP(3–7)GRF (8–27)-NH$_2$
	PACAP type II PVR2 VIP/PACAP1				
VPAC2	VIP2	Helodermin			
	PACAP-3	Ro 25–1553			
	PVR3	Ro 25–1392			
	VIP/PACAP2				

Note. Nomenclature for the PACAP-related receptor superfamily shown in comparison to their previous nomenclature and hormone affinity. Adapted from Harmar *et al.* (1998), with permission.

to inhibit IL-2 transcription in T cells through the reduction of c-Jun. In a recent study, VIP and PACAP were demonstrated to inhibit nuclear factor κB (NF-κB). VIP and PACAP inhibit p65 nuclear translocation and NF-κB DNA binding. In macrophages, VIP and PACAP have been shown to inhibit interferon-γ-induced activation of the Janus kinase 1 (JAK1)/JAK2/signal transactivators and activators of transcription/interferon regulatory signaling cascade.

G. Tumor Biology

The pharmacological characterization of tumor cells expressing PACAP receptors was an integral part of understanding the biology and signal transduction of this hormone and its receptor. Therefore, the majority of the early work on their pharmacology and signal transduction relied on tumor cells such as the rat pancreatic cancer cell line AR-42J, the human neuroblastoma cell line NB-OK1, the human astrocytoma cell line, and the rat pheochromocytoma PC-12 cell line. It has been shown that PACAP stimulates the expression of c-*fos*,c-*myc*, and c-*jun* in a number of tumoral cell lines, indicating that it is a potent stimulator of cell proliferation. In human lung cancer cell lines, PACAP stimulates the growth of tumors injected into nude mice, an effect that can be antagonized by the partial PACAP antagonist PACAP 6–38 (see Table 3). In human tumors, radioligand-binding studies with either ^{125}I-VIP or ^{125}I-acetyl-PACAP-27 show expression of receptor in a large percentage of human tumors including breast,

prostate, pancreas, lung, colon, stomach, and liver as well as lymphomas and meningiomas.

V. CONCLUSIONS

PACAP is one of the most recently described neuropeptides. Its biological relevance is only beginning to be understood. Information thus far indicates that both the hormone and the PAC1 receptor are widely distributed in both the CNS and periphery and that this set of biological mediators is relatively important to normal physiology. With the recent study of genetic knockout mice, more information regarding the function of both the hormone and the receptor will be obtained.

See Also the Following Articles

Amino Acid and Nitric Oxide Control of the Anterior Pituitary ● Cytokines and Anterior Pituitary Function ● Glucagon-like Peptides: GLP-1 and GLP-2 ● Monoaminergic and Cholinergic Control of the Anterior Pituitary ● Neuropeptides and Control of the Anterior Pituitary ● Secretin ● Vasoactive Intestinal Peptide (VIP)

Further Reading

Arimura, A. (1992). Pituitary adenylate cyclase activating polypeptide (PACAP): Discovery and current status of research. *Regul. Pept.* **37**, 287–303.

Delgado, M., and Ganea, D. (2000). Inhibition of IFN-γ-induced Janus kinase-1–STAT1 activation in macrophages by vasoactive intestinal peptide and pituitary adenylate cyclase-activating polypeptide. *J. Immunol.* **165**, 3051–3057.

Delgado, M., and Ganea, D. (2001). Vasoactive intestinal peptide and pituitary adenylate cyclase-activating polypeptide inhibit nuclear factor-κB-dependent gene activation at multiple levels in the human monocytic cell line THP-1. *J. Biol. Chem.* **276**, 369–380.

Harmar, A. J., Arimura, A., Gozes, I., Journot, L., Laburthe, M., Pisegna, J. R., Rawlings, S. R., Robberecht, P., Said, S. I., Sreedharan, S. P., Wank, S. A., and Waschek, J. A. (1998). International Union of Pharmacology. XVIII. Nomenclature of receptors for vasoactive intestinal peptide and pituitary adenylate cyclase-activating polypeptide. *Pharmacol. Rev.* **50**, 265–270.

Leyton, J., Gozes, Y., Pisegna, J., Coy, D., Purdom, S., Casibang, M., Zia, F., and Moody, T. W. (1999). PACAP(6–38) is a PACAP receptor antagonist for breast cancer cells. *Breast Cancer Res. Treat.* **56**, 177–186.

Lyu, R. M., Germano, P. M., Choi, J. K., Le, S. V., and Pisegna, J. R. (2000). Identification of an essential amino acid motif within the C terminus of the pituitary adenylate cyclase-activating polypeptide type I receptor that is critical for signal transduction but not for receptor internalization. *J. Biol. Chem.* **275**, 36134–36142.

Pisegna, J. R., and Wank, S. A. (1993). Molecular cloning and functional expression of the pituitary adenylate cyclase-activating polypeptide type I receptor. *Proc. Natl. Acad. Sci. USA* **90**, 6345–6349.

Pisegna, J. R., and Wank, S. A. (1996). Cloning and characterization of the signal transduction of four splice variants of the human pituitary adenylate cyclase activating polypeptide receptor: Evidence for dual coupling to adenylate cyclase and phospholipase C. *J. Biol. Chem.* **271**, 17267–17274.

Rawlings, S. R., and Hezareh, M. (1996). Pituitary adenylate cyclase-activating polypeptide (PACAP) and PACAP/vasoactive intestinal polypeptide receptors: Actions on the anterior pituitary gland. *Endocr. Rev.* **17**, 4–29.

Reubi, J. C., Laderach, U., Waser, B., Gebbers, J. O., Robberecht, P., and Laissue, J. A. (2000). Vasoactive intestinal peptide/pituitary adenylate cyclase-activating peptide receptor subtypes in human tumors and their tissues of origin. *Cancer Res.* **60**, 3105–3112.

Seki, T., Shioda, S., Izumi, S., Arimura, A., and Koide, R. (2000). Electron microscopic observation of pituitary adenylate cyclase-activating polypeptide (PACAP)-containing neurons in the rat retina. *Peptides* **21**, 109–113.

Vaudry, D., Gonzalez, B. J., Basille, M., Yon, L., Fournier, A., and Vaudry, H. (2000). Pituitary adenylate cyclase-activating polypeptide and its receptors: From structure to functions. *Pharmacol. Rev.* **52**, 269–324.

Wang, H. Y., Jiang, X. M., and Ganea, D. (2000). The neuropeptides VIP and PACAP inhibit IL-2 transcription by decreasing c-Jun and increasing JunB expression in T cells. *J. Neuroimmunol.* **104**, 68–78.

Zeng, N., Athmann, C., Kang, T., Lyu, R. M., Walsh, J. H., Ohning, G. V., Sachs, G., and Pisegna, J. R. (1999). PACAP type I receptor activation regulates ECL cells and gastric acid secretion. *J. Clin. Invest.* **104**, 1383–1391.

Zia, F., Fagarasan, M., Bitar, K., Coy, D. H., Pisegna, J. R., Wank, S. A., and Moody, T. W. (1995). Pituitary adenylate cyclase activating peptide receptors regulate the growth of non-small cell lung cancer cells. *Cancer Res.* **55**, 4886–4891.

Placental Development

MICHAEL T. MCMASTER AND SUSAN J. FISHER

University of California, San Francisco

I. INTRODUCTION
II. MORPHOLOGICAL ASPECTS OF NORMAL HUMAN PLACENTATION/CYTOTROPHOBLAST INVASION
III. MOLECULAR ASPECTS OF PLACENTATION/CYTOTROPHOBLAST INVASION
IV. REGULATION OF CYTOTROPHOBLAST ENDOVASCULAR INVASION

Survival of the eutherian embryo/fetus depends on the formation of a transient but vital organ, the placenta. Therefore, key events early in placental development play a large role in determining the course and outcome of pregnancy.

I. INTRODUCTION

Placentation, the first test of the embryo's differentiative and organogenetic capacity, accomplishes two critical events: attaching the conceptus to the uterus and bringing the fetal and maternal circulations into close proximity to facilitate effective gas, nutrient, and waste exchange. These functions require that fetal placental cells (trophoblasts) acquire an invasive phenotype. In mammals that form a hemochorial placenta (e.g., humans and mice), fetal trophoblasts come in direct contact with maternal blood. Thus, placentation also entails the unique requirement for close cooperation and direct cellular contact between two immunologically distinct organisms.

During implantation and subsequent placental development, fetal trophoblasts and the uterine cells that they encounter intricately regulate the expression of several classes of molecules. These include adhesion receptors and their ligands, proteinases and their inhibitors, growth factors/cytokines and their receptors, immunomodulators, and transcription factors. This article focuses on the profound changes in trophoblast phenotype that occur during placental development, with emphasis on uterine invasion by cytotrophoblasts (CTBs). Data point to the central importance of the intimate relationship that develops between fetal trophoblasts and the maternal vasculature, as well as to strategies for uncovering the regulatory factors that control the formation of these highly unusual connections.

II. MORPHOLOGICAL ASPECTS OF NORMAL HUMAN PLACENTATION/CYTOTROPHOBLAST INVASION

For many reasons, the human placenta has been difficult to study. With its 9-month life span, developmental processes that take months to years to complete in other organs are compressed into a narrow window of time. Within this short period, additional constraints exist: for example, the requirement that a functioning placenta be in place before substantial fetal growth occurs. As a result, the basic elements of placental development occur during the first half of pregnancy, after which additional growth elaborates on these themes. At term, this organ has reached the end of its life span. As a result of an autocrine program of planned obsolescence, pregnancies that continue beyond this point are endangered by complications that are related to a rapid decline in placental function. Accordingly, the concept that embryonic and fetal development occurs along a smooth continuum during the prenatal period applies only to intraembryonic processes. Differentiation of the extraembryonic lineages is by necessity an explosive event that occurs early in pregnancy. As a result, interpreting any picture of placental development depends entirely on when, during its 9-month life span, that snapshot was taken.

The complex anatomy of the placenta has also made this organ difficult to study. Commonly the placenta is depicted as a simple, pancake-shaped sponge connecting the embryo/fetus to the uterus. This portion of the placenta, which is expelled from the uterus during delivery, is easy to obtain and, consequently, frequently studied. But one of the most interesting parts of the placenta is rarely seen. This portion, which lies buried within the uterine wall, separates from the rest of the placenta during pregnancy termination or delivery. As a result, the only way to obtain this tissue is by uterine biopsy of the site where the placenta attached. Thus, special procedures that are similar to the methods used to obtain any other surgical specimen are required to collect this portion of the placenta.

A full understanding of the placenta can be obtained only by studying both its parts. Figure 1 diagrams these two parts and joins them into a single unit to show how they function, together with modified uterine structures, during human pregnancy. The placenta is made up of individual units termed chorionic villi. Each villus has a connective tissue core that contains fetal blood vessels and numerous macrophages, termed Hofbauer cells. The macro-

phages often lie adjacent to a thick basement membrane, which underlies a layer of cytotrophoblast stem cells that are the progenitors of all the trophoblast lineages.

The differentiation pathway that cytotrophoblast stem cells take depends on their location. In floating villi, the CTBs fuse to form a multinucleate syncytium, the syncytiotrophoblast, that covers the villus surface. These villi are attached at only one end to the tree-like fetal portion of the placenta. The rest of the villus floats in a stream of maternal blood, which optimizes exchange, across the syncytium, of substances between the mother and the fetus. In anchoring villi, cytotrophoblast stem cells detach from the basement membrane and form a column of nonpolarized mononuclear cells that invade the uterus. As a result, these villi are attached at one end to the fetal portion of the placenta and at the other end to the uterus. This arrangement anchors the villus to the uterine wall. Invasive CTBs rapidly traverse most of the uterine parenchyma (interstitial invasion). They also breach the uterine veins and arteries that they encounter (endovascular invasion). Their interactions with veins are confined to the portions of the vessels that lie near the inner surface of the uterus, but CTBs migrate in a retrograde direction along much of the intrauterine course of the arterioles. Eventually, these fetal cells completely replace the maternal endothelial lining and partially replace the muscular wall of these vessels. This unusual process diverts uterine blood flow to the floating villi.

III. MOLECULAR ASPECTS OF PLACENTATION/CYTOTROPHOBLAST INVASION

Work from the authors' laboratory has focused on molecular aspects of the cytotrophoblast differentiation pathway that leads to uterine invasion. Given the unusual way in which these cells colonize the uterine blood vessels and channel maternal blood to the floating villi, it was hypothesized that they might replicate portions of standard vasculogenesis and/or angiogenesis programs. As a first test of this theory, the cells' expression of adhesion molecules during interstitial and endovascular invasion was examined. The onset of cytotrophoblast differentiation/invasion was found to be characterized by reduced staining for receptors characteristic of polarized cytotrophoblast epithelial stem cells—integrin $\alpha 6\beta 4$ and E-cadherin—and the onset of expression of adhesion

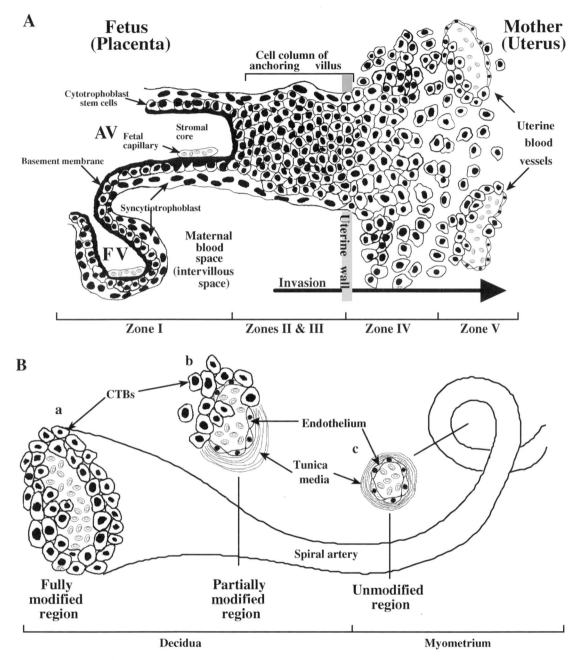

FIGURE 1 (A) Diagram of a longitudinal section of an anchoring chorionic villus (AV) at the fetal–maternal interface at approximately 10 weeks of gestational age. AV functions as a bridge between the fetal and the maternal compartments, whereas floating villi (FV) are suspended in the intervillous space and are bathed by maternal blood. CTBs (cytotrophoblasts) in the AV (Zone I) form cell columns (Zones II and III). CTBs then invade the uterine interstitium (decidua and first third of the myometrium: Zone IV) and maternal vasculature (Zone V), thereby anchoring the fetus to the mother and accessing the maternal circulation. Zone designations mark areas in which CTBs have distinct patterns of adhesion molecule expression. (B) Diagram of a uterine (spiral) artery in which endovascular invasion is in progress (10–18 weeks of gestation). Endometrial and then myometrial segments of spiral arteries are modified progressively. In fully modified regions (a), the vessel diameter is large. CTBs are present in the lumen and occupy the entire surface of the vessel wall. A discrete muscular layer (tunica media) is not evident. (b) Partially modified vessel segments. CTBs and maternal endothelium occupy discrete regions of the vessel wall. In areas of intersection, CTBs appear to lie deep in the endothelium and in contact with the vessel wall. (c) Unmodified vessel segments in the myometrium. Vessel segments in the superficial third of the myometrium will become modified when endovascular invasion reaches its fullest extent (approximately midgestation), whereas deeper segments of the same artery will retain their normal structure. Modified from Zhou *et al.* (1997), with permission.

receptors characteristic of endothelium—VE-cadherin, IgG family members vascular cellular adhesion molecule-1 (VCAM-1) and platelet-endothelial cell adhesion molecule-1 (PECAM-1) and integrins $\alpha V\beta 3$ and $\alpha 1\beta 1$. Accordingly, this phenomenon was termed pseudovasculogenesis. Other investigators showed that additional members of the cadherin family are also up-regulated on invasive CTBs and on decidualizing endometrial stroma. All CTBs in this pathway, regardless of location, stain for Mel-CAM, a melanoma-associated IgG family receptor also expressed on endothelium. Finally, CTBs within the maternal blood vessels turn on the neural cell adhesion molecule (CD56), an adhesion receptor that is also expressed by maternal natural killer cells that home to the pregnant uterus. Thus, as CTBs from anchoring villi invade and remodel the wall of the uterus, these epithelial cells of ectodermal origin acquire an adhesion receptor repertoire characteristic of endothelial cells. It is theorized that this switch permits the heterotypic adhesive interactions that allow fetal and maternal cells to cohabit the uterine vasculature during normal pregnancy.

Changes in the cytotrophoblast adhesion molecule repertoire take place in the context of the cells' equally dramatic modulation of their proteinase and proteinase inhibitor expression. Some aspects of this phenotypic transformation are undoubtedly linked to cytotrophoblast acquisition of an invasive phenotype. For example, expression and activation of matrix metalloproteinase-9 were found to be required for invasion *in vitro*. This observation fits well with recent observations, in other systems, that show that this same proteinase is a key regulator of angiogenesis. It is speculated that CTBs up-regulate the expression of other proteinases/inhibitors in order to present a nonthrombogenic surface to maternal blood. The urokinase-type plasminogen activator and plasminogen activator inhibitor-1, as well as the proteolytically activated thrombin receptor, might function in this manner.

The upstream regulatory factors that control these changes in proteinase and adhesion molecule phenotype include a variety of growth factors. In this regard, vascular endothelial growth factor (VEGF) family members, which are expressed at the maternal–fetal interface, are attractive candidates for regulating pseudovasculogenesis. Other factors, such as hepatocyte growth factor/scatter factor, can promote invasion by interacting with c-Met expressed on invading CTBs.

Finally, invading CTBs up-regulate the expression of other molecules that likely enable them to escape maternal immune rejection. Proteins expressed by trophoblasts that play a role in immunotolerance include human leukocyte antigen G (HLA-G), a unique major histocompatibility class Ib antigen with limited polymorphism, and interleukin-10, a potent immunosuppressive cytokine. HLA-G is expressed by invading CTBs that are in intimate contact with the decidua (which includes abundant maternal immune cells), suggesting a key juxtacrine regulatory role for this molecule. As shown in Fig. 2, HLA-G expression is a very sensitive marker of CTBs that have differentiated toward an invasive phenotype. Interstitial and endovascular CTBs express HLA-G, but syncytiotrophoblast and cytotrophoblast stem cells attached to the villus basement membranes do not. The regulated expression of these molecules by CTBs provides insights into how the placenta, a semiallograft, is able to develop in the context of a fully functional maternal immune system. However, the precise mechanisms whereby the placenta mediates maternal immune tolerance remain poorly understood.

IV. REGULATION OF CYTOTROPHOBLAST ENDOVASCULAR INVASION

How can the knowledge of cytotrophoblast invasion be used to advance the understanding of the regulatory factors that govern placental development? One avenue that is being explored is the extent to which physiological parameters that are known to play important roles in the vasculature operate in the placenta. The first major effort in this direction led to the examination of the role of oxygen tension, one of the major factors at play in the vasculature. In this regard, it is interesting to consider that the placenta is the first organ to function during development. This hierarchy imposes novel requirements on cytotrophoblast growth and differentiation. For example, the critical early stages of placental development occur before the conceptus accesses a supply of maternal blood (≤ 10 weeks of gestation). In accord with this constraint, previous work showed that CTBs proliferate *in vitro* under hypoxic conditions that are comparable to those found during early pregnancy in the uterine lumen and the superficial decidua. As trophoblast invasion of the uterus proceeds, the placental cells encounter increasingly higher oxygen levels, which trigger their exit from the cell cycle and subsequent differentiation.

The discovery that CTBs acquire characteristics of vascular cells during endovascular invasion highlights

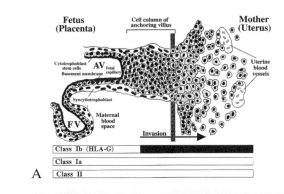

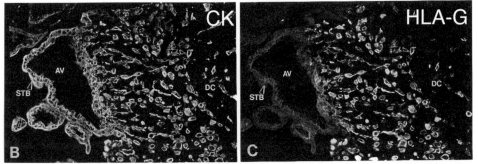

FIGURE 2 Immunostaining of a section of the placental bed shows that HLA-G protein is produced by only invasive CTBs *in vivo*. (A) Summary diagram of the trophoblast populations in anchoring villi and their expression of major histocompatibility class I and II molecules. (B and C) Section of a 14-week placental bed biopsy double-labeled with rat monoclonal antibody 7D3 (anti-cytokeratin) and mouse monoclonal antibody 4H84 (anti-HLA-G). B shows cytokeratin staining, which labels all the trophoblast cells in the section. C shows HLA-G staining detected with fluorescein-conjugated antibodies. The section contains an anchoring villus (AV) with an associated cytotrophoblast cell column and decidua (DC). Note that the invasive CTBs stain strongly for HLA-G, whereas the syncytiotrophoblasts and cytotrophoblast stems cells do not. STB, syncytiotrophoblast.

the potential importance of factors that govern conventional vasculogenesis/angiogenesis in the regulation of placental development. Undoubtedly, this complex differentiation program is controlled by a hierarchy of regulatory factors. At a physiological level, it is already known that oxygen tension, which has profound effects on blood vessels, controls the switch between cytotrophoblast proliferation and differentiation. In these experiments, control anchoring villus explants (6–8 weeks of gestation) were maintained in either a 20 or an 8% O_2 atmosphere, mimicking standard culture conditions and the environment within the uterine interstitium (Fig. 1A, Zone IV), respectively. Other villi were cultured in 2% O_2, mimicking the hypoxic conditions in the fetal compartment near the uterine lumen at this time (Fig. 1A, Zone I; intervillous space). In 20 and 8% O_2, CTBs exit the cell cycle, up-regulate $\alpha 1\beta 1$, and become highly invasive. In hypoxia, CTBs continue to proliferate, but they fail to express $\alpha 1\beta 1$ integrin and do not invade. These observations suggest the

following model. Before CTBs access the maternal blood supply (e.g., at 10 weeks of gestation), the hypoxic environment near the uterine lumen in which early placental development occurs favors cytotrophoblast proliferation, a phenomenon observed *in situ*. As interstitial invasion proceeds, invasive CTBs encounter a positive oxygen gradient that favors differentiation/invasion. Interestingly, hypoxia *in vitro* mimics some of the effects seen in preeclampsia, suggesting the possible consequences of failed endovascular invasion *in vivo*.

It can be envisioned that oxygen acts through a variety of downstream effectors that include molecular families known to play an important role in vasculogenesis/angiogenesis. In this regard, VEGF family members and their receptors are attractive candidates. There are several reports that CTBs, as well as fetal and maternal macrophages, express VEGF. CTBs also express placental growth factor (PlGF), a unique placental form of VEGF. Unlike VEGF, PlGF is not responsive to hypoxia; furthermore, its homodimers are not angiogenic and bind VEGF receptor-1 (Flt-1, Fms-like tyrosine kinase-1) but not VEGF receptor-2 (KDR, kinase insert domain-containing receptor). PlGF also forms heterodimers with VEGF that bind both receptors. VEGF up-regulates the expression of $\alpha 1\beta 1$ and $\alpha V\beta 3$ integrins in endothelial cells. These are the same proinvasive integrins that are up-regulated during cytotrophoblast differentiation, tempting speculation that VEGF family factors play analogous roles in invasive CTBs and angiogenic endothelial cells, a hypothesis that was recently proved. CTBs also express Flt-1 and KDR. Other factors and their cognate receptors that regulate vasculogenesis/angiogenesis, including fibroblast growth factors/receptors, TIEs/angiopoietins, and thrombospondins, are also expressed in the placenta.

Given this complexity, it is likely that the regulated balance of pro- and anti-angiogenic mechanisms is critical to coordinating the development of the hybrid vascular structures, composed of CTBs and maternal cells, that control blood flow to the fetus. Placental development actually requires the coordination of three different vasculogenesis/angiogenesis-like programs. First, fetal blood vessels develop in the stroma of floating chorionic villi (see Fig. 1A, fetal capillary). This process probably employs a vasculogenesis/angiogenesis program similar to that taking place within the embryo proper. Second, differentiating/invading CTBs undergo pseudovasculogenesis, the differentiation program that allows them to take on an endothelial adhesion phenotype (Fig. 1A, Zones II–V). Third, endovascular invasion by CTBs occurs without triggering significant angiogenesis in the maternal vessels, which suggests that CTBs also have novel paracrine mechanisms for rendering quiescent the resident uterine vasculature that they remodel (Fig. 1A, Zone V, uterine blood vessels). How are these different processes coordinated within the same microenvironment? The novel requirements of cytotrophoblast endovascular invasion suggest that known regulatory molecules may have novel actions; alternatively, novel regulatory molecules may control the behavior of these unusual cells.

The importance of trophoblast differentiation to embryonic/fetal development is also revealed by the numerous types of genetically engineered mice with placental defects. In the context of normal and abnormal human cytotrophoblast differentiation/invasion, some of the most interesting molecules implicated in knockout mouse experiments include hepatocyte growth factor/scatter factor and its c-Met receptor, VCAM-1 and the integrin $\alpha 4$ subunit, and the hypoxia-inducible transcription factor HIF-1β (ARNT). Although the discovery that these and other molecules, e.g., Mash-2, Ets-2, Wnt2, and interleukin-11 receptor, play important roles in placentation has for the most part been unexpected, the trophoblast phenotypes of genetically engineered mice, which like humans form a hemochorial placenta, will continue to be extremely informative regarding mechanisms of human placental development and cytotrophoblast pseudovasculogenesis.

In summary, recent advances have uncovered the unexpected finding that specialized fetal cells of the human placenta—CTBs—undergo a novel pseudovasculogenesis differentiation program that enables them to masquerade as the endothelial and smooth muscle components of maternal uterine vessels. Discovery of the regulatory mechanisms that govern this unusual transformation will offer fascinating insights into how the placenta forms. Will the results of these studies be applicable to other normal and abnormal processes that require similar sorts of plasticity? One interesting possibility is that tumor cells, which like CTBs are marauders in search of a blood supply, might co-opt portions of the differentiation program described here. Whether lessons learned from placental development could be used to develop additional anti-angiogenesis cancer therapies, analogous to those described by Folkman and co-workers, remains to be investigated.

Glossary

cytotrophoblast stem cells Mononuclear trophoblast precursors to invasive cytotrophoblasts and syncytiotrophoblasts.

decidua Stromal compartment of the endometrium during pregnancy.

invasive cytotrophoblasts Mononuclear trophoblasts that migrate into the uterine interstitium and vasculature.

syncytiotrophoblasts Multinucleate trophoblasts that line the surface of floating villi.

trophoblast Type of epithelial cell that forms the maternal–fetal interface.

See Also the Following Articles

Angiogenesis • Brain-Derived Neurotropic Factor • Decidualization • Insulin-like Growth Factor (Igf) Signaling • Oxytocin • Placental Gene Expression • Placental Immunology • Uterine Contractility

Further Reading

Burton, G. J., Jauniaux, E., and Watson, A. L. (1999). Maternal arterial connections to the placental intervillous space during the first trimester of human pregnancy: The Boyd collection revisited. *Am. J. Obstet. Gynecol.* **181**, 718–724.

Clark, D. E., Smith, S. K., Licence, D., Evans, A. L., and Charnock-Jones, D. S. (1998). Comparison of expression patterns for placenta growth factor, vascular endothelial growth factor (VEGF), VEGF-B and VEGF-C in the human placenta throughout gestation. *J. Endocrinol.* **159**, 459–467.

Cross, J. C., Werb, Z., and Fisher, S. J. (1994). Implantation and the placenta: Key pieces of the development puzzle. *Science* **266**, 1508–1518.

Damsky, C. H., and Fisher, S. J. (1998). Trophoblast pseudo-vasculogenesis: Faking it with endothelial adhesion receptors. *Curr. Opin. Cell Biol.* **10**, 660–666.

Genbacev, O., Joslin, R., Damsky, C. H., Polliotti, B. M., and Fisher, S. J. (1996). Hypoxia alters early gestation human cytotrophoblast differentiation/invasion *in vitro* and models the placental defects that occur in preeclampsia. *J. Clin. Invest.* **97**, 540–550.

Genbacev, O., Zhou, Y., Ludlow, J. W., and Fisher, S. J. (1997). Regulation of human placental development by oxygen tension. *Science* **277**, 1669–1672.

Guillemot, F., Nagy, A., Auerbach, A., Rossant, J., and Joyner, A. L. (1994). Essential role of Mash-2 in extraembryonic development. *Nature* **371**, 333–336.

Jaffe, R., Jauniaux, E., and Hustin, J. (1997). Maternal circulation in the first-trimester human placenta—Myth or reality? *Am. J. Obstet. Gynecol.* **176**, 695–705.

McMaster, M. T., Librach, C. L., Zhou, Y., Lim, K. H., Janatpour, M. J., DeMars, R., Kovats, S., Damsky, C., and Fisher, S. J. (1995). Human placental HLA-G expression is restricted to differentiated cytotrophoblasts. *J. Immunol.* **154**, 3771–3778.

Norwitz, E. R., Schust, D. J., and Fisher, S. J. (2001). Implantation and the survival of early pregnancy. *N. Engl. J. Med.* **345**, 1400–1408.

Paria, B. C., Reese, J., Das, S. K., and Dey, S. K. (2002). Deciphering the cross-talk of implantation: Advances and challenges. *Science* **296**, 2185–2188.

Rinkenberger, J. L., Cross, J. C., and Werb, Z. (1997). Molecular genetics of implantation in the mouse. *Dev. Genet.* **21**, 6–20.

Roth, I., Corry, D. B., Locksley, R. M., Abrams, J. S., Litton, M. J., and Fisher, S. J. (1996). Human placental cytotrophoblasts produce the immunosuppressive cytokine interleukin 10. *J. Exp. Med.* **184**, 539–548.

Zhou, Y., Fisher, S. J., Janatpour, M., Genbacev, O., Dejana, E., Wheelock, M., and Damsky, C. H. (1997). Human cytotrophoblasts adopt a vascular phenotype as they differentiate. A strategy for successful endovascular invasion? *J. Clin. Invest.* **99**, 2139–2151.

Zhou, Y., McMaster, M., Woo, K., Janatpour, M., Perry, J., Karpanen, T., Alitalo, K., Damsky, C., and Fisher, S. J. (2002). Vascular endothelial growth factor ligands and receptors that regulate human cytotrophoblast survival are dysregulated in severe preeclampsia and hemolysis, elevated liver enzymes, and low platelets syndrome. *Am. J. Pathol.* **160**, 1405–1423.

Placental Gene Expression

AMRITA KAMAT AND CAROLE R. MENDELSON
University of Texas Southwestern Medical Center

I. INTRODUCTION
II. AROMATASE
III. HUMAN PLACENTAL LACTOGEN
IV. CONCLUSIONS

The human placenta is composed of a core of proliferating mononuclear cytotrophoblasts; these trophoblast cells differentiate to form the syncytiotrophoblast layer, which covers the placental villi and has numerous secretory and transport/processing functions. It is this differentiation of cytotrophoblasts to syncytiotrophoblast that generates a cascade of regulatory signals that result in the production of various polypeptide hormones, growth factors, steroid hormones, and steroid-metabolizing enzymes. Cell culture techniques and transgenic technology are used to elucidate molecular events that promote and maintain syncytiotrophoblast differentiation and culminate in expression of different placenta-specific proteins factors.

I. INTRODUCTION

Maintenance of pregnancy and normal growth and development of the fetus are critically dependent on a biomolecular fetal–maternal communication, which is accomplished by the placenta. The placenta is, therefore, a critical organ, not only as the means of exchange of gases, nutrients, and waste products between the fetus and the mother, but also as an important source of hormones, growth factors, and other molecules that maintain uterine quiescence, stimulate fetal growth and development, and contribute to immune privilege. Placental molecules and growth factors include pregnancy-associated hormones (corticotropin-releasing hormone, progesterone, estrogen, and members of the growth hormone/prolactin gene family), enzymes (e.g., aromatase and side chain cleavage enzyme), leptin, interferons, angiogenic growth factors, cell adhesion molecules, and extracellular matrix metalloproteinases. These different molecules play varied but important roles in pregnancy; thus alterations in their expression underlie early pregnancy loss and complications.

In this article, we review work that has elucidated transcriptional regulation of two important human placental molecules, placental lactogen (chorionic somatomammotropin) and the enzyme aromatase, which catalyzes conversion of C_{19} steroids to estrogen.

II. AROMATASE

As normal pregnancy progresses, there is a gradual increase in plasma levels of estrogens and progesterone, which are synthesized primarily by the placenta. Near term in humans, there are extraordinarily high circulating levels of estrogen and progesterone, which decline abruptly with the delivery of the fetus and placenta. Thus, the human placenta, like the placentas of a number of ungulates, including cows, pigs, and horses, is able to synthesize estrogens, a property that is not shared by the placentas of rodent species, such as rats and mice. The physiological significance of the high levels of estrogen production by the human placenta is unclear at this time. However, it is likely that the human placenta has acquired the capacity to synthesize estrogens, in part, to metabolize the high levels of circulating androgens derived from the fetal adrenals, thus preventing their virilizing effects.

The human placenta lacks the enzyme 17α-hydroxylase, thus progesterone cannot be used as a substrate for estrogen biosynthesis. Instead, the high levels of estrogen produced in the human placenta are derived primarily from the C_{19} steroid, 16α-hydroxyandrostenedione, which is secreted by the fetal adrenal. Aromatase P450 is the enzyme responsible for catalyzing the biosynthesis of C_{18} estrogens (17β-estradiol, estrone, and estriol) from C_{19} steroids. Aromatase P450 is expressed exclusively in estrogen-producing cells and is a product of the *CYP19* gene. Homozygous mutations of the single-copy human gene (h*CYP19*) result in virilization of the female fetus *in utero*, conferring subsequent primary amenorrhea.

The h*CYP19* gene spans ~130 kb in the human genome (Fig. 1). It is postulated that expression of h*CYP19* in various estrogen-producing tissues, including the gonads, brain, adipose tissue, and placenta, is driven by tissue-specific promoters that lie upstream of unique first exons, although the aromatase protein synthesized in each of these tissues is identical. Thus, the start site of transcription in placenta (in exon I.1) lies ~100,000 bp upstream of the start site of translation in exon II, whereas the ovary-specific first exon lies immediately upstream of exon II.

Primary cultures of human trophoblast cells transfected with various gene constructs have been used to create functional maps of sequences required for placenta-specific h*CYP19* gene expression. Mononuclear cytotrophoblast cells, which do not express aromatase, are isolated from the midterm placenta. When these cells are placed in culture, they fuse and differentiate to form a multinuclear syncytiotrophoblast. These morphological changes are associated with a marked induction of h*CYP19* gene expression. This primary cell culture system thus provides a physiologically relevant model to study molecular mechanisms in the regulation of h*CYP19* gene expression. Studies using this culture system suggest that 501 bp of exon I.1 5' flanking DNA is sufficient for trophoblast-specific expression of h*CYP19* gene and that sequences between -501 and -246 bp contain silencer elements that may bind inhibitory transcription factors in nonplacental cells. Findings from deletion mapping analysis, site-directed mutagenesis, and electrophoretic mobility-shift assays also indicate that two overlapping hexameric sequences (AGGTCA, -183 to -191 bp), which may bind members of the nuclear receptor superfamily, and a G/C-rich sequence (-233 bp), which binds Sp1 and other as yet unidentified transcription factors, may contribute to the high levels h*CYP19I.1* promoter activity during syncytiotrophoblast differentiation.

In addition to primary cultures of placental cells, choriocarcinoma cell lines such as BeWo and JEG-3 have been used to study regulation of h*CYP19* gene expression. Using transfected JEG-3 choriocarcinoma cells, it has been observed that the proximal 301 bp upstream of exon I.1 is capable of conferring placental cell-specific h*CYP19* gene expression. Within this region, an element has been identified that is capable of binding a "glial cells missing" motif protein, the expression of which is restricted to the placenta. Other studies using BeWo choriocarcinoma cells have also localized a cell-type specific enhancer element between -242 and -166 bp relative to the transcriptional start site in exon I.1, which may play an important role in sustaining high levels of h*CYP19* expression.

In addition to studies in primary cultures of placental cells and choriocarcinoma cell lines, transgenic mice have been used to map h*CYP19* promoter regions required for appropriate tissue-specific and developmental regulation of gene expression. Initially, it was uncertain whether the mouse would serve as an appropriate model, because its placenta

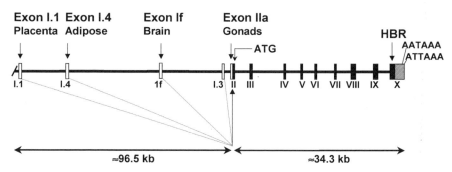

FIGURE 1 Schematic representation of the human *CYP19* gene and its alternative first exons. The protein coding sequences of the human *CYP19* gene, exons II–X (solid bars), and their introns comprise a region of ~ 34 kb. The heme-binding region (HBR) is in exon X, as are two alternative polyadenylation signals. The untranslated exons IIa, I.3/I.4, If, and I.1 (open bars) encoding the 5′ ends of the aromatase P450 mRNAs in the gonads, adipose, brain, and placenta, respectively, encompass a region of ~ 100 kb. These tissue-specific first exons are alternatively spliced onto a common site (shown by the septum) just upstream of the ATG codon in exon II. Based on the Celera Human Genome database (hcg 39857 CYP19GA_x2HTBL5L7WT), the human *CYP19* gene lies on chromosome 15, spanning q14–q15. Reproduced from Kamat *et al.* (2002), with permission from Elsevier Science.

does not express the endogenous *cyp19* gene. It was not known if the lack of estrogen synthesis in the mouse placenta was due to an absence of essential gene regulatory elements or of critical transcription factors. However, expression of hCYP19I.1$_{-2400}$:*hGH* (human growth hormone) or hCYP19I.1$_{-501}$:*hGH* fusion genes in transgenic mice was placenta-specific and developmentally regulated. Thus, just 500 bp of DNA, ~ 100 kb upstream of the coding region of the human *CYP19* gene, is sufficient to mediate placenta-specific expression in transgenic mice. These results clearly indicate that the transcription factors required to activate the human *CYP19* placenta-specific promoter are conserved between human and mouse genes, but that the mouse lacks the critical cis-acting elements required for expression of its endogenous *cyp19* gene.

To localize hCYP19I.1$_{-501}$:*hGH* fusion gene expression within the mouse placenta, *in situ* hybridization was performed using an antisense hGH probe. The main fetal components of the mouse placenta include the trophoblast giant cells, the spongiotrophoblast, and the labyrinthine trophoblast layer. Many of the placental polypeptide hormones and steroidogenic enzymes are expressed in the spongiotrophoblast and the trophoblast giant cells; however, the transgene is not expressed in these cells. On the other hand, the transgene is expressed as early as embryonic day 10.5 (E10.5) specifically in the mouse labyrinthine trophoblast layer (Fig. 2). This trilaminar layer is highly vascularized; its outer cellular layer, which covers two inner layers of syncytial cells, is bathed in maternal blood and thus plays an important role in nutrient and gas exchange.

Therefore, the labyrinthine layer of the mouse placenta appears to be analogous to the human syncytiotrophoblast, which expresses aromatase and also is bathed in maternal blood. Thus, studies using trophoblast cells in culture and transgenic mice indicate that the proximal 501 bp flanking the 5′ end of exon I.1 of the hCYP19 gene is sufficient for placenta-specific expression.

III. HUMAN PLACENTAL LACTOGEN

Placental lactogens (PLs), or chorionic somatomammotropins, play an important role in the regulation of maternal and fetal metabolism and in the growth and development of the fetus. Human *PL* belongs to the growth hormone (*GH*) gene family, which includes the growth hormone gene (*GH-N*) and four growth hormone gene variants (*GH-V, PL-A, PL-B,* and *PL-L*). This five-gene family cluster shares greater than 90% sequence identity and has evolved by gene duplication. However, although *GH-N* is predominantly expressed in the pituitary somatotrophs, the other four genes are expressed selectively in the syncytiotrophoblast layer of the placenta. In addition to the major transcripts encoding the proteins, multiple alternatively spliced products for *GH-V, PL-A, PL-B,* and *PL-L* genes have been observed in the placenta.

Although members of the h*GH/PL* gene family share nearly 91–99% sequence identities throughout their coding regions and within a 500-bp 5′ flanking region just proximal to the transcription start sites, studies conducted over the years indicate that the critical trans-acting factors and the cis-acting

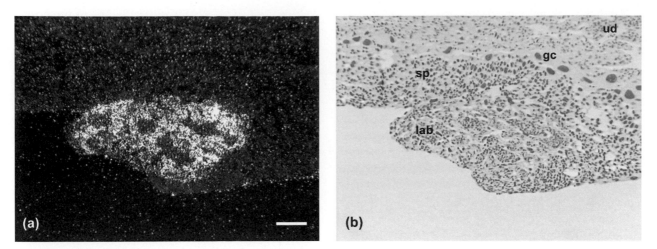

FIGURE 2 Labyrinthine-specific expression of a *CYP19I.1₋₅₀₁:hGH* fusion gene in transgenic mice. Placental tissue obtained from an E10.5 fetal transgenic mouse carrying the *CYP19I.1₋₅₀₁:hGH* fusion gene was processed for *in situ* hybridization using a ³⁵S-labeled antisense hGH cRNA probe and then exposed to photographic emulsion for 1–2 weeks. (a) Darkfield and (b) brightfield micrographs reveal trophoblast giant cells (gc), spongiotrophoblast (sp), labyrinthine trophoblast (lab), and the uterine decidua (ud). Reproduced from Kamat, A., Graves, K. H., Smith, M. E., Richardson, J. A., and Mendelson, C. R. (1999), A 500-bp region, approximately 40 kb upstream of the human CYP19 (aromatase) gene, mediates placenta-specific expression in transgenic mice, *Proc. Natl. Acad. Sci. USA* **96**, 4575–4580, with permission from the National Academy of Science, USA.

elements necessary for placenta-specific expression of *PL* are distinct from those that regulate the expression of h*GH* in the pituitary. Work done mainly in choriocarcinoma cell lines indicates that a ubiquitous Sp1 site, two activator protein-2 (AP-2) sites, and a trophoblast-specific initiator element (InrE) located within the 5′ flanking region are important for the regulation of *PL-A* gene expression. The Sp1 site, although found to be necessary, is not sufficient for maximal basal and enhancer-mediated transcription. However, a 70-kDa InrE-binding protein expressed in human choriocarcinoma cell lines BeWo and JEG-3 is observed to be required for maximal enhancer function and cell-specific h*PL* gene expression. Results also suggest that the InrE elements are required for accurate transcription initiation from the PL promoter in these cells. Expression of h*PL* in the placenta is also regulated by PL enhancers, CSEn1, CSEn2, and CSEn5, located downstream, or 3′, of the *PL-A*, *PL-B*, and *PL-L* genes, respectively. These enhancers are composed of multiple enhansons that work cooperatively to mediate maximal enhancer activity. Work done to characterize the enhancer CSEn2 indicates that several DNA–protein interactions occur within this region. Chorionic somatomammotropin gene enhancer factor-1 (CSEF-1), a 30-kDa protein found in BeWo cells, has been suggested to act through CSEn2 to enhance transcription. Transcriptional enhancer factor-1 (TEF-1) also binds to this element with the same affinity as CSEF-1 but reduces activation of the h*PL* promoter by inhibiting preinitiation complex formation. On the other hand, another member of the TEF family, TEF-5, binds to a unique element in CSEn2 and transactivates the enhancer. Further studies to characterize placenta-specific expression of *PL* genes have also indicated that there are mechanisms to suppress h*PL* gene expression in the pituitary. It has been demonstrated that CSEn2 in conjunction with either CSEn1 or CSEn5 forms a composite silencer in pituitary cells. Additionally, two orientation-dependent repressor elements (PSF-A and PSA-B) that exist in the 5′ flanking region of each of the *PL* and *GH-V* genes, but not in that of the pituitary *GH-N* gene, have been reported to bind pituitary nuclear factors that inhibit transactivation of the placental members of the growth hormone family in the pituitary. Thus, these various *in vitro* studies using both cultured placental cells and choriocarcinoma cell lines have indicated that placenta-specific transcriptional control of the h*PL* gene involves both positive and negative regulation.

Studies have also been conducted to ascertain if the critical cis-acting elements, as defined in cell transfection assays, are able to direct appropriate placenta-specific expression in transgenic mice. In initial studies, a 15-kb transgene fragment containing the *PL-A* gene with 5.4 kb of 5′ flanking sequence and

7.2 kb of 3' flanking sequence was found either not to be expressed or to be expressed at low and variable levels in the mouse placenta. An 87-kb transgene was then created; it contained the majority of the h*GH* gene cluster linked to the entire locus control region, located -15 to -32 kb upstream of the hGH cluster, and was used to determine the expression pattern of the human genes as they exist in the native configuration of their family cluster. In the five transgenic mouse lines that were created, all of the h*GH* cluster genes were appropriately expressed, with h*GH-N* being specifically expressed at relatively high levels in the pituitary and the h*PL* genes being expressed specifically in the placenta. In contrast to the human genome, the mouse genome contains a single pituitary-specific *GH* gene and lacks any *GH*-related *PL* genes. Nonetheless, it is apparent that the mouse placenta has the transcription factors necessary to mediate placenta-specific expression of the human *PL*-containing transgene. Further *in situ* studies have indicated that expression of the h*PL-A*-containing transgene is localized to the labyrinth of the mouse placenta, which, as previously mentioned, is functionally analogous to the syncytiotrophoblast.

IV. CONCLUSIONS

Aromatase and the placental lactogens participate in important placental functions in humans. Whereas aromatase is necessary for the conversion of C_{19} steroids to estrogens, and lack of aromatase expression results in virilization of the fetus, the placental lactogens alter maternal carbohydrate and lipid metabolism to provide for fetal nutrient requirements. However, the biological functions of the products of both of these genes are not fully understood, and individuals with mutations in placental genes for *CYP19* or *PL* genes have had normal pregnancies. Studies on regulation of the h*CYP19* or h*PL* gene have thus far indicated that both negative and positive tissue-specific transcription factors are involved in regulation of the placenta-specific gene expression. Additionally, although the mouse placenta does not express aromatase or PLs, the h*CYP19* and h*PL* transgenes are specifically expressed in the labyrinthine layer of the mouse placenta, which is functionally analogous to the syncytiotrophoblast of the human placenta, where these genes are normally expressed. This suggests that specific cells within the labyrinthine layer of mouse placenta express the appropriate transcription factors required to activate the promoters of the h*CYP19* and h*PL* genes. Future studies in placental cells and in transgenic animals will

likely contribute to our understanding of the positive and negative regulatory elements involved in tissue-specific regulation of aromatase and PL, and to the role that these two important molecules play in human placenta.

Glossary

enhancers DNA sequences that increase the rate of gene transcription from a distance, irrespective of their orientation relative to the transcription start site in the gene.

enhansons Subunits of enhancers; some enhancers are composed of separate 15- to 20-bp elements that cooperate with one another to enhance transcription. These elements are made up of enhansons, which can be duplicated or interchanged to create new enhancer elements. Unlike enhancers, enhansons are sensitive to changes in spacing.

labyrinthine zone Murine placental complex of trophoblast, mesoderm, and vascular derivatives; functionally analogous to the floating chorionic villi in humans.

spongiotrophoblast Intermediate layer in the murine placenta that, like the trophoblast giant cells, arises from the ectoplacental cone; with the giant cell layer, separates the labyrinthine zone from the maternal decidua.

trans-acting factors Transcription factors (specific proteins) that bind to relatively short DNA sequence motifs, or cis-acting elements, to regulate gene transcription. The cis-acting elements can occur in various locations and at different distances and directions relative to the transcriptional start and stop sites within the gene.

trophoblast cells Progenitor cells, important in the formation of the placenta and responsible for various functions, including nutrition of the differentiating embryo and the growing fetus and secretion of hormones indispensable for the maintenance of pregnancy.

trophoblast giant cells Polyploid mouse trophoblast cells that surround the conceptus and lie in direct contact with the maternal decidua.

See Also the Following Articles

Aromatase and Estrogen Insufficiency • Knockout of Gonadotropins and Their Receptor Genes • Oocyte Development and Maturation • Ovulation • Oxytocin • Placental Development • Placental Immunology • Prolactin and Growth Hormone Receptors

Further Reading

Anthony, R. V., Limesand, S. W., and Jeckel, K. M. (2001). Transcriptional regulation in the placenta during normal and compromised fetal growth. *Biochem. Soc. Trans.* **29**, 42–47.

Handwerger, S., and Freemark, M. (2000). The roles of placental growth hormone and placental lactogen in the regulation of human fetal growth and development. *J. Pediatr. Endocrinol. Metab.* **13,** 343–356.

Kamat, A., Hinshelwood, M. M., Murry, B. A., and Mendelson, C. R. (2002). Mechanisms in tissue-specific regulation of estrogen biosynthesis in humans. *Trends Endocrinol. Metab.* **13,** 122–128.

Ringler, G. E., and Strauss, J. F. (1990). *In vitro* systems for the study of human placental endocrine function. *Endocr. Rev.* **11,** 105–123.

Simpson, E. R., Zhao, Y., Agarwal, V. R., Michael, M. D., Bulun, S. E., Hinshelwood, M. M., Graham-Lorence, S., Sun, T., Fisher, C. R., Qin, K., and Mendelson, C. R. (1997). Aromatase expression in health and disease. *Recent Prog. Horm. Res.* **52,** 185–214.

Walker, W. H., Fitzpatrick, S. L., Barrera-Saldana, H. A., Resendez-Perez, D., and Saunders, G. F. (1991). The human placental lactogen genes: Structure, function, evolution and transcriptional regulation. *Endocr. Rev.* **12,** 316–328.

Placental Immunology

JOAN S. HUNT AND MARGARET G. PETROFF

University of Kansas Medical Center

I. INTRODUCTION
II. PLACENTAL REGULATION OF HLA
III. INHIBITORY MOLECULES ON TROPHOBLASTS
IV. UTERINE LEUKOCYTE MODIFICATIONS
V. SUMMARY

Placental immunology may be defined as the study of structural and functional features of the placenta that permit semiallogeneic pregnancy to proceed despite genetic differences between the mother and the fetus. Ordinarily, the presence of "foreign" tissue would stimulate a graft rejection response as is the case in transplantation of organs. In this article, the unique aspects of immune protection at the maternal–fetal interface are presented.

I. INTRODUCTION

In the middle of the past century, immunologists were just beginning to understand the design of the immune system. One general principle emerged; in healthy adults, the immune system is immensely efficient in repelling the invasion of foreign DNA and RNA.

A major enigma is presented by the state of human pregnancy, in which genetically different tissues reside side by side in apparent harmony.

In 1953, P. Medawar was the first to offer ideas for mechanisms that could account for the surprising ability of the fetal semiallograft to survive in a potentially hostile environment. His suggestions included (1) anatomic separation of the mother and fetus; (2) antigenic immaturity of the fetus; and (3) tolerance in the mother. Although somewhat different from Medawar's original ideas, all these mechanisms have now been identified. The blood circulations of the mother and fetus are entirely separate, the major fetal cell surface molecules that stimulate graft rejection appear late, and mothers develop multiple tolerogenic mechanisms.

One of the most impressive features of immunological protection, which may be termed "immune privilege," is the wide range of devices used in maternal endometrium and fetal placenta to ensure tolerance. In humans, these may include (1) tight control over the expression of human leukocyte antigen (HLA) expression by cells in human placentas; (2) production of immunosuppressive substances such as prostaglandin E2, progesterone, and T-helper 2 (T_H2)-type cytokines at the maternal–fetal interface; (3) placental cell expression of the apoptosis-inducing cytokines, Fas ligand (CD95 ligand) and tumor necrosis factor (TNF)-related apoptosis-inducing ligand (TRAIL) (Apo-2 ligand), as well as proteins that inhibit the complement cascade and those that modulate leukocyte proliferation and cytokine secretion (B7-H1); and (4) restriction of migration of antigen-specific T and B lymphocytes into the decidua. Each of these mechanisms is of great interest and will be discussed briefly in this article.

II. PLACENTAL REGULATION OF HLA

A. HLA Class I Antigens

Both beneficial and potentially detrimental effects are exerted by the functionally unique HLA molecules. These cell surface structures are required for host protection against infectious agents but when they are perceived as foreign by the host, as is likely to happen with paternally derived antigens in human pregnancy, they may stimulate graft rejection.

The major histocompatibility complex (MHC) located on the short arm of chromosome 6 encodes the HLA class I antigens. The proteins comprise three ~100 amino acid "domains" with disulfide bonds looping the domains. HLA class I antigens usually have one transmembrane heavy chain (37 to 45 kDa) associated noncovalently with a light chain (β2-microglobulin, ~12 kDa). HLA class I glycoproteins

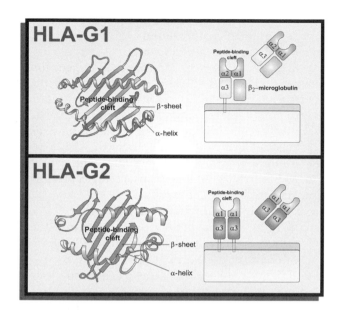

FIGURE 1 Schematic representations of (left) the peptide-binding cleft in HLA-G1 and HLA-G2, as viewed from the top down, and (right) the likely structures of membrane-bound and soluble HLA-G1 and HLA-G2. Note that HLA-G1 is composed of a heavy chain and a light chain (β2-microglobulin), whereas HLA-G2 heavy chains form homodimers and do not bind β2-microglobulin.

carrying foreign peptides within a region called the peptide-binding groove (Fig. 1) are recognized by the T-cell receptor (TCR) on CD8$^+$ precursor cytotoxic T lymphocytes (CTL). The HLA-A, -B, and -C class Ia genes are highly polymorphic and their proteins are co-dominantly expressed on the cell membranes of essentially all eukaryotic cells, the exceptions being germ cells (oocytes, sperm) and placental trophoblast cells. Differences between class I antigens derived from each allele create a major barrier associated with transplantation of donor organs because immune cells recognize nonself alleles as foreign and mount a graft rejection response that includes cytotoxic cells and cytotoxic antibodies.

By contrast, the HLA-E, -F, and -G class Ib genes have few alleles and their proteins are restricted to certain types of cells. Figure 1 shows the probable antigen-binding clefts and stylized isoform structures of soluble HLA-G1 and soluble HLA-G2, two isoforms of HLA-G which are discussed below.

B. HLA Class II (HLA-D) Antigens

The class II antigens have two transmembrane heavy chains, are also highly polymorphic, and also constitute barriers to transplantation. They are expressed primarily on antigen-presenting cells such as macrophages, dendritic cells, and B lymphocytes, but may be expressed on other cells during certain diseases. The class II antigens form homodimers rather than heterodimers. HLA class II (HLA-D) glycoproteins carrying foreign peptides in the homodimeric heavy chain cleft are recognized by TCRs on CD4$^+$ T-helper lymphocytes.

C. HLA on Trophoblast Cells

The surprising success of semiallogeneic pregnancy may be attributed in large part to controlled expression of the HLA molecules in trophoblast cells. These cell surface structures are the main mediators of graft rejection, but HLA is so firmly regulated that there are no known instances of inappropriate expression in fetal tissues as a cause of pregnancy failure where maternal immune cells attack fetal tissues. Trophoblast cells may be subdivided into several subpopulations depending on their stage of differentiation and their anatomic location; regulation of their HLA proteins differs according to need.

D. Trophoblast Subpopulations

Trophoblast cells are derived from the trophectoderm layer of the blastocyst. These cells are not uniform; they differentiate in a stage-specific manner into several subpopulations. The cytotrophoblast is the precursor cell and is driven into one of two pathways of differentiation. In one instance, cytotrophoblast cells coalesce into a multinucleated syncytium. This is an uninterrupted cell layer that, at term, would cover 9 m^2 if spread. The syncytiotrophoblast cell layer modulates bidirectional transport of nutrients and wastes, is responsible for most placental hormone production, and protects the inner cell mass-derived elements (the amnion and chorion membranes, the umbilical cord, and the embryo) from blood-borne maternal immune cells.

A second set of cytotrophoblast cells proliferates and emerges from the floating placental villi to form columns that ultimately contact the maternal decidua (Fig. 2). The extravillous trophoblastic cells invade the spiral arteries and replace the endothelial cells in the vessels. As pregnancy progresses, the extravillous cells cease migrating and regress to form the chorion membrane.

Unlike embryonic cells, trophoblast cells never express normal adult levels or patterns of HLA. As described below, specific HLA class I genes are

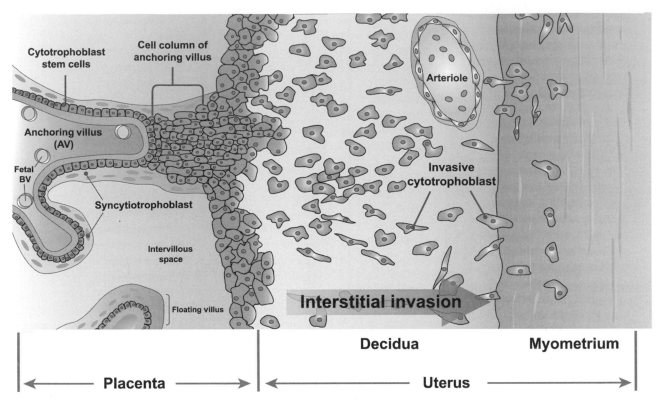

FIGURE 2 A representational drawing of the maternal–fetal interface at the point of contact. Some placental villi form cell columns. Cytotrophoblast cells invade the maternal uterine interstitium and may be found in the myometrium as well as lining maternal spiral arteries. Other villi float in a sea of maternal blood filling the intervillous space.

selected for expression from among the many members of this multigene family, whereas HLA class II genes are essentially unexpressed in trophoblasts. The absence of class II may be due to repressor elements on promoter and other elements in the class II gene sequences. More studies need to be performed to elucidate the nature of the restriction, which is effective even in the presence of class II inducers such as interferon-γ (IFN-γ) and type 1 interferons.

E. HLA Class I in Trophoblasts

The exciting story of how placental expression of the HLA genes and the glycoproteins derived from these genes was revealed has been told frequently. In short, stage of gestation, state of differentiation, and anatomical location dictate expression in this unique cell lineage.

HLA class I message may be present but membrane-bound proteins are difficult to detect in early gestation syncytiotrophoblast and villous cytotrophoblast cells. In late gestation, neither subpopulation contains substantial class I mRNA or membrane-bound HLA class I protein. Although cytotrophoblast cells in early placentas that are proliferating in preparation for column formation are negative for both message and protein, the cytotrophoblast cells distal to the villus in the cytotrophoblastic shell are HLA class I positive. Class I positivity is retained in the chorion membrane cytotrophoblast cells, which are derived from the invasive extravillous cytotrophoblasts.

F. HLA Class I Gene Selection

The ability to select specific members of the HLA class I multigene family for expression is a unique property of trophectoderm-derived cells. Three members of the HLA class I gene family are present in HLA class I positive trophoblasts; one is a class Ia gene, HLA-C, and two are class Ib genes, HLA-E and HLA-G. The highly polymorphic, widely distributed HLA-A and -B antigens are absent.

The function(s) of HLA-C remains unknown. Although the gene is polymorphic and it is clear that proteins derived from this gene are present on trophoblast cells, whether it has any influence on immune cells or the immunobiology of pregnancy is not known. Unlike other class Ia genes, expression is transient and at a comparatively low level. HLA-E is an interesting molecule; it uses the leader sequences of other class I proteins to gain access to the cell surface. Considerable experimentation has led to the idea that HLA-E interacts with natural killer (NK) cell inhibitory receptors and drives these cells into an anergic condition. The decidua in early and mid stages of pregnancy is packed with NK cells that would attack HLA⁻ negative cells, so expression of a class I molecule is very important. HLA-G, which was the first HLA to be discovered on trophoblast cells, has been extensively studied. Much has been revealed about this unusual gene, as described in detail below, although the major functions of the spectrum of protein isoforms derived from this gene remain unclear.

To date, nothing is known of how these three genes are selected for expression in trophoblasts from among the members of the HLA class I multigene family. Their appearance appears to be synchronous, suggesting that whatever mechanism constitutes the "ON" signal influences the expression of all three genes.

G. Immunogenetics of HLA-G

HLA-G is a gene exhibiting several unique features. Its cytoplasmic tail is shortened and may or may not transduce signals. Its promoter region contains a large deletion in the enhancer A/IFN consensus region, which results in crippling of IFN-induced transcription, and the γ-activated site has a single nucleotide substitution that prevents activation. As a consequence and unlike other HLA class I genes, HLA-G is only weakly enhanced by exposure to interferons.

Also in contrast to other HLA class I genes, alternative splicing is a feature of the HLA-G message. Mechanisms underlying the production of multiple transcripts from this gene are unknown. Importantly, some transcripts encode cell surface proteins and others encode soluble proteins. The latter is a consequence of a stop codon in intron 4, which precludes translation into the transmembrane region. All the transcripts are readily identified in placentas and trophoblast cell lines. Because the antibodies to HLA-G are poorly characterized regarding binding site and specificity, expression in adult cells and tissues remains uncertain.

H. Functions of HLA-G

Functions clearly attributable to HLA-G are poorly defined at present. Because expression of this gene, which has few allelic variants, is a prominent feature of the maternal–fetal interface, its substitution for HLA-A or -B is widely believed to be critical to the maintenance of semiallogeneic pregnancy. The gene does express a few alleles, identified as *0101, *0103, *0104, and *0106, that might be immunostimulatory in mismatched couples, but it is not yet known whether mothers recognize the products of the different alleles.

Evidence has been presented for the postulate that HLA-G interacts with macrophage immunoglobulin-like transcript 4 (ILT4) receptors and conveys inhibitory signals to this cell lineage just as HLA-E does to NK cells. If this occurs, it could prevent activation of the macrophages in the decidua and subsequent killing of migrating trophoblastic cells. Presumably, these interactions would be cell–cell involvements and would rely on membrane-bound HLA-G on trophoblasts, but this does not preclude the utilization of soluble HLA-G, which is receiving considerable attention. It is important to remember that other suppressive substances such as progesterone and prostaglandins could have similar effects.

Soluble HLA-G is present in placentas and more recently has been demonstrated in the sera of pregnant women. These proteins could have profound effects on maternal immune cells. Evidence from studies employing soluble HLA-G1 partially purified from trophoblastic tumor cells indicates that this substance stimulates the apoptosis of lectin-activated T lymphocytes through the Fas/FasL pathway, a process that has been identified in immune cells exposed to other soluble HLA class I molecules. An immunoregulatory role for soluble HLA-G is indicated in the finding that levels are higher in mothers who have successful pregnancies following assisted reproductive technology as well as in heart transplant recipients who have less rejection. Furthermore, HLA-G transfected into pig islets increases graft acceptance.

Although it is possible that each of the isoforms derived from alternatively spliced messages has a different function, it seems more likely that there is at least some redundancy; pregnancy proceeds in the absence of HLA-G. The placentas of babies with a homozygous deletion that prevents synthesis of HLA-G1 protein contain other HLA-G isoforms; whether these alternative isoforms are the major players in the spectrum of HLA-G proteins or whether they are simply able to substitute for HLA-G1 remains to be ascertained.

III. INHIBITORY MOLECULES ON TROPHOBLASTS

A. Membrane-Bound Molecules

Since trophoblast subpopulations form the anatomical boundary between maternal blood and tissues and inner cell mass-derived fetal mesenchyme, it is not surprising to find that trophoblast cells display surface-bound proteins that actively participate in defending the fetus from potentially harmful components of the maternal immune system. Toxic entities could include maternal leukocytes as well as cytotoxic antibodies and complement. A number of protective entities on trophoblast membranes have been identified.

1. Tumor Necrosis Factor Superfamily Proteins

Members of the TNF superfamily are emerging as potentially critical mediators of placental immune privilege. Essentially all the ligands may be either membrane-bound or soluble and the same is true of many of the receptors. FasL, which kills activated leukocytes through its receptor, Fas, is expressed discontinuously in villous and extravillous trophoblast cells throughout gestation. Trophoblasts have been shown to mediate apoptosis of leukocytes through the Fas/FasL system *in vitro*. Experiments in mice have shown that the ligand is highly important in protection of the placenta. In FasL-deficient mice, activated maternal leukocytes inappropriately infiltrate the maternal–fetal interface, and viability of the embryos is greatly reduced.

TRAIL is another member of the TNF superfamily that is likely to protect the fetus through expression on trophoblasts. This powerful inducer of apoptosis is incapable of causing death in trophoblasts, most likely because trophoblast cells express high levels of a TRAIL decoy receptor, DcR1. It is generally believed that in a similar fashion, protection against apoptosis by other toxic molecules is effected by receptor blocking. For example, soluble TNF receptor which compete with membrane-bound receptors, are abundant in placentas. FasL, TRAIL, and TNFα are not the only apoptosis-inducing superfamily members in placentas. Messenger RNA encoding other death-inducing ligands in first-trimester placentas include lymphotoxin-β, TNF-like weak inducer of apoptosis (TWEAK), and LIGHT (homologous to lymphotoxin), and term placentas contain these as well as lymphotoxin-α and 4-1B3 ligand (4-1BBL). The distribution of LIGHT protein has now been reported in term placentas, but proteins from most of the other newly identified members have yet to be evaluated systematically.

Importantly, the cytokines that were first identified in the immune system may have other critical functions in placentas such as governing developmental pathways through programmed cell death and perhaps also through effects on gene expression that do not lead to apoptosis. Nearly all the family members that have been examined to date stimulate a protective nuclear factor κB pathway in some cells under specific conditions.

2. Complement Regulatory Proteins

Activation of the complement cascade leads to deposition of complement components on cellular surfaces and formation of lytic pore-forming units termed the membrane attack complexes. The complement system is intended to protect the host against bacteria, parasites, and virus-infected cells. However, damage to host cells can result if they are not protected by a series of complement regulatory proteins, which includes CD59, membrane co-factor protein (MCP, CD46), and decay accelerating factor (DAF, CD55). These complement regulatory proteins are broadly distributed in adult tissues. All three of these membrane-bound proteins are also highly expressed at the apical surface of the syncytiotrophoblast facing the maternal blood space as well by villous (CD59 and MCP) and extravillous (CD59 and DAF) cytotrophoblasts. The presence of these complement regulatory proteins is believed to confer resistance of trophoblasts to antibody-mediated cytotoxicity.

Murine Crry is a transmembrane glycoprotein that functionally resembles DAF and MCP. Crry is absolutely essential to pregnancy in mice. $Crry^{-/-}$ embryos fail to survive in normal mothers due to the spontaneous deposition of complement factor C3 in the developing placenta. Furthermore, $Crry^{-/-}$ embryos remain viable in mothers lacking C3. Activation of the complement system also leads to fetal loss in a murine model of anti-phospholipid syndrome, suggesting that a similar mechanism may occur in women suffering this disorder.

3. B7 Family Proteins

Members of the B7 family of membrane glycoproteins are ligands that interact with receptors belonging to the CD28 family. Of the six known members of the B7 family, five are highly expressed in the human placenta. Expression of one of these, B7-H1 (also known as PD-L1), is relatively restricted, occurring mainly in macrophages, trophoblast cells, and cells constituting some organs. Consistent with the need for immunological protection of the allogeneic fetus, the B7-H1 receptor, PD-1, plays a major role in the maintenance of peripheral immunological tolerance. Mice lacking PD-1 develop severe autoimmune disorders that afflict organs whose cells express B7-H1 and its sister ligand, B7-DC (PD-L2). B7-H1 has been shown to inhibit CD3-activated T lymphocytes stimulate allograft survival, and protect tumor cells from T cell-mediated lysis. B7-H1 also alters their cytokine secretion patterns, possibly driving the T cells into the T_H2-type cytokine production profile that is thought to be important to pregnancy. In addition, B7-H1 induces apoptosis in activated, antigen-specific leukocytes, most likely through a receptor distinct from PD-1. The functional significance of placental B7 family members is not yet known, but their distribution within specific cellular elements of the human placenta indicates that this family of molecules plays an important role in the establishment and maintenance of maternal tolerance to the fetus.

B. Soluble Molecules

Pregnancy is known to require adequate levels of progesterone for both implantation and maintenance. Early on, this hormone is synthesized in the corpus luteum of the ovary and subsequently in the placenta. Progesterone has many functions, one of which may be to discourage the proliferation and cytotoxicity of immune cells. As described below, the maternal–fetal interface is characterized by cells supplying the host (mother) with innate immunity rather than lymphocyte-specific acquired immunity. Progesterone may drive the substitution process, which occurs early following implantation. Furthermore, when exposed to high levels of progesterone, innate immune cells such as macrophages are programmed into a suppressive profile characterized by the absence of T_H1-type inflammatory cytokines (TNFα, IFN-γ) and production of T_H2-type anti-inflammatory cytokines [interleukin-10, transforming growth-β (TGF-β)] as well as the negative regulator of immune cells, prostaglandin E2.

Taken together, these elements probably account in large part for the well-described immunosuppressive environment of the pregnant uterus. However, researchers continue to identify additional protectors

of the placenta; one recent entry is indolamine oxidase, an inhibitor of tryptophan metabolism.

IV. UTERINE LEUKOCYTE MODIFICATIONS

Among the alterations that occur at the maternal–fetal interface, reassortment of leukocytes is one of the most profound. Although the cycling endometrium has lymphoid aggregates composed of T and B lymphocytes, immature NK cells, and randomly distributed macrophages, the antigen-specific T and B cells nearly disappear with the onset of implantation. Thus, the pregnant uterus is populated almost exclusively by cells supplying innate or natural immunity, the NK cells and macrophages. In the human decidua, the NK cells disappear in the second trimester, whereas the macrophages remain throughout pregnancy, providing a measure of host defense against infection.

It is clear that molecules present on the surfaces of migrating trophoblast cells and soluble products of the placenta target decidual immune cells, and there is evidence as well for reciprocal activity, with decidual leukocytes targeting placental cells. For the former, membrane-bound HLA-G and soluble HLA-G represent an excellent example. Decidual macrophages express inhibitory receptors for HLA-G, the ILT proteins termed ILT2 and ILT4. Although as yet untested in decidual macrophages, in other cells, ligand–ILT receptor interactions transduce inhibitory signals that reduce cellular cytotoxicity. Thus, membrane and soluble HLA-G could have a major impact on how leukocytes in the decidua are programmed for the benefit of pregnancy.

For the latter, experiments in gene-deleted mice strongly suggest that TNFα derived from decidual cells influences placental organization. Further, there is considerable information in mice on the interaction between uterine colony-stimulating factor-1 (CSF-1) and its receptor on trophoblast cells. CSF-1-stimulated trophoblast cells become phagocytic and then act as a component of the innate immune system at the maternal–fetal interface. Collectively, these types of studies have contributed to a better understanding of the unique utilization of immune system molecules to promote successful pregnancy.

V. SUMMARY

More than four decades of research have brought reproductive immunologists to the understanding that the placental bed is a dynamic, ever-changing network of maternal–fetal interactions facilitated by a wide range of soluble and cell-surface molecules. Figure 3 illustrates some features of the bidirectional communication that facilitates successful pregnancy. Trophoblast cells secrete powerful soluble molecules such as prostaglandins and progesterone, soluble HLA-G, and immunomodulatory cytokines that include interleukins, members of the TNF supergene family, and members of the TGF-β gene family. Leukocytes are sources of both cytokines and prostaglandins. Membrane-bound molecules on trophoblast cells and leukocytes participate significantly in interactions in the decidua and may also modulate the actions of leukocytes circulating in the mother's blood. These include ILT, c-type lectin, and NK cell immunoglobulin-like receptors for HLA molecules, members of the B7 family of modulators, ligand and receptor proteins for the TNF and TGF-β gene families, and the critically protective complement regulatory proteins.

Identification of the many features of the maternal–fetal interface that circumvent the immune system designed for the destruction of cells carrying foreign DNA and/or RNA has provided the critical framework needed to understand pregnancy failures. Although experiments in women cannot be performed, new approaches to pinpointing the central players in the networks are being conducted in gene-modified mice as well as in nonhuman primates. Both rodent and primate experimental animal systems have attractive features and offer hope for demonstrating proofs of principle that will ultimately lead to new clinical therapies for problem pregnancies.

Acknowledgments

The authors thank their many students and trainees as well as their colleagues for their contributions to this work, which is supported by research grants from the National Institutes of Health.

Glossary

B7 family molecules Cell surface molecules involved in both stimulation and inhibition of immune cells.

complement The collective term for serum proteins that may cause lysis of cells.

cytokines Molecules of 15 to 30 kDa that mediate cellular interactions. They may be either bound to the cell membrane or soluble and are often subdivided by their usual cell of origin, i.e., T-helper 1 (T_H1, pro-inflammatory) and T_H2 (anti-inflammatory) lymphocytes.

cytotoxic T lymphocyte A type of cell that attacks foreign and infected cells.

human leukocyte antigens Glycoproteins encoded by genes within the major histocompatibility complex on human chromosome 6. They are important self-recognition molecules in host defense but, when foreign, constitute targets for cytotoxic T lymphocytes and antibodies.

leukocytes Bone marrow-derived cells involved in innate and immune host defense.

macrophages Leukocytes that reside in tissues and have innate and immune host defense functions.

major histocompatibility complex Genes that encode the human leukocyte antigen class I and class II proteins.

natural killer cells Non-antigen-specific leukocytes that thickly populate the early to mid gestation pregnant uterus.

See Also the Following Articles

Apoptosis ● Decidualization ● Implantation ● Placental Development ● Placental Gene Expression ● Tumor Necrosis Factor (TNF)

Further Reading

Bulmer, J. N. (1995). Immune cells in decidua. *In* "Immunology of Human Reproduction" (M. Kurpisz and N. Fernandez, eds.), pp. 313–334. BIOS Scientific, Oxford.

Freeman, G. J., Long, A. J., Iwai, Y., Bourque, K., Chernova, T., Nishimura, H., Fitz, L. J., Malenkovich, N., Okazaki, T., Byrne, M. C., Horton, H. F., Fouser, L., Carter, L., Ling, V., Bowman, M. R., Carreno, B. M., Collins, M., Wood, C. R., and Honjo, T. (2000). Engagement of the PD-1 immunoinhibitory receptor by a novel B7 family member leads to negative regulation of lymphocyte activation. *J. Exp. Med.* **192**, 1027–1034.

Guleria, I., and Pollard, J. W. (2000). The trophoblast is a component of the innate immune system during pregnancy. *Nat. Med.* **6**, 589–593.

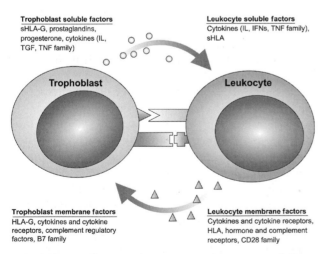

FIGURE 3 Bidirectional interactions between trophoblast cells and leukocytes. Interactions include targeting of soluble molecules supplied by both types of cells as well as direct cell–cell contact and interaction via matching ligands and receptors. IFNs, interferons; IL, interleukins; sHLA-G, soluble HLA-G; TGF, transforming growth factor; TNF, tumor necrosis factor.

Hunt, J. S., Petroff, M. G., Morales, P., Sedlmayr, P., Geraghty, D. E., and Ober, C. (2000). HLA-G in reproduction: Studies on the maternal–fetal interface. *Hum. Immunol.* **61**, 1113–1117.

King, A., Burrows, T., Hiby, V. S., and Loke, Y. W. (1998). Human uterine lymphocytes. *Hum. Reprod. Update* **4**, 480–485.

Le Bouteiller, P., and Mallet, V. (1997). HLA-G and pregnancy. *Rev. Reprod.* **2**, 7–13.

Le Gal, F.-A., Riteau, B., Sedlik, C., Khalil-Daher, I., Menier, C., Dausset, J., Guillet, J.-G., Carosella, E. D., and Rouas-Freiss, N. (1999). HLA-G-mediated inhibition of antigen-specific cytotoxic T lymphocytes. *Int. Immunol.* **11**, 1351–1355.

Mellor, A. L., and Munn, D. (2001). Tryptophan catabolism prevents maternal T cells from activating lethal anti-fetal immune response. *J. Reprod. Immunol.* **52**, 5–13.

Miller, L., and Hunt, J. S. (1996). Sex steroid hormones and macrophage function. *Life Sci.* **59**, 1–14.

Ober, C., and Aldrich, C. L. (1997). HLA-G polymorphisms: Neutral evolution or novel function? *J. Reprod. Immunol.* **36**, 1–21.

Ober, C., Aldrich, C., Rosinsky, B., Robertson, A., Walker, M. A., Willadsen, S., Verp, M. S., Geraghty, D. E., and Hunt, J. S. (1998). HLA-G1 protein expression is not essential for fetal survival. *Placenta* **19**, 127–132.

Petroff, M. G., Chen, L., Phillips, T. A., Azzola, D., Sedlmayr, P., and Hunt, J. S. (2003). B7 family molecules are favorably positioned at the human maternal–fetal interface. *Biol. Reprod.* In press.

Phillips, T. A., Ni, J., and Hunt, J. S. (2001). Death-inducing tumor necrosis factor (TNF) superfamily ligands and receptors are transcribed in human placentae, cytotrophoblasts, placental macrophages and placental cell lines. *Placenta* **22**, 663–672.

Runic, R., Lockwood, C. J., Ma, Y., Dipasquale, B., and Guller, S. (1996). Expression of Fas ligand by human cytotrophoblasts: Implications in placentation and fetal survival. *J. Clin. Endocrinol. Metab.* **81**, 3119–3122.

Xu, C., Mao, D., Holers, V. M., Palanca, B., Cheng, A., and Molina, H. (2000). A critical role for the murine complement regulatory Crry in fetomaternal tolerance. *Science* **287**, 498–501.

Platelet-Derived Growth Factor (PDGF)

CARL-HENRIK HELDIN

Ludwig Institute for Cancer Research, Uppsala, Sweden

I. INTRODUCTION
II. PDGF ISOFORMS
III. PDGF RECEPTORS
IV. FUNCTION OF PDGF *IN VIVO*
V. PDGF IN DISEASE
VI. SUMMARY

Platelet-derived growth factor (PDGF) is of particular importance for the growth, survival, and migration of mesenchymal cell types. It stimulates the differentiation of various cell types of the connective tissue during embryonic development and is important for the formation of blood vessels. In the adult, PDGF regulates the interstitial fluid pressure of the connective tissue and also stimulates the regeneration of connective tissue during wound healing. Over-activity of PDGF is connected with several disorders involving excess cell proliferation, including malignancies, atherosclerosis, and fibrotic conditions.

I. INTRODUCTION

Platelet-derived growth factor (PDGF) constitutes a family of dimeric isoforms, acting on connective tissue cells and certain other cell types. PDGF was originally discovered as a constituent of platelets, which are released into serum in conjunction with blood coagulation. Although the α-granules of platelets are a major storage site for PDGF, PDGF is also produced by many other cell types.

PDGF stimulates the growth of its target cells, but also affects chemotaxis, i.e., directed cell movement, and cell shape through reorganization of the actin filament system. PDGF also affects the differentiation of specific cell types and promotes cell survival. Through these effects, PDGF has important functions in certain organs during embryonic development, as well as in the adult in the stimulation of wound healing and in the maintenance of connective tissue homeostasis.

Overactivity of PDGF has been linked to certain diseases, such as malignancies in which PDGF production may promote tumor growth via autocrine or paracrine stimulation. PDGF is also implicated in other disorders that involve an excess of cell proliferation, e.g., atherosclerosis and fibrotic conditions.

II. PDGF ISOFORMS

The PDGF family contains four different gene products, which are assembled into five different dimeric molecules (Fig. 1). The classical PDGF, purified from human platelets, consists of homo- and heterodimers of structurally related A and B polypeptide chains. More recently, two additional members of the family were discovered, i.e., PDGF C chain and D chain, which appear as homodimeric molecules. The PDGF isoforms are homologous to members of the vascular endothelial growth factor (VEGF) family of angiogenic factors.

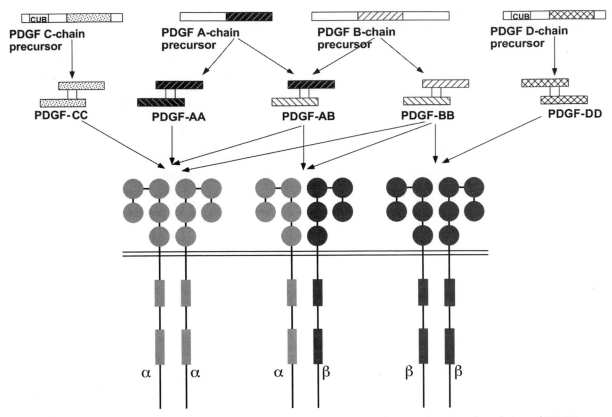

FIGURE 1 Processing and receptor-binding specificities of PDGF isoforms. The A and B chains of PDGF are synthesized as precursors that undergo processing during secretion from the producer cells. The C and D chains are also synthesized as precursors with CUB domains in their N-terminals; these isoforms are processed and activated after secretion from the producer cells. The PDGF isoforms bind to and dimerize α- and β-receptors with different specificities. Each of the receptors has five extracellular Ig-like domains and an intracellular kinase domain that is split into two parts by an intervening sequence.

A. Synthesis of PDGFs

All PDGF isoforms are synthesized as precursor molecules, which undergo processing after synthesis. In the case of the A and B chains, the processing occurs during secretion from the producer cell, resulting in the export of active molecules. In contrast, the C and D chains are secreted as inactive precursors that need to undergo additional cleavage in the extracellular space in order to release the C-terminally located growth factor domain. The cleavages can be performed by plasmin, but the enzymes involved in normal tissues are not known. The N-terminals of the C and D chains contain CUB domains, which are so named because they also are present in complement factor, urchin epidermal growth factor-like protein, and bone morphogenetic protein 1. The CUB domains in PDGF-C and -D keep the growth factor domain inactive.

B. Structure of PDGFs

The crystal structure of PDGF-BB is known; due to sequence conservation, it is likely that the other isoforms are folded similarly. PDGF-BB has a cysteine knot; i.e., one of its internal disulfide bonds passes through the hole formed by two other disulfides and intervening peptide sequences. Cysteine knots, which give a compact structure to the molecules, are also present in the homologous VEGFs, as well as in transforming growth factor-β and nerve growth factor, despite the fact that the latter molecules do not show any sequence similarity to PDGF. In addition to the six cysteine residues involved in the cysteine knot, another two cysteine residues are conserved in the growth factor domain; these residues form interchain disulfide bonds. The C and D chains contain four and two additional cysteine residues, respectively; how they are involved in disulfide bonds is not known.

From the compact cysteine knot of PDGF-BB, two loops (loops I and III) point in one direction and another loop (loop II) points in the other direction. Since the dimer is arranged in an anti-parallel manner, loops I and III from one subunit will be close to loop II of the other subunit; thus, two receptor-binding epitopes occur in the dimeric molecule, each one containing epitopes from loops I and III of one subunit and from loop II of the other subunit.

C. Splice Forms of PDGFs

Certain PDGF isoforms are stored in the extracellular compartment of tissues. The A-chain gene occurs as two splice forms, one with and one without a C-terminal basic sequence, which mediate interactions with components of the extracellular matrix. It is not known whether the splicing of the A-chain gene is regulated, e.g., in response to external signals. A similar basic sequence is also present in the B chain. Whether the CUB domains have effects in addition to keeping the growth factors latent, such as mediating interactions with components of the extracellular matrix and thus providing a mechanism for storage of the PDGF isoforms in the tissues, remains to be elucidated.

Thus, the PDGF family of ligands contains five structurally related members that differ in their processing and other properties. In addition, they differ in their specificity of binding to different receptors, as discussed below.

III. PDGF RECEPTORS

PDGF isoforms exert their cellular effects by binding, with different affinities, to two structurally related protein tyrosine kinase receptors, denoted α- and β-receptors. Each receptor contains five extracellular Ig-like domains and an intracellular kinase domain that is split into two parts by an intervening sequence. The two PDGF receptors form a subfamily among the tyrosine kinase receptors together with the stem cell factor receptor, the colony-stimulating factor 1 receptor, and Flk-1.

A. Receptor Dimerization

Since PDGF isoforms are dimeric and contain two receptor-binding epitopes, they bring together receptors in dimeric complexes on binding. The A and C chains of PDGF bind to α-receptors, the D-chain preferentially to β-receptors, whereas the B chain binds to both α- and β-receptors with high affinity. Therefore, PDGF-AA and -CC cause the formation of αα receptor homodimers, PDGF-DD causes the formation of ββ receptor homodimers, PDGF-AB produces αβ receptor heterodimers as well as αα receptor homodimers, and PDGF-BB produces all three possible combinations of receptor dimers (Fig. 1).

B. Receptor Autophosphorylation

Dimerization is a crucial event in receptor activation, since it brings the intracellular parts of the receptors close to each other so that autophosphorylation *in trans* can occur. The autophosphorylation serves two important functions; i.e., it activates the kinase activity and it creates docking sites for downstream SH2-domain-containing signaling molecules. Activation of the kinase involves autophosphorylation of a tyrosine residue in the activation loop of the kinase, Tyr-849 and Tyr-857 in the α- and β-receptors, respectively. The crystal structures of the PDGF receptor kinases are not known, but solutions of the structures of other kinases have elucidated mechanisms for control of the kinase domain. In the resting state, the activation loop of the kinase is folded over the active site and thereby prevents access to the substrate; phosphorylation causes the activation loop to swing out and thereby allows phosphorylation of the substrates. It is possible that other parts of the receptor, like the juxtamembrane region and the C-terminal tail, also interact with the kinase domain in a negative modulatory manner. Autophosphorylation at tyrosine residues located mainly outside the kinase domain may activate such inhibitory interactions and, in addition, allow binding of downstream signal transduction molecules, initiating a number of signaling pathways. The α- and β-receptors contain at least 9 and 11 such phosphorylation sites that bind, in a specific manner, to different SH2 domain proteins.

C. Docking of SH2 Domain Proteins and Downstream Signaling

Some of the SH2 domain proteins that bind to the PDGF receptors contain intrinsic enzymatic activities, such as the protein tyrosine kinase Src, the protein tyrosine phosphatase SHP-2, phospholipase Cγ, GTPase-activating protein for Ras (RasGAP), and phosphatidylinositol 3'-kinase (PI3-kinase), which consists of a regulatory p85 subunit and a catalytic p110 subunit. Other SH2 domain proteins lack endogenous enzymatic activity and act like adapter molecules, i.e., Shc, Nck, Crk, and Grb2; Grb2 forms a stable complex with Sos1, a nucleotide exchange molecule for Ras.

Much effort has been put into the elucidation of which signaling pathways result in the various cellular effects of PDGF, i.e., cell proliferation, survival, chemotaxis, and actin reorganization. In general, PI3-kinase has been found to be important for the anti-apoptotic and motility responses of PDGF; Src and Ras, which activate the transcription factor Myc and the extracellular signal-related kinase mitogen-activated protein kinase cascade, respectively, are important for the growth-stimulating effect. However, the results depend on the cell type studied and the experimental conditions used for the studies. The difficulties in finding a clear and universal relationship between individual signaling pathways and specific effects can partly be explained by an extensive cross talk between the components in the various signaling pathways.

Both $\alpha\alpha$ and $\beta\beta$ homodimeric receptor complexes transduce mitogenic signals; however, whereas the $\beta\beta$ homodimer stimulates chemotaxis, the $\alpha\alpha$ homodimer inhibits chemotaxis. The molecular mechanism for the difference between the two homodimeric receptor complexes is not known. Moreover, there is evidence that the $\alpha\beta$ heterodimeric complex has unique properties compared to the two homodimers; e.g., it appears to be the complex that causes the most potent mitogenic signal. A possible mechanism for this difference has been elucidated, i.e., the autophosphorylation sites in the PDGF β-receptor differ in a $\beta\beta$ homodimer, compared to an $\alpha\beta$ heterodimer. For example, Tyr-771, which binds RasGAP, is phosphorylated efficiently in the $\beta\beta$ homodimer, but not in the $\alpha\beta$ heterodimer. Thus, the $\alpha\beta$ heterodimer cannot bind RasGAP. Since RasGAP converts active RasGTP to inactive RasGDP, the activation of Ras is therefore more efficient in a heterodimeric receptor than in a $\beta\beta$ homodimeric receptor, which may contribute to its higher mitogenic potency.

D. Internalization of PDGF Receptors

After ligand-induced dimerization, the PDGF receptors are internalized in endosomes. Over time, the pH of the interior of the endosomes becomes acidified, leading to dissociation of the ligand from the receptor. The receptor is then degraded after fusion of the endosomes with lysosomes. An additional degradative route has recently been elucidated, i.e., proteasomal degradation in the cytoplasm, triggered by ubiquitination of the receptor. Alternatively, the receptor is recycled to the plasma membrane after dissociation from the ligand. In the situations that have been studied, the majority of PDGF receptors are degraded after internalization.

IV. FUNCTION OF PDGF *IN VIVO*

PDGF has important functions at specific phases of embryonic development, as well as in wound healing and in control of the homeostasis of the connective tissue compartment in the adult.

A. Embryonic Development

The important function of PDGF during embryogenesis is illustrated by the finding that mice with the A- or B-chain genes or α- or β-receptor genes inactivated die during embryogenesis or perinatally. Data on the phenotypes of mice with the C- or D-chain genes knocked out are not yet available.

A striking effect of knocking out the B-chain or β-receptor genes is that the mesangial cells of the kidney do not develop, causing defective glomeruli with poor filtrating capacity. Moreover, there is a defect in the development of blood vessels in the knockout animals with a dilated aorta. The actual cause of death of the animals is bleeding at the time of birth. The reason for the improper development of the vessels is deficient development of the smooth muscle cells, as well as the inability of the newly formed vessels to attract pericytes.

The major phenotype of animals with the A chain knocked out is emphysema of the lungs, leading to death at approximately 3 weeks of age. The reason for the emphysema is defective distal spreading of alveolar smooth muscle cell progenitors during development.

Since the α-receptor responds to all isoforms containing A, B, and C chains, it is not surprising that knockout of the α-receptor gene gives a more severe phenotype than knockout of the A-chain gene only. The α-receptor knockout animals die during embryogenesis with cranial malformations and deficiency of myotome formation.

Characterization of the expression patterns of PDGF isoforms and their ligands during embryonic development has revealed examples of the expression of a PDGF isoform and the corresponding receptor in the same cell, suggesting autocrine stimulation, as well as in adjacent cell layers, suggesting paracrine stimulation. PDGF receptors are often expressed in mesenchymal cells and PDGF isoforms in adjacent epithelial layers. In this manner, epithelial cells control the development of surrounding mesenchymal structures through the secretion of PDGF isoforms. Although PDGF is of particular importance for the development of connective tissue cells, PDGF receptors are also expressed in cells of nonmesenchymal origin. For instance, the α-receptor is expressed in the ectodermally derived neural crest and the β-receptor in mammary epithelial cells.

B. Central Nervous System

PDGF isoforms and PDGF receptors are expressed in different types of neurons, as well as in the glial cells of the central nervous system (CNS). The importance of PDGF for glial cell differentiation has been particularly well characterized. The α-receptor is expressed on bipotential oligodendroglial–astroglial cell precursors from the rat optic nerve, spinal cord, and other parts of the CNS. PDGF controls the timing of the differentiation of these cells to astrocytes.

PDGF receptors are also expressed on certain postnatal neurons, and PDGF has been shown to have a neurotropic effect on cultured rat dopaminergic neurons.

C. Vascular System

Capillary endothelial cells have been shown to express PDGF β-receptors, and PDGF has been shown to have an angiogenic effect. However, the angiogenic effect appears to be weaker than that of VEGFs or fibroblast growth factors. PDGF appears not to be important for the initial formation of novel vessels, since no apparent vascular abnormality is observed during early embryogenesis in mice with the genes for PDGF or PDGF receptors inactivated. It appears that PDGF isoforms have more important roles in the development of the smooth muscle layer and recruitment of pericytes to the vessels, which is required at later stages of vasculogenesis to give strength to the vessel wall.

PDGF also affects platelet aggregation. On platelet release and aggregation, induced, e.g., by thrombin or collagen, the released PDGF activates PDGF α-receptors present on the platelets, leading to a decreased platelet aggregation. PDGF, which is present in large amounts in platelets, may thus have an autocrine feedback role in the control of platelet aggregation.

D. Tissue Homeostasis

The interstitial fluid pressure in tissues, which is normally slightly negative, is carefully controlled to allow an exchange of fluid and macromolecules between the extracellular compartment and the vascular system. PDGF exerts an important control on the interstitial fluid pressure, probably because of its ability to stimulate the formation of stress fibers in myofibroblasts of the connective tissue and to promote interactions between these cells and molecules of the extracellular matrix.

E. Wound Healing

PDGF stimulates wound healing through actions on several cell types involved in the healing process. It stimulates chemotaxis of neutrophils and macrophages and both chemotaxis and proliferation of fibroblasts and smooth muscle cells. PDGF also stimulates macrophages to secrete other growth factors that are important for various phases of the healing process. Moreover, PDGF acts on connective tissue cells to stimulate the synthesis of matrix molecules, such as fibronectin, collagen, proteoglycans, and hyaluronic acid. PDGF may also be important during later stages of wound healing; for instance, it stimulates the contraction of collagen gels *in vitro*, suggesting that it may stimulate wound contraction *in vivo*.

Topical application of PDGF to large wounds in patients has been shown to increase their rate of healing. It is likely that PDGF also has a role in normal wound healing since it is present in wound fluid from soft tissue. There are several possible sources of PDGF in healing wounds; it has been shown to be released from platelets, activated macrophages, thrombin-stimulated endothelial cells, smooth muscle cells of damaged vessels, activated fibroblasts, and epidermal keratinocytes.

Whereas PDGF has a significant effect on healing of soft tissue wounds, its effect on fracture healing is less clear; there are reports that application of PDGF increases fracture healing, but other reports indicate that PDGF instead induces a soft tissue repair phenotype and response.

V. PDGF IN DISEASE

There is evidence that PDGF is involved in autocrine as well as paracrine stimulation in malignancies. In addition, PDGF overactivity has been linked to other disorders involving an excess cell proliferation, such as atherosclerosis and fibrotic conditions.

A. Malignancies

The finding that the retroviral oncogene v-*sis* is derived from the PDGF B-chain gene and that transformation by v-*sis* involves autocrine stimulation by a PDGF-like growth factor prompted investigations of whether overactivity of PDGF also occurs in human malignancies. Work in recent years has revealed several examples in which overactivity of the PDGF pathway drives the proliferation of tumor cells. There are examples of the classical autocrine situation, in which a PDGF receptor carrying cells starts the production of PDGF. For example, the relatively rare skin tumor dermatofibrosarcoma protuberance (DFSP) is associated with a fusion of the collagen 1A1 gene with the PDGF B-chain gene, causing the production of an excess of a collagen–PDGF fusion protein. The fusion protein is processed to a PDGF-like growth factor that stimulates the producer cell in an autocrine fashion. Other types of sarcomas and glioblastomas are also characterized by overexpression of PDGF, although the mechanisms behind the overexpression are not known.

There are also examples of perturbations of the PDGF signaling pathway intracellularly. Thus, in chronic myelomonocytic leukemia, the gene for the Ets-like transcription factor Tel is fused to the part of the PDGF β-receptor gene coding for the kinase domain. The result is the production of a fusion protein consisting of part of Tel and the PDGF β-receptor kinase. Since Tel forms a dimer, the fusion protein dimerizes, thereby causing a constitutive activation of the kinase. Constitutive PDGF β-receptor dimers can also be formed by interaction of the E5 oncoprotein of bovine papilloma virus with the transmembrane part of the receptor.

In addition to driving the proliferation of the tumor cells themselves, PDGF may be involved in paracrine stimulation of normal cells in tumors. Several types of tumor cells synthesize PDGF. In cases where the tumor cells do not express PDGF receptors, no autocrine stimulation will occur. However, the secreted PDGF may affect other cell types in the tumor. Thus, PDGF has been shown to have a weak angiogenic effect and to stimulate stromal cells. The paracrine effects of PDGF may be of importance for the balanced growth of tumors. Moreover, PDGF is important for the elevated interstitial fluid pressure that often characterizes solid tumors and that makes uptake of chemotherapeutic drugs less efficient.

B. Atherosclerosis

Atherosclerosis is characterized by an inflammatory-fibroproliferative response, which includes an increased expression of PDGF. In experimental models, as well as in naturally occurring lesions, increased expression of PDGF and PDGF receptors is seen. PDGF may be released by platelets trapped in thrombi, by activated macrophages, by smooth muscle cells, or by endothelial cells, and it stimulates the migration of smooth muscle cells from the media of the vessel into the intima layer, where the cells also proliferate in response to PDGF. Such intimal thickening at sites of endothelial cell injury occurs at an early phase of the atherosclerotic process.

C. Fibrotic Conditions

As discussed above, PDGF is important for the development of connective tissue compartments in several organs. In the adult, overactivity of PDGF causes fibrosis of the same organs. Thus, several types of pulmonary fibrosis have been shown to involve overexpression of PDGF. Moreover, intratracheal injection of PDGF-BB has been shown to cause transient proliferation of pulmonary mesenchymal and epithelial cells accompanied by collagen deposition. Overactivity of PDGF is also implicated in several types of glomerulonephritides, liver cirrhosis, and myelofibrosis.

D. PDGF Antagonists

The fact that PDGF is involved in several serious disorders makes the development of clinically useful PDGF antagonists highly warranted. Several types of PDGF antagonists have been developed, including antibodies, DNA aptamers and soluble extracellular receptor domains that sequester PDGF, antibodies that bind to and block PDGF receptors, and low-molecular-weight inhibitors of the receptor kinase. Promising results of such antagonists have been obtained in animal models for malignancies, as well as atherosclerosis and fibrotic conditions; their usefulness in the treatment of patients is currently being evaluated.

VI. SUMMARY

In the human genome, there are four genes encoding PDGF isoforms, PDGF-A, -B, -C, and -D. The four dimeric isoforms, PDGF-AA, -BB, -CC, and -DD, bind with different specificities to two related tyrosine kinase receptors, forming αα, αβ, or ββ receptor dimers.

Important aims of future research will be to elucidate the detailed *in vivo* function of the different PDGF isoforms, in particular, the novel isoforms PDGF-CC and PDGF-DD, and their potential involvement in disease. It will also be important to investigate whether additional receptors are involved in mediating signals from the novel PDGF isoforms. There is preliminary evidence that the different dimeric forms of PDGF α and β receptors transduce different intracellular signals. It will be important to elucidate the *in vivo* significance of such differences.

Acknowledgments

Ingegärd Schiller is thanked for skillful secretarial help.

Glossary

autocrine, paracrine, or endocrine stimulation The process whereby a cell produces a factor(s) that stimulates that cell itself, cells in the immediate environment, or distant cells, respectively.

autophosphorylation A process whereby a kinase phosphorylates itself or kinase-associated receptors in a dimeric complex phosphorylate one another.

chemotaxis Directed cell migration toward a gradient of a chemotactic factor, e.g., a growth factor.

growth factor receptor A transmembrane protein that consists of an extracellular ligand-binding domain and an intracellular effector domain that often is associated with a kinase activity that is activated on ligand binding.

signal transduction pathway A series of molecules activating one another through physical contacts and/or enzymatic modifications, leading to a specific effect, such as cell growth, survival, or migration.

See Also the Following Articles

Cancer Cells and Progrowth/Prosurvival Signaling • Epidermal Growth Factor (EGF) Family • Heparin-Binding Epidermal Growth Factor-like Growth Factor (HB-EGF) • HGF (Hepatocyte Growth Factor)/MET System • Nerve Growth Factor (NGF) • Vascular Endothelial Growth Factor

Further Reading

Betsholtz, C., Karlsson, L., and Lindahl, P. (2001). Developmental roles of platelet-derived growth factors. *BioEssays* **23**, 494–507.

DiMaio, D., Lai, C. C., and Mattoon, D. (2000). The platelet-derived growth factor β receptor as a target of the bovine papillomavirus E5 protein. *Cytokine Growth Factor Rev.* **11**, 283–293.

George, D. (2001). Platelet-derived growth factor receptors: A therapeutic target in solid tumors. *Semin. Oncol.* **28**, 27–33.

Heldin, C.-H., and Westermark, B. (1999). Mechanism of action and *in vivo* role of platelet-derived growth factor. *Physiol. Rev.* **79**, 1283–1316.

Heldin, C.-H., Eriksson, U., and Östman, A. (2002). New members of the platelet-derived growth factor family of mitogens. *Arch. Biochem. Biophys.* **398**, 284–290.

Heldin, C.-H., Östman, A., and Rönnstrand, L. (1998). Signal transduction via platelet-derived growth factor receptors. *Biochim. Biophys. Acta* **1378**, F79–F113.

Mandracchia, V. J., Sanders, S. M., and Frerichs, J. A. (2001). The use of becaplermin (rhPDGF-BB) gel for chronic nonhealing ulcers: A retrospective analysis. *Clin. Podiatr. Med. Surg.* **18**, 189–209, viii.

Östman, A., and Heldin, C.-H. (2001). Involvement of platelet-derived growth factor in disease: Development of specific antagonists. *Adv. Cancer Res.* **80**, 1–38.

Raines, E. W., Bowen-Pope, D. F., and Ross, R. (1990). Platelet-derived growth factor. *In* "Handbook of Experimental Pharmacology: Peptide Growth Factors and Their Receptors" (M. B. Sporn and A. B. Roberts, eds.), pp. 173–262. Springer-Verlag, Heidelberg.

Rosenkranz, S., and Kazlauskas, A. (1999). Evidence for distinct signaling properties and biological responses induced by the PDGF receptor α and β subtypes. *Growth Factors* **16**, 201–216.

Smits, A., and Funa, K. (1998). Platelet-derived growth factor (PDGF) in primary brain tumours of neuroglial origin. *Histol. Histopathol.* **13**, 511–520.

Polycystic Ovary Syndrome

STEPHEN FRANKS

Imperial College London

I. INTRODUCTION
II. ENDOCRINE ABNORMALITIES IN PCOS
III. OVARIAN FOLLICULAR ABNORMALITIES IN PCOS
IV. GENETIC STUDIES OF PCOS
V. CLINICAL MANAGEMENT ISSUES
VI. SUMMARY

Polycystic ovary syndrome (PCOS) is a very common, heterogeneous endocrine disorder that is a major cause of infertility, hirsutism, and metabolic disorders. Its most consistent biochemical feature is hypersecretion of ovarian androgens. PCOS is associated with an increased risk of type 2 diabetes in later life.

I. INTRODUCTION

Polycystic ovary syndrome (PCOS) is the most common endocrine disorder in women, accounting for about three-quarters of all cases of anovulatory infertility and about 90% of the causes of hirsutism. Polycystic ovary syndrome is heterogeneous in its presentation and this has resulted in some discussion about how to define PCOS. The classic definition includes the association of anovulatory menses (or estrogen-replete amenorrhea) with clinical and/or

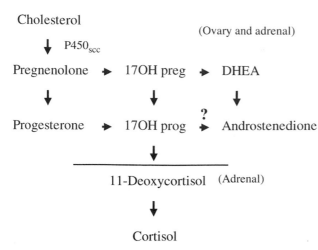

FIGURE 1 The steroidogenic pathway in ovaries and adrenals. Note that cytochrome P450 side chain cleavage enzyme (P450scc) is the key enzyme in the production of pregnenolone, and hence all later stages of steroid production. There is a question concerning the conversion of 17-hydroxy-progesterone (17OH prog) to androstenedione: in the human ovary, it is more likely that androstenedione is derived mainly from conversion of dehydroepiandrosterone (DHEA) by the enzyme 3β-hydroxysteroid dehydrogenase.

biochemical evidence of excess androgen secretion. Using this definition, the estimated prevalence of PCOS is in excess of 5% of the female population of reproductive age. The range of clinical presentation of women with polycystic ovaries—as defined by pelvic ultrasonography—is, however, wide. It includes patients with anovulation who are nonhirsute and those with hirsutism who have regular menstrual cycles. Indeed, polycystic ovaries are found in over 80% of women who would otherwise have been labeled as having "idiopathic hirsutism." The results of ultrasound studies of "normal" populations suggest that polycystic ovaries are present in about 20% of women of reproductive age. The causes of polycystic ovaries (PCOs) and PCOS are not known for certain, but there is strong evidence for a major genetic contribution, as will be discussed in Section IV.

In addition to the reproductive consequences of the syndrome, PCOS is characterized by a metabolic disorder in which hyperinsulinemia and peripheral insulin resistance are the central features. This metabolic dysfunction may play a part in the etiology of anovulation but also has important implications for long-term health. Women with PCOS are two to three times more likely to develop type 2 diabetes mellitus in later life and may also be at increased risk of developing cardiovascular disease.

II. ENDOCRINE ABNORMALITIES IN PCOS

The major endocrine abnormalities in women with PCOS are elevated serum concentrations of androgens and luteinizing hormone (LH) and, particularly in those with the classic definition of PCOS (i.e., including menstrual disturbances), hyperinsulinemia and insulin resistance.

A. Hypersecretion of Androgens

The most common biochemical abnormality in women with polycystic ovaries is hypersecretion of androgens. The ovary appears to be the predominant source of excess androgen production, although many studies have pointed to evidence for an additional adrenal abnormality. Nevertheless, the ovary is clearly the more important contributor to hyperandrogenemia because suppression of LH in women with PCOS leads to a decrease in androgen concentrations to levels that are indistinguishable from those in menopausal or oophorectomized women. Cultured thecal cells from women with polycystic ovaries, regardless of presenting symptoms, produce some 20 times more androstenedione in primary culture than do cells from women with normal ovaries. Increased steroidogenic activity is, however, not confined to androgen production. All stages of the steroidogenic pathway—including progesterone production—appear to be amplified in PCO theca (Figs. 1 and 2). Importantly, these results

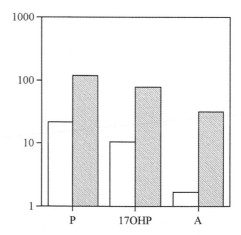

FIGURE 2 Steroid production (in picomoles/1000 cells/48 h) by theca cells from normal (clear bars) and polycystic ovaries (PCO; shaded bars). P, Progesterone; 17OHP, 17-hydroxyprogesterone; A, androstenedione. Note the logarithmic scale. In each case, steroid production by theca cells from polycystic ovaries was significantly greater than that from normal theca (P, $p < 0.01$; 17OHP, $p < 0.01$; A, $p < 0.005$) Redrawn from Gilling-Smith *et al.* (1994).

have recently been confirmed using PCO and normal theca cells that have undergone several passages in culture. This suggests that this biochemical phenotype is an intrinsic feature of the polycystic ovary. Thus, it is unlikely that ovarian hyperandrogenism arises secondary to hypersecretion of LH in PCOS, particularly because this "typical" feature of PCOS occurs in little more than 50% of those with the classic syndrome and in the minority of those with hyperandrogenism and regular cycles.

B. Metabolic Abnormalities in PCOS

In recent years, there has been a great deal of interest in the metabolic associations of PCOS. The classic syndrome is characterized by a distinctive form of insulin resistance. Women with PCOS have higher fasting and glucose-stimulated insulin concentrations and significantly reduced insulin sensitivity compared with weight-matched control subjects (Fig. 3). The cause of this abnormality is unclear, but clinical and laboratory-based studies in PCOS have variously pointed to abnormalities of insulin receptor binding, or, more plausibly, to postreceptor signaling as well as to evidence for a primary abnormality of insulin secretion. It has been demonstrated that weight reduction in obese women with PCOS results in normalization of insulin sensitivity, but "first-phase" insulin secretion in response to an intravenous glucose challenge remains abnormal. These data also illustrate an important principle in understanding the etiology of PCOS, which is that whatever the genetic basis for the syndrome, the phenotype can be influenced by environmental (in this case nutritional) factors.

III. OVARIAN FOLLICULAR ABNORMALITIES IN PCOS

A further phenotypic feature of PCOS is the polycystic ovarian morphology. The polycystic ovary is characterized by the presence of an increased number not only of antral follicles but also of early-growing and preantral follicles. Because these earlier stages of follicular development are thought to be largely independent of gonadotropins, the implication is that local ovarian factors may have a role in genesis of the polycystic ovary. Many growth factors have been shown to have an influence on early folliculogenesis, including those of the transforming growth factor-β superfamily and growth factors signaling through tyrosine kinase coupled receptors such as insulin-like growth factors-I and -II and transforming growth factor α.

Anovulation in PCOS is characterized by arrested development of medium-sized antral follicles. Granulosa cells from these follicles display evidence of premature responsiveness to LH and increased steroidogenesis (indicative of advanced differentiation) compared with similarly sized follicles from normal ovaries. The reason for these

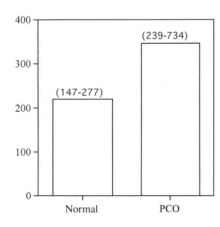

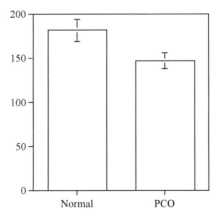

FIGURE 3 (A) Insulin area (median, interquartile range; in milliunits/hour) following a 75-g oral glucose tolerance test dose and (B) insulin sensitivity (in micromoles/minute), measured by the short insulin tolerance test, in 29 women with polycystic ovary (PCO) syndrome and 24 weight-matched control subjects. Insulin area was significantly greater ($p < 0.01$) and insulin sensitivity significantly lower ($p < 0.01$) in women with polycystic ovary syndrome than in controls. Redrawn from Robinson et al. (1993).

differences are not yet entirely clear, but because insulin can greatly enhance the response of the granulosa cell to LH, it seems likely that hyperinsulinemia plays an important part in the mechanism of anovulation.

IV. GENETIC STUDIES OF PCOS

The definition of abnormalities in the ovarian steroidogenic pathway, in the secretion and action of insulin, and in ovarian follicular development has paved the way for the use of a candidate gene approach in the identification of genetic susceptibility loci for PCOS.

A. Genes Involved in the Biosynthesis and Metabolism of Androgens

Genes implicated in the pathway of androgen production and metabolism include those encoding the major endocrine regulator, LH, its receptor, and key P450 steroidogenic enzymes such as cholesterol side chain cleavage (P450scc) and 17α-hydroxylase/17,20 lyase (P450c17 α).

1. CYP11a—Coding for P450 Cholesterol Side Chain Cleavage

A polymorphic sequence [a pentanucleotide repeat—$(tttta)_n$] in the $5'$ regulatory region of CYP11a has been identified, and both case-control association studies and nonparametric linkage analysis have been performed by Gharani and colleagues. Subjects were assigned to two groups according to genotype. The most common genotype, comprising four repeats, occurred with a frequency of 0.59, and was designated 216. Subjects were subdivided according to whether this allele was present (216 +) or absent (216 −). It was found that genotype was associated with serum testosterone concentrations, levels being significantly higher in women with the 216 − genotype (which consists of alleles of six repeats or longer) (Fig. 4). On more detailed analysis, this association held true only in those subjects with clinical evidence of hyperandrogenism. Supportive evidence for the association of PCOS with CYP11a comes from two recent European studies, the first of which has reported a relationship between the $(tttta)_n$ polymorphism and androgen levels in 88 hirsute women. This study found that the CYP11a genotype, together with endocrine markers, predicts the presence of PCO in hirsute women. Another group, in a case-control study, reported that the CYP11a genotype was associated with both PCO and total

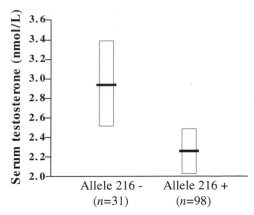

FIGURE 4 Association of CYP11a genotype with serum testosterone in a case-control data set of women with and without PCOS. Note significantly higher serum testosterone concentrations ($p = 0.0009$) in association with the 216 − genotype (more than six pentanucleotide repeats). Data shown are mean and 95% confidence intervals Redrawn from Gharani *et al.* (1997).

testosterone concentrations. Further support for this notion has been obtained from mutation screening of the CYP11a promoter in a 1.85-kb region $5'$ to the start site of translation. Direct sequencing of fragments (amplified by polymerase chain reaction) of DNA samples from affected and unaffected family members has been carried out. Apart from the pentanucleotide repeat polymorphism at position − 466 from the start site of transcription (and a previously identified dinucleotide repeat polymorphism at position − 1314), no variation from the published sequence is found. Structure–function studies of the promoter region using expression systems need to be performed to explore the putative functional role of this element. An alternative explanation is that this polymorphic marker is in linkage disequilibrium with the disease locus, which may be located outside the promoter region.

Segregation of CYP11a has been examined in 20 families. With the aid of a number of polymorphic markers [D15S153, D15S125, CYP11a $(ac)_n$, D15S169, and D15S211], in the region of CYP11a, nonparametric linkage analysis was performed using the GENEHUNTER (multipoint linkage) program. There is evidence for excess allele sharing, i.e., linkage, at the CYP11a locus [nonparametric logarithm of the odds (LOD) (NPL) score, 3.03; $p = 0.003$]. In a parallel parametric analysis, assuming the autosomal dominant model for inheritance, evidence of genetic heterogeneity between families is found, with about 60% of families showing linkage at the *CYP11a* locus. Thus, data from both association and linkage studies suggest that this is a major susceptibility locus for hyperandrogenism in PCOS.

2. CYP17—Coding for 17-Hydroxylase/17,20-Lyase

Because of the reported abnormalities in regulation of 17α-hydroxylase/17,20 lyase in PCOS, initial studies have focused on the role of *CYP17* (coding for P450c17α). Results of a preliminary case-control study suggest that a variant form of *CYP17* is associated with PCOS, but there is no relationship between genotype and serum testosterone levels. Subsequent, larger, case-control studies have also been unable to confirm the putative association. Furthermore, linkage analysis excludes *CYP17* as a major susceptibility gene for PCOS within families.

B. Genes Involved in the Secretion and Action of Insulin

1. The Insulin Gene Variable-Number Tandem Repeat

There is evidence that the insulin gene (*INS*) variable-number tandem repeat (VNTR) is a major susceptibility locus for PCOS. The *INS* VNTR lies in the $5'$ regulatory region of the gene; it has been shown to be involved in regulation of insulin gene expression and has been implicated in the etiology of type 2 diabetes. Class III alleles in the VNTR have been found to be associated with anovulatory PCOS in two independent populations and using two different methods of analysis [case-control studies and by the use of affected family-based controls (AFBAC)]. With the aid of a nonparametric linkage analysis program, it has also been established that there is excess allele sharing at the *INS* VNTR locus. The geometric mean of fasting serum insulin concentrations is significantly higher in families in which linkage is demonstrated than in those families without evidence of linkage. This suggests a functional role for the VNTR variant in the expression of hyperinsulinemia/insulin resistance in PCOS. It is also observed, using transmission disequilibrium (TDT) analysis, that there is a "parent of origin" effect in the transmission of alleles of the VNTR to affected subjects. Class III alleles are transmitted significantly more commonly from fathers than from mothers to the affected daughter. Interestingly, this finding has been mirrored recently in an analysis of families with type 2 diabetes for which PCOS is a known risk factor.

C. Genes Involved in Folliculogenesis

1. The Follistatin Gene

As part of a panel of candidate genes related to gonadotropin action, Urbanek and colleagues examined the follistatin locus on chromosome 5 and, somewhat unexpectedly, found the strongest evidence for linkage with PCOS of any of the 37 candidate genes they had chosen. In their affected sibling-pair analysis, 72% of sisters were concordant for the follistatin genotype, and this remained significant after correction for multiple testing. However, recent follow-up data from the same group suggest that this finding is no longer significant when further families are added to the database. This finding nevertheless remains intriguing, and the possibility arises that this and other genes implicated in folliculogenesis may have a causal role in this disorder, which is, after all, characterized by disordered follicle development.

V. CLINICAL MANAGEMENT ISSUES

A. Diagnosis of PCOS

The diagnosis of PCOS is reached primarily on a clinical basis. A patient presenting with irregular menses, oligomenorrhea, or amenorrhea and who has signs of hyperandrogenism is very likely to have PCOS. Even in the absence of hirsutism, PCOS is the most likely cause of these menstrual symptoms (it accounts for about 30% of cases of amenorrhea overall and about 90% of amenorrheic women with normal estrogen levels).

The majority of patients presenting with hirsutism have polycystic ovaries, irrespective of menstrual history. Much rarer but more serious causes of hirsutism and menstrual disturbances include Cushing's disease, acromegaly, hyperprolactinemia, and tumors of the adrenal or ovary. In such cases, however, there are usually other clues, both clinical and biochemical, to the diagnosis, e.g., short history of increasing hirsutism and significantly elevated serum testosterone (>5 nmol/liter). For this reason, serum testosterone should be measured in all hirsute patients as a screening test to exclude more serious causes of hyperandrogenism. Late-onset ("nonclassical") congenital adrenal hyperplasia due to 21-hydroxylase deficiency may be difficult to distinguish clinically from PCOS, but it is debatable whether this makes much practical difference to management of symptoms. Thus, in a typical situation in which the prevalence of nonclassical

21-hydroxylase deficiency is <5%, for example, routine measurement of 17α-hydroxyprogesterone (the biochemical marker of 21-hydroxylase deficiency) is not necessary.

No single test is diagnostic of the syndrome and choice of investigations should be tailored to the clinical presentation. Serum LH levels are typically elevated in PCOS (follicle-stimulating hormone is normal), but up to 50% of women with all other clinical and biochemical features of the syndrome may have normal serum LH. Measurement of LH is therefore of limited diagnostic value; it is quite specific—elevated LH and normal follicle-stimulating hormone (FSH) essentially occur only in PCOS—but it is not very sensitive. Pelvic ultrasonography will define the polycystic ovarian morphology, but accurate assessment of the ovaries by ultrasound is a particular skill, and false negative results are not uncommon. Conversely, the presence of polycystic ovaries does not necessarily mean that the patient has polycystic ovary syndrome. Polycystic ovaries may be found coincidentally in women who have, for example, hypothalamic, estrogen-deficient amenorrhea.

In summary, pelvic ultrasonography and measurements of LH, FSH, and testosterone may be of some diagnostic value when set in the appropriate clinical context. By contrast, routine measurements of adrenal androgens are not indicated and measurement of sex hormone-binding globulin (which is primarily an index of body weight) is not at all helpful. Because of the increased risk of type 2 diabetes, it is recommended that obese women with PCOS should have a fasting glucose measurement at least once a year and, in view of the associated dyslipidemia, there may also be some merit in checking the lipid and lipoprotein profile at the same time.

B. Management

Because the physiological basis of PCOS is unknown, treatment is largely to alleviate symptoms. Patients with anovulation may require induction of ovulation. The antiestrogen, clomiphene, is usually effective, but even this "simple" treatment should be monitored at a specialist center because of the risk of ovarian hyperstimulation and multiple pregnancy. For those not concerned about fertility, menstrual regulation by means of oral contraceptives or cyclical progestagens should be considered. Nonandrogenic progestagens (e.g., medroxyprogesterone acetate, desogestrel, and gestodene) are obviously preferable to norgestrel and norethisterone for women who may anyway have symptoms of androgen excess.

Symptoms of hyperandrogenism can be managed by antiandrogens such as cyproterone acetate. For women with acne and mild or moderate hirsutism, this can usually be given in the form of Dianette (cyproterone acetate, 2 mg, with ethinylestradiol, 35 mg). Cosmetic advice about removal of hair should not be forgotten, even with administration of antiandrogens.

Obese subjects with PCOS require particular attention. It has been clearly demonstrated that calorie restriction in obese women with PCOS improves insulin sensitivity and glucose tolerance. It also leads to resumption of spontaneous ovulatory cycles and normal fertility in many subjects. Significantly, such improvements in glucose–insulin homeostasis and reproductive function can be achieved with weight reduction of as little as 5% of the initial body weight. Insulin-sensitizing drugs may also have a role in reducing the risk of diabetes and improving ovarian function. The thiazolidinediones (TZDs) are a relatively new class of insulin-sensitizing drugs that have been introduced primarily for the control of type 2 diabetes. In a large randomized, multicenter study, troglitazone has been shown to improve insulin sensitivity and menstrual cyclicity in obese women with PCOS. Unfortunately, this drug has been withdrawn because of serious side effects, and although there are newer, apparently safer preparations available, there are concerns about the wisdom of prescribing TZDs in women of reproductive age. Metformin is a well-established medication in management of type 2 diabetes. Its mechanism of action is complex, but its effects include reduction of insulin receptors and insulin levels. Recent studies in women with PCOS have suggested that this may be a safe and effective means of improving the metabolic profile and reproductive function in both lean and obese women with PCOS. Results so far have been encouraging, but by no means conclusive. Randomized controlled trials have been few and have produced conflicting results.

VI. SUMMARY

PCOS is clinically and biochemically heterogeneous. The major endocrine hallmark is hyperandrogenemia and although it is clear that hypersecretion of adrenal androgens may contribute to the hyperandrogenemia of women with polycystic ovary syndrome, the weight of evidence favors the ovary as the major source of excess androgen secretion.

The biochemical basis for the putative disorder of ovarian androgen biosynthesis remains controversial. There is evidence, from both clinical and *in vitro* studies of human ovarian theca cells, of dysregulation of the rate-limiting enzyme in androgen biosynthesis, cytochrome P450c17α, which catalyzes both 17α-hydroxylase and 17,20 lyase activities. Initial data have suggested that alleles of *CYP17*, the gene encoding P450c17α, are associated with PCOS but this has now been excluded as a candidate gene. However, *CYP11a*, which encodes cholesterol side chain cleavage enzyme, does appear to be a major susceptibility locus for hyperandrogenism in women with PCO. Nevertheless, the finding that the expression of other enzymes in the androgen biosynthetic pathway is also up-regulated suggests that this may not be the only focus for genetic abnormalities of steroidogenesis. The precise nature of the interaction of androgens and genetic loci affecting insulin secretion remains unclear.

From the viewpoint of clinical management, the major issues relate to correction of infertility, menstrual disturbance, and hirsutism. The metabolic abnormalities in PCOS have implications both for management of anovulatory infertility and for the increased risk of type 2 diabetes in later life. Dietary measures are very important in overweight subjects, but there is increasing evidence that insulin-sensitizing agents may have an important role to play in management both of anovulation and of metabolic consequences of PCOS.

Glossary

CYP11a Gene encoding the P450 side chain cleavage enzyme.

insulin gene variable-number tandem repeat Sequence in the regulatory region of the insulin gene.

P450 cholesterol side chain cleavage enzyme Key enzyme in ovarian steroidogenesis.

polycystic ovaries Characteristic ovarian multiple antral follicles, increased stroma, and androgen hypersecretion.

polycystic ovary syndrome Clinical and endocrine abnormalities, typically manifested as anovulation and hyperandrogenism; associated with polycystic ovaries.

See Also the Following Articles

Diabetes Type 2 • Follicle Stimulating Hormone (FSH) • Folliculogenesis • Inhibins, Activins, and Follistatins • Insulin Processing • Insulin Resistance in PCOS

(Polycystic Ovary Syndrome) • Leptin Actions on the Reproductive Axis • Luteinizing Hormone (LH)

Further Reading

Azziz, R., Ehrmann, D., Legro, R. S., Whitcomb, R. W., Hanley, R., Fereshetian, A. G., O'Keefe, M., and Ghazzi, M. N. (2001). Troglitazone improves ovulation and hirsutism in the polycystic ovary syndrome: A multicenter, double blind, placebo-controlled trial. *J. Clin. Endocrinol. Metab.* **86**, 1626–1632.

Dunaif, A. (1997). Insulin resistance and the polycystic ovary syndrome: Mechanism and implications for pathogenesis. *Endocr. Rev.* **18**, 774–800.

Franks, S. (1995). Polycystic ovary syndrome. *N. Engl. J. Med.* **333**, 853–861.

Franks, S., Gharani, N., Waterworth, D., Batty, S., White, D., Williamson, R., and McCarthy, M. (1997). The genetic basis of polycystic ovary syndrome. *Hum. Reprod.* **12**, 2641–2648.

Franks, S., Gharani, N., and McCarthy, M. (2001). Candidate genes in polycystic ovary syndrome. *Hum. Reprod. Update* 7, 405–410.

Franks, S., Mason, D., and Willis, D. (2000). Follicular dynamics in the polycystic ovary syndrome. *Mol. Cell Endocrinol.* **163**, 49–52.

Gharani, N., Waterworth, D. M., Batty, S., White, D., Gilling-Smith, C., Conway, G. S., McCarthy, M., Franks, S., and Williamson, R. (1997). Association of the steroid synthesis gene CYP11a with polycystic ovary syndrome and hyperandrogenism. *Hum. Mol. Genet.* 6, 397–402.

Gilling-Smith, C., Willis, D. S., Beard, R. W., and Franks, S. (1994). Hypersecretion of androstenedione by isolated theca cells from polycystic ovaries. *J. Clin. Endocrinol. Metab.* **79**, 1158–1165.

Legro, R. S., Spielman, R., Urbanek, M., Driscoll, D., Strauss, J. F., and Dunaif, A. (1998). Phenotype and genotype in polycystic ovary syndrome. *Recent Prog. Horm. Res.* **53**, 217–256.

Robinson, S., Kiddy, D., Gelding, S. V., Willis, D., Niththyananthan, R., Bush, A., Johnston, D. G., and Franks, S. (1993). The relationship of insulin insensitivity to menstrual pattern in women with hyperandrogenism and polycystic ovaries. *Clin. Endocrinol.* **39**, 351–355.

Urbanek, M., Legro, R. S., Driscoll, D. A., Azziz, R., Ehrmann, D. A., Norman, R. J., Strauss, J. F., 3rd, Spielman, R. S., and Dunaif, A. (1999). Thirty-seven candidate genes for polycystic ovary syndrome: strongest evidence for linkage is with follistatin. *Proc. Natl. Acad. Sci. U.S.A.* 96, 8573–8578.

Urbanek, M., Legro, R. S., Driscoll, D., Staruss, J. F., Dunaif, A., and Spielman, R. S. (2000). Searching for the polycystic ovary syndrome genes. *J. Pediatr. Endocrinol.* 13(Suppl. 50), 1311–1313.

Pregnancy

See *Decidualization; Implantation; Placental Development*

PRL

See *Prolactin*

Progesterone Action in the Female Reproductive Tract

ORLA M. CONNEELY

Baylor College of Medicine

The biological actions of progesterone in the female reproductive tract are mediated by the specific progesterone receptor, of which there are two isoforms: A and B. These two forms arise from a single gene, and the ratio of the two varies as a function of developemntal and hormonal status and during carcinogenesis. Female mice lacking both forms of the progesterone receptor exhibit impaired sexual behavior, gonadotrophin regulation, ovulation, uterine function, and mammary gland development. The availability of mutant mice lacking either the A or B isoform of the progesterone receptor has allowed the definition of the contribution of each to the reproduction actions of progesterone.

I. INTRODUCTION

Progesterone plays a central role in the establishment and maintenance of pregnancy. The physiological effects of progesterone are mediated by interaction of the hormone with specific intracellular progesterone receptors (PRs) that are expressed as two protein isoforms, PR-A and PR-B. Both proteins arise from the same gene and are members of the nuclear receptor superfamily of transcription factors. Analysis of the structural and functional relationships of each PR isoform using *in vitro* systems has generated compelling evidence to support the conclusion that the PR-A and PR-B proteins have different transcription activation properties when liganded to progesterone (P). Furthermore, the advent of gene targeting approaches to introduce subtle mutations into the mouse genome has allowed researchers to begin to address the significance of the observations made *in vitro* in a physiological context. Selective ablation of PR-A and PR-B proteins in mice using these technologies has allowed researchers to address the spatiotemporal expression and contribution of the individual PR isoforms to the pleiotropic reproductive activities of progesterone. Analysis of the phenotypic consequences of these mutations on female reproductive function has provided proof of concept that the distinct transcriptional responses to PR-A and PR-B observed in cell-based transactivation assays are indeed reflected in the ability of the individual isoforms to elicit distinct physiological responses to progesterone. In PR-A knockout mice in which the expression of the PR-A isoform is selectively ablated (PRAKO), the PR-B isoform functions in a tissue-specific manner to mediate a subset of the reproductive functions of PRs. Ablation of PR-A does not affect the responses of the mammary gland or thymus to progesterone but results in severe abnormalities in ovarian and uterine function, leading to female infertility. These tissue-selective activities of PR-B are due to the ability of this isoform to regulate a subset of progesterone-responsive target genes in reproductive tissues rather than to differences in its spatiotemporal expression relative to the PR-A isoform. More recent studies using PR-B knockout (PRBKO) mice have shown that ablation of PR-B does not affect ovarian, uterine, or thymic responses to progesterone but results in reduced mammary ductal morphogenesis. Thus, PR-A is both necessary and sufficient to elicit the progesterone-dependent reproductive responses necessary for female fertility and the PR-B isoform is required to elicit normal proliferative responses of the mammary gland to progesterone. This article will summarize the current understanding of the selective contribution of the two PR isoforms to progesterone action.

II. PROGESTERONE RECEPTOR ISOFORMS

Receptors for progesterone are expressed as two distinct isoforms, PR-A and PR-B, which arise from a single gene. The expression of both isoforms is conserved in rodents and humans and overlaps spatiotemporally in female reproductive tissues. However, the ratios of the individual isoforms vary in reproductive tissues as a consequence of developmental and hormonal status and during carcinogenesis.

Progesterone receptors have a modular protein structure consisting of distinct functional domains capable of binding steroidal ligand, dimerization of liganded receptors, interaction with hormone-responsive DNA elements, and interaction with co-regulator proteins required for bridging receptors to the transcriptional apparatus. Binding of progestin agonists to the hormone-binding domain induces conformational changes in receptor structure that promote the interaction of co-activator proteins with distinct activation function domains (AFs) located within both the amino- and the carboxy-terminal regions of the receptor. Such co-activators promote chromatin remodeling and bridging with general transcription factors, resulting in the formation of productive transcription initiation complexes at the receptor-responsive promoter. In contrast, binding of receptor antagonist compounds induces receptor conformational changes that render AFs nonpermissive to co-activator binding and instead promote interaction with co-repressor proteins that inhibit the transcriptional activity of the receptor. The ability of progesterone receptors to interact with a variety of co-activator and co-repressor proteins, together with the differing spatiotemporal expression of co-regulators, illustrates a key role of these proteins in mediating different tissue-specific responses of progesterone receptors to steroidal ligand. Importantly, receptors for progesterone can also be activated in the absence of steroidal ligand by phosphorylation pathways that modulate their interactions with co-regulator proteins.

The PR-A and PR-B isoforms differ in that the PR-B protein contains an additional sequence of amino acids at its amino-terminus that is not contained in PR-A. This PR-B-specific domain encodes a third transactivation function region (AF-3) that is absent from PR-A. Recent evidence has demonstrated that the presence of AF-3 allows binding of a subset of co-activators to PR-B that are not efficiently recruited by progestin-bound PR-A. Thus, when expressed individually in cultured cells, PR-A and PR-B display different transactivation properties that are specific to both cell type and target gene promoter context and are associated with the differential ability of PR-A and PR-B to recruit specific co-regulator proteins. Agonist-bound PR-B functions as a strong activator of transcription of several PR-dependent promoters and in a variety of cell types in which PR-A is inactive.

Furthermore, when both isoforms are co-expressed in cultured cells, in cell and promoter contexts in which agonist-bound PR-A is inactive, the PR-A can repress the activity of PR-B. This repressor capability of PR-A also extends to other steroid receptors including estrogen receptor-α (ER-α). Finally, the PR-A and PR-B proteins also respond differently to P antagonists. Whereas antagonist-bound PR-A is inactive, antagonist-bound PR-B can be converted to a strongly active transcription factor by modulating intracellular phosphorylation pathways. Although the sequences of the ligand-binding domains of PR-A and PR-B are identical, the ability of different ligands to induce different conformational changes in PR, together with the synergistic activity of the amino- and carboxy-terminal activation domains, predicts that PR-A or PR-B selective transcriptional regulation can be achieved by manipulating ligand interactions with the carboxy-terminal.

III. PHYSIOLOGICAL ROLE OF PRs

Null mutation of the PR gene encoding both isoforms has provided evidence of an essential role of PRs in a variety of female reproductive and nonreproductive activities. Female mice lacking both PRs exhibit impaired sexual behavior, neuroendocrine gonadotropin regulation, anovulation, uterine dysfunction, impaired ductal branching morphogenesis, and lobuloalveolar differentiation of the mammary gland. PRs also play an essential role in the regulation of thymic involution during pregnancy and in the cardiovascular system through regulation of endothelial and vascular smooth muscle cell proliferation and response to vascular injury. Receptors for progesterone have also been identified in the central nervous system and bone, where progesterone has been implicated in both cognitive function and bone maintenance. However, the essential role of PRs in these regions has not yet been confirmed.

The more recent generation of novel mutant mouse strains in which either the PR-A (PRAKO) or the PR-B (PRBKO) isoform is selectively ablated has facilitated physiological analysis of the individual contributions of these proteins to the reproductive activities of progesterone.

IV. PRs AND OVARIAN FUNCTION

Evidence that ovary-derived progesterone may participate in autocrine regulation of ovarian function first emerged with the demonstration that luteinizing hormone (LH), the primary signal for rupture of preovulatory ovarian follicles leading to ovulation, can stimulate the transient expression of PR mRNA and protein in granulosa cells isolated from preovulatory follicles and that the anti-progestin, RU486, can inhibit ovulation. Definitive proof that PRs are essential mediators of ovulation has been provided by analysis of the ovarian phenotype of the PRKO mouse. Despite exposure to superovulatory levels of gonadotropins, PRKO mice fail to ovulate. Analysis of the histology of these mice has revealed normal development of intraovarian follicles to the tertiary follicular stage. The follicles contain a mature oocyte that is fully functional when isolated and fertilized *in vitro*. However, follicular rupture is effectively eliminated. Despite the ovulatory block, the preovulatory granulosa cells within these follicles can still differentiate into a luteal phenotype and express the luteal marker, P450 side chain cleavage enzyme. Thus, PR is required specifically for LH-dependent follicular rupture leading to ovulation but not for differentiation of granulosa cells to form a corpus luteum (luteinization). Follicular rupture requires induction of a prostaglandin-mediated inflammatory response to LH as well as tissue degradation at the apex of the preovulatory follicle, an event that is mediated by matrix-digesting proteinases. Recent investigations to examine the molecular events associated with ovulation that are mediated by PRs have shown that PRs are induced specifically in the mural granulosa cells of the mature tertiary follicle and are absent from the cumulus granulosa cells that surround the oocyte. Analysis of the expression of potential mediators of ovulation in PRKO mice has demonstrated that LH-induced regulation of COX-2, an enzyme that catalyzes the production of prostaglandins, is unaffected. COX-2 is required for ovulation and is expressed by cumulus granulosa cells. In contrast, the expression of two metalloproteinases, ADAMTS-1 (a desintegrin and metalloproteinase with thrombospondin motifs) and cathepsin-L (a lysosomal cysteine protease), is inhibited in granulosa cells of the mature follicle in PRKO mice. One of these proteases, ADAMTS-1, plays an essential role in ovulation and may represent a critical mediator of the progesterone-induced ovulatory event.

Both the PR-A and the PR-B proteins are induced in preovulatory follicles in response to LH stimulation. Stimulation of immature PRAKO mice with gonadotropins has shown that superovulation is severely impaired in these mice relative to their wild-type counterparts but, in contrast to the findings with PRKO mice, is not completely absent. In contrast, superovulation was unaffected in PRBKO mice expressing only the PR-A protein. Thus, PR-A expression is both necessary and sufficient to mediate the ovulatory response to progesterone.

Histological analysis of the ovaries of PRAKO mice showed numerous mature anovulatory follicles that contained an intact oocyte and were arrested at a stage similar to that previously observed in PRKO mice. Most surprisingly, however, in contrast to PRKO mice, the spatiotemporal regulation of ADAMTS-1 and cathepsin-L by progesterone was unaffected in these mice. Thus, despite its inability to mediate follicular rupture, the PR-B protein is functional in the ovary and capable of regulating a subset of progesterone-responsive target genes.

V. PR ISOFORMS AND UTERINE IMPLANTATION

Female infertility in PRKO mice is also associated with defective uterine implantation and a lack of decidualization of uterine stromal cells in response to progesterone. Consistent with these findings, wild-type embryos failed to implant into the uterus when transferred into uteri of pseudo-pregnant PRKO females. Similarly, mating attempts between superovulated PRAKO females and wild-type males failed to result in successful pregnancies despite the release of small numbers of oocytes from PRAKO females. To determine whether the PRA protein is required for uterine decidualization, ovariectomized PRAKO mice were treated with progesterone and estrogen followed by mechanical stimulation of the left uterine horn of each animal in order to induce decidualization of stromal cells. Decidualization is associated with a marked increase in uterine weight and characteristic histological appearance associated with the differentiation of stromal cells into decidual cells. Both responses were inhibited in PRAKO mice, indicating that expression of the PRA protein in the uterus is required to mediate the decidualization response to progesterone.

The decidualization defect in PRAKO mice was also associated with aberrant regulation of progesterone-responsive target genes associated with implantation. Analysis of the regulation of three genes, calcitonin (CT), histidine decarboxylase (HDC), and amphiregulin (AR), whose expression is increased in the uterine epithelium in response to P in association with uterine receptivity and is abolished in PRKO mice showed that ablation of PR-A resulted in the loss of expression of CT and AR but the regulation of HDC was fully retained. These findings indicated that defective implantation in PRAKO uteri is associated with the loss of P-regulated expression of a subset of genes associated with uterine epithelial receptivity. Importantly, this differential target gene regulation by PR-B was not due to differences in spatiotemporal expression of PR-B relative to PR-A. The expression of PR-B in PRAKO mice showed the same pattern of intrauterine expression and regulation by estrogen as that observed in wild-type mice. Thus, the uterine defects observed in these mice are due to differences in the transcription factor activity of PR-B rather than to differences in the spatiotemporal expression of the protein relative to PR-A.

VI. OPPOSING FUNCTIONS OF PR-A AND PR-B IN THE REGULATION OF UTERINE EPITHELIAL PROLIFERATION

Estrogen is the primary proliferative stimulus for uterine epithelium and its effects are inhibited by progesterone. Ablation of both the PR-A and the PR-B isoforms in PRKO mice results in marked hyperplasia of the lumenal and glandular epithelial tissue due to the unopposed action of estrogen. Selective ablation of PR-A, however, revealed an unexpected capacity of the PR-B protein to contribute to, rather than inhibit, epithelial cell proliferation. Treatment of PRAKO mice with estrogen alone induced epithelial hyperplasia in a manner similar to that observed in PRKO and wild-type mice. However, the addition of progesterone together with estrogen resulted in a marked increase in proliferation over that observed with estrogen alone, a response that was not observed in PRKO mice. These findings indicate that expression of the PR-B protein alone in the uterus results in a gain of proliferative activity. This acquisition of a proliferative activity of progesterone represents a PR-B-dependent gain of function not previously observed in the uterus, indicating that uterine expression of the PR-A isoform is required to oppose not only estrogen-induced proliferation but also that induced by progesterone acting through the PR-B protein.

The discovery that PR-B can contribute to, rather than inhibit, uterine epithelial cell proliferation is likely to have important clinical implications with regard to hormonal management of uterine endometrial dysplasias. Clearly, the relative expression of PR isoforms under these conditions will be an important determinant with regard to the effectiveness of progestin therapy. The results predict that progestin agonists selective for the PR-A protein should improve the effectiveness of progestin therapy for these conditions.

VII. PRs AND MAMMARY GLAND DEVELOPMENT

Estrogen and progesterone are essential for the maintenance of postnatal developmental plasticity of the mammary gland and both hormones play a key role in mammary tumorigenesis. Null mutation of both PR isoforms in PRKO mice has demonstrated that PRs are specifically required for pregnancy-associated ductal proliferation and lobuloalveolar differentiation of the mammary epithelium. The mammary glands of PRKO mice failed to develop the pregnancy-associated side-branching of the ductal epithelium with attendant lobular alveolar differentiation despite normal postpubertal mammary gland morphogenesis of the virgin mice. Ablation of PR expression in these mice also resulted in a significantly reduced incidence of mammary tumor growth in response to carcinogen challenge. These observations underscore a specific role of PRs (as distinct from ERs) as obligate mediators of the intracellular signaling pathways that are essential for the initiation of murine mammary tumors induced by carcinogens.

The use of PRKO mice in combination with mammary gland transplantation techniques has provided important insights into the mechanisms underlying progesterone-dependent mammary gland morphogenesis. Throughout postpubertal mammary gland development, PRs are expressed exclusively in the epithelium. Consistent with these observations, tissue transplantation approaches using wild-type and PRKO mouse tissue to produce mammary gland recombinants that were devoid of PR in either the stromal or the epithelial compartments have provided strong support for the functional involvement of epithelial, rather than stromal, PRs in mediating mammary gland morphogenic responses to progesterone. The expression of PRs is localized to a scattered subset of epithelial cells throughout the ductal epithelium, the majority of which appear to be segregated from proliferating epithelial cells. The hierarchical organization of these receptors and their segregation from proliferating cells are conserved features in rodent and human mammary tissue. Such an expression pattern predicted that regulation of epithelial cell proliferation by progesterone may occur through a paracrine mechanism whereby PRs residing in nonproliferating cells induce the expression of a proliferative signal that promotes the proliferation of neighboring receptor-negative cells. Although PRKO mammary epithelium cannot undergo side-branching, mixing experiments with PRKO and wild-type epithelial cells demonstrate that the branching and differentiation defects can be overcome when PRKO cells are placed in close contact with PR^+ cells. Thus, although lacking PR^+ cells, the PRKO mammary epithelium still retains those PR^- cells that are responsive to PR-mediated paracrine signaling. Recent attempts to uncover downstream mediators of the progesterone response have identified the secreted glycoprotein Wnt-4 as a potential PR target that is co-expressed in PR^+ cells, is regulated by P, and is essential for regulating ductal branching via paracrine regulation of proliferation.

Both isoforms of PR are expressed in the mammary gland of the virgin mouse and during pregnancy, although the levels of PR-A protein exceed those of the PR-B isoform by at least a 2:1 ratio in both cases. To examine the selective contributions of each isoform to the morphogenic responses of the mammary epithelium to progesterone, the morphology of mammary glands of ovariectomized wild-type, PRAKO, and PRBKO mice was compared after exposure to estrogen and progesterone. Ablation of PR-A in PRAKO mice did not affect the ability of PR-B to elicit normal progesterone responsiveness in the mammary gland. The morphological changes in ductal side-branching and lobular alveolar development in these glands were similar to those observed in wild-type mice. Thus, the PRB isoform is sufficient to elicit normal proliferation and differentiation of the mammary epithelium in response to progesterone and neither process appears to require functional expression of the A protein. In contrast, more recent analysis of the mammary glands of PRBKO mice under similar conditions has shown markedly reduced ductal side-branching, whereas lobular alveolar differentiation appeared to be unaffected. Thus, PR-B is the primary mediator of the proliferative response to progesterone, but both the PR-A and the PR-B proteins can provide the differentiative signals associated with alveologenesis.

VIII. SUMMARY

Molecular dissection of progesterone signaling mechanisms using *in vitro* systems has demonstrated that the PR-A and PR-B proteins can respond to the same steroid ligand to induce both overlapping and distinct transcriptional responses that are promoter- and cell context-dependent. The use of genetically manipulated mouse models in which one or both of the PR isoforms are ablated has been pivotal in defining the physiological spectrum of progesterone receptor action as well as the contribution of the individual protein isoforms to the plieotropic activities of the hormone. These approaches have provided compelling evidence that the differences in the transactivation properties of the PR isoforms observed *in vitro* are reflected in a differential capacity to regulate the tissue-selective reproductive activities of progesterone.

Glossary

PRAKO Progesterone receptor A isoform knockout.
PRBKO Progesterone receptor B isoform knockout.
PRKO Progesterone receptor knock-out.

See Also the Following Articles

Co-activators and Corepressors for the Nuclear Receptor Superfamily ● Estrogen and Progesterone Receptors in Breast Cancer ● Estrogen Receptor-α Structure and Function ● Estrogen Receptor-β Structure and Function ● Implantation ● Luteinizing Hormone (LH) ● Ovulation ● Oxytocin ● Progesterone Receptor Structure/Function and Crosstalk with Cellular Signaling Pathways

Further Reading

Conneely, O. M. (2001). Perspective: Female steroid hormone action. *Endocrinology* **142**, 2194–2199.

Conneely, O. M., Mulac-Jericevic, B., DeMayo, F., Lydon, J. P., and O'Malley, B. W. (2002). Reproductive functions of progesterone receptors. *Rec. Prog. Horm. Res.* **57**, 339–355.

Giangrande, P. H., and McDonnell, D. P. (1999). The A and B isoforms of the human progesterone receptor: Two functionally different transcription factors encoded by a single gene. *Rec. Prog. Horm. Res.* **54**, 291–313.

Giangrande, P. H., Kimbrel, E. A., Edwards, D. P., and McDonnell, D. P. (2000). The opposing transcriptional activities of the two isoforms of the human progesterone receptor are due to differential cofactor binding. *Mol. Cell. Biol.* **20**, 3102–3115.

Graham, J. D., and Clarke, C. L. (1997). Physiological action of progesterone in target tissues. *Endocr. Rev.* **18**, 502–519.

Mulac-Jericevic, B., Mullinax, R. A., DeMayo, F. J., Lydon, J. P., and Conneely, O. M. (2000). Subgroup of reproductive functions of progesterone mediated by progesterone receptor-B isoform. *Science* **289**, 1751–1754.

Richer, J. K., Jacobsen, B. M., Manning, N. G., Abel, M. G., Wolf, D. M., and Horwitz, K. B. (2002). Differential gene regulation by the two progesterone receptor isoforms in human breast cancer cells. *J. Biol. Chem.* **277**, 5209–5218.

Progesterone Receptor Structure/Function and Crosstalk with Cellular Signaling Pathways

DEAN P. EDWARDS

University of Colorado Health Sciences Center

Progesterone, a steroid hormone produced in the ovaries, functions primarily in the growth, differentiation, and maintenance of reproductive tissues. The biological effects of progesterone are achieved through activation of specific progesterone receptors, which interact with target DNA either directly or indirectly, via interaction with other DNA-bound proteins.

I. INTRODUCTION

Based on structural and biological properties, steroid hormones are categorized into general families, including female sex steroids (estrogens and progesterone), male sex steroids (androgens), glucocorticoids, mineralocorticoids, and vitamin D metabolites. Progesterone (Fig. 1) is synthesized and secreted cyclically by the ovary and its major biological functions are growth, differentiation, and maintenance of reproductive tract tissues during the menstrual cycle and pregnancy. In the uterus, progesterone is required for differentiation of the glandular epithelium during the luteal postovulatory phase of the menstrual cycle. After fertilization, progesterone prepares the uterus for implantation of the blastocyst and is required for maintenance of pregnancy. In the mammary gland, progesterone is required during pregnancy for development of alveolar glands that synthesize milk proteins; in the ovary, progesterone is required for granulosa cell development. Progesterone has functions as well in certain nonreproductive tract tissues; in the

hypothalamus and pituitary, progesterone is required for regulating synthesis and production of gonadotropin and gonadotropin-releasing hormones, and in the brain, for regulating sexual behavior. Progesterone also plays a role in human diseases, including brain meningiomas, endometriosis, uterine fibroids, and cancers of the uterus and breast.

Steroid hormones exert their biological effects through altering specific networks of gene expression. Target tissues that respond to steroids express receptor proteins that belong to a superfamily of nuclear hormone receptors that function as ligand-dependent transcription factors. Specific receptors exist for each class of steroid hormone, and the basic pathway for receptor-mediated gene regulation is well characterized (Fig. 2). Steroid hormones are lipophilic molecules capable of readily passing across cell membranes. Once inside a target cell, they bind to and convert their cognate receptor from an inactive state to an active state, in which the receptor becomes a transcription factor. Receptor activation involves multiple steps, including a conformational change that promotes dissociation from a multiprotein sequestering complex consisting of molecular chaperones and heat-shock proteins. Receptors then dimerize and bind to specific DNA sequences within the regulatory promoter regions of steroid-responsive genes, referred to as hormone response elements (HREs). Consensus HREs consist of inverted repeat hexanucelotide sequences separated by three unspecified nucleotides to form a 15-bp recognition site, each bound by a symmetric receptor dimer. The DNA-bound receptor can either increase or decrease rates of target gene transcription through additional downstream steps that mediate communication with the general transcriptional machinery. Post-DNA-binding steps include two general pathways: receptor interaction with components of the general transcription machinery, either through direct protein–protein interactions or indirectly through adapter proteins, and recruitment of specific co-activators. Co-activators have no DNA-binding activity and associate with target genes solely through protein interaction with DNA-bound receptors. However, they possess intrinsic enzyme activity for acetylation [such as histone acetyltransferase (HAT)activity] or methylation of core histone proteins. These chemical modifications of core histones can relieve the repressive effects of chromatin on transcription by relaxing nucleosome structure and facilitating access of the general transcription machinery to the promoter. Although steroid hormone receptors do not usually interact with corepressors, certain members of the nuclear

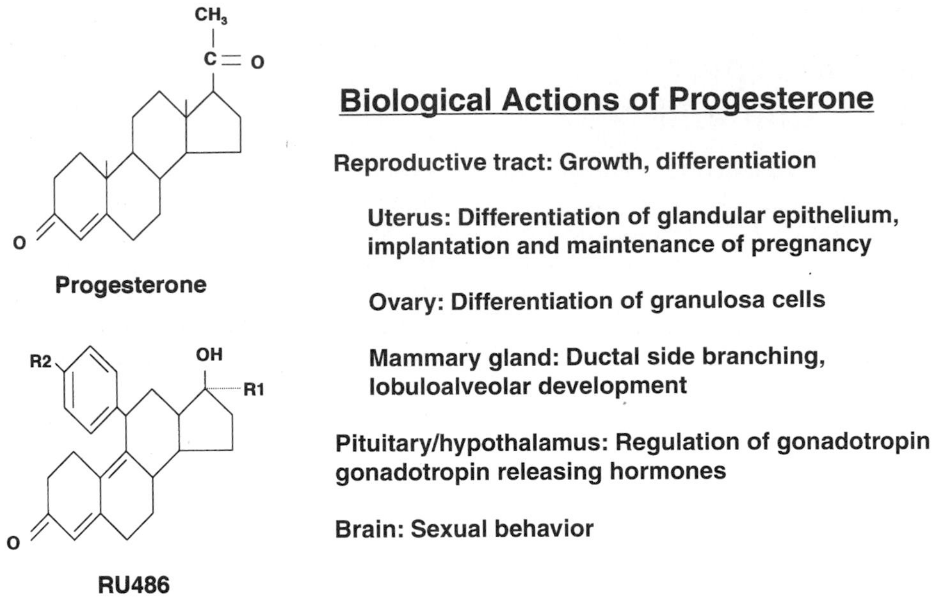

CH3
C=O
O
Progesterone
R2
OH
R1
O
RU486
Biological Actions of Progesterone
Reproductive tract: Growth, differentiation
Uterus: Differentiation of glandular epithelium, implantation and maintenance of pregnancy
Ovary: Differentiation of granulosa cells
Mammary gland: Ductal side branching, lobuloalveolar development
Pituitary/hypothalamus: Regulation of gonadotropin gonadotropin releasing hormones
Brain: Sexual behavior

FIGURE 1 Chemical structures of progesterone and the progesterone antagonist RU486 (Mifapristone) and the major biological actions of progesterone.

hormone receptor superfamily, including retinoid and thyroid hormone receptors, can actively silence gene transcription through recruitment of corepressors that recruit proteins with histone deacetylase (HDAC) enzyme activity. HDACs mediate effects opposite to those of HATs by promoting a condensation of nucleosome structure and impairing access of the general transcription machinery to the promoter.

II. STEROID HORMONE RECEPTORS: GENERAL PROPERTIES

Members of the nuclear receptor superfamily share a similar domain organization consisting of a highly conserved DNA-binding domain (DBD) located in the central part of the molecule, a carboxyl-terminal ligand-binding domain (LBD), and an N-terminal domain that is the most variable region among

DI
NLS
NLS
DI
Hsps
N-
DNA
h
Ligand
-C
AF-1
AF-2
Steroid
Hsp90
p23
SR
p59
Inactive complex
SR
SR
Dimerization
co-activator
SR
SR
General transcript. machinery
TATA
HRE

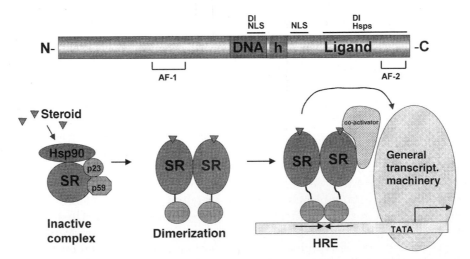

FIGURE 2 General structural organization of steroid receptors as members of the nuclear receptor superfamily of ligand-dependent transcription factors, and activation mechanisms. DI, Dimerization domain; NLS, nuclear localization sequence; h, hinge; Hsps, heat-shock proteins; AF-1, AF-2, transcriptional activation domains; SR, steroid receptor; HRE, hormone response element.

superfamily members (Fig. 2). Three-dimensional atomic structures of isolated DBDs and LBDs have revealed common motifs for these regions. The core DBD contains two asymmetric zinc fingers, each with a zinc ion coordinated by four conserved cysteine residues. An α-helix extends between the two zinc fingers, which makes base-specific contacts in the major groove of HRE DNA. The LBD consists of 10–12 α-helices that fold into a three-layer α-helical sandwich containing a central core positioned between helix bundles on either side. This structure creates a hydrophobic wedge-shaped cavity in which the steroid hormone (ligand) is buried. By comparison, little is known about the structure of the N-terminal domain. Biophysical and biochemical data indicate that the N-terminal domain is in a non-globular extended conformation with little secondary structure. This is the least conserved region among superfamily members with respect to both length and amino acid sequence. The N-terminal domain is functionally important because it is required for full transcriptional activity of steroid hormone receptors and for many cell-specific and target gene-specific responses.

Other functional and structural determinants have been identified within these broader three domains. In addition to binding steroid hormone, the LBD contains determinants for dimerization (DI) in the absence of DNA, for binding of heat-shock proteins (Hsps), and for nuclear localization sequences (NLSs). The DBD contains a second NLS and a dimerization domain that is dependent on DNA binding. DNA-dependent dimerization stabilizes the receptor–DNA complex and facilitates orientation of the receptor dimer with the correct spacing of the HRE. Steroid receptors contain at least two transcription activation function (AF) domains. These are autonomous transferable domains required for the DNA-bound receptor to transmit a transcriptional activation response, and they function as specific binding sites for co-activators. AF-2, located in the LBD, is hormone dependent and becomes activated as a result of the steroid hormone inducing a repositioning of the C-terminal-most α-helix-12 in such a way as to create a specific hydrophobic binding pocket for members of the p160 family of steroid receptor co-activators (SRCs). Little is known about AF-1 in the N-terminus. It can function independently of AF-2 in a constitutive manner or can synergize with AF-2 in a ligand-dependent manner. The co-activators that bind to and mediate the activity of AF-1 are yet not well defined.

III. PROGESTERONE RECEPTOR A AND B ISOFORMS

As a member of the nuclear receptor superfamily, the progesterone receptor (PR) shares the general structural domains, but has several unique features. In most species, PR is expressed as two isoforms, PR-A and PR-B. The exception is rabbits, which express only PR-B. In human tissues, PR-A is a truncated protein lacking the first 164 amino acids from the N-terminal domain; otherwise the two PRs have an identical amino acid sequence throughout the remainder of the protein, including the DBD and LBD (Fig. 3). PR-A and PR-B arise from a single gene by alternate transcription from two promoters. The two forms of PR have similar steroid hormone and DNA-binding activities, but they have distinct transcriptional activities due to differences in the N-terminal region. PR-A and PR-B are capable of forming heterodimers, and in the cell PR can exist in three molecular states of AA, AB, and BB dimers. This ability to produce three molecular forms of PR from a single gene expands the functional range of activities of the receptor without the need for a separate receptor subtype gene. The relative expression of PR-A and PR-B is regulated in a tissue-specific manner and by physiological conditions. The ratio of PR-A to PR-B varies significantly in a regular pattern in the uterus during the menstrual cycle; in some breast tumors, very high PR-A:PR-B ratios have been detected. In normal breast tissue, the ratios are close to 1:1, whereas PR-A appears to be the predominant form of receptor in endometriosis. Thus, a difference in relative expression of PR-A and PR-B is one way for a tissue to regulate response to progesterone. The two promoters responsible for expression of the PR isoforms are estrogen responsive. However, the gene region for these promoters is complex and has potential regulatory sites for multiple other factors, and is not likely to be regulated by estrogen alone.

The transcriptional activities of the two PR isoforms vary, depending on the cell type and the context of the target gene promoter. In general, on classical progesterone response element (PRE) targets, PR-B is a much stronger activator compared to PR-A. However, PR-A can be a strong activator under specific cell and target gene contexts. The stronger activation potential of PR-B is due in part to the existence of a third activation domain (AF-3) within the first N-terminal 164 amino acids that is unique to PR-B (Fig. 3). However, AF-3 is not an autonomous activation domain capable of activating transcription when linked to a heterologous DBD. AF-3 functions

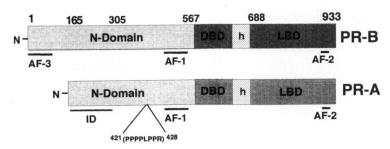

FIGURE 3   Domain organization of human progesterone receptor A and B isoforms (PR-A and PR-B). AF-1, AF-2, AF-3, Transcriptional activation domains; DBD, DNA-binding domain; h, hinge region; LBD, ligand-binding domain; ID, inhibitory domain.

only when linked to the PR DBD, and co-activators that interact with AF-3 have not yet been identified. Thus, AF-3 is thought to facilitate activity of AF-1 and AF-2 through intramolecular domain interactions. In support of this idea, the N- and C-terminal domains of PR (both A and B isoforms) are capable of directly associating with each other in a hormone agonist-dependent manner, but these interactions are more efficient for PR-B than for PR-A.

Under certain cell and target promoter contexts, PR-A is inactive as a transcription factor and can function as a ligand-dependent transdominant repressor of other steroid receptors, including PR-B, estrogen receptor (ER), androgen receptor (AR), glucocorticoid receptor (GR), and mineralocorticoid receptor (MR). PR-A can act in this repressor mode in response to binding either progestin agonists or antagonists. An inhibitory domain (ID) responsible for this transrepressor function has been mapped to the first 140 N-terminal (165–305) amino acids of PR-A (Fig. 3). The ID is functional and transferable to other steroid receptors, such as chicken PR and human ER, which do not exhibit this trans-repressor activity. Truncation of the ID from PR-A increases its transcriptional activity to the level of PR-B. The sequence within the ID is present in both PR isoforms but is active only in the context of PR-B, suggesting that a role of the PR-B-specific N-terminal segment is to suppress the activity of the ID. This is thought to occur through the PR-B N-terminal segment exerting a long-distance effect on the conformation of the PR-A N-terminus.

How PR-A can repress transcriptional activity of other steroid receptors remains unclear. This property does not involve the phenomenon of transcriptional squelching of a common limiting cofactor for PR-B and other steroid receptors. Instead, PR-A and PR-B exhibit a different ability to interact with coregulatory proteins. PR-A inter-

acts more efficiently with the silencing mediator of retinoid/thyroid (SMRT) receptor corepressor than does PR-B, and this difference requires the inhibitory domain of PR-A. Conversely, PR-B interacts more efficiently with members of the SRC family of co-activators than does PR-A. Thus, the A isoform of PR may recruit a distinct coregulatory protein complex to promoters that contains corepressors and is functionally inhibitory to other DNA-bound complexes.

Studies with PR isoform-specific gene knockout mice and transgenic mice that overexpress either PR-A or PR-B have provided evidence that the two forms of PRs have distinct physiological roles *in vivo*. Selective knockout of PR-A in mice has a strong phenotype in the uterus but not in the mammary gland, suggesting that the PR isoforms have tissue-specific roles. Overexpression of PR-A or PR-B results in abnormal mammary gland development, but the phenotypes of the two transgenic mouse lines are not the same.

Transcription factors that harbor both activation and repression domains, or are expressed as truncated forms capable of functioning as dominant transrepressors, have been identified in several different families of transcription factors. Such factors include the Id protein of the MyoD transcription factor family, the jun dimerization proteins (JDP-1 and JDP-2) of the AP-1 (fos/jun) family, and isoforms of the basic-region leucine zipper (bZIP) containing activating transcription factor-2 (ATF-2) and CCAATT/ enhancer-binding protein (C/EBP) transcription factors. These naturally occurring transrepressors have important physiological roles in shutting off activation responses at specific times during development and differentiation or under specific physiological conditions. Among the steroid hormone receptors, PR-A has been suggested to have a similar role that may be particularly relevant in the uterus, in which progesterone is known to antagonize the growth-stimulatory activity of estrogen.

IV. PHOSPHORYLATION OF PR

As with other steroid hormone receptors, PR in human tissues is phosphorylated on multiple serine/threonine residues in a highly specific and hormone-regulated manner. Specific sites of phosphorylation on the PR *in situ* (PR expressed in mammalian cells) that have been confirmed by peptide sequencing are shown in Fig. 4. Most of the sites are located throughout the N-terminal domain; five are unique to PR-B whereas the others are within the N-terminal domain in common with PR-A and PR-B. The exception is phosphorylation of Ser-676 within the hinge region between the DBD and LBD. The PR phosphorylation sites are classified as basal and hormone dependent. Three hormone-dependent sites (Ser-102, Ser-294, and Ser-345) are unphosphorylated in the absence of ligand and become fully phosphorylated in response to hormone *in situ*. Some of the remaining sites are basally phosphorylated without hormone and increase phosphorylation rapidly within 5–10 min after hormone treatment of cells. The hormone dependence of the other sites has not been determined. Most of the phosphorylation sites reside within Ser-Pro motifs and there are at least three kinases capable of phosphorylating human PR, including the cyclin-dependent kinase CDK-2/cyclin A (Ser-130, Ser-162, Ser-190, Ser-213, Ser-400, and Ser-676), mitogen-activated protein kinase (MAPK; Ser-294), and casein kinase II (Ser-81). The kinases that phosphorylate the hormone-dependent sites at Ser-102 and Ser-345 and basal sites at Thr-430, Ser-554 have not yet been identified. The fact that subsets of sites are substrates for different kinases suggests that these groups of phosphorylation sites have distinct roles in PR structure/function and are regulated by different signaling pathways.

The function of PR phosphorylation has not been well defined. Analysis of various phosphorylation site mutants (serine to alanine substitutions) reveal no effect of phosphorylation on PR–DNA binding or steroid-binding activities. However, up to a 50% decrease in hormone-dependent transcriptional activity is observed with two mutants, Ser to Ala-190 and Ser to Ala-676. Other mutations have little to no effect on transcriptional activity of the PR. The Ser-294 phosphorylation site has been reported to be a signal for hormone-dependent down-regulation of the PR that targets the receptor for degradation by proteasomes. The PR from chicken oviduct (cPR) is also phosphorylated on multiple serine/threonine residues in the N-terminal domain and on a single site in the hinge. Phosphorylation site mutations in the N-terminal domain of cPR result in as much as a 75% reduction in transcriptional activity *in situ*, whereas mutation of the hinge region site reduces the hormone sensitivity of cPR-mediated transcription without altering steroid binding affinity. The magnitude of the effect of these phosphorylation site mutations on PR activity varies and is dependent on cell and target gene promoter context, suggesting that phosphorylation has a role in modulating PR interactions with other proteins for which expression may be cell type or target gene specific. Thus, phosphorylation does not appear to be a regulatory on/off switch but seems to have a more subtle role in

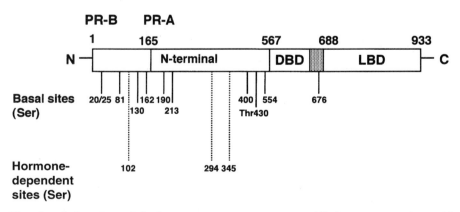

FIGURE 4 Phosphorylation sites of the human progesterone receptor. All sites are on serine residues, with the exception of position 430 (threonine). PR-A, PR-B, Progesterone receptor isoforms A and B; DBD, DNA-binding domain; LBD, ligand-binding domain.

modulating different functional activities of the PR. Additionally, phosphorylation could have a structural role in stabilizing the folded state of the receptor, in particular the N-terminal domain, which is fairly devoid of secondary structure. A physical mapping of the surface structure of the N-terminal domain of the PR by limited proteolysis shows that protease-accessible sites are limited to phosphorylation sites, suggesting that these sites are surface exposed and may stabilize domain interactions or folding within the N-domain.

V. PR CROSSTALK WITH OTHER TRANSCRIPTION FACTORS

Steroid receptors can regulate transcription of genes that lack HREs as a primary response through protein-protein interactions with other DNA-bound transcription factors (Fig. 5). Although this mode of regulation can be either positive or negative, it is more commonly a pathway for negative gene regulation by steroid receptors, and in some cases a mutual repression between steroid receptors and the other transcription factor has been observed. Genes that contain composite response elements consisting of a less than optimal DNA-binding site for the steroid receptor (often a HRE half-site) that overlaps, or is adjacent to, a good binding site for another sequence-specific transcription factor are a variation of this mode of regulation. Regulation of composite elements often involves both receptor–DNA and receptor–protein interactions

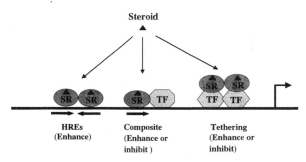

FIGURE 5 Different mechanisms by which steroid receptors activate or inhibit gene transcription as a primary gene regulation response. Left: Direct binding of the steroid receptor (SR) to hormone response elements (HREs) within promoters of steroid-responsive genes. Middle: Composite element consisting of a weak HRE half-site and a neighboring optimal site for another sequence specific transcription factor (TF). Steroid receptors can either enhance or inhibit transactivation mediated by the other transcription factor. Right: Tethering response element. Steroid receptor interacts with another DNA-bound transcription factor through a protein–protein interaction to either enhance or inhibit transactivation.

with other transcription factors. The ability to enhance the activity of other transcription factors arises through recruitment of receptor transcription activation domains; in essence, the receptor acts as a co-activator. Negative regulation can occur via the steroid receptor interfering with activation domains of other transcription factors or competing for DNA-binding sites. Examples of negative PR crosstalk with other transcription factors are repression of nuclear factor κB (NF-κB) activity (through interaction with RelA/p65 subunit), interference with the dioxin arylhydrocarbon receptor (AhR) signaling, inhibition of prolactin-induced Stat5-mediated activation of the β-casein gene, and repression of AP-1 (fos/jun) activity. Not all crosstalk with the PR results in repression; unliganded PR can enhance AP-1 in human endometrial carcinoma cells, although addition of progesterone reverses this enhancement. This positive crosstalk between PR and AP-1 appears to be cell type specific suggesting that other cellular factors are required. Because NF-κB is activated by various cytokines, crosstalk with the PR is thought to be involved in the immunosuppressive effects of progesterone during pregnancy. Progesterone receptor crosstalk with AP-1 and Stat5 is thought to be involved in proliferative and differentiation functions of progesterone, respectively, in the mammary gland and uterus.

VI. PR CROSSTALK WITH CELL SIGNALING PATHWAYS

Steroid receptors as ligand-dependent transcription factors and cell membrane/cytoplasmic signal transduction pathways have traditionally been viewed as completely separate pathways for regulating gene expression in response to external signals. However, it was discovered in the early 1990s that steroid receptors are nuclear targets of certain signal transduction pathways, suggesting a convergence of these two major pathways. Modulation of protein kinases or phosphatases in mammalian cells can either activate steroid receptors in the absence of ligand or potentiate ligand-dependent activity of receptors. Crosstalk with other signal transduction pathways was first reported with cPR and subsequently with human PR and all classes of steroid receptors. Agents that elevate intracellular cAMP (8-bromo-cAMP) to activate protein kinase A (PKA), inhibitors of protein phosphatases 1 and 2A (okadaic acid), and natural peptides that activate membrane receptor-linked signal transduction pathways, including the neurotransmitter dopamine and epidermal growth factor (EGF), can all activate cPR in the absence of progesterone. Although the human PR is not activated in the absence of ligand, 8-bromo-cAMP, okadaic acid, EGF, and activators of protein kinase C, all stimulate hormone-dependent PR transactivation in different cell lines, including breast cancer cells. Activation of cPR in the absence of progesterone by these agents and potentiation of human PR activity in the presence of ligand are not accompanied by changes in receptor phosphorylation. The lack of effect on direct PR phosphorylation suggests that receptor-interacting co-activators are the targets of phosphorylation by these different protein kinase signaling pathways. As evidence for this idea, SRC-1 becomes phosphorylated on two specific MAPK sites (Ser-1179 and Ser-1185) in response to activation of PKA pathways. This phosphorylation does not facilitate direct SRC-1 interaction with the PR; rather, its role is to modulate functional cooperation between SRC-1 and CREB-binding protein (CBP), which is required for activity of a larger multiprotein SRC co-activator complex (Fig. 6).

A reverse crosstalk was recently discovered between human PR and cell membrane/cytoplasmic signaling pathways. The N-terminal region common to PR-A and PR-B contains a short, contiguous polyproline-rich sequence (amino acids 421–428, written as PPPPPLPR using the single-letter code,

where P is proline, L is leucine, and R is arginine) that conforms to a consensus type II motif for binding the Src homology domains (SH3) of cell membrane/cytoplasmic signaling molecules. These polyproline sequences form a left-handed helix conformation that interacts with a binding pocket of SH3 domains. PR interacts *in vitro* and in cells with SH3 domains of various signaling molecules. including c-Src tyrosine kinases. This interaction is stimulated by progestins and is mediated directly by the proline-rich motif in the N-terminus of PR. The consequence of this interaction is a rapid progesterone-dependent stimulation of Src kinase enzyme activity through PR-mediated displacement of an intramolecular SH3 domain interaction that maintains Src kinases in an inactive state. Point mutations in the proline-rich motif that abolish progestin-induced activation of Src do not affect the transcriptional activity of PR. Conversely, point mutations in the DBD or AF-2 that cripple PR as a transcription factor have no effect on the ability of PR to mediate progestin activation of Src kinase. This PR–SH3 domain interaction is of biological consequence. Progestins can rapidly and transiently (10 min) activate the entire Src/ras/MAPK pathway in mammalian cells in a manner that is dependent on the integrity of the proline-rich–SH3 domain interaction motif within the PR. Also, PR–SH3 domain interactions contribute to two known

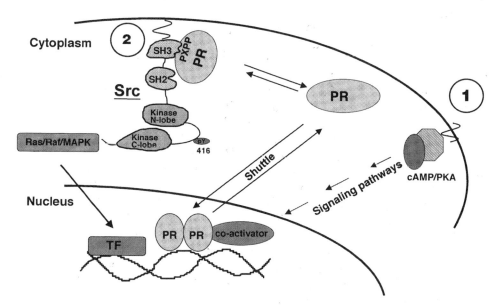

FIGURE 6 Two-way crosstalk between the progesterone receptor (PR) and cell signal transduction pathways. Cell signal transduction pathways can potentiate the transcription activity of nuclear PRs through phosphorylation of receptor-interacting co-activators. (1) Phosphorylation enhances the transcription activity of the receptor–co-activator complex. (2) The PR can modulate other cell-signaling pathways through a direct interaction in the cytoplasm with regulatory SH3 domains of signaling molecules, including Src kinases. This extranuclear function of the PR is rapid (5–10 min) and is not dependent on transcription.

biological responses of progesterone, including inhibition of proliferation of normal breast epithelial cells and induction of meiosis in *Xenopus* oocytes. These data suggest that the PR is a dual-function protein capable of directly interacting with target DNA in the nucleus in its well-established role as a transcription factor, and also interacting with SH3 domains to modulate cytoplasmic signaling pathways (Fig. 6). Although the function of the PR is traditionally thought to take place in the nucleus, it rapidly shuttles between the cytoplasm and nucleus by active nuclear import and export mechanisms. Thus, the PR has the opportunity to encounter signaling molecules in the cytoplasm and to have extranuclear functions.

VII. PROGESTERONE ANTAGONISTS

Several steroid analogues of progesterone that have been developed function as potent PR antagonists. The most important antagonist clinically is RU486 (Mifapristone), which is used as an antifertility agent and in experimental treatment of diseases such as brain meningiomas, endometriosis, uterine fibroids, and breast cancer. The structural features of RU486 that confer antagonist activity are the aromatic ring at the 11β-carbon position and the side chain at the carbon-17 position of the steroid ring structure of progesterone (see Fig. 1). RU486 competes with progesterone for binding to the PR and has a higher affinity for the receptor than does the natural hormone. RU486 binding effectively inactivates the PR by a complex mechanism. The receptor activation steps of dissociation from the sequestering Hsp complex, dimerization, and binding to PREs are not impaired when the PR is occupied by RU486. PR interaction with DNA, however, is nonproductive as a result of RU486 inducing a conformation in the carboxyl-terminal tail of the PR that is distinct from that induced by hormone agonist. This alternate conformation inactivates AF-2 and does not permit interaction with co-activators. However, RU486 is a more potent antagonist than is predicted by a simple inactivation of AF-2 of those PR molecules occupied by RU486. First, PR bound to RU486 is capable of heterodimerization with PR bound to hormone agonist and of inhibiting the activity of the agonist-bound PR *in trans*. Thus, effective inhibition of PR bound to agonist requires less than stoichiometric amounts of RU486. Additionally, the alternate conformation of PR induced by RU486 results in a substantial enhancement of corepressor binding to PR. Thus, in the presence of RU486, PR is capable of actively repressing gene transcription.

As with most steroid antagonists, RU486 is not a pure antagonist and exhibits partial agonist/antagonist activity, dependent on physiological conditions. PR crosstalk with cAMP and protein kinase A signaling pathways results in a dramatic potentiation of the agonist activity of RU486. This antagonist-to-agonist switch appears to be fairly specific to crosstalk with cAMP/PKA signaling pathways. Activation of protein kinase C and growth factor pathways does not cause this functional switch. Only the B receptor responds to cAMP in this manner, suggesting a requirement for both AF-3 and AF-1 together for RU486 to act as an agonist. The mechanism by which the cAMP/PKA pathway potentiates the agonist activity of RU486 involves a decreased association of corepressors (NcoR and SMRT) with PR. However, dissociation of corepressor alone is not sufficient for PR activation. Because AF-2 becomes inactivated by RU486, recruitment of an N-terminal domain co-activator would also be required, but such a co-activator has not yet been identified. Thus, the relative agonist/antagonist activity of RU486 is thought to be a reflection of the balance in the cell between expression and availability of specific N-terminal co-activators and corepressors. This concept is of potential relevance to the clinical use of RU486 and other steroid antagonists and could explain the variable efficacy of steroid antagonists in clinical settings, especially in the treatment of breast cancer.

VIII. SUMMARY

Many biological responses to progesterone are mediated through the PR interacting directly with target DNA, thus acting as a transcription factor, or through the PR interacting with other DNA-bound proteins, thus acting as a transcription cofactor. Transcription activities of PR can be further modulated by variable expression of the A and B isoforms and through crosstalk with other signal transduction pathways. PR-A may also function as a naturally occurring repressor of other members of the steroid hormone group of nuclear receptors. The progesterone receptor also has rapid nontranscription functions through its ability to interact directly with SH3 domains and to activate cytoplasmic signal transduction pathways.

Glossary

DNA-binding domain Region of steroid receptors that makes specific contact with DNA; has a conserved structural motif among members of the nuclear receptor family and can function autonomously.

hormone response elements Specific DNA sequences in the promoter region of steroid-responsive genes; bind and mediate transcriptional responses to steroid receptors.

ligand In the context of the nuclear receptor superfamily, a small lipophilic molecule, in some cases a steroid hormone, that binds to the ligand-binding domain of a receptor.

ligand-binding domain Region of receptor in the C-terminus that binds steroid hormone; has a conserved structural motif and can function autonomously.

progesterone response elements Hormone response elements that are specific for the progesterone receptors.

SH3 domain Src tyrosine kinase homology domain 3; a conserved regulatory region of many signaling molecules that interacts with other proteins.

steroid receptor co-activators Family of proteins of 160,000 molecular weight (p160); interact with transcriptional activation domains of nuclear hormone receptors and act as bridging factors between the DNA-bound receptor and the general transcriptional machinery.

transcriptional activation domain Region of steroid receptors that binds co-activators and mediates transcriptional enhancement activity.

See Also the Following Articles

Androgen Receptor Crosstalk with Cellular Signaling Pathways • Crosstalk of Nuclear Receptors with STAT Factors • Estrogen and Progesterone Receptors in Breast Cancer • Estrogen Receptor-α Structure and Function • Estrogen Receptor-β Structure and Function • Estrogen Receptor Crosstalk with Cellular Signaling Pathways • Progesterone Action in the Female Reproductive Tract • Steroid Receptor Crosstalk with Cellular Signaling Pathways

Further Reading

Boonyaratanakornkit, V., Porter, M., Ribon, V., Sherman, L., Anderson, S. A., Miller, W. T., and Edwards, D. P. (2001). Progesterone receptor contains a proline rich sequence in the amino terminus that directly interacts with SH3 domains and activates Src family tyrosine kinases. *Mol. Cell* 8, 269–280.

Edwards, D. P. (1999). Coregulatory proteins in nuclear hormone receptor action. *Vitam. Horm.* 55, 165–218.

Giangrande, P. H., and McDonnell, D. P. (1999). The A and B isoforms of the human progesterone receptor: Two functionally different transcription factors encoded by a single gene. *Recent Prog. Horm. Res.* 54, 291–313.

Giangrande, P. H., Kimbrel, E. A., Edwards, D. P., and McDonnell, D. P. (2000). The opposing transcriptional activities of the two isoforms of the human progesterone receptor are due to differential cofactor binding. *Mol. Cell. Biol.* 20, 3102–3115.

Knotts, T. A., Orkiszewski, R. S., Cook, R. G., Edwards, D. P., and Weigel, N. L. (2001). Identification of a phosphorylation site in the hinge region of the human progesterone receptor and additional amino-terminal phosphorylation sites. *J. Biol. Chem.* 276, 8475–8483.

Lange, C. A., Shen, T., and Horwitz, K. B. (2000). Phosphorylation of human progesterone receptors at serine-294 by mitogen-

activated protein kinase signals their degradation by the 26S proteasome. *Proc. Natl. Acad. Sci. USA* 97, 1032–1037.

McKay, L. I., and Cidlowski, J. A. (1999). Molecular control of immune/inflammatory responses: Interactions between nuclear factor-κB and steroid receptor-signaling pathways. *Endocr. Rev.* 20(4), 435–459.

McKenna, N. J., Lanz, R. B., and O'Malley, B. W. (1999). Nuclear receptor coregulators: Cellular and molecular biology. *Endocr. Rev.* 20(3), 321–344.

Mulac-Jericevic, B., Mullinax, R. A., DeMayo, F. J., Lydon, J. P., and Conneely, O. M. (2000). Subgroup of reproductive functions of progesterone mediated by progesterone receptor-B isoform. *Science* 289, 1751–1754.

Norman, A. W., and Litwack, G. H. (1997). Estrogens and Progestins. *In* "Hormones" pp. 361–385. Academic Press, San Diego.

Rowan, B. G., Garrison, N., Weigel, N. L., and O'Malley, B. W. (2000). 8-Bromo-cyclic AMP induces phosphorylation of two sites in SRC-1 that facilitate ligand-independent activation of the chicken progesterone receptor and are critical for functional cooperation between SRC-1 and CREB binding protein. *Mol. Cell. Biol.* 20(23), 8720–8730.

Shyamala, G., Yang, X., Cardiff, R. D., and Dale, E. (2000). Impact of progesterone receptor on cell-fate decisions during mammary gland development. *Proc. Natl. Acad. Sci. USA* 97, 3044–3049.

Wagner, B. L., Norris, J. D., Knotts, T. A., Weigel, N. L., and McDonnell, D. P. (1998). The nuclear corepressors NcoR and SMRT are key regulators of both ligand- and 8-bromo-cyclic AMP-dependent transcriptional activity of the human progesterone receptor. *Mol. Cell. Biol.* 18(3), 1369–1378.

Weigel, N. L. (1996). Steroid hormone receptors and their regulation by phosphorylation. *Biochem. J.* 319, 657–667.

Weigel, N. L., and Zhang, Y. (1998). Ligand-independent activation of steroid hormone receptors. *J. Mol. Med.* 76, 469–479.

Pro-inflammatory Cytokines and Steroids

STEPHEN G. HILLIER
University of Edinburgh

I. INFLAMMATION AND REPRODUCTION
II. PRO-INFLAMMATORY CYTOKINES
III. ANTI-INFLAMMATORY STEROIDS
IV. CYTOKINE–STEROID INTERPLAY
V. SUMMARY

Pro-inflammatory cytokines produced by somatic cells and activated macrophages are mediators and modulators of ovulation, menstruation, implantation, and parturition. Each of these hormonally regulated processes is localized to a specialized region of steroid metabolism and action in the female reproductive tract. Steroid hormones synthesized by the adrenal glands (corticosteroids) and ovaries (progesterone) are natural anti-inflammatory agents that are intimately involved in these serial injury-repair processes. The immunoendocrine interplay between pro-inflammatory cytokines and anti-inflammatory steroids is therefore fundamental to reproduction.

I. INFLAMMATION AND REPRODUCTION

Ovulation, menstruation, implantation, and parturition share cardinal features of an acute inflammatory response: vasodilation, increased vascular permeability, and cellular infiltration. Each process involves a tightly controlled phase of local tissue breakdown and regeneration. During ovulation, the wall of the preovulatory follicle and overlying ovarian surface epithelium are breached to release an oocyte for fertilization. Implantation involves invasion of the uterine wall by the embryonic trophoblast to initiate pregnancy. Menstruation, at the conclusion of each nonconceptual ovarian cycle, entails shedding of spent uterine endometrial and vascular tissues. And if pregnancy occurs, parturition culminates in softening of the uterine cervix to permit delivery of the neonate.

In every case, the inflammatory reaction unfolds as a biochemical cascade involving the sequential production of cytokines, lipid mediators (steroids, prostanoids, and leukotrienes), vasoactive mediators, and matrix-degrading proteolytic enzymes. The central role of cytokines is to control the direction, amplitude, and duration of the inflammatory response, thereby localizing and limiting the site of tissue injury and repair.

II. PRO-INFLAMMATORY CYTOKINES

Cytokines serve classic functions in host responses to injury and infection. They also function in the immunoendocrine system during ovulation, implantation, menstruation, and parturition, as paracrine signals that promote tissue remodeling. Cytokines are commonly classified as pro- or anti-inflammatory, as shown in Table 1.

This classification is undoubtedly overly simplistic, since individual cytokines can have multiple, overlapping, and sometimes opposing functions depending on their concentration, site of action,

TABLE 1   Common Pro- and Anti-inflammatory Cytokines

Pro-inflammatory	Anti-inflammatory
Interleukin-1 (IL-1)	IL-4
Tumor necrosis factor-α of GR	IL-10
Interferon-γ	IL-13
IL-6	Interferon-α
IL-8	Transforming
IL-12	growth factor-β
IL-18	
Granulocyte/macrophage colony Stimulating factor	

and the presence of other cytokines and mediators. The best characterized pro-inflammatory cytokines in the female reproductive tract are interleukin-1α (IL-1α), IL-1β, and tumor necrosis factor α (TNFα).

Interleukin-1 and TNFα signal via membrane-associated receptors on target cells to increase the expression of genes with roles in inflammation. The type I IL-1 receptor is a member of the Toll-like receptor (TLR) superfamily involved in signal transduction during inflammation and host defense. The superfamily includes the *Drosophila melanogaster* protein Toll, the IL-18 receptor, and the Toll-like receptors TLR-2 and TLR-4. Ligand binding of the corresponding receptor activates postreceptor signaling networks that in turn activate stress-related transcription factors (SRTFs), such as nuclear factor-κB (NF-κB) and activated protein-1 (AP-1) (Jun/Fos or Jun/Jun dimers), as illustrated for IL-1 in Fig. 1. AP-1 and NF-κB are important in immune and inflammatory responses because they localize the expression of genes encoding chemoattractants, cytokines, cytokine receptors, cell adhesion molecules, and matrix-degrading metalloproteinases (MMPs). They are also molecular targets of anti-inflammatory steroid action. Genes activated by AP-1 and NF-κB include the inducible cyclooxygenase isozyme COX-2, otherwise known as prostaglandin-H synthase-2, which catalyzes the formation of prostanoids essential for ovulation (PGE_2), implantation (PGI_2), and parturition $PGF_{2\alpha}$.

III. ANTI-INFLAMMATORY STEROIDS

The endocrine connection between pro-inflammatory cytokines and steroid hormones is provided by glucocorticoids, which are produced in increased amounts through cytokine action on the adrenal glands as a systemic response to infection. In addition

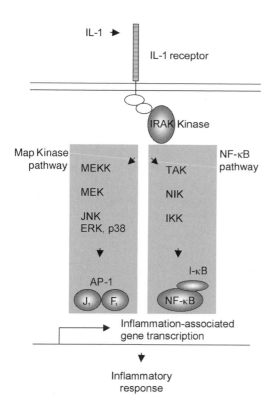

FIGURE 1 Postreceptor mechanisms of inflammatory cytokine action. IL-1, the prototypical inflammatory cytokine, binds to the extracellular domain of the IL-1 receptor, which activates postreceptor signaling via IL-1 receptor-associated kinase (IRAK). IRAK kinases activate at least two major postreceptor signaling pathways, leading to activation of inflammation-associated gene transcription: mitogen-activated protein kinase (MAPK) and nuclear factor κB (NF-κB) pathways. ERK, Extracellular signal-regulated protein kinase; MAPK, p38; MEK, MAPK/ERK kinase; JNK, Jun N-terminal kinase; J, c-Jun; F, c-Fos; AP-1, activated protein-1; TAK, TGF-β-activated kinase; I-κB, inhibitory factor-κB; IKK, I-κB kinase; NIK, NF-κB-inducing kinase.

to classic roles in stress, injury, and nutrition, glucocorticoids exert anti-inflammatory effects via the ligand-activated glucocorticoid receptor (GR) signaling pathway. Mutually negative interactions between the GR and SRTFs underlie the immunosuppressive and anti-inflammatory actions of glucocorticoids.

Progesterone also has immunosuppressive and anti-inflammatory properties that can be explained by transcriptional interference between ligand-activated progesterone receptor (PR) and SRTFs.

A. Glucocorticoid Activation

Reproductive tissues lack expression of key steroidogenic enzymes necessary for glucocorticoid synthesis.

However, like most other tissues in the body, they express GR and are potential sites of glucocorticoid action. Glucocorticoids circulate in the blood in a binding equilibrium with corticosteroid-binding globulin, which sets the concentration of steroid available for interaction with the GR in target tissues. Glucocorticoid action is also influenced by metabolism through 11β-hydroxysteroid dehydrogenase (11β-HSD) activity in target tissues, which determines the relative availability of "active" cortisol or "inactive" cortisone for ligand activation of GR signaling (Fig. 2). Two 11β-HSD isoforms are known to exist in human tissues, both of which are microsomal enzymes belonging to the short-chain alcohol dehydrogenase/reductase superfamily. 11β-HSD type 1 is an $NADP^+$-dependent bidirectional enzyme with predominantly 11-oxoreductase activity, which therefore principally converts cortisone to cortisol. 11β-HSD type 2 (11β-HSD2) is an NAD^+-dependent enzyme with strong dehydrogenase activity, which inactivates cortisol to cortisone. Differential expression of 11β-HSD1 and 11β-HSD2 determines glucocorticoid tissue responsiveness. For example, the high level of 11β-HSD2 relative to 11β-HSD1 expressed in kidney promotes cortisol metabolism to cortisone and protects mineralocorticoid receptors from inappropriate occupation by cortisol. On the other hand, in liver, 11β-HSD1 converts cortisone to cortisol, ensuring that GRs are adequately exposed to cortisol.

Cells of tissues from throughout the body, including the reproductive tract, show increased activation of cortisone to cortisol when challenged with pro-inflammatory cytokines *in vitro*, suggesting a critical paracrine link between glucocorticoid activation and pro-inflammatory cytokine action.

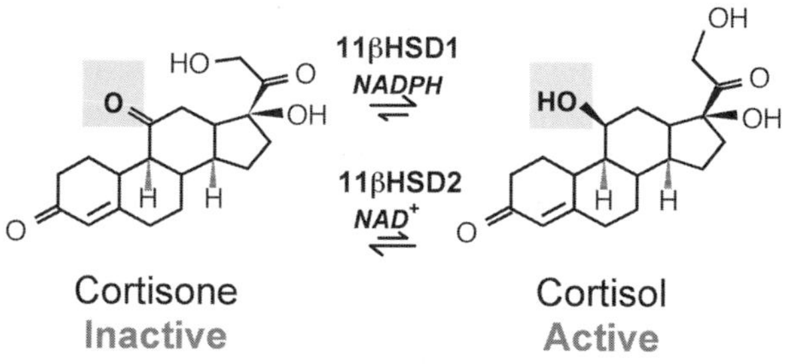

FIGURE 2 Interconversion of cortisone and cortisol catalyzed by 11β-hydroxysteroid dehydrogenases (11β-HSDs). 11β-HSD1 is principally an 11-oxoreductase that reversibly converts "inactive" cortisone to "active" cortisol, which binds and activates glucocorticoid receptors. 11β-HSD2 is a strong 11-dehydrogenase, which inactivates cortisol to cortisone.

IV. CYTOKINE–STEROID INTERPLAY

A. Ovulation

Ovulation in women normally occurs halfway through each menstrual cycle, in response to stimulation of the preovulatory follicle(s) by gonadotropins. The midcycle luteinizing hormone (LH) surge initiates a cascade of biochemical changes in follicular cells and macrophages, leading to dissolution of the follicle wall and shedding of the oocyte. These changes include increased pro-inflammatory cytokine production, progesterone production, activation of COX-2, increased PGE_2 synthesis, histamine release, and increased proteolysis mediated by MMPs. Inhibition of progesterone biosynthesis or pharmacological blockade of the PR prevents ovulation. Mice with null PR mutations are unable to ovulate, demonstrating an absolute need for local progesterone. COX-2 inhibitors also prevent ovulation, and COX-2 and gene knockouts in mice confirm an absolute dependence on COX-2 activation during ovulation. Following follicular rupture, each bout of ovulation-associated damage to the ovary must be rapidly repaired. Inflammation—essential for wound healing—is contained and rapidly resolved. Locally produced progesterone and locally activated cortisol are believed to participate in this compensatory anti-inflammatory process.

Within the preovulatory follicle, a switch in the expression of 11β-HSD isoforms occurs during granulosa cell luteinization. Before induction of ovulation, nonluteinized human granulosa cells express mainly 11β-HSD2 mRNA and little or no 11β-HSD1 mRNA. After exposure to LH or human chorionic gonadotropin, 11β-HSD2 mRNA expression is suppressed and 11β-HSD1 mRNA expression is enhanced. This shift in potential for glucocorticoid metabolism from inactivation to re-activation is reflected in the ability of luteinizing human granulosa cells to undertake predominantly reductive (cortisone → cortisol) metabolism *in vitro* and substantially raised the concentrations of cortisol in follicular fluid. In experiments on cultured rat granulosa cells, treatment with IL-1β mimics the action of LH *in vitro*, up-regulating 11β-HSD1 and down-regulating 11β-HSD2. Treatment of cultured human ovarian epithelial cells with IL-1 also increases the gene expression of 11β-HSD1 and metabolism of cortisone to cortisol *in vitro*. Thus, cytokine-regulated 11β-HSD expression in the follicle wall and on the ovarian surface may determine the local availability of anti-inflammatory cortisol (Fig. 3).

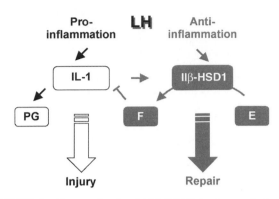

FIGURE 3 Proposed role of 11β-HSD1 in the resolution of LH-induced inflammation at the ovarian surface during ovulation. Ovulation is viewed as a natural injury-repair process. The ovulation-inducing LH surge induces an acute inflammatory response by increasing the local production of inflammatory cytokines (IL-1) and prostaglandins (PG), leading to proteolytic breakdown of the follicle wall and apoptosis of overlying ovarian surface epithelial cells. LH-induced IL-1 simultaneously up-regulates the expression of 11β-HSD1 in granulosa cells and OSE cells, serving to increase the metabolism of "inactive" cortisone (E) into anti-inflammatory cortisol (F). The increased local availability of cortisol is hypothesized to play a role in the resolution of this acute inflammatory event. Reprinted from Yong, P. Y. K., Harlow, C. R., Thong, K. J., Hillier, S. G. (2002). Regulation of 11β-hydroxysteroid dehydrogenase type 1 gene expression in human ovarian surface epithelial cells by interleukin-1. *Human Reproduction* **17** (9), 2300–2306. By permission of Oxford University Press.

B. Menstruation

In the absence of pregnancy, progesterone withdrawal due to regression of the corpus luteum causes menstruation, which is associated with up-regulation of inflammatory mediators in the uterus (IL-8, monocyte chemoattractant peptide-1, and COX-2). Hypoxia due to arteriole vasoconstriction is coincident with progesterone withdrawal and in other body systems is a stimulus for IL-8 expression. IL-8 is not only a powerful leukocyte chemotaxin and secretagogue; it has also been shown to have important roles in neovascularization and mitogenesis and thus may be centrally involved in the local inflammatory and vascular events of menstruation.

The uterus expresses PR and the key components of the glucocorticoid response system, and there is evidence from experiments on rats that both activation of glucocorticoid through 11β-HSD enzyme activity and levels of GR are likely to have roles in modulating glucocorticoid action in the uterus. Although 11β-HSDs and GR are expressed in human endometrium, there are no data on regulation or expression in relation to hormonal status. High concentrations of glucocorticoids inhibit immunologic and inflammatory responses and also inhibit estrogen-stimulated epithelial proliferation. Glucocorticoids can down-regulate uterine estrogen receptors. In the rat, estradiol up-regulates both types of 11β-HSD. Furthermore, 11β-HSD2 mRNA has been localized to the stroma and stratum vasculare of the rat uterus. The physiological significance of the interaction between the GR and the 11β-HSD system in menstruation is as yet unexplored. It remains to be determined whether an altered availability of cortisol to bind to the GR (due to differential expression of 11β-HSD isoforms) is compensated for by activation of the PR by progesterone and vice versa.

C. Implantation

Invasion of the uterine wall by trophoblastic tissue induces a natural inflammatory reaction, which must be contained to allow pregnancy to proceed. Maternal factors secreted into the lumen of the female reproductive tract as well as substances synthesized by the developing embryo itself help to regulate this process. Similar to ovulation, implantation involves increased local production of pro-inflammatory cytokines, dependence on progesterone, up-regulation of COX-2, and increased activity of MMPs that digest collagen as the uterus is penetrated.

During placentation, growth factors and cytokines produced by the placenta and decidual tissues accelerate the production of MMPs by trophoblasts. The release of IL-1β parallels the invasive potential of cytotrophoblasts, being produced in greater amounts by first-trimester cells than term cells. Inflammation-associated IL-1β production and MMP expression are decreased by glucocorticoid treatment *in vitro*. Thus normal trophoblast invasion may be regulated, in part, by the opposing actions of IL-1β and corticosteroids, since both are present in high concentrations at the maternal–fetal interface.

Human placental tissue is a rich source of 11β-HSD activity and a chronic suppressive action of glucocorticoid on cytokine production and nuclear binding of NF-κB and AP-1 proteins in human term placental cytotrophoblasts has been reported. This suggests a potential mechanism through which glucocorticoids may suppress inflammation at maternal–fetal interfaces across gestation.

D. Parturition

Pro-inflammatory cytokines, prostaglandins, anti-inflammatory steroids, and matrix-degrading proteases directly participate in parturition. The pregnant uterus undergoes drastic remodeling during labor and the peripartum period, when the cervix becomes softened, effaced, and dilated to allow expulsion of the neonate. These changes to the cervix can be induced by mechanical trauma (as in "sweeping the membranes") or administration of prostaglandins, anti-progestins, or cytokines, such as IL-1 or IL-8. As in ovulation, menstruation, and implantation, MMPs, up-regulated by pro-inflammatory cytokines and prostaglandins, are instrumental to uterine and cervical tissue remodeling during parturition.

Anti-inflammatory steroids in turn participate in the cytokine- and prostaglandin-mediated mechanisms through which invading cells soften the cervix and initiate the natural onset of birth. Mifepristone, an anti-progestin that ripens the cervix when given during labor, is also a potent anti-glucocorticoid. Combined blockade of PR and GR by this substance presumably impedes ligand-activated anti-inflammatory signaling, thereby promoting the inflammation-associated process of cervical ripening.

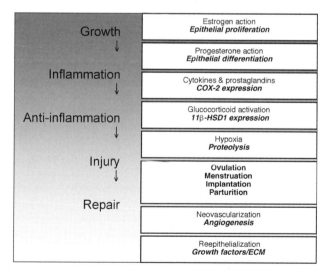

FIGURE 4   Pro- and anti-inflammatory mechanisms common to ovulation, menstruation, implantation, and parturition. All four processes involve locally increased formation of inflammatory cytokines and prostaglandins. Systemic progesterone and glucocorticoids re-activated via local changes in 11β-HSD activity are believed to provide a compensatory anti-inflammatory response. Proteolytic tissue injury is thereby localized, minimized, and promptly healed.

The role of 11β-HSDs in regulating the availability of cortisol to participate in this process remains undetermined but 11β-HSD1 is richly expressed in amniotic membranes, where prostaglandins have been shown to increase the net conversion of cortisone to cortisol *in vitro*.

V. SUMMARY

Locally produced pro-inflammatory cytokines promote inflammation-associated tissue injury and repair during ovulation, menstruation, implantation, and parturition. Each of these critical steps in reproduction depends absolutely on progesterone, which has anti-inflammatory properties. Furthermore, they all occur in regions of the reproductive tract where locally produced pro-inflammatory cytokines and prostaglandins have the potential to alter 11β-HSD enzyme expression, thereby influencing the local availability of cortisol (Fig. 4). Progesterone and cortisol activate anti-inflammatory signaling pathways through binding and activating the PR and GR, respectively. Both types of steroid may serve anti-inflammatory functions in the female reproductive tract, interacting with pro-inflammatory cytokines to localize and contain the natural inflammatory processes on which reproduction depends.

Glossary

corticosteroids Steroid hormones secreted by the adrenal cortex that play crucial roles in nutrition, stress, and tissue responses to injury. In humans, cortisone and its synthetic analogues, such as prednisone and dexamethasone, are used therapeutically to control rheumatism and other inflammatory ailments.

cytokines Polypeptide messenger molecules that mediate cell-to-cell communication through binding to specific receptors on target cells and triggering postreceptor signaling pathways that alter cellular behavior. Cytokines are involved in reproduction, growth and development, injury repair, and the immunoendocrine system. Usually classified as interleukins, interferons, colony-stimulating factors, tumor necrosis factors, or growth factors, their classification is evolving. Interleukins are cytokines produced by leukocytes as part of the immune and inflammatory responses.

inflammation In higher organisms, a defense mechanism that protects the organism from infection and injury by localizing and limiting tissue damage, so that healing can begin. An inflammatory response lasting only a few days is called acute inflammation, whereas a response of longer duration is referred to as chronic inflammation.

prostaglandins Cyclic, unsaturated fatty acids derived from arachidonic acid, a phospholipid that is an integral component of the cell membrane. Inflammatory stimuli induce the rapid release of arachidonic acid, which is converted to prostaglandins, prostacyclin, and thromboxanes by cyclooxygenase (COX) enzyme activity. The inducible form of COX, COX-2, is mainly responsible for the local formation of the prostaglandins necessary for inflammation. Leukotrienes, produced from arachidonic acid due to lipoxygenase enzyme activity, are also important mediators of the inflammatory process, whereas thromboxanes and prostacyclin play roles in blood coagulation.

See Also the Following Articles

Anti-Inflammatory Actions of Glucocorticoids
● Implantation ● Interleukin-1 (IL-1) ● Interleukin-18
● Ovulation ● Tumor Necrosis Factor (TNF)

Further Reading

Adashi, E. Y. (1998). The potential role of interleukin-1 in the ovulatory process: An evolving hypothesis. *Mol. Cell. Endocrinol.* **140**, 77–81.

Andersen, C. Y. (2002). New possible mechanism of cortisol action in female reproductive organs: Physiological implications of the free hormone hypothesis. *J. Endocrinol.* **173**, 211–217.

Arcuri, F., Battistini, S., Hausknecht, V., Cintorino, M., Lockwood, C. J., and Schatz, F. (1997). Human endometrial decidual cell-associated 11β-hydroxysteroid dehydrogenase expression: Its potential role in implantation. *Early Pregnancy* **3**, 259–264.

Bischof, P., Meisser, A., and Campana, A. (2001). Biochemistry and molecular biology of trophoblast invasion. *Ann. N.Y. Acad. Sci.* **943**, 157–162.

Challis, J. R., Lye, S. J., Gibb, W., Whittle, W., Patel, F., and Alfaidy, N. (2001). Understanding preterm labor. *Ann. N.Y. Acad. Sci.* **943**, 225–234.

Espey, L. L. (1994). Current status of the hypothesis that mammalian ovulation is comparable to an inflammatory reaction. *Biol. Reprod.* **50**, 233–238.

Karin, M., and Chang, L. (2001). AP-1—glucocorticoid receptor crosstalk taken to a higher level. *J. Endocrinol.* **169**, 447–451.

Kelly, R. W., King, A. E., and Critchley, H. O. (2001). Cytokine control in human endometrium. *Reproduction* **121**, 3–19.

McKay, L. I., and Cidlowski, J. A. (1999). Molecular control of immune/inflammatory responses: Interactions between nuclear factor-κB and steroid receptor-signaling pathways. *Endocr. Rev.* **20**, 435–4359.

O'Neill, L. A. (2000). The interleukin-1 receptor/Toll-like receptor superfamily: Signal transduction during inflammation and host defense. *Science* **44**, RE1.

Sims, J. E., Nicklin, M. J., Bazan, J. F., Barton, J. L., Busfield, S. J., Ford, J. E., Kastelein, R. A., Kumar, S., Lin, H., Mulero, J. J., Pan, J., Pan, Y., Smith, D. E., and Young, P. R. (2001). A new nomenclature for IL-1-family genes. *Trends Immunol.* **22**, 536–537.

Smith, W. L., and Langenbach, R. (2001). Why there are two cyclooxygenase isozymes. *J. Clin. Invest.* **107**, 1491–1495.

Tetsuka, M., Haines, L. C., Milne, M., Simpson, G. E., and Hillier, S. G. (1999). Regulation of 11β-hydroxysteroid dehydrogenase type 1 gene expression by LH and interleukin-1β in cultured rat granulosa cells. *J. Endocrinol.* **163**, 417–423.

Vadillo-Ortega, F., Sadowsky, D. W., Haluska, G. J., Hernandez-Guerrero, C., Guevara-Silva, R., Gravett, M. G., and Novy, M. J. (2002). Identification of matrix metalloproteinase-9 in amniotic fluid and amniochorion in spontaneous labor and after experimental intrauterine infection or interleukin-1β infusion in pregnant rhesus monkeys. *Am. J. Obstet. Gynecol.* **186**, 128–138.

van der Burg, B., and van der Saag, P. T. (1997). Nuclear factor-β-B/steroid hormone receptor interactions as a functional basis of anti-inflammatory action of steroids in reproductive organs. *Mol. Hum. Reprod.* **2**, 433–438.

Prolactin (PRL)

NIRA BEN-JONATHAN

University of Cincinnati

I. THE PROLACTIN GENE AND PROTEIN
II. PITUITARY AND EXTRAPITUITARY PRL
III. REGULATION OF PRL SYNTHESIS AND RELEASE
IV. PRL RECEPTORS AND SIGNAL TRANSDUCTION
V. BIOLOGICAL FUNCTIONS

Prolactin (PRL) is a 23 kDa protein hormone that is produced and secreted by pituitary lactotrophs. Pituitary PRL synthesis and release are subjected to tonic inhibition by hypothalamic dopamine and are stimulated by many neuropeptides, steroid hormones, and growth factors. PRL binds to a single-span membrane receptor and exerts its action via several interacting signaling pathways. PRL is a multifunctional hormone that affects reproductive, developmental, osmoregulatory, and behavioral functions. In addition to the pituitary, PRL is produced by many tissues throughout the body and is concentrated from the blood into several cell types and fluid compartments. The heterogeneous nature of the PRL-producing cells together with the expression of PRL receptors by almost every tissue in the body supports the role of PRL as both a hormone and a cytokine and underlies its pleiotropic functions.

I. THE PROLACTIN GENE AND PROTEIN

The prolactin (PRL) gene is present as a single copy on human chromosome 6. PRL shares 40% homology with growth hormone (GH) and placental lactogen (PL), and the three hormones were derived by gene duplication from a common ancestral gene some 400 million years ago. Several proteins with similar structural features, generally named PRL-related or PRL-like proteins, are now included as members of the PRL/GH/PL gene family. The rat PRL gene is 10 kb in size and is composed of five exons. The mature mRNA is approximately 1 kb in length and encodes a 227-residue protein that includes a 28-residue signal peptide that is cleaved on entering the endoplasmic reticulum. A 2 to 2.5 kb sequence at the 5′-flanking region of the rat PRL gene (the proximal promoter) controls tissue-specific and hormone-regulated gene expression (Fig. 1). It is made of two distinct domains, a proximal region and a more distal enhancer, both of which are required for pituitary-specific expression. Eight *cis*-acting elements throughout the proximal promoter bind Pit-1, a homeobox transcription factor. Although Pit-1 is expressed only in the pituitary gland, it is not restricted to lactotrophs and requires interactions with other factors to confer the lactotroph phenotype.

The human PRL gene differs from the rat gene in several respects. It is composed of six, rather than five, exons and is more than 15 kb long. The extra noncoding exon, exon 1a, has a transcriptional start site 5.8 kb upstream of the pituitary start site (Fig. 1). In extrapituitary sites such as decidua, myometrium, and lymphoid cells, exon 1a is spliced to exon 1b, generating an mRNA transcript that is approximately 150 bp larger than the pituitary counterpart in the 5′-untranslated region. A superdistal promoter upstream of exon 1a regulates PRL gene expression in extrapituitary sites and is silenced in the pituitary gland. This region does not contain Pit-1-binding sites and its regulation differs from that of the proximal promoter.

The 23 kDa PRL protein is composed of a single chain of 199 residues. It has three intramolecular disulfide bridges between residues 4 and 11, 58 and 174, and 191 and 199, N- or O-linked glycosylation sites, and three phosphorylation sites. A three-dimensional model of PRL predicts that it is arranged in four anti-parallel α-helices organized in an "up-up-down-down" fashion. This bundle motif is shared with hematopoietic factors such as interferon and many interleukins. The 60 to 100% sequence homology between PRL molecules from different species reflects their phylogenetic relationship. Approximately 30 residues, clustered in four distinct regions, are highly conserved and may be important for binding to the receptor.

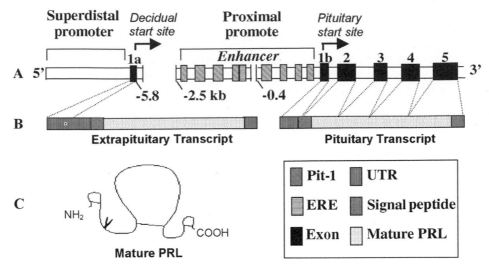

FIGURE 1 Diagram of the human PRL gene (A), extrapituitary and pituitary transcripts (B), and the mature protein (C). Note the use of exon 1a as the transcription start site for extrapituitary PRL and the longer 5'-untranslated region (UTR). The site of N-glycosylation (Y, Asn[31]) is also shown. ERE, estrogen-response element.

Variants of PRL are formed by transcriptional or translational mechanisms and increase the biological specificity as well as the diversity of PRL. Most variants are generated by posttranslational modifications and differ in size or functional groups. Larger variants are formed by dimerization or aggregation and smaller variants are formed by proteolysis, both at the sites of synthesis and at some target tissues. Some variants retain PRL-like activities and others have unique properties or no known functions. Two variants, a 22 kDa isoform and a 16 kDa isoform, are of interest. The 22 kDa form, PRL$_{1-173}$, may be important in female reproduction and is generated by kallikrein, a trypsin-like serine protease. The 16 kDa PRL possesses anti-angiogenic activity and is generated by cathepsin D, an acid protease. The angiostatic activity of 16 kDa PRL may occur via a unique receptor since it has low binding affinity to the classical PRL receptor.

Human PRL is N-glycosylated on Asp[31], adding 2–3 kDa to its molecular mass. Glycosylated PRL is detected in the pituitary and in several body fluids, ranging from 15 to 20% of total PRL in both the pituitary and the plasma to over 50% in the amniotic fluid and milk. The carbohydrate moieties vary among species and tissues and their heterogeneity accounts for differences in bioactivity, immunoreactivity, receptor binding, and metabolic clearance rate of PRL. Although glycosylation often decreases the bioactivity of PRL, unique physiological functions of glycosylated PRL have not been yet identified. PRL

can also be mono- or diphosphorylated on serine and/or threonine residues, a modification that results in charge variability. The ratio of phosphorylated/ nonphosphorylated forms is altered during various physiological states and could be involved in determining the balance between the mitogenic and the anti-mitogenic effects of PRL.

II. PITUITARY AND EXTRAPITUITARY PRL

PRL is the secretory product of the lactotrophs, acidophilic-staining cells of the pituitary. Lactotrophs are the last anterior pituitary cells to differentiate during fetal development and are preceded by GH- and dual GH/PRL-producing cells, the somatolactotrophs. Pit-1 is required for the development of somatotrophs, lactotrophs, and thyrotrophs and its inactivation results in the virtual absence of these cell types. The factors that induce terminal differentiation of lactotrophs are unknown, but several growth factors, including nerve growth factor, epidermal growth factor (EGF), and basic fibroblast growth factor, have been implicated in this process.

Lactotrophs constitute 20–30% of total anterior pituitary cells and are heterogeneous in terms of morphology, basal hormone release, electrical activity, and responsiveness to secretagogues. The dual-secreting cells can be interconverted to somatotrophs or lactotrophs, depending on the nature of the stimulus. This process facilitates the rapid recruitment of PRL-producing cells while bypassing metabolically costly cell division. Unlike most pituitary cells, lactotrophs retain a robust proliferative capacity during adulthood and their number increases during pregnancy and lactation. This proliferative potential also accounts for the higher incidence of lactotroph tumors (prolactinomas) compared to other types of pituitary tumors. Some rat strains are especially sensitive to induction of prolactinomas by estrogens, but a similar role for estrogens in the etiology of human prolactinomas has not been demonstrated.

Although PRL was initially regarded as an exclusive pituitary hormone, many nonpituitary tissues were later found to contain immunoreactive PRL. The widespread distribution of tissues capable of PRL synthesis as well as those that contain PRL is illustrated in Fig. 2. The most established extrapituitary sites that produce PRL are the decidua, immune system, brain, and myometrium, with emerging evidence for PRL synthesis by the skin and

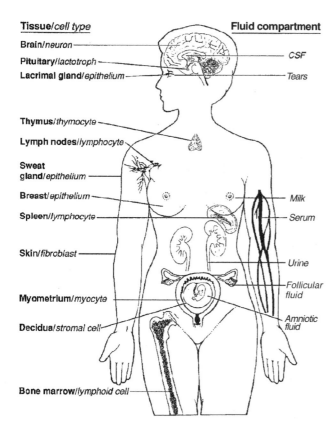

FIGURE 2 Distribution of PRL throughout the human body. Tissues and cells that produce PRL are shown on the left and fluid compartments that contain PRL are shown on the right. Note the heterogeneity of PRL-producing cells (italics) in terms of embryonic origin, morphology, and function.

exocrine glands, including mammary glands, sweat glands, and lacrimal glands. PRL is produced by a wide variety of cells of different embryonic origins, morphology, and physiological functions. Some, e.g., lymphocytes and epithelia, are less differentiated and have a high proliferative capacity, whereas others, e.g., neurons, are postmitotic and terminally differentiated. Immunoreactive PRL is also present in tissues that do not produce PRL but are capable of taking up and concentrating PRL from the blood.

Another remarkable feature of PRL is its presence in most body fluid compartments. Although all hormones are present in serum and most are excreted into urine, PRL is also found in cerebrospinal fluid (CSF) and the amniotic fluid and is secreted into milk, tears, and follicular fluid. Whereas PRL in the amniotic fluid originates from a local source (decidua), that in milk and CSF is derived from both locally produced and circulating PRL. Significant cellular resources must be spent in transporting PRL into these compartments and yet little is currently known about the functions subserved by PRL in these sites.

III. REGULATION OF PRL SYNTHESIS AND RELEASE

Consistent with its function as an adaptive rather than an indispensable hormone, the profile of PRL release varies greatly under many physiological conditions and is dissimilar among species. In humans, serum PRL progressively rises throughout gestation in both the maternal and the fetal circulation and is episodically released in response to suckling during lactation. Adult women have higher serum PRL levels than men but do not exhibit marked changes in the secretory profile of PRL throughout the menstrual cycle. This is in contrast to rodents, in which a clear preovulatory surge of PRL is evident. Stress conditions, including anesthesia, surgery, electric shock, strenuous exercise, and insulin-induced hypoglycemia, also stimulate PRL release in both men and women. PRL is also secreted in an episodic fashion throughout the day with some evidence for sleep-related increases in its circulating levels.

The synthesis and release of PRL by the pituitary lactotrophs are subjected to multiple regulators that can be classified into four broad categories: endocrine, paracrine, juxtacrine, and autocrine (Fig. 3). Endocrine agents originate from the hypothalamus and gonads and reach the lactotrophs via a humoral

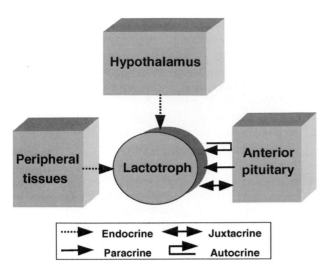

FIGURE 3 Diagram of the four types of regulation of pituitary lactotrophs.

route. Paracrine factors are produced by other pituitary cell types and reach the lactotrophs by diffusion. Juxtacrine interactions emanate from the extracellular matrix and cells adjacent to the lactotrophs. Autocrine agents are synthesized by the lactotrophs themselves. Consequently, the overall secretory activity of the lactotrophs reflects a balance between local and distant releasing and inhibiting factors. In nonhuman species, there is also evidence for PRL-regulating factors that originate from the posterior pituitary.

The pituitary lactotroph is unique in its capacity for constitutive synthesis and secretion of PRL. Unlike pituitary tropic hormones such as luteinizing hormone or adrenocorticotropin hormone, whereby the hypothalamus provides a positive stimulus and peripheral target glands supply negative feedback inhibition, PRL does not have a singular target organ. Hence, its main regulation is provided in the form of tonic inhibition by dopamine, the physiological PRL release-inhibiting factor. Acting via a type 2 dopamine receptor, dopamine exerts multiple actions on the lactotrophs, including suppression of intracellular calcium and cyclic AMP levels, inhibition of PRL gene expression and release, and suppression of cell proliferation. Interruption of dopaminergic input to the lactotrophs caused by physiological inhibition of dopamine release, damage to the pituitary stalk, or dopamine receptor antagonists results in hyperprolactinemia. PRL itself, acting via a short-loop negative feedback mechanism, is the primary regulator of the dopaminergic system. Despite intensive searching, a singular

releasing factor for PRL has not been identified, but several neuropeptides, including thyrotropin-releasing hormone (TRH) and vasoactive intestinal peptide (VIP), are capable of stimulating PRL release under some physiological conditions. In contrast to the pituitary, little is known about the regulation of PRL production/release in extrapituitary sites except that they do not respond to dopamine, neuropeptides, or estrogens but appear to be regulated by local autocrine/paracrine factors.

Pituitary PRL gene expression is affected by many hormones, neurotransmitters, and growth factors. Compounds that bind to G-protein-linked receptors, e.g., TRH, VIP, and dopamine, activate protein kinase A, protein kinase C, and/or calcium/calmodulin-dependent pathways. These are mediated via a variety of transcription factors that bind to consensus sequences within the PRL promoter. Estrogens, on the other hand, freely diffuse into the nucleus, where they bind to either estrogen receptor-α or -β. The activated receptor dimerizes and acts as a transcription factor and binds to a unique DNA sequence called the estrogen-response element that is located in the enhancer region next to a Pit-1-binding site (see Fig. 1). Among the growth factors, insulin and EGF stimulate the PRL gene, whereas transforming growth factor-β suppresses the PRL gene. Many of the growth factors bind to transmembrane receptors with intrinsic tyrosine kinase activity and exert pleiotropic actions such as stimulation of PRL gene transcription, increases in hormone storage, and alterations of lactotroph morphology. Again, details about the control of PRL gene expression in extrapituitary sites are largely unknown.

IV. PRL RECEPTORS AND SIGNAL TRANSDUCTION

PRL exerts its actions by binding to specific, high-affinity plasma membrane receptors. The gene encoding the human PRL receptor is located on chromosome 5 and contains at least 10 exons encompassing over 100 kb. The PRL receptor belongs to the cytokine/GH/PRL receptor superfamily that is characterized by a single-pass transmembrane stretch that divides the receptor into an extracellular ligand-binding domain and an intracellular domain. The extracellular domain contains two disulfide bonds and a WS motif (Trp-Ser-X-Trp-Ser) that is required for correct folding of the receptor and may participate in the formation of a ligand-binding pocket. The cytoplasmic domain has a proline-rich motif (Box 1) near the plasma membrane that couples to intracellular signaling molecules. Another motif (Box 2′) is less conserved.

Humans express primarily one "long" form of the receptor, whereas rats have three: long, intermediate, and short. An intermediate isoform that is uniquely expressed by the rat Nb2 lymphocyte cell line renders these cells dependent on PRL for growth and survival. Given this property, proliferation of Nb2 cells in response to PRL is widely used as a sensitive bioassay for PRL. An intermediate receptor isoform with a deleted segment within the intracellular domain, differentially spliced short receptors, and a soluble receptor form that contains only the extracellular domain have been detected in human tissues, but their exact functions remain to be determined. The PRL receptor is expressed by most tissues, with the highest level of expression in the liver and mammary gland. The PRL receptor concentrations fluctuate under many physiological conditions, especially in response to changes in circulating PRL and steroid hormones. Both PRL and its receptor are also internalized within several cell types but neither the exact intracellular localization nor the function of the internalized receptor or PRL is well understood.

Binding of PRL to its receptor induces sequential receptor dimerization. Two binding sites on the PRL molecule, site 1, comprising helices 1 and 4, and site 2, comprising helices 1 and 3, are required for the induction of receptor homodimerization and formation of an active trimeric complex. The receptor is devoid of intrinsic tyrosine kinase activity, utilizing instead the Janus kinase (JAK)2–signal transducers and activators of transcription (STAT) pathway as its main signaling cascade (Fig. 4). JAK2 (Janus kinase 2), which is constitutively associated with Box 1 on the PRL receptor, is rapidly phosphorylated on receptor dimerization. In turn, the activated JAK2 induces phosphorylation of the receptor, other associated kinases, and Stat proteins. Of the seven known Stat proteins, Stat1, Stat3, and Stat5 are activated by PRL. As revealed by studies with knockout mice, Stat5a and Stat 5b are especially important for mammary gland development and function. The activated (phosphorylated) Stat proteins dimerize and are rapidly translocated into the nucleus, where they bind to specific sequences on target genes. The Ras/Raf/mitogen-activated protein kinase cascade and fyn, a member of the Src kinase family that phosphorylates phosphatidyl inositol 3-kinase, are also activated by PRL in a cell-specific manner but appear to be of lesser importance in

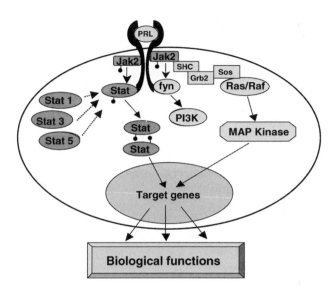

FIGURE 4 Schematic presentation of the PRL receptor and the intracellular signaling pathways that mediate PRL actions.

mediating PRL action than the JAK2–STAT pathway. Notably, all the above-mentioned pathways have been characterized under acute conditions, whereas the mechanism mediating the long-term effects of PRL are not well understood. In addition, human GH and placental lactogens bind to the PRL receptor with high affinity and mimic some of the actions of PRL.

V. BIOLOGICAL FUNCTIONS

PRL is one of the most versatile hormones, with more than 100 functions ascribed to it, far exceeding the number of all known actions of other pituitary hormones combined. These functions are broadly associated with reproduction, growth and development, osmoregulation, metabolism, immunoregulation, brain function, and behavior. Several caveats should be considered, however, when evaluating these functions. First, although both males and females produce PRL and express the PRL receptor, PRL functions have been most extensively studied in females. Second, some PRL effects in lower vertebrates may have been lost during evolution and are recapitulated in higher animals only during certain developmental stages. Third, PRL often exerts species-specific actions among mammals (e.g., luteotropic activity in rodents only), complicating the interpretation of studies with transgenic animals. Fourth, fetal exposure to very high PRL levels via the blood and the amniotic fluid is unique to humans and cannot be carefully examined due to lack of suitable animal models. Fifth, the uneven activity of various PRL isoforms in some functional assays leads to incomplete assessment of the spectrum of actions of PRL. Finally, the ability of related hormones, i.e., GH and placental lactogens, to bind to the PRL receptor and mimic some of the actions of PRL can lead to erroneous interpretations of experimental manipulations.

The effects of PRL on reproduction encompass multiple systems and tissues that differ in their importance in a species-specific manner. The principal target for PRL is the mammary gland. Together with several other hormones, PRL promotes growth and differentiation of the mammary epithelium and is essential for the initiation and maintenance of lactation by increasing the synthesis of all major milk components: the milk proteins α-lactalbumin and casein, lactose, and lipids. In some species, however, continuous lactogenesis is supported by GH rather than by PRL. In rodents, PRL has both luteotropic and luteolytic actions on the ovary and supports progesterone production. Therefore, in these species PRL plays a major role in modulating the reproductive cycle and is crucial for pregnancy and lactation. PRL has well-established mitogenic, secretory, and morphogenic effects on the prostate, but its actions on the testes are not well defined. Under normal conditions, PRL has permissive effects on human reproduction. However, overproduction of PRL (hyperprolactinemia) is one of the major causes of neuroendocrine-related anovulation and infertility in women and impotence in men. The inhibitory effects of excess PRL on these reproductive processes occur at both central (hypothalamic–pituitary) and peripheral (gonadal) sites. Recent evidence indicates that PRL may also play a role as a mitogen/anti-apoptotic factor in breast and prostatic cancer.

PRL plays a major role in regulating water and electrolyte balance in fish and amphibians, with lesser osmoregulatory actions in birds and mammals. Whereas the control of development and body growth is normally ascribed to GH, there are some functional overlaps between GH and PRL, especially in lower vertebrates. Both the metabolic and the immunoregulatory actions of PRL have been matters of controversy. PRL stimulates the proliferation of the pancreatic islets and increases insulin secretion primarily during pregnancy. In the immune system, PRL induces the proliferation and differentiation of functional activity of various lymphoid cells, but transgenic animals lacking PRL or its receptor have little if any immune disturbances. Within the brain, PRL affects the production and release of several hypothalamic releasing/inhibiting hormones, e.g., dopamine and gonadotropin-releasing hormone, and has significant effects on maternal behavior.

Glossary

extrapituitary prolactin sites Several nonpituitary tissues, e.g., decidua, myometrium, brain, and breast, that are capable of *de novo* synthesis of prolactin (PRL). The regulation of PRL synthesis and release from extrapituitary sites differs markedly from that in the pituitary.

Janus kinase (JAK)/signal transducers and activators of transcription (STAT) pathway Intracellular signaling cascade that mediates the action of many cytokines and some growth factors. JAK2 and STAT5 constitute the main pathway that is rapidly activated by prolactin.

lactotrophs A class of anterior pituitary cells that produce prolactin. They constitute over one-third of all pituitary hormone-secreting cells. Lactotrophs are heterogeneous in structure and function and are normally subjected to inhibition by dopamine.

posttranslational modifications Changes in the structure of a protein hormone that include glycosylation, phosphorylation, and cleavage. These modifications affect hormone binding to the receptor or clearance from the circulation and thus alter its biological properties.

prolactin promoter A DNA sequence that is used to regulate the transcription of the prolactin gene. The pituitary proximal promoter is located immediately 5' upstream of the transcription initiation site, whereas the extrapituitary superdistal promoter is located 5.8 kb further upstream.

prolactinomas Nonmalignant tumors of the anterior pituitary that are composed of lactotrophs and result in hyperprolactinemia or abnormally high serum prolactin levels. They usually develop from a single cell (monoclonal) but their etiology is unclear.

See Also the Following Articles

Cytokines and Anterior Pituitary Function ● Endocrine Rhythms: Generation, Regulation, and Integration ● Growth Hormone (GH) ● Neuropeptides and Control of the Anterior Pituitary ● Prolactin and Growth Hormone Receptors

Further Reading

Asa, S. L., and Ezzat, S. (1998). The cytogenesis and pathogenesis of pituitary adenomas. *Endocr. Rev.* **19**, 798–827.

Ben-Jonathan, N., and Hnasko, R. M. (2001). Dopamine as a prolactin inhibitor. *Endocr. Rev.* **22**, 724–763.

Ben-Jonathan, N., Mershon, J. L., Allen, D. L., and Steinmetz, R. W. (1996). Extrapituitary prolactin: Distribution, regulation, functions and clinical aspects. *Endocr. Rev.* **17**, 639–669.

Blackwell, R. E. (1992). Hyperprolactinemia: Evaluation and management. *Reprod. Endocrinol.* **21**, 105–124.

Bole-Feysot, C., Goffin, V., Edery, M., Binart, N., and Kelly, P. A. (1998). Prolactin (PRL) and its receptor: Actions, signal transduction pathways and phenotypes observed in PRL receptor knockout mice. *Endocr. Rev.* **19**, 225–268.

Buntin, J. D. (1993). Prolactin–brain interactions and reproductive function. *Am. Zool.* **33**, 229–243.

Dutt, A., Kaplitt, M. G., Kow, L. M., and Pfaff, D. W. (1994). Prolactin, central nervous system and behavior: A critical review. *Neuroendocrinology* **59**, 413–419.

Freeman, M. E., Kanyicska, B., Lerant, A., and Nagy, G. (2000). Prolactin: Structure, function, and regulation of secretion. *Physiol. Rev.* **80**, 1523–1631.

Gourdji, D., and Laverriere, J. N. (1994). The rat prolactin gene: A target for tissue-specific and hormone-dependent transcription factors. *Mol. Cell. Endocrinol.* **100**, 133–142.

Grimley, P. M., Dong, F., and Rui, H. (1999). Stat5a and Stat5b: Fraternal twins of signal transduction and transcriptional activation. *Cytokine Growth Factor Rev.* **10**, 131–157.

Horseman, N. D. (2001). "Prolactin," pp. 1–404. Kluwer, Boston, MA.

Horseman, N. D., and Yu-Lee, L. Y. (1994). Transcriptional regulation by the helix bundle peptide hormones: Growth hormone, prolactin, and hematopoietic cytokines. *Endocr. Rev.* **15**, 627–649.

Hu, Z.-Z., Zhuang, L., and Dufau, M. L. (1998). Prolactin receptor gene diversity: Structure and regulation. *Trends Endocrinol. Metab.* **9**, 94–102.

Pan, J.-T. (1996). Neuroendocrine functions of dopamine. *In* "CNS Neurotransmitters and Neuromodulators: Dopamine" (T. W. Stone, ed.), pp. 213–231. CRC Press, Boca Raton, FL.

Sinha, Y. N. (1995). Structural variants of prolactin: Occurrence and physiological significance. *Endocr. Rev.* **16**, 354–369.

Vonderhaar, B. K. (1999). Prolactin involvement in breast cancer. *Endocr. Relat. Cancer* **6**, 389–404.

Prolactin and Growth Hormone Receptors

Vincent Goffin and Paul A. Kelly

Faculty of Medicine Necker, Paris

I. INTRODUCTION

II. PRLR AND GHR ISOFORMS HAVE DIFFERENT SIGNALING CAPABILITIES

III. LIGAND-INDUCED RECEPTOR DIMERIZATION: THE FIRST STEP OF SIGNALING

IV. MAJOR SIGNALING PATHWAYS

V. HOW ANIMAL MODELS CAN HIGHLIGHT *IN VITRO* SIGNALING STUDIES

VI. CONCLUSIONS

The prolactin receptor (PRLR) and growth hormone receptor (GHR) are among the class I hematopoietic cytokine receptors. PRLR is expressed is almost all tissues and cell types, although the mammary gland and gonads are the major targets for prolactin (PRL). In primates, both PRL and growth hormone (GH) can activate the PRLR. The GHR bears a strong resemblance to the PRLR but is involved only with the actions of GH, which promotes the growth of several tissue types and has a variety of metabolic functions. Although the Janus kinase/signal transducers and activators of transcription pathway plays a central role in PRLR/GHR signaling, a number of other signaling pathways are also activated by PRLR and GHR < likely relating to the wide spectrum of biological functions carried out by these hormones.

I. INTRODUCTION

It was not until the early 1970s that prolactin (PRL) and growth hormone (GH) were revealed to be two distinct hormones in humans (h). The reason is that in primates, but not in lower species, both PRL and GH are able to activate the PRL receptor (PRLR). The actions mediated by the PRLR (also referred to as the lactogen receptor) are historically linked, but certainly not restricted to milk production and control of reproductive functions; mammary gland and gonads are thus major PRL targets, although the nearly ubiquitous expression of the PRLR renders almost all tissue and cell types potential targets of lactogenic hormones. The GH receptor (GHR) closely resembles the PRLR, but mediates only GH actions (PRL does not bind to the GHR in any species). As suggested by its name, GH exerts growth-promoting activity on several tissues (e.g., soft tissues and long bones) and shows a wide range of metabolic functions.

These two receptors were cloned at almost the same time (in the late 1980s) and are among the five membrane receptors whose sequence analysis led to the identification of a new receptor family, the class I hematopoietic cytokine receptors, which includes receptors for cytokines (e.g., interleukins), erythropoietin, and leptin. Within 5 years after the receptor cDNAs were cloned, biochemical and structural investigations showed that GHR and PRLR must be dimerized to properly transmit signals, which allowed the design of potent PRL and GH antagonists that interfered with the efficient dimerization of these receptors. Until the beginning of the 1990s, however, the downstream mechanisms involved in signal transmission by PRL and GH receptors were only poorly elucidated, and not until the discovery of the Janus tyrosine kinase (JAK) and signal transducers and activators of transcription (STAT) factor families was the JAK/STAT pathway identified as the first major signaling cascade responsible for the effects of PRL and GH. Within the past 6 years, there have been numerous reports describing molecules involved in or interacting with known pathways or even identifying new pathways/molecules.

This article is divided into four sections aimed at elucidating the molecular basis of signaling properties of these receptors: (1) the structure–function relationships of naturally occurring receptor isoforms; (2) the mechanism of ligand-induced receptor activation; (3) the major signaling pathways; and finally (4) the ways in which animal models (knockout, transgenics) can correlate with and highlight molecular studies of PRLR/GHR signaling.

II. PRLR AND GHR ISOFORMS HAVE DIFFERENT SIGNALING CAPABILITIES

PRLR and GHR are single-pass transmembrane receptors with the N-terminal outside the cell (the ligand-binding domain) and the C-terminal inside the cell (the signaling domain). The three structural features conserved among hematopoietic cytokine receptors are found in both the PRLR and the GHR: two pairs of disulfide-linked cysteines in the N-terminal part of the extracellular domain (C12–C22 and C51–C62 in hPRLR), the typical "WS motif" (a double W-S repeat, conservatively mutated into Y-G-E-F-S in the GHR) in the membrane-proximal region of this domain, and finally, the proline-rich region (called Box 1) in the juxtamembrane region of the cytoplasmic domain (Fig. 1). The first two features are required for correct folding and therefore for the functioning of the extracellular domain (including ligand binding and receptor trafficking to the cell surface), whereas Box 1 is required for triggering (all) signaling cascades (see below). These conserved features are thus essential for the PRLR and GHR to elicit their activities.

One of the characteristics of cytokine receptors is that alternative splicing of the primary transcript

(a single gene exists for each receptor) leads to the occurrence of multiple protein isoforms, which in most cases are not correlated with pathological states. These isoforms differ mainly in their cytoplasmic tail, which affects their signaling properties. The classical isoform, called the "long" form, contains ~600 amino acids (591 for hPRLR and 620 for hGHR) and is considered to elicit all the actions attributed to the ligand. The "short" forms are truncated at their C-terminal and lack part of, or almost all of, the cytoplasmic tail. In rat, the short PRLR contains 291 amino acids, and in human cells, a 288-residue PRLR isoform has been recently described. All PRLR isoforms identified thus far from natural sources contain Box 1. Regarding the hGHR, two short isoforms containing 277 or 279 residues and lacking Box 1 have been identified. These short GHRs are thus devoid of signaling properties and act as dominant negatives of the full-length receptor by trapping the ligand and/or by forming inactive heterodimers with long receptor isoforms (see below). Intermediate forms have also been described, such as in rat Nb2 lymphoma cells (393 amino acids, due to a deletion in the PRLR gene) or in human cells (376 amino acids, due to alternative splicing). At least for the Nb2 receptor, none of the major signaling properties displayed by the full-length receptor are affected by this deletion. Finally, soluble receptors corresponding to the extracellular domain of membrane receptors have been identified; they originate either from alternative splicing or from limited proteolysis of full-length receptors (Fig. 1). As deduced from cloned cDNAs encoding these binding proteins (BPs), their overall length is 246 amino acids for the hGHBP and 206 for the PRLBP. Soluble receptors are intrinsically devoid of intrinsic signaling activity, although they may be indirectly involved in PRL/GH functions by controlling the levels of ligand available (BPs increase the hormone's half-life).

III. LIGAND-INDUCED RECEPTOR DIMERIZATION: THE FIRST STEP OF SIGNALING

The extracellular domain is the ligand-interacting region of these receptors. The three-dimensional structure of genetically engineered hPRLR and hGHR extracellular domains has been determined by crystallographic analysis (Fig. 2A). Not only are the GHR and PRLR extracellular domains structurally related (they fold in two antiparallel β-sheets),

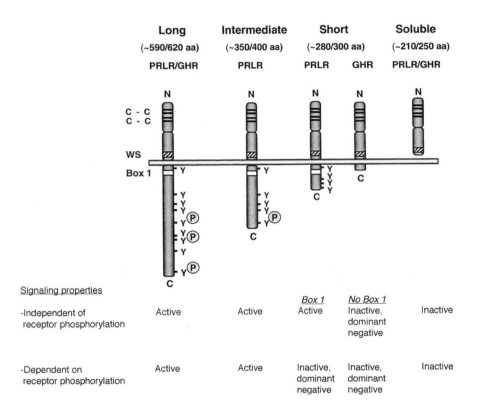

FIGURE 1 Schematic representation of the PRLR and GHR isoforms. The PRLR and GHR exist in various isoforms that differ only in their cytoplasmic tail regions. The four types of receptor isoforms, referred to as long, intermediate, short, or soluble with respect to their overall length, are illustrated. The conserved features among cytokine receptors are indicated: C–C, internal disulfide bonds; WS, for the Trp–Ser repeat, hatched box; and Box 1, for the proline-rich region, white box. "Y" represents tyrosines (number and position of tyrosines are random) of the cytoplasmic domain, some of which are phosphorylated (denoted by "P" in gray circle) by JAK2; short isoforms are not tyrosine-phosphorylated. Signaling properties of each isoform are summarized at the bottom (see text for more details).

their ligands also share a high level of structural similarity since both PRL and GH adopt the antiparallel four-α-helix-bundle fold characteristic of hematopoietic cytokines (Fig. 2B). Thus, it is not surprising that the ligand-induced activation of the PRLR and that of the GHR share very similar mechanisms. PRL and GH interact with two molecules of their receptors via two distinct regions, binding sites 1 and 2 (Fig. 2B). The active hormone–receptor complex is thus a trimer, comprising one molecule of ligand and two (identical) molecules of receptor (homodimer). Thus far, no specific receptor cDNA has been identified for placental lactogen (PL, another member of the PRL/GH hormone family). Interestingly, PRLR/GHR heterodimers have been proposed to constitute such a specific receptor complex, but the physiological relevance of this observation remains to be demonstrated. Since receptor homodimerization is required and is pre-

sumably sufficient to trigger downstream signaling cascades, receptor antagonists that interfere with this process have been designed. Impairing binding site 2 of PRL or GH by introducing sterically hindering mutations within this region leads to ligands that are unable to induce functional dimerization of the receptor and, therefore, act as inhibitors of the natural hormones by competing for receptor-binding sites. In many biological contexts, the ability of PRL or GH antagonists to inhibit PRL- or GH-induced signaling cascades has been clearly demonstrated.

IV. MAJOR SIGNALING PATHWAYS

With the exception of constitutively active N-terminal truncated receptors experimentally engineered for research purposes, all actions mediated by the PRLR and GHR result from their interaction with

A Receptor structure

Extracellular domain

B Ligand structure

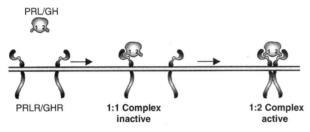

C Ligand-induced receptor homodimerization

FIGURE 2 Mechanism of receptor activation. PRLR and GHR extracellular domains adopt the seven-β-strand sandwich fold typical of cytokine receptors (A), and hormones adopt the four-α-helix-bundle fold typical of hematopoietic cytokines (B). Regions involved in hormone–receptor interactions are indicated. Following ligand binding, receptors are homodimerized in a sequential manner: the first receptor molecule binds to binding site 1 of its ligand, and then the second receptor molecule binds to binding site 2 to form the active trimeric complex (C).

any of their natural ligands, which leads to receptor dimerization and the activation of cascades in the intracellular space. Thus far, in contrast to the majority of cytokine receptors, there is no evidence that any "accessory" membrane protein is required or that the type of ligand (e.g., hPRL, hPL, or hGH for the hPRLR) affects the nature of signals that are transmitted inside the cell.

A. JAK/STAT Pathway

1. Activation of the JAK/STAT Pathway

The PRLR and GHR are devoid of any intrinsic enzymatic activity. In 1993–1994, JAK2 was identified as the Janus tyrosine kinase associated with these receptors. Although the involvement of JAK1 and JAK3 was also proposed later for both receptors, their role is clearly less relevant. In contrast to the

GHR, which recruits JAK2 to the receptor complex on ligand binding, the kinase is constitutively associated with the PRLR; i.e., its recruitment is not induced by ligand binding. For the GHR, SH2-Bβ has been recently identified as a cytoplasmic protein tightly binding to and potentiating the activity of phosphorylated JAK2.

The receptor–JAK2 interaction requires integrity of Box 1, which does not preclude the involvement of additional C-terminal regions of the receptor. Thus, with the exception of short GHR isoforms lacking Box 1 (Fig. 1), all PRL/GH receptor isoforms are able to interact with and activate JAK2 and, therefore, to exhibit some signaling properties. Mutational analysis of Box 1 has assigned a critical role to proline residues in the interaction with JAK2, suggesting an SH3 domain-mediated interaction. However, due to the absence of a typical SH3 domain in the JAK2 sequence, the question of whether the interaction between kinase and the receptors is direct or involves an intermediate protein (adapter) remains unresolved.

JAK2 activation is a prerequisite for triggering many, if not all, downstream signaling cascades (Fig. 3). Accordingly, receptor mutants unable to associate with JAK2, such as engineered Box 1-deleted PRLR or short GHR isoforms (Fig. 1), are unable to trigger tyrosine phosphorylation cascades and downstream activation of target genes. Interestingly, heterodimerization of the short and intermediate PRLR cytoplasmic tails results in complexes that are unable to stimulate JAK2 autophosphorylation, whereas both can associate with and activate the kinase in the context of their respective wild-type receptor. This observation suggests that only "perfect" homodimers can signal properly, which might be important in a physiological context since many tissues express different receptor isoforms, potentially forming heterodimers. Accordingly, short PRL receptors have been assigned a dominant negative role *in vitro* by inhibiting the transcriptional activation of milk protein genes induced by the full-length receptor; the physiological relevance of this observation remains to be demonstrated. Short GHR isoforms have been cloned from patients displaying a novel form of GH insensitivity syndrome, clearly indicating a dominant negative role of this short receptor isoform *in vivo*.

Once it is tyrosine-phosphorylated (i.e., activated), JAK2 phosphorylates the receptor on several tyrosines. No correlation between tyrosines that are preferentially phosphorylated by JAK kinases and their surrounding amino acids has been established

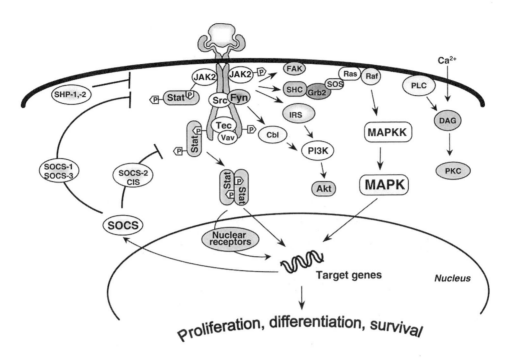

FIGURE 3 Signaling pathways. Major signaling pathways activated by the PRLR and GHR are represented (see text for differences). The JAK/STAT pathway and the MAPK pathway are among the best characterized cascades. In addition to these pathways, several other kinases/adapters have been shown to be involved in PRLR signaling, although their downstream effectors may be less well defined.

(no consensus sequence). Therefore, the reason that the short PRLR isoform does not undergo tyrosine phosphorylation despite its ability to activate JAK2 and the presence of tyrosines in its cytoplasmic domain remains unknown. The phosphotyrosines of receptors, as well as of JAK2, become sites of interaction with signaling molecules containing phosphotyrosine-binding motifs (SH2, PTB). Among these, recruitment of STAT factors to the receptor complex has been extensively studied. Both the PRLR and the GHR activate three of the seven known STATs: Stat1, Stat3, and mainly Stat5 (A and B isoforms). Stat1 and Stat3 bind to phosphotyrosines of the receptors and/or of JAK2; in agreement with these findings, short isoforms containing Box 1 (short PRLR or engineered C-terminal-truncated GHR) activate these STATs although the receptor is not phosphorylated. In contrast, Stat5 interacts only with the phosphotyrosine(s) of full-length and intermediate receptors. Although redundancy between some of these tyrosines has been reported, C-terminal tyrosines play a critical role, at least in the PRLR. Thus, one of the major differences between short and intermediate/long isoforms lies in the ability to activate Stat5-dependent downstream targets, which

is directly correlated with the phosphorylation status of the receptor (Fig. 1).

Once recruited to the receptor complex, STATs are phosphorylated by JAK2 on their C-terminal tyrosine, dissociate from the JAK–receptor complex, and translocate as dimers into the nucleus, where they specifically activate transcription by interacting with consensus DNA sequences within the promoters of PRL or GH target genes. The transcriptional specificity exhibited by identical STAT factors activated by distinct cytokines remains poorly understood. The answer may partly reside in the arsenal of other transcription factors that are also activated and can interact with STATs, modulating their transactivation activity (cross talk). Among these are nuclear receptors (estrogen, progesterone, glucocorticoid, etc.), Sp1 (specificity protein 1), CREB-binding protein/p300, peroxisome proliferator-activated receptor α (PPARα), nuclear factor κB, members of the interferon regulator factor (IRF) family, c-jun, MCM5 (mini-chromosome maintenance protein 5), and BRCA1 (breast cancer 1 gene). Different STATs can also interact with one another; e.g., Stat1 and Stat5 have been reported to exert opposing actions on IRF-I gene transcription.

2. Down-regulation of the JAK/STAT Pathway

The recent discovery of a family of proteins down-regulating the activation of the JAK/STAT pathway has greatly helped in understanding how these activated (phosphorylated) proteins return to their steady state after hormone stimulation. These proteins are denoted SOCS (suppressor of cytokine signaling) or CIS (cytokine-inducible SH2 proteins) and down-regulate the JAK/STAT pathway by interfering with either JAK2 enzymatic activity (SOCS-1, -3) or STAT recruitment to the receptor complex by competing for phosphotyrosine binding (SOCS-2, CIS). Importantly, the SOCS/CIS genes are targets of the cytokine-induced JAK/STAT pathway, meaning that they encode proteins functioning as regulators of this pathway in a feedback manner. Internalization and proteasome-dependent degradation of a GHR/JAK2/CIS complex have been proposed to be important steps in the time-dependent CIS inhibition mechanism. However, not all SOCS proteins inhibit receptor signaling; SOCS-2, which binds directly to the PRLR, potentiates receptor signaling.

In addition to SOCS, SH2-containing tyrosine phosphatases (SHP-1 and SHP-2) are important in signaling down-regulation by dephosphorylating JAK and/or receptors. SIRP (signal-regulated protein), a transmembrane protein interacting with JAK2 on GHR stimulation, recruits signaling molecules to the receptor complex, including the phosphatase SHP-2, which leads to JAK2 dephosphorylation; SIRP is thus currently regarded as a negative regulator of GH signaling. The role of phosphatases remains poorly understood, however, since SHP-2 also appears to be necessary for initiating PRLR and GHR signaling.

B. Other Pathways

The JAK/STAT pathway is undoubtedly one of the major cascades triggered by these receptors. However, many other signaling proteins have been shown to be activated by the PRLR and GHR. This section is aimed at providing an overview, albeit certainly not an exhaustive one, of these additional signaling cascades.

1. Mitogen-Activated Protein Kinase

The well-known mitogen-activated protein kinase (MAPK) pathway involves the Shc (Src homology and containing protein)/SOS (Son of Sevenless)/Grb2 (growth factor receptor-bound protein 2)/Ras/Raf/MAPK cascade. This pathway has been demonstrated

to be activated by both the PRLR and the GHR, including the short PRLR isoform, in agreement with the observation that the membrane proximal Box 1 region is sufficient to activate the MAPK pathway. Shc directly interacts with the receptor complex and becomes tyrosine-phosphorylated, presumably by JAK2. Whether activation of the MAPK cascade requires kinases other than JAK2, e.g., Src kinases, is yet to be elucidated. Also, indirect activation of the MAPK cascade via JAK2-induced phosphorylation of the EGF receptor and subsequent recruitment of Grb2 by phosphorylated EGF receptor have been reported in the case of GH stimulation. More recently, activation of c-jun N-terminal kinase and p38 by PRL has also been described.

2. Src Kinases

At least two members of the Src tyrosine kinase family, namely, Src and Fyn, are activated by the PRLR and this activation seems to occur independent of JAK2. Fyn has been shown to be constitutively bound to the PRLR. Src tyrosine kinases play an important role in PRLR signaling, especially in PRL-induced cell proliferation. There are as yet no reports demonstrating the involvement of Src kinases in GHR signaling.

3. Insulin Receptor Substrate and Phosphatidyl Inositol 3-Kinase

Insulin receptor substrate members (IRS-1, -2, -3) also interact with phosphorylated receptors and themselves become tyrosine-phosphorylated (by JAK2), which creates docking sites for SH2-containing proteins, including the p85 subunit of phosphatidyl inositol 3-kinase (PI3K). One downstream effector of PI3K has been shown to be the serine/threonine kinase Akt, the stimulation of which is involved in the anti-apoptotic effect of GH.

4. Other Molecules

The above-mentioned pathways do not exhaustively summarize the current knowledge in the field of PRLR/GHR signaling, but rather represent a broad overview. Other tyrosine kinases (ZAP-70, Tec), serine/threonine kinases (protein kinase C), phospholipase Cγ and the downstream pathway modulating intracellular calcium concentration, adapters (Cbl, a substrate of Src kinases), guanine nucleotide exchange factors (Vav, complexed to Tec), proteins of the cytoskeleton (FAK), the 17β-hydroxysteroid dehydrogenase/17-ketosteroid reductase (known as PRAP, for PRLR-associated protein), and proteins linked to the apoptotic pathway (including Bax,

Bcl-2, and Bag-1) have also been identified as molecules that are associated with and/or involved in signaling by the PRLR and/or GHR.

V. HOW ANIMAL MODELS CAN HIGHLIGHT *IN VITRO* SIGNALING STUDIES

The analysis of genetically modified animal models (knockout, transgenic) is extremely informative in evaluating the involvement of a particular signaling protein in the physiological development and function of a given organ. For example, the conditional knockout of Stat3 has clearly demonstrated a dramatic delay in the involution process of the mammary gland after weaning, establishing this STAT as a key factor in signaling the initiation of physiological apoptosis *in vivo* in this organ. However, it may prove difficult to correlate this kind of information with the identification of signals involved in upstream activation of signaling proteins in a normal context [e.g., which cytokine(s) or growth factor(s) regulates Stat3 activation in the mammary gland to control involution]. Examples of knockout models that have clearly highlighted the role of signaling proteins involved in PRLR- and GHR-mediated functions are provided below.

Stat5A and Stat5B are two closely related STAT proteins that, although they are encoded by distinct genes, have been often considered to be redundant in most molecular (*in vitro*) studies involving Stat5 analysis. It is only when Stat5A- and Stat5B-deficient mice were shown to exhibit distinct phenotypes that their nonredundant roles began to be understood. Stat5A-deficient mice display alterations of mammary gland development, including defective proliferation of the lobulo-alveolar ductal epithelium during pregnancy and lactation failure. All these phenotypes are very similar to those observed in PRL or PRLR knockout mice, suggesting that Stat5A, originally designated mammary gland factor, is tightly linked to PRLR-mediated signaling. In contrast, Stat5B-deficient mice exhibit a loss of normal sexually dimorphic growth, a phenotype reminiscent of Laron dwarfism in humans, which suggests that Stat5B is presumably more closely linked to GHR- than PRLR-mediated signaling.

Another very interesting knockout is that of SOCS-2, which leads to a gigantism phenotype very similar to that observed in GH transgenic mice. At 6 weeks of age, SOCS-2-deficient mice are 40% heavier than wild-type mice and their long bones are significantly longer, which is strong evidence that SOCS-2 is a natural negative regulator of GH and/or insulin-like growth factor-I (the main second messenger of GH) signaling.

Finally, a negative regulator of PRL signaling, SOCS-1, has recently been proposed as a factor capable of preventing lactation prior to parturition. In fact, mice deficient for SOCS-1 that were rescued from neonatal death by concomitant deletion of the interferon-γ gene were shown to have accelerated mammary lobulo-alveolar development. Interestingly, when a single allele of the SOCS-1 gene was deleted and these animals were crossed with PRLR$^{+/-}$ mice, the lactational defect normally seen in heterozygous mice was rescued. The functional pathways involved in SOCS-1 inhibition of the mammary gland remain to be identified.

VI. CONCLUSIONS

As for all cytokine receptors, the JAK/STAT pathway appears to play a central role in PRLR/GHR signaling, and receptor isoforms unable to activate JAK2 (naturally occurring or experimentally engineered) have been shown to be devoid of signaling properties. However, the variety and multiplicity of signaling pathways activated by PRL and GH receptors are presumably correlated with the unusually extended range of biological functions displayed by these hormones, whose receptors are widespread in the organism. Interconnection (cross talk) of these cascades now appears to be one of the key components to achieving some degree of specificity using a limited set of signaling molecules (JAKs, STATs, MAPKs, etc.) activated by distinct cytokines, hormones, and growth factors. Understanding how these activated protein pathways are organized in space as well as in time is a major challenge for future signaling studies.

Acknowledgments

We thank Nadine Binart for critically reading the manuscript and for helpful suggestions.

Glossary

binding protein In many species, prolactin- and growth hormone-binding proteins are generated and result either from alternative splicing of transcripts encoding full-length receptors or from limited proteolysis of membrane-bound receptors. Soluble binding proteins bind circulating ligands and prolong their half-life. They are devoid of intrinsic signaling properties, but may interfere with membrane-receptor signaling by forming inactive heterodimers (one soluble receptor and one membrane-bound receptor).

cytokine receptor A family of single-pass transmembrane receptors identified in the late 1980s based on sequence comparison of receptors for prolactin, growth hormone, erythropoietin, interleukin-2 (IL-2), and IL-6. Additional members of the class I hematopoietic cytokine receptor superfamily include receptors for leptin, thrombopoietin, and many cytokines regulating the immune system, such as most interleukins. The main conserved features of class I cytokine receptors are two pairs of cysteines and a Trp-Ser repeat (WS motif) in the extracellular domain and a proline-rich region (called Box 1) in the intracellular domain, which is essential for signaling properties. Cytokine receptors are devoid of intrinsic enzymatic activity and signal through associated kinases, the most classical of which are Janus tyrosine kinases (which bind to the Box 1 region of the receptors). Receptors for prolactin and growth hormone are very similar with respect to overall structure and signaling properties.

growth hormone (GH) A polypeptide hormone (191 amino acids in humans) that adopts the α-helix-bundle fold typical of hematopoietic cytokines. GH is secreted mainly by the pituitary gland, although it is also produced by other cell types, such as lymphoid cells. Its actions are related mainly to growth (soft tissues, long bones, etc.) and metabolism. It belongs to a family of hormones that includes prolactin and placental lactogens, as well as other placental factors.

homodimerization Cytokine receptors are activated by clustering of two or more receptor subunits, identical or not. Prolactin and growth hormone receptors are both activated by ligand-induced homodimerization of two identical receptor chains. In fact, a single molecule of ligand (prolactin or growth hormone) contains two binding sites (binding sites 1 and 2), each interacting with one receptor molecule. Based on this homodimerization model for receptor activation, hormone antagonists have been designed by impairing binding site 2 in prolactin or growth hormone, leading to ligands that are able to bind the receptor via their site 1 but unable to induce efficient receptor dimerization.

Janus kinase/signal transducers and activators of transcription (JAK/STAT) The most typical signaling pathway activated by cytokine receptors. This pathway involves a family of four tyrosine kinases designated "Janus" or "JAK" kinases (members are JAK1, JAK2, JAK3, and Tyk2). JAK2 is the main JAK involved in growth hormone and prolactin receptor signaling. Substrates of JAK tyrosine kinases include cytokine receptors and STAT factors. The eight members of the STAT protein family must interact with tyrosine-phosphorylated cytokine receptor complexes to be activated by tyrosine phosphorylation (by JAKs); they then migrate into the nucleus and transactivate cytokine target genes. With respect to growth hormone and prolactin signaling, Stat5 and, to a lesser extent, Stat1 and Stat3 are activated.

mitogen-activated protein kinase (MAPK) pathway One of the major pathways activated by membrane receptors. It involves a cascade of serine/threonine and dual-specificity (Tyr/Ser/Thr) kinases, leading to the activation of several target genes. The MAPK pathway has been historically linked to cell proliferation, but recent data have shown that it is involved in many cell responses and crosstalk with other pathways, including the Janus kinase/signal transducers and activators of transcription pathway. Activation of the MAPK cascade by prolactin and growth hormone receptors involves Box 1 but not the phosphotyrosines of the receptor.

prolactin (PRL) A polypeptide hormone (199 amino acids in humans) that adopts a four-α-helix-bundle fold typical of hematopoietic cytokines. PRL is secreted mainly by the pituitary gland, although it is also produced by other cell types and tissues, such as mammary gland, endometrium, lymphoid cells, and prostate. Its actions are essentially related to reproduction and lactation, but its involvement in an extremely wide spectrum of biological responses has been reported (osmoregulation, immunoregulation, behavior, growth, metabolism, etc.). Prolactin belongs to a family of hormones that includes growth hormone and placental lactogens as well as other placental factors.

receptor isoform Prolactin and growth hormone receptors are encoded by single genes. However, alternative splicing of primary transcripts leads to the existence of many receptor isoforms, which differ in the length of their cytoplasmic domains and are thus referred to as short, intermediate, or long receptors. Short isoforms have a truncated C-terminal tail and are not tyrosine-phosphorylated, which correlates with their inability to exhibit all signaling properties of long (full-length) or intermediate isoforms. In some instances, short isoforms have been suggested to act as dominant negative receptors, presumably because heterodimerization of short and long/intermediate receptors achieves inactive complexes.

suppressor of cytokine signaling (SOCS) A recently identified family of proteins that play an important role in regulating the Janus kinase/signal transducers and activators of transcription (JAK/STAT) pathway. They are currently viewed as negative regulators of this pathway, either by interfering with Janus kinase activity or by competing with STATs for binding to phosphorylated tyrosines of the receptor complex. Since SOCS genes are themselves targets of the JAK/STAT pathway triggered by activated cytokine receptors, they function by negative feedback regulation.

tyrosine phosphorylation Many stages of signaling cascades triggered by cytokine receptors involve tyrosine phosphorylation of various proteins. With respect to the receptor complex, several tyrosine residues within the cytoplasmic domains of prolactin and growth hormone receptors, or on Janus kinase 2 (JAK2) itself, are phosphorylated (by JAK2) and serve as docking sites for downstream effectors containing phosphotyrosine-binding domains (e.g., SH2 domains); candidates are signal transducers and activators of transcription proteins, suppressor of cytokine signaling proteins, phosphatases, or adapters (e.g., Grb2). The short receptor isoforms are not tyrosine-phosphorylated, which prevents some of these interactions from occurring.

See Also the Following Articles

Crosstalk of Nuclear Receptors with STAT Factors • Growth Hormone (GH) • Growth Hormone-Releasing Hormone (GHRH) and the GHRH Receptor • Placental Gene Expression • Prolactin (PRL)

Further Reading

Ayling, R. M., Ross, R., Towner, P., Von Laue, S., Finidori, J., Moutoussamy, S., Buchanan, C. R., Clayton, P. E., and Norman, M. R. (1997). A dominant-negative mutation of the growth hormone receptor causes familial short stature. *Nat. Genet.* **16**, 13–14.

Bole-Feysot, C., Goffin, V., Edery, M., Binart, N., and Kelly, P. A. (1998). Prolactin and its receptor: Actions, signal transduction pathways and phenotypes observed in prolactin receptor knockout mice. *Endocr. Rev.* **19**, 225–268.

Chang, W. P., Ye, Y., and Clevenger, C. V. (1998). Stoichiometric structure–function analysis of the prolactin receptor signaling domain by receptor chimeras. *Mol. Cell. Biol.* **18**, 896–905.

Finidori, J. (2000). Regulators of growth hormone signaling. *Vitam. Horm.* **59**, 71–97.

Herrington, J., Smit, L. S., Schwartz, J., and Carter-Su, C. (2000). The role of STAT proteins in growth hormone signaling. *Oncogene* **19**, 2585–2597.

Hu, Z. Z., Meng, J., and Dufau, M. L. (2001). Isolation and characterization of two novel forms of the human prolactin receptor generated by alternative splicing of a newly identified exon 11. *J. Biol. Chem.* **276**, 41086–41094.

Lee, R. C., Walters, J. A., Reyland, M. E., and Anderson, S. M. (1999). Constitutive activation of the prolactin receptor results in the induction of growth factor-independent proliferation and constitutive activation of signaling molecules. *J. Biol. Chem.* **274**, 10024–10034.

Lindeman, G. J., Wittlin, S., Lada, H., Naylor, M. J., Santamaria, M., Zhang, J. G., Starr, R., Hilton, D. J., Alexander, W. S., Ormandy, C. J., and Visvader, J. (2001). SOCS1 deficiency results in accelerated mammary gland development and rescues lactation in prolactin receptor-deficient mice. *Genes Dev.* **15**, 1631–1636.

Llovera, M., Pichard, C., Bernichtein, S., Jeay, S., Touraine, P., Kelly, P. A., and Goffin, V. (2000). Human prolactin (hPRL) antagonists inhibit hPRL-activated signaling pathways involved in breast cancer cell proliferation. *Oncogene* **19**, 4695–4705.

Sotiropoulos, A., Moutoussamy, S., Renaudie, F., Clauss, M., Kayser, C., Gouilleux, F., Kelly, P. A., and Finidori, J. (1996). Differential activation of Stat3 and Stat5 by distinct regions of the growth hormone receptor. *Mol. Endocrinol.* **10**, 998–1009.

Stofega, M. R., Wang, H., Ullrich, A., and Carter-Su, C. (1998). Growth hormone regulation of SIRP and SHP-2 tyrosyl phosphorylation and association. *J. Biol. Chem.* **273**, 7112–7117.

Wang, X., Darus, C. J., Xu, B. C., and Kopchick, J. J. (1996). Identification of growth hormone receptor (GHR) tyrosine residues required for GHR phosphorylation and JAK2 and STAT5 activation. *Mol. Endocrinol.* **10**, 1249–1260.

Yu-Lee, L., and Jeay, S. (2002). Prolactin and growth hormone receptors. *In* "Hormone Signaling" (V. Goffin and P. A. Kelly, eds.), pp. 121–143. Kluwer Academic, Norwell, MA.

Protein Kinases

ALAIN ENJALBERT AND
CAROLINE LE PECHON-VALLEE

ICNE, Institut Jean-Roche, Université de la Méditerranée, Marseille, France

I. INTRODUCTION
II. DEFINITION OF PROTEIN KINASES
III. STRUCTURE, CLASSIFICATION, AND SUBSTRATE RECOGNITION
IV. REGULATION OF PROTEIN KINASE ACTIVITY
V. TRANSDUCTION MECHANISMS
VI. MAJOR PHYSIOLOGICAL ROLES OF PROTEIN KINASES
VII. PROTEIN KINASES IN HUMAN PATHOLOGIES

Protein kinases are enzymes that catalyze the phosphorylation of proteins. Phosphorylation is an important intracellular signal-generating protein modification used in signal transduction. Protein kinases phosphorylate many proteins and are involved in major cellular processes such as differentiation, proliferation, and cell death.

I. INTRODUCTION

The great importance of the protein kinases within the cell can be understood through review of their function and major physiological roles. This article focuses on the mechanisms that ensure the specificity and tight regulation of protein kinases and their involvement in pathology and disease.

II. DEFINITION OF PROTEIN KINASES

A. The Enzymatic Reaction Catalyzed by Protein Kinases

Protein kinases, members of the family of phosphotransferases, catalyze the transfer of the γ-phosphate of adenosine triphosphate (ATP) to a hydroxyl residue of a protein substrate (see Fig. 1). This covalent

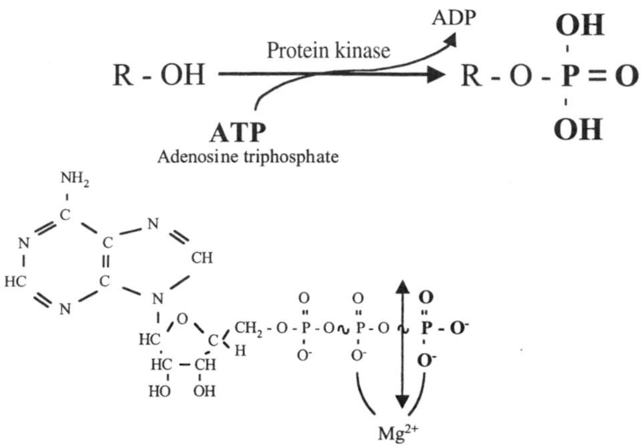

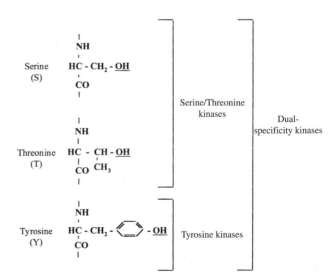

FIGURE I The biochemical reaction catalyzed by the protein kinases, showing the structure of ATP and the γ-phosphate that is transferred to the substrate hydroxyl group.

reaction takes place on the alcoholic aliphatic side chain of serine and threonine residues in the case of serine/threonine kinases. It can also take place on the phenolic group of tyrosine residues with protein–tyrosine kinases and on both serine/threonine and tyrosine residues in the case of dual-specificity kinases (see Fig. 2).

Histidyl kinases transfer the phosphate group onto an aspartate residue in their targets. The phosphate group comes from a histidyl residue that has been previously autophosphorylated within the kinase. These protein kinases have been discovered as a two-component histidine–aspartate phosphorelay in prokaryotes and plants. They are quite distinct from the conventional serine/threonine or tyrosine kinases.

The reverse reaction, or dephosphorylation, catalyzed by protein phosphatases, determines the ratio of phosphorylated and unphosphorylated forms. A vast number of protein phosphatases (PPs) exist, including serine/threonine phosphatases, such as the PP1s, PP2A, and PP2B, and a magnesium-dependent protein phosphatase, PP2C (also called PPM) for. The serine/threonine phosphatases are essentially cytosolic or nuclear. They localize within the cell through their binding to subcellular structures such as the endoplasmic reticulum and the cytoskeleton. Another class of phosphatases is the protein tyrosine phosphatases (PTPs). Some of the PTPs have membrane-spanning domains. They dephosphorylate tyrosine residues but some of them dephosphorylate both tyrosine and serine/threonine residues and are dual-specificity phosphatases. Some protein phosphatases have a very narrow specificity for their

substrate, whereas others dephosphorylate a large number of proteins.

B. The Protein Kinase Superfamily

Protein kinases are part of a huge superfamily. There exist many kinases and isoforms. According to the human genome, there should be more protein kinases than those discovered to date and some of the new kinases should be quite different from the ones already known. Phosphorylation is a primary means of signal transduction. Signal transduction is based on two main principles. First is the posttranslational modification of pre-existing proteins, such as phosphorylation. But isoprenylation, lipidation, methylation, glycosylation, or partial proteolysis also occurs. Second is production of new proteins or second messengers. Nevertheless, phosphorylation is the most common protein modification used in signal transmission, maybe because it is reversible and because protein kinases use a ubiquitous cofactor, ATP.

III. STRUCTURE, CLASSIFICATION, AND SUBSTRATE RECOGNITION

A. Structure

Protein kinase A (PKA), a cyclic adenosine $3',5'$-monophosphate (cAMP)-dependent protein kinase,

FIGURE 2 Phospho-acceptor amino acids. Protein kinases transfer a phosphate group onto the hydroxyl residue of an amino acid according to the specificity of the kinase. Serine/threonine kinases use either serine or threonine amino acids, tyrosine kinases use tyrosine, and dual-specificity kinases use serine, threonine, and tyrosine residues.

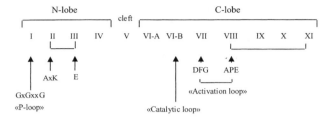

FIGURE 3 Subdomains of the catalytic domain of protein kinase A, showing some of the major residues involved in the structure or catalytic activity of the kinase (see text for discussion).

was one of the first kinases studied and its structure is well known. In the absence of cAMP, PKA enzymes are tetramers composed of two regulatory (R) subunits and two catalytic (C) subunits. Two classes of R subunits, RI and RII, and several isoforms for each class have been identified. The catalytic domain of the PKAs can be divided into 12 subdomains according to the localization of highly conserved regions (see Fig. 3).

The structure of the kinase domain of the PKAs has long served as a model. It folds into a bilobal structure separated by a deep cleft. The smallest N-lobe consists of subdomains I–IV. It is almost a single β-sheet and is involved in proper ATP orientation and binding. The cleft consists of subdomain V and interferes in substrate recognition and catalytic activity promotion. The C-lobe consists of subdomains VI-A, VI-B, and VII–XI and is almost entirely composed of α-helices. Structure and regulatory processes are unique to each kinase but almost every subdomain contains positions in which structurally similar residues are conserved throughout the entire protein kinase superfamily (Fig. 3).

The most important domains for the structure and the function of the protein kinases are subdomains I, II, VI-B, VII, and VIII. Subdomain I (amino acids 43–64; numbering is derived from the PKA sequence) contains the phosphate-anchoring loop, or the P-loop, which is a glycine-rich β-ribbon ATP-binding consensus sequence. This sequence is GxGxxG, in which G represents glycine (in the single-letter amino acid code) and x denotes positions where any residues would be tolerated. Subdomain II (amino acids 65–83) contains the AxK motif, in which the lysine (K) at position 72 is necessary for maximum activity because it is engaged in a salt bridge with the glutamine (E) in position 91 in subdomain III.

Subdomain VI-B (amino acids 161–177) contains the catalytic loop and is directly involved in catalysis.

It is a sequence with at least three conserved residues: an aspartate, a leucine, and an asparagine (DLN). The aspartate residue (D166 in PKA) within the sequence is known as the "catalytic base" because it removes the proton from the hydroxyl group of the phospho-acceptor, producing an anionic oxygen that is involved in the nucleophilic attack of the γ-phosphate of the ATP. In serine/threonine kinases, a lysine (K) is also present (determining a DLKxxN motif) and is thought to be important to neutralize the negative charge of the γ-phosphate and to stabilize the intermediate state during the chemical reaction. In the case of tyrosine kinases, the lysine is replaced by an arginine (R) residue in a DLRAAN (A, alanine) sequence in the case of nonreceptor tyrosine kinases and in a DLAARN sequence in the case of receptor tyrosine kinases. Such conserved features, which characterize subgroups of protein kinases, exist also in other subdomains.

Subdomain VII (amino acids 178–193), also called the "metal-binding loop," referring to the metal ions bound to ATP, contains a DFG triplet (F, phenylalanine). The mutation of the aspartate (D) in this triplet results in an inactive kinase. Subdomain VIII (amino acids 194–210) contains another very important motif for the kinase activity: the APE motif (P, proline). The glutamate (E) is engaged with an arginine residue from subdomain XI in an interaction that contributes to the stability of the C-lobe. The region lying between the DFG and the APE motifs is the activation loop. It is a highly variable sequence but it always contains one or several residues for which phosphorylation induces the conformational rearrangement necessary for kinase activation.

B. Classification

From catalytic domain alignment, Hanks and Quinn, in 1991, provided a general classification of protein kinases. This classification, which is still used, delineates five kinase family groups: (1) AGC, (2) CaMK, (3) GMCC, (4) PTK, and (5) OPK.

1. *AGC group.* This group is so called because it includes protein kinases A, G, and C. The PKA and the PKG families include protein kinases activated by cyclic nucleotides cAMP and cGMP, respectively. The protein kinase C family includes several isoforms, distributed in three subclasses according to their allosteric regulators. The cPKCs (α, βι, βιι, and γ) are the conventional PKCs regulated by calcium, diacylglycerol (DAG), and

phosphatidylserines. The nPKCs (δ, ϵ, η, and θ) are the novel, or nonclassical, calcium-independent PKCs. The aPKCs (ζ and ι/λ) are the atypical calcium- and DAG-independent PKCs. The AGC group also includes the G-protein receptor kinases (GRKs), which phosphorylate G-protein-coupled receptors. These kinases, such as the β-adrenergic receptor kinase (βARK) and the rhodopsin kinase (RK), are involved in desensitization and scaffold construction on the activated receptors (see below).

2. *CaMK group.* The second group of the Hanks and Quinn classification corresponds to the kinases regulated by calcium/calmodulin (CaM). CaMKs are involved in many cellular processes in response to changes of the intracellular calcium concentration. Within the cells, calcium is generally captured by high-affinity calcium-binding proteins such as calmodulin or troponin, which is found in muscles. In the CaMK family of protein kinases (CaM group I, CaM group II, and CaM "other"), the most well-known calcium/CaM-regulated kinases are the CaMKI, CaMKII, and CaMKIV. CaMKI and CaMKIV are closely related and distinct from CaMKII. CaMKII is also called the multiprotein kinase, because it actually comprises a family of closely related enzymes that phosphorylate numerous substrates. Each CaMKII is made of several catalytic subunits. Autophosphorylation may lead to calmodulin trapping, making the kinase calcium independent until it is dephosphorylated by protein phosphorylases or is phosphorylated on additional residues. In the absence of autophosphorylation, the binding of Ca^{2+}/CaM is necessary to promote the transition from an inactive state to a nonactivated state of the CaMK, which has to be phosphorylated to be fully activated.

3. *GMCC group.* The GMCC group is so called because it includes, among others, glycogen synthase kinases (GSKs); mitogen-activated protein kinases (MAPKs), which include the extracellular signal-regulated kinases; cyclin-dependent kinases (Cdks), which are involved in cell cycle progress; and the carboxy-terminal domain (CTD) kinases, which phosphorylate the long carboxy-terminal domain on the largest subunit of RNA polymerase II.

4. *PTK group.* The fourth group is composed of the conventional protein tyrosine kinases (PTKs). It includes nonmembrane (such as Src, Csk, and Fak families) and membrane-spanning protein tyrosine kinases (such as the large growth factor receptor families).

5. *OPK group.* The last group includes various "other protein kinases," i.e., the Raf family from the extracellular signal-related kinase (ERK) cascade and the MAPK/ERK kinase (MEK) family. It includes also other MEK kinases that are intermediates of the c-Jun N-terminal kinase/stress-activated protein kinase (JNK/SAPK) and p38MAPK pathways.

Beyond the distinction based on the catalytic domain amino acid sequence proposed by Hanks and Quinn, protein kinases can be distinguished by the nature of the residues they prefer to phosphorylate or by their subcellular localization. This would lead us either to consider AGC, CaMK, and GMCC kinases plus the other serine/threonine kinases from the OPK group as a unique serine/threonine kinase family, or to view the superfamily of protein kinases as two groups: the cytosolic group and the membrane-spanning protein kinase group. The cytosolic kinase group would include serine/threonine kinases (such as PKAs and PKCs) and tyrosine kinases (such as Src). On the other hand, the group of membrane-spanning protein kinases would include some serine/threonine protein kinases (such as the transforming growth factor-β receptor) and the large group of tyrosine kinase receptors. In addition to membrane or cytosolic localization, subcellular targeting is also important and is different from one kinase to another.

Compartmentalization of protein kinases plays a crucial role in their activity and is frequently determined by specific anchoring proteins. Several of these have already been identified. Several A-kinase-anchoring proteins (AKAPs) target the PKAs to subcellular loci (plasma membrane and mitochondrial surface). AKAPs are characterized by their ability to bind RI or RII regulatory subunits of the PKAs. This binding has two consequences. First, it is supposed to change the catalytic activity of the PKAs. Second, it specifically brings the PKAs into close contact with upstream effectors or downstream substrates via protein–protein or protein–lipid interactions mediated by the AKAPs. In addition, AKAPs can bind several PKAs at once and protein phosphatases as well. Such is the case of AKAP79, which anchors PKA, PKC, and PP2B on the plasma membrane. This mechanism may be useful for the fine and coordinated regulation of signal transduction. Several proteins also regulate PKC anchoring and translocation to particulate fractions, including myristoylated alanine-rich protein kinase C (MAPCK) substrate proteins and the receptors for activated C kinase (RACK) proteins.

C. Substrate Recognition

Protein kinases use proteins as substrates. The phosphorylated residue is identified by the kinase thanks to specificity determinants surrounding it in the substrate sequence. In the case of the PKAs, which are basotropic kinases, the consensus sequence is R-(R/K)-x-S/T-B (where B stands for a hydrophobic residue). Such a small sequence cannot determine by the high specificity needed to select a substrate within the cell. This suggests that additional mechanisms exist, such as the targeting of the substrate and/or the kinase, the accessibility of the substrates, and the existence of a "docking site" on the substrate surface. A docking site corresponds to a larger sequence of amino acids seated astride the phosphorylated residue and an acute three-dimensional folding of the substrate that allows high-affinity interaction with the catalytic core of the kinase and increases the catalytic efficiency. For the moment, only a few docking sites are known. Some kinases are very specific for a protein substrate whereas others phosphorylate a large number of substrates.

IV. REGULATION OF PROTEIN KINASE ACTIVITY

Frequently, the presence of a sequence homologous to the substrate recognition motif in the sequence of the protein kinase forces a refolding of the kinase, which prevents substrate and ATP binding. In the PKA inactive conformation, interaction between regulatory and catalytic subunits is responsible for the autoinhibition of the kinase. In the case of the PKCs, a pseudo-substrate site, located inside the N-terminal conserved "C1" domain of the kinase, interacts with the C-terminal conserved "C4" domain, and the kinase bends back into a closed, inactive conformation. As for the CaMKs, extension of the regulatory domain of the enzyme across the catalytic core leads to multiple inhibitory interactions. In the case of the cytoplasmic tyrosine kinase Src, access to the active site is blocked because of Src homology domain 2 (SH2) and Src homology domain 3 (SH3) intramolecular interactions. Src recruitment via its SH2 domain and dephosphorylation remove the inhibitory constraint from the kinase. In the tyrosine kinase receptor inactive

state, the activation loop obtrudes the substrate and the ATP binding site and leads also to autoinhibition. Thus, almost every protein kinase needs an ultimate rearrangement to achieve the activated state. Several events induce separately or concomitantly this reorganization.

A. Second-Messenger-Mediated Activation

PKA is a prime example of protein kinases regulated by a second messenger. The specific binding of two cAMP molecules onto each PKA regulatory subunit leads to the release of the two catalytic subunits and to the relief of the autoinhibition process. Many of the kinases of the AGC group are activated following production of second messengers. For instance, calcium and diacylglycerol participate in the activation of some PKCs. Others kinases are regulated by the local calcium concentration within the cells. Such is the case of the CaMKs. Indeed, the binding of Ca^{2+}/CaM on the CaMKs releases the constraint of the autoinhibitory domain.

B. Ligand-Mediated Activation of Receptor Protein Kinases

The signal transduction initiated by the ligand binding to tyrosine kinase receptors starts with homo- or heterodimerization. The dimerization results in a conformational change and an auto- or interphosphorylation of several tyrosine residues on the cytoplasmic tail of the transmembrane receptor. Current research suggests that tyrosine kinase receptors can also undergo intracellular transactivation. An example of this is the extracellular growth factor (EGF) receptor transactivation downstream of the G-protein-coupled receptors, but some researchers think that this implies a pseudo-ligand binding. This underlines the importance of the ligand-mediated release of the autoinhibition of protein kinase receptors.

C. Regulation by Phosphorylation

Because protein kinases are proteins, they can be used as a substrate and can then be phosphorylated and activated by other protein kinases. Thus, protein kinase activation in series can take place within cells, as illustrated by activation of the ERK MAPK cascade (Fig. 4). The mitogen-activated protein kinase super-family includes the extracellular signal-regulated kinases, the c-Jun N-terminal kinases/stress-activated protein kinases, and the p38MAPKs. The MAPKs are

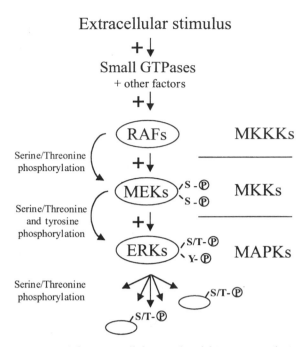

Extracellular stimulus

FIGURE 4 The extracellular-regulated kinase cascade is a prime example of phosphorylations occurring in series within the cell. This cascade is initiated by Raf protein activation (MKKKs). Activated Rafs then phosphorylate MEK proteins (MKKs) on serine (S) residues. MEKs, in turn, phosphorylate extracellular signal-related kinase (ERK) proteins or mitogen-activated protein kinases (MAPKs) on serine/threonine (S/T) and tyrosine (Y) residues. This cascade ends with the phosphorylation on serine/threonine of many substrates by the ERKs.

activated at the very last step of a three-kinase cascade. MAPKs are phosphorylated and activated by the MAP/ERK kinases, or MEKs, also called MAPK kinases (or MKKs), as indicated Fig. 4. The MEKs are phosphorylated and activated by the MEK kinases, also called MAPK kinase kinases (or MKKKs). When considering the ERK MAPK cascade, which ends with the activation of ERK1 or ERK2, MEK kinases are Raf proteins; MEKs are either MEK1 or MEK2. Raf proteins phosphorylate MEKs on serine residues. MEKs, which are dual-specificity kinases, phosphorylate ERKs on serine/threonine and tyrosine residues, and ERKs phosphorylate a large number of substrates on serine and threonine residues.

D. Multifactorial Activation

Raf-1 is one of the MEK kinases. Raf-1 regulation is complex and may illustrate what should be the integrated regulation of most protein kinases. Raf-1 is activated downstream of the small GTPase Ras, but

Ras is not sufficient to activate Raf-1. Raf-1 activation requires protein–protein interactions, binding to phospholipids, and phosphorylations on serine, threonine, and tyrosine residues, as well as appropriate relocalization within the cell. Several protein kinases have been reported to phosphorylate Raf-1, including Src, PKCs, p21PAK, and Akt. The subcellular localization of Raf-1 is dictated by its binding to Ras but also to several other proteins (such as heat-shock protein 90, p50, and 14-3-3 proteins). According to the combination of these regulations, Raf-1 may exhibit graded activity states.

An additional degree of complexity is achieved because of the multiplicity of isoenzymes acting at each level of the MAPK cascade. Ras and Rap-1 are able to promote Raf protein activation. The Raf protein family includes Raf-1, B-Raf, and A-Raf. The fact that several isoenzymes can act at the same step in the cascade could suggest a redundancy, but it is now agreed that it instead involves a precise regulation that results from the great specificity of regulation and function of each isoenzyme.

V. TRANSDUCTION MECHANISMS

As already mentioned, protein kinases can act on the enzymatic activity of other protein kinases, initiating cascades of protein kinases within the cell, as illustrated with the MAPK pathway. In addition, protein kinases can activate or inhibit other enzymes that are not protein kinases. For instance, in hepatocytes (Fig. 5), PKA not only phosphorylates a protein kinase (the phosphorylase kinase) but also phosphorylates and inactivates glycogen synthase I (an enzyme that catalyzes glycogen synthesis).

Protein kinases also phosphorylate nonenzymatic proteins. For instance, ionic channel opening can be regulated by phosphorylation. In addition, cytoskeletal components or adhesion molecules are phosphorylated by protein kinases. Phosphorylation of some proteins blocks their proteolysis, but more generally serine/threonine phosphorylation promotes ubiquitinylation and subsequent degradation of the protein by the proteasome. Phosphorylation of G-protein-coupled receptors by PKAs, PKCs, or the highly specialized G-protein receptor kinases is the first step in G-protein receptor desensitization. Indeed, the receptor phosphorylation induces arrestin binding, G-protein uncoupling, and the receptor internalization. In addition, it is now believed that it may also initiate cross talk with other pathways and even with G-protein-independent pathways.

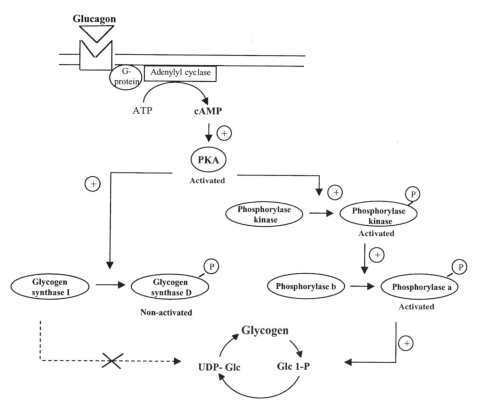

FIGURE 5 The protein kinase cascade regulating glycogen metabolism. In hyperglycemia, glucagon induces protein kinase A (PKA) activation in hepatocytes. PKA activation induces both the inhibition of the glycogen synthase I (a nonkinase enzyme) and the activation of the phosphorylase kinase (a protein kinase). Note that the multiplicity of substrates of PKA renders possible this concomitant effect and prevents a futile cycle from taking place in this metabolic pathway. UDP, Uridine diphosphate; Glc, glucose.

Phosphorylation can affect the activity of transcription factors by modulating their transcriptional activity, but also by regulating their nuclear translocation to the vicinity of DNA. In fact, bidirectional trafficking across the nuclear envelope is tightly regulated for many proteins. The nuclear localization sequence (NLS) targets proteins to the nucleus, whereas the nuclear export sequence (NES) targets proteins to the cytoplasm. The presence of the NLS is not sufficient, however, and a phosphorylation regulatory module for nuclear import (PrNLS), which includes sites in addition to the NLS, has been specified and suggests a significant role of phosphorylation in either promoting or preventing the nuclear localization.

Protein kinases are also involved in the construction of multiprotein scaffolds. Most often they are built on tyrosine kinase receptors through high-affinity phosphotyrosine docking sites. Less frequently, they are built on integrins and on G-protein-coupled receptors. Some investigators

think that these scaffolds are crucial in channeling the signal to the right pathway in the intracellular network of signaling cascades and in determining the quantity of proteins to enter signal transduction by delineating a microenvironment. On the contrary, other workers consider that scaffolds generate a high degree of diversity, because the scaffolds increase considerably the number of outputs by multiplying the number of protein–protein interactions. Most agree that the scaffolds promote cross talk between the linear transduction pathways by recruiting proteins from parallel cascades. Cross talk may be the key for a selective, specific, and efficient signaling. The more signal transduction is studied, the more it is seen to proceed through combinatorial interactions of a limited repertoire of proteins and to depend on a few kinds of protein modifications, such as phosphorylation. Thus, the multiplicity of cross talk between canonical pathways is probably necessary to transmit diverse and specific signals.

VI. MAJOR PHYSIOLOGICAL ROLES OF PROTEIN KINASES

In view of the multitude of substrates they phosphorylate and of the variety of transduction mechanisms they use, it is clear that protein kinases participate in many cellular functions. They are at least involved in shaping cell and adhesion regulation, in cellular metabolism, endocytosis, exocytosis, and cellular growth and differentiation. In particular, protein kinases are implied in the cell cycle and in regulation of apoptosis.

Specific cyclin-dependent kinases complexes regulate transitions between two subsequent phases of the cell cycle. The Cdks are serine/threonine kinases. The Cdk association with cyclins, of which the level of expression is regulated during the cycle, is the major means of regulation of Cdk activity, but phosphorylation also modulates activity. Thus, at least, two phosphorylations steps interfere in the cell cycle regulation. The upstream phosphorylation of the Cdks is followed by the serine/threonine phosphorylation of substrates by the activated Cdks.

Apoptosis is a physiologically and genetically programmed cell death that proceeds both through posttranslational modification of pre-existing factors and through regulation of a specific gene expression level. Thus, every intracellular signaling pathway involving phosphorylation can either inhibit or promote apoptosis at a distance. In addition, some proteins of the apoptotic program are also directly regulated by phosphorylation. Such is the case of caspase 9, for which proteolytic activity is reduced when it is phosphorylated. The unphosphorylated caspase 9 cleaves and activates caspase 3, which is one of the terminal caspases. These caspases are responsible for the cleavage of specific cellular proteins and for the DNA fragmentation seen in the cells committed to apoptosis.

Phosphorylation also takes part in almost every single step of the intracellular signaling pathway, from the membrane to the nucleus. This can be exemplified with the platelet-derived growth factor (PDGF) receptor. The phosphorylation of tyrosine residues on the cytoplasmic tail of such a tyrosine kinase receptor and the binding of PTB- or SH2-domain-containing proteins have already been discussed. Among these proteins, Grb2 is constitutively bound to Sos. Sos is an exchange factor that promotes small GTPase activation. Once the GTPases are activated, the MAPK cascades can continue. Finally, ERKs phosphorylate pre-existing transcription factors (such as Elk-1, CREB, and ATF2), which very quickly stimulate transcription of the so-called early gene products of the Fos/Jun family. Later, Fos and Jun transcription factors, associated in an activator protein 1 (AP-1) complex, the composition of which depends on the previous step, induce transcription of specific target genes.

VII. PROTEIN KINASES IN HUMAN PATHOLOGIES

Because phosphorylation and dephosphorylation play an essential role in almost every regulatable cellular process, any abnormality in protein kinase activity is likely to be a feature in human pathology. For example, current research on diabetes and neurodegenerative and cardiovascular diseases suggests the potential for beneficial spin-offs from the study of protein kinase defects. In particular, the role of tyrosine kinases in cancer is well established. Cancers are characterized by unregulated cell growth, differentiation, and apoptosis, processes in which protein kinases are largely involved. Alteration of protein kinase activity, including tyrosine kinase, can be the result of several mechanisms. First is an abnormal protein kinase expression because of mutation, deletion, or chromosomal translocation. For instance, the activating mutations of Ras proteins, which are upstream protooncogene activators of the MAP/ERK cascade, are encountered in 30% of human neoplasms, including 90% of pancreatic adenomas and 30% of colon adenocarcinomas. In chronic myeloid leukemia (CML), the t(9,22) reciprocal translocation, which causes the Philadelphia chromosome, juxtaposes the sequences of the breakpoint cluster region (BCR) and the c-ABL tyrosine kinase. The resulting fusion protein exhibits an elevated tyrosine kinase activity compared to the normal c-ABL. Second, an overexpression of a normal protein kinase and/or of its endogenous activator is sufficient to induce an adverse autocrine loop. Such is the case in some lung cancers in which a sustained stimulation of the EGF-proliferating pathway has been reported. In addition, a positive correlation between an increased tumor neovascularization, an increased risk of tumor invasion, and a decreased survival is well established. Growth factors such as fibroblast growth factors (FGFs), platelet-derived growth factor β (PDGFβ), and vascular endothelial growth factor (VEGF) are stimulators of angiogenesis. This suggests that the tyrosine kinase pathways that they initiate may be involved in the further growth and invasion or in the switch from a dormant to an active state of the malignant cells.

Nevertheless, the use of protein kinase inhibitors as therapeutic agents is an unfulfilled goal. Most of the protein kinase inhibitors that have been developed are ATP-competitive inhibitors, but because all protein kinases use this nucleotide as a cofactor, it is difficult to get specificity. Adverse toxic effects may result from the inhibition of all of the intracellular phosphorylations and may limit any use of protein kinase inhibitors. It is necessary to target tumoral tissue and to preserve the normal protein kinase activity elsewhere. In addition, cross talk between transduction pathways is likely to render impossible or vain the inhibition of a unique kinase.

A few protein kinase inhibitors and angiosuppressive agents are being used in clinical trials, administered alone or in combination with other anticancer drugs. One example is the c-ABL-specific tyrosine kinase inhibitor, STI571, which is currently being tested for chronic myeloid leukemia. Another is the SU101 PDGF receptor inhibitor, which has already shown promising results in hormonorefractory prostate cancer clinical trials. Moreover, much effort has been made to develop farnesyltransferase inhibitors to prevent Ras protein binding to cell membranes and to block transduction of mitogenic signals.

Considering the crucial role of protein kinases in all major cellular processes, a better knowledge of protein kinase function is essential for a better understanding of cell physiology and pathology. There has been an enormous increase in literature on protein kinases since 1968, when E. G. Krebs first discovered the glycogen phosphorylase kinase and PKA. Ongoing research on protein kinases continues to be a promising field of study. Most efforts likely will continue to focus on discovery of new protein kinases and on gaining insight into the molecular mechanisms of regulation of the protein kinases already known. However, the importance of signal transduction compartmentalization in protein kinase function and the role of protein kinases in establishing cross talk between pathways are already under investigation.

Glossary

enzyme A protein that specifically catalyzes a chemical reaction in order to accelerate the reaction speed.
phosphorylation Binding of a phosphate group onto a molecule.
phosphotransferase An enzyme that catalyzes the transfer of a phosphate group from one molecule to another.

signal transduction A set of events taking place in a cell in response to extracellular stimuli, including input reception, intracellular transmission of the information from the membrane to the nucleus, and integration of concomitant signals, resulting in production of a suitable biological response.
substrate The molecule transformed by the enzyme.

See Also the Following Articles

Angiogenesis • Apoptosis • Cancer Cells and Progrowth/ Prosurvival Signaling • Membrane Receptor Signaling in Health and Disease • Signaling Pathways, Interaction of

Further Reading

Blume-Jensen, P., and Hunter, T. (2001). Oncogenic kinase signaling. *Nature* 411, 355–365.
Bos, J. L., and Zwartkruis, F. J. (1999). Signal transduction. Rhapsody in G proteins. *Nature* 400, 820–821.
Carpenter, G. (2000). EGF receptor transactivation mediated by the proteolytic production of EGF-like agonists. *Science STKE* 15(perspectives), 1–3 (http://www.stke.org).
Edwards, A. S., and Scott, J. D. (2000). A-kinase anchoring proteins: Protein kinase A and beyond. *Curr. Opin. Cell Biol.* 12, 217–221.
Hanks, S. K., and Quinn, A. M. (1991). Protein kinase catalytic domain sequence database: Identification of conserved features of primary structure and classification of family members. *Methods Enzymol.* 200, 38–62.
Kolibaba, K. S., and Druker, B. J. (1997). Protein tyrosine kinases and cancer. *Biochim. Biophys. Acta* 1333, F217–F248.
Luttrell, L. M., Daaka, Y., and Lefkowitz, R. J. (1999). Regulation of tyrosine kinase cascades by G-protein-coupled receptors. *Curr. Opin. Cell Biol.* 11, 177–183.
Miller, W. E., and Lefkowitz, R. J. (2001). Expanding roles for beta-arrestins as scaffolds and adapters in GPCR signaling and trafficking. *Curr. Opin. Cell Biol.* 13, 139–145.
Pearson, G., Robinson, F., Beers Gibson, T., Xu, B. E., Karandikar, M., Berman, K., and Cobb, M. H. (2001). Mitogen-activated protein (MAP) kinase pathways: regulation and physiological functions. *Endocr. Rev.* 22, 153–183.
Protein kinase resource: http://www.sdsc.edu/kinases/pkr.
Schenk, P. W., and Snaar-Jagalska, B. E. (1999). Signal perception and transduction: The role of protein kinases. *Biochim. Biophys. Acta* 1449, 1–24.
Smith, C. M., Radzio-Andzelm, E., Madhusudan, K., Akamine, P., and Taylor, S. S. (1999). The catalytic subunit of cAMP-dependent protein kinase: Prototype for an extended network of communication. *Prog. Biophys. Mol. Biol.* 71, 313–341.

PTH

See *Parathyroid Hormone*

Receptor-Mediated Interlinked Systems, Mathematical Modeling of

DANIEL M. KEENAN* AND JOHANNES D. VELDHUIS†

*University of Virginia • †Mayo Clinic and Foundation, Minnesota

I. INTRODUCTION
II. THE HPT (GnRH–LH–Te) MODEL, AS REPRESENTATIVE OF RECEPTOR-MEDIATED SYSTEMS

Many physiological functions of the body are regulated by endocrine systems, which typically consist of several key nodes, namely, the hypothalamus, the pituitary gland, and various remote target glands.

I. INTRODUCTION

From a "systems" perspective, one can envision three nodes linked by interface functions, which represent the receptor-mediated stimulus–response interactions. Hence, at the macroscopic level, the structure can be viewed as:

Interface functions [$H(\cdot)'s$]

linking
- Hypothalamus
- Pituitary
- Target gland (Testes, Ovaries, Adrenal)

In Fig. 1 are schematic diagrams for three such structures: the male and female reproductive axes and the stress axis. Several major feedback/feed-forward interactions are depicted by arrows. The male reproductive hormone system consists of gonadatropin-releasing hormone (GnRH), produced in the hypothalamus; luteinizing hormone (LH), produced in the pituitary; and testosterone (Te), produced in the testes. The female reproductive hormone system, in addition to GnRH and LH, includes follicle-stimulating hormone (FSH), produced in the pituitary; and estrogen (E), progesterone (P), and inhibin (I), produced in the ovaries. The stress axis consists of corticotropin-releasing hormone (CRH) and arginine vasopressin (AVP), both produced in the hypothalamus; adrenocorticotropic hormone (ACTH),

produced in the pituitary; and cortisol, produced in the adrenal gland.

The above interfaces denote, at each time t, the feedback and/or feed-forward modulation of:

- a rate of pulsing at time t, (a pulse generator), e.g., testosterone and estrogen feedback on GnRH pulsing;
- a rate of hormone synthesis at time t, e.g., GnRH feed-forward/Te feedback on LH synthesis;
- a rate of release at time t (rather than storage) of new synthesis, e.g., GnRH feed-forward on LH.

What is an appropriate formulation of such feedback and feed-forward signals? An appropriate measure must account for lagged and contingent biochemical activities, each with its individual time and strength variabilities, e.g., the degree of saturation of the appropriate receptor sites. The feedback/feed-forward signal of hormone A at the target

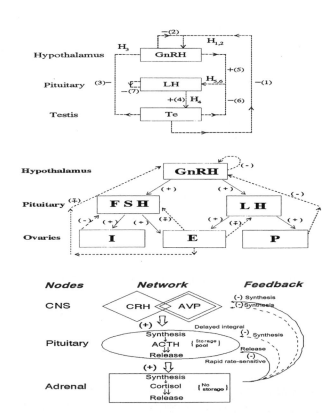

FIGURE 1 Schematic diagrams of the male (top) and female (middle) reproductive axes and the stress-responsive axis (bottom) with specific feedback/feed-forward interactions denoted by arrows. The numbers identify the interactions, a (+) signifies (positive) feed-forward, and a (−) signifies (negative) feedback.

cell (of B) at time t as a concentration time average over a time delay $[l_1, l_2]$ is represented as

$$\int_{t-l_1}^{t-l_2} Y(r)dr = \frac{1}{l_2 - l_1} \int_{t-l_1}^{t-l_2} Y(r)dr,$$

where $Y(r)$ is either a hormone concentration or its rate of change at time r. The effect of a feedback/feedforward signal for a peptide is different from that for a steroid. If hormone A is a steroid, its molecules are able to diffuse through the target cell membrane, whereas if hormone A is a peptide, its molecules do not penetrate but rather attach to receptors on the target cell membrane. Either way, a cascade of biochemical reactions results.

These feedback interactions can be modeled via monotonic logistic dose–response functions

$$H(x_1) = \frac{C}{1 + \exp[-(A + B_1 x_1)]} + D,$$

of one input,

$$H(x_1, x_2) = \frac{C}{1 + \exp[-(A + B_1 x_1 + B_2 x_2)]} + D,$$

of two inputs,

or where the coefficients themselves are described by logistic functions

$$H(x_1, x_2) = \frac{C(x_2)}{1 + \exp[-(A + B_1 x_1 + B_2 x_2)]} + D.$$

If $B_i > 0$, the feedback is positive (i.e., feed-forward effect); if $B_i < 0$, the feedback is negative. For each hormone, its resulting nonbasal rate of synthesis $S(\cdot)$ will depend on time-delayed feedback from the system through some nonlinear dose–response function $H(\cdot)$, plus noise $\xi(\cdot)$. The $H(\cdot)$ function serves the role of an average rate (a "conditional expectation") for all the cells in the endocrine gland; the actual realized rate of synthesis $S(\cdot)$ varies about $H(\cdot)$. Response adaptation and desentization can then be formulated as allowable variation in the parameters of the interfaces.

Whereas dose–response relationships in the above three axes have been largely defined for individual nodes acting in isolation (e.g., GnRH's stimulation of LH secretion, LH's receptor-mediated stimulation of testosterone and estrogen secretion), the implicitly dynamic nature of this network arises from the time-lagged nonlinear feedback and feedforward interactions among all three interconnected loci.

II. THE HPT (GnRH–LH–Te) MODEL, AS REPRESENTATIVE OF RECEPTOR-MEDIATED SYSTEMS

Secretion of a hormone is usually viewed as occurring in two fractions. There is an approximately constant basal secretion as well as nonbasal secretion, the latter being highly variable and fluctuating. For steroid hormones (e.g., Te), nonbasal secretion occurs as a continuous release. For peptide hormones (e.g., GnRH and LH), there is variable mass accumulation within the endocrine gland, which is released in a pulsatile manner. In either case, upon release from a gland, hormones within the capillary bloodstream are immediately subjected to at least two primary dispersive forces: physical diffusion within the plasma space and advective effects of blood flow within the tubular capallaries. The process of irreversible (metabolic) removal of the hormone molecules can take place in the systemic circulation, since blood is delivered to metabolizing tissues, such as the liver, kidneys, and bone marrow macrophages.

Suppose that the systemic circulation can be described topologically as a circle (S^1) of length L. Let $X(x, t)$ be the concentration and $Z(x, t)$ be the rate of secretion at time $0 \leq t \leq T$ and at location $x \in S^1$. Also, let α_i be the elimination rate constant and D_i and A_i the diffusion and advection constants. It is assumed that the concentration dynamics, with initial conditions $X_i(x, 0) = X_i^0(x)$, are described by

$$\frac{\partial X_i(x, t)}{\partial t} = D_i \frac{\partial^2 X_i(x, t)}{\partial t^2} + A_i \frac{\partial X_i(x, t)}{\partial x} - \alpha_i X_i(x, t) + Z_i(x, t)$$

where G denotes GnRH, L denotes LH, and Te denotes testosterone.

The difficulty with that implementation is that blood sampling is ordinarily performed at a single site x_* and for practical reasons probably always will be. Hence, a representation of the above equation applicable to the sampling at a single location (x_*) is needed. The following approximation can be justified (for a given hormone), where the dependency on $x = x_*$ is left implicit; e.g., $X_G(x_*, t)$ and $Z_G(x_*, t)$ are represented as $X_G(t)$ and $Z_G(t)$, respectively, $i = $ G, L, Te,

$$X_i(t) \approx X_i(0)(a_i^{(1)} e^{-\alpha_i^{(1)} t} + a_i^{(2)} e^{-\alpha_i^{(2)} t}) + \int_0^t (a_i^{(1)} e^{-\alpha_i^{(1)}(t-s)} + a_i^{(2)} e^{-\alpha_i^{(2)}(t-r)}) Z_i(s) ds,$$

where $\alpha_i^{(1)}$ can be interpreted as a fast half-life of elimination (primarily diffusion and advection) and $\alpha_i^{(2)}$ as a slow half-life of elimination (irreversible clearance). The $a_i^{(1)}$ and $a_i^{(2)}$ are fractional amounts of secretion, with $a_i^{(1)}$ estimated as 0.63 for LH and 0.76 for Te. The variations among individuals and within a given individual appear to be quite stable, with 0.63 and 0.76 being reasonable representative values. At present, these values have not yet been determined for GnRH.

In order to apply the above model for concentration $(X_i(\cdot))$, models for the rates of secretion for GnRH, L, and Te are formulated in the following sections.

A. GnRH Pulse Generator

The pulsatile nature of GnRH and LH secretion was first discovered in the rhesus monkey and then later in human and other species. There are on the order of 800–1200 GnRH-secreting neurons, each connected to its own individual network of glial cells; the resulting random pulsatile structure is partly modulated by feedback inhibition via testosterone receptors, as well as by a synchronization of network firing frequencies. It is assumed that GnRH signaling dictates the pulse times for LH after a finite time delay τ_L, reflecting hypothalamo–pituitary portal blood transit, and a poststimulus refractory interval, r_L, when further GnRH inputs are ignored. Thus, there will be two corresponding sets of pulse times $T_G^0, T_G^1, T_G^2, \ldots$ and $T_L^0, T_L^1, T_L^2, \ldots$, where

$$T_L^k = Min_j \{ T_G^j | T_G^j \geq T_L^{k-1} + r_L \} + \tau_L,$$

with $T_G^0 = T_L^0 = 0$.

Here the pulse times are viewed as a point process, with $N_i(\cdot)$, $i = G$, L being the associated counting processes (i.e., the number of pulses up to that time). The GnRH pulse times are then assumed to be given by a rate parameter process $\lambda(\cdot)$ (number of pulses/day), modulated by feedback:

$$\lambda(t) = H_{1,2}\left[\int_{(t-l_{1,2})}^{(t-l_{1,1})} X_{Te}(r)dr, \int_{(t-l_{2,2})}^{(t-l_{2,1})} X_G(r)dr \right]$$

and a parameter γ, which controls the regularity of interpulse interval lengths. The conditional probability densities for T_G^k given T_G^{k-1} are

$$p\left[s | T_G^{k-1}, \lambda(\cdot)\right] = \gamma \times \lambda(s) \left(\int_{T_G^{k-1}}^{s} \lambda(r)dr \right)^{\gamma-1}$$
$$\times \exp\left[-\left[\int_{T_G^{k-1}}^{s} \lambda(r)dr \right]^{\gamma} \right].$$

B. Synthesis

A pulsatile rate of secretion means that release is not continuous, but rather at certain times (the pulse times), the rate of secretion rapidly increases, followed by a less rapid decrease; this combined increase and decrease in the rate of secretion will be called a pulse. A pulse at time t, having started at pulse time T^j, is represented by a function $M^j \times \psi(t-T^j)$, where the pulse shape $\psi(\cdot)$ represents the instantaneous rate of secretion per unit mass per distributional volume and M^j is the total mass available for release.

The mathematical effect of cascading target-tissue reactions to a GnRH signal input is (approximately) the multiplication of the initial feedback/feed-forward signal by a linear combination of exponential functions, denoted by $\Gamma_G(\cdot)$, which allows ongoing glandular responses after the signal is withdrawn. Accordingly, synthesis (S), accumulation (C), and fractional mass remaining for later secretion (Ψ) are given as

$$\psi_i(s) = \frac{\beta_i^{(3)}}{\Gamma(\beta_i^{(1)})(\beta_i^{(2)})^{(\beta_i^{(1)}\beta_i^{(3)})}} s^{(\beta_i^{(1)}\beta_i^{(3)})-1}$$
$$\times e^{-(s/\beta_i^{(2)})^{\beta_i^{(3)}}}$$

(normalized rates of secretion for

$i = G, L$) (a 3-parameter gamma

function)

$$\Psi_i(T_i^{j-1}, T_i^j) = \int_{T_i^{j-1}}^{T_i^j} \psi_i(s - T_i^j)ds$$

(fraction of $(j-1) - $ st mass

remaining at time $T_i^j, i = G, L$)

$$S_L(t) = H_{5,6}\left[\int_{T_L^{N_L(t)}-l_{5,2}}^{T_L^{N_L(t)}-l_{5,1}} X_G(s)ds \right.$$
$$\times \Gamma_G\left(t - T_L^{N_L(t)}\right), \left. \int_{t-l_{6,2}}^{t-l_{6,1}} X_{Te}(s)ds + \xi_L(t) \right]$$

(LH synthesis) (expected LH synthesis

rate + allowable variation (ξ))

$$S_G(t) = H_3 \left(\oint_{t-l_{3,2}}^{t-l_{3,1}} X_{Te}(s)ds \right) + \xi_G(t)$$

(GnRH synthesis)

$$A_L^j = \int_{T_L^{j-1}}^{T_L^j} \xi_L(t)dt \text{ and }$$

$$A_G^j = \int_{T_G^{j-1}}^{T_G^j} \xi_G(t)dt$$

(allowable variation in LH
and GnRH mass accumulation)

$$C_L^j = \int_{T_L^{j-1}}^{T_L^j} H_{5,6} \left(\oint_{T_L^{N_L(t)}-l_{5,2}}^{T_L^{N_L(t)}-l_{5,1}} X_G(s)ds \times \Gamma_G(t - T_L^{N_L(t)}), \right.$$
$$\left. \oint_{t-l_{6,2}}^{t-l_{6,1}} X_{Te}(s)ds \right) dt + A_L^j$$

(the storage of newly synthesized LH granules)

$$\approx [\eta_L^{(0)} + \eta_L^{(1)} \times (T_L^j - T_L^{j-1})] + A_L^j$$

$$C_G^j = \int_{T_G^{j-1}}^{T_G^j} H_3 \left(\oint_{t-l_{3,2}}^{t-l_{3,1}} X_{Te}(s)ds \right) dt + A_G^j$$

$$\approx [\eta_G^{(0)} + \eta_G^{(1)} \times (T_G^j - T_G^{j-1})] + A_G^j$$

$$M_i^j = \Psi_i(T_i^{j-1}, T_i^j) M_i^{j-1} + C_i^j$$

(the j-th pulse mass, for $i = L, G$)

$$\approx \Psi_i(T_i^{j-1}, T_i^j) M_i^{j-1} + [\eta_i^{(0)} + \eta_i^{(1)} \times (T_i^j - T_i^{j-1})]$$
$$+ A_i^j$$

$$F_L(t) = \oint_{t-l_{4,2}}^{t-l_{4,1}} X_L(s) \, ds$$

(LH feed-forward signal on Te synthesis)

$$S_{Te}(t) = H_4(F_L(t)) = H_4(\oint_{t-l_{4,2}}^{t-l_{4,1}} X_L(s)ds)$$

C. Secretion

Based upon the above constructions, the corresponding interactively controlled rates of secretion for L, G, and Te are given as

$$Z_L(t) = \beta_L + \sum_{j:T_L^j \le t} [(\eta_L^{(0)} + \eta_L^{(1)} \times (T_L^j - T_L^{j-1})$$

$$+ A_L^j]\psi_L \, (t - T_L^j)$$

$$Z_G(t) = \beta_G + \sum_{j:T_L^j \le t} [(\eta_G^{(0)} + \eta_G^{(1)} \times (T_G^j - T_G^{j-1})$$

$$+ A_G^j]\psi_G \, (t - T_G^j)$$

$$Z_{Te}(t) = S_{Te}(t) = \eta_0 + \frac{\eta_1 + A_{Te}^j}{1 + e^{-(\eta_2 + \eta_3 \times F_L(t))}},$$

$$T_L^{j-1} < t \le T_L^j$$

(A_{Te}^j's, allowable random variations in upper
asymptote (efficacy))

Hence, the basic secretory model for LH and GnRH consists of two components: basal (β) and pulsatile (non-basal) secretion. The amount of mass that accumulates is assumed to be proportional to the previous interpulse interval, plus an allowable random variation (the A_L^j's and A_G^j's). If there were mass accumulation at a rate that randomly varied about a steady-state rate, then the result would be precisely this. Testosterone, also has two components (basal and non-basal), except that the non-basal secretion is assumed to be released continuously, without storage. Moreover, the non-basal component is assumed to be described by a logistic interface function of an LH feed-forward signal, a time-delayed averaging of LH concentration. Again, as in the modeling of the LH and GnRH secretion, flexibility in the structure needs to be allowed. Here, there is allowable pulse-by-pulse variation in the upper asymptote (i.e., efficacy) of the dose-response function, reflecting potential desensitization or adaptation. These models for GnRH, LH, and testosterone secretion reflect the essence of the title: receptor-mediated interlinkages.

D. Concentrations

Incorporating the above secretion rates, the resulting concentration processes are then (approximately) given as: $i = G, L, Te$.

$$X_i(t) = X_i(0)\left[a_i^{(1)}e^{-\alpha_i^{(1)}t} + a_i^{(2)}e^{-\alpha_i^{(2)}t}\right] +$$

$$\int_0^t \left[a_i^{(1)}e^{-\alpha_i^{(1)}(t-s)} + a_i^{(2)}e^{-\alpha_i^{(2)}(t-s)}\right]Z_i(s)ds.$$

What one then observes is a discrete-time sampling of these processes, plus joint uncertainty due to blood withdrawal, sample processing, and hormone measurement errors, $\epsilon_i(k)$, $k = 1, \ldots, n$,

$$Y_i(t_k) = X_i(t_k) + \epsilon_i(k), \quad k = 1, \ldots, n, \quad i = G, L, Te.$$

Using the statistical methods developed, which implement the above models, statistical fits can be obtained for the GnRH, LH, and testosterone

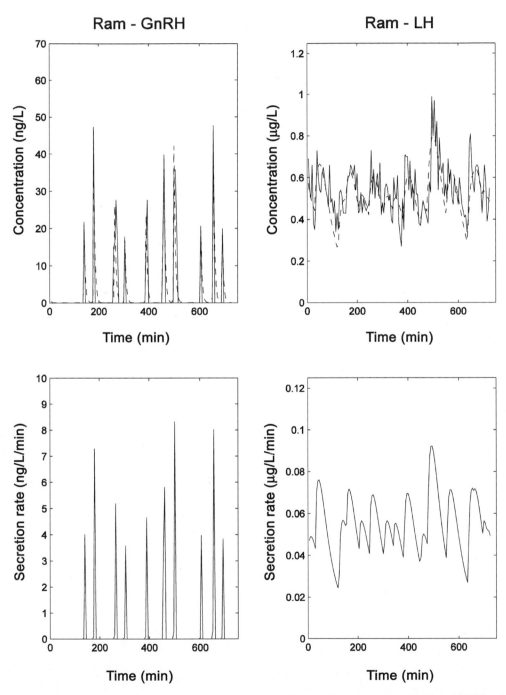

FIGURE 2 GnRH, LH and Te concentrations were obtained in a conscious ram, every 5 min for 12 hours. (Top) GnRH (left) and LH (right) concentrations (continuous line) and their model fits (dashed). (Bottom) Estimated GnRH (left) and LH (right) secretion rates.

concentrations, as well as the estimation of their unobserved secretion rates. The next section presents two applications of the methodology.

E. Applications

For exposition of the above model, data obtained from a ram and a stallion is used. In each, all three of the hormones (GnRH, LH, and Te) were measured. In the ram, blood was sampled every 5 minutes for 12 hours. In the stallion, the sampling was over 6 hours, with GnRH and LH sampled every 5 minutes at the pituitary, and Te and LH sampled every 15 minutes at a jugular. The results are presented in Figs. 2 and 3 for the ram and in Figs. 4 and 5 for the horse. Figure 2 (top) displays the GnRH and LH

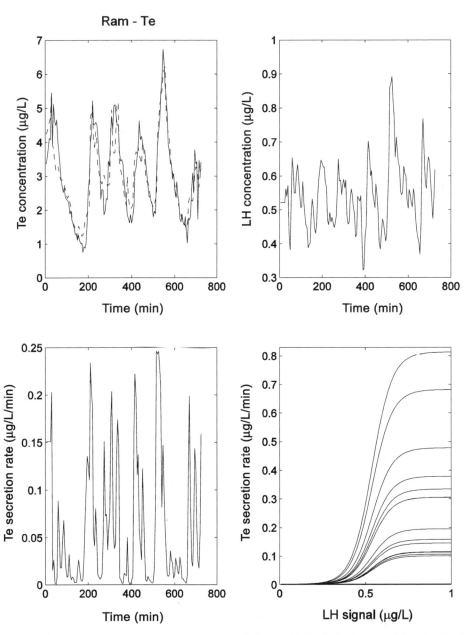

FIGURE 3 (Top left) Te concentration (continuous line) and the model fit (dashed), and (right) the LH feed-forward signal on Te. (Bottom left) The estimated Te secretion right, and (right) the dose-response function, with the allowable, random, pulse-by-pulse responsivity (efficacy) shifts.

concentrations (continuous line) and their respective model fits (dashed line). The bottom half of Fig. 2 shows the corresponding estimated secretion rates for GnRH and LH. Figure 3, top left, shows the observed Te concentrations (continuous line) and the model fit (dashed line) and the LH feed-forward signal is shown in the top right. The bottom

left of Fig. 3 shows the estimated Te secretion rate and in the bottom right is the dose-response function, with the allowable, random, pulse-by-pulse responsitivity (efficacy) shifts. Figures 4 and 5 contain the same plots for the horse, with the addition of LH being observed at both the pituitary and the jugular.

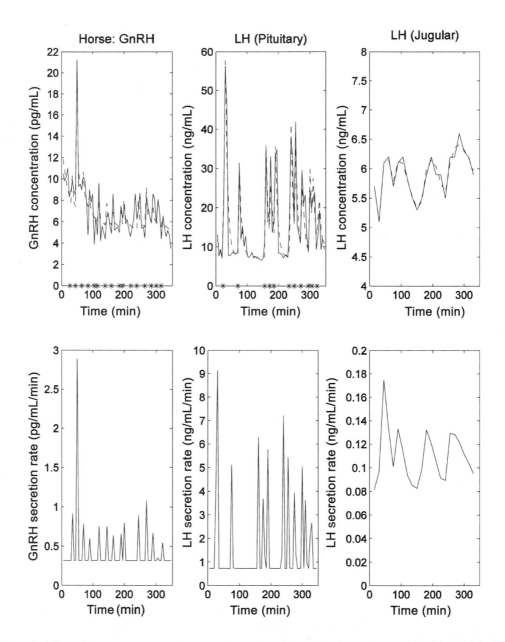

FIGURE 4   GnRH and LH concentration time series monitored every 5 min in pituitary blood, and Te and LH were monitored every 15 min in jugular blood, for 6 hours in an awake stallion. Figures 4 and 5 include the same information format as in Figs. 2 and 3 (with an additional panel for jugular LH). (Top) GnRH (left) and LH (right) concentrations (continuous line) and their model fits (dashed). (Bottom) Estimated GnRH (left) and LH (right) secretion rates.

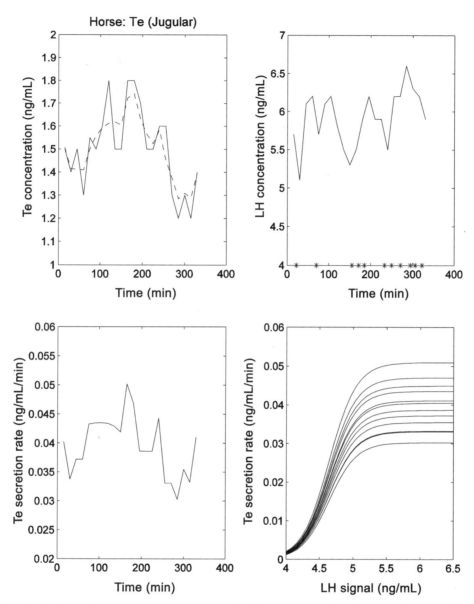

FIGURE 5 (Top) GnRH (left) and LH (right) concentrations (continuous line) and their model fits (dashed). (Bottom) Estimated GnRH (left) and LH (right) secretion rates Figure 5 (Top left) Te concentration (continuous line) and the model fit (dashed), and (right) the LH feed-forward signal on Te. (Bottom left) The estimated Te secretion right, and (right) the dose-response function, with the allowable, random, pulse-by-pulse responsivity (efficacy) shifts.

Acknowledgments

This work was supported by the National Institute of Health (Bethesda, MD) grants K01 AG19164 (DK), R01 AG14799 (JV), and R01 AG19164 (JV).

Glossary

dose–response interface function A function (e.g., a logistic function) whose response output is an instan- taneous rate of hormone synthesis, mass accumulation, or release.

fast and slow elimination Secreted molecules undergo combined diffusion and transport in the bloodstream at very rapid rates (short half-life component, $\alpha^{(1)}$) and are removed more slowly but irreversibly (long half-life component, $\alpha^{(2)}$).

feedback and/or feed-forward signal A signal at time t, constructed as a time-delayed, time-averaging of a hormone concentration (or its rate of change) that serves as an input (driver) to the dose–response interface function.

pulse generator A process, possibly modulated by feedback, that governs the resulting, variable-pulse time-release pattern for a pulsatile secreting gland.

receptor-mediated system A physiological system (e.g., a hormonal axis) whose linkages are interconnected via receptor mechanisms (interface functions).

See Also the Following Article

Receptor–Receptor Interactions

Further Reading

Blum, J. J., Reed, M. C., Janovick, J. A., and Conn, P. M. (2000). A mathematical model quantifying GnRH-induced LH secretion from gonadotropes. *Am. J. Physiol.* **278**, E263–E272.

Keenan, D. M., Licinio, J., and Veldhuis, J. D. (2001). Interactive construct of feedback control in the stress-responsive hypothalamo–pituitary–adrenal axis. *Proc. Natl Acad. Sci. USA* **98**, 4028–4033.

Keenan, D. M., Sun, W., and Veldhuis, J. D. (2000). A stochastic dynamical model of the male reproductive hormone system. *SIAM J. Appl. Math.* **61**, 934–965.

Keenan, D. M., and Veldhuis, J. D. (1997). A stochastic model of admixed basal and pulsatile hormone secretion as modulated by a deterministic oscillator. *Am. J. Physiol.* **273**, R1182–R1192.

Keenan, D. M., and Veldhuis, J. D. (1998). A biomathematical model of time-delayed feedback in the human male hypothalamic–pituitary–Leydig cell axis. *Am. J. Physiol.* **275**, E157–E176.

Keenan, D. and Veldhuis, J. D. (2001). Hypothesis testing of the aging male gonadal axis via a biomathematical construct. *Am. J. Physiol.* **280**, R1755–R1771.

Keenan, D. and Veldhuis, J. D. (2001). Disruptions in the hypothalamic luteinizing-hormone pulsing mechanism in aging men. *Am. J. Physiol.* **281**, R1917–R1924.

Keenan, D. and Veldhuis, J. D. (2002). Statistical reconstruction of hormone secretion rates based upon a composite advection-diffusion-elimination-secretion model. (submitted for publication).

Keenan, D. M., and Veldhuis, J. D. (2000). Explicating hypergonadotropism in postmenopausal women: A statistical model. *Am. J. Physiol.* **278**, R1247–R1257.

Keenan, D. M., Veldhuis, J. D., and Yang, R. (1998). Joint recovery of pulsatile and basal hormone secretion by stochastic nonlinear random-effects analysis. *Am. J. Physiol.* **44**, R1939–R1949.

Veldhuis, J. D. (1999). Male hypothalamic–pituitary–testicular axis. *In* "Reproductive Endocrinology" (S. S. C. Yen, R. B. Jaffe, R. L. Barbieri, ed.), pp. 622–631. Saunders, Philadelphia.

Receptor–Receptor Interactions

Lakshmi A. Devi

Mount Sinai School of Medicine

The function of every cell in the body is regulated by plasma membrane receptors. The dimerization of receptors has been an extensively studied phenomenon. Receptor–receptor associations lead to changes in receptor function by modulating receptor ligand affinity, signaling properties, and trafficking properties. These interactions could be useful to modulate receptor activation and may provide strategies for therapeutic applications.

I. INTRODUCTION

The vast majority of plasma membrane receptors belong to the superfamily of G-protein-coupled receptors (GPCRs), which at current estimates account for ~1% of the genes present in a mammalian genome. Models describing the interaction of GPCRs with their G-protein targets have been based on the assumption that the receptors exist as monomers and couple to G-proteins in a 1:1 ratio. These classical models of receptor/G-protein coupling may be oversimplified, because a number of studies have reported the presence of dimeric and oligomeric arrays in the case of a number of GPCRs. Direct protein–protein interaction (GPCR oligomerization) has not been previously recognized despite a significant amount of indirect evidence derived from cross-linking experiments, target size analysis, and hydrodynamic studies. The availability of GPCR complementary DNAs (cDNAs) now allows direct examination of receptor–receptor association by biochemical and biophysical techniques.

II. METHODS TO STUDY PROTEIN–PROTEIN INTERACTIONS

A. Functional Complementation Assays

One of the techniques used for the study of protein–protein interactions has been functional complementation. For this, mutant receptors that are nonfunctional or partially functional are generated either by site-directed mutagenesis or by exchanging individual domains between two distinct types of receptors (chimeras). If co-expression of these receptors results in increased functional activity as compared to individual receptors, it is taken as a measure of physical association between receptors. Functional complementation studies have documented the association between receptors of the same family as well as between receptors of distantly related families. Such functional complementation studies have been useful in predicting the domains involved in the interaction and have led to modeling studies examining the mechanisms of receptor–receptor interaction.

B. Biochemical Techniques

In order to facilitate physical isolation of the interacting receptor–receptor complexes, differential epitope tagging and immunoisolation have been used. Typically, epitope tags (short peptide sequences from proteins that are not commonly expressed in eukaryotic tissues) are expressed at the N- or C-termini of GPCRs. cDNAs harboring distinct epitopes are co-expressed in heterologous cells. Selective immunoprecipitation of the epitope-tagged complex is achieved using antisera to one of the epitopes. The immunoprecipitate is subjected to size fractionation and the second receptor in the complex is visualized using antisera to the epitope on the second receptor. Depending on the conditions of solubilization and immunoprecipitation, there is a possibility that artifactual aggregation of proteins occurs (due to the inherent hydrophobic nature of GPCRs). This can be overcome by using stringent buffers for solubilization and immunoprecipitation. For example, the presence of a disulfide capping agent (such as iodoacetamide) in the buffers used in the receptor complex isolation process reduces chances of spurious formation of disulfide bonds. Treatment of cells with cross-linking agents followed by extraction with a combination of detergents with diverse physical properties is also helpful to disrupt nonspecific aggregation. An important control for these studies is to mix cells individually expressing receptors that are epitope tagged with distinct epitopes and to subject the mixture to solubilization and immunoprecipitation procedures identical to procedures using cells co-expressing these receptors. In the majority of cases, receptor–receptor interaction is seen only on co-expression of the two receptors. Another control is to co-express GPCRs that are known not to interact. Therefore, when the appropriate controls are used, immunoprecipitation is a valid technique for detecting GPCR dimers.

C. Biophysical Techniques

Proximity-based energy transfer assays have been used to study receptor–receptor interactions in living cells. The bioluminescence resonance energy transfer (BRET) technique measures the transfer of energy between a luminescent donor (luciferase) and a fluorescent acceptor [a mutant form of green fluorescent protein (GFP)]. The catalytic degradation of the substrate coelenterazine, by luciferase, leads to the release of bioluminescent energy that can excite mutant GFP; the resulting fluorescence emission is taken as a measure of physical proximity between the two proteins. Because the Forster energy transfer occurs only when the distance between the donor and acceptor is less than 100 Å, this method is ideally suited to examine receptor–receptor interactions. For this, fusion proteins of GPCRs are generated by genetically fusing luciferase or the mutant GFP to their N- or C-termini.

If a BRET signal is detected on co-expression of these fusion proteins in heterologous cells in the absence of agonist treatment, it is taken as a measure of constitutive dimers in intact cells. The selectivity of the BRET signal is measured by expressing GPCR fusion proteins of different families. BRET signals can detect interactions that occur within the cells as well as on the cell surface. Agonist treatment can cause an increase in the number of receptors in the clathrin-coated pits and this can cause an increase in the BRET signal as a result of increased clustering of receptors. Conditions that block receptor clustering (such as $0.4 M$ sucrose treatment or a dominant-negative mutant of dynamin that is known to block agonist-mediated internalization of GPCRs) have been used to examine receptor–receptor interactions at the cell surface.

Fluorescence resonance energy transfer (FRET) measures the Forster resonance energy transfer between two fluorophores that emit fluorescence at nonoverlapping wavelengths. The efficiency of FRET depends on the overlap in the spectrum of the two fluorophores, their relative orientation, and the distance between them. Typically, fusion proteins of GPCRs (which are fused to two different forms of green fluorescent proteins) are used as donor and acceptor. An external light source is used to excite the donor and the light emitted by the donor excites the acceptor. This method has been used to demonstrate agonist-mediated changes in the level or conformation of receptor–receptor association. A related method, photobleaching FRET, has also been used for examining changes in interactions of receptors on agonist exposure. In this method, antisera conjugated to two different fluorophores (such as fluorescein and rhodamine) are used to bind the receptor. The decrease in the fluorescence intensity of the donor (fluorescein) as a result of photobleaching during prolonged exposure to excitation light is reduced by the acceptor (rhodamine). Because the close proximity of the acceptor slows down the photobleaching process, association between receptors leads to an increase in the photobleaching time constant. Photobleaching FRET is a useful technique to examine the interaction between receptors at the cell surface and has been used to measure changes in interaction mediated by the agonist with a variety of combinations of GPCRs of the rhodopsin family.

BRET and FRET can also be used to measure the strength of interactions between two receptors. For this, increasing amounts of the untagged receptor are co-expressed with a fixed amount of the luciferase-tagged and mutant GFP-tagged GPCR. The concentration of the competitor that decreases the signal by 50% is used to compare the strength of interactions.

III. ROLE FOR RECEPTOR–RECEPTOR INTERACTIONS IN RECEPTOR ACTIVITY

Receptor–receptor interactions have varied effects on the activities of GPCRs. It appears that receptors that are closely related (i.e., members of the same subfamily) as well as distantly related (i.e., members of distinct subfamilies) interact with each other, and this interaction differentially modulates their function (a few examples are shown in Table 1). In some cases, receptor interactions are required for surface expression and generation of functional receptors. In other cases, interactions between two functional receptors lead to the generation of receptors with novel binding properties. Some of these receptors are refractory to selective ligands; activation of both receptors is required for efficient ligand binding and signaling. In some cases receptor–receptor

TABLE I Regulation of GPCR Function by Heteromeric Interactions

Receptor	Modulation of function
Members of the same subfamily	
$GABA_BR_{1a}$–$GABA_BR_2$	Surface expression and signaling
κ–δ opioid	Signaling and trafficking
μ–δ opioid	Signaling
$SSTR_1$–$SSTR_5$ (somatostatin)	Signaling and trafficking
$SSTR_2$–$SSTR_3$ (somatostatin)	Signaling and trafficking
M_2–M_3 (muscarinic)	Signaling
Members of the same family	
$α_{2c}$-adrenergic–M_3 (muscarinic)	Signaling
$SSTR_5$ (somatostatin)–D_2 (dopamine)	Signaling
AT_1(angiotensin)–B_2 (bradykinin)	Signaling and trafficking
δ opioid–$β_2$-adrenergic	Trafficking
κ opioid–$β_2$-adrenergic	Trafficking
Members of different families[a]	
A_1 (adenosine)–$mGluR_1$ (glutamate)	Signaling

[a]Families A and C.

association leads to alterations in the agonist affinity as well as the efficacy and in others only the agonist efficacy is altered. Receptors that couple to distinct G-proteins are able to interact with each other, and this interaction has been shown to differentially affect the signal transduction pathway and/or level of signaling. Receptor–receptor interactions can increase or decrease the level of receptor desensitization due to alterations in agonist-mediated endocytosis of the receptor. Finally, a role for receptor–receptor interaction in the development of pathology has been documented in the case of angiotensin–bradykinin receptor interactions.

IV. FACTORS THAT MODULATE RECEPTOR–RECEPTOR INTERACTIONS

There is a growing body of evidence to support the proposal that GPCRs interact with each other in the absence of agonist. In a large number of cases, receptor–receptor interactions appear to occur in the biosynthetic compartments (i.e., in the endoplasmic reticulum) and to be required for efficient maturation of receptors. However, in some cases, receptors appear to exist as noninteracting units that undergo increased association mediated by the agonist, as evidenced by biochemical and biophysical studies.

In a subset of cases, GPCRs have been shown to interact with other proteins (such as growth factor receptors, ion channels, receptor activity-modifying proteins, and other intracellular signaling molecules), and these interactions result in efficient surface expression, change in the cellular localization, and/or alteration in their functional activity.

V. DOMAINS OF RECEPTOR–RECEPTOR INTERACTIONS

An examination of the possible sites for receptor–receptor interactions has implicated the involvement of extracellular, transmembrane, and/or C-terminal regions in GPCR association. The evidence accumulated thus far points to transmembrane domain-mediated contacts that lead to receptor–receptor interactions. Hydrophobic interactions within the transmembrane domain are thought to provide the proper receptor conformation to facilitate additional interactions at other domains. Hydrophobic interaction via the coiled-coil domain in the C-tail has also been documented in the case of metabotropic γ-aminobutyric acid receptor. Although in the majority of the cases the interactions are mainly hydrophobic in nature, in some cases covalent interactions do occur. Crystallographic studies of the extracellular domain of metabotropic glutamate receptors have identified cysteine residues involved in the covalent homomeric interactions.

VI. SUMMARY

In conclusion, the study of GPCR interactions is a nascent field and studies thus far support the notion that receptor–receptor associations lead to changes in receptor function by modulating their ligand affinity, signaling, and trafficking properties. These interactions could be useful to modulate receptor activation following the corelease of selective endogenous ligands *in vivo*. Alternatively, these interactions could lead to the generation of a hitherto uncharacterized receptor for a unique endogenous ligand. The number of endogenous peptide ligands far exceeds the number of cloned GPCRs. These endogenous peptides could bind and activate interacting receptors that exhibit novel pharmacology; this could explain GPCR subtypes in some cases. Direct physical interactions between GPCRs have enormous ramifications for our understanding of how their actions are regulated. Furthermore, these findings provide a new strategy for the development of novel therapies.

Glossary

BRET/FRET Measures of the bioluminescence/fluorescence energy transfer from the light emitted by catalytic degradation of the substrate coelenterazine, by Renilla luciferase, to the energy acceptor green fluorescent protein. FRET is similar to BRET with the exception that the energy donor molecule, generally a mutant form of green fluorescent protein (cyan fluorescent protein) is excited by an external light source and the emitted energy is used to excite an acceptor, another mutant of green fluorescent protein (yellow or red fluorescent proteins).

differential immunoprecipitation Technique for isolation and visualization of interacting proteins using distinct antisera to individual proteins.

dimers/oligomers Two monomers/multiple monomers in association; a given G-protein-coupled receptor can exist as monomer, homo- or heterodimer, or homo- or heterooligomer.

functional complementation Technique in which coexpression of two receptors that are nonfunctional or partially functional leads to improved functional activity.

G-protein-coupled receptor Heptahelical or serpentine seven-transmembrane-domain receptor.

G-protein-coupled receptor families Three major receptor families: Family A is characterized by a relatively short N-terminal extracellular region, conserved residues in transmembrane helices, and a palmitoylated cysteine in the carboxy-terminal tail. Family B is characterized by the presence of a large N-terminal extracellular domain that contains several well-conserved cysteine residues. Family C is characterized by a very long N-terminal extracellular domain that is sufficient for ligand binding.

homomers/heteromers Physical association between identical proteins leads to homomers and association between nonidentical proteins leads to heteromers.

See Also the Following Article

GPCR (G-Protein-Coupled Receptor) Structure

Further Reading

Bouvier, M. (2001). Oligomerization of G-protein-coupled transmitter receptors. *Nat. Neurosci.* **2**, 274–286.

Cornea, A., Janovick, J. A., Maya-Nunez, G., and Conn, P. M. (2001). Gonadotropin-releasing hormone receptor microaggregation. Rate monitored by fluorescence resonance energy transfer. *J. Biol. Chem.* **276**, 2153–2158.

Devi, L. A. (2001). Heterodimerization of G-protein-coupled receptors: pharmacology, signaling and trafficking. *Trends Pharmacol. Sci.* **22**, 532–537.

Hebert, T. E., Moffett, S., Morello, J. P., Loisel, T. P., Bichet, D. G., Barret, C., and Bouvier, M. (1996). A peptide derived from a β2-adrenergic receptor transmembrane domain inhibits both receptor dimerization and activation. *J. Biol. Chem.* **271**, 16384–16392.

Jones, K. A., Borowski, B., Tamm, J. A., Craig, D. A., Durkin, M. M., Dai, M., Yao, W.-J., Johnson, M., Gunwaldsen, C., Huang, L.-Y., Tang, C., Shen, Q., Salon, J. A., Morse, K., Laz, T., Smith, K. E., Nagarathnam, D., Noble, S. A., Branchek, T. A., and Gerald, C. (1998). GABA$_B$ receptor function as a heterotrimeric assembly of the subunits GABA$_B$R1 and GABA$_B$R2. *Nature* **396**, 674–679.

Jordan, B. A., and Devi, L. A. (1999). G-Protein-coupled receptor heterodimerization modulates receptor function. *Nature* **399**, 697–700.

Kaupmann, K., Malitschek, B., Schuler, V., Heid, J., Froestl, W., Beck, P., Mosbscher, J., Bischoff, S., Kulik, A., Shigemoto, R., Karschin, A., and Bettler, B. (1998). GABA$_B$-receptor subtypes assemble into functional heteromeric complexes. *Nature* **396**, 683–686.

Kunishima, N., Shimada, Y., Tsuji, Y., Sato, T., Yamamoto, M., Kumasaka, T., Nakanishi, S., Jingami, H., and Morikawa, K. (2000). Structural basis of glutamate recognition by a dimeric metabotropic glutamate receptor. *Nature* **407**, 971–977.

Maggio, R., Vogel, Z., and Wess, J. (1993). Coexpression studies with mutant muscarinic/adrenergic receptors provide evidence for intermolecular "cross-talk" between G-protein-linked receptors. *Proc. Natl. Acad. Sci. U.S.A.* **90**, 3103–3107.

Margeta-Mitrovic, M., Jan, Y. N., and Jan, L. Y. (2000). A trafficking checkpoint controls GABA(B) receptor heterodimerization. *Neuron* **27**, 97–110.

Marshall, F. H., Jones, K. A., Kaupmann, K., and Bettler, B. (1999). GABA$_B$ receptors-the first 7TM heterodimers. *Trends Pharmacol. Sci.* **20**, 396–399.

Milligan, G. (2001). Oligomerisation of G-protein-coupled receptors. *J. Cell Sci.* **114**, 1265–1271.

Overton, M. C., and Blumer, K. J. (2000). G-Protein-coupled receptors function as oligomers *in vivo*. *Curr. Biol.* **10**, 341–344.

Romano, C., Yang, W. L., and O'Malley, K. L. (1996). Metabotropic glutamate receptor 5 is a disulfide-linked dimer. *J. Biol. Chem.* **271**, 28612–28616.

Reproductive Stress

See *Stress and Reproduction*

Retinoid Receptors

PETER ORDENTLICH AND RICHARD A. HEYMAN
X-Ceptor Therapeutics, Inc., California

Retinoids are metabolic and synthetic derivatives of vitamin A that have been shown to play an essential role in regulating multiple processes including development, vision, growth, and physiological homeostasis.

I. INTRODUCTION

The majority of these effects are mediated through direct binding to a group of receptors that belong to the nuclear hormone receptor superfamily of proteins. These retinoid receptors fall into two families, retinoic acid receptors (RARs) and retinoid X receptors (RXRs). There are three receptors in each group, RARα, RARβ, RARγ, and RXRα, RXRβ, RXRγ, respectively. The retinoid receptors function as transcriptional regulators in the presence or absence of ligand, through the recruitment of multisubunit regulatory protein complexes to promoter sites. Other factors that influence the action of retinoids include the enzymes and proteins that are required to transport and metabolize retinoids. This article will provide an overview of the RAR and RXR receptors with regard to their structure, mechanism of action, biological activities, and role in disease states.

II. RECEPTOR IDENTIFICATION

Two independent groups identified the first retinoid receptor, RARα, in 1987 using similar approaches. In one case, low-stringency hybridization screening of a cDNA library, with a consensus oligonucleotide sequence based on a highly conserved region of the DNA-binding domain, resulted in successful cloning of a novel sequence with homology to other nuclear hormone receptors. The other group designed a similar screening strategy based upon the finding that in a human hepatocellular carcinoma, the hepatitis B virus genome inserted upstream of a sequence that showed strong homology to other nuclear hormone receptors. Subsequently, it was shown that this receptor, RARα, could bind and be activated by retinoic acid.

Based on sequence homology in the DNA-binding domain, RARβ and RARγ were later identified and also shown to bind and be activated by retinoic acid (Fig. 1). The three RARs are highly conserved in both

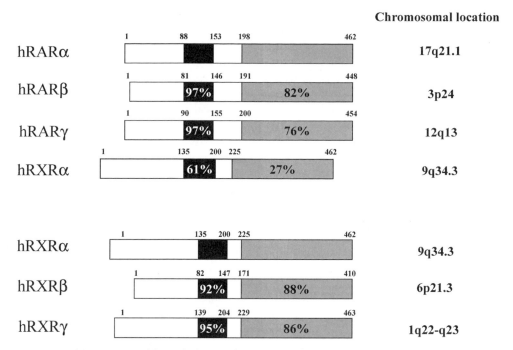

Chromosomal location

Receptor		Chromosomal location
hRARα		17q21.1
hRARβ	97% / 82%	3p24
hRARγ	97% / 76%	12q13
hRXRα	61% / 27%	9q34.3
hRXRα		9q34.3
hRXRβ	92% / 88%	6p21.3
hRXRγ	95% / 86%	1q22-q23

FIGURE 1 Retinoid receptors and homologies A schematic representation of the members of the retinoid receptor family. The diagram provides the amino acid boundaries of the DNA-binding domains (black) and ligand-binding domains (gray) for the receptors. Included also is the amino acid homology of the ligand-binding domains within each class, i.e., RAR and RXR, and also the homology between RXRα and RARα. The DNA-binding domains are generally conserved (greater than 60%) among all the retinoid receptors, whereas the ligand-binding domains are conserved (greater than 75%) within each receptor family, but not between the RAR and RXR (less than 30%) groups. The chromosomal location of each receptor that has been identified in humans is shown as reference.

the DNA-binding domain (97%) and the ligand-binding domain (~75% or greater). The RARs exhibit a broad tissue distribution with the specific isoforms having both overlapping and distinct patterns of tissue and developmental expression. RARα expression is ubiquitous, whereas RARβ is more restricted to neural tissues, heart, lung, and spleen. RARγ is the primary isoform expressed in the skin. In addition to the α, β, and γ subtypes of RAR, differential promoter usage and alternative splicing generate multiple isoforms of each subtype to significantly increase the complexity of retinoid responses. Evolutionarily, the RAR receptors are well conserved and the finding of a retinoid-responsive RAR receptor in ascidians (sea squirts) suggests that retinoid receptor signaling existed early in vertebrate development as long as 500 million years ago.

In an attempt to identify other members of the retinoid receptor family, further screening of cDNA libraries resulted in the isolation of an RARα-related receptor, retinoid X receptor (RXRα). The other isoforms of RXR, β and γ, were subsequently isolated (see Fig. 1 for homologies and chromosomal locations). As with the RARs, multiple splice forms

and transcripts expressed from different promoters add to the multiplicity of RXR isoforms. It is possible that the alternative splicing of retinoid receptor promoters and intron–exon boundaries may result in differential tissue expression, transactivation capabilities, and ligand responsiveness of the individual splice forms. RXRα is highly expressed in liver, kidney, lung, muscle, and spleen. RXRβ is generally found in most tissues and RXRγ is expressed predominantly in muscle and brain. Importantly, RXRs have been shown to be critical heterodimer partners for numerous other nuclear hormone receptors, as discussed in detail below. RXR is also well conserved throughout evolution and is considered one of the parental nuclear hormone receptors from which many of the others have evolved. Functional RXRs have been isolated from organisms as primitive as jellyfish, which indicates that they have existed for 600 million or more years. Unlike RAR, a homologue of RXR called ultraspiracle exists in the fruit fly, *Drosophila melanogaster*, although this receptor does not bind 9-*cis*-retinoic acid (9-*cis*-RA) and may not bind any ligand. It is unclear therefore when retinoid receptors developed the response to retinoids or whether, through evolution, some retinoid receptors lost the ability to respond.

The first natural ligand to be identified for retinoid receptors was all-*trans*-retinoic acid (AtRA), the active metabolite of vitamin A. The AtRA was shown to bind with nanomolar affinity to all three isoforms of RAR. Although the homology of RXRs to RARs in the DNA-binding domain is relatively high (61%), the homology in the ligand-binding domain is less than 30%, suggesting that these receptors respond to different classes of ligands (Fig. 1). In experiments designed to identify RXR ligands, it was therefore surprising to find that AtRA could, at high levels, activate RXRα. Ligand-binding assays could not show binding of AtRA to RXR, and further testing of metabolites of retinoic acid (RA) resulted in the identification of 9-*cis*-RA as a high-affinity ligand for RXRs as well as RARs.

In addition to different ligand specificity, another important finding related to the mechanism of how retinoid receptors function was the identification of RXR as an obligatory heterodimeric partner for a number of nuclear hormone receptors including RARs, thyroid hormone receptor (TR), peroxisome proliferator-activated receptor (PPAR), liver X receptor (LXR), farnesoid X receptor (FXR), pregnane X receptor/steroid and xenobiotic receptor (PXR/SXR), constitutive androstane receptor (CAR), and vitamin D receptor (VDR). Although the consequences of heterodimerization between RXR and these receptors are discussed in greater detail below, it is important to introduce this as a central concept in the identification of ligands that are specific for both RAR and RXR independently as well as those ligands that may regulate heterodimer function through the RXR. Compounds that specifically bind and activate RXR have been termed rexinoids. Supporting the pharmacological importance of rexinoids are findings demonstrating that RXR ligands working through specific heterodimers can recapitulate the activities observed with ligands specific to the heterodimeric partner. One example of this is the result that an RXR ligand, LG100268, can activate a PPARγ/RXR heterodimer and function as an effective insulin sensitizer in animal models of insulin resistance, similar to that observed with the PPARγ-regulating thiazolidinediones. Another example has been the finding that rexinoids such as LG100268, LG100364, and LG101305 can affect both cholesterol levels and atherosclerotic lesion size by virtue of working through another permissive heterodimer partner, LXR. The evidence that rexinoids can control multiple aspects of physiology through the regulation of RXR heterodimers demonstrates the importance of retinoid receptors as tools for pharmacological intervention in a number of diseases. As with RXR, there are also significant efforts to develop synthetic RAR compounds that are isotype specific to both reduce unwanted side effects and focus the pharmacological action of such compounds to specific tissues and disease states. See Fig. 2 for a selection of RAR and RXR ligands.

III. RECEPTOR STRUCTURE

The retinoid receptors exhibit the general modular structure typical of nuclear hormone receptors in that they have five domains separable by sequence, structure, and function (Fig. 3). These domains are termed A/B, C, D, and E. In some receptors, there is also an F domain, for which a clear function has not yet been identified. The N-terminal part of the receptors contains the A/B domain, which harbors an autonomous transcriptional activation function domain termed AF-1. This domain has been shown to be important in regulating cell- and promoter-specific gene expression. The activity of this domain is ligand independent. AF-1 can be regulated by modifications such as phosphorylation in the case of PPARγ and estrogen receptor-β and these modifications result in the recruitment of transcriptional cofactors. The AF-1 can also affect the overall transcriptional activity of the receptor by modulating the activity of the other transcriptional regulator domain, AF-2, which is part of the C-terminal ligand-binding domain. Work by several groups using transgenic and knockout mice has established, among other things, that the primary mediator of many of the effects of RA during development is the RAR/RXRα heterodimer. Based on this observation, the contribution of the AF-1 region in the context of retinoid signaling was assessed by generating transgenic mice expressing wild-type and AF-1 deletion mutants of RXRα. The results indicate that the AF-1 domain is required for the transcriptional activity of the RAR/RXRα heterodimer, but that the ligand-dependent AF-2 domain plays a greater role in effecting most of the RAR/RXRα-mediated downstream events.

The C domain of nuclear receptors contains the DNA-binding domain (DBD) and a weak dimerization function. The approximately 66-amino-acid DNA-binding domain is the most conserved feature among the nuclear hormone receptor family. The DNA-binding domain consists of two zinc-fingers that have been well characterized as protein motifs utilized in many transcription factors for DNA

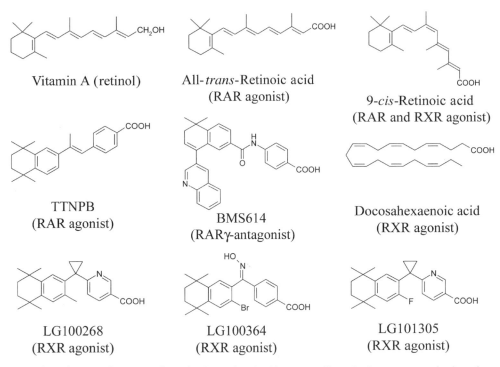

FIGURE 2 Selected retinoid receptor ligands. Several retinoid receptor ligands that represent both endogenous and synthetic small molecule regulators of RAR and RXR are depicted. The structures of vitamin A and the metabolites all-*trans*-retinoic acid and 9-*cis*-retinoic acid are provided as examples of high-affinity endogenous ligands. The other endogenous ligand shown is docosahexaenoic acid, an RXR agonist that may have effects on neural function. Examples of synthetic ligands that are referred to in the text include an RAR agonist, TTNPB, an RAR antagonist, BMS614, and a series of RXR agonists, LG100268, LG100364, and LG101305.

binding and protein–protein interactions. Within the first zinc-finger lies a highly conserved 13-amino-acid region termed the proximal or P box (Fig. 3). The P-box determines the specificity of binding of the receptor to its half-site. In the second zinc-finger, there is a region, termed the distal (D)-box, that contributes to dimerization. A third functionally characterized region within the DNA-binding domain is an approximately 25-amino-acid carboxy-terminal extension (CTE). In the case of RAR/RXR heterodimer DNA binding, the CTE plays a role in promoting both receptor–DNA interactions and receptor–receptor contact. The DBDs of RARα, and RXRα have been crystallized as a heterodimer complex bound to a direct repeat of AGGTCA with spacing of 1 bp. The results of these studies indicate that both the DNA and the receptors induce conformational changes in each other, resulting in a more stable DNA-bound complex. The ability of nuclear receptors, specifically retinoid receptors, to bind and regulate through multiple DNA elements is therefore a function of both the flexibility of the receptor and the DNA site.

The region that connects the DBD and the ligand-binding domain (LBD) has been referred to as the hinge or D region. This is a highly variable domain both in sequence and in length. As the name implies, the main purpose of this part of the receptor is to connect the DNA-binding component to the ligand-binding domain and to allow a high degree of freedom of movement for these domains.

The most important domain for ligand-mediated activity is the LBD, also referred to as the E region. The LBD contains the ligand-binding site, a strong dimerization function, cofactor interaction sites, and a ligand-dependent activation domain (AF-2). The LBD consists of 12 α-helices that form the ligand-binding pocket. Helix 12, which is at the C-terminus of the LBD, contains AF-2. The ligand-binding domains of RARγ and RXRα have been crystallized in the presence of compounds and, in the case of RXRα, also in their absence. The RXRα LBD structure was solved in the presence of 9-*cis* retinoic acid, and the RARγ LBD structure was determined in the presence of both agonists such as all-*trans* retinoic acid and antagonists such as BMS614 (Fig. 2).

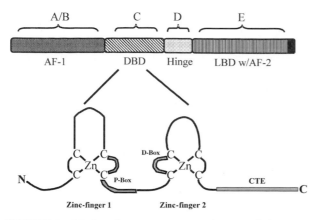

FIGURE 3 Nuclear hormone receptor functional domains. The diagram presents a general view of nuclear hormone receptor structure through delineation of the functional domains. The domains referred to in the text include the N-terminal A/B region that contains a ligand-independent transcriptional activation domain, the C or DNA-binding domain (DBD), the D or hinge region, and the E or ligand-binding domain (LBD). The LBD contains a ligand-dependent transcriptional activation function domain, AF-2 (in black). Shown in greater detail is the structure of the DNA-binding domain. There are two C_2C_2-type zinc-fingers that mediate protein–DNA and protein–protein interactions. Other regions highlighted include the P-box (DNA-binding specificity), the D-box (dimerization), and the carboxy-terminal extension (CTE; DNA and protein interactions).

These studies, along with the structures of other nuclear receptor ligand-binding domains, allowed several conclusions to be made. The 12 α-helices of the LBD form a novel fold termed an anti-parallel α-helical sandwich. In the apo state, helix 12 extends away from the ligand-binding pocket, whereas in the holo state, there is a significant rearrangement of H11, H12, and the region between H1 and H3. The shift in structure of these helices, e.g., H1–H3, H11, and H12, between the ligand-bound active state and the apo- or unbound inactive state has been referred to as a "mouse-trap" mechanism. As implied in this name, once a ligand enters the ligand-binding pocket, H12 is moved into a position in which it essentially traps the ligand in the pocket.

IV. MECHANISM OF ACTION

A. DNA Binding/Heterodimerization

Nuclear hormone receptors have been shown to bind to specific DNA-response element sequences as homodimers or heterodimers. The DNA binding is ligand independent. For RAR and RXR, the retinoid-responsive elements (RAREs and RXREs) that have

been isolated in target gene promoters have the consensus half-site sequence AGGTCA organized in different conformations. One type consists of a direct repeat (DR) of the half-site with an intervening spacer of 1, 2, or 5 (DR1, DR2, or DR5, respectively) bp. The DR5 element is the most common RARE. Another element is a palindromic or inverted half-site repeat, and a third response element is an inverted palindrome or everted half-site repeat (Fig. 4). It is likely as well that sequences flanking the half-sites further contribute to the affinity and specificity of receptor binding to these response elements.

RAR binding to DNA requires formation of a heterodimer with RXR. In the RAR/RXR heterodimer, it is the RAR that determines the ligand-dependent activity of the receptors, so that an RXR ligand is unable to activate the heterodimer in the absence of an RAR ligand. In this situation, RAR is referred to as a nonpermissive partner for RXR activity. As mentioned previously, RXR has also been shown to heterodimerize with many other nuclear hormone receptors including TR, VDR, PPARs, FXR,

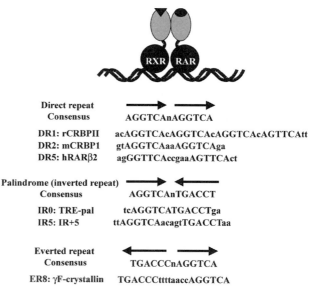

FIGURE 4 Retinoid receptor-response elements. There have been many retinoid receptor-response elements identified in the literature and examples of consensus and selected examples of these elements are shown in this figure. As indicated, the consensus half-site for retinoid receptors is AGGTCA, and the different elements are generated through variable spacing between these half-sites (DR1, DR2, and DR5) or orientation of the half-sites (IR0, IR5, and ER8). The DR1 is taken from the rat cellular retinal-binding protein II (rCRBPII); DR2 from mouse cellular retinal-binding protein I (mCRBPI); DR5 from human RARβ2 gene; IR0 and IR5 are synthetic elements; and ER8 is from the γF-crystallin promoter.

Nurr1, nur77/NGFI-B, and LXRs. Of these, TR and VDR are nonpermissive, and the others are referred to as permissive partners as they can be activated by RXR ligands or the appropriate dimer ligand. In addition to serving as a heterodimeric partner, RXR can bind as a homodimer to DR1 and certain palindrome elements. An important observation relating to how retinoid receptors respond to ligand is that the ternary structure of the receptor bound to DNA dictates the level of response to a given ligand. This is due to the specific RARE contributing to the determination of the affinity and specificity of a compound. This predicts that retinoids and/or small molecules can be synthesized to regulate specific target genes.

Similar to other steroid hormone receptors such as the glucocorticoid receptor, RAR and RXR can also directly or indirectly interact with other transcription factors to regulate target gene expression independent of binding to RAREs or RXREs. This has been demonstrated through inhibition of activator protein-1 (AP-1) and Ca^{2+}/cyclic AMP-response element-binding protein (CREB) activity by RAR and RXR ligands. In the case of RAR, the *trans*-repression can be observed in the absence of the induction of RAR transcriptional activity by certain compounds such as SR11203 and SR11238. It is likely that a combination of retinoid receptor-dependent events contribute to this repression, among which is competition for DNA-binding sites, sequestering of regulatory factors such as CREB-binding protein/p300 (CBP), and direct protein–protein interactions.

B. Transcriptional Regulation

The retinoid receptors function to regulate gene expression through the ability to adapt conformations that induce transcriptional activity in the presence of ligand or repress transcriptional activity in its absence. The gradient of activity that can be achieved, from full repression to full activation, is dependent on the ability of the ligand-binding domain to undergo a series of conformational changes. Much of the work over the past several years has established that large multisubunit protein complexes are recruited to DNA through binding to the receptors. As described previously, in the presence of an agonist, the LBD adopts a conformation in which the AF-2 containing helix 12 moves almost 90° to stabilize the receptor structure and create a binding interface for a class of proteins termed transcription co-activators. Examples of these factors include CBP, p300/CBP-associated factor (pCAF), thyroid hormone receptor-associated

proteins (TRAPs), receptor interacting protein 140 (RIP140), and the p160 proteins including steroid receptor co-activator-1 (SRC-1), SRC-2, and SRC-3. A common characteristic of many of these cofactors is that they have intrinsic histone acetyltransferase activity. Another shared feature is the presence of a protein interaction motif composed of the amino acids Leu-X-X-Leu-Leu (LXXLL). This short peptide sequence is sufficient to promote interaction of the cofactor with the receptor. Amino acids flanking the core sequence have been demonstrated to regulate specificity between cofactor and receptor. The co-activator complex, which is predicted to be approximately 2 MDa, contains an overlapping set of these factors and it is likely that they have regulator functions in addition to acetylating histones. The number, diversity, and expression level of co-activators in different tissues correspond to the tissue- and promoter-specific effects of a given ligand on its receptor. Histone acetylation by the co-activator complex recruited to the receptor in the presence of ligand leads to a loosened and more accessible chromatin structure (Fig. 5). This is expected to facilitate and promote expression of the target gene. The co-activator complex also has been demonstrated to contain kinase and methyltransferase activity.

In the absence of an agonist or in the presence of some antagonists, retinoid receptors, like some other nuclear hormone receptors, have been shown to repress the basal activity of a target gene promoter. This silencing ability is attributed to the presence of another large multifactorial complex. Two co-repressor proteins, nuclear receptor co-repressor (N-CoR) and silencing mediator for retinoid and thyroid hormone receptor (SMRT), have been identified as playing a major role in receptor controlled repression. These proteins share structural similarities, such as multiple repression and receptor interaction domains. Analogous to co-activator proteins, consensus SMRT and N-CoR receptor interaction motifs have been isolated with a minimal shared sequence of Leu/Ile-X-X-Leu/Ile-Leu/Ile. SMRT and N-CoR appear to function partly as platform proteins upon which the remainder of the co-repressor complex is assembled. This complex contains multiple proteins that have intrinsic histone deacetlyase (HDAC) activity. The HDAC activity is expected to maintain the chromatin structure in a tightly bound state that is incompatible with transcription. The ability of nuclear receptors, such as RAR and RXR, to interact in a ligand-dependent manner with at least two large protein complexes with opposing actions helps to explain the wide range of activities of these receptors

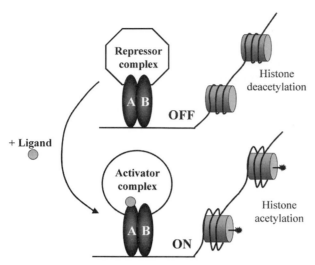

FIGURE 5 Mechanism of transcription regulation by retinoid receptors The diagram illustrates the ligand-mediated activation of transcription by retinoid receptors. A and B refer to any receptor heterodimer or homodimer partner. In the absence of ligand, the receptor dimer is bound to DNA and a large multiprotein co-repressor complex. The co-repressor complex is recruited to the receptors through specific protein–protein interactions between the receptor LBD and short hydrophobic peptide motifs found in various co-repressor proteins, such as SMRT and N-CoR (see text). The repressor complex contains certain enzyme activities, including histone deacetylases, that function to configure the chromatin structure into a state that is inhibitory to transcriptional activation. Upon ligand binding, the repressor complex is displaced through recruitment of a multiprotein activator complex. Similar to co-repressors, the co-activator complex is recruited through protein–protein interactions between the receptors and well-defined peptide motifs in the co-activator proteins. The co-activator complex contains enzyme activities, such as histone acetylases, that alter the chromatin structure to a more transcriptionally permissive state.

and their attractiveness as targets for therapeutic intervention.

The importance of the interaction of RAR with the co-repressors SMRT and/or N-CoR can be seen in the different responses of patients with acute promyelocytic leukemia (APL) to all-*trans*-retinoic acid therapy. Those patients with a translocation of the promyelocytic leukemia (PML) gene with the RARα gene (PML–RAR) respond well to RA, whereas those with a translocation of the promyelocytic leukemia zinc-finger (PLZF) gene with RARα (PLZF–RAR) respond poorly. This can be attributed to the ability of both PLZF and RAR to interact with co-repressors as opposed to just RAR in the PML–RAR fusion. The PLZF–co-repressor interaction is ligand independent and thus treatment by RA has minimal effect. This finding is discussed below in greater detail.

V. RECEPTOR PHYSIOLOGY

Vitamin A and retinoids have been shown to be essential for proper embryonic development and many physiological functions. Some of the characteristics of vitamin A deficiency include blindness, immune system dysfunction, infertility, congenital malformations, heart malformation, and epithelial hyperkeratinization. Vitamin A excess also can be detrimental and lead to birth defects. The effects of retinoids can be classified as receptor mediated and receptor independent. The use of retinoid receptor-specific ligands, cells from receptor null mice, overexpression of receptors, and overexpression of dominant-negative receptors have all contributed experimentally to linking retinoid effects with receptor-mediated effects. This next section provides a brief overview of a selected set of receptor-dependent activities that contribute to proper development and homeostasis, beginning with a review of the phenotypes of the various receptor null mice that have been made.

A. Receptor Mutant Mice

For the RARs, mice lacking the major isotypes have been generated. These mice have also been crossed with one another to generate compound mutants. RARα − /− mice died early after birth and showed signs of degenerative testis. Additional defects include homeotic transformations and congenital defects. RARγ − /− mice also have these defects, leading to improper development of the skull, vertebrae, and ribs. RARγ − /− mice also have decreased viability. RARβ − /− mice display some minor changes including some ocular and long-term memory defects. RARα − /− and RARγ − /− male mice are also sterile. The double mutants of RARα/β and RARα/γ, in which both alleles of a receptor subtype are deleted to maximize phenotypic effects that otherwise may be masked by receptor redundancy, show many more of the expected phenotypes that are observed in vitamin A-deprived animals. RXRα − /− mutant mice exhibit embryonic lethality, due to defects in placenta and heart. These mice also have defects related to eye development. RXRβ − /− mice show male sterility due to improper spermatogenesis, and RXRγ − /− mice exhibit no major phenotypes although long-term memory may be affected. Both RXRβ − /− and RXRγ − /− are viable.

B. Hematopoietic Differentiation

The observation that retinoic acid and its metabolite derivatives could induce differentiation of a number of human leukemic cell lines suggested that retinoids and their receptors would play an important role in physiological myeloid cell development and differentiation. RAR/RXR heterodimers function as modulators of granulocyte differentiation depending on the presence or absence of a ligand. In the presence of retinoic acid, RAR activity promotes granulocyte differentiation, whereas unbound RAR is an inhibitor of promyelocyte differentiation. The role of RARα as a regulator of myeloid differentiation is further supported by the inability of promyelocytes that harbor translocations between RAR and PML and/or PLZF to differentiate, resulting in acute promyelocytic leukemia. The cells with the PML-RAR fusion can be treated with RA and be induced to differentiate, indicating RAR activity as a primary mediator of cellular differentiation in the myeloid system. RAR activity has also been shown to be important in regulation of neutrophil maturation.

C. Cell Proliferation/Apoptosis

The ability of retinoids to regulate cell cycle progression, proliferation, and apoptosis has been well studied, although the mechanisms supporting the observations are not completely known. The inhibitory effect of the RARs and RXRs on cell growth can generally be attributed to their regulation of a number of proteins involved in the process of cell cycle and cell death. The targets of retinoid receptor activity include the AP-1 transcription factor, c-Myc, and retinoblastoma gene product Rb. These proteins are important in controlling the G1 to S phase of the cell cycle, and retinoid inhibition generally occurs at this transition stage.

A primary role for retinoid receptors in apoptosis was found when certain leukemic cells were treated with retinoic acid and other retinoid receptor-selective ligands. It was found that RAR and RXR ligands, when added together to HL60 cells, a promyelocytic cell line, induced apoptosis. These effects were receptor dependent and involved the down-regulation of certain anti-apoptotic proteins. In the development of myeloid cells from bone marrow progenitor cells, RXR also plays an important role through the regulation of apoptosis. In the absence of RXR activation, or down-regulation of RXR expression, myeloid cells undergo less apoptosis. RARs and RXRs have also been shown to regulate apoptosis in T and B lymphocytes. In T cells, rexinoids inhibit T-cell-receptor-mediated apoptosis by inhibiting the expression of the Fas ligand. Proper timing and regulation of cell death are critical in lymphocyte development to eliminate those cellular clones that would otherwise be self-reactive and lead to autoimmunity.

D. Reproduction

Vitamin A has been shown to be important in spermatogenesis and maturation of spermatozoa. Vitamin A deficiency leads to defective spermatogenesis and subsequent sterility. In agreement with this finding, RARα −/−, RARγ −/−, and RXRβ −/− male mice are sterile. These data indicate that the primary mediators of retinoid signaling in the testis are likely to be the RARα and RXRβ receptors and that these receptors are not redundant for proper reproductive development. These mice are sterile due to testicular defects, including degeneration of the seminiferous epithelium, in the case of RARα −/− mice. In the RXRβ −/− mice, the male sterility is due to defective spermatozoa and lipid accumulation in Sertoli cells.

E. Development

The importance of retinoid receptors to proper development and differentiation of tissues is well defined in experiments relating to limb formation as well as the finding that retinoids are teratogenic in humans. Studies in chickens show that placement of beads containing RA into developing limb bud sites can initiate novel developmental programs leading to a new limb structure. Consistent with these results, RAR/RXR antagonists can inhibit limb formation. Multiple limb abnormalities are also seen in RARα −/−, RXRα −/−, and double mutant RARα/RXRα, RARβ/RXRα, and RARα/RARγ mice. The mechanism of retinoid receptor function in limb development involves the induction of a cascade of gene expression, with induction of hox genes Hoxb-6 and Hoxb-8, which in turn lead to up-regulation of Sonic Hedgehog, which consequently up-regulates the bone morphogenic protein BMP-2. These proteins have been shown to be key factors in the process of limb development.

F. Neural Development

Retinoids have been long associated with the differentiation of neurons and the development of the nervous system. The expression patterns of retinoid receptors in the central nervous systems throughout development and into adulthood suggested a role for these receptors in regulating certain neural functions. Data from a variety of sources including phenotypes associated with vitamin A deficiency, RAR/RXR mutant mice, and treatment of animals with retinoid receptor antagonist demonstrate an essential role for retinoid signaling in normal hindbrain development.

The results from RARβ/RXRβ, RARβ/RXRγ, and RXRβ/RXRγ double mutant mice also confirm a role for these receptors in the development of normal locomotor function. This defect in motor function is likely due to a reduction in expression levels of the dopamine receptors D1 and D2. This is consistent with RAR/RXR heterodimers binding to and regulating the promoter of the D2 receptor *in vitro*. These findings also hint at a link between retinoid receptor signaling and such neural disorders as Parkinson's disease and schizophrenia. Recent work that describes the search for endogenous RXR ligands has identified docosahexaenoic acid as a putative ligand. The ability of DHA to activate RXRs and the presence of learning abnormalities in DHA-deficient animals correlate well with the mutant mouse data and further support a role for retinoid receptors in neural development.

G. Retinoid Receptors in Skin

The effects of vitamin A deficiency or excess on skin growth and differentiation have been known for a number of years. A lack of vitamin A leads to hyperkeratosis, which could be reversed upon addition of vitamin A. An excess of vitamin A, however, can result in inhibition of the process of keratinization. Since the levels of vitamin A were shown to be important regulators of skin processes, this led to the use of natural retinoic acids, including AtRA and 13-*cis*-RA, as a treatment for skin disorders including acne and psoriasis and for correcting sun-induced skin damage. The use of retinoic acid, unfortunately also has some undesired side effects including irritation, dryness and peeling of the skin, hair loss, and teratogenicity. Some of the skin-related side effects might be partly due to binding to the intracellular protein cellular retinoic acid-binding protein types I and II. Recent experiments *in vitro* and in animal models has established that the major isoforms of the receptors expressed in adult skin are RARγ and RXRα, although the other isoforms are expressed at varying levels during development. The ability to target RARγ specifically with synthetic agonist or antagonists has the promise of providing the benefits of retinoic acid treatment without the side effects. Indeed, the successful use of RARγ agonists in the treatment of acne and psoriasis has been reported.

VI. RXR HETERODIMERIZATION

As introduced earlier, RXR functions as an obligatory heterodimeric partner for a large number of nuclear hormone receptors. Among the receptors that RXR can heterodimerize with are RARs, TR, VDR, PXR/SXR, PPARs, LXRs, FXR, CAR, and Nurr. Of these, PPARs, LXRs, FXR, PXR/SXR, CAR, and Nurr are permissive to the activation of the heterodimer via binding of an RXR ligand. The other receptors, RAR, TR, and VDR, are not permissive to activation by RXR ligands. The molecular mechanism for whether a heterodimer is permissive or not appears to depend on the recruitment of the co-repressor complex by the RXR partner in the absence of an agonist. In nonpermissive heterodimers such as RAR/RXR, even though an RXR ligand may bind, it is not sufficient to activate the complex, most likely due to an inability to displace the co-repressor from RAR. In this same complex, however, if an RAR agonist is added along with an RXR agonist, the net activation is higher than with the RAR compound alone. In permissive heterodimers, both receptors bind the co-repressor complex weakly so addition of an RXR agonist is sufficient to displace the co-repressor from the heterodimer and thus induce activity. Since these permissive heterodimers represent an important extension of the function of retinoid receptors, this section provides a general overview of the function of the PPAR, LXR, FXR, and xenobiotic receptor (PXR/SXR and CAR) heterodimers. The nonpermissive heterodimer receptors TR and VDR are not discussed, as other than mediating the target specificity through DNA binding of these heterodimers, there is as yet no other physiological role for RXR in these cases. RAR heterodimer function has previously been discussed and the Nurr receptors are also not included, as a physiological role for a Nurr/RXR heterodimer has not yet been established.

A. PPAR/RXR

The PPARs have been shown to be important regulators of lipid metabolism and adipogenesis. There are three isoforms, α, δ, and γ, that activate transcription by binding to promoter elements as heterodimers with RXR. The PPAR/RXR heterodimers can bind primarily to DR1 elements. Natural and synthetic ligands have been identified for all three PPAR isoforms and, along with receptor mutant mice, have allowed for detailed study of the function of these receptors. PPARα is involved in the breakdown of fatty acids and PPARγ has been shown to be important in cellular differentiation of adipocytes and other cell types and to play a role in insulin sensitization, and thus diabetes, as well as atherosclerosis. PPARδ activity has also been linked to lipid metabolism. As PPARs are permissive to RXR ligand activation, it is possible to regulate the heterodimer through either a PPAR-selective agonist or an RXR ligand. Consistent with this, a combination of ligands for both PPAR and RXR leads to synergy in transcriptional activation. Acting presumably through the PPAR/RXR heterodimer, RXR agonists have been shown to have significant effects on insulin sensitization and therefore make RXR a potential therapeutic target for treatment of type II diabetes. Based on the finding that the DNA sequence can influence the activity of a compound, it is also possible that RXR ligands that potentiate the PPARγ/RXR heterodimer activity on specific target genes without activating RXR promiscuously can be found.

B. LXR/RXR

Liver X receptors LXRα and LXRβ function to regulate cholesterol homeostasis and fatty acid metabolism. LXRα −/− mice have been shown to have defects in the process of converting dietary cholesterol to bile acids in the liver due to a lack of activation of expression of the cholesterol-7α-hydroxylase (CYP7A1) enzyme. Additional defects include a reduced expression of genes involved in lipogenesis such as sterol regulatory element-binding protein 1 (SREBP1) and fatty acid synthase. An additional target for LXR/RXR regulation in the macrophage and intestine is the ATP-binding cassette A1 (ABCA1) transporter protein, which is involved in reverse cholesterol transport. Activation of ABCA1 and other genes involved in cholesterol efflux by LXR agonists has been shown to lead to a reduction in cholesterol absorption. Furthermore, LXR agonists have also been demonstrated to increase the circulating levels of high-density lipoprotein cholesterol. Consistent with the various functions of LXRs in regulating cholesterol and lipogenesis, recent results also implicate LXR agonists as having anti-atherosclerotic effects.

As with PPARs, LXRs are permissive to RXR activation and RXR agonists can elicit similar biological responses to LXR-specific agonists including up-regulation of ABCA1 and SREBP1 and inhibition of atherosclerosis in animal models. Consistent with the action of LXR or RXR agonists, both LXR null mutant mice and mice with RXR deleted from hepatocytes exhibit an increase in triglycerides. Additional evidence for a role for retinoid receptors in fatty acid synthesis comes from the observation that patients treated with RXR agonists have elevated triglycerides. The function of the LXR/RXR heterodimer as determined through multiple studies therefore represents an important point of pharmacological intervention, through the LXR receptors and/or RXR receptor, for cholesterol regulation, lipid homeostasis, and control or prevention of atherosclerosis.

C. FXR/RXR

The FXR was identified through homology screening and also by using RXR as bait in a yeast two-hybrid protein interaction assay. FXR functions as a permissive heterodimer with RXR and binds to an inverted repeat-1 DNA element. The finding that bile acids could function as ligands for FXR has established a role for FXR/RXR in bile acid metabolism. Targets for FXR regulation include ileal bile acid-binding protein and bile salt efflux pump in the intestine and CYP7A1 in the liver. FXR inhibits the expression of CYP7A1 and therefore opposes the function of LXR on this target, although the mechanism of how this repression occurs is not clear. Studies have demonstrated that an FXR agonist, when administered to rats, resulted in a lowering of triglycerides. The mechanism of how triglyceride production might be regulated by FXR is not yet known. Further experiments have demonstrated that guggulsterone, a steroid produced by the guggul tree and used for over 2500 years as a treatment for a number of disorders including high cholesterol, functions in the body primarily through FXR. The cholesterol-lowering effects of guggulsterone can be linked to its activity as an antagonist of FXR. The findings with FXR agonists and antagonists indicate that the FXR/RXR heterodimer also represents an important pharmacological intervention point for regulating cholesterol and triglyceride levels.

D. PXR/SXR and CAR

The xenobiotic sensing receptors PXR/SXR and CAR have been shown to regulate responses to foreign chemicals in the body, as well as endogenous compounds such as bile acids. The target genes for these receptors include the cytochrome P450 CYP3 genes for PXR/SXR and CYP2 genes for CAR. There is some overlap between the targets and functions of these receptors, although important pharmacological and species differences exist. Implications for the regulation of these genes include mediating drug–drug interactions and elimination of toxic compounds from the body. As stated previously, these receptors bind to DNA-response elements (DR5) as heterodimers with RXR and are permissive to activation by RXR ligands. Although RXR ligands can activate the heterodimers on isolated response elements in transfection experiments, currently there is no conclusive evidence to suggest that synthetic or endogenous RXR ligands have a physiological role in regulating PXR/SXR or CAR target genes since it is unclear which heterodimer partner the compounds are working through.

As demonstrated in the previous sections, RXR heterodimers play important roles in many natural and disease states. A general statement regarding permissive versus nonpermissive heterodimers based on recent observations is that the RXR-permissive heterodimers appear to be "lipid" sensors that control many metabolic pathways including glucose, fatty acid, bile acid, and cholesterol signaling. Nonpermissive heterodimers alternatively regulate responses to classic endocrine hormones including steroids and nonsteroid hormones.

VII. RETINOID RECEPTORS AND CANCER

A. Acute Promyelocytic Leukemia

As described previously, the role of retinoids and retinoid receptors in regulating cell proliferation and differentiation is well established. As a result of these studies and the finding that translocations of the RARα gene are involved in certain leukemias, a clear link between retinoid signaling and cancer has been established. APL is characterized by abnormal proliferation of promyelocytes in the bone marrow and represents 10–15% of acute nonlymphoid leukemias. Experiments in which APL cells were treated with a variety of compounds demonstrated that AtRA could induce differentiation of these leukemic cells into granulocytes. This key finding has greatly improved the cure rate among patients with this form of leukemia and indicated that retinoid receptor signaling was involved. The majority of APL cases (95%) have been shown to develop as a result of a translocation between the RARα gene, which is on chromosome 17, and the PML gene, which is on chromosome 15. The resulting fusion proteins are shown in Fig. 6. The PML–RARα fusion proteins contain various lengths of the PML

protein fused to a point in the second intron of RARα. The PML–RARα protein contains the N-terminus, the A domain of RARα, and the C-terminal parts of the PML protein. Experiments introducing a transgenic PML–RARα gene into mice result in development of leukemias that are similar to APL and confirm that this gene product is responsible for both the leukemia and the sensitivity of the cells to retinoic acid treatment.

The PML–RAR protein may inhibit myeloid differentiation in several ways. It is possible that PML–RAR inhibits the normal function of retinoic acid signaling by binding to and sequestering RXR, thus inhibiting the function of heterodimers reliant on RXR. Normal PML function may be inhibited through the disruption by PML–RAR of a nuclear structure known as promyelocytic organizing domains (PODs) or PML bodies. PODs have been implicated as sites of protein ubiquitination and turnover as well as storage of cellular factors involved in transcription. One important observation of PML–RAR leukemic cells is that upon treatment with RA, the normal nuclear organization of PODs is regained. Additional studies have demonstrated that the function of PML in regulating apoptosis is also impaired in the PML–RARα-expressing promyelocytes.

In addition to the PML–RARα translocation, APL has been characterized by two other translocations involving RARα that occur in 1–2% of APL cases. Translocation of the RARα gene with the PLZF gene on chromosome 11 results in a PLZF–RARα fusion protein, whereas a translocation with the nucleophosmin (NPM) gene on chromosome 5 results in a NPM–RARα fusion protein. The PLZF–RARα functions in a manner similar to PML–RARα to inhibit normal retinoid signaling and possibly to antagonize the activity of PLZF. Unlike PML–RARα cells, PLZF–RARα cells are unresponsive to retinoic acid treatment. Recent work has implicated the recruitment of a co-repressor protein complex, described in previous sections, to the fusion protein. The co-repressor SMRT has been shown to interact with both PLZF and RARα so that treatment with RA is not sufficient to disrupt the co-repressor–PLZF–RARα complex. Since PML does not interact with co-repressors, the addition of RA can lead to the displacement of the co-repressor complex from PML—RARα and restore transcriptional activity. These data highlight the importance of considering both the retinoid receptors and their cofactors when examining the normal physiology of retinoid signaling as well as the treatment of disease states.

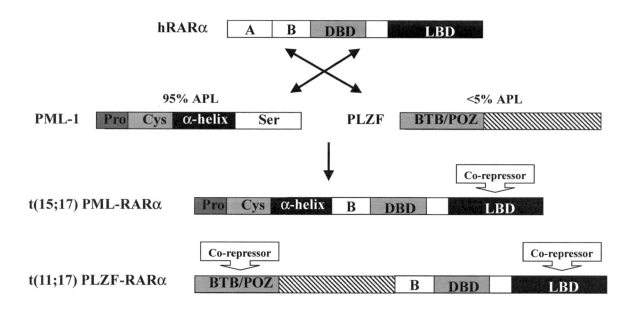

FIGURE 6 RAR translocations and APL. The fusion proteins resulting from translocations between the human RARα (hRARα), PML, and PLZF genes are shown. As indicated, 95% of acute promyelocytic leukemias are the result of a translocation between hRARα and PML-1, generating a fusion protein that contains up to the serine-rich region in PML and all but the A region of RARα. Since the fusion protein contains the RAR LBD, t(15;17) APL can be treated with retinoids such as AtRA. The co-repressor complex is shown bound to the RAR LBD, and presumably retinoids are effective through displacement of this complex. Another 5% of APL is due to a translocation with the PLZF gene. Binding of co-repressor to PLZF is not affected by retinoids, and thus t(11;17) APL patients are resistant to retinoids.

B. Breast Cancer

Based on the role of retinoid receptors in regulating multiple cellular processes, another pharmacological target for retinoids has been the treatment of breast cancer. Both RARs and RXRs are expressed in normal and cancerous breast cells and regulate important functions in these cells including proliferation, differentiation, and apoptosis. Studies using the retinoids AtRA and 9-cis-RA have demonstrated that activation of the RAR/RXR heterodimer in both breast cell lines and in animal models of breast cancer results in an inhibition of tumorigenesis. Based on the promising results obtained with the natural retinoids, synthetic retinoids and rexinoids that have reduced toxicity and unwanted side effects have been tested for breast cancer prevention and treatment. The results from prevention of breast cancer with these compounds in animal models indicate that synthetic, receptor-selective compounds that regulate RAR/RXR will prove to be an important addition to the currently available treatments for this disease.

VIII. SUMMARY

Retinoid signaling is an essential part of normal development and physiology. The discovery that RAR and RXR, members of the nuclear hormone receptor protein family, could mediate many of the *in vivo* effects of vitamin A and its metabolites has helped to uncover the mechanisms by which these effects are generated. The temporal and spatial expression of the retinoid receptors, isoforms, and many splice variants dictates the response to retinoids. It is clear that DNA binding to various response elements and the ability to recruit either co-activator or co-repressor complexes to the DNA are the ultimate result of natural or synthetic ligand addition.

The diversity of responses to retinoids and other physiological ligands is increased by the ability of RXR to function as a master regulator of nuclear receptor signaling through heterodimerization with a number of the receptors. The work identifying the retinoid receptors, characterizing their mechanism of action and role *in vivo*, has greatly influenced the knowledge of how retinoid function may be altered in disease states and how medicine can intervene to correct these defects.

Glossary

dimerization The generation of a multiprotein functional unit comprising proteins of the same class. A monomer is a single unit, and a dimer is two units. In homodimers, the receptors are the same, whereas in heterodimers the receptors are different. This represents a central concept in the function of nuclear hormone receptors, as the majority work as heterodimers or homodimers.

ligand agonist A small molecule that upon binding to the receptor induces a conformation in the ligand-binding domain that results in activation of transcription, leading to an increase in gene expression.

ligand antagonist A small molecule that upon binding to the receptor induces a conformation in the ligand-binding domain that results in an inhibition of transcription activation by agonists, leading to a decrease in gene expression.

ligand inverse agonist A small molecule that upon binding to the receptor induces a conformation in the ligand-binding domain that results in an inhibition of the basal ligand-independent activity of the receptor, leading to a decrease in gene expression.

nuclear hormone receptors These proteins belong to a class of transcription factors that regulate gene expression in response to binding of small molecules called ligands. The ligand-bound receptor can activate or repress gene expression by binding to specific DNA-response elements. In the absence of ligand, these receptors generally repress gene transcription.

response element A short region of DNA that is bound by a transcription factor and the deletion or addition of which affects the transcription of genes containing such elements. For nuclear hormone receptors, most response elements consist of two 6 bp half-sites that have variable spacing and orientation with respect to each other.

retinoids Any of a number of small molecules that can bind to and regulate the activity of the nuclear hormone retinoic acid receptor.

rexinoids Any of a number of small molecules that can bind to and regulate the activity of the nuclear hormone retinoid X receptor.

transcription The process of synthesizing RNA from DNA directed by the activities of the enzyme RNA polymerase. RNA is subsequently made into protein through a process referred to as translation. The transcription process consists of three parts: initiation, elongation, and termination. Transcription factors are those proteins that can bind to specific DNA elements and regulate the process of transcription by activating or repressing RNA polymerase function through different mechanisms.

See Also the Following Articles

Glucocorticoid Receptor Structure and Function ● Ligand Modification to Produce Pharmacologic Agents ● Peroxisome Proliferator-Activated Receptors (PPARs)

Further Reading

Boehm, M. F., Zhang, L., Badea, B. A., White, S. K., Mais, D. E., Berger, E., Suto, C. M., Goldman, M. E., and Heyman, R. A. (1994). Synthesis and structure–activity relationships of novel retinoid X receptor-selective retinoids. *J. Med. Chem.* 37, 2930–2941.

Bourguet, W., Vivat, V., Wurtz, J. M., Chambon, P., Gronemeyer, H., and Moras, D. (2000). Crystal structure of a heterodimeric complex of RAR and RXR ligand-binding domains. *Mol. Cell* 5, 289–298.

Egea, P. F., Mitschler, A., Rochel, N., Ruff, M., Chambon, P., and Moras, D. (2000). Crystal structure of the human RXRalpha ligand-binding domain bound to its natural ligand: 9-*cis* Retinoic acid. *EMBO J.* 19, 2592–2601.

Glass, C. K., and Rosenfeld, M. G. (2000). The coregulator exchange in transcriptional functions of nuclear receptors. *Genes. Dev.* 14, 121–141.

Heyman, R. A., Mangelsdorf, D. J., Dyck, J. A., Stein, R. B., Eichele, G., Evans, R. M., and Thaller, C. (1992). 9-*cis* Retinoic acid is a high affinity ligand for the retinoid X receptor. *Cell* 68, 397–406.

Lin, R. J., Nagy, L., Inoue, S., Shao, W., Miller, W. H., Jr., and Evans, R. M. (1998). Role of the histone deacetylase complex in acute promyelocytic leukaemia. *Nature* 391, 811–814.

Mangelsdorf, D. J., Borgmeyer, U., Heyman, R. A., Zhou, J. Y., Ong, E. S., Oro, A. E., Kakizuka, A., and Evans, R. M. (1992). Characterization of three RXR genes that mediate the action of 9-*cis* retinoic acid. *Genes Dev.* 6, 329–344.

Mangelsdorf, D. J., and Evans, R. M. (1995). The RXR heterodimers and orphan receptors. *Cell* 83, 841–850.

Mangelsdorf, D. J., Ong, E. S., Dyck, J. A., and Evans, R. M. (1990). Nuclear receptor that identifies a novel retinoic acid response pathway. *Nature* 345, 224–229.

Mangelsdorf, D. J., Umesono, K., and Evans, R. M. (1994). The retinoid receptors. *In* "The Retinoids: Biology, Chemistry, and Medicine" (M. B. Sporn, A. B. Roberts and D. S. Goodman, eds.), 2nd ed., pp. 319–349. Raven Press, New York.

Minucci, S., and Pelicci, P. G. (1999). Retinoid receptors in health and disease: Co-regulators and the chromatin connection [see comments]. *Semin. Cell. Dev. Biol.* 10, 215–225.

Nau, N., and Blanar, W. S. (1999). Retinoids: The biochemical and molecular basis of vitamin A and retinoid action. *Handb. Exp. Pharmacol.* 139, 3–619.

Rastinejad, F., Wagner, T., Zhao, Q., and Khorasanizadeh, S. (2000). Structure of the RXR-RAR DNA-binding complex on the retinoic acid response element DR1. *EMBO J.* 19, 1045–1054.

Renaud, J. P., Rochel, N., Ruff, M., Vivat, V., Chambon, P., Gronemeyer, H., and Moras, D. (1995). Crystal structure of the RAR-gamma ligand-binding domain bound to all-*trans* retinoic acid. *Nature* 378, 681–689.

Ross, S. A., McCaffery, P. J., Drager, U. C., and De Luca, L. M. (2000). Retinoids in embryonal development. *Physiol. Rev.* 80, 1021–1046.

Steinmetz, A. C., Renaud, J. P., and Moras, D. (2001). Binding of ligands and activation of transcription by nuclear receptors. *Annu. Rev. Biophys. Biomol. Struct.* 30, 329–359.

Regulators of G-Protein Signaling (RGS) Superfamily

DAVID A. SIERRA AND THOMAS M. WILKIE

University of Texas Southwestern Medical Center, Dallas

I. INTRODUCTION
II. RGS SUPERFAMILY: STRUCTURE AND PHYLOGENETIC RELATIONSHIPS
III. GAP ACTIVITY REGULATES SIGNALING
IV. SUMMARY

G-protein signaling is dependent on a cycle of GTP binding on the G-protein α-subunit and GTP hydrolysis, which activate and inactivate signaling, respectively. Regulators of G-protein signaling (RGS) proteins are GTPase accelerating proteins for specific classes of G-protein α-subunits, serving as feedback inhibitors of G-protein signaling pathways by accelerating the rate of inactivation. RGS proteins may also facilitate signaling by serving as scaffolds and effector proteins. Thus, RGS proteins sharpen the kinetic response of both activation and termination of G-protein signaling in cells.

I. INTRODUCTION

G-protein signaling is regulated by the combined action of receptors and regulators of G-protein signaling (RGS) proteins to control intracellular responses to extracellular signals throughout an animal's lifetime. G-proteins regulate numerous essential functions in higher eukaryotes, including gametogenesis, fertilization, cell motility, feeding behavior, sleep, responses to light, and other environmental and hormonal cues. Signaling via heterotrimeric G-proteins initiates with agonist binding to heptahelical receptors. The role of heterotrimeric G-proteins, composed of α-, β-, and γ-subunits, is to transduce the signal received on agonist binding to the regulation of effector proteins and their downstream second-messenger systems. Signaling specificity is provided by the distinct receptor, G-protein α-subunit, and RGS protein that regulate the pathway.

II. RGS SUPERFAMILY: STRUCTURE AND PHYLOGENETIC RELATIONSHIPS

RGS proteins are expressed in all higher eukaryotes, except for plants, together with all other components of G-protein signaling complexes, including agonists, heptahelical receptors, heterotrimeric G-protein α-, β-, and γ-subunits, and effector proteins. The first RGS protein was discovered in baker's yeast and found to be an important feedback inhibitor of the mating response to pheromone. Yeast of the opposite mating types recognize each other's proximity and initiate the first steps of conjugation via a G-protein signaling pathway. In the absence of the RGS protein termed Sst2 (supersensitive to pheromone), yeast could not recover from pheromone-induced cell cycle arrest in preparation for mating. Several years later, sequence similarity to the yeast Sst2 protein was independently discovered in several RGS proteins by three groups studying B-cell maturation, vesicular transport, and roundworm motility and egg laying. Similarity within these proteins was restricted to a region of approximately 130 amino acids, termed the RGS domain (Figs. 1 and 2). Subsequent experiments demonstrated that the RGS domain of RGS proteins displayed GTPase accelerating protein (GAP) activity toward the corresponding G-protein α-subunits expressed in yeast, worms, and mammals.

The superfamily of RGS proteins expressed in metazoan organisms now contains five families of RGS-like proteins, including RGS, rgRGS, RGS-PX, GPRK, and AKAP-RGS (Fig. 1 and Table 1). Proteins in the RGS and rgRGS families have very similar three-dimensional structures but the amino acid sequences are only distantly related between the families (Fig. 2). Interestingly, the GAP activity of proteins within each RGS-like family is restricted to a specific class of G-protein α-subunit, indicative of regulatory specificity within different G-protein signaling pathways (Table 1).

A. The RGS Domain

Mammals express 22 RGS proteins that can be grouped into five subfamilies based on sequence

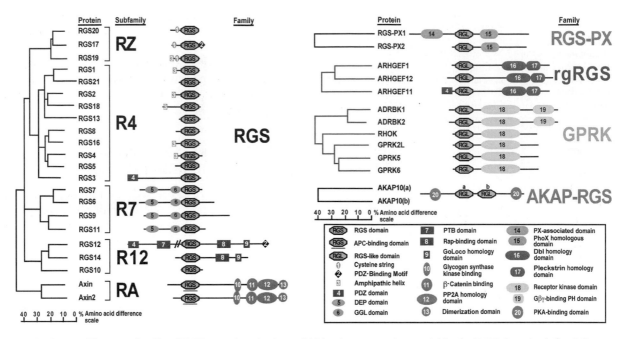

FIGURE 1 The superfamily of RGS proteins. Amino acid identity comparisons within the RGS domain defined five families of RGS and RGS-like proteins: *RGS, RGS-PX, rgRGS, GPRK,* and *AKAP-RGS.* The RGS family is further subdivided into five subfamilies: *RZ, R4, R7, R12,* and *RA.* Human RGS domains contain between 127 and 130 amino acids. Branch junctions approximate the values calculated by DNAStar for sequence identity for each pair of sequences calculated as 100% minus the sum of the horizontal distance to and from the common branch point. Protein domains flanking the RGS domain are identified in the figure, and functions are summarized in Table 2. Common aliases for *RGS* genes are indicated in Table 1.

similarity within the RGS domain (Fig. 1). RGS proteins in the RZ, R4, R7, and R12 subfamilies all display GAP activity (Table 1). By contrast, the RA subfamily proteins lack GAP activity; they are scaffold proteins that help assemble components of the wnt signaling pathway during development and cancerous growth.

The structure of the RGS domain was solved by both X-ray crystallography and nuclear magnetic resonance. Interestingly, even though the entire RGS4 protein was crystallized (complexed with a $G_{\alpha i}$ subunit), only the RGS domain of RGS4 was resolved, whereas the N- and C-terminal residues were disordered. The correspondence of the ordered structure to the evolutionarily conserved RGS domain, which conveys GAP activity, indicates that the RGS domain is a discrete unit of folding and function. The RGS domain is a globular structure composed of two four-helical bundles. Residues within three loops on one surface are important for GAP activity and substrate specificity (Fig. 2). This surface has been termed the "A" or active site. However, RGS proteins do not have residues that directly contribute to catalysis, but rather appear to

stabilize the transition state of GTP hydrolysis on the G_{α} subunit. RGS proteins with amino acid substitutions, deletions, or insertions within this region (from experimental mutagenesis or found naturally, as in the RA subfamily) lack GAP activity. A potential regulatory or "B" site occurs within an acidic domain in helices 4 and 5; in axin, this region binds a peptide fragment of adenomatous polyposis coli (APC), and R4 family RGS proteins are thought to alternatively bind phosphatidylinositol 3,4,5-triphosphate (PIP_3) and Ca^{2+}/calmodulin to regulate GAP activity. Other regions of RGS proteins bind additional proteins and lipids (Table 2). Interestingly, the most highly conserved residues within the RGS domain face inward and maintain structure. Several outward-facing residues are conserved within subfamilies and, together with flanking domains, may interact with other proteins or lipids in the signaling complexes that convey specific regulatory functions.

B. Superfamily of RGS Domain Proteins

Sequence homology between families of RGS-like proteins is low and difficult to detect. The different

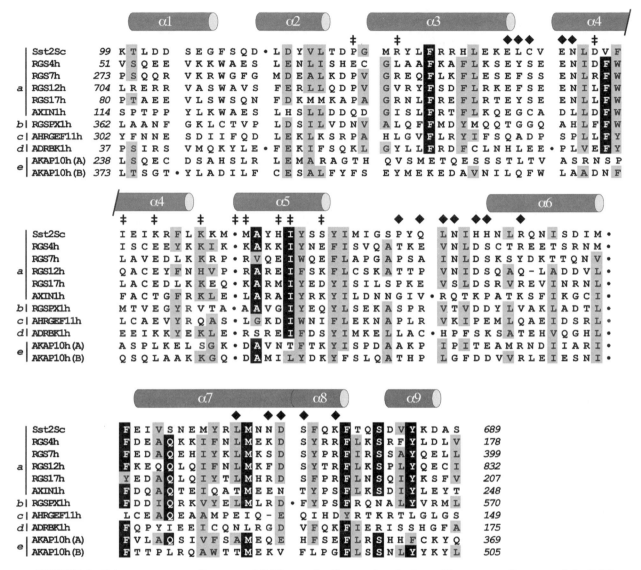

FIGURE 2 Primary structure alignment of RGS superfamily proteins. Amino acid sequence alignment of the RGS domains from a representative member of each RGS subfamily, *R4, R7, R12, RZ,* and *RA,* and the yeast RGS protein Sst2 (*a*) and the four families of RGS-like domains (*b, RGS-PX; c, rgRGS; d, GPRK; e, AKAP-RGS*). The features noted in the RGS domain include the position of the α-helices in RGS4, AXIN, and ARHGEF11 (rods), G$_\alpha$ contact residues in RGS4 (diamonds), residues in AXIN that bind APC (double dagger), highly conserved, inward-facing amino acid identities (black), and amino acids of similar chemical function (gray). Dots signify amino acid insertions that were omitted from the alignment, spaces show where other proteins in the RGS superfamily have amino acid insertions, and dashes signify that an amino acid is not present in that RSG subfamily at that position within the alignment.

families are so divergent that only a few inward-facing residues important for structural integrity are conserved (Fig. 2). On the other hand, the crystal structures of RGS and rgRGS proteins are very similar, with the conserved residues identically placed within the RGS domain structure, supporting the notion that these RGS-like proteins are evolutionarily related. Presumably, members of the RGS-PX, GPRK, and AKAP-RGS families also have similar structures,

but this is yet to be determined. As a cautionary note, the first protein demonstrated to have G$_\alpha$-GAP activity, the effector protein phospholipase C-β (PLC-β), is structurally unrelated to the RGS proteins. Thus, G$_\alpha$-GAP activity has evolved independently at least twice.

Within the superfamily of RGS domain proteins, GAP activity is observed in some but not necessarily all of the proteins of the RGS, rgRGS, RGS-PX, and

GRPK families and not in either RGL domain of AKAP10 (Table 1). Interestingly, the different RGS-like GAPs accelerate GTP hydrolysis on distinct types of G_α subunits. This substrate selectivity may help provide specificity in the regulation of G-protein signaling pathways.

Mammals, flies, and roundworms express four classes of G_α subunits, termed G_i, G_q, G_{12}, and G_s. The four classes are defined on the basis of similarity in sequence, gene structure, and regulation of effector proteins. The G_q class activates phospholipase C-β, and thus regulates the production of the second messengers inositol 1,4,5-triphosphate (IP$_3$), diacylglycerol (DAG), and oscillations in the concentration of intracellular Ca^{2+}. The G_i class regulates diverse effectors, including the inhibition of adenylyl cyclase, activation of cyclic GMP (cGMP) phosphodiesterase, potassium channel opening, and activation of phospholipase C-β. The G_{12} class activates a guanine nucleotide exchange factor on the small GTP-binding

TABLE 1   RGS Superfamily G_α-GAP Activity

Family	Subfamily	Locus (alias)	G_α-GAP	LocusLink ID No.
RGS	R4	RGS1 (BL34)	$G_{i/q}$	5996
		RGS2 (GOS8)	$G_q > G_i$	5997
		RGS3 (RGS15, PDZ-RGS)	$G_{i/q}$	5998
		RGS4	$G_{i/q}$	5999
		RGS5	$G_{i/q}$	8490
		RGS8	$G_{i/q}$	85397
		RGS13	$G_{i/q}$	6003
		RGS16 (RGS-r)	$G_{i/q}$	6004
		RGS18	$G_{i/q}$	64407
		RGS21	[a]	[b]
	R7	RGS6	$G_{i/q}$	9628
		RGS7	$G_{i/q}$	6000
		RGS9	$G_{i/q}$	8787
		RGS11	$G_{i/q}$	8786
	R12	RGS10	$G_{i/q}$	6001
		RGS12	$G_{i/q}$	6002
		RGS14	$G_{i/q}$	10636
	RZ	RGS17 (RGSZ2)	$G_z > G_i$	26575
		RGS19 (GAIP)	G_i	10287
		RGS20 (RGSZ1, Ret-RGS1)	$G_z > G_i$	8601
	RA	AXIN1	—	8312
		AXIN2 (AXIL, CONDUCTIN)	—	8313
RGS-PX		RGS-PX1 (SNX13, KIAA0713)	G_s	23161
		RGS-PX2 (MSTP043)	[a]	83891
rgRGS		ARHGEF1 (P115-RHOGEF, LSC)	G_{12}	9138
		ARHGEF11 (GTRAP48, KIAA0380, PDZ-RHOGEF)	G_{12}	9826
		ARHGEF12 (LARG, KIAA0382)	G_{12}	23365
GPRK		ADRBK1 (GRK2, BARK1)	G_q	156
		ADRBK2 (GRK3, BARK2)	G_q	157
		GPRK2L (GRK4, GPRK4)	ND	2869
		GPRK6 (GRK6)	ND	2870
		RHOK (RK, GRK1)	ND	6011
AKAP-RGS		AKAP10 (PRKA10, D-AKAP2)	—	11216

Note. LocusLink (http://ncbi.nlm.nih.gov).

[a]GAP activity untested.

[b]LocusLink number not assigned; ND, not done; —, no GAP activity.

TABLE 2 RGS Protein Domains and Functions

Family	Subfamily		Domain number and name	Function
RGS	RZ	RGS	RGS domain	G_Z-, G_i-GAP
	R4, R7, R12	RGS	RGS domain	G_i-, G_q-GAP
	RZ	1	Cysteine string	Membrane localization
	RZ, R12	2	PDZ-binding motif	Scaffold binding
	R4, RZ	3	Amphipathic helix	Membrane localization and receptor selectivity
	R4, R12	4	PDZ domain	Scaffold/protein-binding motif
	R7	5	DEP domain	Unknown function: possible membrane protein and phospholipid binding
	R7	6	GGL domain	$G_{\beta 5}$ binding
	R12	7	PTB domain	Scaffold–phosphotyrosine binding
	R12	8	Rap-binding domain	Binds small GTPase Rap
	R12	9	GoLoco homology domain	Binds $G_{\alpha i}$-GDP, $G_{\alpha o}$-GDP
	RA	RGS	APC-binding domain	Scaffold function: binds adenomatous polyposis coli protein
	RA	10	GSK-binding domain	Scaffold function: binds glycogen synthase kinase
	RA	11	β-Catenin-binding domain	Scaffold function: binds β-catenin, prevents nuclear translocation
	RA	12	PP2A homology domain	Scaffold function: binds protein phosphotase PP2A
	RA	13	Dimerization domain	Homodimerization domain
RGS-PX		RGL	RGS-like domain	G_s-GAP
		14	PX-associated domain	Unknown
		15	PhoX homologous domain	Vesicle binding
rgRGS		RGL	RGS-like domain	G_{12}-GAP
		4	PDZ domain	Scaffold function
		16	Dbl homologous domain	Rho guanine nucleotide exchange factor (GEF)
		17	Pleckstrin homology domain	Unknown function: possible membrane localization
GPRK		RGL	RGS-like domain	G_q-GAP
		17	Pleckstrin homology domain	Unknown function: possible membrane localization
		18	Receptor kinase domain	Phosphorylates activated G-protein-coupled receptors
		19	Gβγ-binding PH domain	Binds βγ-subunit of G-protein
AKAP-RGS		RGL	Rgs-like domain	Unknown
		20	PKA-binding domain	Binds PKA regulatory subunit

protein Rho (RhoGEF). G_α subunits of the G_s class activate the effector protein adenylyl cyclase, which stimulates the production of the second messenger cyclic AMP (cAMP). The activity of these four classes of G-proteins is opposed by the GAP activity of proteins in the RGS superfamily. G_q and G_i proteins are substrates for proteins in the RGS family, G_{12} proteins are regulated by rgRGS proteins, and G_s proteins are substrates for RGS-PX proteins (Table 1). An aspect of signaling specificity is that RGS proteins in the RGS, rgRGS, and RGS-PX families have no GAP activity on the G-protein substrates of the other two RGS families. G_q proteins are exceptional because GTP hydrolysis on these α-subunits can be accelerated by RGS and GPRK proteins within the RGS superfamily and the unrelated effector protein PLC-β.

At least two other families of proteins that contain RGS-like domains are expressed in metazoans (Table 2). AKAP10 contains two RGS-like domains; although the function of this protein is not known, it is tempting to speculate that it regulates protein kinase A (PKA) activity in response to G_s-stimulated cAMP production. GPRK is the fifth family of RGS-like proteins, including at least two proteins, ADRBK1 and ADRBK2, that have weak G_q-GAP activity. It is not known whether ADRBK1 and ADRBK2 interact with RGS G_q-GAPs to regulate G_q signaling complexes or whether GAP activity by GPRKs, RGS-PX, and/or RGS may influence receptor desensitization and internalization. Several of the GPRK genes have been deleted in mice, leading to a wide range of defects including light-dependent retinal degeneration, embryonic cardiomyocyte hypoplasia, and increased sensitivity and/or lack of desensitization to physiologically relevant doses of pharmacological agents.

C. Multidomain RGS Proteins

Proteins in the RGS superfamily are defined by their RGS domains, but each has additional flanking domains with distinct functions. These modules mediate protein or lipid interactions that are unique to individual families and even subfamilies of RGS proteins (Fig. 1). A brief description of protein domains specific to different RGS protein families and their functions is presented in Tables 2 and 3. These groupings suggest that the functional domains contribute to subfamily-specific catalytic activities, subcellular localization, and/or regulation (summarized in Fig. 3). For example, the kinase domain in GPRK family proteins phosphorylates activated heptahelical receptors, leading to their internalization and down-regulation. A different family of RGS-like proteins, the rgRGS proteins, are distinguished by a dbl homology domain that binds and activates its effector protein Rho, thereby regulating cell shape changes and motility. The RGS-PX proteins have a PX domain, which is usually found in proteins called nexins, involved in vesicular trafficking within cells. Genetic and biochemical evidence from vertebrates and invertebrates indicates that RGS, GPRK, and rgRGS proteins regulate G_q, G_i, and G_{12} signaling via G-protein-coupled receptors but it is unclear whether the G_s-GAPs of the RGS-PX family regulate hormonal signaling or vesicular transport.

Some RGS proteins serve as scaffolds that bring proteins into proximity to allow specific interactions. For example, the RA protein axin is a scaffold protein that negatively regulates the wnt signaling pathway. The RGS domain of axin has no GAP activity but binds another scaffold protein on the wnt pathway, APC. Flanking the axin RGS domain are additional domains that bind the serine/threonine kinase GSK, its phosphorylation target β-catenin, and its negative regulator, protein phosphatase 2A. Axin and APC together assemble a signaling complex that regulates the stability and activity of the transcription factor β-catenin, thereby influencing development and tumor progression.

Scaffolding functions can also serve to bring the RGS domain into a particular receptor complex where it can act on the G_α subunit and serve to

TABLE 3   RGS Deficiencies in Eukaryotes

Species	RGS family	Gene	Phenotype of genetic deficiency
Saccharomyces cerevisiae	RY[a]	*Sst2*	Supersensitive to pheromone, delayed recovery from cell cycle arrest
		Rgs2	Enhanced glucose response
Schizosaccharomyces pombe		*Rgs1*	Increased sensitivity to mating factor, mating defects
A. nidulans		*FlbA*	No conidiophore formation or asexual reproduction
Caenorhabditis elegans	R7	*Egl-10*	Hypokinesis and delayed egg-laying
		Eat-16	Hyperkinesis and precocious egg-laying
	RC[b]	*Rgs1*	Rgs1;Rgs2 double-mutant delayed recovery from fasting
		Rgs2	
Drosophila melanogaster	R12	*Loco*	Impaired glial cell function and dorsal–ventral axis formation
	rgRGS	*DRhoGEF*	Gastrulation defects
Mus musculus	R7	*RGS9*	Delayed recovery to light in photoreceptor cells
	R4	*RGS2*	Reduced male aggression, T-cell defects, hypertension
	RA	*axin*	Duplication of anterior structures during embryogenesis
	GPRK	*GRPK2*	Embryonic lethality from cardiomyocyte hypoplasia
		GRPK3	Reduced olfactory desensitization, increased muscarinic-evoked airway response

[a]RY is an RGS subfamily found in fungi.
[b]RC is an RGS subfamily found only in *C. elegans*.

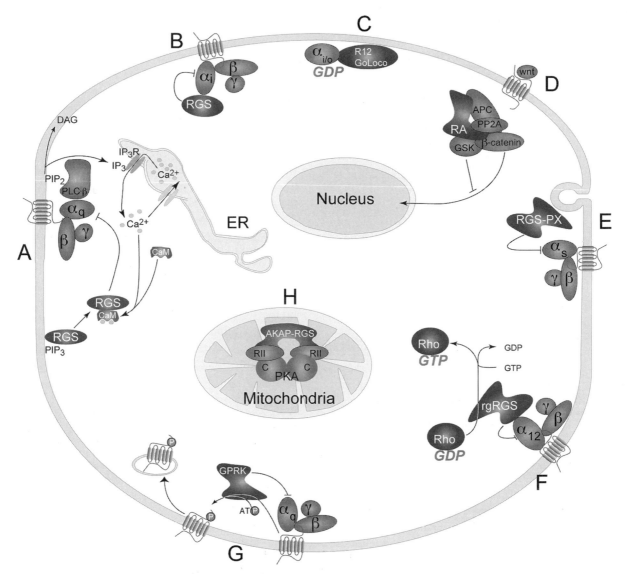

FIGURE 3 Actions of RGS superfamily proteins in cellular signaling complexes. (A) G_q class G-proteins activate PLC-β to produce DAG and IP_3. IP_3 causes the release of the second messenger Ca^{2+} from intracellular stores. Ca^{2+}/calmodulin (CaM) displaces PIP_3 on RGS proteins of the R4 subfamily, which acts as a GAP on the G_α subunit. (B) G_i class G-proteins are negatively regulated by RGS proteins of the R4, R7, R12, and RZ subfamilies. (C) The GoLoco domain of R12 RGS proteins interacts with $G_{\alpha i/o}$-GDP. (D) RA RGS proteins function as structural components of the wnt signaling pathway, bringing β-catenin into proximity of its negative regulator, GSK kinase, which phosphorylates β-catenin, marking it for proteosome-mediated degradation. (E) RGS-PX proteins function as GAPs for $G_{\alpha s}$ and also bind to vesicles. (F) rgRGS serve as GAPs for G_{12} class G-proteins and as guanine nucleotide exchange factors for small Rho G-proteins. (G) GPRKs can serve as GAPs for G_q class G-proteins and also phosphorylate activated receptors, promoting their internalization and down-regulation. (H) AKAP10 contains two RGS-like domains of unknown function and two domains that bind the regulatory subunit of PKA, and it is highly enriched in mitochondria.

distinguish hormonal signals sent through different receptors that couple to the same G-protein. For example, in pancreatic acinar cells, RGS4 has been shown to preferentially inhibit signaling through m3-muscarinic receptors, relative to cholecystokinin receptors, despite the fact that they both couple to

$G_{\alpha q}$. RGS4 contains an N-terminal domain shared by some other R4 subfamily members that is responsible for this receptor selectivity. This allows the cell to regulate signaling specificity through a combination of receptor-dependent activation by agonists and attenuation by RGS proteins.

III. GAP ACTIVITY REGULATES SIGNALING

A. G-Proteins Transduce Extracellular Signals to Regulate Intracellular Responses

All higher eukaryotes, including yeast, *Dictyostelium discoides*, plants, and animals, utilize G-protein signaling to mediate intracellular responses to extracellular stimuli. G-protein signaling systems have several components, each encoded by distinct multigene families. Extracellular signals received by heptahelical receptors are coupled by heterotrimeric G-proteins to the regulation of effector proteins that generate intracellular second messengers. Following agonist stimulation, cells must recover to maintain homeostasis. RGS proteins can rapidly attenuate G-protein signaling through feedback regulatory mechanisms. Thus, G-proteins act as signal transducers under the positive and negative regulation of receptors and RGS proteins, respectively. Activation and inactivation may occur within a G-protein signaling complex, composed of perhaps six distinct proteins, which acts like a molecular machine to convey extracellular signals and coordinate intracellular responses. All of the molecular components of G-protein signaling cascades, from ligands to effector proteins, are required to relay information from the outside of the cell to the inside.

B. Regulation of GTP Binding and Hydrolysis

The essential regulatory feature of G-protein signaling is the cycle of GTP binding and hydrolysis on the G_α subunit. Many of the proteins that interact with the G_α subunit regulate its transit through this cycle. Signaling is initiated on receptor binding of extracellular agonists, such as nucleotides or small peptides, or the activation of a prebound chromophore by light. RGS proteins may help assemble a signaling complex that brings receptor, G-protein, and effector protein into proximity to stimulate rapid activation on ligand binding. The GAP activity of RGS proteins accelerates GTP hydrolysis and thereby can rapidly terminate signaling. The balance of activation by hormone binding and inactivation by RGS GAP activity controls the signaling flux through G-proteins.

The heterotrimeric $G_{\alpha\beta\gamma}$ protein complex is required for the receptor to stimulate intracellular signaling (Fig. 4). G_α is the largest subunit in the complex, ranging from 41 to 45 kDa, and binds the guanine nucleotide. $G_{\beta\gamma}$ forms a stable heterodimer of 35 and 7 kDa subunits, respectively. In the inactive state, G_α binds GDP to assume a conformation with high affinity for $G_{\beta\gamma}$. G_α-GDP$\beta\gamma$ can interact with the intracellular loops and tail of the receptor. Agonist binding to receptor on the outside of the cell conveys conformational changes to the intracellular surfaces of the receptor that catalyze the dissociation of GDP from the G_α subunit. In the open state, the G_α subunit will bind GDP or GTP with equal affinity but the cytosolic concentration of GTP is 100-fold higher that GDP, which promotes GTP binding and progression of the activity cycle. GTP binding induces a conformational change in the switch regions of the G_α protein. The switch regions bind at least three different proteins ($G_{\beta\gamma}$, effector proteins, and RGS proteins) at different times during the cycle of GTP binding and hydrolysis. Conformational changes in the switch regions favor dissociation of the previous binding partner and association of the next partner in the cycle. GTP binding to the G_α subunit weakens its interaction with $G_{\beta\gamma}$ and receptor but induces a conformational change that favors interaction with effector proteins. Both G_α-GTP and $G_{\beta\gamma}$ can regulate independent effector proteins. Thus, information is transduced from extracellular ligand binding to effector proteins that regulate the production of intracellular second messengers, such as cAMP and Ca^{2+}. G_α remains active until GTP is hydrolyzed. Conformational changes in G_α-GDP drive the dissociation of the effector protein, thus terminating signaling and favoring reassociation of $G_{\beta\gamma}$. The cycle of GTP binding and hydrolysis can be repeated in the presence of persistent agonist.

RGS proteins are important regulators of G-protein activity because they are GAPs for G_α subunits, thereby inactivating or attenuating signaling. GAP activity is conveyed by the RGS domain. The RGS domain from several different RGS proteins can stimulate GTP hydrolysis up to 2000-fold above the basal activity of the G_α subunit, with all of the catalytic residues being supplied by the G_α subunit. Additionally, recent studies have shown that some RGS proteins also serve as scaffolds to help assemble active receptor complexes that are tightly coupled to effector proteins. Thus, RGS proteins regulate the kinetics of the G-protein activity cycle, and some apparently can accelerate both the activation and the inactivation of signaling. Current models of G-protein signaling suggest that signaling initiates within a multiprotein complex including receptor, G-protein, effector, RGS protein, and perhaps membrane lipids and other proteins (Figs. 3 and 4).

The duration and intensity of G-protein signaling can be modulated by posttranslational modifications of the receptors and RGS proteins that regulate the cycle of GTP binding and hydrolysis. Signaling is

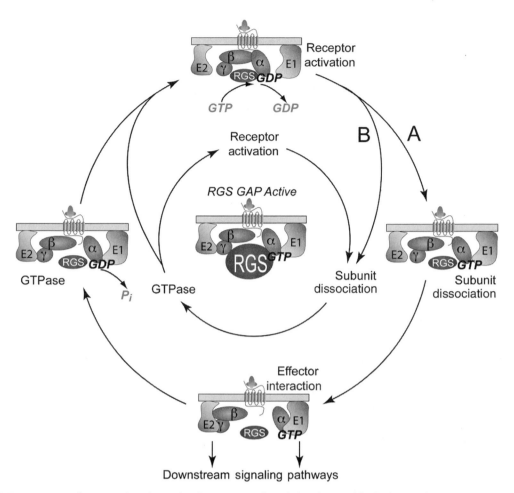

FIGURE 4 Action of RGS within the cycle of guanine nucleotide binding and hydrolysis in heterotrimeric G-protein signaling complexes. In the presence of hormone agonist, receptor activation causes the exchange of GDP for GTP on the α-subunit. In the presence of low or rising second-messenger levels, RGS is inactive, promoting pathway A, where subunit dissociation is followed by effector interaction, and the activation of downstream signaling pathways, causing an increase in second messenger levels. Intrinsic GTPase activity of G_α cleaves the terminal phosphate from GTP, and the cycle is poised for another round in the continued presence of hormone agonist. When second-messenger levels are high, pathway B is promoted, where receptor activation is followed by subunit dissociation, and the GAP activity of RGS accelerates GTP hydrolysis before effector interaction can take place. In the continued presence of hormone agonist, multiple cycles of pathway B can uncouple hormone binding from effector protein activation, thereby terminating signaling. Repeating switches between pathways A and B can initiate oscillations in the production of second messengers, as observed in Ca^{2+} oscillations evoked by G_q-coupled agonists.

activated by agonist (Fig. 4, pathway A) and can be terminated when agonist is depleted or overwhelmed by antagonist. Signaling can also be terminated by constitutively active RGS GAP activity, despite agonist stimulation of the G-protein. Thus, RGS proteins can uncouple effector protein activation even in the presence of persistent agonist (Fig. 4, pathway B). If RGS GAP activity is transiently activated and inactivated in response to the rise and fall of intracellular second messengers, then second-messenger production and downstream signaling can oscillate. RGS proteins have been proposed to play an

important role in generating Ca^{2+} oscillations in response to G_q-coupled agonists and thus regulate diverse biological processes such as the release of peptides from neuroendocrine cells and the proliferation and growth of cardiomyocytes during development and progression to heart disease.

C. Effectors as GAPs

At least three G-protein-coupled effectors have GAP activity or stimulate an associated GAP. Although this accelerates the rate of return to the basal state, effector activation, and thereby signaling, is maintained by persistent agonist stimulation. However, signaling can rapidly terminate on agonist dissociation from the receptor. Thus, effector GAP activity allows a rapid response to both activating and inhibitory inputs.

The rgRGS proteins are both GAPs and effector proteins for G_{12} class α-subunits. These proteins mediate cell shape changes during development and cell migration. Cell shape changes are regulated by the small GTPase Rho, which controls the assembly of actin stress fibers. Rho can be activated by a variety of guanine nucleotide exchange factors (GEFs). rgRGS proteins are RhoGEFs that are uniquely responsive to activation of G_{12} class α-subunits. The rgRGS proteins have an RGS-like domain that binds and accelerates GTP hydrolysis on G_{12} class α-subunits and a dbl-homology domain with RhoGEF activity. This signaling pathway, which couples heterotrimeric G-proteins to the small GTPase Rho, is conserved in vertebrates and invertebrates.

A second example of an effector with GAP activity was discovered in vertebrate photoreceptor cells. In this case, the G-protein transducin interacts with separate GAP and effector proteins, RGS9 and the γ-subunit of cGMP phosphodiesterase (PDE), respectively. RGS9 GAP activity on transducin is intrinsically weak but is augmented by both PDEγ and a recently discovered protein termed R9AP. Thus, a multiprotein complex of G-protein, RGS effector, and ancillary proteins serves the signaling requirements of vertebrate photoreceptor cells.

The regulation of G_q class proteins is a third variation on this theme of multiprotein signaling complexes. As mentioned previously, like rgRGS, PLC-β is both a $G_α$-GAP and an effector protein, but its sequence and structure are unrelated to those of RGS proteins. In addition to PLC-β, several RGS proteins also have G_q-GAP activity and appear to regulate PLC-β activity within a signaling complex composed of receptor, G-protein, RGS, and PLC-β. Currently under debate is why G_q signaling is regulated by both PLC-β and RGS GAPs. One proposal is that GAP activity of PLC-β is constitutive, and this drives a rapid cycle of GTP binding and hydrolysis in the presence of persistent agonist. This is sufficient to maintain $G_α$ and $G_{βγ}$ in proximity to the active receptor, acting like a kinetic scaffold to prevent G-protein dissociation from the receptor complex. Despite G_q-GAP activity, PLC-β still generates second messengers in the presence of persistent agonist, but only while the RGS GAP is inactive. By contrast, the GAP activity of many RGS proteins appears to be regulated by the rise and fall of second messengers inside the cell. Thus, GAP activity drives a repeating cycle of GTP binding and hydrolysis; PLC-β generates second messengers, whereas RGS proteins act as feedback inhibitors to uncouple G-protein activation from effector protein activation (Fig. 3). The combined action of these two GAPs may initiate pulses, or oscillations, of second messenger, as observed in many cell types during the initiation of Ca^{2+} signaling by G_q-coupled agonists.

IV. SUMMARY

GTP binding and hydrolysis on G-proteins drive cycles of protein–protein interactions that mediate signaling inside cells in response to extracellular signals. Heterotrimeric G-protein α- and/or βγ-subunits can independently regulate effector proteins, and thus, a single stimulus can generate a bifurcating signal. G-protein signaling via both $G_α$ and $G_{βγ}$ is subject to feedback regulation through their attendant RGS proteins. The five families of RGS proteins in the RGS superfamily bind, and often accelerate GTP hydrolysis, to distinct types of G-proteins via interactions through their RGS domains. In addition to their catalytic properties, several RGS proteins function like scaffolds to organize multiprotein complexes that rapidly initiate and terminate signaling (summarized in Fig. 3). Each subfamily of RGS protein has protein domains, in addition to the RGS domain, that bind proteins and/or lipids that convey distinct regulatory properties. Thus, regulatory specificity is achieved by the combination of G-protein substrate specificity, cellular targeting, and accessory protein interactions with RGS proteins. Regulation of G-protein signaling by RGS proteins is found in fungi, *Dictyostelium*, and metazoan organisms at all stages of their life cycles and is fundamental to intercellular communication in higher eukaryotic organisms.

Glossary

effector protein $G_α$ and $G_{βγ}$ bind and regulate proteins that either increase or decrease the intracellular concentration of small molecules, termed second messengers, that stimulate cellular responses to extracellular hormones.

G-protein Proteins that are composed of three subunits; the α-subunit binds GTP and has GTPase activity, the β- and γ-subunits form stable heterodimers, and both $G_α$ and $G_{βγ}$ can independently activate effector proteins in response to hormone stimulation.

G-protein-coupled receptors Heptahelical transmembrane proteins that bind hormones, chromophores, or other extracellular ligands to promote G-protein signaling inside the cell.

GTPase accelerating proteins (GAPs) Proteins that accelerate the hydrolysis of GTP on distinct types of G-protein α-subunits. GAPs occur in four of the five families of RGS-like proteins and the effector protein phospholipase C-β.

regulators of G-protein signaling proteins GTPase accelerating proteins for the α-subunit of heterotrimeric G-proteins.

second messenger Small molecules, such as cyclic AMP, inositol 1,4,5-triphosphate, diacylglycerol, or Ca^{2+}, that alter the activity of target enzymes and ion channels to influence cellular responses to extracellular hormones, neurotransmitters, and other stimuli.

See Also the Following Articles

Further Reading

Barrett, K., Leptin, M., and Settleman, J. (1997). The Rho GTPase and a putative RhoGEF mediate a signaling pathway for the cell shape changes in *Drosophila* gastrulation. *Cell* **91**, 905–915.

Carman, C. V., Parent, J. L., Day, P. W., Pronin, A. N., Sternweis, P. M., Wedegaertner, P. B., Gilman, A. G., Benovic, J. L., and Kozasa, T. (1999). Selective regulation of Gαq/11 by an RGS domain in the G protein-coupled receptor kinase, GRK2. *J. Biol. Chem.* **274**, 34483–34492.

Chase, D. L., Patikoglou, G. A., and Koelle, M. R. (2001). Two RGS proteins that inhibit Gαo and Gαq signaling in *C. elegans* neurons require a Gβ5-like subunit for function. *Curr. Biol.* **11**, 222–231.

Chen, C. K., Burns, M. E., He, W., Wensel, T. G., Baylor, D. A., and Simon, M. I. (2000). Slowed recovery of rod photoresponse in mice lacking the GTPase accelerating protein RGS9-1. *Nature* **403**, 557–5560.

Gilman, A. G. (1987). G proteins: Transducers of receptor-generated signals. *Annu. Rev. Biochem.* **56**, 615–649.

Kimple, R. J., Kimple, M. E., Betts, L., Sondek, J., and Siderovski, D. P. (2002). Structural determinants for GoLoco-induced inhibition of nucleotide release by Gα subunits. *Nature* **416**, 878–881.

Kozasa, T., Jiang, X., Hart, M. J., Sternweis, P. M., Singer, W. D., Gilman, A. G., Bollag, G., and Sternweis, P. C. (1998). p115 RhoGEF, a GTPase activating protein for Gα12 and Gα13. *Science* **280**, 2109–2111.

Ross, E., and Wilkie, T. M. (2000). GTPase-activating proteins for heterotrimeric G proteins: Regulators of G protein signaling (RGS) and RGS-like proteins. *Annu. Rev. Biochem.* **69**, 795–827.

Sierra, D. A., Gilbert, D. J., Householder, D., Grishin, N. V., Yu, K., Ukidwe, P., Barker, S. A., He, W., Wensel, T. G., Otero, G., Brown, G., Copeland, N. G., Jenkins, N. A., and Wilkie, T. M. (2002). Evolution of the regulators of G protein signaling multigene family in mouse and human. *Genomics* **79**, 177–185.

Snow, B. E., Krumins, A. M., Brothers, G. M., Lee, S. F., Wall, M. A., Chung, S., Mangion, J., Arya, S., Gilman, A. G., and Siderovski, D. P. (1998). A G protein γ subunit-like domain shared between RGS11 and other RGS proteins specifies binding to Gβ5 subunits. *Proc. Natl. Acad. Sci. USA* **95**, 13307–13312.

Tesmer, J. J., Berman, D. M., Gilman, A. G., and Sprang, S. R. (1997). Structure of RGS4 bound to AlF4⁻-activated Gαi1: Stabilization of the transition state for GTP hydrolysis. *Cell* **89**, 251–261.

Wang, L., Sunahara, R. K., Krumins, A., Perkins, G., Crochiere, M. L., Mackey, M., Bell, S., Ellisman, M. H., and Taylor, S. S. (2001). Cloning and mitochondrial localization of full-length D-AKAP2, a protein kinase A anchoring protein. *Proc. Natl. Acad. Sci. USA* **98**, 3220–3225.

Wilkie, T. M., Gilbert, D. J., Olsen, A. S., Chen, X. N., Amatruda, T. T., Korenberg, J. R., Trask, B. J., de Jong, P., Reed, R. R., Simon, M. I., Jenkins, N. A., and Copeland, N. G. (1992). Evolution of the mammalian G protein α subunit multigene family. *Nat. Genet.* **1**, 85–91.

Zheng, B., Ma, Y. C., Ostrom, R. S., Lavoie, C., Gill, G. N., Insel, P. A., Huang, X. Y., and Farquhar, M. G. (2001). RGS-PX1, a GAP for Gαs and sorting nexin in vesicular trafficking. *Science* **294**, 1939–1942.

Salicylic Acid

D'MARIS AMICK DEMPSEY AND DANIEL F. KLESSIG

Boyce Thompson Institute for Plant Research, New York

Salicylic acid, a phenolic compound synthesized by plants, plays an important role in signaling mechanisms that regulate plant defenses against pathogens. Plant genetic studies show that salicylic acid regulates components of its own signaling pathway and is involved in cross talk with other pathways involved in mediating disease resistance and thermogenesis.

I. INTRODUCTION

Salicylic acid (SA) and its derivatives, collectively known as salicylates, are just some of the many phenolic compounds synthesized by plants.

Until recently, the function of salicylates in plants was obscure; thus, they have traditionally been classified as secondary metabolites. By contrast, the pharmacological benefits of salicylates in humans are well documented. Aspirin (acetylsalicylic acid), for example, at various doses, protects against heart attack and stroke, inhibits blood clotting, and reduces pain, fever, and joint swelling. Only during the past 15 years have researchers discovered that SA serves important functions in plants. It is a signaling molecule that activates heat production, induces disease resistance, and, possibly, stimulates flowering.

II. SA-REGULATED PROCESSES IN PLANTS

The first conclusive demonstration that SA functions as an endogenous signaling molecule came from Raskin and co-workers, who were studying thermogenesis in the voodoo lily (*Sauromatum guttatum*). On the day of flowering, there are two distinct periods during which the temperature of the spadix (floral spike) can increase by approximately 14°C. Prior to each thermogenic event, a large, transient increase in endogenous SA levels is detected. Confirming the role of SA as the signal for this phenomenon, it has been shown that exogenously supplied SA, as well as its derivatives acetylsalicylic acid (ASA) (Fig. 1) and 2,6-dihydroxybenzoic acid, can induce thermogenesis in explants of the voodoo lily spadix, whereas 31 structurally similar compounds do not have this effect.

SA also has been shown to play an important signaling role in plant disease resistance, and the mechanisms through which it activates this phenomenon have been studied extensively. The ability of a plant to recognize a pathogen is sometimes regulated by the direct or indirect interaction between the products of a plant resistance (*R*) gene and a pathogen avirulence (*avr*) gene. If either of these gene products is lacking, the plant fails to activate defenses in a timely and/or effective manner and the pathogen colonizes the plant. By contrast, when both gene products are present, a wide variety of resistance responses are activated in the inoculated leaf. These may include increases in reactive oxygen species (ROS), strengthening of cell walls, and synthesis/activation of various defense-associated proteins, such as the pathogenesis-related (PR) proteins. In addition, resistant plants frequently develop a hypersensitive response (HR) (Fig. 2). Subsequent to these local responses, uninoculated leaves usually exhibit increased *PR* gene expression and systemic acquired resistance (SAR).

It has been known for many years that treatment of tobacco with SA or ASA enhances resistance to tobacco mosaic virus (TMV) and induces PR protein accumulation. SA has more recently been shown to activate *PR* gene expression in several plant species and to enhance resistance to a variety of pathogens. The first direct evidence that SA is an endogenous signal for disease resistance came from studies of pathogen-infected tobacco and cucumber plants. In tobacco resisting infection by TMV, SA levels increased 20- to 50-fold in inoculated leaves, with these increases preceding or paralleling the accumulation of *PR* gene transcripts. SA levels also increased 2- to 10-fold in the uninoculated leaves, and this rise correlated with increased systemic *PR* gene expression. Similarly, in cucumber infected with *Colletotrichum lagenarium*, *Pseudomonas syringae*, or tobacco necrosis virus, 10- to 100-fold increases in SA levels were detected in the phloem sap of infected leaves prior to SAR development and activation of a defense-associated peroxidase in the uninoculated tissue.

Analyses of SA-deficient tobacco and *Arabidopsis* plants [due to inhibition of the SA biosynthetic pathway or expression of the salicylate hydroxylase (SH)-encoding *nahG* transgene] have further confirmed that SA plays an important role in activating disease resistance. These plants fail to develop SAR or express *PR* genes in the uninoculated leaves following pathogen infection. Furthermore, they are susceptible to infection by pathogens that they normally would resist and exhibit heightened susceptibility to those that cause disease. HR development is also delayed in TMV-infected SH-expressing tobacco and the lesions that form grow substantially larger than do those on comparable wild-type (wt) plants. Based on these results, SA may also regulate cell death and pathogen containment. Consistent with this possibility, inhibition of the SA biosynthetic enzyme phenylalanine ammonia lyase (PAL) in soybean suspension cells blocks pathogen-induced HR cell death. Additionally, genetic analyses of certain *Arabidopsis* mutants reveal that SA is required for expression of a constitutive cell death phenotype that mimics an HR.

Whether SA is a mobile signal that induces defense responses in uninfected tissues has been the subject of much debate. The timing at which SA levels increase and SAR develops in both tobacco and cucumber is consistent with this possibility. Furthermore, SA clearly is mobile; it has been detected in the phloem

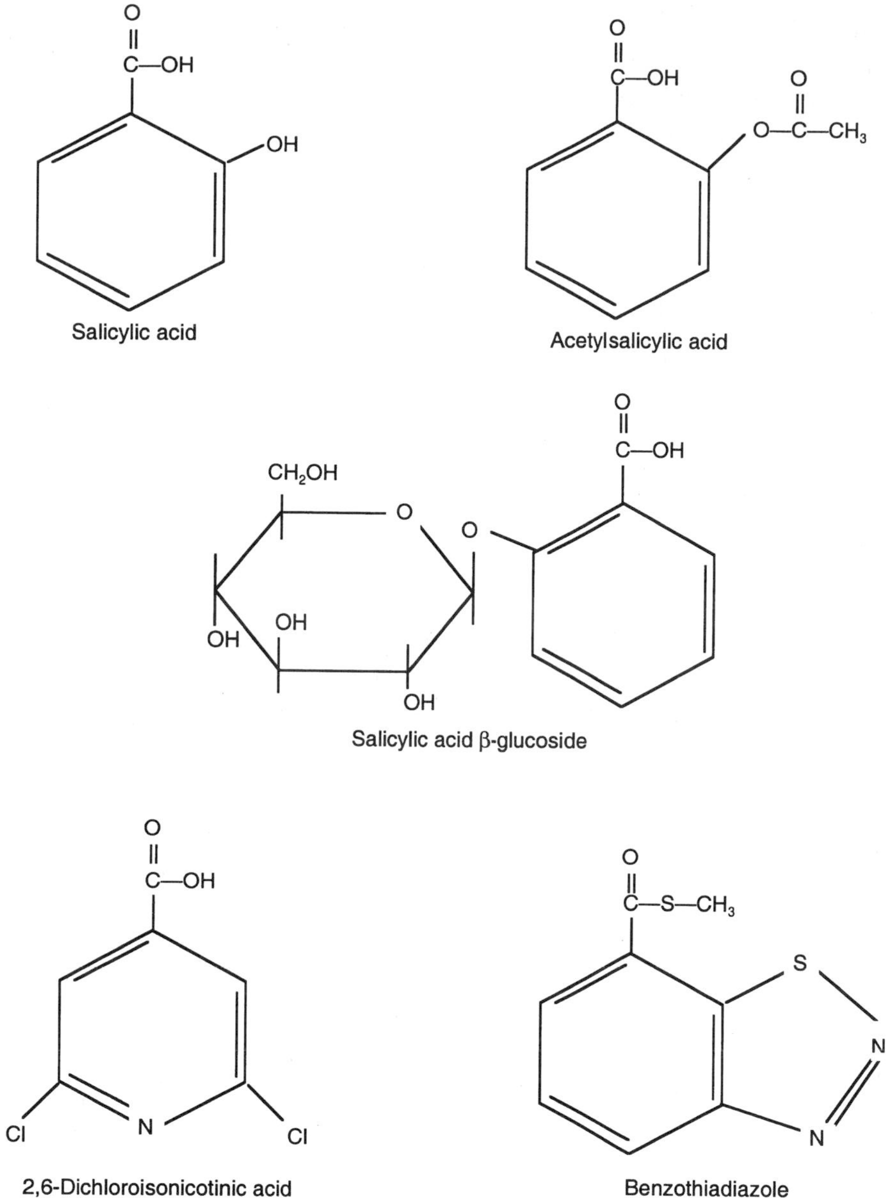

FIGURE 1 Salicylic acid and its derivatives or functional analogues. Salicylic acid and its derivative acetylsalicylic acid (aspirin) induce *PR* expression and systemic acquired resistance in plants; in contrast, salicylic acid β-glucoside is thought to be a storage form of salicylic acid. The synthetic compounds 2,6-dichloroisonicotinic acid and benzothiadiazole *S*-methyl ester, which exhibit structural similarity to salicylic acid, also induce defense responses in plants. In particular, benzothiadiazole *S*-methyl ester has been used commercially in the field to protect crop plants against certain pathogens.

sap of pathogen-infected cucumber and tobacco leaves. Tracer studies using $^{18}O_2$ or the SA precursor [^{14}C]benzoic acid (BA) also have suggested that much of the SA in the uninoculated leaves is transported there from the inoculated leaves. Alternatively, SA may be converted into methylsalicylate, a volatile compound that could serve as an airborne SAR signal.

A growing body of evidence, however, suggests that SA is not the long-distance SAR signal. In *P. syringae*-infected cucumber, the SAR signal is transmitted from the inoculated leaf several hours

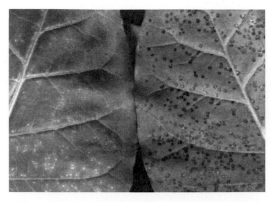

FIGURE 2 The hypersensitive response (right) and systemic acquired resistance in tobacco following TMV infection. Tobacco plants resisting infection by TMV initially develop a hypersensitive response, characterized by necrotic lesions at the sites of pathogen entry. Subsequently, a broad-based, long-lasting systemic acquired resistance develops in uninoculated tissues. A secondary viral infection of the uninoculated leaves, occurring several days after the initial infection, results in much smaller lesions (left) as compared with those induced by the primary infection. The leaves are shown 4 days after infection. Reprinted from *Trends in Plant Science*, Vol. 2, pp. 266–274 (1997) (Durner *et al.*), with permission from Elsevier Science.

before an increase in SA levels can be detected in the petiole of the inoculated leaf. In addition, wild-type scions (the grafted tops of chimeric tobacco plants) develop SAR and express *PR* genes following TMV infection of SH-expressing or PAL-suppressed rootstocks. Because SA accumulation is not completely abolished in these rootstocks, it is possible that a small amount of SA travels to the scion and induces SAR. However, transgenic tobacco rootstocks that constitutively accumulate SA due to expression of the cholera toxin A1 subunit do not induce *PR* expression or SA accumulation in wt scions. Although these results suggest that SA is not the long-distance SAR signal, SA clearly plays an important downstream role in the defense pathway. SA-deficient scions fail to exhibit *PR* gene expression and/or SAR following infection of wt rootstocks.

Induction of flowering in various *Lemna* species, as well as in *Arabidopsis thaliana*, *Impatiens balsamina*, *Onacidium*, and *Pisita stratiotes* L, and flower bud formation in tobacco tissue cultures have been associated with SA treatment, thus SA has been proposed to be the inductive signal for flowering. However, other evidence does not support this conclusion. For example, SA levels are comparable in flowering and vegetative *Lemna* plants, and

the ability of SA to stimulate flowering in several plant species appears to be a nonspecific effect. Thus, whether SA plays any role in flowering remains unclear.

III. SA METABOLISM

A large body of evidence suggests that SA, many phytoalexins, and lignin are synthesized by the shikimate–phenylpropanoid pathway. The first step of this pathway, which is rapidly induced following pathogen infection, is the conversion of phenylalanine (Phe) to *trans*-cinnamic acid (*t*-CA) by PAL. Depending on the plant species, SA is then generated from *t*-CA through one of two intermediates, benzoic acid or *ortho*-coumaric acid. Both tobacco and cucumber appear to utilize the BA intermediate. The mechanism through which BA is generated from *t*-CA is poorly understood. An oxidative pathway, analogous to β-oxidation of fatty acids, and a nonoxidative pathway, involving the intermediate benzaldehyde, have both been proposed. Supporting the former possibility, no labeled benzaldehyde is detected in TMV-infected tobacco supplied with $3\text{-}[^{13}C_1]$Phe. Once BA is formed, it can be converted to SA by BA 2-hydroxylase (BA2H). Characterization of partially purified BA2H reveals that its activity is strongly induced by exogenously supplied BA or TMV infection. Because this activation is blocked by cycloheximide (CHX), *de novo* synthesis of BA2H appears to be required. Alternatively, a recent study has suggested that BA is not the direct precursor of SA. Rather, a conjugate of BA, consisting of BA and a glucose (BAG) molecule, may be converted to SA.

Like BA, SA also can be conjugated to a glucose molecule. The predominant SA conjugate in many plant species is SA 2-O-β-D-glucoside (SAG); the BAG recently identified in tobacco is benzoylglucose. In tobacco and *Arabidopsis*, free SA and SAG can be detected at low levels. After infection, SA and SAG levels rise, with SAG predominating in both the inoculated and uninoculated leaves. The kinetics of accumulation for free BA parallel those of SA; however, there are conflicting reports as to whether BAG levels increase following infection or are constitutively elevated. The enzyme responsible for conjugating SA, and possibly BA and other phenolics, is uridine diphosphate (UDP)-glucose:SA glucosyltransferase. This enzyme has been characterized in several plant species, and genes encoding this enzyme have been recently cloned from tobacco.

The role of SAG during the resistance response is unclear. Chemically synthesized SAG activates *PR-1* expression in tobacco leaves. However, this induction probably is mediated by free SA, which is released from SAG by a nonspecific cell-wall-associated β-glucosidase. Thus, SAG does not appear to be the signal for defense responses. An alternative role for SAG is to serve as a storage form for SA. Conjugation of phenolic acids, as well as other phytohormones (e.g., auxin), to sugar molecules is a common and potentially reversible mechanism for the storage of various highly active or toxic compounds. In TMV-infected tobacco, deconjugation of SAG in the uninfected tissues of plants exhibiting SAR might therefore provide a rapid source of SA. In conjunction with other SAR-associated defenses, this SA might superinduce resistance, thereby ensuring the extremely rapid restriction of pathogen spread that is the hallmark of SAR.

In addition to the phenylpropanoid pathway, SA can be synthesized from isochorismate, which is derived from chorismate. This isochorismate pathway is utilized in microorganisms, and recent evidence suggests that it also functions in plants. Isoforms of isochorismate synthase have been purified and characterized from *Catharanthus roseus*. Furthermore, the *eds16* (also known as *sid2*) mutant of *Arabidopsis*, which exhibits enhanced disease susceptibility and fails to accumulate high levels of SA after pathogen attack, was recently found to contain a lesion in isochorismate synthase 1 (ICS1). Consistent with this possibility, transgenic tobacco and *Arabidopsis* expressing the two bacterial enzymes involved in the chorismate/isochorismate pathway exhibit elevated SA levels and enhanced disease resistance to viral, fungal, and oomycete pathogens.

IV. MECHANISMS OF SA ACTION

The mechanisms through which SA signals thermogenesis and disease resistance have been studied intensely. In voodoo lilies, SA has been shown to induce alternative oxidase (Aox) expression, which in turn activates the alternative respiratory pathway, thereby generating heat. By contrast, SA appears to utilize multiple mechanisms to induce defense responses.

In tobacco, some defense-associated responses, such as expression of *PR* genes, enhancement of disease resistance, activation of the SA-inducible protein kinase (SIPK), which is a mitogen-activated protein kinase (MAPK), and increases in cytosolic calcium levels, are directly induced by exogenously supplied SA. Interestingly, the ability of SA to enhance disease resistance appears to be mediated by at least

two pathways. One pathway, which regulates resistance to several viruses, including TMV, potato virus X, and cucumber mosaic virus, is sensitive to the Aox inhibitor salicylhydroxyamic acid (SHAM). By contrast, the pathway conferring resistance to a bacterial pathogen (*Erwinia caratovora*) and a fungal pathogen (*Botrytis cinerea*), as well as activating *PR-1* gene expression, is SHAM insensitive.

In addition to the defenses directly activated by SA, some responses, including generation of ROS, activation of HR-like cell death, and induction of certain defense genes, are poorly, if at all, activated by SA alone. Rather, SA potentiates these responses; they are induced more rapidly and/or to a greater extent when SA is supplied prior to or at the time of pathogen infection or treatment with elicitors (biotic or abiotic compounds/factors that induce various defense responses). The relationship between the SA-activated and SA-potentiated response pathways is unclear. However, they may be linked by a proposed positive feedback loop that involves SA, the ROS H_2O_2, and cell death.

In an effort to elucidate the mechanisms through which SA signals defense responses, several SA-interacting proteins or SA-binding proteins (SABPs) have been identified in tobacco. The first SABP identified was the H_2O_2-degrading enzyme catalase (CAT). Because SA and its functional analogues (i.e., those capable of inducing *PR* expression and enhanced resistance) inhibit CAT activity, it has been proposed that SA-mediated CAT inhibition leads to elevated levels of ROS, which might play a role in HR and SAR. Consistent with this possibility, SA also inhibits ascorbate peroxidase (APX), the other major H_2O_2-scavenging enzyme found in plant cells. However, subsequent studies suggest that H_2O_2 functions upstream, rather than downstream of SA in the defense pathway. These conflicting results may yet be reconciled by the presence of a putative self-amplifying feedback loop involving SA and H_2O_2. Alternatively, SA-mediated CAT inhibition might signal resistance through the generation of SA free radicals, which could initiate lipid peroxidation and thereby activate defenses.

To date, at least two other tobacco SABPs have been identified and characterized. SABP2 exhibits high affinity for SA ($K_d = 90$ nM) and has been recently purified. SABP3 exhibits moderate affinity for SA ($K_d = 3-4$ μM) and has been shown to be the chloroplast carbonic anhydrase (CA). The ability of CA to reversibly convert carbon dioxide to bicarbonate is unaffected by SA, suggesting that its recently identified antioxidant activity is critical for defense signaling. It is striking that three of the five SA-interacting proteins currently identified (CAT, APX, and CA) exhibit antioxidant activity. In addition, cytosolic aconitase has been shown to interact with SA. The SA-mediated inhibition of this enzyme may increase citrate levels, which are known to induce *Aox* gene expression. This induction, along with the ability of SA to activate *Aox* expression directly, may play a role in activating the SHAM-sensitive pathway for viral resistance.

It is interesting to note that several SA-interacting proteins, notably CAT, APX, and aconitase, are also regulated by nitric oxide (NO). This small molecule, which signals a wide variety of processes in animals, has been recently shown to regulate aspects of plant growth, development, and disease resistance. In particular, NO is required for pathogen-induced defense gene expression in tobacco and *Arabidopsis*. NO is also needed for HR development in pathogen-infected *Arabidopsis* and it synergizes with ROS to induce cell death in pathogen-treated soybean suspension cells. These findings, combined with the observation that NO induces SA accumulation in tobacco and that SA induces NO accumulation in soybean, suggest that NO, SA, ROS, and cell death are all part of a self-amplifying feedback loop that regulates defense responses. Whereas NO induces *PR-1* expression in tobacco via an SA- and cyclic adenosine diphosphate-ribose (cADPR)-dependent pathway, it activates *PAL* expression via an SA-independent, but cADPR- and cyclic guanosine monophosphate (cGMP)-dependent pathway. Thus, both SA-independent and SA-dependent pathways mediate NO-induced defense responses. Moreover, several critical players in the animal NO signaling pathway are also utilized in plants.

Beyond regulating components of the SA signaling pathway, SA also cross-modulates the activity of the ethylene-mediated and jasmonic acid (JA)-mediated defense pathways. Some of the defenses regulated by ethylene and/or JA include expression of the defensin (*PDF1.2*) and thionin (*Thi2.1*) genes, resistance to certain pathogens, and development of induced systemic resistance (ISR) following infection by nonpathogenic root-colonizing rhizobacteria. Although these pathways do not require SA, there is growing evidence that SA influences them in either a positive or a negative manner. For example, SA antagonizes ethylene/JA-induced defense gene expression in pathogen-inoculated tobacco and *Arabidopsis*; it also antagonizes JA-mediated resistance to herbivorous insects in tobacco. By contrast, SA works in conjunction with ethylene or JA to superinduce *PR*

gene expression in tobacco. Furthermore, SA, ethylene, and JA are all required for the induction of apoptotic (HR-like) cell death in *Arabidopsis* protoplasts treated with the fungal toxin fumonisin B1. All of these signals also may be involved in mediating resistance to *B. cinerea* in *Arabidopsis*. The mechanisms by which SA positively interacts with ethylene and/or JA to induce defenses are not known; however, the ability of SA (or certain SA analogues) to inhibit JA synthesis or action in several plant species provides at least one mechanism for the negative regulation.

V. SA-INDUCED GENE EXPRESSION

SA treatment induces many of the same plant defense genes that are activated by pathogen attack. Traditionally, the SA-induced genes have been divided into one of two categories, immediate-early or late, depending on how rapidly they are activated by SA treatment and whether protein synthesis is required for their activation. Expression of the immediate-early genes, such as those encoding several gluta-thione *S*-transferases and the ethylene response element binding protein 1 (EREBP1), can be detected within 30 min of SA treatment. Expression of the *Agrobacterium tumefaciens* octopine (*ocs*) and nopaline (*nos*) synthase genes and activation of the cauliflower mosaic virus (CaMV 35S) promoter also are rapidly detected following SA treatment. Because induction of these genes is insensitive to the protein synthesis inhibitor CHX, their expression is probably regulated by preformed transcription factors. The promoters of genes belonging to this class contain an activator sequence-1 (*as-1*) or an *as-1*-like element; these cis-acting sequences partially mediate gene induction following SA, auxin, jasmonate, or H_2O_2 treatment. A family of basic leucine zipper (bZIP)-containing transcription factors that bind TGACG motifs, called TGA or OBF factors, binds these elements. SA treatment has been shown to enhance an *as-1* binding activity [presumed to be activation sequence factor-1 (ASF-1), a member of the TGA family] whereas phosphatase treatment of nuclear extracts decreases it. Based on these results, regulation of *as-1* binding activity by a phosphorylation event could provide a mechanism for the rapid, CHX-insensitive induction of immediate-early genes by SA. A MAPK (SIPK) that is rapidly activated in tobacco by TMV infection and SA treatment has been purified and characterized. Whether SIPK plays a role in activating the *as-1* binding activity following SA treatment is not known.

In contrast to the immediate-early genes, the late-response SA-induced genes are activated several hours after SA treatment and their induction is more sustained and is sensitive to CHX. Although the promoters for this class of genes, which includes the acidic *PR* genes, have been studied intensively, no common SA-responsive element has been identified. Analysis of the tobacco *PR-2d* promoter identified a TCA element that is common to several acidic *PR* promoters. However, this element is not required for SA inducibility of the *PR-2d* gene *in vivo*. Rather, a 25-bp element that contains sequences similar to W boxes is involved in SA-induced *PR-2d* expression. The W boxes are found in the promoters of several elicitor- and wound-induced genes. In addition, microarray analysis has revealed that they are found in the promoters of many genes induced during SAR development. The W boxes are bound by WRKY proteins; these proteins have been identified in parsley, tobacco, and *Arabidopsis*. They are a family of zinc-finger-type transcription factors, found exclusively in plants, that bind specifically to W box-type [(T)TGAC(C/T)] DNA sequence elements. The recent discovery that SA treatment and TMV infection induce a tobacco WRKY protein that binds an element in the basic class 1 chitinase (*PR-3*) gene provides an additional link between W boxes and SA-induced gene expression.

In the tobacco *PR-1a* promoter, researchers have identified an *as-1*-like motif that modulates, although is not obligately required for, SA-induced expression. Possibly, a second factor that is synthesized *de novo* after SA treatment works in conjunction with the *as-1* binding factor to induce this late class gene. By contrast, the *as-1*-like TGA binding site identified in the *Arabidopsis PR-1* promoter is required for SA-induced gene expression. The tobacco and the *Arabidopsis PR-1* genes also contain potential nuclear factor κB (NF-κB) binding sites. The significance of this element in tobacco is not known; however, mutations in the *Arabidopsis* sequence abolish inducibility of this promoter by the SA analogue 2,6-dichloroisonicotinic acid (INA). Analysis of the *Arabidopsis PR-1* promoter indicates that it also contains a W box. Because mutations in this box cause elevated levels of basal and induced gene expression, this element appears to regulate *PR-1* expression negatively. Finally, Myb binding sites have been identified in the tobacco *PR-1a* promoter. However, because overexpression or antisense expression of a TMV- and SA-inducible Myb gene (*myb1*) fails to affect SA-induced *PR-1a* expression, the importance of these sequences remains unclear.

VI. GENETIC ANALYSIS OF THE SA SIGNALING PATHWAY

To elucidate the SA signaling pathway, numerous mutants of *Arabidopsis* have been generated. Based on their phenotype, these mutants can be divided into several broad categories; due to space constraints, only some are discussed here. The first category, which includes the *lsd* (lesion-simulating disease resistance response), *cpr* (constitutive expresser of *PR* genes), *acd2* (accelerated cell death), *cim3* (constitutive immunity), and *dnd1* (defense with no HR cell death) mutants, exhibits constitutive *PR* expression and enhanced disease resistance. These mutants also accumulate elevated levels of SA, and several develop spontaneous HR-like lesions. Whether all of these mutations represent genes in the SA signaling pathway is unclear. Many stimuli, such as ozone, ultraviolet light, and the over- or underexpression of various transgenes, also induce constitutive SA accumulation, spontaneous lesion formation, elevated *PR* expression, and enhanced resistance. Thus, activation of these defense responses may result from perturbations in cellular metabolism. Consistent with this possibility, the *acd2* mutation has been recently shown to alter red chlorophyll catabolite reductase and the *dnd1* mutation affects a cyclic nucleotide-gated ion channel.

By contrast, another class of mutants, named *npr1* (nonexpresser of *PR* genes) or *nim1* (noninducible immunity), fails to express *PR* genes or develop SAR following treatment with SA or its analogues. Cloning of the *Npr1* gene revealed that this critical SA signal transducer contains ankyrin repeats and a broad-complex, tamtrack, and bric-à-brac/potxvirus, zinc finger (BTB/POZ) domain. These domains, which are involved in protein–protein interactions, are required for NPR1 to be functional. NPR1 was subsequently shown to accumulate in the nucleus following SA treatment, and this nuclear localization is necessary but not sufficient for *PR* gene activation. A direct link between NPR1 and *PR* gene expression was established by the discovery that NPR1 differentially binds various members of the TGA transcription factor family.

In addition to the NPR1-dependent pathway, there is growing evidence that SA can signal defenses via an NPR1-independent pathway. For example, crossing an *npr1* mutant allele into enhanced disease resistance mutants (*cpr5*, *cpr6-1*, *cpr22*, or *acd6*) has either no effect or only a partial effect on constitutive defense gene expression and/or disease resistance. Furthermore, several suppressors of the *npr1* mutation have been identified. Some of these, including *ssi1*, *ssi2*, and *ssi4* (suppressor of SA insensitivity of *npr1–5*), constitutively express *PR* genes and exhibit enhanced disease resistance to bacterial and/or oomycete pathogens. By contrast, the *sni1* (suppressor of *npr1-1*, inducible) mutation restores the ability of INA to induce *PR* gene expression and resistance in the *npr1* background. Based on these observations, the SNI1 protein, which shares limited homology with the mammalian tumor suppressor retinoblastoma (Rb), may function as a negative regulator of SAR. Following SA treatment, SNI1-mediated suppression of the SAR signaling pathway would be alleviated by activated NPR1.

A category of mutants that affect SA synthesis has also been identified. These mutants, including *eds1*, *eds5*, and *eds16* [enhanced disease susceptibility; *eds5* and *eds16* correspond to *sid1* and *sid2* (SA induction deficient), respectively] and *pad4* (phytoalexin deficient), also exhibit increased pathogen susceptibility and/or depressed defense response activation following pathogen infection. The *EDS1* and *PAD4* genes encode proteins with some similarity to triacylglycerol lipases; their function in the SA signaling pathway is currently obscure. By contrast, *EDS16* encodes ICS1, which may catalyze SA synthesis via the chorismate/isochorismate pathway, as previously discussed.

VII. SUMMARY

Over the past 15 years, our understanding of the role of SA in plants has been transformed from the assumption that SA mimics an endogenous signal to the realization that SA is a *bona fide* signal that regulates thermogenesis, disease resistance, and possibly flowering. In addition, it has been demonstrated that SA is synthesized via the phenylpropanoid pathway, and possibly the chorismate/isochorismate pathway. Analyses of the mechanisms of action of SA have revealed that SA induces thermogenesis by activating *Aox* gene expression. How SA activates disease resistance is less clear, but the discovery that CAT, APX, aconitase, and CA are SA-interacting proteins provides several interesting leads to follow. The observation that several SA-interacting proteins also are regulated by H_2O_2 and NO suggests there is significant interplay between these signals. Moreover, these findings argue that parallel defense signaling strategies are used in plants and animals. Combined with the mounting evidence revealing positive and negative cross talk between the SA-, JA-, and ethylene-mediated defense pathways, there are multiple avenues yet to be explored in our quest to understand how SA signals disease resistance in plants.

Glossary

alternative oxidase The terminal oxidase of the alternative respiratory pathway; unlike the cytochrome respiratory pathway, which conserves energy from electron flow as chemical energy (ATP), the alternative respiratory pathway releases this energy as heat.

hypersensitive response Manifested by the formation of necrotic lesions at the site of pathogen entry; thought to play a role in reducing pathogen growth and spread.

pathogenesis-related proteins Encompass several families of proteins that are expressed first in the inoculated and subsequently in the uninoculated leaves of plants resisting pathogen attack; due to the correlation between *PR* gene expression and development of hypersensitive response and systemic acquired resistance, increased *PR* expression is frequently used as a marker for these phenomena.

phytoalexins Low molecular-weight compounds that exhibit antimicrobial activity.

salicylate hydroxylase Enzyme encoded by the bacterial *nahG* gene; converts salicylic acid into catechol, a compound that does not induce defense responses.

systemic acquired resistance Long-lasting enhanced resistance to a wide variety of pathogens; developed in the uninoculated tissues of a plant following a primary infection.

thermogenesis Generation of heat; occurs in certain plants during the flowering process; in voodoo lilies, the increased temperature of the spadix (the central column of the flower) volatilizes compounds, releasing a foul odor that attracts pollinating insects.

See Also the Following Articles

Abscisic Acid • Auxin • Brassinosteroids • Cytokinins • Ethylene • Gibberellins • Jasmonates • Systemins

Further Reading

Asai, T., Stone, J. M., Heard, J. E., Kovtun, Y., Yorgey, P., Sheen, J., and Ausubel, F. M. (2000). Fumonisin B1-induced cell death in *Arabidopsis* protoplasts requires jasmonate-, ethylene-, and salicylate-dependent signaling pathways. *Plant Cell* **12**, 1823–1835.

Chong, J., Pierrel, M.-A., Atanassova, R., Werck-Reichart, D., Fritig, B., and Saindrenan, P. (2001). Free and conjugated benzoic acid in tobacco plants and cell cultures. Induced accumulation upon elicitation of defense responses and role as salicylic acid precursors. *Plant Physiol.* **125**, 318–328.

Dempsey, D. A., Shah, J., and Klessig, D. F. (1999). Salicylic acid and disease resistance in plants. *Crit. Rev. Plant Sci.* **18**, 547–575.

Dong, X. (2001). Genetic dissection of systemic acquired resistance. *Curr. Opin. Plant Biol.* **4**, 309–314.

Kachroo, P., Shanklin, J., Shah, J., Whittle, E. J., and Klessig, D. F. (2001). A fatty acid desaturase modulates the activation of defense signaling pathways in plants. *Proc. Natl. Acad. Sci. U.S.A.* **98**, 9448–9453.

Kinkema, M., Fan, W., and Dong, X. (2000). Nuclear localization of NPR1 is required for activation of *PR* gene expression. *Plant Cell* **12**, 2339–2350.

Klessig, D. F., Durner, J., Noad, R., Navarre, D. A., Wendehenne, D., Kumar, D., Zhou, J. M., Shah, J., Zhang, S., Kachroo, P., Trifa, Y., Pontier, D., Lam, E., and Silva, H. (2000). Nitric oxide and salicylic acid signaling in plant defense. *Proc. Natl. Acad. Sci. U.S.A.* **97**, 8849–8855.

Maleck, K., Levine, A., Eulgem, T., Morgan, A., Schmid, J., Lawton, K. A., Dangl, J. L., and Dietrich, R. A. (2000). The transcriptome of *Arabidopsis thaliana* during systemic acquired resistance. *Nat. Genet.* **26**, 403–410.

Mauch, F., Mauch-Mani, B., Gaille, C., Kull, B., Haas, D., and Reimmann, C. (2001). Manipulation of salicylate content in *Arabidopsis thaliana* by the expression of an engineered bacterial salicylate synthase. *Plant J.* **25**, 67–77.

Murphy, A. M., Chivasa, S., Singh, D. P., and Carr, J. P. (1999). Salicylic acid-induced resistance to viruses and other pathogens: A parting of the ways? *Trends Plant Sci.* **4**, 155–160.

Raskin, I. (1992). Role of salicylic acid in plants. *Annu. Rev. Plant Physiol. Plant Mol. Biol.* **43**, 439–463.

Ribnicky, D. M., Shulaev, V., and Raskin, I. (1998). Intermediates of salicylic acid biosynthesis in tobacco. *Plant Physiol.* **118**, 565–572.

Slaymaker, D. H., Navarre, D. A., Clark, D., del Pozo, O., Martin, G. B., and Klessig, D. F. (2002). The tobacco salicylic acid-binding protein 3 (SABP3) is the chloroplast carbonic anhydrase, which exhibits antioxidant activity and plays a role in the hypersensitive defense response. *Proc. Natl. Acad. Sci. U.S.A.* **99**, 11640–11649.

Verbern, M. C., Verpoorte, R., Bol, J. F., Mercado-Blanco, J., and Linthorst, H. J. (2000). Overproduction of salicylic acid in plants by bacterial transgenes enhances pathogen resistance. *Nat. Biotechnol.* **18**, 779–783.

Wendehenne, D., Pugin, A., Klessig, D. F., and Durner, J. (2001). Nitric oxide: comparative synthesis and signaling in animal and plant cells. *Trends Plant Sci.* **6**, 177–183.

Yang, P., Chen, C., Wang, Z., Fan, B., and Chen, Z. (1999). A pathogen- and salicylic acid-induced WRKY DNA-binding activity recognizes the elicitor response element of the tobacco class 1 chitinase gene promoter. *Plant J.* **18**, 141–149.

Secretin

SEBASTIAN G. DE LA FUENTE AND
THEODORE N. PAPPAS

Duke University Medical Center

Secretin, a 27-amino-acid peptide hormone produced by intestinal S cells, is released into the duodenum primarily in response to pH changes following food ingestion. Its major target organs include the pancreas, stomach, and gallbladder. Secretin affects pancreatic bicarbonate secretion, gastric acid secretion, and motility and augmentation of bile flow. Secretin has been found to be altered in some clinical conditions and is currently used as a diagnostic tool for assessing pancreatic function in chronic pancreatitis, in identification of the main pancreatic duct, and in diagnosis of gastrinoma (Zollinger–Ellison syndrome).

I. INTRODUCTION

The polypeptide hormone secretin was discovered in 1902 by Starling and Bayliss as a substance capable of stimulating pancreatic bicarbonate secretion. Based on purified intestinal mucosa extracts, secretin is structurally a linear sequence of 27 amino acids. The advent of highly sensitive radioimmunoassay techniques has help to identify the physiological stimulus that triggers cellular release of secretin as well as its major biological effects. The homology between secretins of different species has facilitated the understanding of its actions and roles in gastrointestinal physiology.

Secretin is synthesized by the intestinal S cells and is secreted into the bloodstream when the upper segments of the small intestine are exposed to the acidic contents of the emptying stomach. The main target organ of the hormone is the pancreas, which is stimulated to discharge bicarbonate into the intestinal lumen, neutralizing the contents of the intestines. In addition, secretin augments the release of digestive enzymes from the pancreas and inhibits further production of acids in the stomach.

The stimulatory properties of secretin that impact the pancreas are pharmacologically useful as a diagnostic tool to examine pancreatic exocrine function and to assist in the recognition of the main pancreatic duct in imaging studies. Secretin is also a valuable tool in the diagnosis of gastrinoma. Of clinical importance is the fact that altered levels of secretin have been found in various pathological conditions, thus making secretin a possible target for future therapeutic approaches.

II. STRUCTURE AND CHEMICAL PROPERTIES

The linear 27-amino-acid secretin polypeptide has a molecular weight of 3055. The amino acid sequence has been determined in pigs, cows, dogs, chickens, humans, and rats (Fig. 1). Bovine secretin is identical to porcine secretin, whereas chicken and porcine secretins are similar at only 14 amino acid positions. The secretin precursor structure consists of the secretin sequence, a signal peptide, an amidation–cleavage sequence, a 72-amino-acid carboxyl-terminal extension peptide, and a short N-terminal peptide (Fig. 2). The NH_2-terminal sequence seems to be required for full bioactivity. Alteration of this segment results in significant loss of secretin capacity to stimulate exocrine pancreatic secretion.

Secretin shares structural homology with many other peptides present in the gut and brain. These include vasoactive intestinal peptide (VIP), gastric inhibitory peptide (GIP), glucagon gene-related products (glucagon, GLP-1, GLP-2), and peptide histidine–isoleucine amide (PHI). Other compounds, such as growth hormone-releasing hormone (GHRH), pituitary adenylate cyclase-activating polypeptide (PACAP), and peptide HM (PHM), are also members of the secretin family. Prealbumin is somehow homologous to the secretin sequence. The similarities between some of these peptides are shown in Fig. 3.

Secretin is thermally stable at neutral pH, but at acidic pH it is labile and can be converted into β-aspartyl peptide. Secretin tends to be adsorbed by glass and plastic, thus it is necessary to add albumin to secretin solutions to avoid adsorption to these surfaces. Secretin has a short plasma half-life of 2–4 min and a metabolic clearance rate of approximately 13–15 $ml^{-1} kg^{-1}$. The kidneys are responsible for most of its clearance.

III. GENE COMPOSITION AND EXPRESSION

The human secretin gene has been recently found to be located in chromosome 11p15.5. The locus is composed of four exons with a coding sequence spanning 713 bp of genomic DNA and encoding 123 amino acids. The human gene shares similarities to the gene in pigs and rodents, and all have a common four-exon structure. The first exon encodes a signal peptide and a segment of the N-terminal peptide; the bioactive secretin is encoded in the second exon. The third and four exons encode the C-terminal peptide of prosecretin. Although the posttranslational processing of secretin is not known in detail, a precursor has been isolated from the porcine intestine consisting of secretin plus 41 amino acids at the C terminus. The hormone-coding regions are highly comparable within secretin genes of different species; however, the C-terminal peptide differs substantially, suggesting that this portion is not of physiological importance. The secretin gene is also comparable to other genes of the secretin family. Among gene family members, VIP, glucagon, and secretin are all encoded in one exon. In contrast, GIP and growth hormone-releasing hormone peptides are encoded in separated exons.

IV. SYNTHESIS OF SECRETIN

Immunoreactive methods have identified the small intestine of most species as the major site of secretin production. Immunoreactivity of secretin is highest in the duodenum and decreases along the horizontal axis, reaching insignificant levels in the ileum; however, low-level immunoreactivity has also been found in the porcine colon. Biosynthesis of secretin takes place in intestinal S cells. These are enteroendocrine cells that are interspersed among other epithelial cells, occurring at a frequency of approximately 6 cells per 1000 epithelial cells. A majority of the S cells are distributed within the intestinal villi, with small numbers in the

Human synthetic secretin structure
H-His-Ser-Asp-Gly-Thr-Phe-Thr-Ser-Glu-Leu-Ser-Arg-Leu-Arg-*Glu-Gly*-Ala-Arg-Leu-
-Gln-Arg-Leu-Leu-Gln-Gly-Leu-Val-NH_2

Porcine secretin structure
H-His-Ser-Asp-Gly-Thr-Phe-Thr-Ser-Glu-Leu-Ser-Arg-Leu-Arg-*Asp-Ser*-Ala-Arg-Leu-
-Gln-Arg-Leu-Leu-Gln-Gly-Leu-Val-NH_2

FIGURE 1 Amino acid sequences of synthetic human and porcine secretins. The two structures differ only at amino acids 15 and 16 (Glu-Gly vs Asp-Ser).

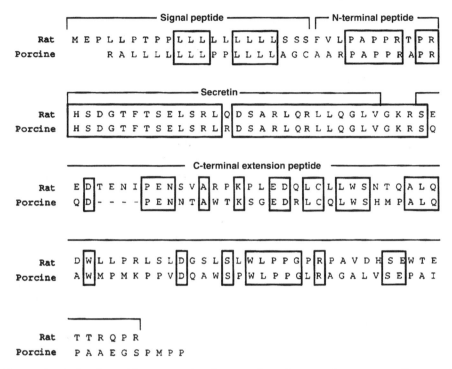

FIGURE 2 Comparison of amino acid sequences for the rat and porcine secretin precursors. Boxes enclose identical amino acids. Predicted functional domains are indicated above the amino acid sequences. Reproduced from "Comprehensive Endocrinology—Gut Peptides Biochemistry and Physiology" (J.H. Walsh and G.J. Dockray), p. 150 (1994), Raven Press, with permission from the publisher and the authors.

middle and upper crypt region. Ultrastructurally, S cells are characterized by a pear-shaped cytoplasm containing small, irregular granules of 200 nm displaying slight argyrophilia. Serotonin and substance P have been shown to be co-expressed in some duodenal S cells; however, this co-expression depends on the species studied and occurs in a small percentage of cells. The renewal time of S cells has been estimated to be 5 days. Guinea pigs and rodent secretin levels are relatively high at birth, falling in the postnatal period. Secretin cells have been identified in the rat duodenum as early as day 17 of gestation. Secretin mRNA is present in the developing pancreas, reaching maximal levels at day 19 of gestation.

Although extraintestinal sources of secretin have been experimentally located throughout the central nervous system, it is generally accepted that only the small intestine produces significant amounts.

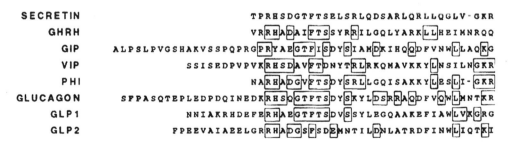

FIGURE 3 Alignment of the amino acid sequences encoded by the coding exons of the secretin family of genes. Amino acids identical to the corresponding exon in the secretin gene (top line) are enclosed in boxes. Sequences shown are encoded by the respective rat genes, with the exception of human gastric inhibitory peptide (GIP). GHRH, Growth hormone-releasing hormone; VIP, vasoactive intestinal peptide; PHI, peptide histidine–isoleucine amide; GLP, glucagon-like peptide. Reproduced from "Comprehensive Endocrinology—Gut Peptides Biochemistry and Physiology" (J. H. Walsh and G. J. Dockray), p. 152 (1994), Raven Press, with permission from the publisher and the authors.

Early experiments have demonstrated small concentrations in pituitary and pineal glands, hypothalamus, thalamus, and olfactory lobe. Secretin-like immunoreactivity has also been reported in the gastric antrum and pancreatic islets; however, these findings have not been corroborated. Measurements of secretin mRNA have failed to demonstrate significant concentrations in locations other than the intestines, but very low levels may simply be below the detection limits of Northern blot analysis techniques.

V. STIMULATORY RELEASE OF SECRETIN

Among the known factors that trigger the release of secretin (Table 1), intralumenal acidification of the duodenum and proximal jejunum results in the strongest stimulus for secretion. Considerable amounts of hydrochloric acid (HCl) are normally produced in the stomach, facilitating digestion of large pieces of ingested foods. Most of this gastric acid production is buffered by the food and by alkaline secretions, but a considerable quantity of acid enters the duodenum, reducing duodenal intralumenal acidity to a pH range of 3.0–5.0. Experimental studies have calculated the pH threshold for secretin release to be approximately 4–5 in humans and 4.5 in dogs. Experimentally, infusing acid into the intestinal lumen stimulates secretin release. The increase in plasma secretin concentration levels depends on the acid load delivered to the duodenum and parallels the increase in secretion of bicarbonate from the pancreas.

Many substances stimulate the release of secretin (see Table 1), including bile salts, fatty acids, and herbal extracts. Intralumenal infusion of bile salts triggers the pancreas to release bicarbonate-rich secretions in animals and humans; however, little is known about the physiological role of endogenous bile in stimulating secretin release. Fatty acids, specifically oleic acid, also stimulate secretin release. Additionally, geranyl-geranyl acetone (a cyclic polyisoprenoid experimentally used to heal ulcers) and L-phenylpentanol, which is used as a condiment in some cultures, when administered intraduodenally, increase plasma secretin concentrations and pancreatic bicarbonate secretion.

The role of the nervous system in controlling secretin secretion has long been a controversial issue. Based on animal studies, some investigators have proposed that secretin's actions depend heavily on cholinergic input; however, the fact that atropine (an anticholinergic drug) fails to inhibit secretin secretion in humans in response to duodenal acidification suggests a minor vagal control in secretin release. To date, the mechanisms by which a decreased duodenal pH stimulates secretin production remain unclear; nevertheless, in vitro studies have shown that secretin can be released after induction by Ca^{2+} and cAMP.

Three substances are known to inhibit the release of secretin: oxethazine, somatostatin, and Met-enkephalin. Oxethazine is a substance with local anesthetic properties; when infused in the duodenum of dogs, it suppresses the plasma concentration increment of secretin and bicarbonate secretion in response to acidification. Little is known about the mechanism of action of this drug. In addition, both somatostatin and Met-enkephalin have been shown to reduce secretin levels and pancreatic response to duodenal acidification, but it is unclear if this inhibition occurs at physiological concentrations.

VI. BIOLOGICAL AND PHYSIOLOGICAL ACTIONS

A. Receptor Structure

Characterization of the secretin receptor in pancreatic acinar cells of guinea pigs has led to distinguish two different receptor types—high affinity and low affinity-depending on the receptor avidity for secretin. Secretin is a potent agonist for the high-affinity receptor whereas VIP weakly stimulates it. The low-affinity receptor shows much lower affinity for secretin and higher affinity for VIP. Both are G-protein-linked receptors that activate the adenylyl cyclase enzyme, resulting in augmentation of intracellular cyclic AMP (cAMP). The receptor is composed of seven putative hydrophobic transmembrane domains with a 427-amino-acid sequence; the molecular weight is 48,696.

TABLE 1   Substances That Influence Sectretin Release

Stimulants	Inhibitors
Acid[a]	Oxethazine
Bile salts	Somatostatin
Long-chain fatty acids	Met-enkephalin
Oligopeptides (in rats)	
Sodium oleate	
Herbal extracts	
Geranyl-geranyl acetone	

[a]Intraduodenal acid is the strongest stimulus for secretin release.

Secretin receptor mRNAs have been detected in several tissues in addition to the pancreas, including heart, stomach, and nervous system. Autoradiographic examination of rat pancreatic tissue demonstrates high-affinity binding sites in both acinar and ductal cells, with no binding on islets and vascular structures.

B. Secretin Effects and Mechanisms of Action

Secretin activity can be grouped into two categories: actions occurring at physiological levels and actions occurring at supraphysiological levels. Most of these actions are included in Table 2. Secretin effects can also be grouped into stimulatory or inhibitory actions.

Stimulation of pancreatic water and bicarbonate secretion represents the main physiologic action of secretin, resulting in neutralization of the acidic chyme entering the proximal intestines. Low intraduodenal pH triggers secretin secretion, which results in an incremental release of pancreatic water and bicarbonate. Among the components of the gastric chyme, titratable acid appears to be the main stimulant for secretin secretion. Immunoreactive levels of secretin are also significantly increased after ingestion of a meal of mixed types of foods. Additionally, fatty acids and the digestive by-products of fat cause release of significant amounts of immunoreactive secretin. It is well established that actions of secretin on the exocrine pancreas are potentiated by cholecystokinin (CCK) in dogs and humans. The concomitant release of CCK along with secretin produces a greater response, compared to the sum of their individual actions, because both hormones act together.

Animal studies have shown that secretin exerts inhibitory effects on gastric acid secretion and gastric motility, therefore acting as an enterogastrone. It is not clear whether these inhibitory actions result from a direct secretin effect on the stomach or as a consequence of various hormones and/or peptides acting in concert. Several hormones (serotonin, somatostatin, and peptide YY) are known to be released postprandially and modify acid secretion and gastric emptying rates. Interactions between such hormones and secretin may explain the inhibitory actions of secretin on gastric physiology. In rodents, for example, secretin strongly inhibits basal acid output by stimulating both somatostatin and prostaglandin release, thus indirectly influencing gastric secretion. However, these effects are less clear in humans; infusion of exogenous secretin at doses similar to levels seen following acidified meals fail to inhibit acid secretion. Furthermore, inhibition of acid output has not been achieved after administration of fivefold higher doses of exogenous secretin. On the other hand, both continuous and intermittent infusions of secretin have shown to retard gastric emptying of solid meals in humans. Pure secretin has shown to stimulate pepsin release in cats, dogs, and humans. Very small doses of secretin increase serum group pepsinogen I and pepsin output in young, healthy human volunteers. Gastric mucous secretion has been found to be increased by secretin in cats, dogs, and humans, but the physiological significance of these findings remains to be elucidated.

Biliary secretion is influenced by administration of supraphysiological doses of exogenous secretin. Pharmacological administration of secretin augments bile flow and bicarbonate concentration in bile, but it is unclear to date whether these effects are produced by endogenous secretin.

Other actions attributed to secretin include induction of bicarbonate secretion from duodenal

TABLE 2   Actions of Secretin

Level	Stimulation	Inhibition
Physiological	Secretion of water and electrolytes from pancreas Secretion of water and electrolytes in bile	Gastric emptying Gastric acid secretion Intestinal motility
Supraphysiological[a]	Bile flow Lower esophageal sphincter Release of insulin Secretion from Brunner's glands in the duodenum Renal excretion of water and electrolytes Cardiac output Splanchnic blood flow Lipolysis in fat cells	

[a]Pharmacological doses.

Brunner's glands, inhibition of lower esophageal sphincter tone, and lipolysis. Several studies have suggested a tropic effect of secretin on the pancreas. Pharmacological doses of secretin increase pancreatic weight, protein, DNA content, and thymidine incorporation in animals. These actions have been attributed to a costimulatory effect of secretin and CCK, which is known to have tropic properties. It is not known if theses actions take place in humans.

Secretin has also been found to mediate relaxation of intestinal smooth muscle in rats and to inhibit upper small intestinal motility in humans. Exogenous secretin influences the release of insulin, glucagon, parathyroid hormone, calcitonin, somatostatin, and pancreatic polypeptide (PP). Exogenous nonphysiologic secretin infusion rates can also produce incremental increases in pancreatic enzyme secretion. Most of these actions have been observed either at supraphysiological concentrations or in experimental models.

VII. CLINICAL APPLICATIONS OF SECRETIN/PATHOLOGICAL CONDITIONS

A. Pharmacological Uses of Secretin

Secretin has been used clinically for assessment of pancreatic exocrine function, identification of minor papilla during endoscopic retrograde cholangiopancreatography (ERCP), and diagnosis of gastrinoma (Zollinger–Ellison syndrome). Secretin is an adjunct to ultrasound and resonance magnetic imaging in inflammatory conditions of the pancreas, such as chronic pancreatitis. The periductal fibrosis present in the chronically inflamed pancreas limits the dilatation of the main duct after maximal secretin stimulation, which is used to distinguish chronic pancreatitis from the normal pancreas. The sensitivity, specificity, and efficacy of functional secretin studies have been estimated to be 67, 90, and 81%, respectively, as compared to histological evaluation. Pancreatic insufficiency can also be evaluated after administration of secretagogues (i.e., secretin and CCK). Secretin stimulatory effects are also used to collect pancreatic juices during ERCP. Concomitant utilization of secretin and ultrasound has been reported to be useful in selection of patients with pancreas divisum for accessory duct sphincteroplasty. In these patients, secretin is used to localize the site where the main pancreatic duct drains.

The differential effects of secretin on normal and gastrin-producing tumors are use to distinguish between hypergastrinemic conditions and patients with Zollinger–Ellison syndrome (ZES). ZES is characterized by gastrin-producing neuroendocrine tumors that are usually located in the pancreas or proximal duodenum; the tumors release excessive amounts of gastrin into the circulation. Intravenous administration of secretin in these patients produces an exaggerated gastrin response that is useful to identify ZES. Both synthetic porcine secretin and human synthetic secretin have been shown to be adequate testing agents. Additionally, secretin tests have been used to localize gastrinomas within the gut and to ensure a correct extirpation of the tumor during surgery. The two methods have been described for these purposes: selective intra-arterial secretin injection with successive recollection of venous hepatic sampling and intra-operative secretin testing to confirm resection of the tumor. Postoperatively, secretin tests have been used to detect subclinical disease recurrence. However, with the advent of octreotide scanning and intraoperative ultrasound, the secretin-dependent localization techniques are no longer commonly utilized. Secretin has recently elicited considerable attention due to alleged benefits of secretin in treating autism in children. Unfortunately, however, double-blind studies have found no evidence of such effectiveness.

B. Pathophysiology of Secretin: Conditions of Excess or Deficiency

Plasma secretin concentration levels have been found altered in various clinical conditions. Hypersecretinemia (blood secretin levels above normal) is seen in ZES, in some cases of duodenal ulcers with marked hypersecretion of acid, and in patients with advanced renal failure. One case has been reported in the medical literature of a patient with a pancreatic tumor secreting five different hormones, one of which included secretin; however, no cases of isolated secretin production have been documented. Patients with ZES present abnormally elevated plasma secretin levels, with fasting concentrations above 15 pg/ml, which is rarely seen in healthy persons. In healthy subjects, plasma secretin concentrations are elevated after a prolonged fast or with extenuated physical exercise. In both instances, oral or intravenous administration of glucose reduces secretin blood levels.

Hyposecretinemia, or a blood secretin level below normal, has been found in patients with untreated adult celiac disease or achlorhydria. Secretin concentrations in patients with celiac disease fail to increase after exogenous duodenal acidification or after a mixed meal. In contrast, patients with achlorhydia present reduced secretin levels after a mixed meal, although the response to duodenal acidification remains normal.

Glossary

chyme Semifluid mixture consisting of partly digested food and gastric juices; passes from the stomach into the small intestine.

exon Portion of DNA that encodes a section of the mature messenger RNA.

intron Portion of DNA that lies between two exons; it is transcribed into RNA, but is not expressed in the final product.

locus Position in a chromosome of a particular gene or allele.

peptide Compound formed by two or more amino acids, in which a carboxyl group of one is united with the amino group of another.

See Also the Following Articles

Cholecystokinin (CCK) • Gastrin • Gastrointestinal Hormone (GI) Regulated Signal Transduction • Gastrointestinal Hormone-Releasing Peptides • Glucagon Gene Expression • Glucagon-like Peptides: GLP-1 and GLP-2 • Peptide YY • Vasoactive Intestinal Peptide (VIP)

Further Reading

Geoghegan, J., and Pappas, T. N. (1997). Clinical uses of gut peptides. *Ann. Surg.* **225**(2), 145–154.

Henriksen, J. H., and Shaffalitzky de Muckadell, O. B. (2000). Secretin, its discovery, and the introduction of the hormone concept. *Scand. J. Clin. Lab. Invest.* **60**, 463–472.

Metz, D. C., Buchanan, M., Purich, E., and Fein, S. (2001). A randomized controlled study comparing synthetic porcine and human secretins with biologically porcine secretin to diagnose Zollinger–Ellison syndrome. *Aliment. Pharmacol. Ther.* **15**, 669–676.

Mutoh, H., Ratineu, C., Ray, S., and Leiter, A. B. (2000). Review article: Transcriptional events controlling the terminal differentiation of intestinal endocrine cells. *Aliment. Pharmacol. Ther.* **14**(Suppl. 1), 170–175.

Nussdorfer, G. G., Bahcelioglu, M., Neri, G., and Malendowicz, L. K. (2000). Secretin, glucagon, gastric inhibitory polypeptide, parathyroid hormone, and related peptides in the regulation of the hypothalamus–pituitary–adrenal axis [review article]. *Peptides* **21**(2), 309–324.

Solomon, T. E., Varga, G., Zeng, N., Wu, S. V., Walsh, J. H., and Reeve, J. R. (2001). Different actions of secretin and Gly-extended secretin predict secretin receptor subtypes. *Am. J. Physiol. (Gastrointest. Liver Physiol.)* **280**, G88–G94.

Ulrich, C. D., Holtmann, M., and Miller, L. (1998). Secretin and vasoactive peptide receptors: Members of a unique family of G protein-coupled receptors [review article]. *Gastroenterology* **114**, 382–397.

Whitmore, T. E., Holloway, J. L., Lofton-Day, C. E., Maurer, M. F., Chen, L., Quinton, T. J., Vincent, J. B., Scherer, S. W., and

Lok, S. (2000). Human secretin (SCT): Gene structure, chromosome location, and distribution of mRNA. *Cytogenet. Cell Genet.* **90**, 47–52.

Selective Estrogen Receptor Modulators

See *SERMs*

SERMs (Selective Estrogen Receptor Modulators)

DONALD P. MCDONNELL
Duke University Medical Center

I. INTRODUCTION
II. THE EMERGENCE OF THE SERM CONCEPT
III. THE MECHANISM OF ACTION OF SERMs

Although estrogen was initially considered solely a reproductive hormone, extensive clinical findings have indicated that its influence extends to a variety of target tissues not generally considered to be involved in reproduction. Specifically, estrogen has positive actions in the skeleton, the cardiovascular system, and the central nervous system. Interestingly, the mechanism by which this hormone manifests its biological activities in different tissues is dissimilar, enabling the development of selective estrogen receptor modulators (SERMs), compounds whose relative estrogenic/antiestrogenic activities vary between cells.

I. INTRODUCTION

Despite the medical benefits afforded by estrogen replacement therapy, the number of women who initiate or remain on therapy for greater than 1 year is relatively small. This is due in part to the fear that estrogens increase the risk of developing breast cancer. Consequently, it was anticipated several years ago that there was an unmet medical need for novel estrogen receptor modulators that would retain the beneficial effects of estrogens in most target organs but which would be inactive in the breast.

The emergence of selective estrogen receptor modulators (SERMs), compounds whose agonist/antagonist activities are manifest in a cell-selective manner, indicates that considerable progress toward this goal has been made. It is likely that a clearer understanding of the mechanisms that determine the pharmacological activities of the currently available SERMs will assist in the discovery and development of additional compounds of this class for use in the treatment of conditions associated with long-term estrogen deprivation.

With few exceptions, the clinical studies supporting nonreproductive actions of estrogens have not been performed in a double-blinded, placebo-controlled manner. Therefore, it has been difficult to establish, in a definitive manner, whether estrogens have clinically important, beneficial activities in postmenopausal women outside of their utility to treat climacteric symptoms. In the absence of these definitive studies, there has been some reluctance on the part of the pharmaceutical industry to invest in the development of improved "estrogens." Some resolution to this issue was provided by the recent publication of the interim results of the National Institutes of Health-sponsored Women's Health Initiative (WHI). This trial was set up to examine the long-term effects of the most popular hormone replacement regimens in the cardiovascular system and in breast although many other secondary outcomes were considered. One arm of this trial, a combination of conjugated equine estrogens and the progestin medroxyprogesterone acetate (HRT), was terminated early because an interim analysis demonstrated a clear increase in the incidence of breast cancer and cardiovascular events. This was a disappointing result considering the general belief, based on multiple retrospective studies, that postmenopausal estrogen supplementation would be beneficial in the cardiovascular system. Although overshadowed by an enormous amount of negative media coverage, this study also proved in a definitive manner that estrogens reduced the incidence of hip fractures by approximately 40% and significantly reduced the incidence of colorectal cancer. However, aside from the established effects of estrogen on the quality of life of menopausal women, the additional positive and negative effects highlighted by the WHI study appear to cancel each other out and do not support long-term use of HRT. It remains to be determined whether estrogen alone (the second ongoing arm of the WHI study) provides an improved risk–benefit profile in women without a uterus.

From the perspective of drug discovery, the results from the WHI are very useful. It demonstrated conclusively that estrogens were beneficial in the skeleton and that they reduced the incidence of colorectal cancer. Furthermore, it made it clear that compounds that could manifest estrogenic activities in a tissue-selective manner would have utility in menopausal medicine. Although far from optimal, the clinical profiles of the first-generation SERMs have suggested that it will be possible to generate compounds that provide only the beneficial effects of estrogens and which significantly improve the health of postmenopausal women. As will be discussed below, the currently available SERMs arose from the accidental discovery that compounds designed as anti-estrogens could exhibit estrogenic activity in some tissues. It is likely that elucidation of the mechanisms of this tissue selectivity will enable the rational development of improved SERMs. Thus, although some consider the findings of the WHI study to signal the end of HRT, others see it as an impetus to develop compounds with improved specificity and share in the expectation that such medicines will have a positive impact on the health of menopausal women.

II. THE EMERGENCE OF THE SERM CONCEPT

Considering the classical models of estrogen action, it was initially difficult to understand how, beyond taking advantage of fortuitous pharmacokinetic properties, it would be possible to develop therapeutically useful SERMs. However, in the early 1990s a landmark study demonstrated that the "anti-estrogen" tamoxifen could actually function as an estrogen in the lumbar spine. Specifically, this placebo-controlled trial demonstrated that like estrogen, tamoxifen could increase bone mineral density in the lumbar spine of postmenopausal women who were being administered tamoxifen as adjuvant therapy for breast cancer. Indeed, were it not for the fact that this drug also functioned as an estrogen in the uterus and that this activity has been associated with an increased risk of endometrial cancer, it may have been used as a treatment for osteoporosis. Regardless, it was this finding that birthed the field of SERMs and provided the impetus to search for compounds that functioned like tamoxifen in bone but lacked uterotrophic activity. To date, these efforts have led to the development of one compound, raloxifene, which is approved for the treatment and prevention of osteoporosis. Several additional SERMs, with pharmaceutical properties superior to

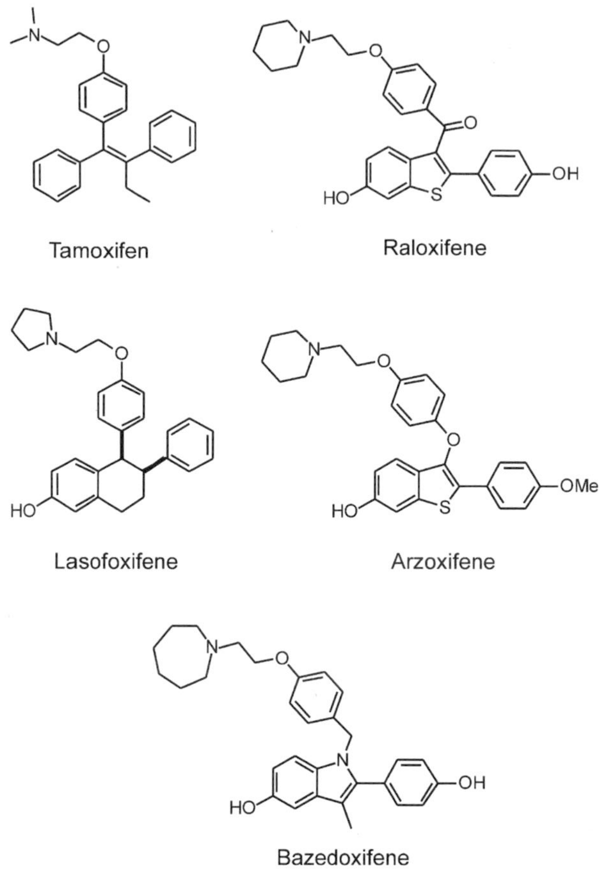

FIGURE 1 Structures of the most clinically important SERMs.

those of raloxifene, i.e., lasofoxifene, bazedoxifene, and arzoxifene, are in the late stages of clinical development and will likely emerge on the market in the near future (Fig. 1).

III. THE MECHANISM OF ACTION OF SERMS

The observation that the SERM tamoxifen could manifest estrogenic activities in some cells but oppose estrogen action in others suggested that a reevaluation of the classical models of ER pharmacology was needed. In the established models of estrogen action, the unoccupied nuclear estrogen receptor (ER) resides in the nuclei of target cells in an inactive form. Upon binding to an agonist, such as estradiol, the biochemical properties of the ER are altered in a way that allows the interaction of a receptor dimer with specific DNA sequences [estrogen-response elements (EREs)] within the promoters of responsive genes. The DNA-bound ER can then regulate target gene transcription, either positively or negatively. In this

model, agonists function as "switches" that facilitate the conversion of ER from an inactive to an active form, whereas antagonists function by competitively inhibiting the binding of agonists. However, the realization that the relative agonist/antagonist activity of ER ligands can differ between cells and even between different promoters in the same cell suggests that the pharmacology of this class of compounds is more complex than originally anticipated. This complexity has allowed the development of SERMs, compounds whose agonist and antagonist activities are manifest in a cell- and promoter-restricted manner. Although SERMs are a relatively new classification, the observation that the biological character of ER ligands could differ between cells was first observed in the late 1960s when it was demonstrated that tamoxifen, then classified as an ER antagonist, could function as a partial agonist in the reproductive systems of rodents. Since that time, other SERMs that display unique agonist/antagonist profiles have emerged, leading to the realization that different compounds acting through the same receptor can manifest different activities in different cells. The explanation for this cellular discrimination is slowly being unraveled, providing a molecular mechanism to explain the differential activity of SERMs and suggesting ways to develop improved compounds of this class in the future.

A major advance in understanding estrogen action was the discovery and cloning in 1996 of a second estrogen receptor (ER-β) that is genetically distinct from ER-α, which was cloned in 1986. The expression patterns of these receptors and the phenotypic consequences of their disruption differ, indicating that each has a distinct role in ER pharmacology. It has been shown that ER-β can heterodimerize with ER-α and inhibit ER-α action *in vitro*, suggesting that differences in the relative expression levels of the two receptors may dictate cellular sensitivity to estrogens. Although the roles of these two receptors in SERM action remain to be established, raloxifene and tamoxifen have been shown to bind to both receptors. On classical ERE-containing genes, these SERMs function as pure antagonists when acting through ER-β but can function as partial agonists when acting through ER-α. However, it now appears that in certain circumstances tamoxifen and other SERMs, acting through ER-β, may manifest robust agonist activity. For instance, on some promoters ERs do not interact directly with EREs but rather are tethered to promoters through protein–protein interactions with transcription factors prebound to promoters.

When ER-β interacts with promoters in this manner, its transcriptional activity is suppressed by estrogens and activated by SERMs, and the reverse is true for ER-α. These indirect ER–promoter interactions have been demonstrated conclusively only *in vitro*; thus, although these findings are intriguing, the physiological significance of these alternate pathways remains to be established. Regardless, it is clear that the actions of estrogens and SERMs *in vivo* represent their composite activities through these two receptors as homo- or heterodimers.

In the uterus, a tissue that predominantly expresses ER-α, tamoxifen but not raloxifene (a second-generation SERM) manifests agonist activity, indicating that SERM pharmacology cannot be explained solely by differential receptor activation. This finding, which has been confirmed in several *in vitro* systems, suggests that some cells are able to distinguish between ER-α–tamoxifen and ER-α–raloxifene complexes. Using protein crystallography and techniques that evaluated the surface changes of the receptor that occur upon ligand binding, it was demonstrated that the structure of the ER was influenced by the nature of the bound ligand. Cumulatively, these studies indicate that the conformations of the tamoxifen–ER, raloxifene–ER, and estradiol–ER complexes are different from one another and from the unbound receptor. The relevance of receptor conformation to biological activity was strengthened recently by the observation that the structure of ER-α in the presence of the pure antagonist ICI164,384 is distinct from that observed in the presence of agonists or SERMs. Thus, receptor conformation appears to be the primary determinant of the pharmacological activity of SERMs, estrogens, and anti-estrogens.

The full significance of the differential effect of estrogens and SERMs on ER structure was not realized until the discovery of co-activators and co-repressors, proteins that interact with and modulate ER function. Co-activators such as SRC-1 (steroid receptor co-activator-1), GRIP1 (glucocorticoid receptor interacting protein-1), and AIB-1 (amplified in breast cancer-1) (p160 family), preferentially interact with agonist-activated ER and potentiate transcriptional activation by coupling the receptor to the transcription apparatus and by altering the architecture of the target promoter, thus facilitating transcription. Much of what is known about the role of the known co-activators in SERM action has come from studies of tamoxifen. Some studies have demonstrated that overexpression of the p160 co-activators (SRC-1, GRIP-1, and AIB-1) in target cells can convert tamoxifen from an antagonist into an

agonist. Additional studies have indicated that tamoxifen-activated ER is capable of interacting, in an ectopic manner, with cofactors with which estradiol–ER would not normally couple. Whether these types of interactions occur when ER is occupied by other SERMs remains to be determined. In contrast to co-activators, co-repressors like nuclear receptor co-repressor (NCoR) and silencing mediator for retinoid and thyroid hormone receptor (SMRT) interact preferentially with antagonist-activated ER and suppress activation by altering the structure of the responsive promoter in such a way as to reduce its ability to be transcribed. The importance of co-repressors in SERM action was confirmed in studies demonstrating that tamoxifen could function as a full agonist in cells derived from mice bearing a genetic disruption of NCoR. It is not yet clear whether the co-repressors are physiologically important regulators of ER action or whether they are engaged only when the receptor is bound to a synthetic antagonist. To date, over 20 different ER-interacting co-activators and co-repressors have been identified. These have different relative and absolute expression levels among cells and display distinct preferences for different ER–ligand complexes. It appears that differential cofactor recruitment is a key determinant of SERM pharmacology and that progress will be made in the near future in ascribing the different activities of these compounds to specific ER–cofactor interactions.

It is not likely that differential cofactor recruitment alone is the only determinant of the agonist/antagonist activity of SERMs. For example, in cultured cells, ligand binding to ERs can activate extranuclear signaling pathways in a transcription-independent manner. Although the physiological importance of these activities is unclear, they highlight the extreme complexity of ER action and the multiplicity of the systems and signaling pathways that may be modulated by the ERs and their ligands.

To summarize, the complex pharmacological activities of SERMs are the result of at least three different factors (Fig. 2): (1) differential receptor expression; (2) receptor conformation (an activity that influences cofactor recruitment); and (3) differential expression of cofactors. Globally, these activities explain most of the tissue-selective activities of SERMs, although the specific contribution of each activity and the particular components that are important for a given tissue remain to be determined.

Upon binding to an agonist or an antagonist, the ER (α- and/or β-isoforms) undergoes a conformational change that permits its spontaneous dimerization

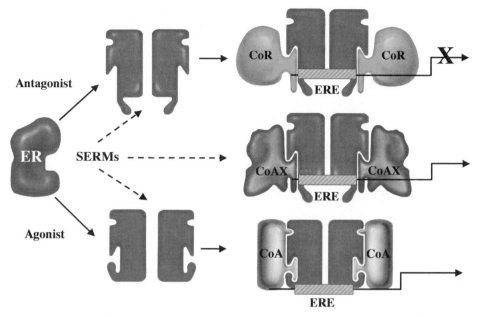

FIGURE 2 An updated model of estrogen receptor action may help to explain the activity of SERMs. CoA, co-activator; CoAX, co-activator X (yet to be identified); CoR, co-repressor.

and facilitates the subsequent interaction of the dimer with specific DNA sequences, EREs, located within the regulatory regions of target genes. It has now been determined that receptors activated with full agonists, such as 17β-estradiol, can couple with any one of a number of transcription co-activators. The resulting biological response will be determined by the cofactors that are available in a given cell and which of these proteins actually dock with the receptor. In the presence of a pure antagonist such as ICI182,780, it has been demonstrated that ER interacts preferentially with a co-repressor protein. Upon binding SERMs, however, the receptor has been shown to adopt overall conformations that make these complexes distinct from agonist- or antagonist-activated receptor. These complexes can interact with either co-activators or co-repressors and are very sensitive to the expression levels of these proteins. When co-repressors dominate, SERMs function as antagonists, whereas when co-activators dominate, partial agonist activity is observed. To complicate things further, it has also been shown that in certain circumstances SERM-activated ERs can interact in an ectopic manner with co-activators with which the ER–estradiol complex does not normally interact. The implication of this model is that the major determinants of SERM activity are receptor shape and the relative and absolute levels of co-activators in target cells.

Glossary

co-activators Proteins that interact with activated transcription factors at target gene promoters and facilitate their contact with the general transcription apparatus in cells. In addition, co-activators nucleate the assembly of a large complex of proteins at target gene promoters that enhance transcriptional activation by enzymatically modifying histones and effecting a local decondensation of chromatin.

co-repressors Proteins that interact with inactive transcription factors and help to inhibit the activity of these proteins by nucleating a large complex of proteins, which functions to condense chromatin structure and repress transcription.

See Also the Following Articles

Co-activators and Corepressors for the Nuclear Receptor Superfamily • Environmental Disruptors of Sex Hormone Action • Estrogen and Progesterone Receptors in Breast Cancer • Estrogen Receptor-α Structure and Function • Estrogen Receptor-β Structure and Function • *In Vitro* Fertilization • Osteoporosis: Hormonal Treatment • Osteoporosis: Pathophysiology

Further Reading

Brzozowski, A. M., *et al.* (1997). Molecular basis of agonism and antagonism in the oestrogen receptor. *Nature* **389**, 753–758.
Delmas, P. D., *et al.* (1997). Effects of raloxifene on bone mineral density, serum cholesterol concentrations, and uterine

endometrium in postmenopausal women. *N. Engl. J. Med.* **337**, 1641–1647.

Kraichely, D. M., Sun, J., Katzenellenbogen, J. A., and Katzenellenbogen, B. S. (2000). Conformational changes and coactivator recruitment by novel ligands for estrogen receptor-α and estrogen receptor-β Correlations with biological character and distinct differences among SRC coactivator family members. *Endocrinology* **141**, 3534–3545.

Love, R. R., *et al.* (1992). Effects of tamoxifen on bone mineral density in postmenopausal women with breast cancer. *N. Engl. J. Med.* **326**, 852–856.

McDonnell, D. P. (1999). The molecular pharmacology of SERMs. *Trends Endocrinol. Metab.* **10**, 301–311.

McDonnell, D. P., and Norris, J. D. (2002). Connections and regulation of the human estrogen receptor. *Science* **296**, 1642–1644.

McKenna, N. J., and O'Malley, B. W. (2000). An issue of tissues: Divining the split personalities of selective estrogen receptor modulators. *Nat. Med.* **6**, 960–962.

McKenna, N. J., Lanz, R. B., and O'Malley, B. W. (1999). Nuclear receptor coregulators: Cellular and molecular biology. *Endocr. Rev.* **20**, 321–344.

Norris, J. D., *et al.* (1999). Peptide antagonists of the human estrogen receptor. *Science* **285**, 744–746.

Shang, Y., and Brown, M. (2002). Molecular determinants for the tissue specificity of SERMs. *Science* **295**, 2465–2468.

Shang, Y., Hu, X., DiRenzo, J., Lazar, M. A., and Brown, M. (2000). Cofactor dynamics and sufficiency in estrogen receptor-regulated transcription. *Cell* **103**, 843–852.

Shiau, A. K., *et al.* (1998). The structural basis of estrogen receptor/coactivator recognition and the antagonism of this interaction by tamoxifen. *Cell* **95**, 927–937.

Tzukerman, M. T., *et al.* (1994). Human estrogen receptor transactivational capacity is determined by both cellular and promoter context and mediated by two functionally distinct intramolecular regions. *Mol. Endocrinol.* **8**, 21–30.

Women's Health Initiative Investigators (2002). Risks and benefits of estrogen plus progestin in healthy postmenopausal women: Principal results from the Women's Health Initiative Randomized Controlled Trial. *J. Am. Med. Assoc.* **288**, 321–333.

Sex Hormone-Binding Globulin (SHBG)

Geoffrey L. Hammond and Kevin N. Hogeveen
University of Western Ontario, Canada

Sex hormone-binding globulin (SHBG) transports androgens and estrogens in the blood and regulates the access of these sex steroids to their target tissues. Plasma SHBG is produced by the liver and is structurally identical to the androgen-binding protein (ABP) produced in Sertoli cells. A single *SHBG* gene encodes both SHBG and ABP, and its expression in the liver and testis responds differently to developmental, hormonal, and external cues. The *SHBG* gene is expressed in several other tissues, as well as in cancer cell lines that contain alternatively spliced *SHBG* transcripts of unknown function. Genetic variants of human *SHBG* that influence its expression and/or the plasma levels of SHBG have been identified. The biological significance of *SHBG* expression in the testis may vary between species, and this article will review the current understanding of the structure and function of SHBG in the context of its proposed roles in male reproduction.

I. STRUCTURE AND FUNCTION OF PLASMA SEX HORMONE-BINDING GLOBULIN AND TESTICULAR ANDROGEN-BINDING PROTEIN

Plasma sex hormone-binding globulin (SHBG) and testicular androgen-binding protein (ABP) are homodimeric glycoproteins, and each monomeric subunit comprises two laminin G-like (LG) domains (Fig. 1). These two laminin G-like domains are also found in several other proteins with diverse and unrelated functions, including protein S, GAS 6 (product of the growth arrest-specific gene 6), and several extracellular matrix-associated proteins (e.g., laminin, merosin, and agrin). The significance of these structural similarities is unknown but several of these proteins are ligands for plasma membrane receptors or interact in some way with other proteins. The amino-terminal LG domain of each subunit contains a steroid-binding site, the dimerization domain, and several metal-binding sites. Contrary to previous assumptions, it is now known that each subunit of the SHBG homodimer contains a functional steroid-binding site that may exist in different states of occupancy by various ligands. The structure and functional properties of the carboxyl-terminal LG domain of SHBG are less well understood but it normally contains two consensus sites for N-linked glycosylation, one of which is conserved phylogenetically and likely provides a specialized function. Although glycosylation is not necessary for steroid binding or dimerization, it may influence the biological half-life of the protein and/or its partitioning

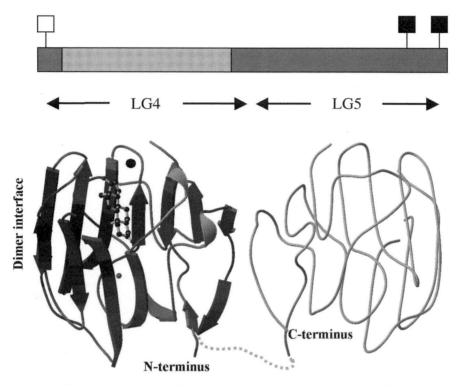

FIGURE 1 Structure of human sex hormone-binding globulin. Linear diagram of the 373 amino acid residues that constitute the mature human SHBG monomer (top) showing the positions of one O-linked (open box) and two N-linked (solid boxes) carbohydrate chains. The internal shaded region corresponds to the minimal sequence required to produce a truncated form of SHBG that contains a fully active steroid-binding site and dimerization domain. Each human SHBG monomer includes two laminin G-like domains (LG4 and LG5). The crystal structure of the amino-terminal LG4 domain (bottom) shows 5α-dihydrotestosterone in the steroid-binding site, the position of the homodimer interface, and a Ca^{2+} ion (small shaded ball). Also shown is a Zn^{2+} ion (solid ball) that occupies a potential zinc-binding site within a region (between residues P130 and P137) of disorder (not visible), which lies over the entrance of the steroid-binding site. Occupancy of this zinc-binding site specifically reduces the binding affinity of estradiol without changing the binding affinity of androgens. The predicted structure and relative position of the carboxy-terminal LG5 domain within the context of the overall SHBG monomer tertiary structure are also shown, with a dashed line corresponding to a short 5-residue sequence of unresolved structure connecting the LG4 and LG5 domains.

within extravascular compartments of sex steroid hormone-sensitive tissues.

In the blood, human SHBG binds biologically active androgens and estrogens with high affinity, and the plasma concentrations of SHBG play a key role in regulating the distribution of these steroids between the protein-bound (primarily SHBG-bound and albumin-bound) and the non-protein-bound or "free" fractions. This finding is considered to be important because only free steroids are generally considered to be available to target tissues. However, there is evidence that SHBG can enter the extravascular compartments of some tissues and may therefore exert a local effect on the access of steroids to their target cells. Human SHBG is also a zinc-binding protein, and occupancy of a zinc-binding site within the amino-terminal LG domain influences its steroid-binding specificity. This may be important in tissues where zinc concentrations are particularly high and where SHBG may accumulate, such as in the male reproductive tract.

Plasma SHBG and ABP interact with cell membranes of steroid-dependent tissues within the male reproductive tract. Although the significance of these interactions is not well understood, they may serve different functions. For instance, after being secreted into the seminiferous tubule fluid of male rats, ABP is actively taken up by epithelial cells within the epididymis. This is believed to facilitate the entry of testosterone into these cells and enhance the activation of androgen-responsive genes encoding proteins involved in sperm development. By contrast, only unliganded SHBG is capable of binding specific "receptor" sites within human prostate plasma

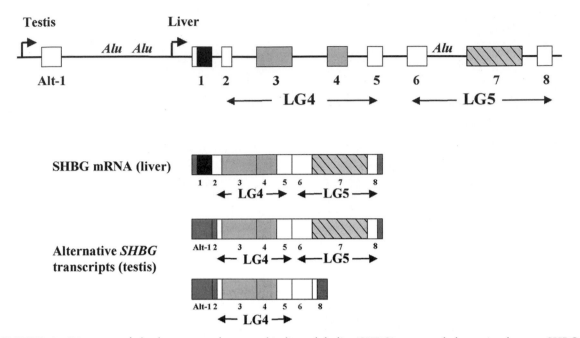

FIGURE 2 Diagrams of the human sex hormone-binding globulin (*SHBG*) gene and the major human *SHBG* transcripts in the liver and testis. The structure of the human *SHBG* gene (top) shows the positions of repetitive *Alu* sequences and the major transcription start sites (arrows) utilized in the liver and testis. The exons that produce SHBG mRNA in the liver and the alternative *SHBG* transcripts found in the testis are shown below the diagram of the *SHBG* gene structure with respect to sequences that encode the LG4 and LG5 domains of human SHBG. Boxes within the diagrams of these transcripts correspond to exon sequences. Exons (3 and 4) that encode sequences that constitute the steroid-binding site and dimerization domain are shaded in the gene sequence (top) and transcript sequences (bottom). The exon 1 sequence included within the SHBG mRNA found in the liver shows the sequence that encodes the secretion signal polypeptide (black area), which is removed during production of the mature form of plasma SHBG. In the testis, the two major *SHBG* transcripts contain an alternative exon 1 (Alt-1) sequence that replaces the exon 1 sequence present in the SHBG mRNA found in the liver, and they either contain or lack sequences corresponding to exon 7 (diagonally striped rectangles). The dark gray shaded areas within the exon 1 and exon 8 sequences present within the liver SHBG mRNA correspond to 5′ and 3′ noncoding sequences, respectively. Similarly, the dark gray shaded areas within Alt exon 1 and exon 2 sequences within the alternative transcripts found in the testis represent 5′ noncoding regions, whereas the dark gray shaded regions in exon 8 sequences correspond to the 3′ sequences that follow the termination of the major open reading frames.

membranes. In these circumstances, the membrane-bound SHBG can interact with biologically active androgens or estrogen, and if this occurs, SHBG appears to dissociate from the receptor, resulting in an increase in intracellular cyclic AMP levels and the activation of a signal transduction cascade. Although this receptor system has been characterized extensively at the biochemical level, the receptor itself has not been identified and its biological significance remains obscure.

II. CONTROL OF *SHBG* GENE EXPRESSION

Plasma SHBG and testicular ABP are encoded by eight exons within a single 4 kb gene (*SHBG*), which is located on the short arm (p12–p13) of human chromosome 17 (Fig. 2). The temporal and spatial expression of *SHBG* varies considerably between species, as does its sensitivity to various hormonal stimuli. Little is known about how *SHBG* is regulated during fetal life but it is expressed transiently in the livers of fetal rodents, resulting in fluctuations of plasma SHBG levels during critical periods of sexual development, and this likely occurs in other species including humans. In rats and mice, however, *SHBG* is not expressed in the liver during postnatal life and the very small amount of SHBG in the blood of mature rats most likely originates from gonadal sources. By contrast, *SHBG* expression in the livers of most other mammalian species increases after birth and represents the major source of plasma SHBG throughout life. In humans, changes in plasma SHBG levels occur during puberty, leading to approximately twofold higher levels in women than in men. Plasma SHBG levels in humans are also under complex hormonal and metabolic control. For instance, exogenous estrogens and thyroid hormone markedly increase plasma SHBG levels, whereas anabolic androgens and androgenic progestins reduce plasma SHBG levels. Low plasma SHBG levels are found in obese men and women and this may in some way be related to the effects of insulin on reducing SHBG production by hepatocytes. The latter are of interest because several reports have indicated that low plasma SHBG levels are an early indicator of predisposition to diabetes and associated cardiovascular disease. However, it is not known whether any of these effects are mediated at the level of gene expression or reflect changes in the plasma half-life of SHBG.

The expression of *SHBG* in rat Sertoli cells has been studied extensively and is controlled directly by follicle-stimulating hormone and indirectly by testosterone through intermediary effects involving factors produced by the myoid cells surrounding the seminiferous tubules. The promoter responsible for controlling the production of ABP mRNA in Sertoli cells has been examined but the molecular mechanisms responsible for its regulation remain to be defined.

When the human *SHBG* proximal promoter sequence is compared with the corresponding regions of *SHBG* proximal promoter sequences in several other mammalian species, there is one major difference. The human *SHBG* promoter includes a region that contains two nuclear factor-binding sites that are not present in the promoters of other species. One of these sites binds hepatocyte nuclear factor-4, whereas the other binds the upstream stimulatory factor, and it is possible that this difference contributes to some of the species differences in *SHBG* expression.

III. SIGNIFICANCE OF ALTERNATIVE *SHBG* TRANSCRIPTS AND *SHBG* VARIANTS

The rat and human *SHBG* genes produce several other transcripts in addition to those encoding plasma SHBG and testicular ABP. These transcripts invariably contain alternative noncoding exon 1 sequences that replace the exon 1 that contains the translation initiation codon for the SHBG and ABP precursor polypeptides. The human alternative *SHBG* transcripts also often lack exon 7 sequences, and repetitive *Alu* sequences are located upstream of both the exon 1 and the exon 7 sequences that are

either replaced or removed from these transcripts (Fig. 2). This may be significant because exons within the rat ABP that are differentially utilized are also preceded by repetitive DNA sequence elements. A rat *SHBG* transcript with an alternative exon 1 sequence has been shown to encode an ABP-related product containing a localization signal that directs it to the nucleus. However, the coding sequence for the unique amino-terminal sequence associated with this protein is not conserved in the alternative human *SHBG* transcripts identified to date. It has also been reported that *SHBG* is expressed in a variety of other tissues and cell types including rodent kidney, gut, and brain, the human uterus, placenta, and prostate, and several human cancer cell lines. The identity of the *SHBG* transcripts in most of these tissues and cell lines has not been defined but most of them are alternatively spliced transcripts with alternative exon 1 sequences.

Several human *SHBG* variants have been reported. The most common is a single-nucleotide polymorphism in exon 8, which results in a D327N substitution and introduces an additional N-glycosylation site in the carboxy-terminal laminin G-like domain. Although the steroid-binding affinities of this variant protein are normal, it may have an increased plasma half-life. However, even homozygous carriers of this allele display no obvious phenotype. A $(TAAAA)_n$ polymorphism in the human *SHBG* proximal promoter has been identified. The number of these repeats influences its transcriptional activity but it remains to be determined whether this polymorphism is associated with clinical disorders attributed to low plasma SHBG levels. It is likely that other variations in the coding and regulatory sequences of human *SHBG* exist and may explain the interindividual variations in plasma SHBG levels that may contribute to the etiology of diseases associated with inappropriate exposure to either androgens or estrogens.

IV. ROLE(S) OF *SHBG* GENE EXPRESSION IN MALE REPRODUCTION

The ABP produced by rat Sertoli cells is secreted into the lumen of the seminiferous tubule and accompanies the developing sperm as they migrate to the *caput* epididymis, where it is internalized by lumenal epithelial cells. Although it has been assumed that this plays an important role in maintaining a highly androgenic environment during sperm maturation, there is no evidence that this role is conserved across species, and it may simply be restricted to mammals that lack SHBG in their blood circulation. Moreover, the mouse testis produces much less ABP than the rat testis, and transgenic mice that overexpress rat ABP in their Sertoli cells tend to become infertile due to meiotic arrest and a marked increase in germ cell apoptosis. The reason for this is not known but there is evidence that immunoreactive ABP produced in Sertoli cells is internalized by germ cells.

Early reports indicated that SHBG isolated from human testis homogenates differed from plasma SHBG in terms of its carbohydrate composition. However, it is virtually impossible to exclude the plasma contamination of SHBG from such extracts and there is evidence that plasma SHBG can readily enter the interstitial compartments of the testis. Thus, this difference in SHBG glycoforms between plasma and testis extracts might simply reflect the sequestration of a particular glycoform of plasma SHBG by the testis. Moreover, although *SHBG* transcripts can be readily detected in the human testis, what proportion of these transcripts encode an SHBG molecule with a leader sequence for secretion is not known. In fact, all of the near-full-length SHBG cDNAs isolated from human testis libraries contain alternative exon 1 sequences, and the testes of mice that express human *SHBG* transgenes contain only these same alternative transcripts. The biological significance of the alternative transcripts is obscure, but their abundance is tightly regulated throughout the spermatogenic cycle. These observations raise obvious questions about whether SHBG and ABP play distinct species-specific roles in controlling sex steroid hormone action in the testis and accessory reproductive tissues, and whether *SHBG* transcripts with alternative exon 1 sequences have some other function that remains to be defined.

In some human reproductive tissue, such as the prostate, there is evidence that plasma SHBG accumulates within extravascular compartments and within the stroma in particular. The mechanism responsible for this is unknown but SHBG in the extravascular compartments of these tissues might play a more direct role in regulating either the entry of active steroids into their target cells or the removal of metabolites. For instance, human SHBG not only binds testosterone with high affinity but also binds its major metabolites and with either higher (5α-dihydrotestosterone) or equal (5α-androstanediols) affinity. Furthermore, the possible interaction between SHBG and specific extracellular components within these locations may represent an additional means of modulating the actions of androgens and/or estrogens in reproductive tissues.

Glossary

androgen-binding protein A protein identical in sequence to the plasma sex hormone-binding globulin that is produced in the Sertoli cells of the testis. In rats, this protein displays a preference for biologically active androgens.

sex hormone-binding globulin A homodimeric plasma glycoprotein composed of two 42 kDa polypeptide subunits encoded by the *SHBG* gene. Each subunit contains a high-affinity steroid-binding site, which in humans binds both biologically active androgens and estrogens.

See Also the Following Articles

Androgen Effects in Mammals ● Androgen Receptor-Related Pathology ● Dihydrotestosterone, Active Androgen Metabolites and Related Pathology ● Phytoestrogens ● Sex Hormones and the Immune System

Further Reading

Avvakumov, G. V., Grishkovskaya, I., Muller, Y. A., and Hammond, G. L. (2001). Resolution of the human sex hormone-binding globulin dimer interface and evidence for two steroid-binding sites per homodimer. *J. Biol. Chem.* **276**, 34453–34457.

Avvakumov, G. V., Muller, Y. A., and Hammond, G. L. (2000). Steroid-binding specificity of human sex hormone-binding globulin is influenced by occupancy of a zinc-binding site. *J. Biol. Chem.* **275**, 25920–25925.

Grishkovskaya, I., Avvakumov, G. V., Sklenar, G., Dales, D., Hammond, G. L., and Muller, Y. A. (2000). Crystal structure of human sex hormone-binding globulin: Steroid transport by a laminin G-like domain. *EMBO J.* **19**, 504–512.

Hammond, G. L. (1997). Determinants of steroid hormone bioavailability. *Biochem. Soc. Trans.* **25**, 577–582.

Hogeveen, K. N., Talikka, M., and Hammond, G. L. (2001). Human sex hormone-binding globulin promoter activity is influenced by a (TAAAA)$_n$ repeat element within an *Alu* sequence. *J. Biol. Chem.* **276**, 36383–36390.

Jänne, M., Deol, H. K., Power, S. G. A., Yee, S.-P., and Hammond, G. L. (1998). Human sex hormone-binding globulin gene expression in transgenic mice. *Mol. Endocrinol.* **12**, 123–136.

Jänne, M., and Hammond, G. L. (1998). Hepatocyte nuclear factor-4 controls transcription from a TATA-less human sex hormone-binding globulin gene promoter. *J. Biol. Chem.* **273**, 34105–34114.

Joseph, D. R. (1994). Structure, function, and regulation of androgen-binding protein/sex hormone-binding globulin. *Vitam. Horm.* **49**, 197–280.

Rosner, W. (1996). Sex steroid transport: Binding proteins. *In* "Reproductive Endocrinology, Surgery, and Technology" (E. Y. Adashi, J. A. Rock and Z. Rosenwaks, eds.), pp. 605–625. Lippincott–Raven, Philadelphia.

Sex Hormones and the Immune System

DANIELA VERTHELYI

Food and Drug Administration, Maryland

I. INTRODUCTION
II. ESTROGENS
III. PROLACTIN
IV. PROGESTERONE
V. ANDROGENS
VI. PREGNANCY AND THE IMMUNE SYSTEM
VII. SEX HORMONES AND AUTOIMMUNE DISEASE

The immune response is dimorphic, with females mounting stronger immune responses following infection or immunization and being more susceptible to autoimmune diseases than males. Sex hormones play an important role in this dimorphism by influencing the development, maturation, activation, and death of immune cells. The flow of information, however, is not unidirectional, with cytokines acting directly and indirectly on the pituitary axis and the gonads to affect the release of sex hormones. Knowledge about the physiology of the integration between the endocrine system and the immune system is rapidly increasing and creating new treatment modalities for both endocrine and immune diseases.

I. INTRODUCTION

The immune system consists of an array of cells that develop and mature in bone marrow and thymus. Mature T lymphocytes, B lymphocytes, monocytes, dendritic cells, and Langerhans cells then enter the circulation and home to peripheral lymphoid organs (lymph nodes, spleen, tonsil) and the gut-associated lymphoid tissue (Peyer's patches and appendix) as well as the skin and mucous membranes and await activation by "danger" (infections, transformed cells, etc.) with the task of recognizing and defending "self" from "nonself."

The immune system is integrated with the endocrine system through a network of signaling molecules including cytokines, chemokines, and hormones. Although this is a bidirectional interaction, this article will address only the effects of sex hormones on the cells of the immune system. One of the consequences of this interaction is a dimorphic

immune response, with females having higher levels of circulating immunoglobulins (Ig) and stronger antibody responses to immunization and infection than males, as seen in different species. Sex hormones modulate the immune response by influencing lymphocyte development, maturation, and selection; cell trafficking; cytokine and chemokine production; lymphocyte proliferation; expression of adhesion molecules and HLA receptors; and death by apoptosis. This myriad of effects may result from direct binding of sex hormones to receptors on the immune cells or indirectly by acting on somatic cells at the site of lymphocyte maturation and differentiation. The potential for sex hormones to regulate the immune system is especially evident during pregnancy when the high estrogen and progesterone levels mediate the down-regulation of delayed-type hypersensitivity (DTH), thus protecting the fetus—an hemiallograft—from rejection, while inducing higher Ig levels. Of great clinical importance, females can mount stronger immune responses after trauma. Together with their greater immune responsiveness, females also are at a greater risk of developing autoimmune diseases. For the purpose of this article, sex hormones, their precursors, and their metabolites will be addressed as one. In addition, whereas this article will attempt to tease out the effects of individual sex hormones on the immune system, it is the changes in hormonal milieu as a whole, and not any individual hormone, that modulate the immune response.

II. ESTROGENS

17β-Estradiol and several of its precursors and metabolites act directly on immune cells, alter the sites of lymphocyte development, and modify the immune milieu (see Table 1). Estrogens modulate both the adaptive and the innate immune systems. The presence of estrogen receptors (estrogen receptor-α and estrogen receptor-β) has been demonstrated in immune cells (macrophages and CD8$^+$ T cells) and various stromal cells of hematopoietic and lymphoid organs (bone marrow, thymus, and spleen).

Women of reproductive age tend to have higher Ig (both IgM and IgG) levels in peripheral blood and mount a stronger humoral immune response to most microbial (e.g., *Escherichia coli*, *Brucella abortus*, measles, rubella, and hepatitis B) and nonmicrobial antigens than men. Estrogens also modify T-cell-mediated responses, reducing delayed-type hypersensitivity responses, and delaying graft rejection. *In vitro*, low concentrations of estrogen promote—whereas

TABLE 1   Effects of Estrogen on the Immune System (Animal Model Data)

On sites of immune cell development

On bone marrow
- Increased estrogen levels reduce bone marrow mass and increase death of pre-B cells
- Hypogonadal mice (HPG/Bm–hpg/hpg or ovariectomized) have increased bone marrow cellularity with accumulation of B-cell precursors that reverts with estrogen treatment

On thymus
- Increased estrogen leads to thymus atrophy with apoptosis of $CD4^+$ $CD8^+$ T-cell precursors
- Prepubertal gonadecomy leads to thymus hypertrophy

Chronic administration of estrogen leads to development of alternative sites of lymphopoiesis in liver and spleen

In peripheral blood

On B cells
- Increased percentage of B cells in S and G2/M phases
- Reduced susceptibility to apoptosis, partly due to increased expression of Bcl/2
- Increased number and activity of plasma cells in peripheral blood and bone marrow, leading to elevated antibody levels
- Increased expression of autoantibodies (e.g., anti-dsDNA, cardiolipin phosphatidyl serine)

On T cells
- Decreased delayed-type hypersensitivity response in mice
- Reduced proliferation when stimulated *in vitro* with PHA or Con A

On the cytokine milieu
- Hormone-responsive elements identified upstream of IL-6 and IFN-γ-encoding genes
- Elevated estrogen levels increased frequency of IL-6 and IL-10 and reduced TNF-α-secreting cells in spleen
- Both increased and reduced IFN-γ and IL-2 reported in different mouse models
- Reduced IL-1 and TNF-α reported with anti-estrogens

On innate immunity
- Increased estrogen levels reduce NK-cell activity
- Increased estrogen levels reduce phagocytic and cytostatic activity of macrophages
- Elevated serum estrogens reduce macrophage production of reactive oxygen intermediates and IL-1
- At low concentrations, estrogen increased, TNF-α release by LPS-stimulated macrophages, whereas the opposite was evident at higher concentrations

---

high concentrations reduce—mixed lymphocyte reactions. Estrogens inhibit proliferation and facilitate apoptosis (by down-regulating Bcl-2) of $CD4^+$ T cells in a dose-dependent manner.

Cytokines have dramatic effects on the regulation of immune responses and the pathogenesis of a variety of diseases. Pro-inflammatory cytokines, such as interleukin-1 (IL-1), IL-6, and tumor necrosis factor α (TNFα), are produced primarily by phagocytic monocytes in response to an infectious agent. The cytokines secreted by T cells have been categorized as type 1 or Th1 [secreting interferon-γ (IFN-γ)] and type 2 or Th2 (secreting IL-4, IL-5, and IL-10) and promote an adaptive response to the pathogen that is mainly cellular (type 1) or antibody (type 2) mediated. Estrogens favor a type 2 immune response by increasing the secretion of type 2 cytokines and by protecting type 2 $CD4^+$ T cells from death by apoptosis. Premenopausal women have larger numbers of cells secreting TNFα and IFN-γ than postmenopausal women and estrogen levels in their sera correlate with the number of cells secreting IL-4 on stimulation with phytohemagglutinin (PHA). In human $CD4^+$ Jurkat T-cell lines, estrogens suppress IL-2 secretion and receptor expression. This reduction is associated with decreased nuclear binding of nuclear factor kappa B and activator protein 1.

Estrogens modulate the innate immune response by altering the phagocytic and antigen-presenting properties of macrophages and dendritic cells. At low concentrations, estrogen increases TNFα release by lipopolysaccharide-stimulated macrophages, whereas the opposite is evident at higher concentrations. In addition, estrogens modulate the maturation of $CD14^+$ monocytes into dendritic cells by granulocyte/macrophage colony-stimulating factor (GM-CSF) and IL-4. With regard to natural killer (NK) cells, in mice, treatment with estrogens leads to stimulation of NK-cell activity during the first month, but prolonged exposure reduces NK-cell activity, both *in vivo* and *in vitro*. A similar reduction in NK-cell activity is observed in prostate cancer patients treated with estrogens.

III. PROLACTIN

A variety of immune cells express receptors for prolactin. Estrogen stimulates pituitary production of prolactin through its inhibition of hypothalamic dopaminergic suppression. In addition, several lines of evidence suggest that lymphohematopoietic cells in the periphery secrete prolactin. Prolactin stimulates both cellular and humoral immunity. On T cells, it promotes type 1 responses by increasing the secretion of IL-2 and IFN-γ and the expression of IL-2 receptors. On B cells, prolactin appears to synergize with estrogen to promote Ig production. Hyperprolactinemia, created by the transplantation of syngeneic pituitary glands, accelerates the mortality from immune complex glomerulonephritis in autoimmune B/W [(New Zealand Black × New

Zealand White)F1] mice, suppresses T-cell proliferation, and increases autoantibody concentrations.

IV. PROGESTERONE

Studies have shown that high levels of progesterone *in vivo* prolong the survival of allogeneic skin grafts as well as xenogenic tumor cell implants in hamster uteri. Progesterone, in contrast with estrogen or testosterone, inhibits spontaneous or glucocorticoid-induced thymocyte apoptosis *in vivo* and *in vitro*. In addition, treatment of T cells with pharmacological concentrations of progesterone blocks T-cell activation and killing by PHA or concanavalin A (Con A).

The identification of progesterone receptors on B cells, plasma cells, and macrophages suggests a direct effect on lymphocytes. Interestingly, the progesterone receptors are at low to undetectable levels in lymphocytes from nonpregnant women. Lymphocyte expression of progesterone receptors is up-regulated on cell activation either by a mitogen (e.g., PHA) or by allogeneic stimuli (such as the fetus). In addition, progesterone induces the secretion of progesterone-induced blocking factor, which blocks NK-cell activity, augments the secretion of IL-3, IL-4, IL-5, and IL-10, and inhibits the secretion of IL-12 by $CD4^+$ and $CD8^+$ T cells. The resulting shift in the cytokine balance toward type 2 is required for a successful pregnancy (see below).

V. ANDROGENS

Expression of the androgen receptor has been documented in lymphoid and nonlymphoid cells of thymus and bone marrow, but its expression in mature peripheral lymphocytes remains controversial. This expression pattern suggests that the major impact of androgens must be on the developmental maturation of T and B lymphocytes rather than on the mature effector cells. Like estrogens, androgens induce thymus involution with apoptosis of $CD4^+CD8^+$ (DP) thymocytes that is mediated by increased local $TNF\alpha$ and reduced IL-3. Prepubertal castration of male mice induces hypertrophy of the thymus. The resulting thymus retains its normal architecture but has increased cellularity (mainly due to proliferation of DP immature thymocytes). Administration of androgens blocks the proliferation of immature T cells. Castration of male mice also results in expansion of the pre-B-cell population in the bone marrow that may be reversed by testosterone or dehydrotestosterone treatment. Despite the apparent lack of androgen receptor in peripheral mature immune cells, a 40% increase in spleen weight is observed in castrated male mice.

In vitro, androgens enhance the activity of $CD8^+$ T cells as demonstrated by the reduced proliferation of spleen cells in response to PHA. In addition, higher levels of IFN-γ and IL-2 and lower levels of IL-4 and IL-10 are secreted by phytohemagglutinin-stimulated lymphocyte culture supernatants of men compared with women. In mice, treatment *in vivo* or direct exposure of lymphocytes to androgens leads to increased production of IL-2. Androgens also reduce at high doses (or increase at low doses) $TNF\alpha$ secretion and nitric oxide synthesis by macrophages. On B cells, androgens reduce Ig secretion and proliferative responses to pokeweed mitogen. This effect is partially dependent on IL-10 secretion but independent of the hormonal status of the cell donor (male or female; luteal or follicular phase of menstrual cycle; postmenopausal).

In contrast to estrogens, androgens have favorable effects on the course of several autoimmune diseases. This has been shown in animal models of experimental autoimmune encephalitis, adjuvant arthritis, and systemic lupus erythematosus (SLE). The protective effects are mediated by the shift toward a type 1 immune response, the reduced B-cell activity with lower Ig secretion, and the reduced secretion of pro-inflammatory cytokines by macrophages. These encouraging results have led to several ongoing clinical trials in patients with multiple sclerosis and SLE.

VI. PREGNANCY AND THE IMMUNE SYSTEM

A special event in hormonal status, pregnancy, is known to down-regulate cell-mediated immune responses, especially of the Th1 type, to safeguard the fetus. The cytokine milieu is important during implantation and contributes to the maintenance of the feto-placental unit. Low doses of IL-4, IL-5, GM-CSF, IL-3, or anti-$TNF\alpha$ improve implantation and reduce resorption rates whereas administration of $TNF\alpha$, IFN-γ, or IL-2 causes abortion. In addition, during pregnancy there is an increase in γ/δ T cells and reduced NK-cell activity. These changes in the immune milieu are partly mediated by sex hormones. As a result, the pregnant woman has reduced DTH and allograft rejection, increased susceptibility to intracellular infections, and higher immunoglobulin levels than nonpregnant women.

VII. SEX HORMONES AND AUTOIMMUNE DISEASE

Autoimmune diseases are disorders in which the immune system attacks self in an uncontrolled manner. The phenomenon of gender bias in the susceptibility to autoimmune diseases has been recognized for many years. The data on the incidence of human autoimmune disease in adulthood show that females account for 65–75% of rheumatoid arthritis, Addison's disease, and myastenia gravis patients; for 85% of Hashimoto thyroiditis and Grave's disease patients; and for >90% of SLE patients. Changes in sex hormone levels such as during puberty, pregnancy, and menopause impact on the course of these diseases. Although sex hormones alone do not cause autoimmune disease, abnormal hormone levels or an altered response to these sex hormones may provide fertile ground for other factors (genetic, infectious) to trigger disease. Abundant clinical evidence connects estrogen to the pathogenesis of SLE; SLE patients, in general, have increased levels of estrogen or active estrogen metabolites and reduced levels of androgens in sera. The majority of the symptomatic episodes in women with regular menstrual cycles occur during the luteal phase of the menstrual cycle. Flares commonly take place during or immediately after pregnancy. In postmenopausal women, the impact of hormonal replacement on the incidence and course of SLE remains controversial and has led to a large ongoing multicenter trial. Additional evidence for the pathogenic role of steroid hormones on SLE includes a report describing three cases of previously healthy women who developed SLE after repeated cycles of ovulation induction. Moreover, repeated cycles of ovulation induction therapy in SLE patients have resulted in severe (even fatal) flares in SLE patients with anti-cardiolipin antibodies. It should be noted, however, that SLE is a multifactorial disease and hundreds of women undergo repeated cycles of ovulation induction every year without developing autoimmune diseases.

Several lines of investigation suggest a pathogenic role for the reduced levels of dehydroepiandrosterone sulfate (DHEAS) in female SLE patients, including an association with reduced levels of IL-2 and IFN-γ that are characteristic of SLE. Recent clinical trials showed that supplementation with exogenous DHEAS resulted in a modest clinical improvement in patients with moderate disease. The proposed mechanistic basis for their therapeutic success is the modulation of T-cell activity and cytokine secretion *in vivo*.

Glossary

adaptive immunity Branch of the immune system that mediates antigen-specific immune responses and immunologic memory. It consists of two limbs, cellular immunity and humoral immunity, which are mediated respectively by T and B cells expressing rearranged clonotypic antigen receptors capable of specifically recognizing the diverse antigens of the myriad infectious agents in the environment.

cytokines Soluble proteins that are involved in the regulation of the growth and activation of immune cells and mediate normal and pathologic inflammatory and immune responses.

innate immunity Branch of the immune system that is activated by conserved pathogen-associated molecular patterns, mediates immediate pathogen elimination, and presents the pathogen's antigens to the adaptive immune system. Its effector cells include natural killer cells, monocytes/macrophages, dendritic cells, neutrophils, basophils, eosinophils, tissue mast cells, and epithelial cells.

See Also the Following Articles

Androgens: Pharmacological Use and Abuse • Corticotropin-Releasing Hormone, Stress, and the Immune System • Glucocorticoids and Autoimmune Diseases • Placental Immunology • Progesterone Action in the Female Reproductive Tract • Prolactin (PRL) • Sex Hormone-Binding Globulin (SHBG)

Further Reading

Angele, M. K., Xu, Y. X., Ayala, A., Schwacha, M. G., Catania, R. K., Cioffo, W. G., Bland, K. L., and Chaudry, I. H. (1999). Gender dimorphism in trauma-hemorrhage-induced thymocyte apoptosis. *Shock* 12, 316–322.
Derkesen, R. H. W. M. (1998). Dehydroepiandrosterone (DHEA) and systemic lupus erythematosus. *Semin. Arthritis Rheum.* 27, 335–347.
Kanda, N., and Tamaki, K. (1999). Estrogen enhances immunoglobulin production by human PBMCs. *J. Allergy Clin. Immunol.* 103, 282–288.
McMurray, R. W. (2001). Estrogen, prolactin and autoimmunity. *Int. Pharmacol.* 1, 995–1008.
McMurray, R. W., Suwannarj, S., Ndebele, K., and Jenkins, J. K. (2001). Differential effects of sex steroids on T and B cells: Modulation of cell cycle phase distribution, apoptosis and bcl-2 protein levels. *Pathobiology* 69, 44–58.
Szekeres-Barho, J., Barakonyi, A., Par, G., Polgar, B., Palkovics, T., and Szereday, L. (2001). Progesterone as an immunomodulatory molecule. *Int. Immunopharmacol.* 1, 1037–1048.
Verthelyi, D. (2001). Sex hormones as immunomodulators in health and disease. *Int. Immunopharmacol.* 1, 983–994.
Verthelyi, D., and Ansar Ahmed, S. (1998). Estrogen increases the number of plasma cells and enhances their autoantibody production in nonautoimmune C57BL/6 mice. *Cell. Immunol.* 189, 125–134.

Encyclopedia of Hormones.

Sexual Differentiation, Molecular and Hormone Dependent Events in

PAUL-MARTIN HOLTERHUS AND OLAF HIORT
University of Lübeck, Germany

Sexual differentiation is the result of complex mechanisms involving developmental genetics and endocrinology. The advancements of molecular genetics have permitted a new insight into the understanding of the control of gonadal development, the synthesis of gonadal hormones, as well as the disposition of hormone action. This is further enhanced by the study of molecular abnormalities in humans in the genes encoding for developmental proteins, enzymes, and receptors within this cascade.

I. INTRODUCTION

The genetic sex is mediated through the chromosomal set, which is usually 46,XY or 46,XX. This chromosomal pattern is the beginning of a cascade of genetic events leading to the development of the male gonads (the testes) or the female gonads (the ovaries), which represent the gonadal sex (Fig. 1). The gonads, in turn, secrete steroidal and peptide hormones that are essential for development of the internal and external genitalia, i.e., the phenotype. The phenotypic sex, however, is mediated by means of androgen action only, regardless of the genetic or gonadal sex. The term "sexual determination" is used to describe developmental processes leading to global gonadal function. In contrast, "sexual differentiation" describes the specific hormone actions leading to the sexual phenotype of an individual. This accounts both for the development of internal and external genitalia and for the progression of sexual maturation during puberty. The gender of an individual is the sex of assignment and usually depends on normal sexual determination and differentiation.

It has long been recognized that the presence of the Y chromosome is usually associated with male development and that the lack of the Y chromosome will mediate female development. However, rarely, sex reversal may occur, meaning that there is a male phenotype with a 46,XX karyotype or a female phenotype with a 46,XY karyotype. Even more rarely, there is differentiation of both gonadal structures—testicular and ovarian tissue—resulting in true hermaphroditism. In such cases, the chromosomal set may be 46,XX, 46,XY, or a chromosomal mosaic or chimera, such as 46,XX/46,XY.

II. SEXUAL DETERMINATION

The developmental pathways of gonadal, adrenal, urinary, and renal systems are closely linked. Several genes are known to be involved in the processes leading to creation of the undifferentiated gonad (Table 1). Abnormalities in the Wilms' tumor 1 (*WT1*) gene are associated with failure of gonadal differentiation, nephropathy, development of Wilms' tumors (Denys–Drash syndrome and Frasier syndrome), and WAGR syndrome, which also involves anomalies of the eye (aniridia) and mental retardation. The role of the *WT1* gene in gonadal differentiation is not sex specific, because gonadal dysgenesis occurs in both 46,XX and 46,XY individuals. This suggests the importance of the gene in formation of the bipotential gonad rather than in testicular or ovarian development. However, abnormalities of the external genitalia are limited to 46,XY patients.

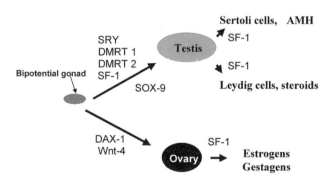

FIGURE 1 Molecular events in gonadal differentiation. From the bipotential gonad, either testis or ovary develops under tight control of specific genes. These genetic events have to occur in a distinct time frame and control each other. Gonadal differentiation leads to development of steroid-producing cells, which, in turn, are the key for further sexual differentiation.

TABLE 1 Genes Involved in Sexual Determination

Gene	Gene localization	Protein	Protein function	Affected pathway/metabolite synthesized
WT1	11p13	WT1	Transcription factor	Development of bipotential gonad
FTZ1-F1	9q33	Steroidogenic factor-1	Receptor	Gonadal development; steroidogenesis
DAX-1	Xp21	DAX-1	Transcription factor	Adrenal and gonadal development
SRY	Yp11.3	TDF	Transcription factor	Testicular development
SOX-9	17q24	SOX-9	Transcription factor	Testicular and cartilage development
DMRT1 and DMRT2	9p24	DMRT1 and DMRT2	Unknown	Testicular development
Wnt-4	1p31	Wnt-4	Growth factor	Ovarian development
AMH	—	Amh	Peptide hormone	Regression of Müllerian ducts
AMH II R	12	AMH receptor type 2	Receptor	Regression of Müllerian ducts
LHR	2p21	LH receptor	Receptor	Induction of testosterone synthesis
StAR	8p11	Steroidogenic acute regulatory protein	Transporter protein	Regulator of rapid steroid synthesis
CYP11A	15q23–24	P450 side chain cleavage	Enzyme; gonads and adrenals	Pregnenolone
CYP17	10q24	P450c17	Enzyme; gonads and adrenals	17α-OH pregnenolone, 17α-OH progesterone, dehydroepiandrosterone, androstenedione
HSD3B2	1p11	3β-Hydroxysteroid dehydrogenase type 2	Enzyme; gonads and adrenals	Progesterone, 17α-OH, progesterone, androstenedione
CYP21B	6p21	21-Hydroxylase	Enzyme; adrenals	11-Deoxycortisol, deoxycorticosterone
HSD17B3	9p22	17β-Hydroxysteroid dehydrogenase type 3	Enzyme; testis	Testosterone
SRD5A2	2p23	5α-Reductase type 2	Enzyme; androgen target tissues	Dihydrotestosterone
CYP19	15q21	Aromatase	Enzyme	Estradiol formation
AR	Xq12	Androgen receptor	Receptor	Androgen action

Another gene involved in the development of the bipotential gonad and the kidneys is the recently cloned *LIM1* gene. Homozygous deletions in this gene in mice lead to developmental failure of both gonads and kidneys. To date, no human mutations in this gene have been described, although a phenotype of renal and gonadal developmental defects in association with brain abnormalities might be anticipated. The role of steroidogenic factor-1 (SF-1) in gonadal formation is not yet clear. SF-1 is the product of the *FTZ1-F1* gene and is believed to be a nuclear orphan hormone receptor due to the presence of two zinc fingers and a ligand-binding domain in its molecular structure. *FTZ1-F1* mRNA is expressed in the urogenital ridge, which forms both the gonads and the adrenals, and is also found in developing brain regions. Mice lacking SF-1 fail to develop gonads, adrenals, and the hypothalamus. In humans, SF-1 mutation leads to adrenal insufficiency and sex reversal in 46,XY individuals. However, SF-1 is probably also involved in other aspects of sexual development, because it regulates expression of steroidogenic enzymes as well as transcription of the anti-Müllerian hormone (AMH).

Progression of gonadal differentiation beyond the bipotential gonad stage is mediated through gonosomal and autosomal genes. It was long believed and has been proved that a specific testis-determining factor (TDF) is essential for testicular development and that the encoding gene is located on the Y chromosome. This gene, named *sex-determining region of the Y chromosome (SRY)*, is a single-exon gene; it encodes a protein with a DNA-binding motif that acts as a transcription factor and in turn regulates the expression of other genes. There is evidence that *SRY* binds to the promoter of the *AMH* gene and also controls expression of steroidogenic enzymes. Thus, *SRY* probably induces expression of *AMH*, preventing the formation of Müllerian duct derivatives. Genetically engineered mice with a normal male phenotype have been produced by introducing the mouse homologue *sry* into female mouse embryos, evidence that *SRY* is the TDF. Furthermore, naturally occurring mutations of *SRY* have been described in humans.

Autosomal genes that are structurally related to *SRY* genes have been described. These "*SRY*-box-related," or *SOX*, genes are to some extent involved in testicular development. *SOX-9* is connected with chondrogenesis and gonadal differentiation. This gene is transcribed especially following *SRY* expression in male gonadal structures. Additionally, *SOX-9* is an activator of the type II collagen gene, which is essential for formation of the extracellular matrix of cartilage. Defects in *SOX-9* therefore lead to skeletal malformations known as campomelic dysplasia as well as to sex reversal in 46,XY species.

The *DAX-1* gene is involved in adrenal, ovarian, and testicular development. This gene is located on the X chromosome; the name *DAX-1* derives from the gene location: the dosage-sensitive sex reversal locus (adrenal hypoplasia congenital critical region) on X gene 1. *DAX-1* is expressed during ovarian development but is silent during testis formation, implying a critical role in ovarian formation. Interestingly, *DAX-1* is repressed by *SRY* during testicular development. However, if a duplication of the *DAX-1* region on Xp21 is present in a 46,XY patient, and, thus, the activity of its gene product is enhanced, testicular formation is impaired. In contrast, mutations in *DAX-1* diminishing its activity lead to a lack of adrenal formation and also to hypogonadal hypogonadism in congenital adrenal hypoplasia. Additional genes involved in testicular differentiation have been localized on chromosome 10 and on chromosome 9 (*DMRT1* and *DMRT2*).

Until recently, the genetic events leading to ovarian development have not been well understood. Ovarian differentiation has been presumed to be a passive event, dependent on the absence of the dominant effects of the genes involved in testicular differentiation. However, there is a role for an active genetic pathway mediating ovarian development. Wnt-4 is an example of a member of the Wnt family of locally acting secreted growth factors. The corresponding gene is located on chromosome 1. In mice, deletion of *Wnt-4* causes virilization of XX animals. In contrast, it has been recently demonstrated that a duplication of 1p31–p35, which includes the *Wnt-4* locus in a 46,XY human, is associated with sex reversal and hence a female phenotype. *Wnt-4* is known to up-regulate *DAX-1*, which in turn antagonizes *SRY*. These findings suggest that *Wnt-4* has a key role in gonadal development and is also actively involved in ovarian differentiation.

III. SEXUAL DIFFERENTIATION

In early gestation, the anlagen for the Wolffian and Müllerian ducts are present in the fetus, regardless of the karyotype. If testicular formation is unhindered, the Sertoli cells will produce AMH. High concentrations of AMH and active binding to membrane receptors in the mesenchymal cells surrounding the Müllerian ducts are necessary to exert the action of AMH. Reduced AMH excretion due to reduced Sertoli cell numbers is thus responsible for partial uterus formation in sex determination disorders. The AMH gene is under transcriptional control of several proteins involved in sexual differentiation. SF-1 binds directly to the AMH gene promoter and activates its transcription in Sertoli cells. A regulatory effect of SRY on AMH receptor expression has also been reported. Both lack of AMH and insensitivity to this hormone have been described in human disease. In persistent Müllerian duct syndrome (PMDS), 46,XY males are characterized by the presence of fallopian tubes and a uterus. The external genitalia are unequivocally male because steroid hormone formation is normal. Mutations within the AMH gene have been demonstrated in AMH deficiency. Although patients with AMH deficiency may have low serum AMH levels, in approximately 50% of the cases, AMH is within the normal limit or even elevated. This is assumed to be due to a defect of the type II AMH receptor, which is necessary for binding of ligand and exertion of AMH action. This receptor has been cloned and functionally relevant mutations have been demonstrated in patients with PMDS. The AMH type II receptor gene has been localized on chromosome 12. PMDS due to both AMH and AMH type II receptor gene mutations is inherited in an autosomal recessive fashion.

IV. ENZYMATIC PATHWAYS OF SEX STEROID SYNTHESIS

Unhindered steroid hormone formation and action are necessary for normal development of the external genitalia. Furthermore, defects in cholesterol synthesis may also lead to distinct sex phenotypes, including defects in genital development. The Smith–Lemli–Opitz syndrome is an autosomal recessive disorder with several congenital abnormalities and mental retardation. In addition to genital malformations, polydactyly, cardiac abnormalities, and growth disorders are noted. This syndrome is caused by defects in 7-dehydrocholesterol reductase, with elevated levels of the cholesterol precursor 7-dehydrocholesterol and low serum cholesterol levels. Analysis of mutations in the 7-dehydrocholesterol reductase gene in patients with biochemically proved Smith–Lemli–Opitz syndrome has for the first time demonstrated the importance of intact cholesterol synthesis for steroid production.

The first steps of steroid biosynthesis are common pathways for glucocorticoids, mineralocorticoids,

and sex steroids. Testosterone synthesis in the developing testes is controlled during early fetal life by human chorionic gonadotropin (hCG) and only later by the fetal luteinizing hormone (LH). Both hCG and LH stimulate testosterone synthesis via the LH receptor (LHR). The LHR belongs to a family of G-protein-coupled receptors with seven transmembrane helices. It has a long extracellular domain involved in ligand binding, in contrast to other receptors of this family, e.g., the thyroid-stimulating hormone (TSH) receptor. The genetic organization of LHR was elucidated in 1995. The gene is localized on chromosome 2p21 and spans over 90 kb, with a coding region divided into 11 exons. Naturally occurring mutations within the LHR, depending on their localization, have been demonstrated to result both in loss as well as gain of function. Inactivating mutations of the LHR are associated with gonadotropin unresponsiveness and lead to Leydig cell agenesis and subsequently to defective sexual differentiation. More often the result is a completely female phenotype, but incomplete virilization due to partial receptor responsiveness with subnormal androgen synthesis has been described. These mutations are typically located in the transmembrane domain of the receptor, but mutations within the extracellular domain have also been reported to result in loss of function. These molecular abnormalities imply an active role of the LHR in Leydig cell growth and differentiation. In contrast, constitutive activation of the LHR leads to normal male phenotype, although precocious pseudopuberty occurs due to mutation of the LHR, with excessive secretion of testosterone by the Leydig cells (familial testotoxicosis). Microscopically, Leydig cell hyperplasia is evident in the testes of these patients. Activating mutations of the LHR are also located in the transmembrane domain, frequently near the third intracellular loop of the receptor.

Defects within the first steps of steroid synthesis will affect either all or at least two of the final metabolites within the gonads and the adrenals. Steroid hormones are synthesized from cholesterol within the mitochondria. The acute stimulation of steroid synthesis is mediated by the steroidogenic acute regulatory (StAR) protein, which is an active transporter of cholesterol through the inner mitochondrial membrane. Mutations within StAR lead to severe lack of adrenal steroidogenesis as well as lack of virilization in 46,XY individuals in lipoid congenital adrenal hyperplasia. Intrauterine survival of affected embryos is possible, because placental steroidogenesis is not StAR dependent. Due to accumulation of cholesterol, the adrenals and testes are further damaged and the residual non-StAR-dependent steroid synthesis is also diminished. Therefore, at birth, low levels of steroids may be measurable, but these may be depleted later. The StAR gene has been cloned and several mutations have been characterized in patients with lipoid congenital adrenal hyperplasia. StAR mutations, as are all other genetic defects of steroid biosynthesis, are inherited in an autosomal recessive fashion, and both genetic female and male individuals can be affected.

The first enzymatic step in steroid synthesis from cholesterol to pregnenolone is mediated by the mitochondrial cytochrome P450 enzyme, which cleaves the cholesterol side chain. Until recently, only one naturally occurring mutation in this enzyme had been described in association with human disease. It was hypothesized that although the mutation did not exert a dominant negative effect, it would still cause 46,XY sex reversal and adrenal insufficiency because haploinsufficiency would lead to slow accumulation of cholesterol in the target organs, and hence to their destruction. It has been postulated that homozygous P450 side chain cleavage (P450scc) mutations would also—in contrast to defects in StAR—affect placental steroid synthesis and therefore these fetuses would not survive. This does not hold true for the other enzymes of early androgen biosynthesis. The P450c17 enzyme is a qualitative regulator of steroid synthesis with two distinct activities. The activities of both 17α-hydroxylase and 17,20 lyase can be differentially regulated. Although 17α-hydroxylase catalyzes the conversion of pregnenolone to 17-OH pregnenolone and progesterone to 17-OH progesterone, the 17,20 lyase activity is necessary for the enzymatic reaction from 17-OH pregnenolone to dehydroepiandrosterone and 17-OH progesterone to androstenedione. P450c17 is encoded by a single-copy gene on chromosome 10q24.3 and mutations within this gene can inhibit both functions, or, selectively, only the 17,20 lyase activity, of the resulting protein. Patients with isolated 17,20 lyase deficiency have been described only recently. The underlying molecular abnormalities within the P450c17 protein result in a severely diminished 17,20 lyase activity but only moderately inhibited 17α-hydroxylase function. Interestingly, 17,20 lyase activity depends largely on phosphorylation of the protein, and dephosphorylation of P450c17 may be a major factor in isolated 17,20 lyase deficiency. To date, only two mutations in the P450c17 gene fulfill the criteria for causing isolated

17,20 lyase deficiency. Differentiation of the two enzyme activities is important in diagnosing human disorders of P450c17 deficiency, because a combined defect will cause hyperaldosteronism and endocrine hypertension, whereas patients with isolated 17,20 lyase deficiency will have normal glucocorticoid synthesis.

The third important enzyme of ubiquitous steroidogenesis is 3β-hydroxysteroid dehydrogenase (3β-HSD), which also plays a major role in androgen biosynthesis. 3β-HSD catalyzes the formation of Δ^4 steroids, thus also the synthesis of androstenedione, the major precursor of testosterone. Two isoforms of the human enzyme have been cloned. The type 1 enzyme catalyzes the formation of progesterone, androstenedione, and 17-OH progesterone from pregnenolone, dehydroepiandrostenedione, and 17-OH pregnenolone. Type 2 3β-HSD shares a 90% sequence homology with the type 1 form, but has a lower catalytic efficiency. Genes for both types are located on chromosome 1p13.1 and consist of four exons. In 3β-HSD deficiency, mutations within the gene encoding for the type 2 enzyme have been found. Type 2 3β-HSD is predominantly expressed in the adrenals and gonads, hence its blockade results in congenital adrenal hyperplasia. In males, defective virilization due to diminished testosterone synthesis is also noted. Females may demonstrate signs of excessive virilization due to elevated adrenal androgens.

The classic form of congenital adrenal hyperplasia and the most common cause of intersex disorders in 46,XX individuals is 21-hydroxylase deficiency. The enzymatic step from 17α-hydroxyprogesterone to 11-deoxycortisol is inhibited in the glucocorticoid pathway, and this inhibition occurs in part also in the synthesis of deoxycorticosterone from progesterone in mineralocorticoid synthesis. Patients with severe 21-hydroxylase deficiency will have excessively high adrenal androgen levels and 46,XX children will display severe virilization of the external genitalia. In children with the 46,XY karyotype, the phenotype is not altered. The CYP21 gene has been determined to be involved; CYP21 is localized on chromosome 6p21.3 and direct genetic analysis is performed on a regular basis for diagnostic purposes. This is the prerequisite not only for genetic counseling, but also for approaches for experimental prenatal maternal therapy with glucocorticoids.

Late sex steroid synthesis defects comprise enzymatic reactions that do not inhibit glucocorticoid and mineralocorticoid formation. Although 17β-hydroxysteroid dehydrogenase (17β-HSD)

converts androstenedione to testosterone within the testes, 5α-reductase (5α-R) catalyzes the conversion of testosterone to dihydrotestosterone (DHT) in the peripheral target cells. At least five different 17β-HSD isoenzymes exist. Only mutations in the type 3 enzyme have been demonstrated to be responsible for defective sex differentiation in patients with 17β-HSD deficiency. This disorder is characterized by a severe virilization defect in 46,XY individuals, although they show strong signs of virilization during puberty, with marked phallic enlargement. The type 3 17β-HSD gene is located on chromosome 9p22, spanning over 11 exons and encoding a protein of 310 amino acids. This enzyme is expressed only in the testes, compatible with its important role in testicular androgen formation. However, no strict genotype–phenotype correlation has been demonstrated in 17β-HSD deficiency. It remains to be investigated whether the other 17β-HSD isoenzymes play a critical role in the phenotypic expression of 17β-HSD deficiency due to decreased peripheral conversion of testosterone to androstenedione.

Further conversion of testosterone to DHT is catalyzed in the peripheral target tissues and not within the gonads. The two isoenzymes of 5α-reductase are expressed in diverse tissues, but type 2 5α-reductase is more abundant in genital structures. The type 1 enzyme is necessary for reduction of androgens to inhibit excess formation of estrogens, and thus mice lacking this enzyme fail to maintain normal pregnancies. A specific role of the 5α-reductase type 1 enzyme in male sexual differentiation has not been demonstrated. In contrast, several mutations have been described in the type 2 enzyme in patients with defective virilization. The underlying gene has been localized to chromosome 2p23 and is divided into five exons. In 5α-reductase deficiency, DHT formation is severely diminished. However, testosterone levels are normal or even elevated. Affected 46,XY individuals are usually born with ambiguous external genitalia, but the phenotype may be highly variable. The differentiation of Wolffian structures, which is largely dependent on testosterone, is not impaired. At the time of puberty, strong virilization may occur due to high endogenous testosterone levels. Gynecomastia due to estrogen excess has rarely been described.

In 46,XX patients, a rare cause for virilization is a defect in the aromatization of estradiol from testosterone. The aromatase complex belongs to the cytochrome P450 enzymes and is expressed in the gonads and in a variety of other tissues. There is only one corresponding gene, localized on chromosome 15q21. The mother carrying a fetus with aromatase deficiency may suffer from excessive masculinization. Biochemical analysis showing low or absent estradiol in conjunction with elevated androstenedione and testosterone is diagnostic. In males, aromatase deficiency will not lead to a genital abnormality, but due to the diminished estradiol, skeletal maturation is delayed extensively.

V. MECHANISMS OF ANDROGEN ACTION

The final biological steps in the cellular cascade of normal male sexual differentiation are initiated by the molecular interaction of testosterone and dihydrotestosterone with the androgen receptor (AR) in androgen-responsive target tissues. The AR is a ligand-activated transcription factor of androgen-regulated genes. It is commonly assumed, though not experimentally proven to date, that a controlled temporal and spatial expression of androgen-regulated genes during early embryogenesis provokes a distinct spectrum of functional and structural alterations of the internal and external genitalia, ultimately resulting in the irreversible formation of the normal male phenotype. However, the AR is also expressed in females during embryogenesis, and elevated androgens during this stage, as in congenital adrenal hyperplasia, will lead to virilization in genetic females.

The AR belongs to the intracellular family of structurally related steroid hormone receptors. Transcriptional regulation through the AR is a complex multistep process involving androgen binding, conformational changes of the AR protein, receptor phosphorylation, nuclear trafficking, DNA binding, cofactor interaction, and, finally, transcription activation. The human AR gene was cloned more than a decade ago by several groups and has been mapped to Xq11–q12. It spans approximately 90 kilobases (kb) and comprises eight exons(1–8, or A–H). Transcription of the AR gene and subsequent splicing usually results in distinct AR mRNA populations in genital fibroblasts. Translation of the mRNA to the AR protein usually leads to a product migrating at about 110 kDa in Western immunoblots, comprising between 910 and 919 amino acids.

The AR shares its particular modular composition of three major functional domains with the other steroid hormone receptors. A large N-terminal domain precedes the DNA-binding domain, followed by the C-terminal ligand-binding domain. Additional functional subdomains can be identified by *in vitro* studies of artificially truncated, deleted, or point-mutated ARs. Upon entering target cells, androgens interact very specifically with the ligand-binding pocket of the AR. This initiates an activation cascade with conformational changes and nuclear translocation of the AR. Prior to receptor binding to target DNA, homodimerization of two AR proteins occurs in a ligand-dependent manner. This is mediated by distinct sequences within the second zinc finger of the DNA-binding domain as well as through specific structural N–C-terminal interactions. The AR homodimer binds to hormone response elements (HREs) that usually consist of two palindromic (half-site) sequences within the promoter of androgen regulated genes. Through chromatin remodeling, direct interaction with other transcription factors, and specific co-activators and corepressors, a steroid receptor-specific modulation of the assembly of the preinitiation complex is achieved, resulting in specific activation or repression of target gene transcription.

Defective androgen action due to cellular resistance to androgens causes the androgen insensitivity syndrome (AIS). The end-organ resistance to androgens results in a wide clinical spectrum of defective masculinization of the external genitalia in 46,XY individuals. Müllerian duct derivatives are usually completely absent because of the normal ability of the fetal testes to produce AMH. Cloning of the AR gene made it obvious that inactivating mutations of the AR gene represent the major molecular genetic basis of AIS. Due to the X-chromosomal recessive inheritance, female carriers may typically be conductors. Partial impairment of AR function is usually associated with partial androgen insensitivity syndrome (PAIS). The considerable variability in the degree of impaired AR activity accounts for a wide clinical spectrum of external undervirilization observed in PAIS. In the complete androgen insensitivity syndrome (CAIS), any *in vivo* androgen action is abolished due to complete inactivation of *in vivo* AR signaling. Therefore, these patients have normal female external genitalia with a short and blind-ending vagina. At puberty, CAIS patients acquire a normal female body shape and they show normal breast development. This is due to increasing estradiol levels that accompany elevated pubertal testosterone biosynthesis and conversion to estradiol by aromatization. Usually, pubic or axillary hair is absent.

More than 300 different mutations have been identified in AIS to date. Extensive structural alterations of the AR can result from complete or partial deletions of the AR gene. Smaller deletions may introduce a frameshift into the open reading frame, leading to a premature stop codon downstream of the mutation. Similar molecular consequences arise from the direct introduction of a premature stop codon due to point mutations. Such alterations usually lead to severe functional defects of the AR and are associated with CAIS. Extensive disruption of the AR protein structure can also be due to mutations leading to aberrant splicing of the AR mRNA. However, because aberrant splicing can be partial, thus enabling expression of the wild-type AR, the AIS phenotype is not necessarily CAIS but may also present as PAIS. The most common molecular defects of the AR gene are missense mutations. They may result either in CAIS or in PAIS because of complete or partial loss of AR function. Mutations within the ligand-binding domain may alter androgen binding but may also influence dimerization due to disruption of N–C-terminal structural interactions. Mutations within the DNA-binding domain can affect receptor binding to target DNA. The functional role of mutations within the N-terminal domain is not completely understood. Moderate extension of the polyglutamine trinucleotide segment (> 30) may cause a moderate inhibition of transcriptional activity and therefore result in mild androgen insensitivity, i.e., gynecomastia. Isolated male infertility due to impaired spermatogenesis may be a symptom of mild AIS as well. Increasing knowledge about the cofactors of AR signaling continue to influence the concept of the pathogenesis of AIS on the molecular level. Recently, the first female patient with complete AIS without an AR gene mutation, but with clear experimental evidence for an AR co-activator deficiency as the only underlying molecular mechanism of defective androgen action, has been reported. Cofactors of the AR will presumably play a pivotal role in understanding the phenotypic variability in AIS. So far, only a few mechanisms contributing to the phenotypic diversity in AIS have been identified in affected individuals. A striking phenotypic variability in a family with partial AIS has been attributed to differential expression of the 5α-reductase type 2 enzyme in genital fibroblasts. Another mechanism may be the combination of varying androgen levels during early embryogenesis and partially inactivating mutations of the ligand-binding domain.

Moreover, postzygotic mutations of the AR gene resulting in a somatic mosaicism of mutant and wild-type AR genes can contribute to modulation of the phenotype. This can result in a higher degree of virilization than expected from the AR mutation alone, because of the expression of the wild-type AR in a subset of somatic cells. Because at least one-third of all *de novo* mutations of the AR gene occur at the postzygotic stage, this mechanism is not only important for phenotypic variability in AIS but also crucial for genetic counseling.

Further decoding of the molecular and biochemical pathways is necessary for a comprehensive understanding of normal and abnormal sexual determination and differentiation. Based on the known molecular defects involved in impaired human sexual development, recent achievements in the fields of functional genomics and proteomics offer unique opportunities to identify the genetic programs downstream of these pathways, which are ultimately responsible for the structure and function of a normal or abnormal genital phenotype.

Glossary

gonads Testes and ovaries; develop from the urogenital ridge through a bipotential gonad. This process is mediated through differentiated genetic control.

hormone receptor A mediator for hormone action. In sexual differentiation, receptors for peptide hormones and steroid hormones play an active role.

sexual determination Gonadal development via genetically determined pathways.

steroid biosynthesis Synthetic pathways that start with cholesterol; defined enzymatic steps produce the final products, glucocorticoids, mineralocorticoids, and sex steroids. Intermediate products may induce distinct hormonal actions, as is seen in enzymatic pathway defects that lead to abnormal hormonal profiles and defined disorders in humanz.

See Also the Following Articles

Androgen Effects in Mammals • Anti-Müllerian Hormone • Dihydrotestosterone, Active Androgen Metabolites and Related Pathology • Environmental Disruptors of Sex Hormone Action • Gonadotropin-Releasing Hormone and Puberty • Gonadotropin-Releasing Hormone Ontogeny • Sexual Differentiation of the Brain • Spermatogenesis, Hormonal Control of • Testis Descent, Hormonal Control of

Further Reading

Adachi, M., Takayanagi, R., Tomura, A., Imasaki, K., Kato, S., Goto, K., Yanase, T., Ikuyama, S., and Nawata, H. (2000). Androgen-insensitivity syndrome as a possible coactivator disease. *N. Engl. J. Med.* **343**, 856–862.

Auchus, R. J. (2001). The genetics, pathophysiology, and management of human deficiencies of P450c17. *Endocrinol. Metab. Clin. N. Am.* **30**, 101–119.

Brinkmann, A. O. (2000). Lessons to be learned from the androgen receptor. *Eur. J. Dermatol.* **11**, 301–303.

Hiort, O., and Holterhus, P. M. (2000). The molecular basis of male sexual differentiation. *Eur. J. Endocrinol.* **142**, 101–110.

Holterhus, P. M., Wiebel, J., Sinnecker, G. H., Bruggenwirth, H. T., Sippell, W. G., Brinkmann, A. O., Kruse, K., and Hiort, O.

(1999). Clinical and molecular spectrum of somatic mosaicism in androgen insensitivity syndrome. *Pediatr. Res.* **46**, 684–690.

Jenster, G. (1998). Coactivators and corepressors as mediators of nuclear receptor function: An update. *Mol. Cell. Endocrinol.* **143**, 1–7.

Jordan, B. K., Mohammed, M., Ching, S. T., Délot, E., Chen, X. N., Dewing, P., Swain, A., Rao, P. N., Elejalde, B. R., and Vilain, E. (2001). Up-regulation of WNT-4 signalling and dosage-sensitive sex reversal in humans. *Am. J. Hum. Genet.* **68**, 1102–1109.

Lee, M. M., and Donahoe, P. K. (1993). Müllerian inhibiting substance: A gonadal hormone with multiple functions. *Endocr. Rev.* **14**, 152–164.

Lim, H. N., and Hawkins, J. R. (1998). Genetic control of gonadal differentiation. *Baill. Clin. Endocrinol. Metab.* **12**, 1–16.

Quigley, C. A., De Bellis, A., Marschke, K. B., El-Awady, M. K., Wilson, E. M., and French, F. S. (1995). Androgen receptor defects: Historical, clinical, and molecular perspectives. *Endocr. Rev.* **16**, 271–321.

White, P. C., and Speiser, P. W. (2000). Congenital adrenal hyperplasia due to 21-hydroxylase deficiency. *Endocr. Rev.* **21**, 245–291.

Sexual Differentiation of the Brain

CHARLES E. ROSELLI

Oregon Health and Science University

The hormonal environment that exists during perinatal development is thought to be the predominant determinant for sex differences in reproductive endocrinology and behavior. In this way, the brain and the reproductive system appear to follow the same rules of sexual differentiation, and, as such, the brain conforms to the hormonal theory of sexual differentiation that was first elaborated by the classic work of Alfred Jost. Specifically, in mammals, sex chromosomes specify differentiation of the bipotential gonads into either testes or ovaries.

Subsequent sexual development of the genitalia and the brain is dependent on the influence of gonadal hormones.

I. INTRODUCTION

Males and females have evolved to have distinct reproductive potentials marked by profound gender differences in the control of gonadal function and behavior by the central nervous system. Females exhibit cyclic ovarian cycles characterized by fluctuating levels of gonadotropins and gonadal steroids that lead to periodic ovulation. In many species, the expression of female reproductive behaviors is synchronized to occur at or around the time of ovulation by the sequential secretion of high levels of estradiol followed by progesterone. Males, on the other hand, exhibit tonic steady-state levels of gonadotropins and gonadal steroids that maintain an uninterrupted production of sperm and an unconstrained potential for fertilization.

II. INFLUENCE OF TESTOSTERONE ON THE DEVELOPING BRAIN: GONADOTROPIN SECRETION

Specific regions of the brain play important roles in controlling reproductive behavior, gonadal function, and ovulation. The concept of sexual differentiation of the brain began with studies of reproductive functions. Early studies on rats by Carroll Pfeiffer showed that testicular implants into neonatal female rats permanently blocked ovulation. Pfeiffer concluded, incorrectly, that anterior pituitary function was altered by exposure to testicular secretions. It was later shown through transplantation experiments that the pituitary from a male rat could support ovulation and that the sex difference resides in the brain, not in the pituitary. Subsequent studies demonstrated unequivocally that the ability of rats to ovulate is related to the absence of testes in neonatal life. Males castrated within the first few days of life are able to sustain estrogen-stimulated gonadotropin secretion necessary for cyclic gonadotropin secretion and ovulation. Females exposed to exogenous testosterone within a week of birth become permanently anovulatory. These studies in rats demonstrate that the secretion of gonadotropins is regulated by both a tonic and a cyclic neural feedback system. Both genetic males and neonatally androgen-exposed (androgenized) females lack the neural mechanisms that control the ovulatory discharge or surge of gonadotropin. In contrast, these neural mechanisms are functional in genetic females and in neonatally castrated males.

The surge mechanism for the control of gonadotropin is not sexually differentiated in nonhuman primates, as it is in rodents. Castrated male monkeys secrete surge levels of luteinizing hormone in response to an estrogen challenge, and ovulation can be sustained when ovarian implants are placed subcutaneously into castrated male monkeys.

III. INFLUENCE OF TESTOSTERONE ON THE DEVELOPING BRAIN: SEXUAL BEHAVIOR

Gonadal hormone exposure during development is also responsible for dimorphisms in neural mechanisms that regulate sexual behavior. Charles Phoenix and colleagues demonstrated that the exposure of fetal female guinea pigs to testosterone permanently suppressed the expression of female sexual receptivity and facilitated malelike mounting behavior in adulthood. Similar studies performed on rats demonstrate that exposing neonatal females to testosterone will suppress feminine sexual behavior and enhance masculine sexual behavior. Conversely, castration of male rats soon after birth permanently suppresses masculine sexual behavior and enhances feminine sexual behavior. Exogenous testosterone treatment during early pregnancy masculinizes the genitalia and behaviors of female rhesus monkeys in infancy and adulthood. These studies suggest that gonadal steroids influence the differentiation of the brain in nonhuman primates as well as in rodents.

Phoenix referred to the permanent developmental effects of gonadal steroids as organizational effects to distinguish them from the activational effects that steroids exert to influence behavior temporarily during adulthood. At the time that this terminology was proposed, there was no evidence for hormone-dependent structural or chemical sex differences in the central nervous system. However, scientists have now identified many hormone-dependent sex differences in the anatomy and chemistry of the brain, some of which may underlie the differences in neuroendocrine function and sexual behavior that have been described. Any sex difference in brain structure or function established during sexual differentiation should remain after gonadectomy in adulthood or after adults of either sex are exposed to equivalent hormone doses. On the other hand, sex differences that are the result of activational steroid effects should be eliminated after gonadectomy or in the presence of similar hormone environments.

IV. CRITICAL PERIODS

Steroid hormones have an organizational effect only when present during a sensitive developmental period, commonly referred to as the critical period for sexual differentiation. The critical period is an empirical concept that differs depending on the species and the various brain functions being considered. For rats, which are born in an immature state, androgens given just after birth can affect adult sexual behavior. Other species, such as guinea pigs and nonhuman primates, must be exposed to androgens prenatally for adult behaviors to be modified.

These landmark studies established the thesis that the sexual phenotype of the brain is caused by the differentiating actions of testosterone during early development. In this way, sexual differentiation of the brain is comparable to that of other components of the reproductive system. Moreover, like the reproductive system, the female-typical brain appears to develop in the relative absence of hormonal exposure. It is increasingly apparent that a diverse set of brain functions is sexually differentiated. Some, such as regulation of gonadotropin and prolactin secretion, sexual behavior, maternal behavior, and aggression, are closely related to reproductive function. Others, such as taste preference, play behavior, and learning behavior, are not directly related to reproduction but are influenced by early hormone exposure.

V. ROLE OF ESTROGENIC METABOLITES OF TESTOSTERONE

When newborn female rats are treated with estradiol they develop a pattern of anovulatory sterility in adulthood that is very similar to that observed with perinatal testosterone exposure. In fact, the neonatal brain is much more sensitive to estrogen than to androgen and the effects of neonatal androgen exposure can be blocked by antiestrogens. Although these results were at first puzzling, it is now known that the developing rat brain has the capacity to convert circulating androgen to estrogen because of the presence of cytochrome P450 aromatase within neurons. This evidence led to the formulation of the aromatization hypothesis, which suggests that circulating androgens are converted into estrogens by aromatase in the brain, and that these estrogens are responsible for masculinizing the developing nervous system. If estrogen is the masculinizing hormone, then what protects the fetal brain from maternal estrogens? In rats, a protein found in the blood, called alphafetoprotein, binds estrogen but not testosterone

in the first few weeks after birth. Alphafetoprotein traps circulating estrogen and thus protects the female brain from steroid exposure. In males, testicular testosterone is not bound by alphafetoprotein. Testosterone readily enters the neonatal brain of the male and is converted to estradiol to exert masculinizing effects.

There is little evidence that aromatized metabolites of testosterone play a role in sexual differentiation in other animal models, including guinea pigs and nonhuman primates. In these species, testosterone or its major androgenic metabolite, dihydrotestosterone, masculinizes the central nervous system and behavior. Nonetheless, high levels of aromatase are present in developing brains of every species so far studied, suggesting that locally produced estrogen may be needed for neural growth. Alphafetoprotein does not protect the fetus from maternal steroids in nonrodent species; instead, the placenta is thought to be important as a barrier that regulates the exposure of the fetus to maternal as well as exogenous steroids.

VI. SEXUAL DIMORPHISMS IN THE MAMMALIAN BRAIN

Sex differences in brain function are thought to derive, in part, from structural or morphological differences in the central nervous system. Sex differences in neural morphology are referred to as sexual dimorphisms. Over the past 30 years, sexual dimorphisms in the nervous system have been described at virtually every anatomical level—molecular, ultrastructural, cellular, and neural. Moreover, structural and cellular differences leading to sex differences in neural function and behavior appear to be distributed throughout the nervous system rather than concentrated in a single structure or circuit.

The first demonstration of a sexual dimorphism in the brain was the discovery by Raisman and Field that the number of synapses in the preoptic area was greater in male rats than in females. More apparent sexual dimorphisms in the number, size, and shape of neurons were soon described in the song control circuits of zebra finches. The song control nuclei are five to six times larger in males than in females. Moreover, it is believed that early exposure to androgen or estrogen organizes the larger masculine song system.

In rats, there is an obvious sex difference in a group of neurons called the sexually dimorphic nucleus of the preoptic area (SDN-POA). Roger Gorski was first to note that the volume of the

SDN-POA is about five times larger in the male than in the female. Most of this difference arises because there are greater numbers of neurons in the male nucleus. Like the song control nuclei in zebra finches, the volume of the SDN-POA is controlled by perinatal exposure to gonadal steroids but is not affected by circulating hormones in adulthood. Males castrated at birth have much smaller SDN-POAs in adulthood, whereas females treated with testosterone perinatally have larger malelike SDN-POAs as adults. Thus, perinatal exposure to androgens permanently alters the structure of the SDN-POA. Moreover, development of the nucleus conforms to the aromatase hypothesis because it has been demonstrated that conversion of testosterone to estradiol in the brain is required to masculinize the SDN-POA. Further support for this hypothesis was provided when it was shown that the SDN-POA in androgen-insensitive rats is masculinized. These rats have nonfunctional androgen receptors and thus masculinization cannot be mediated through this pathway. However, androgen-insensitive neonatal rats have normal levels of aromatase and estrogen receptor function, suggesting that the aromatization pathway mediates sexual differentiation of the SDN-POA.

Perinatal steroid hormones seem to act, in part, by preventing apoptotic cell death in the SDN-POA. Studies have shown that the incidence of apoptosis in SDN-POA between postnatal day 7 (P7) and P10 is higher in female rats than in male rats. Administration of testosterone or estradiol reduces the incidence of apoptosis in the SDN-POA of female rats or neonatally castrated male rats. The exact function of the SDN-POA is not yet completely understood. An indication of its function is the positive correlation between volume of the SDN-POA of rats and quantitative measures of adult male copulatory behavior. However, lesions of SDN-POA in rats cause only a transitory decline in male copulatory behavior. The function of the SDN-POA is much better understood in gerbils, which have a similar sexually dimorphic area (SDA) within the preoptic hypothalamus. Bilateral lesions of this region eliminate mating behavior in male gerbils.

Sexual dimorphisms have been identified in homologous medial preoptic nuclei of many species, including rats, gerbils, mountain voles, guinea pigs, ferrets, quail, macaques, and humans (see Section VII). In each case, males exhibit a larger volume and cell density than do females. The presence of sexually dimorphic nuclei within the medial preoptic area of so many species supports the idea that these structures are evolutionarily homologous. Other sexual dimorphisms are evident in several regions of the rat nervous system that are associated with sexual behavior and gonadotropin secretion. Most, but not all, of these nuclei are larger in males than in females. In particular, a cell group in the preoptic area of the hypothalamus known as the anteroventral periventricular preoptic nucleus (AVPv) is larger and has more cells in females than in males. The AVPv has extensive projections throughout the hypothalamus and is thought mediate the feedback of ovarian hormones to control the release of gonadotropin-releasing hormone by the hypothalamus. The development of sex differences in AVPv appears to be due to the organizational effects of perinatal hormone exposure. The nuclear size differences can be reversed by castration of newborn males or administration of testosterone or its aromatized metabolites to females within the first week of life. In contrast to SDN-POA, testosterone and estradiol increase cell death in AVPv during perinatal development, accounting for the smaller nuclear size in males.

Another well-studied model of sexual differentiation is found in the spinal cord. A small cluster of motoneurons in the lower lumbar spinal cord form the spinal nucleus of the bulbocavernosus (SNB). These motoneurons innervate the striated bulbocavernosus muscle at the base of the penis and play a role in erection and ejaculation. This nucleus and its target musculature are absent in the adult female. The musculature and SNB are present in both sexes at birth. The sexual dimorphism arises as the result of perinatal steroid hormone exposure. The results of several studies show that exposure to testosterone or the nonaromatizable androgen dihydrotestosterone maintains the bulbocavernosus musculature. Moreover, estrogen is not effective, so aromatization seems to be unimportant for the masculine development of this system. In the absence of androgen exposure, the muscles and the motoneurons in females begin to die. Androgens, either endogenous or exogenously administered, enhance muscle differentiation, which in turn appears to promote the survival of SNB motoneurons. No one knows yet what neurotropic substance the bulbocavernosus muscles provide to keep the SNB neurons alive.

Aside from the critical role of steroid hormones and programmed cell death, other factors may contribute to sexual differentiation of the nervous system. The behavior of rat dams with their male pups constitutes an example of how experience might interact with steroids to alter neural systems and behavior. During the postnatal period, the dam grooms the anogenital region of her pups to stimulate urination and defecation. Male pups are groomed more often than female pups. Injecting females with testosterone attracts more attention from the dam, suggesting that the dam may detect androgenic metabolites in the pup's urine. This maternal attention contributes directly to the expression of normal male sexual behavior and the size of the SNB in adult males.

In summary, steroid hormones play a pivotal role in the sexual differentiation of the nervous system. In most models that have been studied, one can manipulate the sexual dimorphism in the nervous system by manipulating steroid hormones. Steroids, powerful regulators of gene expression and cellular function, act during early life to control cell survival, synapse formation, cell migration, and cell differentiation within the nervous system. Most likely steroid hormones act together with neurotransmitters and growth factors to sculpt neural development. In addition, social and environmental factors have been shown to play a role in shaping sex differences in the nervous system. Collectively these mechanisms act together to determine the final sexual phenotype of the brain. Recent evidence suggests that steroids also produce temporary structural changes in the brain of the adult, highlighting the notion that some neural sexual dimorphisms require steroid hormone both during development and in adulthood to display sex differences fully in neuroendocrine function and behavior.

VII. SEXUAL DIFFERENTIATION OF THE HUMAN BRAIN

Male and female humans, like other animals, are exposed to different hormonal environments during early development. Males have elevated levels of testosterone toward the end of the first trimester and into the first few weeks of the second trimester and again during the first 6 months after birth. Females probably produce estrogens prenatally, although it is not clear that this contributes to development. The question of whether these hormonal differences influence sexual differentiation of the human brain and behavior cannot yet be answered unequivocally. This results, in part, from obvious ethical restrictions on hormonal manipulations in human fetuses. In addition, human males and females experience a very different process of socialization that undoubtedly contributes to behavioral sex differences. Consequently, it is difficult to determine the relative contribution that hormones and social environment make to psychosexual development in humans.

Sex differences have been reported in a variety of human behaviors. Males are typically more aggressive, exhibit more rough-and-tumble play behavior, and perform better on visuospatial tasks. Females typically excel at verbal skills, especially verbal fluency and perceptual speed. Although these differences are statistically significant, they are based on a large number of subjects and there is usually more variation within each sex than between sexes for most human behaviors. The largest behavioral sex differences are seen in childhood play, sexual orientation, and gender identity.

A number of structural sexual dimorphisms in the human brain have been described, but many of the reports are controversial and their functional significance is less well established than in animal models. The sexually dimorphic nucleus identified in the preoptic area of humans was named the SDN-POA because it was thought to be the analogue of the SDN-POA found in rats and is larger in males than in females. Two subsequent studies have failed to replicate this finding, although both reported a sex difference in a separate subregion of the preoptic area, i.e., the anterior hypothalamus, known as the third interstitial nucleus of the anterior hypothalamus (INAH-3). The INAH-3 is larger in males than in females. Although controversial, the size of INAH-3 has also been related to sexual orientation, with homosexual and bisexual men having smaller (i.e., female-typical) INAH-3s than presumed heterosexual men. Other hypothalamic regions reported to show sex differences in humans include the suprachiasmatic nucleus and the bed nucleus of the stria terminalis. Midline brain structures showing sex differences include portions of the corpus collosum, anterior commissure, and massa intermedia. The anterior commissure has been related to sexual orientation and the corpus collosum has been related to language lateralization.

An informative approach for asking whether fetal steroids affect neural development in humans is to study individuals with clinical conditions that disturb the normal relationship between genetic sex and hormonal sex. It must be remembered, however, that these studies are not true experiments, and data derived from them are not conclusive on their own. Nonetheless, one interesting set of patients is females that are exposed to excessive androgens *in utero*, typically due to congenital adrenal hyperplasia (CAH). Individuals with CAH lack synthetic enzymes needed to produce corticosteroids and as a consequence large amounts of precursor androgens are produced prenatally. The external genitalia may be mildly or extensively virilized. CAH girls behave more like boys, showing a pattern of behavior consisting of rough active outdoor play and interest in toys generally preferred by boys, with less interest in feminine clothing and doll play. In adulthood, CAH women are usually attracted to men, but are more likely to be homosexual or bisexual than are non-CAH women. Although some researchers attribute the behavioral masculinization in CAH girls to influences of androgens on brain development, others have noted that many other influences exist in this condition, such as psychological and social issues associated with chronic illness, ambiguous genitalia, and reduced fertility.

A clinical condition that has provided information on the behavioral consequences of androgen deficiency is androgen insensitivity. Genetic males with androgen insensitivity produce androgens but exhibit a defect in the androgen receptor that makes the receptor incapable of responding. Completely androgen-insensitive individuals look like normal females at birth, are raised as females, and develop feminine secondary sexual characteristics at puberty; however, they fail to menstruate because they lack female internal reproductive organs. These individuals act like normal females, displaying feminine spatial learning behavior and verbal behavior, and are sexually attracted to men. The fact that androgen-insensitive humans exhibit unambiguous feminine behaviors and gender identity argues that, unlike the case of androgen-insensitive rats, aromatized metabolites of androgens cannot be playing a major role for masculinizing the human brain. In agreement, it has been reported that males having congenital estrogen deficiency due to mutation of the aromatase gene assume a heterosexual sexual orientation and male sexual identity. There is evidence that *in utero* exposure of females to the synthetic estrogen diethylstilbestrol (DES) can masculinize the development of language lateralization, but this effect is small. Taken as a whole, these observations suggest that estrogen does not have the critical effect on nervous system sexual differentiation described in some rodent models.

VIII. SUMMARY

Gonadal steroids have profound effects on the sexual development of the brain in many nonhuman species. Testosterone secretion by fetal testes in males during the critical period is both necessary and sufficient to masculinize and defeminize gonadotropin feedback and the expression of adult sexual behaviors. In some rodent species, the intracellular aromatization of testosterone to estradiol is critical for these events to occur. In contrast, females develop in the absence of high androgen exposure. Developmental exposure to androgens has a permanent influence over the cell morphology and circuitry of the brain, i.e., the size of specific regions, the patterns of synaptic connections, the distribution of various neurotransmitters, and the expression of steroid receptors and signaling molecules. However, in some cases the functional significance of these sexual dimorphisms remains to be established. The cellular and molecular processes by which androgens and estrogens act to organize sex specific brain functions are not completely understood, but have been shown to include the regulation of cell migration, neuronal growth and axonal branching, and programmed cell death. Steroid hormones have also been shown to interact with social and environmental factors ultimately to determine the final sexual phenotype of the brain. Because of the dramatic effects of perinatal androgens in lower species, it has been generally assumed that similar processes occur in humans. Indeed, a number of behaviors and morphological brain features are sexually dimorphic in humans. Studies of humans with clinical syndromes in which fetuses are exposed to too much or too little androgen provide some support for these suppositions. However, because social environment plays such a crucial role in human psychosocial development, the question of whether and to what degree hormones influence the sexual differentiation of the human brain and behavior cannot yet be answered.

Glossary

activational effect Postpubertal process by which sex steroids exert an effect that transiently activates preexisting hormone-sensitive neural circuits.

aromatase Cytochrome P450 enzyme that converts androgens to estrogens; an important signaling pathway by which testosterone affects neural development and function.

critical period Time during development when sex steroids exert their organizational effects.

organizational effect Early developmental process by which sex steroids exert an effect that causes permanent, hard-wired differences in the structure and function of the central nervous system.

sexual dimorphism Sex difference in brain structure or function.

sexual differentiation Developmental process by which the two sexes become different.

See Also the Following Articles

Androgen Effects in Mammals • Aromatase and Estrogen Insufficiency • Dihydrotestosterone, Active Androgen Metabolites and Related Pathology • Environmental Disruptors of Sex Hormone Action • Estrogen in the Male: Nature, Sources and Biological Effects • Oxytocin • Sexual Differentiation, Molecular and Hormone Dependent Events in • Spermatogenesis, Hormonal Control of • Testis Descent, Hormonal Control of

Further Reading

Arnold, A. P. (1997). Sexual differentiation of the zebra finch song system: Positive evidence, negative evidence, null hypotheses, and a paradigm shift. *J. Neurobiol.* **33**, 572–584.

Auger, A. P., Perrot-Sinal, T. S., and McCarthy, M. M. (2001). Excitatory versus inhibitory GABA as a divergence point in steroid-mediated sexual differentiation of the brain. *Proc. Natl. Acad. Sci. U.S.A.* **98**, 8059–8064.

Breedlove, S. M. (1994). Sexual differentiation of the human nervous system. *Annu. Rev. Psychol.* **45**, 389–418.

Collaer, M. L., and Hines, M. (1995). Human behavioral sex differences: A role for gonadal hormones during early development. *Psychol. Bull.* **118**, 55–107.

Cooke, B., Hegstrom, C. D., Villeneuve, L. S., and Breedlove, S. M. (1998). Sexual differentiation of the vertebrate brain: principles and mechanisms. *Front. Neuroendocrinol.* **19**, 253–286.

Davis, E. C., Popper, P., and Gorski, R. A. (1996). The role of apoptosis in sexual differentiation of the rat sexually dimorphic nucleus of the preoptic area. *Brain Res.* **734**, 10–18.

Forger, N. G. (1999). Sexual differentiation, psychological. *In* "Encyclopedia of Reproduction" (E. Knobil and J. D. Neill, eds.), Vol. 4, pp. 421–430. Academic Press, San Diego.

Gorski, R. A. (1985). Sexual differentiation of the brain: Possible mechanisms and implications. *Can. J. Phys. Pharm.* **63**, 577–594.

Grumbach, M. M., and Auchus, R. J. (1999). Estrogen: Consequences and implications of human mutations in synthesis and action. *J. Clin. Endocrinol. Metab.* **84**, 4677–4694.

Haseltine, F. P., and Ohno, S. (1981). Mechanisms of gonadal differentiation. *Science* **211**, 1272–1277.

Henderson, R. G., Brown, A. E., and Tobet, S. A. (1999). Sex differences in cell migration in the preoptic area/anterior hypothalamus of mice. *J. Neurobiol.* **41**, 252–266.

McCarthy, M. M. (1994). Molecular aspects of sexual differentiation of the rodent brain. *Psychoneuroendocrinology* **19**, 415–427.

Nilsen, J., Mor, G., and Naftolin, F. (2000). Estrogen-regulated developmental neuronal apoptosis is determined by estrogen receptor subtype and the Fas/Fas ligand system. *J. Neurobiol.* **43**, 64–78.

Resko, J. A., and Roselli, C. E. (1997). Prenatal hormones organize sex differences of the neuroendocrine reproductive system: Observations on guinea pigs and nonhuman primates. *Cell Mol. Neurobiol.* **17**, 627–648.

Tobet, S. A., and Hanna, I. K. (1997). Ontogeny of sex differences in the mammalian hypothalamus and preoptic area. *Cell Mol. Neurobiol.* **17**, 565–601.

Wilson, J. D. (2001). Androgens, androgen receptors, and male gender role behavior. *Horm. Behav.* **40**, 358–366.

Sgk Protein (Serum- and Glucocorticoid-Inducible Protein Kinase)

GARY L. FIRESTONE

University of California, Berkeley

I. INTRODUCTION
II. Sgk PROTEIN STRUCTURE–FUNCTION
III. CELLULAR AND PHYSIOLOGICAL FUNCTIONS OF STIMULUS-INDUCED Sgk
IV. REGULATION OF Sgk EXPRESSION DURING DEVELOPMENT AND IN ADULT TISSUE
V. STIMULUS REGULATION OF Sgk PROMOTER ACTIVITY AND GENE TRANSCRIPTION
VI. REGULATION OF Sgk PHOSPHORYLATION AND ENZYMATIC ACTIVITY THROUGH THE GROWTH FACTOR-ACTIVATED PI3-KINASE PATHWAY
VII. Sgk SUBSTRATE SPECIFICITY AND TARGET PROTEINS
VIII. HORMONE AND STIMULUS-DEPENDENT CONTROL OF Sgk SUBCELLULAR COMPARTMENTALIZATION
IX. POTENTIAL CONNECTIONS OF Sgk WITH HUMAN DISORDERS

Serum- and glucocorticoid-inducible protein kinaseSerum- and glucocorticoid-inducible protein kinase (Sgk) is a unique point of crosstalk that is targeted by diverse hormone signaling cascades. Cell surface receptor, nuclear receptor, and cellular stress signal transduction pathways converge on Sgk to alter cellular function, control cell proliferation, activate osmoregulatory pathways, and/or determine whether a cell survives or undergoes apoptosis. An important biological feature of Sgk is that this protein kinase is regulated at three distinct levels of cellular control. Unlike most other protein kinases, the transcription, enzymatic activity, and subcellular localization of Sgk can be acutely controlled in a stimulus-dependent manner. Sgk mediates its downstream effects through phosphorylation of specific proteins and by its specific binding to certain target proteins, although only a limited number of Sgk substrates and nonsubstrate target proteins have been identified.

The list of hormone- and stimulus-dependent cascades that include Sgk as a key integrator of receptor signaling events continues to expand, and Sgk has been implicated in the pathology of several human endocrine disorders.

I. INTRODUCTION

In vertebrates and other multicellular organisms, individual cells are inundated with many types of hormonal cues and other extracellular stimuli that activate a diverse array of intracellular signal transduction pathways. The ability of cells to sense dynamic changes in their environment and then mount physiologically appropriate responses requires communication with regulatory molecules that can coordinately integrate the intracellular signals that emanate from different receptor signaling cascades. One such critical intracellular component is the serum- and glucocorticoid-inducible protein kinase, Sgk. This protein kinase was originally isolated in a differential screen for glucocorticoid-inducible transcripts from rat mammary epithelial tumor cells as a novel protein kinase that is under acute transcriptional control by serum and glucocorticoids.

Emerging evidence implicates Sgk as an important focal point by which cell surface receptors, nuclear receptors, and cellular stress signaling pathways converge to alter cellular function and the proliferative state and/or determine whether a cell survives or undergoes apoptosis. For example, in different cell and tissue types, Sgk can act as a stimulus-dependent switch in cellular responses to glucocorticoids, mineralocorticoids, follicle-stimulating hormone, growth factor-/insulin-activated cell survival and proliferative pathways, hyperosmotic shock, and transforming growth factor-β (TGF-β). Furthermore, Sgk has been implicated in the pathology of endocrine disorders such as diabetic nephropathy and in physiological abnormalities associated with alterations in the mineralocorticoid control of renal sodium transport.

The various hormone receptor-activated cascades regulate Sgk availability and function at three distinct levels of cellular control. First, an expanding set of hormonal and nonhormonal extracellular cues strongly stimulate Sgk gene expression. Second, Sgk is phosphorylated and enzymatically activated as a downstream component of the phosphatidylinositol 3-kinase (PI3-kinase) signaling cascade that mediates the mitogenic and cell survival response to many growth factors and insulin. Finally, the nuclear–cytoplasmic shuttling of Sgk is controlled by the cell cycle, as well as by exposure to specific hormones and to environmental stress. Thus, a biologically significant feature of Sgk is the simultaneous and stringent stimulus-dependent regulation of its transcription, subcellular localization, and enzymatic activity (Fig. 1).

II. Sgk PROTEIN STRUCTURE–FUNCTION

The *sgk* gene encodes a 431-amino-acid, 50 kDa protein, and its catalytic domain shows strong homology (45–55% identity) to the catalytic domains of several well-characterized members of the "AGC" family of serine/threonine protein kinases that are constitutively expressed. The protein kinases most closely related to Sgk are Akt/protein kinase B (PKB), protein kinase A, protein kinase C-ζ, and the rat $p70^{S6K}/p85^{S6K}$ kinases. In addition, two other Sgk isoforms have been uncovered (Sgk-2 and Sgk-3), although their cellular functions have not been well studied. This article will restrict its discussion to the originally isolated isoform of Sgk. Members of the related family of mammalian protein kinases that includes Sgk propagate cell signaling cascades associated with the control of cell growth, differentiation, and cell survival and are highly conserved between metazoans and mammals. For example, in addition to humans, rats, and mice, Sgk homologues have been identified in the genomes of diverse species such as frogs, the nematode *Caenorhabditis elegans*, and the budding yeast *Saccharomyces cerevisiae*. One rationale for the evolutionary conservation of Sgk is its role in allowing unicellular and multicellular organisms to adapt and survive environmental stresses such as extreme changes in nutrient levels, temperatures, or osmolarity. In this regard, the two yeast Sgk homologues can be functionally complemented with mammalian Sgk, which strengthens the notion of an evolutionarily important role for Sgk in integrating hormone-activated cellular signals.

As shown in Fig. 2, Sgk has several distinctive structural features that are likely to control aspects of Sgk function in a stimulus-specific context. Sgk has three general regions, a relatively short (70 amino acids) unique amino-terminal domain, a central region containing the catalytic domain, and a unique carboxy-terminal domain. Each of these subregions contains important structural features required for the cellular regulation of Sgk. The N-terminal domain contains a phosphorylation site at serine 78 (P-P-S78-P) that fits the P-x-S/T-P consensus requirements for certain proline-directed kinases and has been shown to be phosphorylated by the big mitogen

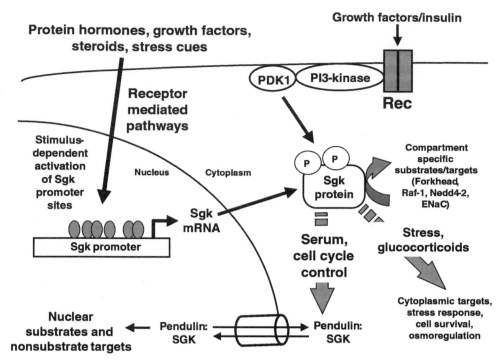

FIGURE 1 Hormone and stimulus control of Sgk expression, enzymatic activity, and subcellular localization. Sgk is regulated at three distinct levels of cellular control. The activation of hormone receptor-dependent cascades, as well as environmental stress, regulates Sgk expression by targeting distinct elements in the Sgk promoter. The growth factor/insulin activation of the PI3-kinase pathways results in the phosphorylation of Sgk and the generation of an enzymatically active Sgk. Under proliferative conditions, Sgk is imported by the actions of pendulin/importin-α into the nucleus, where Sgk has access to its nuclear target proteins. After treatment with glucocorticoids or exposure to environmental stress, Sgk resides in a cytoplasmic compartment and mediates the cell survival response.

activative protein kinase 1 (BMK1)/extracellular signal-related kinase 5 (ERK5) member of the mitogen-activated protein kinase (MAPK) family. There are several proline-rich tracts in the N-terminal domain that could conceivably be recognition sites for Sgk target proteins, as well as a putative mitochondrial import signal that may localize cytoplasmic Sgk to this organelle as part of the hormone-dependent cell survival response.

The central domain of Sgk contains all of the essential amino acid sequences necessary to be a functional serine/threonine protein kinase including lysine 127 in the ATP-binding region and threonine 256 in the activation loop. Mutation of lysine 127 (to methionine) forms a kinase-dead version of Sgk. As described in more detail in Section VI and diagrammed in Fig. 2, Sgk is enzymatically activated by phosphorylation of threonine 256 in the activation loop of Sgk, as well as by phosphorylation of serine 422 in the carboxy-terminal domain, by the PI3-kinase-dependent pathway through the direct actions of phosphoinositide-dependent protein kinase 1

(PDK1). The central domain also contains a nuclear localization signal between amino acids 131 and 138 in the central domain (see Section VIII) that controls the signal-dependent nuclear import of Sgk, as well as specific recognition sites for other proteins such as Nedd4-2 at a PY domain (see Section III). Similarly, the carboxy-terminal domain contains a putative PDZ-binding motif that is likely to be involved in Sgk recognition of target proteins. The Sgk structure domains suggest that this protein kinase acts through phosphorylation of specific substrates (see Section VII) and through specific sets of regulated protein–protein interactions.

III. CELLULAR AND PHYSIOLOGICAL FUNCTIONS OF STIMULUS-INDUCED Sgk

A. Role of Sgk in Glucocorticoid and Growth Factor Regulation of Cell Proliferation

Sgk is a transcriptionally induced component of glucocorticoid- and growth factor-regulated gene

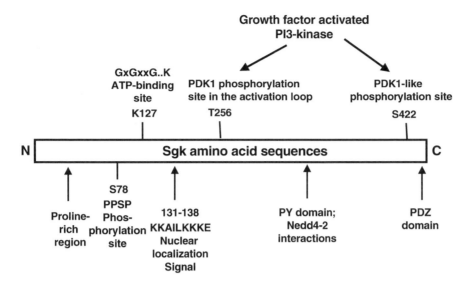

FIGURE 2 Sgk protein structure and functions. The Sgk protein contains three phosphorylation sites. Serine 78 is a proline-directed phosphorylated site that is recognized by members of the mitogen-activated protein kinase family. Threonine 256 and serine 422 are phosphorylated by PDK1 through a PI3-kinase-dependent cascade and are required for the growth factor/insulin activation of Sgk enzymatic activity. Lysine 127 is needed for ATP binding and protein kinase activity. Sgk also contains a proline-rich region in the N-terminal domain, a nuclear localization signal at 131–138, a PY domain required for the Sgk interactions with Nedd4-2, and a putative PDZ site that likely is involved in the recognition of Sgk target proteins.

networks that are highly associated with the control of cellular proliferation. In mammary tumor cells, the serum-induced expression and S-phase nuclear import of Sgk (see Section VIII) are necessary for cell cycle progression of mammary epithelial cells. The BMK1/ERK5 member of the mitogen-activated protein kinase gene family was shown to induce cell proliferation through its interaction with and phosphorylation of Sgk. Consistent with a role for Sgk in proliferative control in normal cells, the sgk gene resides in a single chromosomal locus assigned to band 6q23, a region frequently affected by deletion in various human neoplasias. Sgk appears to also be involved in certain hormone-regulated growth inhibitory responses. The glucocorticoid-induced G1 cell cycle arrest of mammary tumor cells is accompanied by and partially dependent on the stimulated expression of cytoplasmic localized Sgk in mammary tumor cells. Ectopic expression of Sgk in this cell system inhibits cell proliferation. Given that glucocorticoids are considered a physiological stress hormone, it is tempting to consider that the induction of Sgk by this steroid allows cells to mount physiologically appropriate responses to changes in the external milieu resulting from mitogenic cues and/or stress stimuli.

B. Role of Sgk in the Cellular Stress Response and in Cell Survival Cascades

Sgk has been shown to be a cell survival component of the responses to cellular stressors such as hyperosmotic shock in various epithelial cells. Subsequent to the original cloning of Sgk, this protein kinase was revealed in a screen for an osmotic shock-inducible gene from hepatocytes, and sgk transcripts have been shown to be induced by hyperosmolarity and secretagogues in shark rectal gland. Hyperosmotic shock strongly induces Sgk transcription in mammary epithelial cells by a pathway that utilizes the p38/MAPK cascade, which is the mammalian homologue of the stress-activated S. cerevisiae HOG1 proline-directed protein kinase. Expression of the wild-type enzymatically active Sgk, but not the kinase-dead forms of Sgk, protects the transfected cells from stress-induced apoptosis, whereas expression of kinase-dead forms of Sgk had no protective effects. Sgk was also shown to be an important component of the glucocorticoid cell survival response to growth factor deprivation in a human breast cancer cell line. The Sgk-3 isoform has been implicated in the interleukin-3-mediated survival of hematopoietic cells, suggesting that a subset of cellular responses are likely be Sgk isoform-specific.

C. Role of Sgk in Mineralocorticoid and Insulin Regulation of Sodium Homeostasis and in Osmotic Control of Cell Volume

Sgk stimulates epithelial sodium channel (ENaC) activity and enhances its membrane abundance in co-injected *Xenopus laevis* oocytes, suggesting that one function of Sgk is to control cell volume and sodium homeostasis following osmotic stress of cells. Evidence from several studies indicates that Sgk plays a central role in integrating mineralocorticoid and insulin signals as part of the osmoregulatory mechanism in the kidney. The current viewpoint is that aldosterone regulates sodium homeostasis by stimulating the expression of Sgk, which in turn causes an increase in total renal cell membrane ENaC activity. Sgk directly binds to the ENaC β-subunit, but does not phosphorylate this ion channel. Recent evidence shows that Sgk does phosphorylate the ubiquitin ligase Nedd4-2, which reduces the binding of Nedd4-2 to the C-terminal tail domain of the ENaC β-subunit. The Sgk-dependent phosphorylation of Nedd4-2 appears to require a PY domain recognition site within Sgk (see Fig. 2). As a result, the degradation of ENaC is reduced, with the net effect being an elevation in the steady state level of membrane-associated ENaC and subsequent stimulation of sodium transport in response to mineralocorticoids. Insulin signaling plays a role in the process, and in renal cells insulin can synergize with mineralocorticoids to regulate sodium transport. Insulin has been proposed to activate Sgk enzymatic activity through the PI3-kinase cascade (see Section VI), and consistent with this notion, an inhibition of PI3-kinase activity blocks insulin-stimulated sodium transport. This response, which has been generally observed in cell systems, has a physiological impact because in one study, decreased sodium excretion during sodium depletion was observed in Sgk knockout mice compared to littermate controls.

D. Other Biological Functions of Sgk

Although not directly linked to stimulus-regulated mechanisms, Sgk has been implicated in a variety of cellular functions that may eventually prove to be associated with hormonal mechanisms of action. For example, Sgk has been linked to the function and cellular utilization of several other ion channels, such as the cystic fibrosis transmembrane regulator-dependent chloride channel and certain voltage-gated potassium channels. The control of potassium ion channel activity suggests a role for Sgk in neuronal excitability. Consistent with this concept, a recent study has implicated Sgk in facilitating memory consolidation of spatial learning in rats. Sgk transcripts were shown to be expressed at significantly higher levels in the hippocampus, an area of the brain with a high level of glucocorticoid receptors, of fast learners compared to slower learners. Thus, it is likely that many functions of Sgk will eventually be revealed, beyond the stimulus-dependent control of proliferation, cell survival, and osmoregulatory processes.

IV. REGULATION OF Sgk EXPRESSION DURING DEVELOPMENT AND IN ADULT TISSUE

Sgk expression is under stringent developmental control during mouse embryogenesis. Sgk transcripts are first observed at embryonic day 8.5 (E8.5) in the decidua and yolk sac, and then during developmental stages E9.5 through E12.5, this kinase is highly localized in the heart chamber, otic vesicle, blood vessels surrounding the somites, and lung buds. At later stages of mouse embryogenesis, E13.5 through E16.5, sgk expression becomes highly concentrated in brain (choroid plexus), distal epithelium, terminal bronchi/bronchioles, adrenal gland, liver, thymus, and intestines, remains high in heart tissue, and is expressed at a low level in the other embryonic tissues. In the adult, Sgk is concentrated in the choroid plexus of the brain, which is involved in osmotic and pH regulation of cerebral spinal fluid. Sgk is also concentrated in specific areas of the adult kidney (glomeruli and nephrons in the cortical region, as well as in the medulla, papilla, and calyces), suggesting a role in regulating osmotic balance. Consistent with this concept, Sgk is induced by the mineralocorticoid aldosterone in the cortical collecting ducts of the rodent kidney. In adult rat tissue, Sgk is also highly expressed in the thymus, ovary, and lung. A high level of Sgk has been reported in phagocytes, which is consistent with Sgk being involved in the inflammatory response. The tissue-specific and temporal pattern of *sgk* expression during mouse embryogenesis suggests that *sgk* has a potential role in heart development and/or vasculogenesis at early developmental stages and may function in tissues involved in osmoregulation and other physiological stress pathways at later developmental stages and in the adult.

V. STIMULUS REGULATION OF Sgk PROMOTER ACTIVITY AND GENE TRANSCRIPTION

Sgk expression can be acutely regulated by a variety of hormones and extracellular stress cues that are known to target specific DNA elements in gene promoters. Only a few studies have used the Sgk promoter to rigorously establish the transcriptional control of Sgk gene expression. Glucocorticoids, the p53 tumor suppressor gene, follicle-stimulating hormone, and hyperosmotic stress have been shown to induce Sgk gene products by pathways that target specific DNA elements in the promoter (Fig. 3). In addition to these stimuli, Sgk transcript levels have been to shown to be stimulated in a tissue-specific manner by mineralocorticoids, TGF-β, cytokines such as granulocyte/macrophage colony-stimulating factor and tumor necrosis factor α, ischemic injury of the brain, growth factors such fibroblastic growth factor and platelet-derived growth factor, diabetic nephropathy, changes in hepatocyte cell volume, inflammatory disease, and fibroblast wound repair, whereas heparin suppresses Sgk expression. Although

these studies have not characterized the precise level of regulation, it is likely that these responses involve selective changes in Sgk transcription through the control of Sgk promoter activity. In this regard, based on sequence analysis, a variety of intriguing putative DNA elements exist in this promoter for transcription factors known to play a role in cellular differentiation, proliferation, and stress responses and may thereby account for hormone-regulated changes in Sgk expression.

A. Sgk Is the Primary Glucocorticoid-Responsive Gene Containing a Glucocorticoid-Response Element in Its Promoter

Sgk expression is stimulated by glucocorticoids in a variety of cells and tissues, and the Sgk promoter contains a functional glucocorticoid-response element (GRE) that accounts for its glucocorticoid inducibility. A combination of mutagenesis, transfection of Sgk promoter-driven reporter plasmids, and DNA–glucocorticoid receptor-binding assays revealed the presence of the Sgk GRE, which is located at approximately − 1000 bp of the Sgk promoter (Fig. 3). The Sgk GRE is highly homologous to the consensus glucocorticoid-response element and is sufficient to confer glucocorticoid responsiveness to a heterologous promoter in a manner that requires a functional receptor. Mutation of the Sgk GRE eliminates glucocorticoid responsiveness of the Sgk promoter. These decisive promoter studies support the notion that Sgk is a primary glucocorticoid-responsive gene. Given that glucocorticoid and mineralocorticoid receptors bind to the same DNA element, it is likely that the GRE in the Sgk promoter accounts for the aldosterone induction of Sgk transcripts in mammalian and amphibian renal cells.

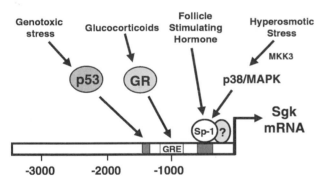

FIGURE 3 Hormone and environmental stress pathways target distinct elements in the Sgk promoter. Sgk is a primary glucocorticoid-responsive gene and contains a functional glucocorticoid-response element (GRE) in its promoter. The Sgk GRE is similar to consensus GREs in other systems and binds to the glucocorticoid receptor (GR) with high affinity. The Sgk promoter is also targeted by the p53 tumor suppressor gene as a downstream response to genotoxic stress. Follicle-stimulating hormone activates a receptor signaling pathway that simulates Sgk transcription through a Sp-1 transcription factor. Hyperosmotic stress activates a p38/mitogen-activated protein kinase (p38/MAPK) pathway through the actions of MKK3 (MAPK kinase kinase-3), which also targets Sp-1 in the Sgk promoter. Sp-1 interacts with other transcription factors in a tissue-dependent manner to stimulate Sgk transcription. The Sgk promoter contains many other putative transcription factor sites that likely account for the regulation of Sgk gene expression of other hormones and extracellular stimuli.

B. Regulation of Sgk Promoter Activity by the p53 Tumor Suppressor Protein, Hyperosmotic Stress, and Follicle-Stimulating Hormone

The Sgk promoter is a transcriptional target of the p53 tumor suppressor protein, a known target of genotoxic stress. Using both functional and DNA-binding strategies, the wild-type p53 tumor suppressor protein was shown to strongly stimulate Sgk promoter activity in mouse mammary epithelial cells, but repressed Sgk promoter activity in Rat2 fibroblasts. The Sgk p53 sequences at − 1380 bp and at − 1345 bp were sufficient to confer p53-dependent transactivation or transrepression to a heterologous promoter in a cell type-specific manner. Interestingly, both the murine and the human wild-type p53 tumor suppressor proteins, but not a mutant p53, can functionally interfere with the glucocorticoid receptor transactivation of the Sgk promoter through events converging on the Sgk GRE.

Sgk promoter activity can be stimulated by follicle-stimulating hormone in adult rat ovarian granulosa cells through activation of the Sp-1 transcription factor in the Sgk promoter. This response is also dependent on activation of the cyclic AMP pathway, although the precise upstream pathways that target Sp-1 have not characterized. A systematic mutagenic analysis of the Sgk promoter activity revealed a hyperosmotic stress-regulated element that is located between positions -50 and -40 in the Sgk promoter and that mediates the hyperosmotic response to the organic osmolyte 0.3 M sorbitol. This region of the Sgk promoter contains a consensus Sp-1 DNA element, and the stimulus-regulated binding of the Sp-1 transcription factor to this site accounts for the stimulation of Sgk transcription. The hyperosmotic stress cascade targets Sp-1 in the Sgk promoter by activating the p38/MAPK stress kinase. For example, incubation with the SB202190- or SB203580-specific inhibitors of p38/MAPK dampens the hyperosmotic stress stimulation of the Sgk promoter and Sgk protein production. Active MAPK kinase kinase-3 acts upstream of p38/MAPK to stimulate Sgk promoter activity in a sorbitol-dependent manner (Fig. 3). Sp-1 is known to interact with other transcription factors, and it is likely that the follicle-stimulating hormone and the hyperosmotic stress control of Sgk promoter activities require different Sp-1 protein–protein interactions.

VI. REGULATION OF Sgk PHOSPHORYLATION AND ENZYMATIC ACTIVITY THROUGH THE GROWTH FACTOR-ACTIVATED PI3-KINASE PATHWAY

The stimulus-dependent control of Sgk phosphorylation and enzymatic activity through a PI3-kinase cascade represents a second level of Sgk regulation in the cell (Fig. 1). The PI3-kinase-activated signal transduction pathway enhances cell survival and proliferation in response to a variety of growth factors. PI3-kinase directly binds to tyrosine kinase receptors (or to insulin substrate-1) via a SH2 domain in its p85 subunit. PI3-kinase converts phosphatidylinositol 4,5-biphosphate to phosphatidylinositol 3,4,5-triphosphate, which binds to the pleckstrin homology domain

contained within PDK1, resulting in its activation. Active PDK1 then directly phosphorylates and enzymatically activates several serine/threonine protein kinases, including Sgk and several protein kinases most homologous to Sgk, such as Akt/PKB. Full stimulation of Sgk enzymatic activity requires the PDK1-dependent phosphorylation at threonine 256, which is located within the activation loop of Sgk, and at serine 422, in the carboxy-terminal domain. Ablation of both phosphorylation sites by mutation of threonine 256 and serine 422 to alanines inhibits Sgk enzymatic activity and in some systems forms a potent dominant negative form of Sgk. Furthermore, substitution of the PI3-kinase-dependent phosphorylation sites with aspartate to mimic the charge effects of phosphorylation generates a constitutively active protein kinase. Treatment of cells with the LY294002 chemical inhibitor of PI3-kinase abolishes the hormone activation of Sgk enzymatic activity and prevents the production of the hyperphosphorylated forms of Sgk in the cell systems that have been examined.

Sgk phosphorylation and enzymatic activity have been shown to be regulated as a downstream component of the PI3-kinase cascade in response to a variety of extracellular signals, such as serum growth factors, insulin-like growth factor-I, insulin, oxidative stress, and hyperosmotic stress. Importantly, the disruption of PI3-kinase-dependent phosphorylation and activation of Sgk abolishes many Sgk cellular functions, such as insulin-stimulated sodium transport, glucocorticoid-dependent effects on cell proliferation and cell survival, mitogenic cell survival responses, and the cellular response to osmotic changes. The precise role of Sgk in many of these cellular functions has not been established because the same sets of extracellular signals that activate the stimulus-induced Sgk enzymatic activity also activate constitutively expressed Akt/PKB, which is highly related to Sgk and contains analogous PDK-1-dependent phosphorylation sites. In studies examining its downstream targets, Akt/PKB, like Sgk, has been indicated to play roles in maintaining cell survival in response to growth factors, in insulin-regulated glucose metabolism, in transcriptional control, and in regulation of apoptosis after environmental stress in many different cell types. Although Sgk and Akt/PKB are highly homologous in their catalytic domains and have similar activation profiles, they display unique features that suggest that they provide complementary rather than redundant cell functions.

VII. Sgk SUBSTRATE SPECIFICITY AND TARGET PROTEINS

By screening of a peptide library, consensus Sgk substrate sites that are generally similar to the Akt/PKB enzymatic specificity (RXRXXS/T) and that suggest some overlap in protein substrates have been identified. Sgk phosphorylates several peptides, and the most selective peptide substrate for Sgk is KKRNRRLSVA, which was named Sgktide. Arginines at the $-2/-3$ and the $-5/-6$ positions, relative to the phosphorylated serine, were found to be required for Sgk activity. In mostly *in vitro* assays, several substrates for Sgk have been revealed. Both Sgk and Akt/PKB have been shown to phosphorylate *in vitro* glycogen synthase kinase 3, the apoptotic component Bad, the forkhead transcription factor FKHRL1, and the Raf-1 component of mitogen signaling cascades. In transfected cells, the T256A/S422A mutant Sgk acts as dominant negative for phosphorylation of the forkhead transcription factor and attenuates the cell survival response to extracellular stress. These results directly implicate Sgk in the hormone-dependent control of cell survival. There are subtle differences in the substrate specificity of Sgk and Akt/PKB that are likely to be biologically significant. The best example with an endogenous substrate is with the FKHRL1 forkhead transcription factor in that Sgk and Akt/PKB display preferences for different phosphorylation sites in this protein. Given the important role of forkhead transcription factors in controlling cell survival and apoptotic responses, one viewpoint is that this dual phosphorylation causes a more enhanced cell survival response. It is likely that hormone-regulated activation of both Sgk and Akt/PKB, for example, by insulin and other growth factors, similarly enhances the corresponding downstream cascades through the complementary actions of Sgk and Akt/PKB.

As mentioned earlier, Sgk phosphorylates the ubiquitin ligase Nedd4-2, which causes a significant reduction in the interaction of this ligase with the ENaC, resulting in a net mineralocorticoid-dependent elevation in ENaC levels in the membrane of renal cells. ENaC is a direct protein-binding target of Sgk, and although the precise mechanism underlying these interactions has not been established, it is tempting to consider that Sgk–ENaC protein–protein interactions allow the efficient access of Sgk to its Nedd4-2 substrate. Sgk was also shown to bind to, but not phosphorylate, the nuclear import receptor pendulin/importin-α, and the hormone-regulated implications of this observation are described below.

Only a limited number of Sgk substrates and nonsubstrate target proteins have been identified, and a key future direction for the field will be to identify the many unknown Sgk target proteins that account for the stimulus-dependent responses associated with Sgk.

VIII. HORMONE AND STIMULUS-DEPENDENT CONTROL OF Sgk SUBCELLULAR COMPARTMENTALIZATION

Emerging evidence suggests that the regulated subcellular localization of Sgk, a third level of cellular control of Sgk, is a physiologically important process that helps the cells integrate extracellular proliferative, stress, and differentiation signals. The control of Sgk compartmentalization provides Sgk access to its critical targets and is particularly important for integrating intracellular signaling pathways when different hormonal cues with opposite cellular functions can induce enzymatically active Sgk. Depending on the extracellular stimuli, the regulated compartmentalization of Sgk can be viewed as controlling the accessibility of this protein kinase to its substrates and nonsubstrate protein targets.

A. Stimulus and Cell Cycle Regulation of Sgk Localization to the Nucleus or the Cytoplasmic Compartment

The subcellular distribution of Sgk between the nucleus and the cytoplasm is stringently controlled in a stimulus-dependent manner in mammary epithelial cells and in ovarian cells. In serum-stimulated proliferating mammary tumor cells, a nuclear form of Sgk can be detected, whereas in glucocorticoid growth-arrested cells or in hyperosmotically stressed cells, enzymatically active Sgk is localized exclusively to the cytoplasmic compartment. During the *in vivo* transition from granulosa cells in the proliferative stage of growing follicles in the ovary to terminally differentiated nongrowing luteal cells, the subcellular distribution of Sgk changes from being predominately nuclear to almost entirely cytoplasmic.

Laser scanning cytometry, which simultaneously monitors Sgk localization and DNA content in individual mammary tumor cells of an asynchronously growing population, revealed that Sgk actively shuttles between the nucleus and the cytoplasm in synchrony with the cell cycle. Sgk is predominantly nuclear in S and G2/M phase cells and resides in the cytoplasmic compartment during the G1 phase of the cell cycle. Immunofluorescence and biochemical studies showed that treatment with glucocorticoids, which induce a G1 cell cycle arrest, or exposure to hyperosmotic stress results in a cytoplasmic form of Sgk. The precise cytoplasmic compartment in which Sgk resides has not been fully characterized, although some evidence indicates a mitochondrial location for the stressed-induced Sgk. In cells synchronously released from the G1/S boundary, Sgk exclusively localizes to the nucleus during progression through the S phase. The forced retention of exogenous Sgk in either the nucleus or the cytoplasm suppresses the growth and DNA synthesis of serum-stimulated cells. This result indicates that a key proliferative signal in mammary tumor cells is the continuous shuttling of Sgk between the nucleus and the cytoplasm. In the ovarian system, on treatment with FSH, Sgk resides in the nucleus of proliferating granulosa cells, and in terminally differentiated luteal cells, Sgk is located in the cytoplasmic compartment.

Taken together, these results suggest that the spatial and temporal regulation of Sgk is vital for executing complex growth and differentiation programs, which suggests the existence of specific regulatory mechanisms for localizing Sgk to distinct cellular compartments. Conceivably, the signal-dependent sequestration of Sgk in different subcellular locations also entails interactions with particular cellular proteins that target Sgk to specific intracellular destinations and thereby control accessibility to its protein targets.

B. Mechanism of Stimulus Regulation of Sgk Nuclear-Cytoplasmic Shuttling

A yeast two-hybrid screen demonstrated that the nuclear receptor pendulin/importin-α is a highly specific Sgk-interacting protein. *In vitro* binding assays and co-immunoprecipitations of cell extracts demonstrated that pendulin/importin-α strongly binds to Sgk. Pendulin/importin-α recognizes nuclear localization signals in its cargo proteins and then through the interactions with importin-β, the receptor–cargo protein complex is imported into the nucleus through nuclear core complexes. Mutagenesis of Sgk identified a "bipartite-like" nuclear localization signal sequence, KKAILKKKE, between amino acids 131 and 139 in Sgk. This sequence mediates the *in vitro* binding of Sgk to pendulin/importin-α and the nuclear import of Sgk. For example, mutation of the Sgk nuclear localization signal by amino acid substitutions (K to A) in the context of the full-length Sgk ablates the *in vitro* interaction of Sgk with pendulin/importin-α.

Subcellular localization studies documented that pendulin/importin-α co-localizes with Sgk to the nucleus in serum-stimulated cells and to the cytoplasmic compartment in dexamethasone-treated mammary tumor cells. One viewpoint is that the selective interactions between Sgk and pendulin/importin-α control the cell cycle-dependent nuclear localization of Sgk in serum-treated cells and play a role in distributing Sgk to the cytoplasm in glucocorticoid-treated or stressed cells. Thus, the Sgk–pendulin/importin-α interactions provide a mechanistic basis for the stimulus-regulated compartmentalization.

IX. POTENTIAL CONNECTIONS OF Sgk WITH HUMAN DISORDERS

The central role of Sgk in integrating the cross talk between nuclear receptor and plasma membrane receptor signals would predict that many physiological abnormalities would be associated with the dysfunctional regulation of expression, activity, and subcellular localization of Sgk. Indeed, recent evidence has indicated that Sgk plays a role in the pathology of certain human disorders. Alterations in Sgk expression, in combination with its cellular role in osmoregulation, suggest a role for Sgk in the nephropathy that is associated with the diabetic disease state, conceivably as part of the hyperosmotic response in the kidney to high plasma glucose levels. Similarly, Sgk has been implicated in the salt-sensitive hypertension associated with the insulin-resistance syndrome. Transforming growth factor-β stimulates Sgk expression, and this response suggests that Sgk plays a role in the fibrogenic actions of this hormonal cue and by extension is involved in fibrosing disease. Consistent with this notion, Sgk expression is elevated in fibrosing pancreatitis and in inflammatory bowel disease. The stimulus-dependent cell survival and proliferative functions of Sgk directly suggest that defects in the cellular control of Sgk signaling may be associated with a subset of human disorders with dysfunctional growth control and apoptotic mechanisms, such as cancer. The control of Sgk nuclear–cytoplasmic shuttling may be a particularly important facet of Sgk control because the nuclear form of Sgk is associated with proliferative conditions, whereas after cellular stress the cytoplasmic form of Sgk is important for cell survival and anti-proliferative responses. Thus, it is tempting to consider that the nuclear Sgk substrates could provide potential targets for therapeutic intervention to selectively dampen cell proliferation or to modulate pathological states of cells associated with the nuclear localization of Sgk. In a complementary manner, small-molecule inhibitors of Sgk kinase activity have the potential to be developed as novel therapeutic agents to control certain neoplasias by selectively regulating proliferative, survival, and/or apoptotic signaling pathways that are dependent on Sgk.

Glossary

hormone receptor signaling cascade The chain of intracellular events beginning from the activation of a hormone receptor that ends in the final response to the hormone. Also known as a signal transduction pathway.

phosphatidylinositol 3-kinase (PI3-kinase) Kinase that directly binds to tyrosine kinase receptors (or to insulin substrate-1) via a SH2 domain in its p85 subunit. PI3-kinase converts phosphatidylinositol 4,5-biphosphate to phosphatidylinositol 3,4,5-triphosphate. The PI3-kinase signal transduction pathway mediates cell survival and proliferative responses to a variety of growth factors and insulin.

phosphoinositide-dependent protein kinase-1 Protein kinase that is activated by phosphatidylinositol 3-kinase and in turn directly phosphorylates and enzymatically activates serum- and glucocorticoid-inducible protein kinase.

serum- and glucocorticoid-inducible protein kinase Protein kinase that is regulated by hormones and other extracellular signals at three distinct levels of cellular control and is a unique point of cross talk in hormone signaling cascades.

stress response The ability of cells to survive or undergo apoptosis in response to environmental stress conditions, such as changes in osmolarity, nutrient deprivation, or extreme temperatures. Generally considered to be initiated by receptor-mediated events.

See Also the Following Articles

Apoptosis ● Membrane Receptor Signaling in Health and Disease ● Receptor–Receptor Interactions ● Signaling Pathways, Interaction of ● Stress

Further Reading

Alliston, T. N., Gonzalez-Robayna, I. J., Buse, P., Firestone, G. L., and Richards, J. S. (2000). Expression and localization of serum/glucocorticoid-induced kinase in the rat ovary: Relation to follicular growth and differentiation. *Endocrinology* **141**, 385–395.

Bell, L. M., Leong, M. L., Kim, B., Wang, E., Park, J., Hemmings, B. A., and Firestone, G. L. (2000). Hyperosmotic stress stimulates promoter activity and regulates cellular utilization of the serum- and glucocorticoid-inducible protein kinase (Sgk) by a p38 MAPK-dependent pathway. *J. Biol. Chem.* **275**, 25262–25272.

Brunet, A., Park, J., Tran, H., Hu, L. S., Hemmings, B. A., and Greenberg, M. E. (2001). Protein kinase SGK mediates survival signals by phosphorylating the forkhead transcription factor FKHRL1 (FOXO3a). *Mol. Cell. Biol.* **21**, 952–965.

Buse, P., Tran, S. H., Luther, E., Phu, P. T., Aponte, G. W., and Firestone, G. L. (1999). Cell cycle and hormonal control of nuclear–cytoplasmic localization of the serum- and glucocorticoid-inducible protein kinase, Sgk, in mammary tumor cells: A novel convergence point of anti-proliferative and proliferative cell signaling pathways. *J. Biol. Chem.* **274**, 7253–7263.

Casamayor, A., Torrance, P. D., Kobayashi, T., Thorner, J., and Alessi, D. R. (1999). Functional counterparts of mammalian protein kinases PDK1 and SGK in budding yeast. *Curr. Biol.* **9**, 186–197.

Chen, S. Y., Bhargava, A., Mastroberardino, L., Meijer, O. C., Wang, J., Buse, P., Firestone, G. L., Verrey, F., and Pearce, D. (1999). Epithelial sodium channel regulated by aldosterone-induced protein sgk. *Proc. Natl. Acad. Sci. USA* **96**, 2514–2519.

Debonneville, C., Flores, S. Y., Kamynina, E., Plant, P. J., Tauxe, C., Thomas, M. A., Munster, C., Chraibi, A., Pratt, J. H., Horisberger, J. D., Pearce, D., Loffing, J., and Staub, O. (2001). Phosphorylation of Nedd4–2 by Sgk1 regulates epithelial Na$^{(+)}$ channel cell surface expression. *EMBO J.* **20**, 7052–7059.

Faletti, C. J., Perrotti, N., Taylor, S. I., and Blazer-Yost, B. L. (2002). sgk: An essential convergence point for peptide and steroid hormone regulation of ENaC-mediated Na$^+$ transport. *Am. J. Physiol. Cell. Physiol.* **282**, C494–C500.

Kobayashi, T., and Cohen, P. (1999). Activation of serum- and glucocorticoid-regulated protein kinase by agonists that activate phosphatidylinositide 3-kinase is mediated by 3-phosphoinositide-dependent protein kinase-1 (PDK1) and PDK2. *Biochem. J.* **339**, 319–328.

Lee, E., Lein, E. S., and Firestone, G. L. (2001). Tissue-specific expression of the transcriptionally regulated serum and glucocorticoid-inducible protein kinase (Sgk) during mouse embryogenesis. *Mech. Dev.* **103**, 177–181.

Maiyar, A. C., Phu, P. T., Huang, A. J., and Firestone, G. L. (1997). Repression of glucocorticoid receptor transactivation and DNA binding of a glucocorticoid response element within the serum/glucocorticoid-inducible protein kinase (sgk) gene promoter by the p53 tumor suppressor protein. *Mol. Endocrinol.* **11**, 312–329.

Park, J., Leong, M. L., Buse, P., Maiyar, A. C., Firestone, G. L., and Hemmings, B. A. (1999). Serum and glucocorticoid-inducible kinase (SGK) is a target of the PI 3-kinase-stimulated signaling pathway. *EMBO J.* **18**, 3024–3033.

Pearce, D. (2001). The role of SGK1 in hormone-regulated sodium transport. *Trends Endocrinol. Metab.* **12**, 341–347.

Waldegger, S., Barth, P., Raber, G., and Lang, F. (1997). Cloning and characterization of a putative human serine/threonine protein kinase transcriptionally modified during anisotonic and isotonic alterations of cell volume. *Proc. Natl. Acad. Sci. USA* **94**, 4440–4445.

Wang, J., Barbry, P., Maiyar, A. C., Rozansky, D. J., Bhargava, A., Leong, M., Firestone, G. L., and Pearce, D. (2001). SGK integrates insulin and mineralocorticoid regulation of epithelial sodium transport. *Am. J. Physiol. Renal Physiol.* **280**, F303–F313.

SHBG

See *Sex Hormone-Binding Globulin*

Signaling Pathways, Interaction of

GUANGNAN LI AND RAVI IYENGAR

Mount Sinai School of Medicine, New York

A large group of eukaryotic genes encode proteins that span the cell membrane and function as cell surface receptors. On engagement by cognate ligands, membrane receptors initiate a variety of signaling pathways that control diverse biological processes. It is already clear that signal pathways starting from membrane receptors are interconnected with one another via protein networks that are subjected to multiple positive and negative feedback mechanisms. Within these networks, a specific biological response can be generated by an array of diverse signaling pathways.

I. INTRODUCTION

This article will first explore the cell proliferation pathways controlled by receptor tyrosine kinases (RTKs) and then elaborate on the functional interactions between signaling pathways initiating from G-protein-coupled receptors (GPCRs) and RTKs in regulation of cell proliferation (see Fig. 1). Finally, the mechanisms for controlling the specificity of signaling pathways will be discussed.

II. RTKS AND MAPK PATHWAY

Members of one large family of cell surface receptors with intrinsic protein tyrosine kinase (PTK) activity, the receptor tyrosine kinases, catalyze the transfer of the γ phosphate of ATP to hydroxyl groups of tyrosines on target proteins. All receptor tyrosine kinases contain an extracellular ligand-binding domain that is usually glycosylated. The ligand-binding domain is connected to the cytoplasmic domain by a single transmembrane helix. The cytoplasmic domain contains a conserved PTK core and additional regulatory sequences that are subjected to autophosphorylation and phosphorylation by heterologous protein kinases. The initial search for candidate molecules mediating the mitogenic effects of growth factors such as epidermal growth factor (EGF) and platelet-derived growth factor (PDGF), which stimulate RTKs, led to the identification of the tyrosine-phosphorylated proteins of 42 and 44 kDa, which are referred to as MAPK1/2 (mitogen-activated protein kinase 1/2) or ERK1/2 (extracellular signal-regulated kinase 1/2). MAPKs are believed to be central components of proliferative pathways. Their enzymatic activity increases in response to mitogenic stimulation. Inhibition of their function prevents cell proliferation in response to many growth factors, whereas constitutive activation of molecules acting upstream of MAPKs often induces tumorigenesis.

The general mechanisms for the activation of MAPKs by growth factor receptors of the tyrosine kinase class were established during the past decade. Binding of EGF to its cognate receptors leads to the tyrosine phosphorylation of several substrates including the EGF receptor (EGFR) itself. Such phosphorylation sites serve as docking sites for the binding of adapter proteins that contain structural motifs involved in protein–protein interactions.

Adapter protein Grb2 (growth factor receptor-binding protein 2), which possesses a Src homology 2 (SH2) domain and two SH3 domains, forms a complex with guanine nucleotide exchange factor for Ras and Sos (son of sevenless), via its SH3 domains. The Grb2/Sos complex is recruited to an activated RTK through binding of the Grb2 SH2 domain to specific phosphotyrosine sites of the receptor, thus translocating Sos to the plasma membrane where it is close to Ras and can stimulate the exchange of GTP for GDP. The PH

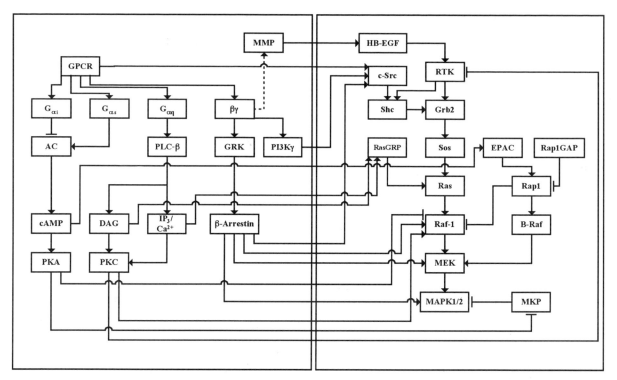

FIGURE 1 Regulation of the RTK–MAPK cascade by GPCR signaling pathways. In the right box are the components and related regulators of the RTK–MAPK cascade, and in the left box are the effectors and components of GPCR and heterotrimeric G-proteins. Within the signaling circuits, lines with arrows represent stimulation and lines with vertical bars at the end represent inhibition. Dotted lines indicate indirect regulation or regulation by unknown mechanisms. GPCR, G-protein-coupled receptor; MMP, matrix metalloproteinase; AC, adenylyl cyclase; PLC-β, phopholipase C-β; GRK, G-protein-coupled receptor kinase; PI3Kγ, phosphatidylinositol 3-kinase γ; DAG, diacylglycerol; IP₃, inositol 1,4,5-trisphosphate; PKA, protein kinase A; PKC, protein kinase C; HB-EGF, heparin-binding epidermal growth factor; RTK, receptor tyrosine kinase; Shc, Src homology and collagen; Grb2, growth factor receptor-binding protein 2; RasGRP, guanyl nucleotide-releasing protein for Ras; Sos, son of sevenless; EPAC, exchange protein directly activated by cAMP; MAPK, mitogen-activated protein kinase; MEK, MAPK kinase/ERK kinase; MKP, MAPK phosphatase.

(pleckstrin homology) domain of Sos is also essential for membrane translocation and for complete activation of Ras.

Membrane recruitment of Sos can be also accomplished by binding of Grb2/Sos to Shc (Src homology and collagen), another adapter protein that possesses a phosphotyrosine-binding (PTB) domain, a SH2 domain, and a SH3 domain. Shc forms a complex with many receptors through its PTB domain. Shc is a substrate for the RTKs and, on tyrosine phosphorylation, binds to the SH2 domain of Grb2.

Alternatively, Grb2/Sos complexes can be recruited to the cell membrane by binding to membrane-linked docking proteins, such as insulin receptor substrate 1 or fibroblast growth factor (FGF) receptor substrate 2, which become tyrosine phosphorylated in response to activation of certain RTKs.

Once in the active GTP-bound state, Ras stimulates MAP kinase kinase kinases (MAPKKKs) Rafs, which include Raf-1, A-Raf, and B-Raf. Activated Raf stimulates MAPK kinase (MAPKK), which is also called MEK (MAPK kinase/ERK kinase), by phosphorylating a key Ser residue in the activation loop. MEK then phosphorylates MAPK on Thr and Tyr residues at the activation loop, leading to its activation. Activated MAPKs phosphorylate and regulate the activity of key enzymes and nuclear proteins, which can ultimately regulate the expression of genes essential for cell proliferation.

III. G-PROTEIN-COUPLED RECEPTORS AND CELL PROLIFERATION

GPCRs are involved in diverse important biological activities, from cellular functions (cell proliferation, cell transformation, cell differentiation, endocytosis, exocytosis, neurotransmission, chemotaxis, etc.), to physiological functions (photo- and chemoreception, secretion from endocrine and exocrine glands, blood pressure control, etc.), to morphogenesis (embryogenesis, angiogenesis, tissue regeneration, etc.).

The proliferative effect of GPCRs was recognized by the initial finding that the serotonin and muscarinic acetylcholine receptors can trigger the transformation of fibroblast cells. It also has been shown that DNA viruses encoding functional GPCRs, including human cytomegalovirus, Herpesvirus saimiri, and Kaposi's sarcoma-associated herpes virus, can contribute to malignant transformation and ultimately to human cancer due to their persistent activity. The ability of GPCRs to affect cell growth was further confirmed by the identification of the naturally occurring activated mutants of G_α in various cancers. The activated mutants $G_{\alpha s}$, $G_{\alpha i2}$, and $G_{\alpha 12}$ are referred to as the *gsp*, *gip2*, and *gep* oncogenes, respectively.

The signaling pathways mediating the proliferative effects of GPCRs and heterotrimeric G-proteins are still under intensive study. The RTK–MAPK pathway appears to play an essential role in cell proliferation. The emerging picture is that GPCRs achieve their mitogenic effect through the regulation of the RTK–MAPK pathway at different levels by multiple mechanisms.

IV. HETEROTRIMERIC G-PROTEINS AND THEIR SECOND MESSENGER-GENERATING SYSTEMS

Approximately 20 mammalian G-protein α-subunits have been identified. Based on their primary sequence similarity, they are divided into four families: G_s, G_i, G_q, and G_{12}. These G-protein α-subunits regulate the activity of several second-messenger-generating systems. The members of the G_q family control the activity of phosphatidylinositol-specific phospholipases, such as phospholipase C-β, which hydrolyzes phosphatidylinositol 4,5-bisphosphate (to generate two second messengers, inositol 1,4,5-trisphosphate (IP_3) and diacylglycerol (DAG). IP_3 and DAG in turn lead to an increase in the intracellular concentrations of free calcium $[Ca^{2+}]_i$ and the activation of a number of protein kinases, including protein kinase C (PKC). The members of the G_s family activate adenylyl cyclases, whereas G_i family members can inhibit a subset of these enzymes, thereby controlling the intracellular concentrations of cyclic AMP (cAMP).

cAMP can further activate protein kinase A (PKA) and the recently identified guanine nucleotide exchange factor for small GTPase Rap1, EPAC (exchange protein directly activated by cAMP). G_α subunits of the G_i family, which includes $G_{\alpha i1}$, $G_{\alpha i2}$, $G_{\alpha i3}$, $G_{\alpha o}$, transducin ($G_{\alpha t}$), and gustducin ($G_{\alpha gust}$), also activate a variety of phospholipases and phosphodiesterases and promote the opening of several ion channels. The members of the $G_{\alpha 12}$ family stimulate small GTPase Rho through Rho guanine nucleotide exchange factors (RhoGEF), which include p115-RhoGEF, PDZ-RhoGEF, and leukemia-associated RhoGEF.

Thus far, 6 G-protein β-subunits and 12 G-protein γ-subunits have been cloned. On GPCR activation, dimers are released from the heterotrimeric complex and regulate the activity of many signaling molecules, including ion channels, phosphatidylinositol 3-kinases (PI3Ks), phospholipases, adenylyl cyclases, and receptor kinases. Distinct pools of $G_{\beta\gamma}$ subunits may play different roles in signal transmission.

V. SIGNALING BY GPCRs TO MAPK PATHWAY THROUGH SECOND MESSENGERS

A. PKA

In NIH 3T3 cells, activated $G_{\alpha s}$ and 8-Br-cAMP inhibit H-Ras-stimulated DNA synthesis and MAPK activity. Phosphorylation of Raf-1 at multiple serine residues by PKA on cAMP activation reduces the affinity of Raf for Ras and thus decreases Raf kinase activity. Also, PKA-mediated phosphorylation of a negative regulatory phosphatase of MAPKs is required for agonist-induced activation of MAPKs in T cells.

B. PKC

Activation of PKC by G-protein-coupled receptors results in EGFR phosphorylation on multiple Ser and Thr residues, including Thr-654 in the juxtamembrane domain of EGFR. PKC-induced phosphorylation of EGFR results in an inhibition of its PTK activity and in strong inhibition of EGF binding to the extracellular ligand-binding domain. PKC-mediated phosphorylation of the juxtamembrane domain of EGFR thus appears to provide a negative feedback mechanism for the control of receptor activity. Moreover, PKC can phosphorylate and activate Raf-1 and thus stimulate MAPK activity. Thus, PKC can have different effects in connecting the GPCR to RTK pathways, depending on its sites of action.

C. RasGRP

In addition to the catalytic domain, RasGRP, a guanyl nucleotide-releasing protein for Ras, consists of an atypical pair of "EF hands" that bind calcium and a DAG-binding domain. RasGRP activates Ras and causes transformation in fibroblasts. ERK1 and ERK2 are activated in rat2 cells expressing RasGRP in response to increases in membrane DAG and free cytoplasmic calcium induced by GPCR agonist endothelin-1. Sustained ligand-induced signaling and membrane partitioning of RasGRP are absent when the DAG-binding domain is deleted. RasGRP is expressed in the nervous system, where it may couple changes in DAG and possibly calcium concentrations to Ras activation.

D. Rap1 and EPAC

1. Control of the MAPK Pathway by Rap1

Ras-related protein Rap1 was identified in a screen for proteins that can suppress the transformed phenotype of fibroblasts oncogenically transformed by one of the mutated Ras genes, K-ras. Rap1 can interact with members of the Raf subfamily, Raf-1 and B-Raf. Its effect on the MAPK pathway depends on the interaction partners.

2. Inhibition of Raf-1 by Rap1

Rap1 binds to the serine/threonine kinase Raf-1 *in vitro*, through an interaction with both the Ras-binding domain and the adjacent cysteine-rich region of Rap1 and, in addition, the two proteins co-immunoprecipitate. It has been proposed that Rap1 inhibits Ras/ERK signaling by trapping Raf-1 in an inactive complex.

3. Activation of B-Raf by Rap1

In some cell types, Rap1 is implicated in the activation of the MAPK pathway. The mechanism may be that Rap1 binds to and activates the Raf family member B-Raf. The evidence for this interaction includes the direct binding of Rap1 to, and activation of, B-Raf *in vitro* and the fact that inhibitors of Rap1, such as Rap1 GTPase-activating protein (Rap1GAP) and Rap1N17, abolish the activation of the B-Raf–MAPK pathway. The different effect of Rap1 on B-Raf (activating) and Raf-1 (inactivating) is thought to reside in the interaction of Rap1 with the cysteine-rich region of the two kinases, as swapping the two domains reverses the effect of Rap1 on the two proteins.

4. EPAC

Rap1 is activated in response to a range of stimuli through a number of second-messenger molecules, including cAMP, Ca^{2+}, and diacylglycerol. PKA is activated by cAMP. However, by using inhibitors and mutants, it was found that PKA is not involved in the cAMP-induced activation of Rap1. Indeed, although PKA phosphorylates Rap1 near its carboxy-terminus, this phosphorylation is not required for cAMP-dependent activation. The search of sequence databases for possible Rap1 GEFs that might be directly regulated by cAMP led to the discovery of EPAC. In addition to containing homologies to other GEFs for Ras-like proteins, EPAC possesses sequences related to the regulatory subunit of PKA. EPAC is activated both *in vitro* and *in vivo* by direct binding of cAMP. Also, EPAC mutant with deletion of the cAMP-binding domain activates Rap1 *in vitro*. This indicates that the cAMP-binding domain normally inhibits the exchange activity of EPAC until cAMP binds, most likely causing a conformational change that relieves the inhibition.

VI. SIGNALING BY GPCRs TO MAPK PATHWAY THROUGH OTHER HETEROTRIMERIC G-PROTEIN EFFECTORS

A. RTK

RTK can be transactivated through an extracellular pathway on GPCR stimulation. It has been shown that a chimeric RTK consisting of the EGFR ectodomain and the transmembrane and intracellular portion of the PDGF receptor (PDGFR) is transactivated by treatment of Rat1 fibroblasts with GPCR ligands but endogenous PDGFR is not. Hence, GPCR-induced transactivation of the artificial RTK does not involve an intracellular pathway and is dependent on the extracellular ligand-binding domain of the EGFR. In the presence of diphtheria toxin mutant CRM197 that specifically blocks heparin-binding EGF (HB-EGF) function or the matrix metalloprotease inhibitor batimastat (BB94), lysophosphatidic acid (LPA)-, carbachol-, or tetradecanoyl-phorbol-13-acetate (TPA)-induced transactivation of the EGFR and tyrosine phosphorylation of SHC are completely abrogated in COS-7 and HEK 293 cells. Flow cytometric analysis directly confirms cell surface ectodomain shedding of proHB-EGF on treatment with GPCR agonists or TPA. Therefore, it has been proposed that activation of heterotrimeric G-proteins by agonist-occupied GPCR induces the extracellular activity of a transmembrane metalloproteinase, which leads to the extracellular processing of a transmembrane growth factor precursor and release of the mature factor, and consequently stimulates RTKs and MAPKs.

B. PI3Kγ

Overexpression of PI3Kγ in COS-7 cells activates MAPK in a $G_{\beta\gamma}$-dependent fashion. Wortmannin, an inhibitor of PI3Ks, or expression of a catalytically inactive mutant of PI3Kγ abolishes the stimulation of MAPK by $G_{\beta\gamma}$ or in response to stimulation of M2 muscarinic G-protein-coupled receptors.

Expression of a mutant Sos protein lacking the domain involved in Ras-specific guanine nucleotide exchange activity, a dominant negative mutant N17-Ras, or a dominant negative mutant of Raf-1 inhibits MAPK stimulation by PI3Kγ without affecting MAPK stimulation by the activated form of MEK. Therefore, signaling from G-protein-dependent receptors, $G_{\beta\gamma}$, and PI3Kγ to the MAPK pathway occurs upstream of Sos. Expression of PI3Kγ in COS-7 cells stimulates tyrosine phosphorylation of Shc and enhances the association of Shc with Grb2, whereas a mutant of Shc lacking the tyrosine phosphorylation site, Y317F, suppresses the stimulation of MAPK induced by LPA, the expression of $G_{\beta\gamma}$ and carbachol in m2-transfected cells, the expression of PI3Kγ, or the expression of the Src-related tyrosine kinase Fyn. The nonspecific tyrosine kinase inhibitor genistein or the Src-like specific inhibitor PP1 potently blocks MAPK activation by PI3Kγ. Thus, stimulation of MAPK by PI3Kγ requires a tyrosine kinase that, in turn, phosphorylates Shc and induces its association with Grb2. Therefore, receptors coupled to heterotrimeric G-proteins can stimulate the MAPK pathway through $G_{\beta\gamma}$ subunits, PI3Kγ, a tyrosine kinase, and Shc.

VII. SIGNALING BY HEPTAHELICAL RECEPTORS TO MAPK PATHWAY THROUGH HETEROTRIMERIC G-PROTEIN-INDEPENDENT PATHWAYS

A. β-Arrestin-Mediated Recruitment of Src Kinase and Activation of MAPK Pathway

Stimulation of β_2 adrenergic receptors (β_2ARs) results in the dissociation of heterotrimeric G-proteins into $G_{\alpha s}$-GTP and $G_{\beta\gamma}$ subunits. The release of $G_{\beta\gamma}$ facilitates GRK (G-protein-coupled receptor kinase)-mediated phosphorylation of the agonist-occupied receptor. β-Arrestin-1 functions as an adapter, binding to both GRK-phosphorylated receptor and c-Src.

β-Arrestin-1 mutants, disrupted either in c-Src binding or in the ability to target receptors to clathrin-coated pits, block β_2AR-mediated activation of the MAP kinases Erk1 and Erk2. β-Arrestin-1 binding, which terminates receptor–G-protein coupling, can initiate a second wave of signal transduction in which the "desensitized" receptor functions as a critical structural component of a mitogenic signaling complex.

In HEK-293 cells expressing angiotensin II type 1a receptors (AT1aR), angiotensin stimulation triggers β-arrestin-2 binding to the receptor and internalization of AT1aR-β–arrestin complexes. Within these complexes, β-arrestin-2 acts as a scaffold to assemble component kinases of the MAPK cascade, Raf-1, MEK1, and ERK2.

B. c-Src

The β_3AR can directly recruit c-Src. Unlike the other GPCRs, the β_3AR is not phosphorylated by G-protein receptor kinases and thus does not bind to β-arrestin and undergo internalization. Interestingly, β_3AR contains proline-rich sequences in both the third intracellular loop and the carboxyl-tail, which appear to mediate the interaction with the SH3 domain of c-Src and activate the MAPK cascade. Disruption of these proline-rich sequences abolishes the ability of the receptor to bind c-Src and to stimulate the MAPK pathway without affecting the signaling by the heterotrimeric G-proteins.

VIII. MECHANISMS FOR CONTROLLING THE SPECIFICITY OF SIGNALING PATHWAYS

It is apparent that signaling pathways are intertwined with one another to form a large network that is subjected to stimulatory and inhibitory inputs. Such complexity is essential for mediating the pleiotropic biological processes in response to the myriad of extracellular cues. However, it also poses an enormous challenge for the cell to maintain the specificity of the signaling pathways. Several mechanisms have been proposed for the control of specificity in cell signaling.

A. Cell-Specific Profiling of Signaling Components

As more and more signaling pathways and downstream effectors have been identified, each receptor may activate many potential pathways and effectors. However, the biological outcome of signals generated at the cell surface in response to receptor stimulation is strongly dependent on the developmental stages and cell types. For instance, in early development, FGFR1 plays an important role in the control of cell migration, a process that is crucial for mesodermal patterning and gastrulation, whereas stimulation of FGFR1 in fibroblasts leads to cell proliferation. Moreover, activation of a given membrane receptor by a specific ligand transduces a unique biological response, even though these pathways utilize a common repertoire of proteins. PDGF and EGF, for instance, stimulate unique biological responses in their target tissues, although the intracellular signaling pathways that are activated by PDGF and EGF are very similar indeed.

In addition, activation of the same signaling molecules in different cells leads to distinct responses. For example, stimulation of PI3K by insulin in muscle cells results in the enhancement of metabolic processes, whereas stimulation of PI3K by nerve growth factor (NGF) in neuronal cells leads to an anti-apoptotic signal. Similarly, when cAMP increases on GPCR activation, the MAPK pathway is stimulated in neuronal PC12 cells but inhibited in fibroblast NIH 3T3 cells.

The most plausible explanation for these observations is that there is cell type- and stage-specific expression of signaling components, such as effector proteins and transcription factors, in different cell types and at different developmental stages. Therefore, a similar input can lead to a different output in a different cellular context.

B. Combinatorial Control

Signal specificity can be defined in part by a combinatorial recruitment during signaling processes. For instance, even though every RTK contains a core PTK, there exist some other regulatory elements that recruit and activate a unique set of signaling proteins via their own tyrosine autophosphorylation sites and by means of the tyrosine phosphorylation sites on closely associated docking proteins. The combinatorial recruitment of a particular complement of signaling proteins from a common preexisting pool of signaling cassettes is one mechanism for control of signal specificity. This process is further regulated by differential recruitment of stimulatory and inhibitory proteins by the different receptors and downstream effector proteins, leading to fine-tuning of cellular responses.

C. Scaffold Proteins

It has been shown that scaffolding proteins that bind simultaneously to several proteins are able to insulate common components of signaling pathways from closely related signaling cascades. In yeast, Sterile 11 (Ste11) is shared by two signaling pathways and functions as the MAPKKK. The scaffolding protein Ste5 has been shown to interact with a pheromone-activated G-protein and with components of the MAP kinase cascade. Ste5 forms a complex with Ste11, Ste7, and Fus3, leading to insulation of the pheromone-induced MAP kinase cascade from the closely related osmolarity response pathway, in which MAPKK Pbs2 acts as both the scaffolding protein and the intermediate kinase that relays signal from MAPKKK Ste11 to downstream MAP kinase Hog1.

Of note, the output of signaling cascades through scaffold protein is determined by a balance of all components. Too much or too little of any component in the scaffolded complexes may decrease the output of the pathway. Therefore, a scaffolded pathway is in principle more sensitive to fluctuations in the concentrations of pathway components, even though scaffolds have the advantage of facilitating efficient signaling with specificity.

D. Cellular Compartmentalization

In recent years, it has become apparent that the cellular localization of signaling components involved in cell signaling has a profound impact on their biological activity. As mentioned above, AT1aR activation can lead to $G_{\beta\gamma}$ release, which facilitates GRK-mediated phosphorylation of the receptor. The phosphorylated residues on the receptor function as docking sites for β-arrestin translocation from the cytoplasm; the β-arrestin further acts as a scaffolding protein for the assembly of c-Src, Raf-1, MEK1, and ERK2. For RTK signaling, many of the targets of RTKs are located at the cell membrane, and membrane translocation is required for activation of many cellular processes. Binding of SH2, PTB, or SH3 domains to activated receptors or to membrane-linked docking proteins leads to membrane translocation. In addition, membrane translocation is regulated in part by PH or FYVE domains, two protein modules that bind to different phosphoinositides.

The translocation of activated ERK1/2 proteinss from the cytoplasm into the nucleus is another example of the role of protein localization in cell signaling.

E. Signal Duration and Amplitude

Signal duration and signal strength are essential determinants of signal transmission and biological responses. For instance, RTKs that induce transient stimulation of MAPK (e.g., EGFR) stimulate PC12 cell proliferation, whereas RTKs that stimulate a sustained and robust MAPK response (e.g., NGF receptor, FGFR) promote neuronal differentiation of the same cells. Alternatively, overexpression of EGFR in PC12 cells leads to sustained MAPK response, resulting in cell differentiation, although the same receptors give a proliferative response when expressed at lower levels. These experiments show that the biological outcome (proliferation versus differentiation) is determined by the integrative amplitude of various inputs over time. Signal threshold can be determined by the specific activity of a given RTK and by the balanced action of the various inhibitory or stimulatory signals that are regulated by other pathways. For example, the signal generated by an RTK can be prolonged by increasing the intracellular cAMP level that enhances B-Raf activity by activation of Rap1. Signaling pathways are also subjected to multiple negative feedback mechanisms at the level of the receptor itself by inhibitory protein tyrosine phosphatases and by receptor endocytosis and degradation. In addition, the specific activity of key effector proteins can be negatively regulated by inhibitory signals. The balance between the various stimulatory and inhibitory responses will ultimately determine the strength and duration of the signals that are transmitted through the networks of signaling cascades following their initiation at the cell surface in response to receptor stimulation.

IX. SUMMARY

It is very common for signaling pathways activated from membrane receptors to be interconnected with one another via complicated intracellular protein networks. As an example, the proliferative response generally controlled by the RTK–MAPK pathway can be regulated by GPCR signaling pathways at multiple levels by different mechanisms. The frequently applied tool of targeted gene disruption used by geneticists for analyzing signaling pathways is complicated by the existence of redundant signaling pathways and multi-tasking components shared by multiple signaling cascades. Consequently, more sophisticated tools should be developed and applied for the analysis of cellular signaling pathways. To understand the control of the specificity among signaling networks, there is a need for new techniques for determination of protein localization and measurement of kinetics of cellular signaling events in the context of living cells and even in the live animal. In addition, detailed analyses of gene expression patterns by microarray analysis of genes that are expressed in response to growth factor stimulation of cells derived from normal or pathological tissues will reveal new links between signaling pathways. Finally, for the future study of cellular signaling networks, the modern biochemists, geneticists, and transductionists will benefit from the adoption of approaches that have been developed by engineers to describe complicated networks.

Glossary

G-protein-coupled receptor Seven-transmembrane protein that is usually (but not always) coupled to heterotrimeric G-proteins to achieve its biological functions.

mitogen-activated protein kinase (MAPK) cascade MAPKs constitute a family of kinases that are activated by phosphorylation in response to extracellular stimuli. MEKs, the kinases that phoshorylate MAPKs, are themselves regulated by phosphorylation. Such sequential chains of kinase phosphorylation and activation are called kinase cascades.

receptor tyrosine kinase Transmembrane receptor with a single membrane-spanning region that possesses intrinsic protein tyrosine kinase activity in its cytoplasmic domain and ligand-binding ability in its extracellular domain.

scaffold protein A protein capable of binding to multiple signaling components, thereby providing a platform to relay signals and achieve specificity of communication among components.

See Also the Following Articles

Activating and Inactivating Receptor Mutations ● Co-activators and Corepressors for the Nuclear Receptor Superfamily ● GPCR (G-Protein-Coupled Receptor) Structure ● Heterotrimeric G-Proteins ● Membrane Receptor Signaling in Health and Disease ● Membrane Steroid Receptors ● Receptor–Receptor Interactions ● Steroid Receptor Crosstalk with Cellular Signaling Pathways

Further Reading

Blume-Jensen, P., and Hunter, T. (2001). Oncogenic kinase signalling. *Nature* **411**(6835), 355–365.

Bos, J. L., de Rooij, J., and Reedquist, K. A. (2001). Rap1 signalling: Adhering to new models. *Nat. Rev. Mol. Cell. Biol.* **2**(5), 369–377.

Ferrell, J. E., Jr (2000). What do scaffold proteins really do? *Science* (52), E1. Available at http://www.stke.org/cgi/content/full/OC_sigtrans;2000/52/pe1.

Gschwind, A., Zwick, E., Prenzel, N., Leserer, M., and Ullrich, A. (2001). Cell communication networks: Epidermal growth factor receptor transactivation as the paradigm for interreceptor signal transmission. *Oncogene* **20**(13), 1594–1600.

Jordan, J. D., Landau, E. M., and Iyengar, R. (2000). Signaling networks: The origins of cellular multitasking. *Cell* **103**(2), 193–200.

Marinissen, M. J., and Gutkind, J. S. (2001). G-protein-coupled receptors and signaling networks: Emerging paradigms. *Trends Pharmacol. Sci.* **22**(7), 368–376.

Miller, W. E., and Lefkowitz, R. J. (2001). Expanding roles for β-arrestins as scaffolds and adapters in GPCR signaling and trafficking. *Curr. Opin. Cell. Biol.* **13**(2), 139–145.

Schlessinger, J. (2000). Cell signaling by receptor tyrosine kinases. *Cell* **103**(2), 211–225.

Smith, F. D., and Scott, J. D. (2002). Signaling complexes: Junctions on the intracellular information super highway. *Curr. Biol.* **12**(1), R32–R40.

Somatostatin

MALCOLM J. LOW

Oregon Health and Science University

I. INTRODUCTION
II. EVOLUTION OF THE SOMATOSTATIN GENE FAMILY
III. SOMATOSTATIN GENE ORGANIZATION AND REGULATION
IV. SOMATOSTATIN RECEPTORS
V. REGULATION OF HORMONE SECRETION BY SOMATOSTATIN
VI. EXTRAHYPOTHALAMIC SOMATOSTATIN AND BRAIN FUNCTION
VII. DIAGNOSTIC AND THERAPEUTIC USES OF SOMATOSTATIN
VIII. SUMMARY

Somatostatins are cyclic neuropeptides that exert a broad array of inhibitory and modulatory activities in the endocrine, gastrointestinal, nervous, and immune systems. The archetypal somatostatin, somatotropin release-inhibiting factor, inhibits secretion of pituitary growth hormone. It interacts with five known somatostatin subtypes. The recent development of small-molecule receptor-subtype-specific ligands and new genetic models of somatostatin peptide and receptor mutations promises to provide more definitive answers to the unresolved questions of somatostatin function in extrahypothalamic brain tissue.

I. INTRODUCTION

A peptide that potently inhibited growth hormone (GH) release from cultured pituitary cells was unexpectedly identified during the early efforts to isolate a GH-releasing factor from hypothalamic extracts. The factor responsible for both this inhibition of GH secretion and the inhibition of insulin secretion by a pancreatic islet extract was eventually purified from porcine hypothalamus and its amino acid sequence determined by Brazeau and colleagues in 1973. This cyclic peptide containing 14 amino acids was named somatostatin (SS14). Subsequently, a second N-terminal extended form, SS28, was identified as a secretory product from various tissues. Both forms of mammalian somatostatin are derived posttranslationally from a common prohormone by the action of specific prohormone convertases. In addition, the isolation of SS28(1–12) in some tissues suggests that SS14 can also be secondarily processed from SS28. SS14 is the predominant form of somatostatin produced in the brain (including the hypothalamus) and most other tissues, whereas SS28 is found in highest concentrations in the gastrointestinal tract, especially the small intestine.

The biological activities of somatostatin are much wider than the inhibition of GH secretion for which it was named. Somatostatin also inhibits thyrotropin secretion from the pituitary and has nonpituitary roles, including neurotransmitter or neuromodulator activity in the central and peripheral nervous systems and regulatory functions in the gut and pancreas. As a pituitary regulator, somatostatin is a true neurohormone, i.e., a neuronal secretory product that enters the blood (hypophyseal–portal circulation) to affect cell function at remote sites. In the gut, somatostatin is present in both the myenteric plexus (where it acts as a neurotransmitter) and in epithelial cells, where it influences the function of adjacent cells by a paracrine mechanism. Somatostatin can influence its own secretion from pancreatic delta cells (an autocrine function) in addition to acting as a paracrine factor on other endocrine cell types in pancreatic islets. Gut exocrine secretion can be modulated by intralumenal action, so somatostatin can also be considered to be a lumone. Because of its wide distribution, broad spectrum of regulatory effects, and evolutionary history, this peptide can be regarded as an archetypal gut–brain peptide.

II. EVOLUTION OF THE SOMATOSTATIN GENE FAMILY

The genes that encode somatostatin in humans and a number of other species exhibit striking sequence homology, even in primitive jawless fish (Fig. 1).

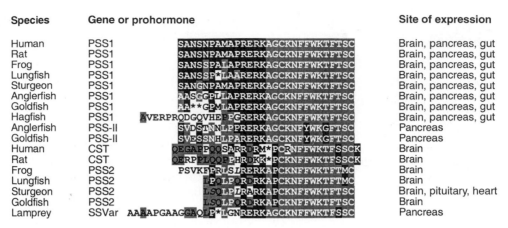

FIGURE 1 Amino acid sequence comparisons of somatostatin-like peptides in species of different vertebrate taxa. The conserved mammalian sequence of SS28 derived from prosomatostatin 1 (PSS1) is shown for humans and rats. The cyclic SS14 peptide (gray shading) at the C-terminus of SS28 has been conserved in all vertebrate PSS1 genes. Teleost fish have a second gene encoding PSS-II that is proteolytically processed to a SS28-like peptide characterized by the C-terminal sequence of [Tyr^7, Gly^{10}]SS14. A mammalian cortistatin (CST) gene encodes either human CST17 (DRMPCRNFFWKTFSSCK) or rat CST14 (PCKNFFWKTFSSCK), both of which have 11 amino acid homologies with SS14. Frog, lungfish, sturgeon, and goldfish have a PSS2 gene that may be the orthologue of mammalian CST. Lampreys (*Lampetra fluviatilis*) produce a variant of SS14 (SSVar) containing the [Ser^{12}] but not the [Pro^2] substitutions present in CST. Amino acid identity among sequences is indicated by the different combinations of font shading. An asterisk (*) has been inserted in some sequences to maximize alignment.

Furthermore, the amino acid sequence of SS14 is identical in all vertebrates. Until recently, it was accepted that all tetrapods have a single gene encoding both SS14 and SS28 whereas teleost fish have two nonallelic prosomatostatin genes (PSS1 and PSS-II), each of which encodes only one form of the mature somatostatin peptides. Comparative endocrinologists have inferred that a common ancestral gene underwent a gene duplication event after the split of teleosts from the ancestors of tetrapods.

However, both lampreys and amphibians, which pre- and postdate the teleost evolutionary divergence, respectively, have now been shown to contain at least two distinct PSS genes. A more distantly related gene identified in mammals encodes cortistatin (CST), a somatostatin-like peptide that is highly expressed in cortex and hippocampus. Rat CST14 differs from SS14 by three amino acid residues but has high affinity for all known subtypes of somatostatin receptors (see later). The human gene sequence predicts a tripeptide-extended CST17 and a further N-terminally extended CST29 (Fig. 1). A revised evolutionary concept of the somatostatin gene family is that a primordial gene underwent duplication during or before the advent of chordates and the two resulting genes subsequently underwent differing rates of mutation to produce the distinct prosomatostatin and procortistatin genes in mammals.

A second gene duplication likely occurred in teleosts to generate PSS1 and PSS-II from the ancestral somatostatin gene.

III. SOMATOSTATIN GENE ORGANIZATION AND REGULATION

The mammalian gene has a relatively simple organization consisting of two coding exons separated by one intron (Fig. 2). A single promoter directs transcription of the PSS1 gene in all tissues and there are no known alternative mRNA splicing events. Apart from its expression in neurons of the periventricular and arcuate hypothalamic nuclei and involvement in GH secretion, somatostatin is highly expressed in the cortex, lateral septum, extended amygdala, reticular nucleus of the thalamus, hippocampus, and many brain stem nuclei in human and rat brain tissue. Cortistatin, present in the brain at a small fraction of the levels of somatostatin and in a more limited distribution, is primarily confined to the cortex and hippocampus.

The molecular mechanisms underlying the developmental and hormonal regulation of somatostatin gene transcription have been most extensively studied in pancreatic islets and islet-derived cell lines. Less is known concerning the regulation of somatostatin

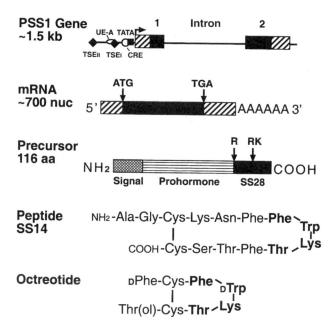

FIGURE 2 Summary of somatostatin biosynthesis in mammals. Structures of the mammalian PSS1 gene, mRNA, precursor protein, mature SS14 peptide, and the synthetic SSTR agonist octreotide are presented schematically. The promoter elements in the PSS1 gene (TSE, UE-A, CRE, and TATA) are discussed in the text. The 5' and 3' untranslated regions of exons 1 and 2 and within the corresponding polyadenylated mRNA are indicated by diagonal stripes. ATG, Translation initiation codon; TGA, translation stop codon; R, arginine; K, lysine.

gene expression in neurons, except that activation is strongly controlled by binding of the phosphorylated transcription factor cyclic adenosine monophosphate (cAMP) response element binding protein (CREB) to its cognate CRE contained in the promoter immediately 5' to a consensus TATA sequence. Experiments performed in transgenic mice suggest that accurate neural-specific somatostatin gene expression requires distal genomic elements in addition to the proximal 300 nucleotides that are sufficient for islet cell expression. The proximal enhancer elements in the somatostatin gene promoter that bind complexes of homeodomain-containing transcription factors (PAX6, PBX, and PREP1) and up-regulate transcription in pancreatic islets may actually represent gene silencer elements in neurons (promoter elements TSE$_{II}$ and UE-A). Conversely, another related cis-element in the somatostatin gene (promoter element TSE$_I$) apparently binds a homeodomain transcription factor PDX1 (also called STF1/IDX1/IPF1) that is common to developing brain, pancreas, and foregut

and regulates gene expression in both the central nervous system (CNS) and gut.

Similar to other genes encoding polypeptide precursors, the posttranslational intracellular trafficking and processing of PSS represent additional control points in the expression of somatostatin (Fig. 2). A peptide motif assuming an amphipathic α-helical conformation near the N-terminus of PSS appears to play an essential role in targeting the prohormone through the endoplasmic reticulum and Golgi compartments that constitute part of the regulated secretory pathway. A second highly conserved amino acid motif, NPAMAP (in single-letter code: N, asparagine; P, proline; A, alanine; M, methionine) within the SS28(1–12) sequence is important for directing the endoproteolytic processing of PSS1 to either SS28 at the 5' single basic amino acid (Arg) residue or to SS14 at the 3' paired basic amino acid (Arg-Lys) residues by appropriate prohormone convertases.

IV. SOMATOSTATIN RECEPTORS

Five somatostatin receptor subtypes (SSTR1–SSTR5) have been identified by gene cloning techniques, and one of these (SSTR2) is expressed in two alternatively spliced forms, SSTR2a and SSTR2b. The SSTRs are members of the rhodopsin-like G-protein-coupled receptor clan, and their unique amino acid signature is provided by a seven-element fingerprint of peptide sequences located in conserved regions of the N- and C-termini, extra- and intracellular loops, and transmembrane domains. They are most closely related to the vertebrate opioid receptors and the invertebrate allatostatin receptor family. The five SSTR subtypes are encoded by separate genes located on different chromosomes, are expressed in unique or partially overlapping distributions in multiple target organs, and differ in their coupling to second-messenger signaling molecules, and therefore in their range and mechanism of intracellular actions. The subtypes also differ in their binding affinity to specific somatostatinergic ligands. Some of these differences have important implications for the use of somatostatin analogues in diagnostic imaging and in pharmacotherapy.

All SSTR subtypes are coupled to pertussis-toxin-sensitive G-proteins and bind SS14 and SS28 with high affinity in the low-nanomolar range, although SS28 has a modestly higher affinity for SSTR5. SSTR1 and SSTR2 are the two most abundant subtypes in brain and probably function as both postsynaptic receptors and presynaptic autoreceptors in the hypothalamus and limbic forebrain, respectively. SSTR4 is most highly expressed in the hippocampus. SSTR3 is uniquely localized on nonmotile neuronal cilia, structures that have an unknown role in neuronal signaling. All the subtypes are expressed in the pituitary, but SSTR2 and SSTR5 are the most abundant receptors on somatotrophs. These two subtypes are also the most physiologically important in pancreatic islets. SSTR5 is responsible for inhibition of insulin secretion from beta cells and SSTR2 is essential for inhibition of glucagon from alpha cells (Table 1).

Binding of somatostatin to its receptors leads to activation of one or more inhibitory G-proteins (G_i/G_o), which in turn inhibit adenylyl cyclase activity and decrease the concentration of intracellular cAMP. Other G-protein-mediated actions common to all SSTRs are activation of a vanadate-sensitive phosphotyrosine phosphatase (PTP) and modulation of mitogen-activated protein kinases (MAPKs). MAPK activity has been reported to be increased by SSTR1 and SSTR4, decreased by SSTR2 and SSTR5, and modulated in both directions by SSTR3. Different subsets of SSTRs can activate inwardly rectifying K^+ channels and/or inhibit voltage-dependent Ca^{2+} channels. The net effects of SSTR coupling to these membrane conductances include hyperpolarization of the resting membrane potential, decreased frequency of action potentials, and decreased probability of vesicle release from nerve terminals. SSTR1 also activates a Na^+/H^+ exchanger and α-amino-3-hydroxy-5-methyl-4-isoxazole propionic acid (AMPA)/kainate glutamate receptors, whereas SSTR2 inhibits non-N-methyl-D-aspartate (NMDA) glutamate receptors in some cells. SSTR2 and SSTR4 have been reported to couple positively to phospho-

lipase C/inositol 1,4,5-trisphosphate and phospholipase A_2 activities, respectively.

The lowering of intracellular cAMP and Ca^{2+} are the most important mechanisms for the inhibition of hormone secretion from endocrine cells, whereas actions on PTP and MAPK are postulated to play a role in antiproliferative effects of somatostatin on tumor cells. Recent provocative data suggests that SSTRs may form oligomeric complexes, including in some cases heterodimers with non-SSTRs, greatly increasing the possible signaling complexity of somatostatin ligands.

V. REGULATION OF HORMONE SECRETION BY SOMATOSTATIN

A. Inhibition of GH Secretion and GH Negative Feedback

In the pituitary, somatostatin directly inhibits secretion of GH and thyrotropin and, under limited conditions, of prolactin and adrenocorticotropic hormone (ACTH), from their respective cell types. However, the full role of somatostatin in the regulation of GH secretion is much more complex and involves a constant interplay with hypothalamic growth hormone-releasing hormone (GHRH), circulating hormones, and additional modulatory peptides at the level of both the pituitary and the hypothalamus. The predominant hypothalamic influence on GH release is stimulatory, thus section of the pituitary stalk or lesions of the ventromedial hypothalamus cause reductions of basal and induced GH release. When the somatostatinergic component is inactivated (e.g., by antisomatostatin antibody injection in rats), basal GH levels and GH responses to the usual provocative stimuli are enhanced. Negative feedback

TABLE 1 Diverse Inhibitory Functions of Somatostatin on Nervous, Endocrine, Gastrointestinal, and Immune System Cell Secretion[a]

Organ	Cell type	Factor inhibited	SS receptor
Brain (hypothalamus)	SS neuron	Somatostatin	SSTR1
Brain (hypothalamus)	GHRH neuron	GHRH	SSTR2
Brain (hippocampus)	CA1 pyramidal	Glutamate	SSTR4
Pituitary gland	Somatotroph	Growth hormone	SSTR2, SSTR5
Pancreatic islet	β cell	Insulin	SSTR5
Pancreatic islet	α cell	Glucagon	SSTR2
Stomach	Parietal cell	HCl	SSTR2
Immune system	T lymphocyte	Interferon γ	SSTR2

[a]Abbreviations: SS, somatostatin; GHRH, growth hormone-releasing hormone; SSTR, somatostatin receptor.

control of GH release is mediated by GH and by insulin-like growth factor-I (IGF-I), which is synthesized in the liver under control of GH. Direct GH effects on the hypothalamus act by short-loop feedback, whereas those involving IGF-I and other circulating factors influenced by GH, including free fatty acids and glucose, are long-loop systems analogous to the pituitary–thyroid and pituitary–adrenal axes. Control of GH secretion thus includes two closed-loop systems (GH and IGF-I) and one open-loop regulatory system (neural) (Fig. 3).

Although most of the evidence for a direct role of GH in its own negative feedback has been derived from animals, an elegant study in normal men demonstrated that GH pretreatment blocks the subsequent GH secretory response to GHRH by a pathway that is dependent on somatostatin. The mechanism responsible for this GH feedback via the hypothalamus has been largely elucidated in rodent models. GH receptors are selectively expressed on somatostatin neurons in the hypothalamic periventricular nucleus and on neuropeptide Y (NPY) neurons in the arcuate nucleus. Expression of the

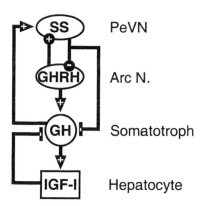

FIGURE 3 Regulatory feedback loops in the hypothalamic control of pituitary growth hormone secretion. Growth hormone-releasing hormone (GHRH) and somatostatin (SS) are the principal stimulatory and inhibitory factors mediating GH secretion. GH stimulates the synthesis and release of insulin-like growth factor-I (IGF-I) from hepatocytes, which inhibits GH secretion from the pituitary. GH also inhibits its own secretion by a short-loop feedback circuit involving the stimulation of somatostatin neurons in the periventricular nucleus (PeVN) of the hypothalamus. A common neural mechanism leading to the inhibition of GH secretion is the activation of somatostatin neurons. Stimulatory and inhibitory neuronal synapses are represented by circular terminals marked with a plus or minus sign, respectively. Stimulatory and inhibitory hormonal pathways are represented by arrows with a plus sign or bars with a minus sign, respectively. Arc N, Arcuate nucleus.

c-*fos* gene in both populations of GH receptor-positive neurons is acutely elevated by GH administration, indicating an activation of hypothalamic circuitry that includes these neurons. Data from many experiments strongly support a model of GH negative feedback regulation that involves the primary activation of periventricular somatostatin neurons by GH. These tuberoinfundibular neurons then inhibit GH secretion directly by release of somatostatin in the median eminence, but in addition they indirectly inhibit GH secretion by way of collateral axonal projections to the arcuate nucleus that synapse on and inhibit GHRH neurons (Fig. 3).

B. Neural Regulation of Tuberoinfundibular Somatostatin and GHRH

GHRH-containing nerve fibers that terminate adjacent to portal vessels in the external zone of the median eminence arise principally from within, above, and lateral to the infundibular nucleus in the human hypothalamus, corresponding primarily to the rodent arcuate nucleus. Perikarya of the tuberoinfundibular somatostatin neurons are located almost completely in the medial periventricular nucleus and parvocellular component of the anterior paraventricular nucleus. Neuroanatomical and functional evidence suggests a bidirectional synaptic interaction between the two peptidergic systems.

Multiple extrahypothalamic brain regions provide efferent connections to the hypothalamus and regulate GHRH and somatostatin neuronal activity. Somatosensory and affective information are integrated and filtered through the amygdaloid complex. The basolateral amygdala provides an excitatory input to the hypothalamus whereas the central extended amygdala, which includes the central and medial nuclei of the amygdala together with the bed nucleus of the stria terminalis, provides a γ-aminobutyric acid (GABA)ergic inhibitory input. Many intrinsic neurons of the hypothalamus also release GABA, often with a peptide cotransmitter. Excitatory cholinergic fibers arise to a small extent from forebrain projection nuclei, but mostly from hypothalamic cholinergic interneurons, which densely innervate the external zone of the median eminence. Similarly, the origin of dopaminergic and histaminergic neurons is local, with their cell bodies located in the hypothalamic arcuate and tuberomammillary bodies, respectively. Two important ascending pathways to the medial basal hypothalamus regulate GH secretion and they originate from serotonergic neurons in the raphe nuclei and adrenergic neurons in the nucleus of the tractus solitarius and ventral lateral nucleus of the medulla.

Both GHRH and somatostatin neurons express pre- and postsynaptic receptors for multiple neurotransmitters and peptides. The α2-adrenoreceptor agonist clonidine reliably stimulates GH release, and for this reason a clonidine test has been a standard diagnostic tool in pediatric endocrinology. The net stimulatory effect on GH secretion appears to involve a dual mechanism of action—inhibition of somatostatin neurons and activation of GHRH neurons—and is blocked by the specific α2 antagonist yohimbine. In addition, a partial attenuation of the effects of clonidine by 5-hydroxytryptamine (5-HT$_1$/5-HT$_2$) antagonists suggests that some of the relevant α2 receptors are located presynaptically on serotonergic nerve terminals and increase serotonin release. Both norepinephrine and epinephrine play physiological roles in the adrenergic stimulation of GH secretion. Adrenergic α1 agonists have no effect on GH secretion in humans but β2 agonists such as the bronchodilator salbutamol inhibit GH secretion by stimulating the release of somatostatin from nerve terminals in the median eminence. These effects are blocked by propranolol, a nonspecific β antagonist. Dopamine generally has a net effect of stimulating GH secretion, but the relative importance of different dopamine receptor subtypes and their localization on specific neuronal structures in the hypothalamus is not known.

The effect of serotonin (5-hydroxytryptamine) on GH release in humans has been difficult to decipher because of the large variety of 5-HT receptor subtypes. However, clinical studies with the receptor-selective agonist sumatriptan clearly implicate the 5-HT$_{1D}$ receptor subtype in the stimulation of basal GH levels. The drug also potentiates the effect of a maximal dose of GHRH, invoking in its mechanism of action the recurring theme of GH disinhibition by inhibition of hypothalamic somatostatin neurons. Histaminergic pathways acting through H1 receptors play only a minor, conditional stimulatory role in GH secretion in man.

Acetylcholine (ACh) appears to be an important physiological regulator of GH secretion. Blockade of muscarinic (m1) ACh receptors reduces or abolishes GH secretory responses to GHRH, glucagon, arginine, morphine, and exercise. In contrast, drugs that potentiate cholinergic transmission increase basal GH levels and enhance GH response to GHRH in normal individuals or in patients with obesity or Cushing's disease. *In vitro*, acetylcholine inhibits somatostatin release from hypothalamic fragments, and acetylcholine can act directly on the pituitary to inhibit GH release. There may even be a paracrine cholinergic control system within the pituitary. However, the sum of evidence suggests that the primary mechanism of action of m1 agonists is to inhibit somatostatin neuronal activity or the release of peptide from somatostatinergic terminals.

Many neuropeptides in addition to GHRH and somatostatin are involved in the modulation of somatotroph activity in the human. GH secretion is stimulated by galanin, opioid peptides, and ghrelin, the endogenous ligand for the growth hormone secretagogue receptor (GHS-R), each of which act at least in part by a GHRH-dependent mechanism. A larger number of neuropeptides are known or suspected to inhibit GH secretion in humans, at least under certain circumstances. The list includes NPY, corticotropin-releasing hormone (CRH), calcitonin, oxytocin, neurotensin, vasoactive intestinal peptide (VIP), and thyrotropin-releasing hormone (TRH). Inhibitory actions of NPY are well established in the rat. Its effect on GH secretion is secondary to stimulation of somatostatin neurons and is of particular interest because of the presumed role in GH autofeedback (discussed earlier) and the integration of GH secretion with regulation of energy intake and expenditure.

C. Somatostatin and GH Secretory Rhythms

GH secretion in young adults exhibits a true circadian rhythm over a 24-h period, characterized by greater nocturnal secretion that is independent of sleep onset. However, GH release is further facilitated when slow-wave sleep coincides with the normal circadian peak. Under basal conditions, GH levels are low most of the time, with an ultradian rhythm of about 10 (men) or 20 (women) secretory pulses per 24 h, as calculated by deconvolution analysis. Both sexes have an increased pulse frequency during the nighttime hours, but the fraction of total daily GH secretion associated with the nocturnal pulses is much greater in men. Overall, women have more continuous GH secretion and more frequent GH pulses that are of more uniform size compared to men. These sexually dimorphic patterns in the human are actually quite similar to those in the rat, although not as extreme.

The neuroendocrine basis for sex differences in the ultradian rhythm of GH secretion is not fully understood. Gonadal sex steroids play both an organizational role during development of the hypothalamus and an activational role in the adult, in which they regulate gene expression of many of the peptides and receptors central to GH regulation. In the human, unlike the rat, the hypothalamic actions of testosterone appear to be predominantly due to its aromatization to 17β-estradiol and interaction with estrogen receptors. Hypothalamic somatostatin appears to play a more prominent role in men than in women for the regulation of pulsatile GH secretion, and this difference is postulated to be a key factor in producing the sexual dimorphism.

D. Somatostatin Effects on Gastrointestinal and Immune Systems

Somatostatin exerts inhibitory effects on virtually all endocrine and exocrine secretions of the pancreas, gut, and gallbladder (Table 2). Somatostatin also inhibits secretion by the salivary glands and, under some conditions, the secretion of parathyroid hormone and calcitonin. Somatostatin blocks hormone release in many endocrine-secreting tumors, including insulinomas, glucagonomas, VIPomas, carcinoid tumors, and some gastrinomas. Somatostatin and SSTR expression are coinduced by inflammatory and immune reactions in macrophages, T lymphocytes, splenocytes, and synovial fibroblasts in rheumatoid arthritis, consistent with paracrine or autocrine modulation of proliferative and hormonal responses in these cells.

TABLE 2 Physiologic Effects of Somatostatin In the Gastrointestinal Tract and Other Tissues

Inhibits hormone secretion from	Inhibits other gastrointestinal actions
Stomach and intestine	Gastric acid secretion
Gastrin	Gastric and jejunal fluid secretion
Secretin	Gastric emptying
Gastrointestinal polypeptide	Pancreatic bicarbonate secretion
Motilin	Pancreatic enzyme secretion
Glicentin (enteroglucagon)	(stimulates intestinal absorption of water and electrolytes)
Vasoactive intestinal peptide	Gastrointestinal blood flow
Pancreatic islets	Vasopressin-stimulated water transport
Insulin	Bile flow
Glucagon	Extragastrointestinal actions
Somatostatin	Inhibits the function of activated immune cells
Genitourinary tract	Induction of apoptosis
Renin	Inhibition of tumor growth

VI. EXTRAHYPOTHALAMIC SOMATOSTATIN AND BRAIN FUNCTION

The physiological actions of somatostatin in extrahypothalamic brain tissue remain the subject of active investigation. In the striatum, somatostatin increases the release of dopamine from nerve terminals by a glutamate-dependent mechanism involving SSTR2. In the pontine reticular formation, somatostatin blocks fear-potentiated acoustic startle responses and attenuates the increase of neuronal activity produced by the application of glutamate. Somatostatin is widely coexpressed with NPY in the limbic cortex and hippocampus GABAergic interneurons that modulate the excitability of pyramidal neurons. Temporal lobe epilepsy is associated with a marked reduction in somatostatin-expressing neurons in the hippocampus, consistent with a putative inhibitory action on seizures. Somatostatin has general arousal properties and induces rapid eye movement (REM) sleep whereas cortistatin, in contrast, has neuronal depressant actions and stimulates slow-wave sleep. A wealth of correlative data has linked reduced forebrain and cerebrospinal fluid concentrations of somatostatin with Alzheimer's disease, major depression, and other neuropsychiatric disorders, raising speculation about the role of somatostatin in modulating neural circuits underlying cognitive and affective behaviors.

VII. DIAGNOSTIC AND THERAPEUTIC USES OF SOMATOSTATIN

A. Somatostatin Analogues and Pharmacotherapy

An extensive pharmaceutical discovery program has been ongoing to synthesize somatostatin analogues with receptor subtype selectivity and improved pharmacokinetics and oral bioavailability compared to the native peptide. Initial efforts focused on the rational design of constrained cyclic peptides that incorporated D-amino acid residues and included the $[Trp^8-Lys^9]$ dipeptide of somatostatin, which structure-function studies demonstrated is necessary for high-affinity binding of the peptide to its receptor. Many such analogues have been studied in clinical trials, including octreotide (Fig. 2), lanreotide, vapreotide, and the hexapeptide MK678. Each of these compounds is an agonist with similarly high-affinity binding to SSTR2 and SSTR5, moderate binding to SSTR3, and no (or low) binding to SSTR1 and SSTR4. More recently, a combinatorial chemistry approach has led to a new generation of nonpeptidyl somatostatin agonists that bind selectively and with subnanomolar affinity to each of the five SSTR subtypes. In contrast to the marked success in development of potent and selective somatostatin agonists, there is a relative paucity of useful antagonists.

The actions of octreotide (SMS 201-995, or Sandostatin) illustrate the general potential of somatostatin analogues in therapy. This compound controls excess secretion of GH in acromegaly in most patients and shrinks tumor size in about one-third. Octreotide is also indicated for the treatment of thyrotropin-secreting adenomas that recur after surgery. It is used to treat other functioning, metastatic neuroendocrine tumors, including carcinoid, VIPoma, glucagonoma, and insulinoma, but is seldom of use for the treatment of gastrinoma. It is also useful in the management of many forms of intractable diarrhea (acting on salt and water excretion mechanisms in the gut) and to reduce external secretions in pancreatic fistulas (thus permitting healing). A decrease in blood flow to the gastrointestinal tract is the basis of its use in bleeding esophageal varices associated with hepatic cirrhosis and portal hypertension, but it is not effective in the treatment of bleeding from peptic ulcers.

The only major undesirable side effect of octreotide is reduction of bile production and of gallbladder contractility, leading to "sludging" of bile and an increased incidence of gallstones. Other common adverse effects, including nausea, abdominal cramps, flatulence, and diarrhea secondary to malabsorption of fat, usually subside spontaneously within 2 weeks of continued treatment. Long-term octreotide therapy is not associated with impaired glucose tolerance, despite an inhibitory effect on insulin secretion, presumably because of compensating reductions in carbohydrate absorption and GH and glucagon secretion that are also caused by the drug.

B. Somatostatin Receptor Imaging and Cytotoxic Therapies

Somatostatin analogues labeled with a radioactive tracer have been used as external imaging agents for a wide range of disorders. A ^{111}In-labeled analogue of octreotide (Octreoscan) has been approved for clinical use in the United States and several other countries. A majority of the neuroendocrine tumors and many pituitary tumors that express SSTRs are visualized by external imaging techniques after administration of this agent; a variety of nonendocrine tumors and inflammatory lesions are also visualized, all of which have in common the expression of SSTRs. Such tumors include non-small-cell cancer of the lung, meningioma, breast cancer, and astrocytomas. Because activated T cells of the immune system display SSTRs, inflammatory lesions that take up the tracer include sarcoidosis, Wegener's granulomatosis, tuberculosis, and many cases of Hodgkin's disease and non-Hodgkin's lymphoma. Although the tracer lacks specificity in differential diagnosis, its ability to identify the presence of abnormality and the extent of the lesion provides important information for management, including tumor staging. The use of a portable radiation detector in the operating room makes it possible to ensure the completeness of removal of medullary thyroid carcinoma metastases. New developments in the synthesis of positron emission tomography (PET) tracers chelated to octreotide have allowed for the sensitive detection of meningiomas less than 1 cm in diameter and located beneath osseous structures at the base of the skull.

The ability of somatostatin to inhibit the growth of normal and some neoplastic cell lines and to reduce the growth of experimentally induced tumors in animal models has stimulated interest in somatostatin analogues for the treatment of cancer. Somatostatin's tumorostatic effects may be a combination of direct actions on tumor cells due to inhibition of growth factor receptor expression, inhibition of MAPK, and stimulation of PTP. SSTR1, SSTR2, SSTR4, and SSTR5 can all promote cell cycle arrest associated with induction of the tumor suppressor retinoblastoma (Rb) and p21, whereas SSTR3 can trigger apoptosis accompanied by induction of the tumor suppressor p53 and the proapoptotic protein Bax. In addition, somatostatin has indirect effects on tumor growth by its inhibition of circulating, paracrine, and autocrine tumor growth-promoting factors and it can also modulate the activity of immune cells and influence tumor blood supply. Despite this promise, the therapeutic utility of octreotide as an antineoplastic agent remains controversial.

Two new treatment approaches in preclinical trials may yet effectively utilize somatostatin receptors in the arrest of cancer cells. The first is receptor-targeted radionuclide therapy using octreotide chelated to a variety of γ- or β-emitting radioisotopes. Theoretical calculations and empirical data suggest that radiolabeled somatostatin analogues can deliver a tumoricidal radiotherapeutic dose to some tumors after receptor-mediated endocytosis. A variation on this theme is the chelation of a cytotoxic chemotherapeutic agent to a somatostatin analogue. A second approach involves somatic-cell gene therapy to transfect SSTR-negative pancreatic cancer cells with an SSTR gene. Therapeutic results could occur from the creation of autocrine or paracrine inhibitory growth effects or with the addition of targeted radionuclide treatments.

VIII. SUMMARY

Somatostatin is a phylogenetically ancient peptide that occupies numerous regulatory niches in diverse organ systems. Comparative genomic analyses suggest that at least two gene duplications of a primordial somatostatin gene have occurred in the past 500 million years of vertebrate evolution, yielding a family of related peptides that signal through five different subtypes of somatostatin receptors. In the simplest terms, somatostatin can be considered a paninhibitory factor for a large number of hormones, including pituitary growth hormone, cytokines, and exocrine secretions, in addition to its roles in modulating neuronal activity and regulating cell proliferation. A great deal of largely circumstantial evidence points to widespread activity of somatostatin within neural circuits underlying locomotor, cognitive, and emotional processes.

Glossary

cAMP response element Consensus nucleotide sequence 5′-TGACGTCA-3′; found in the promoter of many hormone-regulated genes, including somatostatin; a specific binding site for the transcriptional activator cAMP response element binding protein (CREB).

hypophyseotropic hormones Neurotransmitters, including neuropeptides, dopamine, and γ-aminobutyric acid; secreted from tuberoinfundibular neurons and conveyed as hormones through the long portal vessels, acting at a distance on pituitary cells and regulating their function.

mitogen-activated protein kinases Protein serine/threonine kinases that mediate intracellular signaling through three major mitogen-activated protein kinase cascades: ERK1/ERK2, JNK/SAPK, and p38.

octreotide A commonly used eight-residue peptidyl analogue of SS14 with a long biological half-life and efficacy as an agonist at SSTR2 and SSTR5.

phosphotyrosine phosphatase Enzyme that catalyzes the dephosphorylation of tyrosine residues from signaling molecules and thereby opposes the action of protein tyrosine kinases, which are key mediators of cellular responses such as proliferation and differentiation.

prohormone A precursor (either peptide or steroid) to an active hormone; produced in significant amounts as an intermediate in the pathway of production of the active hormone.

somatostatins Cyclic neuropeptides, the archetype being SS14, or somatotropin release-inhibiting factor, so named for one of its biological activities, inhibition of the secretion of pituitary growth hormone.

somatostatin receptors, types 1–5 Five subtypes of G-protein-coupled, seven-transmembrane-domain somatostatin receptors.

tuberoinfundibular neurons Located in several nuclei of the medial basal hypothalamus; project axons to the median eminence and infundibulum (pituitary stalk) and release their neurotransmitters adjacent to the fenestrated, tuberohypophyseal portal blood vessels supplying the pituitary gland.

See Also the Following Articles

Ghrelin • Glucagonoma Syndrome • Growth Hormone-Releasing Hormone (GHRH) and the GHRH Receptor • Growth Regulation: Clinical Aspects of GHRH • Peptide YY • Peptidomimetics

Further Reading

Andersen, F. G., Jensen, J., Heller, R. S., Petersen, H. V., Larsson, L. I., Madsen, O. D., and Serup, P. (1999). Pax6 and Pdx1 form a functional complex on the rat somatostatin gene upstream enhancer. *FEBS Lett.* **445**, 315–320.

Giustina, A., and Veldhuis, J. D. (1998). Pathophysiology of the neuroregulation of growth hormone secretion in experimental animals and the human. *Endocr. Rev.* **19**, 717–797.

Goudet, G., Delhalle, S., Biemar, F., Martial, J. A., and Peers, B. (1999). Functional and cooperative interactions between the homeodomain PDX1, Pbx, and Prep1 factors on the somatostatin promoter. *J. Biol. Chem.* **274**, 4067–4073.

Lamberts, S. W., van der Lely, A. J., de Herder, W. W., and Hofland, L. J. (1996). Octreotide. *N. Engl. J. Med.* **334**, 246–254.

Low, M. J., Otero-Corchon, V., Parlow, A. F., Ramirez, J. L., Kumar, U., Patel, Y. C., and Rubinstein, M. (2001). Somatostatin is required for masculinization of growth hormone-regulated hepatic gene expression but not of somatic growth. *J. Clin. Invest.* **107**, 1571–1580.

Montminy, M., Brindle, P., Arias, J., Ferreri, K., and Armstrong, R. (1996). Regulation of somatostatin gene transcription by cyclic adenosine monophosphate. *Metabolism* **45**, 4–7.

Muller, E. E., Locatelli, V., and Cocchi, D. (1999). Neuroendocrine control of growth hormone secretion. *Physiol. Rev.* **79**, 511–607.

Patel, Y. C. (1999). Somatostatin and its receptor family. *Front. Neuroendocrinol.* **20**, 157–198.

Rohrer, S. P., Birzin, E. T., Mosley, R. T., Berk, S. C., Hutchins, S. M., Shen, D. M., Xiong, Y., Hayes, E. C., Parmar, R. M., Foor, F., Mitra, S. W., Degrado, S. J., Shu, M., Klopp, J. M., Cai, S. J., Blake, A., Chan, W. W., Pasternak, A., Yang, L., Patchett, A. A., Smith, R. G., Chapman, K. T., and Schaeffer, J. M. (1998). Rapid identification of subtype-selective agonists of the somatostatin receptor through combinatorial chemistry. *Science* **282**, 737–740.

Schwartz, P. T., Perez-Villamil, B., Rivera, A., Moratalla, R., and Vallejo, M. (2000). Pancreatic homeodomain transcription factor IDX1/IPF1 expressed in developing brain regulates

SPERMATOGENESIS, HORMONAL CONTROL OF

somatostatin gene transcription in embryonic neural cells. *J. Biol. Chem.* **275**, 19106–19114.

Slooter, G. D., Mearadji, A., Breeman, W. A., Marquet, R. L., de Jong, M., Krenning, E. P., and van Eijck, C. H. (2001). Somatostatin receptor imaging, therapy and new strategies in patients with neuroendocrine tumours. *Br. J. Surg.* **88**, 31–40.

Spier, A. D., and de Lecea, L. (2000). Cortistatin: A member of the somatostatin neuropeptide family with distinct physiological functions. *Brain Res. Brain Res. Rev.* **33**, 228–241.

Strowski, M. Z., Parmar, R. M., Blake, A. D., and Schaeffer, J. M. (2000). Somatostatin inhibits insulin and glucagon secretion via two receptor subtypes: An *in vitro* study of pancreatic islets from somatostatin receptor 2 knockout mice. *Endocrinology* **141**, 111–117.

Trabucchi, M., Tostivint, H., Lihrmann, I., Jegou, S., Vallarino, M., and Vaudry, H. (1999). Molecular cloning of the cDNAs and distribution of the mRNAs encoding two somatostatin precursors in the African lungfish *Protopterus annectens*. *J. Comp. Neurol.* **410**, 643–652.

Spermatogenesis, Hormonal Control of

SARAH MEACHEM AND ROBERT MCLACHLAN

Prince Henry's Institute of Medical Research, Australia

The process of spermatogenesis in the adult testis depends on two pituitary hormones, follicle-stimulating hormone and luteinizing hormone; luteinizing hormone, in turn, stimulates the production of androgens, notably testosterone. Specific cellular sites during spermatogenesis are specifically and conjointly regulated by hormonal activities. Production of viable, healthy sperm is a complex process that requires a high degree of cellular, hormonal, and molecular interactions; understanding the precise mechanisms of hormonal interaction is significant in developing a strategy for the design of an effective male hormonal contraceptive.

I. INTRODUCTION

Production of fertile sperm, a testicular process under the control of follicle-stimulating hormone (FSH) and luteinizing hormone (LH), is necessary for reproductive viability. LH stimulates the production of androgens, notably testosterone, which is required for the attainment of male secondary sexual characteristics. Results from a wide array of animal and human experiments have identified specific cellular sites during spermatogenesis that are specifically and conjointly regulated by FSH and testosterone. It appears, however, that FSH is not essential for sperm production, because animals congenitally lacking FSH can be fertile, although their testis size and total sperm output are diminished. It seems that FSH plays an important role in establishing the foundations for full adult spermatogenesis by controlling the population of Sertoli cells, which determine adult spermatogenic capacity. In addition, FSH acts to optimize sperm production via involvement in multiple steps of spermatogenesis, most notably the steps involving the earliest germ cell forms, the spermatogonia. Testosterone is essential for spermatogenesis, particularly in supporting spermatid meiosis and maturation. Understanding the basic physiology of sperm production has important ramifications for understanding the common problem of male infertility and, conversely, in the design of a hormonal contraceptive. Thus far, clinical studies of androgen-based contraception have shown that there are two sites of inhibition, both dependent on gonadotropin suppression, at the level of the spermatogonia and sperm release. The following brief review of the basic endocrine control and organization of the testis prefaces a more detailed discussion of the hormonal control of spermatogenesis.

II. OVERVIEW OF THE HYPOTHALAMIC–PITUITARY–TESTICULAR AXIS

The adult testis has two main functions, to produce sperm for fertility and to produce androgens for maintaining secondary sexual traits. Sperm and androgen production are dependent on stimulation by the gonadotropins LH and FSH. The gonadotropins are produced by and secreted from the anterior pituitary in response to gonadotropin-releasing hormone (GnRH) stimulation from the hypothalamus. LH exerts its effects on testicular Leydig cells to stimulate the production and secretion of androgens, most notably testosterone. Testosterone is essential for the initiation and maintenance of spermatogenesis and exerts its effects on the germ cells via receptors on Sertoli, Leydig, and peritubular cells. FSH acts via specific G-protein-coupled surface receptors located exclusively on Sertoli cells and is important for normal testicular growth and sperm production (see Fig. 1).

The process of sperm production, or spermatogenesis, in many mammals is a continuous process that takes place throughout the reproductive life span of the animal. However, in some mammals, spermatogenesis shows marked seasonal variation; in others, a single wave of spermatogenesis is followed by sterility. Spermatogenesis is a compli-

cated process in which stem cells (called spermatogonia) undergo a complex sequence of proliferative and differentiation steps before they give rise to mature sperm (Fig. 1). Spermatogonia must proceed through three main phases before giving rise to mature sperm: (1) spermatogonia first undergo mitosis; (2) cells called spermatocytes then undergo reduction of a diploid chromosome number by the process of meiosis; (3) haploid, round spermatids are finally transformed into highly organized motile spermatozoa, a process termed spermiogenesis. The last event in spermiogenesis is the release of spermatozoa from the seminiferous epithelium into

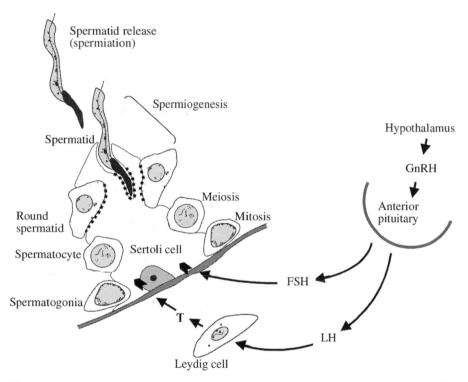

FIGURE 1 The hormonal control of spermatogenesis and structural organization of the testis. Follicle-stimulating hormone (FSH) and luteinizing hormone (LH) are secreted from the anterior pituitary under the influence of gonadotropin-releasing hormone (GnRH) from the hypothalamus. FSH targets the developing germ cells via specific G-protein-coupled receptors (●) on the Sertoli cell plasma membrane; LH stimulates the Leydig cells to produce and secrete androgens, predominantly testosterone (T), which in turn exerts its effects on the developing germ cells via nuclear receptors (●) in the Sertoli cell. Spermatogenesis is an elaborate process by which spermatogonia must proceed through multiple mitotic divisions, then meiosis, to produce haploid, round spermatids; these steps are followed by a complex sequence of morphological transformations that give rise to spermatozoa (spermiogenesis), ending in release of the spermatozoa from the Sertoli cell, into the tubule lumen (spermiation). In humans, the total time for spermatogonia to develop into mature sperm is 65 days; this time varies depending on the species. Extensive animal studies have shown that spermatogenesis depends on both FSH and T, each having both independent and synergistic effects on spermatogenesis. Although FSH is not essential for spermatogenesis, it plays a key role establishing the size of the Sertoli cell population during testicular development and in supporting spermatogonial development in adult animals. In contrast, T is required for the complete maturation of spermatids, and both FSH and T have been shown to play an important role in promoting spermatocyte and spermatid survival and in maintaining specialized junctions (···) involved in the adhesion of spermatids to the Sertoli cell.

the tubule lumen, a process termed spermiation. These phases of spermatogenesis occur along similar lines in all mammals and have been well described.

III. ORGANIZATION OF THE TESTIS

The mammalian testis is encapsulated by a dense connective tissue called the tunica albuginea. The testis is composed of two major compartments, the seminiferous tubules, containing the nurturing Sertoli cells and the developing germ cells, and the interstitium, where Leydig cells and other interstitial cells reside. The testis contains many seminiferous tubules, which are convoluted loops connected at both ends to the excurrent duct system, also known as the rete testis. The mature spermatozoa pass from the tubules into the rete testis and then pass through the efferent ducts to the epididymis for final maturation before being capable of fertilizing an egg. The seminiferous tubules consist of the seminiferous epithelium and the lumen. Within the epithelium, the Sertoli cell provides structural and nutritional support for the developing germ cells; the lumen allows sperm and secretory products to be transported out of the testis. The interstitium contains the blood and lymphatic vessels responsible for the supply of nutrients into and out of the testis. Leydig cells are responsible for the generation of testosterone and other steroids.

The seminiferous epithelium has three compartments with different functions. Tight junctional complexes connecting the adjacent Sertoli cells form two permanent (basal and adlumenal) compartments and a temporary, intermediate compartment. Spermatogonia and early spermatocytes reside in the basal compartment. These cells have relatively free access to nutrients coming from the lymphatic and vascular systems. The intermediate compartment is formed during transit of spermatocytes from the basal to the adlumenal compartment, which involves the successive breakdown and formation of tight junctions. The adlumenal compartment contains all later stage germ cell types and is stringently controlled by the Sertoli cells via the tight junctional complexes, which limit the passage of macromolecules into the adlumenal environment. The junction is commonly referred to as the blood–testis barrier and becomes functional in early postnatal life. Numerous other Sertoli cell attachments to the developing germ cells assist in maintaining the structural integrity of the epithelium and provide a link for the cells to communicate. The success of spermatogenesis relies on the communication between all testicular cells.

IV. HORMONAL DEPENDENCY OF SPERMATOGENESIS

The hormonal control of spermatogenesis has been studied extensively for many years, and differing emphasis has been placed on the relative roles of endocrine, paracrine, and autocrine factors. It must be understood that the complexity of germ cell development and the intricate intercellular relationships make it difficult to define clearly the exact control of each step in sperm production. In a wide range of experimental paradigms, different species have been used, different approaches to manipulating hormone levels have been employed, and, most importantly, there have been many different methods for describing or quantifying changes in germ cell production. Broadly speaking, hormone withdrawal and replacement have been used to dissect out the factors that regulate initiation, maintenance, and restoration of the spermatogenic process. This has varied from the complete withdrawal of pituitary factors by hypophysectomy, to active immunization with GnRH, to treatment with GnRH antagonists, and to the use of congenitally GnRH-deficient mice. The relatively selective withdrawal of testosterone has been achieved by sex steroid treatment (which causes gonadotropin suppression and a resultant decrease in testicular testosterone levels to $<5\%$ of normal), treatment with antiandrogens, and immunization against LH. FSH withdrawal has been achieved by disrupting FSH action by genetically modifying mice and by passively immunizing animals against FSH. A diverse range of qualitative and quantitative end points has been used to evaluate the effects of hormone on spermatogenesis. The advent of sophisticated stereological methods for quantitative analysis of cell populations has led to major advances in defining the sites of hormone action.

The precise mechanism by which FSH and testosterone exert their effects on the developing germ cells has not been elucidated but involves a highly orchestrated molecular and genomic response. Studies on the role of FSH and testosterone indicate that both hormones have independent and synergistic effects on germ cell development.

V. FSH DEPENDENCY

FSH plays a key role in the development of the immature testis, particularly by controlling the size of the Sertoli cell population, which is set early in postnatal life. This is of particular importance for the adult animal because Sertoli cell number dictates sperm output. After debating many conflicting data from animal models, there is agreement that some degree of complete spermatogenesis can be initiated and maintained in the absence of FSH; however, quantitatively normal spermatogenesis depends on FSH. FSH acts at multiple sites in the spermatogenic pathway by promoting spermatogonial proliferation and survival and viability of later germ cell types by presumably maintaining structures and proteins involved in attachment of the germ cell to the Sertoli cell. More specifically, rat and monkey studies have shown that FSH plays a major role in supporting spermatogonial development, with FSH having more pronounced effects on certain subpopulations. FSH has been shown to play a role in later germ cell types, supporting spermatocytes and round spermatid development presumably by supporting cell survival. The specialized Sertoli cell junctional apparatus has been shown to be a hormone-sensitive structure; the structures are found between Sertoli cells and at stages from mature round spermatids to mature sperm before spermiation. This specialized apparatus has been shown to be disorganized in long-term gonadotropin-deplete rats and can be restored by FSH treatment, suggesting that FSH is important for the maintenance of the junctional apparatus. *In vitro* experiments on Sertoli and round spermatid cultures suggest that FSH is important for adherence of the round spermatids to the Sertoli cells. Finally, FSH may be involved in the release of mature sperm from the epithelium, based on reports that more sperm are retained within the seminiferous epithelium following acute FSH withdrawal. Another way that FSH can support germ cell development is via the Leydig cells. FSH has been shown to regulate Leydig cell products that play a role in spermatogenesis and promote maturation of the Leydig cell population.

VI. TESTOSTERONE DEPENDENCY

Spermatogenesis has an absolute requirement for testosterone, particularly for the maturation of spermiogenic cells. Data from rodent models of testosterone replacement provide no evidence that testosterone supports spermatogonial development, although rodent models expressing high levels of testicular testosterone appear to have a detrimental effect on spermatogonial development. The viability of spermatocytes and spermatids is enhanced in the presence of testosterone and there are marked increases in cell degeneration in the absence of testosterone. The major lesion following selective testosterone withdrawal is during rat spermiogenesis, wherein sperm production is ablated as a consequence, at least in part, of the premature release of round spermatids from the seminiferous epithelium. Hence, round spermatid maturation is dependent on testosterone, which promotes the attachment of round spermatids to the Sertoli cells, possibly by induction of structures and proteins involved in cell adhesion. Finally, sperm release (spermiation) is also partly dependent on testosterone, because when testicular testosterone is reduced, mature sperm are retained and phagocytosed within Sertoli cells.

It has been established that testosterone is the active androgen supporting spermatogenesis in the normal testis; however, within the testis, testosterone can be metabolized by 5α-reductase enzymes to a more potent androgen, dihydrotestosterone (DHT). There is some evidence to support the notion that when testosterone levels are low (such as during LH suppression, when the level falls to $<5\%$ of normal), metabolism of testosterone to DHT may be important in maintaining some degree of spermatogenesis.

VII. FSH AND TESTOSTERONE SYNERGY

There are many reports suggesting that FSH and testosterone act synergistically and that they exert the same biological effect. For example, it is clear that germ cell apoptosis/viability can be regulated by FSH and testosterone. Acute models of gonadotropin suppression/replacement in rats have revealed that both FSH and testosterone affect spermiation but that both are required for normality. FSH and testosterone can stimulate Sertoli cell products such as androgen-binding protein and transferrin. Synergy has been shown to play a role in maintaining proteins involved in cell adhesion. Sertoli cell N-cadherin, one such protein, has been shown to be maximally produced *in vitro* in the presence of both FSH and testosterone. Furthermore, *in vitro* studies of round spermatids and Sertoli cells show that binding of round spermatids to Sertoli cells is dependent on testosterone only in the presence of FSH. In addition, *in vivo* studies show that spermiogenesis is restored in hypophysectomized testosterone-replaced rats when FSH is administered. Monkey and human studies have demonstrated the relevance of several of these hormonally sensitive steps, notably spermatogonial development and sperm release, which are disrupted following gonadotropin suppression. Whether these are the results of independent or synergistic actions of FSH and testosterone in these species is unclear.

VIII. RELEVANCE TO MALE CONTRACEPTIVE DEVELOPMENT

Studies in animals and humans have improved our understanding of the physiological basis of male contraception based on testosterone administration to suppress gonadotropins. Two major sites of spermatogenesis in humans have been identified as hormone sensitive, i.e., spermatogonial development and spermiation. Given the data from animal models, it appears that FSH withdrawal is important for spermatogonial development and that both FSH and testosterone are critical for spermiation. Clinical studies have shown that the extent of spermatogenic suppression and time of onset vary among individuals and between racial groups. Although not proved, it is thought that these differences may be attributed to differences in the degree and onset of gonadotropin suppression, and that faster and deeper suppression of both FSH and testosterone will lead to a more profound inhibition of spermatogenesis and thus create an effective contraceptive. Some studies provide evidence indicating that administration of progestins in combination with androgens may provide this desired effect, although further investigation is necessary. Another issue relating to variations in the degree of spermatogenic suppression between racial groups may be differences in androgen metabolism by 5α reduced enzymes; whether these differences are genetic or environmental, such as diet, is unclear.

IX. CONCLUSION

Control of sperm production is mediated by FSH and LH via testosterone. A wide variety of animal models, most notably rodent models, coupled with quantitative analyses of testicular cell populations, have recognized that the sperm generation pathway contains steps sensitive to the independent action of FSH and testosterone and steps requiring synergistic actions. It is apparent that FSH is particularly important for early testicular growth, particularly in establishing the size of the Sertoli cell population and in supporting spermatogonial development in adulthood. Testosterone, however, is critical for maturation of round spermatids, because FSH is unable to

complete this vital step; sperm release seems to require both hormones. Limited monkey and human studies have shown that gonadotropin suppression results in inhibition of spermatogonial development and sperm release. Further elucidation of the precise mechanisms by which these hormones affect sperm production will be significant for the design of the first effective hormonal contraceptive strategy for men.

Glossary

follicle-stimulating hormone Pituitary hormone that induces germ cell production and development of their supporting cells in the ovary and testis.

hormone Substance released by an endocrine gland; travels through the bloodstream to exert an effect on remote cells, tissues, and organs.

luteinizing hormone Pituitary hormone that acts with follicle-stimulating hormone to stimulate sex hormone release.

Sertoli cells The "nurse" cells of the seminiferous epithelium; provide nutritional and structural support for developing germ cells.

spermatids Haploid germ cells produced by the second meiotic division in spermatogenesis; differentiate into mature spermatozoa.

spermatocytes Tetraploid germ cells that undergo two meiotic divisions, yielding haploid spermatids.

spermatogenesis Process whereby spermatogonia divide and differentiate into mature spermatozoa.

spermatogonia Diploid germ cells that divide and differentiate; the most immature germ cell type.

stereological Methodology that allows structural information (for instance, estimation of cell number) to be derived from sections of a structure.

testosterone Male sex hormone (androgen) secreted by interstitial Leydig cells of the testis; responsible for triggering development of sperm and secondary sexual characteristics.

See Also the Following Articles

Anti-Müllerian Hormone ● Dihydrotestosterone, Active Androgen Metabolites and Related Pathology ● Estrogen and Spermatogenesis ● Follicle Stimulating Hormone (FSH) ● Male Hormonal Contraception ● Sexual Differentiation, Molecular and Hormone Dependent Events in ● Testis Descent, Hormonal Control of

Further Reading

Anderson, R. A. (2000). Hormonal contraception in the male. *Br. Med. Bull.* **56**, 717–728.
Huhtaniemi, I., and Bartke, A. (2001). Perspective: male reproduction. *Endocrinology* **142**, 2178–2183.
Kumar, T. R., Wang, Y., Lu, N., and Matzuk, M. M. (1997). Follicle stimulating hormone is required for ovarian follicle maturation but not male fertility. *Nat. Genet.* **15**, 201–204.

McLachlan, R. I., O'Donnell, L., Stanton, P. G., Balourdos, G., Frydenberg, M., deKretser, D. M., and Robertson, D. M. (2002). Effects of testosterone plus medroxyprogesterone acetate on semen quality, reproductive hormones and germ cell populations in normal young men. *J. Clin. Endocrinol. Metab.* **87**, 546–556.

McLachlan, R. I., O'Donnell, L., Meachem, S. J., Stanton, P. G., deKretser, D. M., Pratis, K., and Robertson, D. M. (2002). Identification of specific sites of hormonal regulation in spermatogenesis in rats, monkeys and man. *Recent Prog. Horm. Res.* **57**, 149–179.

Meachem, S. J., McLachlan, R. I., Stanton, P. G., Robertson, D. M., and Wreford, N. G. (1999). FSH immunoneutralization acutely impairs spermatogonial development in normal adult rats. *J. Androl.* **20**, 756–762; discussion, 755.

Muffly, K. E., Nazian, S. J., and Cameron, D. F. (1994). Effects of follicle-stimulating hormone on the junction-related Sertoli cell cytoskeleton and daily sperm production in testosterone-treated hypophysectomized rats. *Biol. Reprod.* **51**, 158–166.

O'Donnell, L., Pratis, K., Stanton, P. G., Robertson, D. M., and McLachlan, R. I. (1999). Testosterone-dependent restoration of spermatogenesis in adult rats is impaired by a 5α-reductase inhibitor. *J. Androl.* **20**, 109–117.

O'Donnell, L., Narula, A., Balourdos, G., Gu, Y. Q., Wreford, N. G., Robertson, D. M., Bremner, W. J., and McLachlan, R. I. (2001). Impairment of spermatogonial development and spermiation after testosterone-induced gonadotropin suppression in adult monkeys (Macaca fascicularis). *J. Clin. Endocrinol. Metab.* **86**, 1814–1822.

Russell, L. D., Kershaw, M., Borg, K. E., El Shennawy, A., Rulli, S. S., Gates, R. J., and Calandra, R. S. (1998). Hormonal regulation of spermatogenesis in the hypophysectomized rat: FSH maintenance of cellular viability during pubertal spermatogenesis. *J. Androl.* **19**, 308–319; discussion 341–342.

Singh, J., O'Neill, C., and Handelsman, D. J. (1995). Induction of spermatogenesis by androgens in gonadotropin-deficient (hpg) mice. *Endocrinology* **136**, 5311–5321.

Sinha Hikim, A. P., and Swerdloff, R. S. (1999). Hormonal and genetic control of germ cell apoptosis in the testis. *Rev. Reprod.* **4**, 38–47.

Sinha Hikim, A. P., Rajavashisth, T. B., Sinha Hikim, I., Lue, Y., Bonavera, J. J., Leung, A., Wang, C., and Swerdloff, R. S. (1997). Significance of apoptosis in the temporal and stage-specific loss of germ cells in the adult rat after gonadotropin deprivation. *Biol. Reprod.* **57**, 1193–1201.

Weinbauer, G. F., Schlatt, S., Walter, V., and Nieschlag, E. (2001). Testosterone-induced inhibition of spermatogenesis is more closely related to suppression of FSH than to testicular androgen levels in the cynomolgus monkey model (*Macaca fascicularis*). *J. Endocrinol.* **168**, 25–38.

Wreford, N. G. (1995). Theory and practice of stereological techniques applied to the estimation of cell number and nuclear volume in the testis. *Microsc. Res. Tech.* **32**, 423–436.

StAR Protein

See *Steroidogenic Acute Regulatory Protein*

Stem Cell Factor[1]

DIANA LINNEKIN, TANYA JELACIC, AND SHIVAKRUPA
National Cancer Institute, Maryland

I. INTRODUCTION AND HISTORICAL PERSPECTIVE
II. THE SCF LIGAND
III. THE SCF RECEPTOR
IV. BIOLOGY
V. MECHANISMS OF ACTION
VI. PATHOPHYSIOLOGY
VII. SUMMARY

Stem cell factor (SCF) is a growth factor that binds the receptor tyrosine kinase Kit, leading to the activation of multiple signal transduction components, including members of the Src family. SCF is essential for the survival, growth, and maturation of stem cells involved in gametogenesis, hematopoiesis, and melanogenesis.

I. INTRODUCTION AND HISTORICAL PERSPECTIVE

Although stem cell factor (SCF) was cloned in 1990, this growth factor has a remarkably rich history. The receptor for SCF is the receptor tyrosine kinase (RTK) Kit. In mice, the c-Kit gene product maps to the *White Spotting* (*W*) locus on chromosome 5 and SCF maps to the *Steel* (*Sl*) locus on chromosome 10. Mice with mutations in the *W* locus were first identified in 1927. These animals were characterized by alterations in coat pigmentation, abnormalities in reproduction, and macrocytic anemia. In 1956, mice with the identical defects were found to have mutations in the *Sl* locus. The complementary nature of the phenotypes of these animals suggested that the *W* and *Sl* gene products were a receptor and its ligand. The isolation of the v-Kit oncogene from the Hardy–Zuckerman 4 strain of feline sarcoma virus by Peter Besmer and co-workers in 1986 set the stage to test this possibility formally. In 1987, the c-Kit proto-oncogene was cloned and the following year it was mapped to the *W* locus. Multiple groups then cloned the ligand for Kit and demonstrated that it mapped to the *Sl* locus. The cloning of SCF allowed

[1] The content of this publication does not necessarily reflect the views or policies of the Department of Health and Human Services, nor does mention of trade names, commercial products, or organizations imply endorsement by the U. S. Government.

rigorous assessment of its biological activities. Indeed, this growth factor proved to be critical for stem cells involved in gametogenesis, hematopoiesis, and melanogenesis. Although clinical use of SCF may be limited by its capacity to activate mast cells, gain-of-function mutations in Kit are associated with a variety of diseases in humans. Thus, understanding the cellular and molecular biology of the SCF receptor may be useful in designing approaches for treatment of these disorders, as well as harnessing the considerable biological potency of the ligand.

II. THE SCF LIGAND

SCF, also termed mast cell growth factor, Kit ligand, and Steel factor, is the ligand for the receptor tyrosine kinase Kit. The human SCF gene is located on chromosome 12q22–q24, is 50 kb in length, and consists of eight exons. The murine SCF gene has been mapped to chromosome 10 in a region flanked by genes encoding peptidase-2 and phenylhydroxylase. The cDNA for SCF has been cloned and sequenced from a variety of species including human, mouse, rat, pig, and chicken [Accession Nos. (mouse) U44725; (human) M59964; (rat) M59966; (pig) L07786; and (chicken) D13516]. The first exon of the human SCF gene codes for the signal peptide required for membrane anchoring of SCF. Exons 2 through 6 code for the transmembrane region. Exon 7 codes for the extracellular region and exon 8 encodes the cytoplasmic tail. SCF protein is found as both a soluble form (sSCF or SCF^{165}) and a membrane-bound form (mSCF or SCF^{220}). These forms are generated by alternate splicing of a primary transcript at exon 6. One splice product gives rise to a protein of 275 amino acids containing a cleavable amino-terminal signal peptide. The cleavage of the signal peptide gives rise to SCF^{248}, also designated KL-1 or SCF-1. It contains an extracellular domain, a 22-amino-acid transmembrane domain, and a 36-amino-acid cytoplasmic domain. SCF^{248} undergoes proteolytic cleavage at Ala-165 to generate the soluble form of SCF, SCF^{165}. The other splice variant of SCF lacks the proteolytic cleavage site and gives rise to a membrane-bound form of SCF, SCF^{220}, also termed KL-2 or SCF-2.

Soluble SCF exists as a heavily glycosylated 50 to 60 kDa noncovalent homodimer that can dissociate and reassociate in solution. The recently described crystal structure revealed a large dimerization region and a charged receptor-binding region that includes hydrophobic crevices. The concentration of soluble SCF in human serum is approximately 3 ng/ml.

Consequently, it exists primarily as a monomer. In contrast, the close proximity of mSCF in the plasma membrane results in the dimerization of this molecule. Dimerization of membrane-bound SCF facilitates signaling through the Kit receptor. Both forms of SCF are biologically active, with distinct as well as overlapping functions. Membrane-bound SCF induces more persistent tyrosine kinase activation than soluble SCF. This is likely due to the slower internalization of Kit after binding this form of the growth factor.

SCF is expressed by stromal cells, fibroblasts, and endothelial cells and is also present at low levels in the circulation. SCF is also expressed along the migratory pathway of stem cells in embryos and this plays an important role in development. Sertoli cells, ovarian follicular cells, brain, and olfactory bulb also express SCF. The ratio of membrane SCF to soluble SCF varies considerably in different tissues. Fibroblasts, brain, thymus, spleen, and bone marrow express higher levels of SCF^{248}, whereas placenta, cerebellum, and testis have higher levels of SCF^{220}. The exact mechanism of regulation of the levels of different SCF proteins is unknown.

III. THE SCF RECEPTOR

The receptor for SCF is Kit, a receptor tyrosine kinase sharing homology with receptors for platelet-derived growth factor (PDGF) and colony-stimulating factor-1 (CSF-1). Kit has also been designated as stem cell factor receptor and CD117. The gene for human c-Kit has been mapped to 4q11–q34, spans approximately 70 kb of DNA, and has 21 exons [GenBank Accession Nos. (human) X06182 and (mouse) Y00864]. Human Kit encodes a 145 kDa glycosylated protein (GenBank Accession No. 1817733) containing an extracellular domain of approximately 500 amino acids, a 30-amino-acid juxtamembrane domain, a cytoplasmic kinase domain divided into two parts by a 77-amino-acid kinase insert region, and a 50-amino-acid carboxy-terminal tail region. The extracellular domain contains five immunoglobulin-like repeat regions, the first three of which constitute the ligand-binding domain. The fourth immunoglobulin-like domain is involved in receptor dimerization and the function of the fifth domain has not been defined. Some of these features are illustrated in Fig. 1. An alternative splice form of Kit, termed KitA, has a four-codon insertion (GNNK) in the extracellular domain just proximal to the membrane-spanning region. Both forms are co-expressed in most tissues. Another variant of Kit that consists of only the second

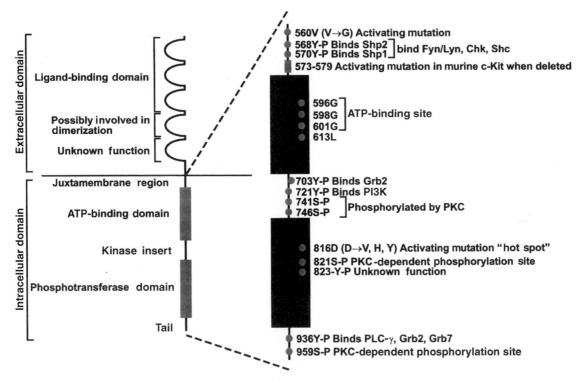

FIGURE 1 Structure—function relationships of the Kit receptor tyrosine kinase. The extracellular domain of Kit is divided into five immunoglobulin-like regions. The intracellular domain is composed of the juxtamembrane region, the catalytic domain, a kinase insert, and a carboxy-tail. Amino acids that contribute to the activation of Kit or that interact with specific signaling molecules are designated by small circles.

catalytic domain and the carboxy-terminal tail is expressed in spermatids. Full-length Kit is proteolytically cleaved in a process dependent on the fifth immunoglobulin-like domain, to give rise to a soluble form of Kit. The function of soluble Kit is not fully defined; however, it binds to SCF and may act as a receptor antagonist *in vivo*.

Kit is expressed in a variety of different cells. In hematopoietic tissue, it is expressed in stem cells, progenitor cells (pluripotent as well as progenitors committed to the myeloid, lymphoid, erythroid, and megakaryocytic lineages), bone marrow mononuclear cells with lymphoid markers, and mast cells. In most hematopoietic lineages, Kit expression decreases during maturation. However, mast cells, activated platelets, and some subsets of NK cells are exceptions. Nonhematopoietic cells expressing Kit include melanocytes, spermatozoa, vascular endothelium, interstitial cells of Cajal (ICCs), breast glandular epithelial cells, sweat glands, astrocytes, oocytes, theca cells, and renal tubules. Kit is also expressed in the human endometrium and placenta during pregnancy.

Surface expression of Kit is regulated by multiple mechanisms. Interaction with SCF induces internalization of the receptor through clathrin-coated pits. Kit is also ubiquitinated and can be degraded in either the lysosome or the proteasome pathway. In addition, certain cytokines regulate surface expression of Kit. Transforming growth factor-β can induce the downregulation of Kit through reductions in mRNA stability. This is also seen with interleukin-3 (IL-3) stimulation in mast cells. The processing of membrane-bound receptor to generate the soluble form also determines the surface expression levels of Kit in umbilical endothelial cells, mast cells, and human plasma.

IV. BIOLOGY

Kit and SCF are expressed in many tissues. The correct function of these proteins is necessary for maintenance of gastrointestinal motility, hematopoiesis, melanogenesis, gametogenesis, and some aspects of central nervous system (CNS) function. The following section will summarize the biological role of SCF and Kit in each of these organ systems.

A. Central Nervous System

The widespread expression of Kit and SCF in the CNS of adult animals was a surprising finding since the *W* and *Sl* mutant mice do not exhibit gross CNS abnormalities. However, a subtle abnormality has recently been demonstrated in *Ws/Ws* adult rats, which express a Kit mutant with impaired kinase activity. These rats have reduced long-term potentiation (LTP) in the mossy fiber–CA3 pathway of the hippocampus. Impaired spatial learning and memory in the Morris water maze test were also observed in these animals. *Sl/Sl*^{d} mice, which express the soluble but not the transmembrane form of SCF, are also known to have impaired hippocampal learning, but have normal LTP.

B. Gastrointestinal Tract

The ICCs are unusual cells in that they have characteristics of smooth muscle cells, fibroblasts, and neuronal cells. These are the only cells in the gastrointestinal tract (GI) tract that express Kit. The discovery of this exclusive expression of Kit revolutionized the study of these cells. Immunostaining for Kit *in situ* allowed visualization of the complex network that ICCs form throughout the GI tract. Although expression of Kit is universal among the ICCs, expression of other proteins varies, and there are different subpopulations of ICCs within the different regions of the GI tract.

ICCs have characteristics similar to cells of both neural crest and mesenchymal origins. However, studies in the late 1990s revealed that ICCs and the surrounding smooth muscle cells are both derived from mesenchymal precursors that express Kit. Precursors that contact SCF maintain Kit expression and develop into ICCs. Precursors that do not interact with SCF lose Kit expression and develop into smooth muscle cells. Mature smooth muscle cells express SCF, which is necessary for the maintenance of the ICC phenotype of their neighbors.

The ICCs are the pacemaker cells of the GI tract, generating and propagating the slow waves that control the frequency of contraction. Thus, the ICC network is essential to GI motility. These cells also integrate motor signals from the enteric nervous system. Kit signaling is essential to pacemaker function. Chronic exposure to antibodies specific for Kit or to inhibitors of signaling molecules

downstream of Kit [i.e., the phosphatidylinositol 3-kinase (PI3K) inhibitors Wortmannin and LY-294002] lead to the loss of slow waves and eventually reductions in the number of ICCs. Interestingly, some subpopulations of ICCs are more resistant to these treatments than others. Similarly, subpopulations of ICCs are altered to differing extents in mice with different *W* or *Sl* mutations.

C. Hematopoietic Cells

Expression of Kit and SCF is necessary for hematopoiesis in the fetal liver and in adult bone marrow. Kit is expressed primarily on hematopoietic stem cells, pluripotential progenitor cells, and early myeloid, lymphoid, erythroid, and megakaryocytic progenitors, whereas SCF is expressed by supporting stromal cells. SCF supports the survival of the stem cells and pluripotential progenitors, but induces only limited increases in proliferation as a single factor. However, SCF, in combination with certain other growth factors, strongly induces the proliferation of progenitors leading to a variety of lineages. SCF and erythropoietin stimulate the growth of erythroid progenitors. SCF and IL-3 induce the proliferation of progenitors that can differentiate into granulocytes, macrophages, and mast cells. SCF and thrombopoietin stimulate the growth of megakaryocytic progenitors. Expression of Kit decreases as differentiation progresses and is eventually lost altogether on most mature hematopoietic cells. Mast cells, activated platelets, and a subset of natural killer cells are the only fully differentiated hematopoietic cells that express Kit. SCF has a potent effect on mast cells and can induce them to migrate, proliferate, and degranulate.

D. Melanocytes

Expression of Kit and SCF is necessary for normal pigmentation of skin and hair. The precursors of melanocytes, the pigment-producing cells, arise in the neural crest in the embryo and migrate to the epidermis. The migratory path of the Kit-expressing melanocyte precursors is defined by SCF-expressing mesenchymal cells. Injection of pregnant mice with antibody that blocks binding of SCF during this phase of melanocyte migration leads to offspring that are almost completely lacking in pigmentation. However, injections that do not coincide with melanocyte migration do not alter pigmentation.

After birth, Kit is expressed in melanocytes in the hair follicles and skin, and SCF is expressed in keratinocytes. Hair follicles cycle between states of rest (telogen), active growth (anagen), and regression (catagen). Kit signaling is necessary for the replacement of melanocytes when the follicles progress from telogen to anagen. Injection of antibody specific for Kit into hair follicles at this stage leads to the growth of unpigmented hairs. However, if the injection is not repeated, the follicles produce fully pigmented hairs during their next anagenic phase. In addition to maintaining normal pigmentation in the skin, Kit signaling plays a role in hyperpigmentation in response to ultraviolet B (UVB) light. Both Kit expression and SCF expression increase in response to UVB light. Although the expression of other enzymes involved in melanin production is not dependent on Kit signaling, the expression of tyrosinase, the critical rate-limiting enzyme, is dependent on an increase in cyclic AMP levels mediated by Kit signaling. Thus, injection of anti-Kit antibodies into the skin prevents the hyperpigmentation response to UVB light.

E. Germ Cells

Expression of Kit and SCF is essential for the formation of primitive gonads in the embryo and for normal fertility in adult animals. Primordial germ cells (PGCs) in both sexes originate outside the genital ridge. PGCs express Kit, whereas cells in and on the way to the genital ridge express SCF. The PGCs follow a "trail" of SCF-expressing cells from their point of origin to the genital ridge. Along the way and at their destination, they proliferate. After the expansion of PGCs in the genital ridge, the primitive gonads differentiate into ovaries or testes, and Kit expression decreases and remains at low levels until the onset of puberty. Although Kit and SCF are crucial for the establishment of primitive gonads in both sexes, their role in adult reproductive function varies with sex. Certain *W* and *Sl* mutations cause infertility in one sex but not in the other.

In adult males, Kit is expressed by spermatogonia and primary spermatocytes, and SCF is expressed by Sertoli cells. Mature spermatozoa express a unique form of Kit that is severely truncated. This form of the protein may be involved in releasing the oocyte from arrest at fertilization. Injection of this protein into oocytes induces parthenogenesis. The necessity of both Kit and SCF is demonstrated by the infertility of male W^v and Sl^d mutant mice, which have reduced Kit function and a lack of transmembrane SCF, respectively.

In adult females, Kit is expressed in oocytes and theca cells, and SCF is expressed by the surrounding granulosa cells. Interaction between Kit and SCF is necessary for follicular development and maturation, but not ovulation and luteinization. There is also evidence that Kit signaling is involved in driving oocytes into meiotic arrest.

V. MECHANISMS OF ACTION

A. Receptor Dimerization and Autophosphorylation

As described above, Kit is a RTK. As a monomer, Kit is essentially inactive. Similar to other RTKs, the conformation of the juxtamembrane region imposes structural constraints that reduce spontaneous activation. This may be due to the formation of an α-helical structure by the unoccupied Kit monomer. Consequently, mutations in this region can activate Kit in the absence of ligand. Binding of SCF induces the rapid dimerization of Kit. This is likely promoted by interaction with noncovalently bound ligand dimers. *In vitro*, the first, second, and third Ig-like regions are sufficient to induce the dimerization of soluble forms of Kit. Biochemical data suggest that portions of the fourth immunoglobulin domain contribute to the dimerization of full-length Kit protein in cells. Ligand binding to wild-type Kit induces rapid increases in receptor autophosphorylation. Although the intracellular domain of Kit contains 22 tyrosine residues, autophosphorylation of only tyrosines 568, 570, 703, 721, 823, and 936 of human Kit has been confirmed.

B. Autophosphorylation of Kit and Initiation of Downstream Signaling Pathways

Multiple signal transduction components are activated after autophosphorylation of Kit. This occurs, in part, through recruitment of SH2-containing proteins to the Kit receptor complex via phosphorylated tyrosine residues. Two important residues in the recruitment of adapter proteins and signaling components to the human Kit receptor complex are tyrosines 568 and 570 in the juxtamembrane region. These are docking sites for Src family members, Shc and Chk (Csk-homologous kinase). In addition, the protein tyrosine phosphatases Shp1 and Shp2 have been reported to interact with tyrosines 569 and 567 on murine Kit, respectively. These correspond to tyrosines 570 and 568 on human Kit. Although most reports indicate that mutation of either of these residues has minimal effects on SCF-mediated growth, the mutation of both residues dramatically impairs growth. Thus, the juxtamembrane region is critical in providing docking sites for a variety of proteins involved in SCF signal transduction as well as maintaining inactive Kit monomers.

Of the signaling components shown to interact with the Kit juxtamembrane region, Src family members have been studied most extensively. Those activated by SCF include Lyn, Fyn, and likely Src and Yes, as well as others. Tyrosine 568 of human Kit is the predominant binding site for Src family members. Interestingly, mutation of this residue results in only subtle alterations in responses to SCF. In contrast, Lyn-deficient mast cells and hematopoietic progenitors have more dramatic abnormalities in SCF-mediated responses. Furthermore, data obtained with Src family inhibitors and dominant inhibitory mutants support an important role for this kinase family in Kit stimulus-response coupling mechanisms. This likely occurs through signaling components activated independent of tyrosine 568. Src family members contribute to the activation of the Jnk family of serine/threonine kinases. Jnks 1 and 2 contribute to the SCF-induced proliferation of mast cells.

Activation of the Ras–Raf–mitogen-activated protein (MAP) kinase cascade may also be initiated through the Kit juxtamembrane region in a Src-dependent manner. In transfected porcine aortic endothelial cells, mutation of tyrosine 570 reduces SCF-induced activation of ERKs and mutation of tyrosine 568 nearly eliminates it. Concomitant with this are decreases in the phosphorylation of Shc that are dependent on Src family members. In contrast, SCF has been reported to activate ERKs in mast cells expressing Y567F murine Kit. Thus, initiation of the ERK signaling pathway likely occurs through multiple sites on Kit. For example, in vitro studies have shown that growth factor receptor-binding protein 2 (Grb2) can bind tyrosine 703 or 936 in the kinase insert or carboxy-tail, respectively. Furthermore, ERKs may be activated through different mechanisms in distinct cell lineages

Tyrosine 721 in the kinase insert domain is another important autophosphorylation site on human Kit. Mutation of tyrosine 719, the corresponding residue in murine Kit, does not significantly impair Kit activity, but does eliminate recruitment of PI3K to the Kit receptor complex. Infection of mast cells with this mutant results in a reduction of SCF-induced adhesion of mast cells to fibronectin, as well as minor alterations in survival and growth. Similar defects have been observed in mast cells derived from mice engineered to express this mutant. In addition, significant defects in spermatogenesis occur in transgenic mice expressing Y719F Kit, but no alterations in pigmentation or steady state hematopoiesis were observed. Therefore, direct interaction of Kit and PI3K is essential for maturation of sperm and contributes to some aspects of SCF-mediated responses in mast cells, but is not required for Kit-dependent pigmentation or hematopoiesis. Interestingly, bone marrow mast cells derived from mice deficient for p85α PI3K had dramatic decreases in SCF-induced proliferation in vitro. Thus, PI3K also contributes to SCF-mediated responses through mechanisms independent of tyrosine 719.

Two signaling components activated downstream of PI3K are Akt and Jnks. Activation of Akt is dependent on the interaction of PI3K and Kit. Similar to numerous other growth factors, Akt contributes to the capacity of SCF to promote viability. In contrast, activation of Jnk1 and Jnk2 is involved in SCF-induced proliferation.

In the second catalytic domain, phosphorylation of tyrosine 821 of murine Kit (corresponding to tyrosine 823 of human Kit) makes critical contributions to the SCF-induced survival and proliferation of mast cells. Signaling components that interact with this site remain to be identified. Interestingly, tyrosine 821 is not required for SCF-induced activation of PI3K, Ras, or ERKs or for induction of c-myc, c-myb, c-fos, or junB.

Tyrosine 936 is an autophosphorylation site in the carboxy-tail of Kit. In vitro studies have shown that it binds to phospholipase Cγ (PLC-γ) and Grb7. The role of the interaction of these proteins with Kit in SCF-mediated responses is not known. Phosphorylation of PLC-γ requires tyrosine 728 in the kinase insert region of murine Kit. This is not critical for proliferation induced by soluble SCF but is required for responses to membrane-bound SCF.

C. Serine Phosphorylation of Kit

In addition to the important role of autophosphorylated tyrosine residues in Kit signaling, this receptor is also heavily phosphorylated on serine residues. A series of elegant studies by Lars Rönnstrand and co-workers demonstrated that protein kinase C (PKC) isoforms are responsible for serine phosphorylation of Kit at multiple sites. Serines 741 and 746 on human Kit are directly phosphorylated by PKC, and serines 821 and 959 are PKC-dependent sites. Serine phosphorylation reduces interaction of Kit with multiple SH2-containing proteins and is associated with decreased mitogenic responses to SCF as well as increased migration. Increased association with PI3K and increases in Akt activity have been observed in cells expressing Kit with serines 741 and 746 mutated.

D. Kit Signaling and the Janus Kinase/Signal Transducers and Activators of Transcription Pathway

The Janus kinase/signal transducers and activators of transcription (JAK/STAT) pathway is critical for responses mediated by ligands interacting with cytokine receptor superfamily members. Less is known about the activation of this pathway by RTKs such as Kit. We have shown that SCF rapidly and transiently activates JAK2. In addition, reduction in expression of JAK2 using antisense oligonucleotides partially impairs SCF-induced growth. The region of Kit coupling to activation of JAK2 remains to be identified. SCF also activates Stat family members, including Stat1 and Stat5. Stat1 interacts with tyrosine residues in the second catalytic domain of Kit, whereas full activation of Stat5 requires the carboxy-tail of Kit. Stat3 is also phosphorylated on serine residues after stimulation with SCF. Importantly, activation of the JAK/STAT pathway is extremely rapid, transient, and lineage-specific. One means of negatively regulating this pathway could be through Socs1 (suppressor of cytokine signaling). This protein interacts with Kit and constitutive expression reduces SCF-induced growth. Shp1 is also a negative regulator of Kit signaling that may down-regulate JAK2 activity. A summary of the structure–function relationships of the intracellular region of Kit is summarized in Fig. 1. Furthermore, some of the signaling pathways activated by Kit are shown in Fig. 2.

E. Signaling through Different Receptor and Ligand Isoforms

Two isoforms of human Kit result from alternate splicing of mRNA. This results in the insertion of a 4-amino-acid sequence just proximal to the membrane-spanning region in the extracellular domain. Although the biological significance of this insert remains unclear, recent studies suggest differences in internalization, signaling, and possibly transforming activity of these isoforms. Differences in the signaling of soluble and membrane-bound SCF have also been reported. The kinetics of ligand-induced phosphory-

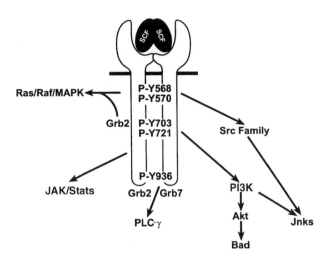

FIGURE 2 Signaling pathways activated by Kit. SCF binds Kit, induces dimerization, and increases autophosphorylation activity of this receptor tyrosine kinase. The indicated autophosphorylation sites recruit signaling components coupled to the biochemical pathways indicated.

lation of Kit are more protracted after stimulation with membrane-bound SCF than with soluble SCF. Thus, this isoform may be more biologically potent. Furthermore, PI3K and PLC-γ may make different contributions to biological responses mediated by soluble SCF versus membrane-bound SCF.

F. Transcription Factors: Activation and/or Induction

As described above, Stat family members phosphorylated after stimulation with SCF include Stat1, Stat3, and Stat5. SCF-induced increases in the DNA-binding activity of both Stat1 and Stat5 have also been reported. Both of these proteins interact with Kit, but it remains to be determined whether Kit directly activates Stat family members or whether nonreceptor kinases such as JAK2 or a Src family member are upstream activators. *In vitro* studies have shown that Kit can phosphorylate Stat1 directly. The role of these events in SCF-mediated responses is yet to be established.

The micropthalmia transcription (Mi) factor is a member of the basic/helix-loop-helix/leucine zipper family. It is highly tissue-specific and expressed in both melanocytes and mast cells. Mice or humans lacking this protein have defects in pigmentation and a reduction in mast cell numbers. Signaling through Kit results in serine phosphorylation of Mi via activation of ERKs. This increases the transcriptional activity of Mi by increasing association with the transcriptional co-activator p300/CREB-binding protein (where CREB is Ca^{2+}/cAMP-response element-binding protein).

One family of transcription factors regulated downstream of Akt is the forkhead family. Recent studies indicate that SCF induces the phosphorylation of FOXO1a, 3a, and 4. This did not require the activation of ERKs, p38, or PKC but did require PI3K.

SCF also induces the expression of a variety of immediate-early response genes that are transcription factors. These include c-myc, c-fos, junB, c-myb, and egr-1.

VI. PATHOPHYSIOLOGY

A. Preliminary Comments

As discussed above, Kit makes important contributions to the development and function of hematopoietic, germ cell, and pigmented tissues. It is also important in terms of the function of different aspects of the CNS and the GI tract. The critical nature of Kit in normal physiology is highlighted by the aberrations resulting from the absence of functional Kit or its ligand SCF. In addition, a number of diseases are associated with overexpression or gain-of-function mutations.

B. Gain-of-Function Mutations

The Kit proto-oncogene was identified after the discovery of the v-*Kit* oncogene in the Hardy–Zuckerman strain of feline sarcoma virus. The v-Kit protein contains the catalytic domain and kinase insert region of Kit, but is missing the extracellular domain, as well as portions of the carboxyl-tail and juxtamembrane region. The capacity of Kit to be usurped by a retrovirus as a transforming protein suggested that alterations in the expression or activity of this kinase could be involved in other disease processes. Indeed, in the past decade, gain-of-function mutations in Kit have been identified and associated with a variety of human diseases including gastrointestinal stromal cell tumors (GISTs), mastocytosis, leukemia, lymphoma, germ cell tumors, and small cell carcinoma of the lung.

Two regions of Kit where gain-of-function mutations occur with high frequency are the juxtamembrane region and the second catalytic domain. As described earlier, the secondary structure of the juxtamembrane region maintains the unoccupied receptor in a conformation that inhibits catalytic activity. Mutations in this region alter this configuration and often result in increases in Kit kinase activity in the absence of ligand. The second catalytic domain is the ATP-binding pocket and is another hotspot for activating mutations of Kit. Mutations in the analogous region of Flt3, Met, Ron, and Ret also activate these RTKs.

Gain-of-function mutations in the second catalytic domain of Kit were originally described in mastocytoma cell lines of human, mouse, and rat origin in the early 1990s. More recently, mutations in this region have been found in patients with a variety of different diseases, many of which involve hematopoietic cells. In 1995, mutations in codon 816 of Kit were first described in patients with mastocytosis. Mutations in this region have also been found in some patients with core binding factor leukemias, sinonasal lymphomas, and germ cell tumors. Interestingly, patients with more than one of these conditions have been reported. Mastocytosis can be associated with myeloproliferative disease. Patients with both mastocytosis and germ cell tumors have also been reported.

In 1998, mutations in the juxtamembrane region of Kit were found in patients with GISTs. Interestingly, these mutations occur at higher frequencies in patients with malignant GIST than in those with benign tumors. Malignant GIST is extremely resistant to chemo- and radiotherapy. In 2001, astonishing improvement in a patient with malignant GIST was reported after treatment with STI571, an inhibitor of bcr-abl, Kit, and the PDGF receptor. Subsequent to these findings, the results of several clinical trials indicate that this drug is tremendously beneficial in the treatment of patients with malignant GISTs. *In vitro*, STI571 inhibits the kinase activity of Kit juxtamembrane mutants at lower concentrations than wild-type Kit. Furthermore, cells expressing this form of mutant Kit undergo apoptosis after exposure to this drug. Thus, targeted inhibition of mutant Kit shows great promise in the treatment of GIST.

C. Alterations in Expression of Kit

In acute myeloid leukemia (AML), large percentages of patients express Kit on leukemic blast cells. This has led to speculation that Kit may be a molecular target for the treatment of AML. Treatment of one AML patient refractory to standard chemotherapy regimens with the Kit inhibitors SU5416 and SU6668 induced remission. However, it remains to be determined whether this approach will be helpful in the management of this disease in the majority of patients.

Inappropriate expression of Kit, SCF, or both has been reported in patients with breast cancer, small cell carcinoma of the lung (SCCL), melanoma, and some tumors of the CNS. Among these diseases, the role of Kit and SCF expression in SCCL and melanoma have been studied most extensively. Therefore, the remainder of this section will focus on studies relating to these two diseases.

Although Kit plays an important role in the development of melanocytes, expression in mature melanocytes may lead to apoptosis. Interestingly, decreases in Kit expression have been observed in tissues from melanoma patients. A strong correlation between reductions in the transcription factor activator protein-2 (AP-2) and Kit expression have been reported. Since the Kit reporter contains multiple AP-2 sites, the loss of AP-2 may lead to a reduction in the expression of Kit and facilitate the escape of melanoma cells from SCF-induced apoptosis. Ectopic expression of Kit in a melanoma cell line dramatically reduced metastatic potential *in vivo*.

In contrast to melanoma, co-expression of Kit and SCF contributes to autocrine growth of SCCL.

Seventy percent of SCCL cell lines or primary tumor specimens co-express Kit and its ligand. The role of this putative autocrine loop in the growth of these cells has been illustrated by several approaches. Ectopic expression of a dominant-inhibitory Kit mutant, as well as treatment with drugs that inhibit Kit activity such as AG1296, STI571, SU5416 and SU6597, dramatically inhibits the growth of SCCL cells.

D. Loss-of-Function Mutations

The phenotypes of the various *W* and *Sl* mutant mice demonstrate the critical role of SCF and Kit in germ cell development, pigmentation, and hematopoiesis, as well as in the functioning of the intestinal tract and portions of the CNS. Reviews extensively describing these animals are listed under Further Reading. This section will briefly summarize the effect of mutations in the Kit or SCF genes in each of these organ systems in mice and indicate whether corresponding defects have been noted in humans.

Mutations in Kit have been associated with defects in pigmentation in mice, rats, pigs, and humans. This may also contribute to roan coloring in horses. In humans, loss-of-function mutations in one allele of Kit are associated with autosomal

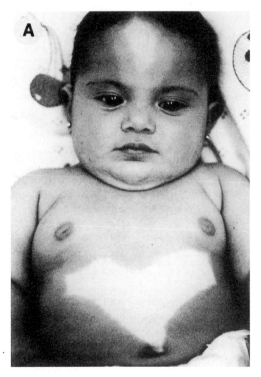 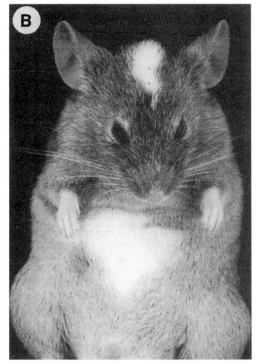

FIGURE 3 Loss-of-function mutations in one allele of Kit cause alterations in pigmentation in humans and mice. Reprinted from Fleischman *et al.* (1991) *Proc. Natl. Acad. Sci. USA* **88**, p. 10885, with permission.

dominant piebaldism. Mutations in the first catalytic domain of human Kit have been observed in many of these patients. Similar to *W* and *Sl* mice, which are heterozygotes for dominant inhibitory mutations, white spots are observed on the ventral trunk, forehead, and extremities. Shown in Fig. 3 are a child and a mouse that are both heterozygotes for the identical loss-of-function mutation in Kit.

Kit contributes to the development of the interstitial cells of Cajal and these cells are important in the pacemaker activity of the gastrointestinal tract. The importance of Kit in normal intestinal function is highlighted by the abnormality in intestinal pacemaker activity in *W* mice. In humans with autosomal dominant piebaldism, there is an increased frequency of megacolon and other gastrointestinal difficulties. Loss of ICCs is associated with motility disorders in human (e.g., Hirschsprung's disease) and other animals (e.g., grass sickness in horses).

W and *Sl* mice also have dramatic alterations in hematopoietic tissue. The more severe variants are mast cell deficient and have macrocytic anemia. The anemia results from decreases in numbers of erythroid progenitors, particularly those corresponding to CFUe (colony forming unit erythroid). No dramatic defects in hematopoiesis have been noted in humans with mutations in Kit. However, the patients examined have had mutations in only one allele of the Kit gene. Similarly, heterozygotic *W* mice have very mild alterations in hematopoietic tissue. Thus, it is unknown whether Kit plays the same nonredundant role in hematopoiesis in humans as it does in mice.

The gene products for both Kit and SCF are expressed at high levels in the murine hippocampus. As discussed previously, mice and rats with mutations in SCF or Kit have deficits in hippocampal-dependent learning. In addition, there are reductions in numbers of sensory nerves in some *W* and *Sl* mice, as well as reports of auditory deficiencies in rats with mutations in Kit. In humans, retardation and sensorineural deafness have been reported in patients with autosomal dominant piebaldism.

The development of both sperm and oocytes requires functional Kit and SCF. Mice with severe defects in either gene product are sterile. Exciting recent studies demonstrate that the interaction of Kit with PI3K is required for spermatogenesis in mice. More subtle alterations in oogenesis may also depend on the association of PI3K and Kit. In humans, reductions in Kit may be linked to defects in sperm development. Kit is also a candidate gene for contributions to ovarian failure.

VII. SUMMARY

SCF binds the receptor tyrosine kinase Kit. Interaction of this ligand and receptor induces rapid autophosphorylation of Kit, dimerization, and activation of multiple signaling components, including Src family members, the JAK/STAT pathway, the Ras–Raf–MAP kinase cascade, PI3K, and PLCγ. SCF promotes the survival, growth, and maturation of stem cells from multiple lineages. In addition, when combined with other growth factors, SCF is potently synergistic. Loss of expression of either Kit or SCF is lethal in mice. Mice with mutations resulting in reductions in expression or function of Kit or SCF have defects in pigmentation and hematopoiesis, are mast cell deficient, and have reproductive difficulties. Mutations resulting in the activation of Kit in the absence of ligand are associated with human diseases, including GISTs, mastocytosis, sinonasal lymphomas, germ cell tumors, and some myeloid leukemias. Inappropriate co-expression of Kit and SCF has been implicated in SCCL, and down-regulation of Kit on melanocytes may contribute to metastatic melanoma.

Glossary

hematopoiesis Development of multiple lineages of blood cells from a pluripotential stem cell. These include red blood cells, platelets, lymphocytes (T and B), natural killer cells, monocytes, and granulocytes (neutrophils, eosinophils, and mast cells). This process is regulated by soluble and membrane-bound growth factors, cell contact, and interaction with the extracellular matrix.

receptor tyrosine kinase Membrane-spanning protein that binds ligand via the extracellular domain and contains a protein tyrosine kinase in the intracellular domain. Interaction with ligand promotes dimerization and subsequent increases in the catalytic activity of the kinase.

signal transduction The process of transferring information from the extracellular milieu to the cellular interior and ultimately into the nucleus. This biochemical process is integral to the control of cellular survival, growth, development, and function.

See Also the Following Articles

Angiogenesis ● Erythropoietin, Biochemistry of ● Protein Kinases

Further Reading

Blume-Jensen, P., and Hunter, T. (2001). Oncogenic kinase signaling. *Nature* **411**, 355–365.

Broudy, V. C. (1997). Stem cell factor and hematopoiesis. *Blood* **90**, 1345–1364.

Downward, J. (2001). The ins and outs of signalling. *Nature* **411**, 759–762.

Galli, S. J., Zsebo, K. M., and Geissler, E. N. (1994). The kit ligand, stem cell factor. *Adv. Immunol.* **55**, 1–97.

Heinrich, M. C., Blanke, C. D., Druker, B. J., and Corless, C. L. (2002). Inhibition of KIT tyrosine kinase activity: A novel molecular approach to the treatment of KIT-positive malignancies. *J. Clin. Oncol.* **20**, 1692–1703.

Keller, J. R., and Linnekin, D. M. (2000). Stem cell factor. *In* "The Cytokine Reference: A Compendium of Cytokines and Other Mediators of Host Defense" (J. J. Oppenheim, M. Feldmann, S. K. Durum, T. Hirano and N. Nicola, eds.), pp. 877–897. Academic Press, London.

Linnekin, D. (1999). Early signaling pathways activated by c-Kit in hematopoietic cells. *Int. J. Biochem. Cell Biol.* **31**, 1053–1074.

Linnekin, D., and Keller, J. R. (2000). Stem cell factor receptor. *In* "The Cytokine Reference: A Compendium of Cytokines and Other Mediators of Host Defense" (J. J. Oppenheim, M. Feldmann, S. K. Durum, T. Hirano and N. Nicola, eds.), pp. 1913–1934. Academic Press, London.

Longley, J. B., Reguera, M. J., and Yongsheng, M. (2001). Classes of c-kit activating mutations: Proposed mechanisms of action and implications for disease classification and therapy. *Leukemia Res.* **25**, 571–576.

Steroid Hormone Receptor Family: Mechanisms of Action

Milan K. Bagchi

University of Illinois, Urbana-Champaign

The steroid hormones, which include the sex steroids (estrogen, progesterone, and androgens) and adrenal steroids (glucocorticoids and mineralocorticoids), have long been known to control the growth, development, and homeostasis of various mammalian tissues.

I. INTRODUCTION

The biological action of a steroid hormone is mediated by its cognate intracellular receptor, which regulates the expression of a specific set of genes in the nucleus. The steroid receptors belong to a large, evolutionarily related family of transcription factors, known as the nuclear receptor (NR) superfamily. This family, which has 48 members, also includes the receptors for thyroid hormones, retinoic acids, and vitamin D as well as receptors for a variety of other metabolic ligands. Many orphan receptors, for which the ligands remain undiscovered, also belong to this family. The signal transduction pathway of the NRs has been studied extensively as a model system to investigate the fundamental mechanisms of eukaryotic gene regulation. These studies have provided a blueprint for the mechanism of action of these important cellular regulatory molecules. The goal of this article is to provide a brief overview of the current mechanistic concepts and emerging models of the NR pathway.

II. FUNCTIONAL DOMAINS OF NUCLEAR RECEPTORS

Biochemical, molecular genetic, and structure–function analyses during the mid to late 1980s revealed that the NRs possess a modular structure containing discrete functional domains consistent with their role as ligand-inducible transcription factors (Fig. 1). Generally, the receptor structure is composed of three principal modules: (1) an evolutionarily conserved DNA-binding domain (DBD), which anchors the NR to its target DNA, (2) a somewhat less conserved carboxy-terminal ligand-binding domain (LBD), and (3) a poorly conserved amino-terminal activation function region, AF-1. A flexible hinge region (D) joins the DBD and LBD. Mutational analysis of the LBD led to the identification of a highly conserved second activation function region, AF-2, which is

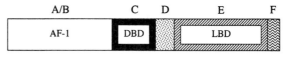

FIGURE 1 Functional domains (A/B, C, D, E, and F) of a prototype nuclear hormone receptor. The DBD (C) and LBD (EF) represent DNA- and ligand-binding domains, respectively. AF-1 (A/B) and AF-2 (F) indicate constitutive and ligand-inducible transcriptional activation function regions, respectively.

essential for ligand-dependent activation by NRs. In certain receptors, such as thyroid hormone and retinoic acid receptors, the LBD functions as a repression domain in the absence of ligand. In addition, the LBD contains signals for receptor homo- and/or heterodimerization and nuclear localization. The LBD is, therefore, a uniquely important domain involved in many aspects of receptor function.

III. HORMONE-INDUCED ACTIVATION

Hormones play a pivotal role in activating NRs. A steroid receptor is functionally inactive in cells in the absence of its cognate hormone. Several lines of evidence suggest that the unliganded receptor exists in an oligomeric complex in association with several heat-shock proteins, which are thought to function as chaperone proteins. In this inactive state, the receptor does not interact with DNA. Hormone binding leads to the disaggregation of the receptor from heat-shock proteins and converts it to a form that is able to bind DNA. For certain steroid receptors, such as the glucocorticoid and mineralocorticoid receptors, ligand binding occurs in the cytoplasm of target cells, inducing nuclear translocation of the ligand–receptor complex. Although the hormone-occupied receptors are always localized in the nucleus, many of the NRs are found in the nuclear compartment even in the absence of their cognate ligands. Certain NRs, such as thyroid hormone receptor (TR) and retinoic acid receptor (RAR), bind to DNA in the unliganded state and function as transcriptional repressors of target genes.

Hormone binding triggers a striking conformational change in the LBD of the receptor. Crystal structures of various NR LBDs complexed with agonist or antagonist ligand have thrown considerable light on the molecular nature of this structural change. In the absence of ligand, the LBD structure, which is composed of 12 contiguous α-helices, has a fairly open conformation. The hormone fits into a hydrophobic pocket formed by different layers of helices and directly contacts several amino acid residues of the receptor. On hormone binding, the LBD assumes a rather compact conformation. Comparison of the crystal structures of unliganded and liganded NRs suggested that hormone binding induces a dramatic repositioning of helix 12. Whereas in the unliganded NR, helix 12 extends away from the LBD, in the liganded receptor, this helix folds back tightly against the body of the LBD and makes contacts with the ligand itself. This ligand-induced rearrangement creates a surface consisting of residues contributed by helices 3, 4, and 12 that is utilized by the hormone-bound receptor for interaction with transcriptional co-regulators, such as co-activators (see below), which play critical roles in the hormonal signal transduction pathways.

IV. TARGET DNA RECOGNITION

A critical step in the hormone-response pathway of NRs is the recognition of the target gene by the receptor. This may occur through direct interaction of the DBD with specific enhancer sequences referred to as hormone-response elements (HREs) or through protein–protein interactions with other classes of DNA-bound transcription factors, such as activating protein 1 (AP-1) or Sp1, at the target promoter. For the classical steroid receptors, estrogen receptor (ER), glucocorticoid receptor (GR), progesterone receptor (PR), androgen receptor (AR), and mineralocortocoid receptor (MR), the response elements contain a 15 bp core sequence, composed of two half-sites of 6 bp (AGAACA for GR, PR, AR, and MR; AGGTCA for ER) arranged in a dyad axis of symmetry (palindromic). The half-sites are separated by 3 bp of random composition. These receptors bind to their response elements as head-to-head homodimers. DNA recognition by these NRs involves contacts of amino acids present in two interdependent zinc-finger structures in the DBD with specific base pairs within the major groove of the core HRE motif and the phosphate backbone.

Nonsteroid receptors, such as the TR, RAR, and vitamin D receptor (VDR), bind to response elements that contain direct repeats of a core recognition motif, AGGTCA. These receptors bind mostly as heterodimers with the retinoid X receptor (RXR). A RXR–TR heterodimer can bind to response elements consisting of direct repeats or inverted palindromes of the core AGGTCA motif. The number of base pairs separating the direct repeats of the core recognition motif determines DNA-binding specificities of different heterodimeric pairs. For example, direct repeats separated by 3, 4, and 5 bp represent response elements for VDR, TR, and RAR, respectively.

V. TRANSCRIPTIONAL ACTIVATION

In a target cell, a DNA- and hormone-bound NR is thought to regulate gene expression by influencing local chromatin structure and enhancing the transcription initiation process at the target promoter. Studies exploiting steroid receptor-regulated *in vitro* gene expression systems indicated that the promoter-bound receptor stimulates transcriptional initiation by facilitating the formation of a stable preinitiation complex containing RNA polymerase II and other basal transcription factors. The precise mechanism by which the receptor achieves this effect remains to be determined. The receptor may promote transcription initiation by facilitating recognition of the promoter by a certain initiation factor(s) or simply by stabilizing the promoter DNA–protein complex once it is formed or perhaps by influencing both reactions. Recent work from a number of laboratories indicates that a class of mediator proteins, termed co-activators, is recruited by the receptor to modify chromatin structure. The co-activators may also function as signaling intermediates between the hormone-occupied receptors and the RNA polymerase II transcription machinery.

A surprisingly large number of nuclear receptor-interacting proteins that may serve as co-activators have been isolated using yeast two-hybrid screening, far Western cloning, and biochemical methods based on NR affinity chromatography. A hallmark of these putative co-activators is that they interact with the nuclear receptors in a ligand-dependent manner and enhance their transcriptional activity. The steroid receptor co-activator-1 (SRC-1), which stimulates transactivation by several nuclear hormone receptors, was the first co-activator reported for the NR superfamily. Additional receptor-interacting proteins, TIF2/GRIP1 and pCIP/ACTR/RAC3/AIB1, which show striking structural similarity to SRC-1, were soon isolated by other laboratories. The remarkable similarity in amino acid sequence among these proteins, all of which exhibit an approximate molecular size of 160 kDa, indicates the existence of a p160 family of nuclear receptor co-activators.

In addition to the p160 family of proteins, several other potential co-activators have been described. Prominent among these is the transcriptional co-activator CREB-binding protein (CBP, where CREB denotes Ca^{2+}/cyclic AMP response element-binding protein) and its homologue p300. It is believed that CBP/p300 is recruited as a secondary co-activator of NRs through its direct interaction with primary p160 co-activators. There is strong biochemical evidence that CBP/p300 co-exists with one or more p160 proteins in a large receptor-co-activation complex. These co-activators work together in a synergistic fashion to enhance ligand-dependent transactivation mediated by nuclear receptors. Microinjection of an anti-SRC-1 or anti-CBP antibody into cultured cells partially blocked ligand-dependent gene activation by

PR, ER, and other nuclear receptors. Most importantly, gene knockout studies show that loss of SRC-1 function partially impaired the physiological actions of several NRs.

A CBP-associated factor (p/CAF), the mammalian homologue of yeast GCN5, is reported to interact with CBP and the p160 proteins, as well as directly with NR LBDs. p/CAF is also reported to function as a co-activator of several NRs. Interestingly, all three co-activators, p160s, CBP, and p/CAF, possess intrinsic histone acetyltransferase (HAT) activities, suggesting that they might function as chromatin remodelers. Furthermore, CBP has been shown to interact directly with the components of the RNA polymerase II machinery. Collectively, these results indicate that the p160 family of proteins, CBP/p300, and possibly additional co-factors like p/CAF act in unison with the activated nuclear receptors to remodel chromatin structure and then directly recruit the basal transcription apparatus to effect steroid-dependent gene activation.

Another class of co-activator that plays a critical role in NR-mediated transactivation is the thyroid receptor-associated protein/vitamin D receptor-interacting protein (TRAP/DRIP) complex, comprising 13–15 polypeptides. This complex interacts with the LBD of many NRs in a hormone-dependent manner. A single subunit, TRAP220/DRIP205, anchors the entire complex to the LBD and enhances NR-mediated transactivation in an *in vitro* chromatin-free transcription system. Additional protein–protein interactions between the TRAP/DRIP150 subunit and the AF-1 of GR have been documented. Unlike the p160/CBP complex, the TRAP/DRIP complex is devoid of HAT activity. Several subunits of the TRAP/DRIP complex are also present in a mammalian complex corresponding to the yeast mediator complex that associates with the RNA polymerase II holoenzyme. These findings raise the possibility that the TRAP/DRIP complex, once recruited by a NR, may stimulate transcription by directly contacting and influencing the activity of the RNA polymerase II machinery at the core promoter.

The fact that the p160/CBP complex possesses HAT activity but the TRAP/DRIP complex does not has led to the proposal that these co-activator complexes interact with the receptor in a two-step sequential manner to effect transcriptional activation. According to this hypothesis, the NR initially recruits the SRC/CBP complex, which remodels and opens up the chromatin. This is followed by the recruitment of the TRAP/DRIP complex, which interacts with and stimulates the activity of the RNA polymerase II initiation apparatus. Although this is an attractive model, it is not clear how a strict temporal order of recruitment can be maintained or an efficient exchange of co-activators can be achieved. Furthermore, one also needs to consider the possibility that these co-activators function in parallel pathways of receptor-dependent activation, which might be operative in a promoter-specific manner.

Ligand binding to a NR acts as a switch for co-activator recruitment. For steroid receptors such as the GR, ER, and PR, ligand-induced release of receptor-associated heat-shock proteins likely precedes co-activator binding. For certain other receptors such as TR and RAR, ligand-dependent displacement of co-repressors might be a necessary prerequisite for co-activator action. In both cases, the ligand-induced conformational change in the receptor LBD generates a surface to which the co-activator protein docks. Recent studies in several laboratories indicated that multiple conserved leucine-rich sequences, termed NR boxes, exist in the p160 family of co-activators. These NR boxes contain the signature LXXLL motif, where L is leucine and X is any amino acid. An amphipathic helical peptide containing a LXXLL motif mediates the interaction of the co-activator with the LBDs of various nuclear receptors. The leucine residues 1 and 5 form intimate contacts with well-conserved amino acids within the core hydrophobic pocket of the LBD. The residues immediately surrounding the LXXLL motif determine receptor specificity. Crystal structure data support the view that two LXXLL motifs of a single SRC-1 molecule may interact with the individual AF2 domains of both subunits of a NR homo- or heterodimer. Recent studies also indicate that the AF-1 domains of several steroid receptors have the ability to interact with and recruit p160 co-activators, although the molecular basis of this interaction is unclear. One can envision that the co-activator molecule, once docked via interaction with AF-1 or AF-2, may then function as a physical bridge between the transactivation domain of the receptor and the RNA polymerase II transcription machinery during gene activation. Further studies are clearly necessary to test this plausible mechanism.

VI. TRANSCRIPTIONAL REPRESSION

Transcriptional repression by ligand-bound NRs is well documented. Typically, overexpression of a given nuclear receptor ("interfering receptor") in a transient transfection system often results in the repression of ligand-induced transcriptional activation of target genes by another member of the superfamily ("activating receptor"). Such mutually antagonistic interactions have been described between various pairwise combinations of the steroid receptors ER, GR, PR, and TR and also between NRs and AP-1. No DNA binding by the interfering receptor is required for this effect. Conceptually, transcriptional interference or "squelching" occurs due to the interaction of the activation domains of nuclear receptors with a common but limiting target protein, such as a co-activator, in their signaling pathways. Consistent with this hypothesis, overexpression of SRC-1 appears to alleviate the antagonistic competition between liganded ER and PR in a cell. Similar overexpression of CBP/p300 was also noted to partially overcome the antagonistic interplay between GR and AP1, indicating that this co-activator could be a limiting component common to both signal transduction pathways.

Another mode of transcriptional repression, termed silencing, is displayed by certain nuclear receptors, such as TR and RAR. These receptors actively repress the transcription of cellular genes bearing the cognate hormone-response elements. In the absence of hormone, TR or RAR binds to its response element in a ligand-independent manner and functions as a silencer of basal level transcription from the target promoter. Ligand binding to the receptor releases transcriptional silencing and leads to the activation of target gene expression. The mechanism of this ligand-induced switch from repression to activation of gene expression is a topic of intense investigation in many laboratories.

Recent studies indicated that transcriptional silencing by TR or RAR is dictated, in part, by the association of the receptor with cellular co-repressors. A number of candidate co-repressors have been described among which two distinct but structurally related co-repressors, NR co-repressor (NCoR) and silencing mediator of retinoid and thyroid receptors (SMRT), have been studied most extensively. NCoR/SMRT harbors multiple independent repression domains, which contribute to its overall repression function. The co-repressor uses its carboxy-terminal receptor interaction domain to interact with unliganded TR or RAR but fails to interact with the ligand-occupied receptors. Within the receptor interaction domain of the co-repressor, two CoRNR boxes containing I/LXXI/VI signature motifs mediate interactions with the unliganded LBD. These amphipathic helical sequences are reminiscent of the LXXLL motifs found in the co-activator. It is likely that one NCoR/SMRT molecule is bound per DNA-bound heterodimer, with each CoRNR box contacting a single NR LBD.

The critical determinants of receptor–co-repressor interaction appear to be the presence of the I/LXXI/VI motifs in the co-repressor and the structure of the NR LBD. Although the co-repressor uses the same hydrophobic pocket in the NR LBD that is used by the co-activator, there are important differences. The AF-2 helix is clearly inhibitory to co-repressor binding. In the unliganded receptor, this helix is displaced outside the ligand-binding pocket, allowing the co-repressor to bind. Ligand binding triggers a dramatic change in the position of helix 12, resulting in the displacement of the co-repressor and formation of the co-activator-binding surface. Ligand-induced exchange of co-repressors with co-activators can conceivably take place without the receptor coming off the DNA.

Recent biochemical studies indicate that NCoR/SMRT exists in a large multiprotein complex containing histone deacetylase 3 (HDAC3) and additional polypeptides such as WD40 repeat protein TBL1 and G-protein suppressor 2. Although HDAC3 is the most prevalent histone deacetylase that was found biochemically to be associated with the co-repressor complex, there are reports that NCoR/SMRT associates with Sin 3, HDAC1, and HDAC2. Once anchored to the DNA-bound NR, the co-repressor complex apparently utilizes the histone deacetylase to maintain a repressive chromatin state. In addition, one can envisage that one or more repression domains of the recruited co-repressor may directly contact critical components of the basal transcription machinery and negatively impact the assembly of a functional initiation complex.

NCoR and SMRT are also involved in the transcriptional repression pathway of nuclear receptors other than TR and RAR. Most interestingly, estrogen or progesterone receptor complexed with certain antagonist ligands recruits these co-repressors to the target promoter to block transcription. In tamoxifen- or raloxifen-bound estrogen receptor, due to the presence of an additional side chain in the antagonist, helix 12 is positioned improperly. Helix 12, instead of packing normally as in the hormone-bound LBD, overlaps with the surface that docks the co-activator. This ligand-specified variation prevents co-activator interaction and facilitates co-repressor binding. The recruited co-repressor then negatively modulates the transcriptional activity of the target promoter.

VII. REGULATION OF CHROMATIN STRUCTURE

In the cell, the transcription units are packaged into nucleosomes and remain in a repressed state. An essential first step in the NR-dependent gene activation pathway is, therefore, chromatin remodeling. Several multisubunit ATP-dependent chromatin-remodeling complexes, such as yeast SWI/SNF or *Drosophila* ISWI, which use the energy of ATP to alter nucleosome structure, have been characterized. Brg1, a subunit of human SWI/SNF, interacts with the GR and is required for efficient receptor-dependent activation of a MMTV (mouse mammary tumor virus) promoter stably integrated into chromosomal DNA. Brg1 is also recruited to an ER-regulated promoter in response to the hormone and critically regulates the transcriptional activity of the receptor. Furthermore, the addition of purified Brg1 to an *in vitro* transcription system reconstituted from chromatinized templates facilitated RAR-dependent transactivation. Taken together, these results point to an important role of ATP-dependent chromatin remodelers in NR-mediated gene activation.

NR-associated factors can also remodel chromatin by modulating acetylation of histones in nucleosomes. Whereas certain co-activators are found to possess intrinsic histone acetyltransferase activity, the co-repressors are associated with histone deacetylases. It is known that hyperacetylation of the lysine-rich tails of histones H3 and H4 on a chromatin DNA can destabilize nucleosomes and facilitate the binding of transcription factors to the promoter regulatory elements, leading to gene activation. Hypoacetylation of acetylated H3 and H4 by deacetylases, on the other hand, creates a repressive chromatin conformation, leading to gene repression. It is therefore postulated that targeted recruitment of acetyltransferase or deacetylase to a particular gene may modulate its transcriptional activity. The recruitment of a co-repressor by a promoter-bound receptor is thought to induce local hypoacetylation of histones to create a repressive chromatin conformation, leading to gene repression. The recruitment of a co-activator, in contrast, would lead to local hyperacetylation of histones, which may destabilize nucleosomes on a chromatin DNA. This, in turn, is likely to allow the binding of a RNA polymerase II transcription initiation complex at the core promoter, leading to gene activation. Consistent with this hypothesis, many of the candidate nuclear receptor co-activators, such as CBP, p/CAF, and SRC-1/p160, are known to possess intrinsic histone acetyltransferase activity. Additionally, recent reports suggested that CBP/p300 or SRC-1 enhanced steroid receptor-dependent transactivation from a chromatinized hormone-responsive template. It has been shown that this effect involves the acetylation of histones and is critically dependent on HAT activity of CBP/p300.

Unliganded TR functions as a repressor of a target promoter by recruiting a co-repressor complex containing histone deacetylase to the promoter. In the presence of thyroid hormone, the co-repressor complex containing the deacetylase is released from the promoter-bound receptor, thereby relieving the transcriptional repression. The receptor then recruits a co-activator complex, which consists of one or more histone acetyltransferases, to promote gene activation. The co-activators and co-repressors appear to act by regulating histone acetylation at the target promoter in an opposing fashion (Fig. 2).

In addition to acetylation, other covalent modifications, such as phosphorylation, methylation, and ubiquitination of histones and nonhistone proteins, have been known to modulate NR function at the target promoter. There is ample evidence that phosphorylation via various kinase cascades influences the transactivation activity of several members of the steroid receptor superfamily such as the GR, PR, and ER. There is now evidence that specific phosphorylation events may modulate co-activator recruitment and function. For example, mitogen-activated protein kinase (MAPK)-induced phosphorylation of specific

serine residues in the AF-1 of ER-β facilitates SRC-1 recruitment by the tamoxifen-complexed receptor. In contrast, MAPK-induced phosphorylation in the amino-terminus of peroxisome proliferator-activated receptor-γ leads to inhibition of receptor function.

Most striking among the hormone- and NR-induced chemical modifications at the target promoter is the methylation of nucleosome and transcriptional co-factors by a family of arginine-specific methyltransferases. The p160 co-activators, anchored to promoter-bound NRs, recruit the co-activator-associated methyltransferase 1 (CARM1). Interestingly, the carboxy-terminal region of p160 proteins contains distinct binding sites for both CARM1 and CBP/p300. Consistent with this scenario, CARM1 and p300 synergistically stimulate transactivation by ER and this synergism is dependent on the presence of a p160 co-activator. Whereas CARM1 methylates specific arginine residues in histone H3, CBP/p300 possesses intrinsic HAT activity. It is therefore conceivable that CARM1 and p300 cooperate to induce multiple concurrent histone modifications to induce efficient chromatin remodeling, which allows subsequent recruitment of the transcription machinery. It is also interesting to note that CARM1 and CBP/p300 can undergo direct protein–protein interaction with each other. A functional consequence of this interaction is methylation of CBP/p300 by CARM1. Although the methylated CBP/p300 retains HAT activity and can still act as a co-activator for NR-mediated

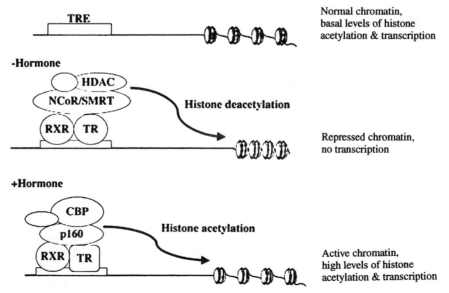

FIGURE 2 A model of nucleosomal remodeling of a TR-responsive promoter by co-repressor and co-activator complexes containing HDAC and HAT activities, respectively. TRE indicates thyroid hormone-response element.

transcription, it fails to interact with CREB, resulting in a block in CREB activation. These results unveil a new regulatory mechanism involving co-factor methylation and stress the point that a combinatorial network of various NRs, their ligands, and co-regulatory proteins underlie the complexity of hormonal signaling.

VIII. SUMMARY

The research on the NR pathway, which was initiated with the discovery of the concept of steroid receptors by Elwood Jensen and colleagues more than 40 years ago, has made tremendous progress through the years and led to the development of the best-understood model of eukaryotic gene regulation to date. The recent discovery of the co-activators and co-repressors has added additional layers of complexity to this regulatory pathway. Many details of the biochemistry, structure, function, and biology of these new molecules remain to be explored. A better mechanistic understanding of how the interplay of these co-regulatory molecules regulates the expression of specific NR-regulated genes during development and homeostasis in living cells will likely emerge from future studies.

Glossary

AF-1 and AF-2 Amino-terminal and carboxyl-terminal activation function regions of a nuclear receptor.
chromatin DNA packaged into nucleosomes or histone octamers.
co-activator A cellular co-regulatory protein that facilitates gene activation by a transcription factor.
co-repressor A cellular co-regulatory protein that facilitates gene repression by a transcription factor.
histone acetyltransferase An enzymatic activity that transfers an acetyl group from acetyl coenzyme A to histones.
histone deacetylase An enzymatic activity that removes an acetyl group from histones.
hormone antagonist A drug that counteracts the action of a hormone by binding to a nuclear receptor.
hormone-response element Short DNA sequences bound by nuclear receptors.
in vitro **transcription** Study of RNA synthesis from a DNA template in cell extracts.
methyltransferases Enzymes that promote methylation of substrates.
nuclear receptors A family of ligand-inducible transcription factors.

See Also the Following Articles

Co-activators and Corepressors for the Nuclear Receptor Superfamily ● Crosstalk of Nuclear Receptors with STAT Factors ● Effectors ● Orphan Receptors, New Receptors, and New Hormones ● Steroid Nomenclature ● Steroid Receptor Crosstalk with Cellular Signaling Pathways

Further Reading

Bagchi, M. K. (1998). Molecular mechanisms of nuclear receptor-mediated transcriptional activation and basal repression. In "The Molecular Biology of Steroid and Nuclear Hormone Receptors" (L. P. Freedman, ed.), pp. 159–190. Birkhauser, Boston, MA.
Chen, H., Lin, R. J., Schiltz, R. L., Chakravarty, D., Nash, A., Nagy, L., Privalsky, M. L., Nakatani, Y., and Evans, R. M. (1997). Nuclear receptor coactivator ACTR is a novel histone acetyltransferase and forms a multimeric activation complex with P/CAF and CBP/p300. Cell 90, 569–580.
Chen, H., Lin, R. J., Xie, W., Wilpitz, D., and Evans, R. M. (1999). Regulation of hormone-induced histone hyperacetylation and gene activation via acetylation of an acetylase. Cell 98, 675–686.
Chen, D., Ma, H., Hong, H., Koh, S. S., Huang, S.-M., Shurter, B. T., Aswad, D. W., and Stallcup, M. R. (1999). Regulation of transcription by a protein methyltransferase. Science 284, 2174–2177.
Darimont, B. D., Wagner, R. L., Apriletti, J. W., Stallcup, M. R., Kushner, P. J., Baxter, J. D., Fletterick, R. J., and Yamamoto, K. R. (1998). Structure and specificity of nuclear receptor–coactivator interactions. Genes Dev. 12, 3343–3356.
Dilworth, F. J., Fromental-Ramain, C., Yamamoto, K., and Chambon, P. (2000). ATP-driven chromatin-remodeling activity and histone acetyltransferases act sequentially during transactivation by RAR/RXR. Mol. Cell 6, 1049–1058.
Freedman, L. P. (1999). Increasing the complexity of coactivation in nuclear receptor signaling. Cell 97, 5–8.
Glass, C. K., and Rosenfeld, M. G. (2000). The coregulator exchange in transcriptional functions of nuclear receptors. Genes Dev. 14, 121–141.
Guenther, M. G., Lane, W. S., Fischle, W., Verdin, E., Lazar, M. A., and Shiekhattar, R. (2000). A core SMRT corepressor complex containing HDAC3 and TBL1, a WD40-repeat protein linked to deafness. Genes Dev. 14, 1048–1057.
McKenna, N. J., and O'Malley, B. W. (2002). Combinatorial control of gene expression by nuclear hormone receptors and coregulators. Cell 108, 465–474.
Nolte, R. T., Wisely, G. B., Westin, S., Cobbs, J. E., Lambert, M. H., Kurokawa, R., Rosenfeld, M. G., Willson, T. M., Glass, C. K., and Milburn, M. V. (1998). Ligand binding and coactivator assembly of the peroxisome proliferator-activated receptor-γ. Nature 395, 137–143.
Perissi, V., Staszewski, L. M., McInerney, E. M., Kurokawa, R., Krones, A., Rose, D. W., Lambert, M. H., Milburn, M. V., Glass, C. K., and Rosenfeld, M. G. (1999). Molecular determinants of nuclear receptor-corepressor interaction. Genes Dev. 13, 3198–3208.
Shang, Y., Xiao, H., DiRenzo, J., Lazar, M. A., and Brown, M. (2000). Cofactor dynamics and sufficiency in estrogen receptor-regulated transcription. Cell 103, 843–852.

Shiau, A. K., Barstad, D., Loria, P. M., Cheng, L., Kushner, P. J., Agard, D. A., and Green, G. L. (1998). The structural basis of estrogen receptor/coactivator recognition and the antagonism of this interaction by tamoxifen. *Cell* **95**, 927–937.

Tremblay, A., Tremblay, G. B., Labrie, F., and Giguere, V. (1999). Ligand-independent recruitment of SRC-1 to estrogen receptor β through phosphorylation of activation function AF-1. *Cell* **3**, 513–520.

Zhang, X., Jeyakumar, M., Petukhov, S., and Bagchi, M. K. (1998). A nuclear receptor corepressor modulates transcriptional activity of antagonist-occupied steroid hormone receptor. *Mol. Endocrinol.* **12**, 513–524.

Steroid Nomenclature

ANTHONY W. NORMAN AND HELEN L. HENRY
University of California, Riverside

I. BASIC RING STRUCTURE
II. CLASSES OF STEROIDS
III. STRUCTURAL MODIFICATION
IV. ASYMMETRIC CARBONS

Steroids are relatively complex organic molecules with approximately 18–27 carbon atoms. To accurately describe the nature and position of the functional groups attached to steroids (and other organic molecules), chemists have devised a formal system of nomenclature. This article provides an introduction to steroid nomenclature and provides the systematic names of some common steroids as well as the structures of several steroid hormones.

I. BASIC RING STRUCTURE

Steroids are derived from a phenanthrene ring structure (1) to which a pentano ring has been attached; this yields in the completely hydrogenated form cyclopentanoperhydrophenanthrene or the sterane ring structure (2).

Steroid structures are not normally written with all the carbon and hydrogen atoms as illustrated in 2 of Fig. 1; instead, the shorthand notation as presented for sterane (3, Fig. 1) is usually employed. In this representation, the hydrogen atoms are not indicated and unless specified otherwise it is assumed that the cyclohexane (A, B, C) or cyclopentane (D) rings are fully reduced; that is, each carbon has its full complement of carbon and/or hydrogen bonds. Also indicated in sterane (3) is the standard numbering

system for all the carbon atoms in the four rings as well as the letter designation of each ring of a steroid.

II. CLASSES OF STEROIDS

In vertebrate systems, there are six families of steroid hormones that can be classified both on a

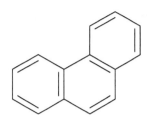

Phenanthrene
(1)

Cyclopentanoperhydrophenanthrene (sterane)
(2)

Sterane
(3)

FIGURE 1 Parent ring structures of steroids. Phenanthrene (1) is the building block to generate the two 4-ring structures **2** and **3**. The structures for cyclopentanoperhydrophenanthrene (**2** and **3**) represent the same molecule; in **2**, all the hydrogen atoms are indicated, whereas in **3** the tetrahedral bonding of all carbons is assumed (no double bonds are present) and for the sake of convenience the hydrogen atoms are not shown. In (3), the standard numbering system for the carbons of the A, B, C, and D rings of the steroid nucleus is indicated.

structural basis and on a biological (hormonal) basis. They are the estrogens (female sex steroids), the androgens (the male sex steroids), the progestins, the mineralocorticoids, the glucocorticoids, and vitamin D along with its daughter metabolites. The bile acids, structurally related to cholesterol, constitute a seventh class of steroids. All of these steroids are biologically derived from cholesterol (Fig. 2).

III. STRUCTURAL MODIFICATION

The basic steroid ring structures illustrated in sterane (3) can undergo an array of modifications by introduction of hydroxyl or carbonyl substituents and by introduction of unsaturation (double or triple bonds). In addition, heteroatoms such as nitrogen or sulfur can replace the ring carbons, and halogens and or amino groups may replace steroid hydroxyl moieties. Ring size can be expanded or contracted by addition or removal of carbon atoms. The consequences of these structural modifications are

TABLE 1 Steroid Nomenclature Conventions

Modification	Prefix	Suffix
Hydroxyl group (–HO)	Hydroxy	-ol
Hydroxyl above plane of ring	β-OH	—
Hydroxyl below plane of ring	α-OH	—
Keto or carbonyl group (C=O)	Oxo-	-one
Aldehyde (–CHO)	—	-al
Carboxylic acid (COOH)	Carboxy	-oic acid
Double bond (–C=C–)	—	-ene
Triple bond (–C≡C–)	—	-yne
Saturated ring system	—	-an
One less carbon atom	-Nor	—
One additional carbon atom	-Homo	—
One additional oxygen atom	-Oxo	—
One less oxygen atom	-Deoxy	—
Two additional hydrogen atoms	-Dihydro	—
Two less hydrogen atoms	-Dehydro	—
Two groups on same sides of plane	Cis	—
Two groups on opposite sides of plane	Trans	—
Other ring forms (rings A and B trans, as in allopregnane)	Allo	—
Opening of a ring (as in vitamin D)	Seco-	—
Conversion at a numbered carbon from conventional orientation (as in epicholesterol or 3α-cholesterol)	-Epi	—

designated by application of the standard organic nomenclature conventions of steroids. The pertinent aspects of this system are summarized in Table 1. Prefixes and suffixes are used to indicate the type of structural modification. Any number of prefixes may be employed (each with its own appropriate carbon number and specified in order of decreasing preference of acid, lactone, ester, aldehyde, ketone, alcohol, amine, and ether); however, only one suffix is permitted.

The formal names of steroids are devised in accordance with the official nomenclature rules for steroids laid down by the International Union of Pure and Applied Chemistry. Table 2 lists the trivial and systematic names of a number of common steroids.

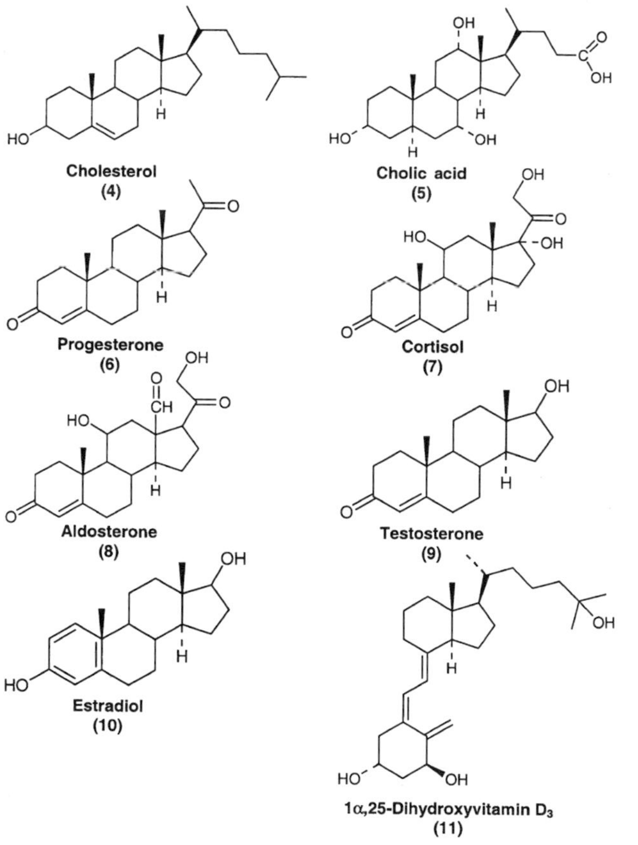

FIGURE 2 Structure of cholesterol (4) and cholic acid (a bile acid) (5) and representative structures of a steroid hormone from each steroid family (structures 6–10). The hormone form of vitamin D₃ is 1α,25(OH)₂ vitamin D₃ (11).

IV. ASYMMETRIC CARBONS

An important structural feature of any steroid is the presence of asymmetric carbon atoms and designation in the formal nomenclature of the structural isomer that is present. For example, reduction of pregnane-3-one (12) to the corresponding 3-alcohol (13) will produce two epimeric steroids (14) and (15) (see Fig. 3). The resulting hydroxyl may be above the plane of the A ring and is so designated on the structure (**14**) by a solid line; it is referred to as a -3β-ol. The epimer or -3α-ol (**15**) has the hydroxyl below the plane of the A ring and is so designated by a dotted line for the −C···OH bond. If the α or β orientation of a substituent group is not known, it is designated with a wavy −C−OH line.

Another locus where asymmetric carbon atoms play an important role in steroid structure determination is the junction between each of the A, B, C, and D rings. Figure 4 illustrates these relationships for cholestanol and coprostanol. In the 5α form, the 19-methyl and the α-hydrogen on carbon 5 are on opposite sides of the plane of the A:B ring; this is referred to as a *trans* fusion. When the 19-methyl and β-hydrogen on carbon 5 are on the same side of the A:B ring fusion, this is denoted *cis* fusion. In this case, the steroid structure can no longer be drawn in one plane (as in **24**). Thus, in all 5β steroid structures that

TABLE 2   Trivial and Systematic Names of some Common Steroids

Trivial name	Systematic name
Aldosterone	18,11-Hemiacetal of 11β,21-dihydroxy-3,20-dioxopregn-4-ene-18-al
Androstenedione	Androst-4-ene-3, 17-dione
Androsterone	3α-Hydroxy-5a-androstan-17-one
Cholecalciferol (vitamin D₃)	9,10-Secocholesta-5,7,10(19)-trien-3β-ol
Cholesterol	Cholest-5-ene-3β-ol
Cholic acid	3α,7α,12α,-Trihydrozy-5b-cholan-24-oic acid
Corticosterone	11β,21-Dihydroxypregn-4-ene-3, 20-dione
Cortisol	11β,17,21-Trihydroxypregn-4-ene-3,20-dione
Cortisone	17,21-Dihydroxypregn-4-ene-3, 20-dione
Dehydroepiandrosterone	3β-Hydroxy-5-androstene-17-one
Deoxycorticosterone	21-Hydroxypregn-4-ene-3,20-dione
Ergocalciferol (vitamin D₂)	9,10-5-eco-5,7,10(19), 22-ergostatetraen-3β-ol
Ergosterol	5,7,22-Ergostatrien-3-β-ol
Estriol	Estra-1,3,5(10)-triene-3,16α, 17β-triol
Estrone	3-Hydroxyestra-1,3,5(10)-triene-17-one
Etiocholanolone	3α,-Hydroxy-5b-androstane-17-one
Lanosterol	8,24-Lanostadiene-3β-ol
Lithocholic acid	3α,-Hydroxy-5β-cholan-24-oic acid
Progesterone	Pregn-4-ene-3,20-dione
Testosterone	17β-Hydroxyandrost-4-ene-3-one

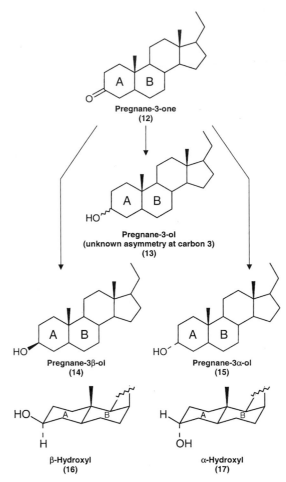

FIGURE 3 Structural consequences resulting from reduction of pregnane-3-one (**12**). The orientations of the α- and β-hydroxyls of compounds pregnane-3β-ol and pregnane-3α-ol as equatorial (**16**) or axial (**17**) substituents, respectively, on the chair version of the A rings are shown in the bottom row.

have *cis* fusion between rings A and B, the A ring is bent into a second plane that is approximately at right angles to the B:C:D rings (see **24** of Fig. 4). Thus, each of the ring junction carbons is potentially asymmetric and the naturally occurring steroid will have only one of the two possible orientations at each ring junction. Although there are two families of naturally occurring steroids with either *cis* or *trans* fusion of the A:B rings, it is known that the ring fusions of B:C and C:D in virtually all naturally occurring steroids are *trans*.

The chemical determination and designation of the absolute configuration of asymmetric carbon atoms on the side chain according to formal rules of nomenclature are complex. The "sequence rules" of Cahn *et al.* must be applied. These rules describe operational procedures to generate an unambiguous nomenclature specification of the absolute configu-

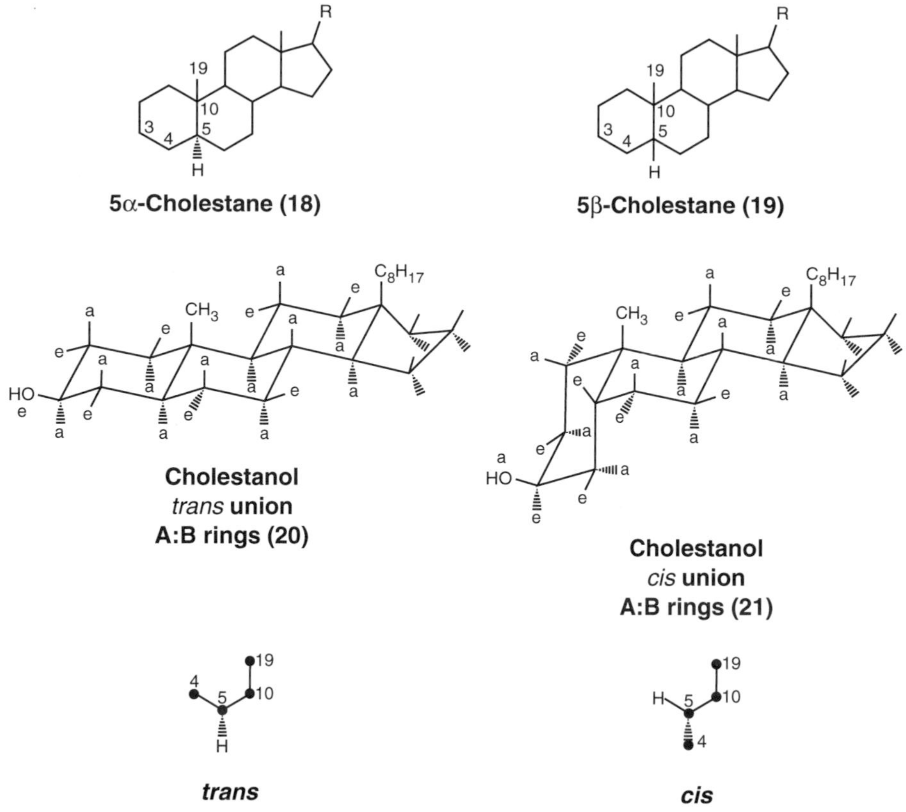

FIGURE 4 Structural relationships resulting from *cis* or *trans* A:B ring fusion in two typical steroids. In 5α-cholestane and cholestanol, the A:B ring fusion is *trans*, whereas in 5β-cholestane and coprostanol, the A:B ring fusion is *cis*. The orientation of substituents around carbon 5 for the *cis* and *trans* circumstances is illustrated in the bottom row. a, axial orientation; e, equatorial orientation; ●–●, carbon–carbon bonds.

ration of all chemical compounds whether they be steroids, sugars, amino acids, thiopolymers, or other compounds.

Glossary

asymmetric carbon A carbon atom in a complex molecule that is chemically bonded to four different substituents.

chirality The right- or left-handedness of an asymmetric carbon of organic molecules.

steroid A member of the lipid class of compounds composed of the four-ring cyclopentanoperhydrophenanthrene nucleus, it is the basic structural component of steroid hormone families such as estrogens, progestogens, androgens, mineralocorticoids, glucocorticoids, and vitamin D and its metabolites.

Further Reading

Barton, D. H. R., and Cookson, R. D. (1956). Steroid conformational analysis. *Q. Rev. Chem. Soc.* 10, 44–53.

Cahn, R. S., Ingold, C. K., and Prelog, V. (1966). Specification of molecular chirality. *Angew. Chem. Int. Ed.* 5, 385–415.

Fieser, L., and Fieser, M. (1959). "Steroids." Van Nostrand-Reinhold, Princeton, NJ.

IUPAC Rules of Steroid Nomenclature (1972). *Pure Appl. Chem.* 31, 285–322.

Norman, A. W., and Litwack, G. (1997). "Hormones," pp. 1–558. Academic Press, San Diego, CA.

Steroidogenic Acute Regulatory (StAR) Protein, Cholesterol, and Control of Steroidogenesis

JEROME F. STRAUSS, III

University of Pennsylvania Medical Center

I. INTRODUCTION
II. THE CRITICAL ROLE OF StAR
III. MOLECULAR GENETICS OF CONGENITAL LIPOID
   ADRENAL HYPERPLASIA

Steroidogenic acute regulatory protein (StAR) plays an essential role in controlling the rate-determining step of steroid hormone synthesis. StAR is a 30 kDa protein and its mRNA is found at high levels in tissues that are involved in steroidogenesis: human adrenal cortex, ovary, and testis. It is also found at lower levels in other tissues (e.g., kidney). This article discusses the role of StAR, its structure and activity, the regulation of the *StAR* gene, and possible models for the mechanism of action of the protein.

I. INTRODUCTION

Cholesterol is the substrate for steroid hormone synthesis, and in humans, circulating lipoproteins are the major source of cholesterol used for steroidogenesis. Low-density lipoproteins (LDLs) are a primary reservoir of steroidogenic cholesterol, although other lipoproteins including very-low-density lipoproteins and high-density lipoproteins (HDLs) also contribute to the steroidogenic pool. The LDL receptor family and HDL (SR-BI) receptors are highly expressed on cells that produce large amounts of steroids, and tropic hormones up-regulate the expression of these receptors, ensuring that an adequate supply of substrate is available for steroid biosynthesis. *De novo* synthesis provides cholesterol for steroidogenesis when lipoprotein-derived substrate is insufficient. Excess cholesterol accumulated by steroidogenic cells is esterified and stored in cytoplasmic lipid droplets ready for mobilization by cholesterol ester hydrolase, which is activated by protein kinase A in response to tropic hormone stimulation. Thus, in contrast to protein hormone-secreting glands, which store preformed hormone, steroidogenic glands store hormone precursors.

The initial step in steroid hormone synthesis is the cleavage of the cholesterol side chain to form pregnenolone. This reaction is catalyzed by an enzyme system located on the matrix side of the inner mitochondrial membranes consisting of cytochrome P450 side chain cleavage ($P450_{scc}$); adrenodoxin, an iron sulfur protein electron shuttle; and adrenodoxin reductase, a flavoprotein that transfers electrons from NADPH to adrenodoxin. Cholesterol must be translocated from the relatively cholesterol-rich outer mitochondrial membrane to the inner mitochondrial membrane to come into contact with $P450_{scc}$, requiring it to traverse the aqueous space separating the two membranes. The acute regulation of steroidogenesis is due largely to the increased delivery of the hydrophobic cholesterol to the inner mitochondrial membrane. This acute mode of regulation of steroidogenesis is superimposed on the longer-term control that includes changes in the transcription of genes involved in steroid biosynthesis, cellular cholesterol uptake, and intracellular sterol trafficking.

In vivo and *in vitro* studies from more than 30 years ago demonstrated that cycloheximide and other inhibitors of translation block tropic hormone-stimulated pregnenolone production and cause cholesterol to accumulate in the outer mitochondrial membranes. These observations led to the concept that the acute increase in steroidogenesis requires a short-lived, cycloheximide-sensitive protein that is activated or synthesized in response to tropic hormone stimulation. Orme-Johnson and colleagues and Stocco and colleagues reported the induction of an ~30 kDa phosphoprotein in cells stimulated by tropic hormones or cyclic AMP (cAMP) analogues. The 30 kDa protein was localized to mitochondria and shown to be derived from a larger precursor molecule. The 30 kDa protein was subsequently isolated from MA-10 Leydig tumor cells and partial amino acid sequences were obtained, allowing the cloning of the cDNA for the murine protein and later the human protein. The protein was named steroidogenic acute regulatory protein (StAR) and it was proposed to be the cycloheximide-sensitive factor controlling the rate-determining step in steroidogenesis.

II. THE CRITICAL ROLE OF StAR

The following evidence supports the notion that StAR has a critical role in steroid hormone synthesis: (1) Expression of StAR in MA-10 Leydig tumor cells correlates with the enhanced steroidogenesis. (2) In monkey kidney COS-1 cells, which are not steroidogenic, co-transfection of StAR and the cholesterol side-chain cleavage system results in enhanced steroidogenesis. In the absence of StAR, COS-1 cells expressing the cholesterol side-chain cleavage system produce substantial amounts of pregnenolone only when a polar hydroxysterol precursor that readily enters into mitochondria is provided as an exogenous substrate. However, COS-1 cells expressing both StAR and the cholesterol side-chain cleavage enzyme are capable of producing large amounts of pregnenolone from endogenous cholesterol. StAR also increases cholesterol flux through other mitochondrial P450 enzymes that oxidize cholesterol including P450c27, the enzyme that synthesizes 27-hydroxycholesterol, a bile acid precursor and potent regulator of cellular sterol homeostasis. (3) Mutations that inactivate StAR cause congenital lipoid adrenal hyperplasia, a rare autosomal recessive disorder in which the synthesis of all adrenal and gonadal steroid hormones is severely impaired at the cholesterol side-chain cleavage step, resulting in massive accumulation of cholesterol in the adrenal cortex and testicular Leydig cells. (4) Targeted deletion of the murine StAR gene results in a phenotype in nullizygous mice that mimics human congenital lipoid adrenal hyperplasia.

III. MOLECULAR GENETICS OF CONGENITAL LIPOID ADRENAL HYPERPLASIA

The clinical phenotype of congenital lipoid adrenal hyperplasia includes the onset of profound adrenocortical insufficiency shortly after birth, hyperpigmentation reflecting increased production of proopiomelancortin, elevated plasma renin activity as a consequence of reduced aldosterone synthesis, and male pseudo-hermaphroditism resulting from deficient fetal testicular testosterone synthesis. The affected offspring are the products of uneventful pregnancies, delivered at term. Early in the disease, the steroidogenic cells of the enlarged adrenal cortices in affected individuals are engorged with lipid droplets containing cholesterol esters, giving rise to the condition's name. Administration of adrenocorticotropic hormone or human chorionic gonadotropin to subjects with congenital lipoid adrenal hyperplasia does not elicit the normal acute increase in serum levels of adrenal or gonadal steroid hormones.

Congenital lipoid adrenal hyperplasia is a rare disease, except in Japan and Korea, where it accounts for 5% or more of all cases of congenital adrenal hyperplasia. Mutations in the StAR gene have been identified in more than 60 unrelated patients with congenital lipoid adrenal hyperplasia. Analysis of DNA from the parents of several patients confirmed that this disease is inherited in an autosomal recessive pattern. Mutations found in the StAR gene, which is composed of seven exons and is located on chromosome 8p11.2, include frameshifts caused by deletions/insertions, splicing errors, and nonsense and missense mutations, all of which lead to the absence of StAR protein or the production of functionally inactive protein. Several nonsense mutations were shown to

result in C-terminal truncations of StAR. One of these mutations, Q258X, which results in the deletion of the final 28 amino acids of the StAR protein, accounts for 80% of the known mutant alleles in the affected Japanese population. All of the known point mutations that produce amino acid substitutions occur in exons 5–7 of the gene, the exons that encode the C-terminus. The metabolic defect in congenital lipoid adrenal hyperplasia is progressive, with adrenal and gonadal steroidogenesis becoming increasingly impaired with time after birth. A model has been proposed to explain the disease process that postulates the existence of some StAR-independent steroidogenesis prior to the severe cellular damage resulting from cholesterol accumulation and cholesterol oxidation, which ultimately results in a nonfunctional steroidogenic cell (Fig. 1). Comparison of the clinical course of 46,XX females with congenital lipoid adrenal hyperplasia to that of 46,XY subjects reinforced the proposed pathophysiological mechanism. 46,XX females underwent spontaneous puberty and secondary sexual development, whereas 46,XY patients were unable to undergo spontaneous puberty and had insufficient testicular androgen production in utero to masculinize the external genitalia. The sparing of some ovarian function in the face of mutations that inactivate StAR reflects the presence of modest StAR-independent steroidogenesis in follicles that is sufficient to sponsor estradiol synthesis. Because the ovary is essentially steroidogenically quiescent during fetal life and because follicles produce steroids only when they are recruited to mature, most follicles are spared from the ravages of cholesterol engorgement, leaving a source of viable, albeit impaired, steroid-producing cells at the time of puberty.

IV. STRUCTURE AND ACTIVITY OF StAR

Human StAR is synthesized as a 285-amino-acid protein in the cytoplasm. The N-terminus of StAR is characteristic of proteins imported into mitochondria: the first 26 amino acid residues are predicted to form an amphipathic helix. Pulse–chase studies reveal that newly synthesized StAR pre-protein (37 kDa) is rapidly imported into mitochondria and processed to the mature 30 kDa form. The pre-protein has a very short half-life (minutes) but the mature form is longer-lived (hours). Drugs that collapse the mitochondrial proton gradient inhibit StAR import, and agents that block mitochondrial matrix metalloendoproteinases prevent the cleavage of the StAR N-terminal mitochondrial targeting sequence from imported protein.

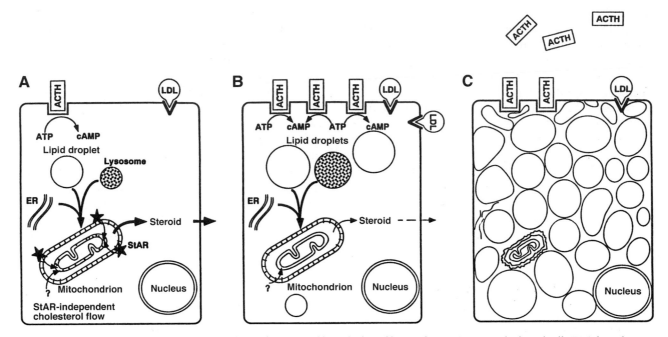

FIGURE 1 Model of the pathophysiology of congenital lipoid adrenal hyperplasia. (A) Normal adrenal cell. (B) Adrenal cell deficient in StAR at an early stage of the disease. The efficient flow of cholesterol to the inner mitochondrial membranes is impaired, leaving only a modest StAR-independent steroidogenesis. Consequently, corticotropin secretion is increased, resulting in adrenal cortical hyperplasia and increased uptake of LDL cholesterol, with accumulation of internalized cholesterol in lipid droplets due to inefficient movement of the substrate to P450scc. (C) Late stage of the disease, with massive accumulation of cholesterol in cytoplasmic lipid droplets, leading to organelle compression and auto-oxidation of cholesterol with subsequent peroxidative damage to proteins and organelles and a severe impairment of steroidogenesis.

To identify the domains of StAR critical for steroidogenesis, Arakane *et al.* generated StAR mutants and examined their activity in COS-1 cells transfected with the cholesterol side-chain cleavage enzyme. Deletion of the C-terminal 28 amino acids ablated StAR's steroidogenic activity, whereas removal of the last 10 amino acids reduced steroidogenic activity by 50%. These experiments indicated that residues in the C-terminus are critical for StAR's activity. The location of critical domains in the C-terminus of StAR is consistent with the analysis of gene mutations causing congenital lipoid adrenal hyperplasia in which mutations that inactivate StAR result from amino acid replacements located in exons encoding the C-terminal half of the protein.

It has been suggested that StAR takes on a molten globule configuration at pH 3.5–4.0, a pH that may be generated in the immediate vicinity of mitochondria. The molten globule configuration may facilitate the unfolding of StAR in preparation for action on the mitochondria and the subsequent movement through the import pore into the mitochondrial matrix. As discussed below, the crystal structure of a protein with a C-terminal domain similar to that of StAR has

been determined. The crystal structure reveals that the StAR C-terminus contains a hydrophobic tunnel that can bind cholesterol.

V. THE ROLE OF PHOSPHORYLATION

The mature StAR protein contains two consensus sequences for cAMP-dependent protein kinase phosphorylation at serine 57 and serine 195. Tropic hormones act via cAMP-mediated signaling cascades to rapidly increase the production of steroids. The cAMP second-messenger system activates protein kinase A, which phosphorylates proteins on either threonine or serine residues in a specific sequence context. Phosphorylation of StAR is a plausible mechanism by which preexisting or newly synthesized StAR can be rapidly activated.

Serine 195 of human StAR must be phosphorylated for maximal steroidogenic activity. cAMP promotes the incorporation of phosphorus into this residue within minutes of stimulation. The other consensus protein kinase phosphorylation site at serine 57 does not appear to be essential for StAR's steroidogenic activity. In contrast, mutation of serine 195 to an aspartic acid residue, which mimics the charge effect of phosphorylation, modestly increased the steroidogenic activity of the protein. These observations suggest that post- or co-translational modification of StAR can increase the activity of existing or newly made StAR protein, providing a mechanism by which tropic hormones acting through the intermediacy of cAMP can rapidly increase steroidogenesis.

VI. THE TISSUE-SPECIFIC EXPRESSION OF StAR

Tissues that express StAR at high levels carry out tropic hormone-regulated mitochondrial sterol hydroxylations through the intermediacy of cAMP. StAR mRNA is abundant in human adrenal cortex, ovary, and testis. It is also found in lower abundance in kidney and monocytes, findings consistent with the fact that 1α-hydroxylation of vitamin D takes place in the kidney as well as monocyte/macrophages, a reaction catalyzed by a mitochondrial P450 enzyme. The brain also expresses StAR in some species, which may reflect a role in neurosteroid production. StAR mRNA was not detected in the human placenta, an observation that is consistent with the fact that pregnancies hosting a fetus affected with congenital lipoid adrenal hyperplasia go to term. Although estrogen production is impaired in these pregnancies as a result of diminished fetal adrenal androgen production, placental progesterone synthesis is not significantly affected, indicating that the trophoblast cholesterol side-chain cleavage reaction is independent of StAR.

StAR protein is detectable in thecal cells of human ovarian follicles in the adult ovary, but only in granulosa cells of luteinized follicles. Theca and granulosa cells of the fetal ovaries do not stain for StAR. StAR is prominent in fetal and adult testicular Leydig cells and present at low levels in Sertoli cells of adult testis. In the kidney, StAR is localized to the distal convoluted tubules. These observations are consistent with the clinical phenotype of congenital lipoid adrenal hyperplasia in which fetal adrenal and testicular steroidogenesis is markedly affected, whereas ovarian steroidogenic activity is spared to some extent because the ovaries are relatively quiescent until puberty.

VII. THE StAR GENE AND ITS REGULATION

The abundance of StAR protein in steroidogenic cells is determined primarily by the rate of StAR gene transcription. In differentiated cells, StAR transcrip-tion is rapidly (within 15 to 30 min) activated by the cAMP signal transduction cascade. In differentiating cells (e.g., luteinizing granulosa cells), the induction of StAR transcription takes a longer time (hours) and requires on-going protein synthesis. StAR gene transcription is controlled, in part, by steroidogenic factor-1 (SF-1), also known as Ad4BP, an orphan nuclear receptor. The human StAR promoter contains three cooperative cis elements that bind SF-1 and are required for cAMP stimulation of StAR transcription. In addition to SF-1, CCAAT enhancer-binding protein-β, Sp1, GATA-4, and SREBP-1a (a member of the transcription factor family that governs the expression of many genes involved in lipid metabolism) contribute to the transcriptional control of StAR expression in a positive fashion, whereas DAX-1, another orphan nuclear receptor, inhibits StAR transcription, probably through interactions with SF-1.

VIII. HOW DOES StAR WORK?

StAR was originally thought to stimulate cholesterol movement from the outer to the inner mitochondrial membrane as it was imported into the mitochondria. The importation process was proposed to create contact sites between the two membranes, allowing cholesterol to flow down a chemical gradient. However, a StAR mutant lacking the N-terminal 62 amino acids (N-62 mutant) that contain the mitochondrial targeting sequence was as effective as wild-type StAR in stimulating steroidogenesis. The overexpressed N-62 StAR protein was distributed throughout the cytoplasm of the transfected cells, whereas wild-type StAR was almost exclusively located inside mitochondria. Recombinant human N-62 StAR stimulated pregnenolone production by isolated ovarian mitochondria in a dose- and time-dependent fashion, with significant increases in steroid production observed within minutes with nanomolar concentrations. A mutant recombinant protein in which the A218V mutation, which is found in subjects with congenital lipoid adrenal hyperplasia, was completely inactive. The recombinant N-62 StAR also stimulated the transfer of cholesterol but not phosphatidylcholine from cholesterol-rich phosphatidylcholine vesicles to sterol-poor acceptors. The transfer of sterols in these assays could not be ascribed to fusion of the donor vesicles and acceptor membranes. These experiments are most consistent with the idea that StAR enhances the desorption of cholesterol from sterol-rich donor membranes (Fig. 2). The desorption process may involve the

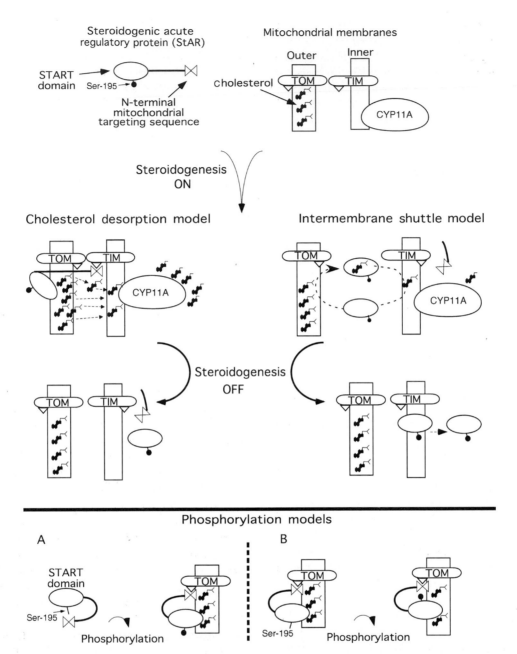

FIGURE 2 Models of StAR action. The StAR N-terminal mitochondrial targeting sequence binds to one or more of the known transmembrane outer mitochondrial transporters (TOM) and transmembrane inner mitochondrial transporters (TIM), linking it to the importation machinery. Cholesterol desorption model: The C-terminus of the protein (START domain) stimulates cholesterol desorption. The importation of the START domain removes the protein from its site of action, terminating sterol movement to the inner membrane. During or following importation, the StAR pre-protein is processed to yield the mature StAR form. Intermembrane shuttle model: The StAR protein is imported into the intermembrane space [the StAR-related lipid transfer (START) domain predicted model], and the targeting sequence is proteolytically cleaved, leaving the START domain in the intermembrane space, where it rapidly oscillates from the outer to the inner mitochondrial membranes, delivering cholesterol one molecule at a time. StAR is removed from the intermitochondrial space by an undetermined mechanism, thereby terminating sterol movement. Phosphorylation models: (A) Cyclic AMP-mediated phosphorylation of serine 195 located in the START domain of StAR reduces an inhibitory action of the N-terminal targeting sequence on StAR function, allowing more efficient interaction with the mitochondria. Alternatively (B), cyclic AMP-mediated phosphorylation of serine 195 might reduce an inhibitory action of the N-terminal targeting sequence on the START domain, allowing greater activity of this sterol transporter domain.

binding of cholesterol by the StAR C-terminus, which forms a hydrophobic tunnel, as predicted from the crystal structure of a StAR-like protein (MLN64), that can accommodate cholesterol molecules. Although the ability of StAR to bind cholesterol might suggest that it functions as shuttle, the relatively small amount of StAR in cells and its short functional life cannot account for the needed flux of cholesterol to P450scc if StAR can move only one or two moles of sterol per mole of StAR. Consequently, a "catalytic" role for the protein is required.

The observations reviewed above suggest a mechanism of StAR action that entails the efficient targeting of newly synthesized StAR pre-protein to the mitochondria by the protein's N-terminus. On reaching the mitochondria, the StAR C-terminus interacts with the relatively sterol-rich outer membrane, causing cholesterol to desorb from the outer membrane and transit to the relatively sterol-poor inner membrane, perhaps through preexisting contact sites. The import of StAR into the mitochondria and its subsequent processing remove the protein from its locus of action, effectively terminating sterol movement from the outer to the inner mitochondrial membranes. Thus, the mature protein represents a record of the past action of StAR.

It has been attractive to postulate that a "receptor" for StAR on the mitochondrial outer membrane is involved in the cholesterol translocation process. The hypothetical receptor, which could be a protein or a lipid, is evidently not specific for mitochondria of steroidogenic cells, since StAR works in the context of COS-1 cells, which are not normally steroid hormone-producing cells. The fact that immunohistochemical and electron microscope studies suggest that N-62 StAR mutants are not selectively accumulated by mitochondria argues against an abundance of high-affinity receptors for the StAR C-terminus on the mitochondria. Hence, either very few high-affinity sites or transient interactions are sufficient to promote cholesterol movement.

IX. StAR PARALOGUES

When StAR was first identified, it was thought to be a unique molecule. It is now evident that a family of proteins sharing a domain that is similar to the C-terminus of StAR exist, the so-called StAR-related lipid transfer (START) domain proteins. The absence of StAR from the human placenta, an organ that produces a significant amount of pregnenolone, documented the existence of StAR-independent ster-

oidogenesis but raised the possibility that another protein might subserve StAR's function in the placenta. MLN64, a gene discovered to be amplified in breast and ovarian cancer cells, shares significant structural homology with StAR. MLN64 was shown to increase pregnenolone production in COS-1 cells expressing the cholesterol side-chain cleavage enzyme system. MLN64 is anchored to late endosomes through N-terminal membrane-spanning domains; freeing the C-terminus of MLN64, which is homologous to StAR, from the membrane-spanning domains increases steroidogenic activity. Cleavage of the MLN64 protein releasing its C-terminus apparently occurs in various tissues, including the human placenta. Thus, the MLN64 C-terminus may replace StAR's function in the placenta. The roles of other START domain proteins in intracellular sterol trafficking and in steroidogenesis remain to be explored.

Acknowledgments

Work in the author's laboratory was supported by NIH Grant HD-06274.

Glossary

congenital lipoid adrenal hyperplasia Inherited metabolic disease characterized by markedly impaired adrenal and gonadal steroid hormone synthesis due to mutations in the *StAR* gene.

cytochrome P450scc (CYP11A) The catalytic component of the cholesterol side-chain cleavage system that performs three cycles of oxidation and reduction on the cholesterol side chain, resulting in the formation of pregnenolone and isocapraldehyde.

steroidogenic factor 1 An orphan nuclear receptor that plays a key role in controlling the transcription of the *StAR* gene.

See Also the Following Articles

Glucocorticoid Biosynthesis: Role of StAR Protein ● **Lipoprotein Receptor Signaling** ● **Luteinizing Hormone (LH)** ● **Neuroactive Steroids**

Further Reading

Arakane, F., Kallen, C. B., Watari, H., Foster, J. A., Sepuri, N. B. V., Pain, D., Stayrook, S. E., Lewis, M., Gerton, G. L., and Strauss, J. F., III (1998). The mechanism of action of steroidogenic acute regulatory protein (StAR): StAR acts on the outside of mitochondria to stimulate steroidogenesis. *J. Biol. Chem.* **273**, 16339–16345.

Arakane, F., King, S. R., Du, Y., Kallen, C. B., Walsh, L. P., Watari, H., Stocco, D. M., and Strauss, J. F., III (1997). Phosphorylation of steroidogenic acute regulatory protein (StAR) modulates its steroidogenic activity. *J. Biol. Chem.* **272**, 32656–32662.

Bose, H. S., Sugawara, T., Strauss, J. F., III, and Miller, W. L. (1996). The pathophysiology and genetics of congenital lipoid adrenal hyperplasia. *N. Engl. J. Med.* **335**, 1870–1878.

Caron, K. M., Soo, S.-C., Clark, B. J., Stocco, D. M., Wetsel, W., and Parker, K. L. (1997). Targeted disruption of the mouse gene encoding the steroidogenic acute regulatory protein provides insight into congenital lipoid adrenal hyperplasia. *Proc. Natl. Acad. Sci. USA* **94**, 11540–11545.

Christenson, L. K., and Strauss, J. F., III (2000). Steroidogenic acute regulatory protein (StAR) and the intramitochondrial translocation of cholesterol. *Biochim. Biophys. Acta* **1529**, 175–187.

Kallen, C. B., Billheimer, J. T., Summers, S. A., Stayrook, S. E., Lewis, M., and Strauss, J. F., III (1998). Steroidogenic acute regulatory protein (StAR) is a sterol transfer protein. *J. Biol. Chem.* **273**, 26285–26288.

Lin, D., Sugawara, T., Strauss, J. F., III, Clark, B. J., Stocco, D. M., and Miller, W. L. (1995). Role of steroidogenic acute regulatory protein in adrenal and gonadal steroidogenesis. *Science* **267**, 1828–1831.

Petrescu, A. D., Gallego, A. M., Okamura, Y., Strauss, J. F., III, and Schroeder, F. (2001). Steroidogenic acute regulatory protein binds cholesterol and modulates mitochondrial membrane sterol domain dynamics. *J. Biol. Chem.* **276**, 36970–36982.

Stocco, D. M. (2001). StAR protein and the regulation of steroid hormone biosynthesis. *Annu. Rev. Physiol.* **63**, 193–212.

Strauss, J. F., Kallen, C. B., Christenson, L. K., Watari, H., Devoto, L., Arakane, F., Kiriakido, M., and Sugawara, T. (1999). The steroidogenic acute regulatory protein (StAR): A window into the complexities of intracellular cholesterol trafficking. *Rec. Prog. Horm. Res.* **54**, 369–395.

Tsujishita, Y., and Hurley, J. H. (2000). Structure and lipid transport mechanism of a StAR-related domain. *Nat. Struct.* **7**, 408–414.

Watari, H., Arakane, F., Moog-Lutz, C., *et al.* (1997). MLN64 contain a domain with homology to the steroidogenic acute regulatory protein (StAR) that stimulates steroidogenesis. *Proc. Natl. Acad. Sci. USA* **94**, 8462–8467.

Steroid Receptor Crosstalk with Cellular Signaling Pathways

Nancy L. Weigel and Irina U. Agoulnik

Baylor College of Medicine

Steroid hormone receptors are hormone-activated transcription factors. Regulated by a wide variety of cell signaling pathways, steroid hormone receptors alter phosphorylation of target proteins. Conversely, steroids and their receptors act at many levels to regulate diverse cell signaling pathways and their target transcription factors. Thus, the actions of steroids and other cellular regulators are intricately intertwined.

I. INTRODUCTION

As hormone-activated transcription factors, the steroid hormone receptors and the cell signaling-regulated transcription factors such as activator protein 1 (AP-1) can regulate components of each other's pathways at the transcriptional level. The focus here, however, is on the cross-regulation of the activities of the signaling pathway components. Three major mechanisms are of importance: (1) regulation of steroid receptor phosphorylation and function by cellular signaling pathways, (2) interactions between steroid receptors and transcription factors that have activities regulated by cellular signaling pathways, and (3) activation of cellular signaling pathways by steroids.

II. STEROID RECEPTOR STRUCTURE AND FUNCTION

The steroid hormone receptors belong to a large family of ligand-activated transcription factors; the family includes steroid receptors such as the estrogen and androgen receptors, receptors for thyroid hormone and retinoic acid, and a large number of receptors for other small, hydrophobic molecules. In the absence of hormone, steroid receptors associate with heat-shock protein complexes, which hold the receptor in a conformation capable of binding hormone and protect the receptor from degradation (Fig. 1). The location of the receptor in the absence of hormone is specific to the receptor and sometimes to the cell type. Glucocorticoid and androgen receptors are predominantly cytoplasmic in the absence of hormone, whereas the estrogen and progesterone receptors are predominantly nuclear. The steroid hormones are hydrophobic cholesterol derivatives and can freely pass through the cell membrane. Binding of hormone causes conformational changes in the hormone-binding domain that favor dissociation from the heat-shock protein complexes. The receptors form dimers and associate with DNA

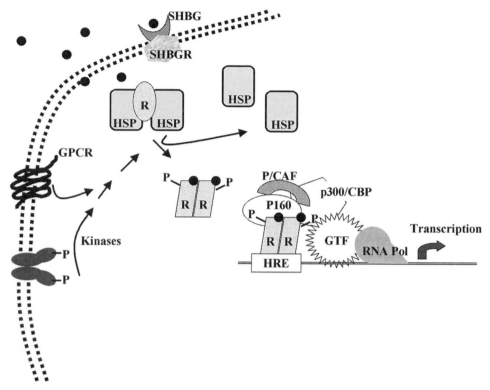

FIGURE 1   In the absence of hormone, steroid receptors (R) associate with heat-shock proteins (HSP). Binding of steroid (●) results in dissociation from heat-shock proteins, dimerization, and binding to specific hormone response elements (HRE) in the promoters of target genes. The receptor recruits co-activators, including the p160 (also called steroid receptor co-activator) family of proteins, P/CAF, and p300/CBP. These proteins perform a variety of functions, including acetylation of histones, and interact with general transcription factors (GTF) to stimulate transcription of target genes. Activation of a variety of membrane receptors, including G-protein-coupled receptors (GPCR) and growth factor receptors, stimulates a cascade of phosphorylations; this results in enhanced phosphorylation (P) of steroid receptors and their associated proteins, altering the resulting transcriptional activity. Among the signaling pathways that can be induced is steroid-mediated activation of steroid hormone-binding globulin (SHBG) and its receptor, steroid hormone-binding globulin receptor (SHBGR), which elevates cAMP levels, activating protein kinase A. In some cases, altered cell signaling is sufficient to activate a steroid receptor in the absence of any hormone, a pathway termed ligand-independent activation.

containing sequences (hormone response elements) specifically recognized by the receptor; these sequences are in the promoters of target genes. In addition, the receptors recruit complexes of proteins, termed co-activators, which serve a variety of functions to enhance the transcriptional activity of the receptor. Among the best characterized activities of the co-activators is the ability to acetylate histones at target genes, opening up chromatin and allowing access for RNA polymerase and other factors needed for transcription. The receptors and their co-activators are phosphoproteins. Signals emanating from membrane receptors, including growth factor receptors and G-protein-coupled receptors, regulate the phosphorylation and activity of the steroid receptors. Sometimes these changes in cell signaling are suffi-

cient to activate a steroid receptor in the absence of hormone, a process termed ligand-independent activation.

The general structures of the steroid receptors are very conserved; the structure of the estrogen receptor-α is depicted in Fig. 2. Steroid receptors contain highly conserved DNA-binding domains, which consist of two Zn^{2+} finger motifs (region C) and less well-conserved hormone-binding domains (region E) linked to the DNA-binding domain by the hinge region (D). The hormone-binding domains also contain a region important for transcriptional activity, activation function-2, (AF-2), which binds co-activators, facilitating transcription. The hinge region contains a nuclear localization signal. Some receptors contain an additional carboxyl-terminal

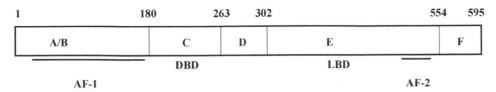

FIGURE 2 The general structural organization of a steroid receptor, depicting the structure of the human estrogen receptor-α. All receptors contain regions A–E. The numbering indicates the amino acid positions bordering the functional domains in estrogen receptor-α. Regions C and E of steroid receptors contain the DNA-binding domain (DBD) and the ligand-binding domain (LBD), respectively. Within the A/B domain and the E domain, each steroid receptor contains a region important for transcriptional activity (AF-1 and AF-2). Region D, termed the hinge region, contains a nuclear localization signal. Although estrogen receptor-α contains an F domain, which is not required for hormone binding, some receptors lack this region.

segment (F), which is not required for hormone binding. The amino-terminal regions of the receptors (A/B) are the least conserved and are the most variable in length, ranging from less than 200 amino acids in the estrogen receptor to more than 500 in the progesterone receptor. This region contains an additional activation function (AF-1). The relative importance of AF-1 and AF-2 in inducing transcription is dependent on receptor, promoter, cell type, and activation signal.

III. REGULATION OF STEROID RECEPTOR FUNCTION BY CELLULAR SIGNALING PATHWAYS

Two major approaches have been utilized to assess the role of cellular signaling in the activity of steroid receptors. The first method is to modulate the activity of cellular signaling pathways and to determine the effect on receptor activity. The advantage of this scheme is that one can rapidly identify cellular signaling pathways that contribute to the regulation of steroid receptors. However, it is frequently difficult to identify the means by which the alterations in cell signaling modulate the receptor activity. The target of the kinases may be the receptor, associated proteins, or both. The second technique is to mutate phosphorylation sites in the steroid receptors and to determine the roles of the individual phosphorylation sites. This approach is limited by the necessity of first identifying the phosphorylation sites in the steroid receptors, a difficult undertaking that has not been completed for the majority of the steroid receptors.

A. Activation of Steroid Receptors by Cellular Signaling Pathways

Investigators have known for a long time that some steroid-regulated genes are also regulated by signal transduction pathways. Initially, it was assumed that the cell signaling pathways were acting independently of steroid receptors through proteins such as cAMP response element binding protein (CREB), the activation of which is dependent on phosphorylation. However, it is now evident that alterations in kinase activity can activate some steroid receptors in the absence of hormone. This was first shown by introducing into cells lacking the progesterone receptor a plasmid encoding the chicken progesterone receptor and a reporter plasmid containing progesterone response elements linked to the coding region of chloramphenicol acetyltransferase (CAT). CAT activity, induced in response to progesterone or 8-Br cyclic adenosine monophosphate (cAMP) (an activator of protein kinase A), was then measured. Surprisingly, both treatments induced CAT activity and both were dependent on the progesterone receptor. Subsequent studies revealed that activators of diverse signal transduction pathways cause ligand-independent activation of chicken progesterone receptor. These include epidermal growth factor (EGF), which acts through a membrane-bound receptor that induces its tyrosine kinase activity, and dopamine, which acts through a serpentine membrane receptor that causes activation of G-protein-coupled pathways. Responses of steroid receptors to signal transduction pathways are receptor, activator, and cell type specific. The estrogen receptor appears to be the most responsive of the receptors. Although there are unique genes for most of the steroid receptors, the discovery of a second gene encoding an estrogen receptor has altered the nomenclature in the field. The estrogen receptor that was cloned originally and is the best studied is now termed ER-α; the more recently discovered receptor is termed ER-β. Discussions of the estrogen receptor in literature prior to 1996 refer to ER-α. Many stimuli, including dopamine, 8-Br cAMP, EGF, and other growth factors, activate ER-α, and there is evidence that ER-β can also be activated by cell signaling pathways in the absence of hormone. Most studies of ligand-independent activation have been done in cells transfected with expression plasmids for receptors and with artificial reporters, raising the question of whether such activation can occur *in vivo*. Two types of studies support the belief that these are pathways that contribute to biological activity *in vivo*. First, EGF can induce responses (such as DNA synthesis) that are also induced by estrogen in the uteri of ovariectomized mice; the EGF action is blocked by the estrogen receptor antagonist, ICI 164384, indicating that EGF is acting through the estrogen receptor. Moreover, EGF fails to induce DNA synthesis in the uteri of mice that lack ER-α. Second, dopamine can induce a sexual receptivity response in rats (lordosis) that is normally progesterone dependent. Administration of a progesterone receptor antagonist, mifepristone, inhibits this response, confirming that dopamine is acting through the progesterone receptor.

Other steroid receptors are less responsive to changes in cell signaling. Although the human androgen receptor can be activated under specific circumstances by treatments that elevate cAMP levels or by growth factors, in many cases the changes in cell signaling are insufficient to activate the receptor, although they do increase the response to hormone. Although avian and rodent progesterone receptors can be activated in the absence of ligand, comparable conditions fail to activate the human progesterone receptor. However, treatment with growth factors or activation of protein kinase A does enhance hormone-dependent activity. Moreover, treatment with 8-Br cAMP causes the antagonist mifepristone to act as an agonist. The glucocorticoid receptor responds similarly. It is resistant to ligand-independent activation, but altered cell signaling enhances activity either in combination with agonists or with the antagonist mifepristone.

B. Role of Phosphorylation in Steroid Receptor Action

All of the steroid receptors, as well as some, if not all, of the co-activators, are phosphoproteins. Although the identification of the phosphorylation sites is incomplete, most have been identified. The number of sites in each receptor ranges from as few as four in chicken progesterone receptor to more than a dozen in the human progesterone receptor. The sites are predominantly serines, although phosphothreonine has been identified in the glucocorticoid receptor and in the human progesterone receptor. Tyrosine phos-

phorylation in these proteins occurs rarely. Under some conditions, phosphorylation of Tyr-537 in the hormone-binding domain of the estrogen receptor is detected. A majority of the phosphoserines and phosphothreonines are followed by prolines, implicating proline-directed kinases, such as the cyclin-dependent kinases and the mitogen-activated kinases, in the regulation of their phosphorylation. Almost all the phosphorylation occurs in the amino termini of the receptors. The major exception is a Ser-Pro motif in the hinge region of the steroid receptors. In contrast to the other sites, this site appears to be conserved among all receptors, and phosphorylation has been demonstrated in chicken and human progesterone receptors, mouse estrogen receptor, and human androgen receptor. Typically, the receptors exhibit some phosphorylation in the absence of hormone, but the degree of phosphorylation is enhanced upon hormone treatment. The phosphorylation of some sites such as Ser-118 in the estrogen receptor and several of the sites in the progesterone receptor is almost exclusively dependent on hormone or an activating signal such as EGF.

The roles of the phosphorylation sites are diverse and have not been fully elucidated. Reported functions range from increasing response to low levels of hormone, to altering affinity for DNA, regulating transcriptional activity, and playing a role in the stability of the receptors. One of the best characterized sites is Ser-118 in human ER-α. This site is phosphorylated either in response to hormone or to treatment with EGF. Mutation of this site to an alanine modestly reduces the transcriptional activity of the receptor in response to hormone. However, a negative charge (provided either by a phosphate or an artificially substituted glutamic acid) at this position is absolutely required for EGF-induced activation of ER-α in some cell lines. Substitution of a glutamic acid for the serine is insufficient to produce a constitutively active receptor. Thus, EGF must induce phosphorylation either of other sites in ER-α or, more likely, on associated proteins to induce ligand-independent activation.

The receptors are substrates for a variety of kinases. Although most of the sites are proline-directed kinase sites, the human progesterone receptor contains a casein kinase II site, and Ser-167 in the human estrogen receptor is a potential target of multiple kinases, including casein kinase II, Rsk, and Akt. Estrogen, progesterone, and glucocorticoid receptors are all substrates for the cyclin-dependent kinase 2 (Cdk2); activation of Cdk2 enhances the transcriptional activity of estrogen and glucocorticoid receptors. On treatment with EGF, Ser-118 in the estrogen receptor is phosphorylated by mitogen-activated protein kinase (MAPK; also called extracellular signal-regulated kinase, or ERK), contributing to ligand-independent activation. However, hormone-induced phosphorylation of Ser-118 is not dependent on MAPK; instead, cyclin H Cdk7 plays a role in hormone-dependent phosphorylation.

There are receptor-specific effects on steroid receptors of the MAPK family of proline-directed kinases, which includes the ERK, Jun N-terminal kinase (JNK) or stress-activated protein kinase, and p38/HOG signaling cascades. Activation of JNK stimulates the activity of ER-α whereas it inhibits the activity of the glucocorticoid receptor through phosphorylation of Ser-246 in the glucocorticoid receptor. Activation of ERK stimulates the activity of estrogen and progesterone receptors, but inhibits glucocorticoid receptor activity. Thus, the activities of the steroid receptors are regulated by many kinases and the consequences are receptor specific.

In addition to altering the activities of the steroid receptors through phosphorylation of the receptors, signal transduction pathways alter phosphorylation and activity of co-activators. This aspect of receptor function is less well studied, but there is good evidence that the steroid receptor co-activator (SRC) family of nuclear receptor co-activators is phosphorylated by ERK and that these phosphorylations modulate the ability of the SRC proteins to serve as co-activators.

IV. STEROID RECEPTOR INTERACTIONS WITH REGULATED TRANSCRIPTION FACTORS

Although steroid receptor activities, which result from binding directly to specific DNA sequences, are the best characterized of steroid receptor actions, there is ample evidence that steroid receptors also regulate transcription of target genes through interactions with other transcription factors, independently of a direct interaction of the receptor with the DNA. These activities may be stimulatory or inhibitory, depending on the target gene, receptor, and interacting transcription factor. Conversely, these transcription factors influence the activities of the steroid receptors. In some cases, the cross talk involves DNA-independent protein/protein interactions, and in others, the response is dependent on the sequence including and surrounding the element to which the transcription factor binds in its target gene. Steroid receptors influence several of the

transcription factors for which expression, subcellular localization, and activity are highly dependent on cellular signaling pathways.

A. NF-κB

Steroid receptors modulate the function of nuclear factor κB (NF-κB), a ubiquitously expressed transcription factor. Five members of the family have been identified, with the most well-characterized active complex being a heterodimer of the p50 and p65 (RelA) subunits. Prior to activation, p50 and p65 are located in the cytoplasm and are bound to an inhibitory κB subunit, IκB. Activating signals such as growth factors or inflammatory cytokines such as tumor necrosis factor α (TNFα) induce phosphorylation of IκB, leading to its degradation by the proteasome pathway. This frees the p50/p65 complex, permitting nuclear translocation, binding to DNA, and activation of target genes. Steroid receptors interact with NF-κB through the p65 subunit and can reciprocally modulate transcriptional activity. Both ER-α and androgen receptor-dependent mutual repression of NF-κB activity have been reported. Repression may occur either through direct physical interaction or through competition for a limited pool of co-activators. The best studied example of mutual repression between a steroid receptor and NF-κB is the functional interaction between glucocorticoid receptor and NF-κB. Studies of glucocorticoid receptor repression of NF-κB-induced activation of intercellular adhesion molecule or interleukin (ICAM-1 or IL-8) genes, for example, reveal that the glucocorticoid receptor interacts with RelA at the promoter, but does not block binding of RelA to DNA or formation of the preinitiation complex. However, the presence of the glucocorticoid receptor blocks phosphorylation of Ser-2 in the carboxyl-terminal domain (CTD) of RNA polymerase, a step required for transcription of target genes.

B. AP-1

The proteins that bind to AP-1 response elements are diverse, consisting of complexes containing either a heterodimer of Fos and Jun transcription factors or homodimers of Jun proteins alone. These proteins are regulated both at the level of transcription and by posttranslational modification. Originally characterized as proteins that are activated by protein kinase C, these proteins are regulated by numerous cell signaling pathways. Among these is the JNK pathway. Functional interactions between AP-1 proteins and steroid receptors are numerous and the response is

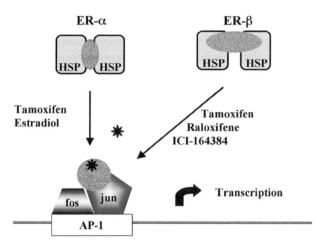

FIGURE 3 Estrogen receptor-mediated activation of transcription through an activator protein (AP-1) site. Estrogen receptors can promote transcription of a target gene through binding to the Jun partner of a Fos/Jun heterodimer bound to an AP-1 site. Although both estrogen receptor-α (ER-α) and ER-β are capable of activating transcription through AP-1 sites, the hormone specificity of the activation differs. HSP, Heat-shock protein complex.

receptor and promoter specific. Both ER-α and ER-β interact with AP-1 complexes. ER-α stimulates AP-1 activity on treatment with either an agonist such as estradiol or an antagonist such as tamoxifen (Fig. 3). Surprisingly, ER-β stimulates AP-1 activity only on binding antagonists. ER interacts with the Jun partner of the heterodimer. The finding that antagonists of conventional hormone response element-dependent transcription can stimulate estrogen receptor-dependent transcription through AP-1 elements complicates the simple model of antagonists as compounds that block the actions of steroid receptors. The ability of a specific compound to antagonize receptor activity is clearly not universal, but is dependent on the function measured.

In contrast to the estrogen receptor, the glucocorticoid receptor frequently inhibits the activity of AP-1 on activation by agonists, although this is, again, dependent on the promoter. The glucocorticoid receptor inhibits the activity of the AP-1 element in the proliferin gene when a Fos/Jun heterodimer binds to the site, but stimulates the activity of Jun homodimers. Similar to the ER, the glucocorticoid receptor binds to Jun; mutations in the glucocorticoid receptor that abrogate binding to conventional hormone response elements do not eliminate regulation of AP-1 proteins either *in vitro* or in a transgenic mouse expressing only the mutant receptor. The striking difference in phenotype between

glucocorticoid receptor null mice (embryonic lethal) and mice expressing only a glucocorticoid receptor that lacks the ability to bind to a hormone response element provides strong evidence that many glucocorticoid receptor actions do not require binding to a conventional response element. For example, the glucocorticoid effects on the immune system are retained in mice with the mutant receptor.

Although studies of the androgen receptor have not been as extensive, there is evidence that AP-1 complexes acting through the Jun partner can inhibit the activity of the androgen receptor and that the androgen receptor inhibits the activity of the AP-1 complex.

C. Interactions with Other Transcription Factors

The functional interaction of steroid receptors with other transcription factors is an active area of research. Among the other transcription factors that interact with steroid receptors are a member of the signal transducer and activator of transcription (STAT) family of transcription factors, STAT5. STAT proteins are cytoplasmic prior to activation. Activation of membrane-bound receptors, including cytokine receptors, causes activation of the Janus family tyrosine kinases (Jak kinases), which, in turn, phosphorylate cytoplasmic STAT proteins, promoting dimerization of the STAT proteins, translocation to the nucleus, and transcriptional activation. Both STAT proteins and glucocorticoid receptors are cytoplasmic in the absence of activating signals. Activation of either can promote nuclear localization of the other. These interactions can stimulate or inhibit the activities of the transcription factors. Activation of the glucocorticoid receptor stimulates STAT-dependent transcription of the β-casein gene, but STAT can also inhibit glucocorticoid receptor activity. Another example of a steroid receptor influencing transcription of target genes through other transcription factors is the activation of the cathepsin D gene by estradiol through interaction of estrogen receptor with the transcription factor Sp-1.

V. STEROID-INDUCED ACTIVATION OF CELLULAR SIGNALING PATHWAYS

Steroids, acting through classical steroid receptors as well as through other means, induce the activation of a variety of signal transduction pathways. Although there has been evidence for a role of steroids in the activation of cellular signaling pathways for many years, elucidation of the precise mechanisms by which steroids transmit signals to activate kinases is a relatively new and active field of research. The actions of steroids are transmitted by diverse means, including through classical steroid receptors associated with membranes or acting in the cytoplasm, through steroid hormone-binding globulin, and through G-protein-coupled receptors. In addition, there is evidence for membrane receptors, which are structurally unrelated to classical steroid receptors, but these have not yet been cloned and little is known about these proteins.

A variety of studies have provided evidence that either the classical steroid receptor proteins or closely related proteins function as activators of cell signaling pathways. Membrane-bound glucocorticoid and estrogen receptors contain regions on the extracellular surface that cross-react with antibodies to the well-characterized estrogen and glucocorticoid receptors. Binding of estradiol by the membrane estrogen receptor in GH3 pituitary cells induces release of prolactin and subsequent activation of its signaling cascade. Interestingly, one of the ER-α antibodies blocks estradiol-induced prolactin response whereas another induces prolactin release in the absence of estradiol. Finally, reduction in ER-α expression in these cells using antisense oligonucleotides inhibits membrane estrogen receptor expression.

Steroid hormones acting through estrogen, androgen, or progesterone receptors can activate ERK through interaction with and activation of Src kinase, a tyrosine kinase. Although the result, i.e. activation of Src kinase, is similar, estrogen receptors and progesterone receptors interact with different regions of Src. Downstream actions of estradiol, such as activation of endothelial nitric oxide synthase (NOS), are blocked by inhibitors of ERK activation, suggesting a role for ERK in many estradiol-dependent nongenomic actions. In many instances steroids induce rapid alterations in calcium flux and/or induce the activities of a variety of kinases. Some of these actions appear to be independent of classical steroid receptors, although the mechanisms that induce the changes in signaling molecules have not been identified. In one case, a G-protein-coupled receptor (GPCR) is activated.

One steroid pathway that has been partially elucidated is the sex hormone-binding globulin (SHBG) pathway. SHBG serves as a carrier for steroids in the blood. In addition, it has the capacity to bind to a specific membrane receptor. When receptor-bound SHBG binds to an appropriate steroid, such as estradiol or dihydrotestosterone (DHT),

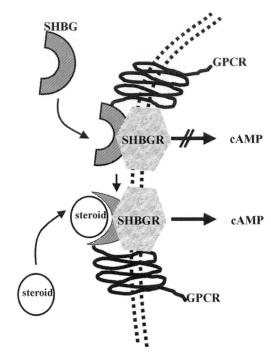

FIGURE 4 Steroids increase cAMP levels through activation of steroid hormone-binding globulin receptor (SHBGR). In the absence of an activating steroid, the steroid hormone-binding globulin (SHBG) can bind to SHBGR, but does not induce production of cAMP. Binding of steroid activates the receptor, which may be a G-protein-coupled receptor (GPCR), or associates with a GPCR to stimulate synthesis of cAMP.

the levels of cAMP are increased (Fig. 4). The receptor for SHBG has not been cloned, but there is indirect evidence that it is a G-protein-coupled-receptor because compounds or proteins that inhibit G-protein signaling block SHBG-mediated induction of cAMP.

VI. SUMMARY

Steroid hormone action and cellular signaling pathways intersect at many levels of the signaling pathways, providing many opportunities for mutual regulation and feedback between steroid receptors, kinases, and downstream transcription factors regulated by signal transduction pathways. For example, when an estrogen receptor-containing cell is exposed to estradiol, the result is a plethora of signaling events, including classical gene regulation through estrogen response elements, regulation of a subset of genes regulated by other transcription factors, such as AP-1 and Sp-1, and direct induction of a variety of cell signaling pathways leading to kinase activation.

Glossary

agonist Compound that binds to a cellular receptor, stimulating its biological activity.

antagonist Compound that binds to a cellular receptor and blocks agonist-dependent induction of biological activity.

co-activator Molecule that binds to a transcription factor and stimulates the transcription of the target gene to which the factor is bound.

G-protein-coupled receptors Seven-transmembrane-spanning regions (also termed serpentine regions) that interact with heterotrimeric GTP-binding proteins, resulting in alterations in downstream signaling.

proteasome Large protein complex responsible for degrading proteins that have typically been modified by ubiquitination.

See Also the Following Articles

Androgen Receptor Crosstalk with Cellular Signaling Pathways • Co-activators and Corepressors for the Nuclear Receptor Superfamily • Crosstalk of Nuclear Receptors with STAT Factors • Estrogen Receptor Crosstalk with Cellular Signaling Pathways • GPCR (G-Protein-Coupled Receptor) Structure • Progesterone Receptor Structure/Function and Crosstalk with Cellular Signaling Pathways • Steroid Hormone Receptor Family: Mechanisms of Action

Further Reading

Boonyaratanakornkit, V., Scott, M. P., Ribon, V., Sherman, L., Anderson, S. M., Maller, J. L., Miller, W. T., and Edwards, D. P. (2001). Progesterone receptor contains a proline-rich motif that directly interacts with SH3 domains and activates c-Src family tyrosine kinases. *Mol. Cell* **8**, 269–280.

Falkenstein, E., Tillman, H.-C., Christ, M., Feuring, M., and Wehling, M. (2000). Multiple actions of steroid hormones—A focus on rapid, nongenomic effects. *Pharmacol. Rev.* **52**, 513–555.

Herrlich, P. (2001). Cross-talk between glucocorticoid receptor and AP-1. *Oncogene* **20**, 2465–2475.

Kousteni, S., Bellido, T., Plotkin, L. I., O'Brien, C. A., Bodenner, D. L., Han, L., Han, K., DiGregorio, G. B., Katzenellenbogen, J. A., Katzenellenbogen, B. S., Roberson, P. K., Weinstein, R. S., Jilka, R. L., and Manolagas, S. C. (2001). Nongenotropic, sex-nonspecific signaling through the estrogen or androgen receptors: Dissociation from transcriptional activity. *Cell* **104**, 719–730.

Lechner, J., Welte, T., Tomasi, J. K., Bruno, P., Cairns, C., Gustafsson, J., and Doppler, W. (1997). Promoter-dependent synergy between glucocorticoid receptor and Stat5 in the activation of beta-casein gene transcription. *J. Biol. Chem.* **272**, 20954–20960.

McKenna, N. J., Lanz, R. B., and O'Malley, B. W. (1999). Nuclear receptor coregulators: Cellular and molecular biology. *Endocr. Rev.* **20**, 321–344.

Nissen, R. M., and Yamamoto, K. R. (2000). The glucocorticoid receptor inhibits NFκB by interfering with serine-2 phosphorylation of the RNA polymerase II carboxy-terminal domain. *Genes Dev.* **14**, 2314–2329.

Rogatsky, I., Logan, S. K., and Garabedian, M. J. (1998). Antagonism of glucocorticoid receptor transcriptional activation by the c-Jun N-terminal kinase. *Proc. Natl. Acad. Sci. U.S.A* **95**, 2050–2055.

Rogatsky, I., Trowbridge, J. M., and Garabedian, M. J. (1999). Potentiation of human estrogen receptor α transcriptional activatiton through phosphorylation of serines 104 and 106 by the cyclin A–CDK2 complex. *J. Biol. Chem.* **274**, 22296–22302.

Rosner, W., Hryb, D. J., Khan, M. S., Nakhla, A. M., and Romas, N. A. (1999). Androgen and estrogen signaling at the cell membrane via G-proteins and cyclic adenosine monophosphate. *Steroids* **64**, 100–106.

Rowan, B. G., Garrison, N., Weigel, N. L., and O'Malley, B. W. (2000). 8-Bromo-cyclic AMP induces phosphorylation of two sites in SRC-1 that facilitate ligand-independent activation of the chicken progesterone receptor and are critical for functional cooperation between SRC-1 and CREB binding protein. *Mol. Cell. Biol.* **20**, 8720–8730.

Safe, S. (2001). Transcriptional activation of genes by 17 beta-estradiol through estrogen receptor–Sp1 interactions. *Vit. Horm.* **62**, 231–252.

Tremblay, A., Tremblay, G. B., Labrie, F., and Giguère, V. (1999). Ligand-independent recruitment of SRC-1 to estrogen receptor β through phosphorylation of activation function AF-1. *Mol. Cell* **3**, 513–519.

Weigel, N. L. (1996). Steroid hormone receptors and their regulation by phosphorylation. *Biochem. J.* **319**, 657–667.

Weigel, N. L., and Zhang, Y. (1998). Ligand-independent activation of steroid hormone receptors. *J. Mol. Med.* **76**, 469–479.

Stress

PAUL J. ROSCH

New York Medical College, Valhalla, and American Institute of Stress

I. ORIGINS OF THE STRESS CONCEPT
II. THE GENERAL ADAPTATION SYNDROME AND DISEASES OF ADAPTATION
III. STRESS-RELATED DISORDERS AND MECHANISMS OF ACTION

Stress, a term used interchangeably to refer to stimuli and to the psychophysiologic responses and pathologic consequences when such stimuli are severe or prolonged, is a highly personalized phenomenon. It is thus difficult to define, much less measure. Our current concepts of stress derive from early studies of physiologic responses to stressors, but technological advances have provided new insights into the mechanisms that may be involved in mediating the role of stress in different disorders.

I. ORIGINS OF THE STRESS CONCEPT

A. Claude Bernard's Milieu Intérieur and Walter Cannon's "Homeostasis"

Although the word "stress" has been used for over five centuries as a synonym for distress, its current meaning dates back only six decades, when the term was essentially coined by the brilliant Canadian investigator Hans Selye. Selye's concept of stress had its roots in the research of Claude Bernard, who first demonstrated the mechanisms responsible for maintaining blood sugar levels and body temperature within a physiologic range whenever normalcy was threatened. In his 1865 "Introduction to the Study of Experimental Medicine", Bernard wrote that "all the vital mechanisms, however buried they may be, have only one object: that of preserving constant the conditions of life in the milieu intérieur (internal environment). ...It is a fixity of the *milieu intérieur* which is the condition of free and independent life." Bernard also identified the existence of ductless (endocrine) glands, as opposed to those with ducts (exocrine), and originated the term "internal secretion."

A half-century later, Walter Cannon referred to this "fixity of the milieu intérieur" as the "steady state" and coined the term "homeostasis" to describe the numerous balancing mechanisms necessary to maintain the steady state. In studying the motor activities responsible for progressively propelling food through the gut, he noted that when his experimental animals were hungry, peristaltic waves increased in frequency and amplitude; however, if they became frightened, no such increases were seen and there was a diminution or even transient cessation of peristalsis. His further investigations revealed that this and other responses during fright were due to an outpouring of adrenaline and stimulation of the sympathetic nervous system. By 1915, Cannon had concluded that the greatest stimulation occurred under conditions of extreme hunger, thirst, fear, or rage, and during sexual activity. All of these situations automatically and immediately precipitated a cascade of coordinated nervous system and metabolic responses throughout the body. Cannon theorized that these integrated activities had been exquisitely honed over the lengthy course of evolution to facilitate "fight or flight" life-saving measures. He summarized the mechanisms responsible for maintaining heart rate, blood pressure, temperature, and blood concentrations of sugar, protein, fat, calcium, and oxygen during normal and emergency conditions in "The Wisdom of the Body," first published in 1932.

B. Hans Selye and "They Just Looked Sick"

As a medical student, Selye had noted that patients who subsequently developed very different diseases often exhibited identical signs and symptoms during the first few days of their illness. They all had low-grade fevers, feelings of malaise, fatigue, generalized aches, and "they just looked sick." He was 18 and excited about the possibility of using his weekends to study the mechanisms that might be responsible for these common nonspecific signs and symptoms, but was advised that this would be fruitless and that he should devote any spare time to his studies. Selye graduated first in his class; he later earned a doctorate in organic chemistry and received a Rockefeller scholarship in 1931, which he used to study under the renowned biochemist, J. B. Collip, at McGill Medical School. At the time, only two ovarian hormones had been identified, but Collip thought there was a third and Selye was sent to the Montreal slaughterhouses to retrieve as many cow ovaries as possible. Collip processed these into an extract for Selye to inject into female rats; the rats were subsequently examined for any changes in tissues that might be attributed to a new ovarian hormone. Not only were no such effects detected, but most of the rats became very sick and several died.

Although Selye found no gross or microscopic changes in the ovaries or breasts of the injected rats, he observed that all of the animals showed ulcerations in the stomach, enlargement of the adrenals, and shrinkage of the thymus and lymphoid tissues. The most plausible cause seemed to be some contaminant in Collip's chemical concoction. There was a bottle of formaldehyde used to fix tissues for microscopic study in front of him; on a whim, he injected liberal amounts of this toxic substance into several rats and was amazed to find that it produced results identical to those observed with Collip's new extract. Injecting other toxic chemicals produced these same changes; he subsequently demonstrated (in experiments that would be impossible to perform today) that noxious physical and/or emotional stimuli could produce these same pathologic changes. Selye viewed these common pathologic findings, as well as the very early similar symptoms in sick patients he had observed as a medical student, as a nonspecific response to what he chose to call "biologic stress."

In 1936, Selye submitted his findings to the editor of *Nature*, in the form of a 74-line letter; the editor agreed to publish the letter if Selye omitted the word "stress," because at the time, in colloquial speech, the word had the connotation of "nervous strain." Also,

Selye was unaware that stress had been used for centuries by engineers and physicists to describe something quite different from what Selye was proposing. Hooke's Law (1658) stated that the magnitude of stress (an external force) would produce a proportional amount of strain (deformation) in a metal, depending on its degree of malleability. Therefore, "strain" would have been preferable, and Selye later complained on several occasions that, had he been aware of this, he would have gone down in history as the father of the "strain" concept. Considerable confusion was created when his research had to be translated into other languages. In 1946, when invited to explain his theories at the prestigious Collège de France, where 100 years previously, the great Claude Bernard had presented his concept of *the milieu intérieur*, the academicians responsible for maintaining the purity of the French language were unable to find a suitable word or phrase to convey Selye's concept of biologic stress. After several days of debate, they decided that a new word would have to be created and *le stress* was born, quickly followed by *el stress, il stress, lo stress, der stress* in other European languages, with similar neologisms in Russian, Japanese, Chinese, and Arabic. Stress is one of the few words still preserved extant in languages that do not use the Latin alphabet.

Other difficulties arose as "stress" was increasingly incorporated into vernacular speech and eventually became a popular buzzword; it was used interchangeably to refer to both physical and emotional challenges, the body's response to these stimuli, as well as to the pathological consequences of such interactions. Even Selye had difficulties when he tried to extrapolate his laboratory research to humans. In helping him to prepare his *First Annual Report on Stress* 1951, I included a critical letter that had appeared in the *British Medical Journal*. Using verbatim citations from Selye's own writings, one physician had concluded that "stress, in addition to being itself, was also the cause of itself, and the result of itself." Because it was apparent that most people viewed stress as some unpleasant threat, Selye had to create a new word, "stressor," to differentiate stimulus from response. Another problem was that all of his experiments had been conducted in laboratory animals and had focused only on the damaging effects of stress. It was apparent that stress was not always necessarily harmful for humans. Increased stress results in increased productivity—up to a certain level that differs for each of us. It is only when this level is exceeded that damage is apt to

occur. Nor is stress always a synonym for something bad. Winning a race or election may be just as stressful as losing, or more so. A passionate kiss and contemplating what might follow could be described as stressful but hardly comparable to the feeling experienced during a root canal procedure. Were the physiological changes associated with "good" stress different? Could good stress negate the effects of bad stress? Selye subsequently created "eustress" to refer to good stress that might promote health.

II. THE GENERAL ADAPTATION SYNDROME AND DISEASES OF ADAPTATION

Selye viewed the initial stereotyped response to stress described in his 1936 *Nature* report as a "call to arms" of the body's defense mechanisms and referred to it as an "alarm reaction." If a state of stress persisted, a "stage of resistance" ensued, during which there was increased adaptation to the noxious stimulus. When prolonged further, resistance/adaptation became inadequate or disappeared in a third and final stage of exhaustion. He termed this three-phased response the General Adaptation Syndrome, the initial component being the alarm reaction, when adaptation had not yet been acquired, a subsequent stage of resistance, during which adaptation to the offending stimulus was maximal, and a final stage of exhaustion, when all resistance was lost.

Autopsy findings during various phases of the General Adaptation Syndrome revealed pathologic changes in the cardiovascular system, kidneys, gastrointestinal tract, soft tissues, and other structures reminiscent and often indistinguishable from those seen in patients with rheumatoid arthritis, disseminated lupus, gastrointestinal ulcers, and cardiovascular and kidney disorders. Selye reasoned that if stress could produce this type of pathology in his laboratory animals, perhaps it could contribute to these and other diseases in humans; he referred to these as "diseases of adaptation." These pathologic changes were influenced by various factors, including the nature and severity of the stressor, the duration of exposure, and prior sensitization through dietary alterations or the administration of certain steroids. He subsequently discovered how to produce consistently different disorders such as myocardial necrosis or nephrosclerosis by placing the animals on a high-sodium diet and administering desoxycorticosterone acetate (DOCA). Conversely, a high-potassium diet and strategies that conserved potassium minimized myocardial damage.

III. STRESS-RELATED DISORDERS AND MECHANISMS OF ACTION

Selye identified over two dozen different steroids in the adrenal venous effluent, but it was difficult to distinguish between those with physiologic hormonal activities and others that represented metabolites or precursors having little clinical significance. After numerous experiments, he concluded that there were three main types of adrenal cortical hormones, which he classified as glucocorticoids, mineralocorticoids, and testoids. Glucocorticoids, or "sugar hormones," produced in the zona fasciculata had a pronounced influence on carbohydrate metabolism because they promoted gluconeogenesis by breaking down protein to provide glucose. Other catabolic or antianabolic effects included lympholysis, eosinopenia, and inhibition of inflammation. Whereas these anti-inflammatory effects delayed wound healing and increased susceptibility to infection, glucocorticoids such as cortisone were later found to provide clinical benefits, especially in patients with rheumatoid arthritis. Mineralocorticoids, or "salt hormones," such as DOCA, manufactured in the zona glomerulosa, had their major effects on electrolytes by promoting the reabsorption of sodium and the excretion of potassium. The testoids, or sex steroids, also known as "protein" hormones, originated in the zona reticularis and appeared to have similar but much weaker effects than testosterone on secondary sex characteristics and protein anabolism. Selye's categorizations were somewhat deceptive because the close structural similarity of all adrenal cortical steroids resulted in overlapping effects. Glucocorticoids had some sodium retention properties and mineralocorticoids could mimic certain glucocorticoid carbohydrate responses. When 9a-halogenated and 2-methylated analogues of cortisone were subsequently synthesized, it was found that they had very potent glucocorticoid and mineralocorticoid actions. Conversely, compounds with a double bond in the 1 and 2 positions separated these effects.

In 1937, Selye tried to determine what stimulated the adrenal cortex during stress. Until the late nineteenth century, the human pituitary was thought to be a vestigial organ and no pituitary hormone had yet been isolated. After many complicated surgical interventions, he discovered that only removal of the anterior pituitary prevented the adrenal cortical response to stress. Experiments designed to elucidate the role of the pituitary showed that administering crude lyophilized anterior pituitary extract (LAP), the only hypophyseal product that was available at the time, definitely caused enlargement of the adrenal cortex. Of equal interest was the observation that LAP tended to simulate the damaging effects of DOCA with respect to the production of nephrosclerosis and myocardial damage during stress. When subsequent advances led to the isolation and purification of pituitary hormones, it became obvious that adrenocorticotropic hormone (ACTH) was not responsible for these LAP effects. On the other hand, somatotropic hormone (STH) or growth hormone could, under certain conditions, produce changes similar to those observed with DOCA and LAP. Further investigations revealed that STH could antagonize or reverse the catabolic effects of ACTH and tended to prevent the weight loss and susceptibility to infection seen following the administration of ACTH and glucocorticoids. For example, the rat's normal resistance to tuberculosis could be temporarily lost by pretreatment with ACTH but was restored when STH was administered concomitantly. ACTH clearly stimulated the production of glucocorticoids and STH augmented mineralocorticoid activities either by increasing their production or by exaggerating their effects. This suggested that there were checks and balances between ACTH and STH in the pituitary and between glucocorticoids and mineralocorticoids in the adrenal. ACTH and glucocorticoids had strong anti-inflammatory effects whereas STH and mineralocorticoids stimulated inflammatory and proliferative connective tissue responses. How these activities were influenced by emotional stress in humans or could contribute to "diseases of adaptation" was not clear.

When DOCA was used to treat patients with adrenal insufficiency due to adrenalectomy or Addison's disease, there were reports of focal areas of necrosis in the heart and skeletal muscle, evidence of periarteritis nodosa, nephrosclerosis, worsening of joint distress, and even the development of incapacitating arthritis, as had been seen in experimental animals. The tendency to develop hypertension even with very small doses of DOCA was also a frequent problem encountered during the treatment of adrenal insufficiency. DOCA is not manufactured in any appreciable amount in humans. When aldosterone, the naturally occurring human mineralocorticoid, became available, attempts to demonstrate its ability to counter the anti-inflammatory effects of cortisone or produce the pathology seen with DOCA in laboratory studies were disappointing. It seemed unlikely that aldosterone caused significant pathology in humans but subsequent evidence supports Selye's theory. Researchers have now confirmed that aldosterone can contribute to cardiovascular and renal pathology as well as to fibrosis and collagen formation by promoting sodium influx and hypertrophy in vascular smooth muscle cells, generation of oxygen free radicals, and stimulation of growth factors and by potentiating the pressor effects of angiotensin II.

Extrapolating the results of animal studies to humans can be hazardous. This is especially true when dealing with stress-related research. Contemporary stress is most often due to a variety of emotional challenges that can occur several times a day, rather than to the physical threats primitive man was subjected to on a sporadic basis. Although "flight or fight" responses to severe stress can occur, we are much more apt to experience other signs and symptoms that are subtler and cover a wide range of emotional and physical responses, as illustrated in Table 1.

Although there is a great deal of anecdotal evidence that stress can contribute to emotional and physical disorders, attempting to prove this by delineating the mechanisms of actions that may be involved is difficult. There are numerous confounding influences and no animal models that reflect the wide range of emotions that humans experience. The consensus of opinion is that when secreted in response to acute stress, hormones such as adrenaline and cortisol stimulate protective body defense mechanisms and

help the body adapt, but when repeatedly invoked or produced in excess for sustained periods, the resultant physiologic responses become damaging. The most relevant research has focused on the cardiovascular system, showing that stress due to lack of control on the job, for example, results in hypertension and coronary heart disease. Other factors, such as social instability, can also cause changes in clotting factors that contribute to heart attacks and strokes. One report has revealed that the 40% spike in mortality rates seen in Russian men following the fall of communism was largely due to cardiovascular disease.

Chronic stress has been shown to reduce immune system resistance to the common cold and has been implicated in other viral-linked disorders, ranging from herpes and autoimmune disease syndrome (AIDS) to certain malignancies. Repeated and/or long-term stress can also affect how we age, especially with respect to neuronal brain damage. Memory loss for recent events, one of the hallmarks of aging, is due to progressive atrophy of the hippocampus, which is responsible for memory retrieval and learning. As the old adage goes, "You can't teach an old dog new tricks." Stress hormones such as cortisol cause the same type of hippocampal shrinkage seen in the elderly. Studies show that patients suffering from depression or posttraumatic stress disorder often

TABLE 1 Common Signs and Symptoms of Stress

1. Frequent headaches, jaw clenching, or pain	26. Insomnia, nightmares, or disturbing dreams
2. Gritting and grinding teeth	27. Difficulty concentrating; racing thoughts
3. Stuttering or stammering	28. Trouble learning new information
4. Tremors; trembling of lips or hands	29. Forgetfulness, disorganization, or confusion
5. Neck ache, back pain, or muscle spasms	30. Difficulty in making decisions
6. Light headedness, faintness, or dizziness	31. Feeling overloaded or overwhelmed
7. Ringing, buzzing or "popping" sounds	32. Frequent crying spells or suicidal thoughts
8. Frequent blushing or sweating	33. Feelings of loneliness or worthlessness
9. Cold or sweaty hands or feet	34. Little interest in appearance or punctuality
10. Dry mouth or problems swallowing	35. Nervous habits; fidgeting or feet tapping
11. Frequent colds, infections, or herpes sores	36. Increased frustration, irritability, or edginess
12. Rashes, itching, hives, or "goose bumps"	37. Overreaction to petty annoyances
13. Unexplained or frequent "allergy" attacks	38. Increased number of minor accidents
14. Heartburn, stomach pain, or nausea	39. Obsessive or compulsive behavior
15. Excess belching or flatulence	40. Reduced work efficiency or productivity
16. Constipation, diarrhea, or loss of bowel control	41. Lies or excuses to cover up poor work
17. Difficulty breathing or frequent sighing	42. Rapid or mumbled speech
18. Sudden attacks of life-threatening panic	43. Excessive defensiveness or suspiciousness
19. Chest pain, palpitations, or rapid pulse	44. Problems in communication or sharing
20. Frequent urination	45. Social withdrawal and isolation
21. Diminished sexual desire or performance	46. Constant tiredness, weakness, or fatigue
22. Excess anxiety, worry, guilt, or nervousness	47. Frequent use of over-the-counter drugs
23. Increased anger, frustration, or hostility	48. Weight gain or loss without dietary changes
24. Depression or frequent or wild mood swings	49. Increased smoking, alcohol, or drug use
25. Increased or decreased appetite	50. Excessive gambling or impulse buying

complain of memory loss for recent events and difficulties in learning and concentration that correlate with increased cortisol levels. An increase in blood sugar, insulin, and cholesterol levels and a decrease in bone density and muscle mass have also been linked to chronic stress. These and other adverse effects can be aggravated by poor lifestyle habits, such as alcohol, drug, and tobacco abuse, faulty diet, and lack of exercise, all of which are also often stress related.

To test the hypothesis that allostatic load reflected the effects of stress on the body and contributed to disease, a group of healthy elderly people were studied; their blood pressure, blood glucose, and cholesterol levels were correlated with cortisol measurements. Follow-up 3 years later confirmed that those with the highest allostatic loads were the ones most apt to develop newly diagnosed cardiovascular disease and were significantly more likely to show declines in mental as well as physical functioning.

Advances in our understanding of how the body responds to stress or to any attempt to change the status quo have always depended on the information available about biochemical and physiologic functions. Although Claude Bernard first described the existence of endocrine glands, he had scant knowledge of their activities. Walter Cannon knew little about the functions of the adrenal cortex, nor was Hans Selye aware of the host of neurotransmitters (such as endorphins, dopamine, and serotonin) that play an important part in the response to stress. The endorphins, which have powerful effects on mood and pain perception, are secreted simultaneously with ACTH in amounts that are proportional to the magnitude of the stressful stimulus. Measurements following the removal of the pituitary or adrenal, or following the administration of dexamethasone, confirm that the production and release of endorphins are regulated by the same adrenal steroid feedback mechanisms that control the secretion of ACTH, the premier stress hormone.

There are far more questions than answers about how the body responds to stress or how emotions can contribute to disease. As René Dubos noted, "what happens in the mind of man is always reflected in the diseases of his body." Selye's proposal that stress-related hormones caused different diseases was criticized as being simplistic because the available data supported other interpretations, such as a "permissive" or "conditioning" role. It was pointed out that interactions between stress and the adrenal could include the following effects:

- Nonspecific effects due to overproduction of corticoids.
- Nonspecific effects due to decreased elimination of corticoids.
- Nonspecific effects due to conditioning of the target by corticoids, causing increased sensitivity.
- Nonspecific effects due to the stressor, but requiring the presence of corticoids to maintain tissue reactivity.
- Specific effects due to the stressor, and not influenced by adrenal factors.
- Specific effects due to the stressor, and requiring adrenal activity.
- Any combination of the above.

The stress saga is far from over. Many of Selye's theories may be incorrect or incomplete based on subsequent observations. However, as he often reminded me, "Theories don't have to be correct, only facts do. Some theories are valuable for their heuristic merit, in that they encourage others to discover new facts that lead to better theories." Selye's concepts of stress and its effects on health are a good example of this and are likely to be his greatest legacy.

Glossary

alarm reaction First stage of the General Adaptation Syndrome in which gastric ulcerations, adrenal hypertrophy, and shrinkage of the thymus and lymphatic tissues are consistently seen within 48 h following exposure to noxious stimuli.

desoxycorticosterone acetate Adrenal cortical steroid with predominant effects on electrolytes such as sodium and potassium.

diseases of adaptation Maladies observed during the course of the General Adaptation Syndrome in experimental animals; Selye believed the maladies were the counterpart of diseases in humans with similar pathologic changes.

eustress Selye's term for "good" stress that promotes health.

General Adaptation Syndrome Selye's term for the manifestations of stress in the whole body following prolonged stress exposure; the syndrome develops over time in three phases: the alarm reaction, the stage of resistance, and the stage of exhaustion.

homeostasis Walter Cannon's term for the body's tendency to maintain physiological stability in response to influences that threaten to disturb the steady state.

milieu intérieur Claude Bernard's term for the internal environment of the body, or the "soil" in which all biologic reactions occur.

stage of exhaustion Third and final stage of the General Adaptation Syndrome, during which the ability to adapt to stress is exhausted and death often ensues.

stage of resistance Second stage of the General Adaptation Syndrome, during which the body's resistance to stress is maximized.

stressor Selye's term for any stimulus that produces a state of stress.

See Also the Following Articles

Adrenocorticotropic Hormone (ACTH) and Other Proopiomelanocortin (POMC) Peptides ● Corticotropin-Releasing Hormone Receptor Signaling ● Corticotropin-Releasing Hormone, Stress, and the Immune System ● Endocrine Rhythms: Generation, Regulation, and Integration ● Glucocorticoid Biosynthesis: Role of StAR Protein ● Mineralocorticoids and Hypertension ● Stress and Reproduction

Further Reading

Bernard, C. (1865). [Greene, H.C., (transl.) (1957)]. "An Introduction to the Study of Experimental Medicine." Dover, New York.

Cannon, W. B. (1939). "The Wisdom of the Body." W.W. Norton, New York.

Epstein, M. (2001). Aldosterone as a determinant of cardiovascular and renal dysfunction. *J. R. Soc. Med.* **94**, 378–383.

Rosch, P. J. (1958). The growth and development of the stress concept and its significance in clinical medicine. *In* "Modern Trends in Endocrinology" (H. Gardiner-Hill, ed.), pp. 278–298. Butterworths, London.

Selye, H. (1950). "Stress." Acta, Inc., Montreal.

Selye, H., and Rosch, P. J. (1954). Integration of endocrinology. *In* "Glandular Physiology and Therapy" (American Medical Association Council on Pharmacy and Chemistry, ed.), pp. 1–10. J. B. Lippincott, Philadelphia.

Selye, H., and Rosch, P. J. (1954). The renaissance in endocrinology. *In* "Medicine and Science" (I. Galdston, ed.), pp. 30–43. International Universities Press, New York.

Selye, H. (1976). "Stress in Health and Disease." Butterworths, Boston.

Stress and Reproduction

JUDY L. CAMERON

Oregon National Primate Research Center, Oregon Health and Science University

I. INTRODUCTION
II. REPRODUCTIVE CONSEQUENCES OF STRESS
III. MULTIPLE FORMS OF STRESS
IV. MECHANISMS OF STRESS ACTION

Many forms of stress, including energetic stresses (e.g., undernutrition, exercise, temperature stress, and lactation), stresses associated with injury and illness (e.g., pain and infection), and psychosocial stresses (e.g., fear, anxiety, and discomfort), can lead to a suppression of reproductive hormone secretion and, if sustained, a suppression of fertility. Exposure to stress in the adolescent period can delay the onset of puberty. Stress-induced reproductive dysfunction can occur in both females and males.

I. INTRODUCTION

All forms of stress act primarily at the level of the central nervous system (CNS) to lead to a suppression of the activity of the hypothalamic neurons that provide the central neural drive to the reproductive axis [i.e., gonadotropin-releasing hormone (GnRH) neurons]. Not all stresses cause a suppression of reproductive axis activity in all animals. Multiple factors, including dominance rank, magnitude of the stress, perception of the stress, aggressiveness of the animal, and level of activity of the reproductive axis prior to stress exposure, play important roles in modulating the response of the reproductive axis to both acute and chronic stresses. The neural mechanisms by which stress signals modulate the function of GnRH neurons are in the early stages of being mapped. Although some neural systems, such as the hypothalamic–pituitary–adrenal axis, are activated by many stresses, they do not play a causal role in all forms of stress-induced reproductive dysfunction.

II. REPRODUCTIVE CONSEQUENCES OF STRESS

Stress exposure can be acute, chronic, or intermittent and vary from mild to severe. The reproductive consequences of stress exposure depend on both the severity of the stress and the duration of the stress. Individual differences in stress sensitivity also play an important role in determining the outcome of stress exposure. In females, mild or acute forms of stress can lead to a suppression of circulating gonadotropin secretion, which in turn can lead to a lengthening of the menstrual cycle (primarily due to a lengthening of the follicular phase due to slow follicular development), a suppression of ovulation, or impaired luteal function (characterized by low progesterone secretion and in more severe cases a shortening of the luteal phase). Exposure to more severe or chronic forms of stress can result in impaired ovarian cyclicity with the occurrence of irregular menstrual cycles (oliogomenorrhea) or the complete loss of menstrual cyclicity (amenorrhea). As ovarian steroid production is decreased, there is also a decline in secondary sexual characteristics, including breast size and amount of subcutaneous fat. In males, stress-induced reproductive impairment is characterized by a decrease in testosterone secretion and thus a loss of libido and a decrease in spermatogenesis and hormonal support for secondary sexual characteristics. Chronic stress occurring during the process of pubertal development can impair the progression of puberty, leading in some cases to a very marked delay in the pubertal development of reproductive capacity and the accompanying development of secondary sexual characteristics.

The primary site of stress-induced disruption of the reproductive axis appears to be at the level of the GnRH neurons, which provide the central neural drive to the reproductive axis (Fig. 1). Using animal models of various stresses, it has been shown for at least some stresses that GnRH secretion is impaired. However, more typically, it is inferred that GnRH secretion is impaired by measuring a suppression in pituitary gonadotropin secretion. This conclusion is further supported by the finding that in all conditions of stress-induced reproductive dysfunction studied to date, administration of exogenous GnRH can stimulate the function of the reproductive axis, indicating that stress is not acting to directly suppress pituitary or gonadal activity. In some forms of acute stress, a fall in gonadotropin secretion can be noted within minutes to hours. With more subtle stresses, impairment of gonadotropin secretion is generally noted when the stress is present on a chronic basis.

III. MULTIPLE FORMS OF STRESS

A. Energetic Stresses

1. Undernutrition

Much of what is known about mechanisms by which nutritional status modulates the activity of the reproductive axis comes from the clinical study of patients with the psychiatric disorder anorexia nervosa. This syndrome involves an obsessive fear of being fat and leads to a profound decrease in food intake and extreme weight loss that can become life-threatening. Nearly all women who develop anorexia nervosa show a loss of ovarian cyclicity and amenorrhea. Gonadotropin secretion during the weight loss phase of anorexia nervosa is very low and often nonpulsatile in nature or pulsatile only during the nighttime period, as it is in the early pubertal period. Anorexia can often start in the teenage years, and if it starts prior to menarche, it can delay menarche for many years, holding the girl in a prepubertal state long beyond the normal time of puberty. This delay in activation of adult-like gonadotropin secretion and

ovarian function is accompanied by minimal secretion of the ovarian steroid hormones, and thus development of secondary sexual characteristics is delayed. Such a prolongation of childhood and maintenance of a girlish body habitus can be advantageous in certain sports, such as ballet, and the prevalence of anorexia in girls participating rigorously in such sports is much higher than in the normal population. Although over 90% of anorexic patients are female, the incidence of this disease is increasing in males, and they too show a profound suppression of reproductive hormone secretion and a loss of fertility and sexual function when low body weight is sustained.

A number of studies with experimental animals show that brief periods of severe undernutrition (such as fasting) can also lead to a suppression of reproductive hormone secretion. In addition, decreased reproductive hormone secretion has been documented in humans after several days of fasting. However, in general, fertility would not be expected to be compromised by brief periods of undernutrition because sperm production and development of oocytes take place over a prolonged period (weeks to months). There is evidence in rodents that acute undernutrition in the late follicular phase can block ovulation, but this has not been demonstrated in larger species.

The relationship between chronic mild-to-moderate undernutrition and activity of the reproductive axis is more controversial. There is generally little animal research addressing this question, probably because maintaining animals on diets for a prolonged period of time would be a rather inefficient method of determining the mechanisms by which energy availability modulates reproductive function, in terms of both time and money. Livestock that are maintained with suboptimal nutritional support have compromised fertility, but again, most of the experimental work examining the mechanisms by which nutrition impairs fertility in these species has utilized rather severe forms of undernutrition. In human populations in which mild to moderate undernutrition is relatively common, minimal impact on adult fertility has been reported. However, there are stronger correlations between moderate nutritional compromise and later timing of puberty onset, as well as poorer pregnancy outcome. Overall, it would appear that although prolonged periods of mild to moderate undernutrition do have some impact on function of the reproductive axis and fertility, the impact is relatively weak compared to either acute or chronic forms of severe undernutrition.

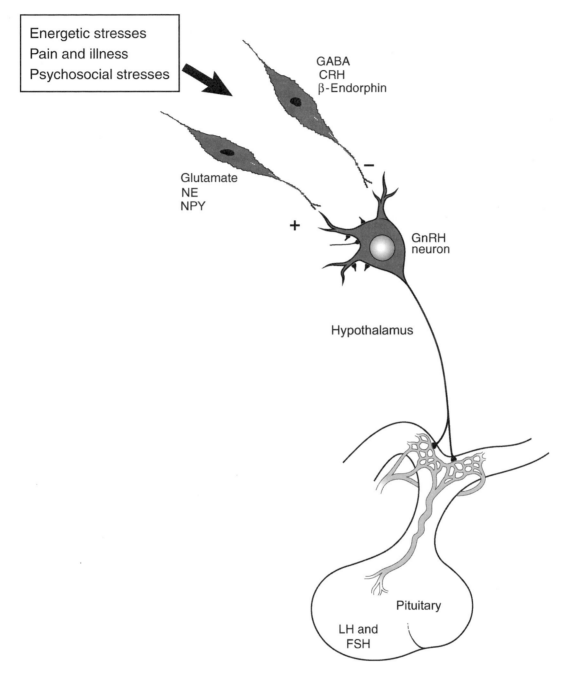

FIGURE 1 Schematic diagram showing that stresses act to suppress the activity of the reproductive axis by affecting neural systems that modulate the activity of hypothalamic GnRH-containing neurons.

2. Exercise

Women participating in vigorous exercise training programs have an increased incidence of menstrual disorders. These range from irregular cyclicity to a complete loss of menstrual cycles for prolonged periods of time. The more marked forms of exercise-induced reproductive dysfunction are associated with low circulating levels of luteinizing hormone (LH), follicle-stimulating hormone, and estrogen. If exercise regimens are very heavy in the adolescent years, individuals can experience a delay in puberty, which can be quite extensive in length. Exercise-induced reproductive dysfunction can be very rapidly reversed by a brief hiatus in the exercise regimen, as often occurs in athletes when they experience an injury or take a vacation. Exercise-induced reproductive dysfunction can also be rapidly reversed by increasing food intake, indicating that the mechanism by which exercise impairs reproductive function involves decreases in energy availability. Moreover, reproductive dysfunction in athletic women is often associated with the presence or history of eating disorders or an abnormal preoccupation with weight and diet. Exercise-induced reproductive dysfunction is more prevalent in females participating in sports where emphasis is put on a lean body image, such as ballet, compared to sports where increased body mass in encouraged. Exercise-induced reproductive dysfunction is less commonly reported in men, perhaps in part because of the lower emphasis on leanness and in part because changes in reproductive hormones in men are less readily detected compared to loss of menstrual cycles in women.

3. Lactation

Energetic stress occurring during lactation is also an important regulator of fertility and has the potential to profoundly suppress the activity of the reproductive axis. Suppression of the hypothalamic–pituitary–gonadal axis stems both from the energetic drain associated with milk production and from other neuroendocrine signals that occur with lactation, including increased prolactin and oxytocin release. As with other energetic stresses, the degree of reproductive suppression is directly related to the energy stress; thus, in animals there is good evidence that nursing a greater number of offspring has more of a suppressive effect on reproductive function than nursing one or two offspring. In humans, provision of breast milk as the sole source of nutrition for an infant, with no bottle supplementation, generally leads to a longer period of postpartum amenorrhea. Other important variables that play a role in determining the effects of lactation on reproduction include the frequency of nursing and the amount of food available to the mother.

4. Pain, Illness, and Immunological Stresses

Chronic illness and exposure to pain, such as in patients with fibromyalgia, can be associated with an increased incidence of reproductive dysfunction. Inflammation and other conditions associated with activation of the immune system can also lead to a suppression of reproductive function, particularly when CNS levels of cytokines are elevated. Much of the experimental work examining the interactions between immune activation and the activity of the reproductive axis has utilized acute administration of endotoxin. This inflammatory-like stress is

accompanied by a suppression of LH secretion, a delay in folliculogenesis, and decreases in luteal function. However, the response of the reproductive axis is influenced by the endocrine environment at the time of the inflammatory challenge. For example, an elevation in CNS interleukin-1α levels can rapidly suppress LH secretion in nonhuman primates when estrogen levels are low, but leads to an elevation of LH secretion in the presence of significant estrogen concentrations.

5. Psychosocial Stress

The effects of behaviorally induced stresses, that is, psychological and social stresses involving elicitation of anxiety, fear, and discomfort, on reproductive function have been studied extensively in animal models. Both restraint stress and the expectation of mild footshock (as a conditioned stimulus) can lead to rapid suppression of reproductive hormone secretion in rodent models. In human populations, it has been more difficult to selectively study the impact of psychosocial stress on reproductive function because these stresses rarely occur in isolation from other stresses or in a timely fashion so that they can be easily studied. One of the best characterized forms of psychosocial stress-induced reproductive dysfunction comes from studies of women who present to infertility clinics with functional hypothalamic amenorrhea (FHA). By definition FHA is a state of subfertility that is not associated with substantial undernutrition or exercise, does not involve lactation, and is not associated with any organic or structural causes of decreased fertility. Studies of women with FHA show that they experience more psychological stress than other women, although they do not experience more stressful life events, but rather react more profoundly to the stressful events they do experience. They also show increased activation of physiological systems that respond to stress, including increased activation of the hypothalamic–pituitary–adrenal axis. Treatment of these patients with cognitive behavior therapy or with drugs that reduce the activity of some central neural systems that are activated by stress can restore fertility, although not in all cases. For example, both opiate antagonists and metaclopromide, a dopamine agonist, have been shown to stimulate reproductive hormone secretion and restore menstrual cyclicity in some, but not all women with FHA.

Although the majority of studies examining the effects of psychosocial stress on reproduction have documented stress-induced suppression of reproductive function, there are a handful of human studies that have reported that girls who have grown up under conditions of family stress, such as in homes where the father is absent, in homes where there has been family conflict, or in homes where the parents have divorced, enter puberty at a significantly earlier age. However, mechanisms by which such stress exposure would advance the onset of puberty have not been established. Moreover, there is the possibility that early stress exposure does not cause advancement of puberty, but rather, that the likelihood of early puberty and exposure to early life family stresses may simply be correlated because they are both influenced by a common factor(s). For example, one of the factors governing the age of menarche in a girl is the age of her mother at menarche. Thus, it is possible that mothers who experienced early menarche are more likely to have family conflict or divorce when their children are young and to have daughters who exhibit early menarche.

A more detailed understanding of how psychosocial stress can impact on reproduction comes from animal studies, with investigations in nonhuman primates having particular relevance to understanding this human condition. Nonhuman primates live in complex social groups and have higher cortical brain areas similar to those of humans; moreover, the anatomical and functional organization of their reproductive axis is very similar to that of humans. A number of studies have shown that acute stresses (i.e., restraint, receipt of aggressive attacks, and placement in an unfamiliar social situation) can rapidly suppress reproductive hormone secretion in a variety of nonhuman primates. However, not all acute stresses have this effect, particularly those that are associated with less direct threat to the individual. Thus, the perception of severity of stress appears to be an important factor in determining whether a stress will lead to a suppression of reproductive hormone secretion. Chronic exposure to social stresses (such as

troop reorganization or being placed in a new social environment) can lead to a marked and sustained suppression of reproductive hormone secretion. However, not all individuals respond to chronic stresses with suppressed reproductive function. Studies have shown a high degree of correlation between aggressiveness and testosterone titers, with the more aggressive males showing higher circulating levels of testosterone. Dominance rank, particularly in times of social instability, is also often correlated with circulating testosterone levels in males. It has also been hypothesized that social status (i.e., dominance rank) plays an important role in determining lifetime reproductive success in primates, with subordinate animals experiencing a greater degree of social stress and having a lesser degree of reproductive success. However, the support for this hypothesis is not uniform and this remains a controversial notion. It would appear that multiple factors, including dominance rank, magnitude of stress, perception of the stress, aggressiveness of the animal, and level of activity of the reproductive axis prior to stress exposure, can play important roles in modulating the response of the reproductive axis to both acute and chronic stresses (Fig. 2).

IV. MECHANISMS OF STRESS ACTION

There are two general ways in which stress exposure is thought to be able to suppress GnRH neuronal activity, by increasing the activity of neural systems that are inhibitory to GnRH neurons or decreasing the activity of neural systems that are stimulatory to GnRH neurons (Fig. 1). To date, most attention has been focused on the activation of inhibitory systems; however, the complete neural mechanisms by which stress modulates the reproductive axis for any of the stresses discussed in this article are far from being understood. The mechanisms by which various forms

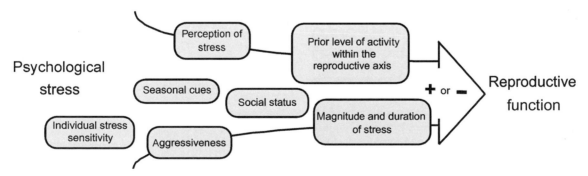

FIGURE 2 Schematic diagram showing modulatory factors that play an important role in determining whether stress exposure will lead to reproductive dysfunction within an individual.

of stress impair reproductive axis activity appear to have some common elements, but there also appear to be mechanisms that are specific to each type of stress. For example, many forms of stress can activate the hypothalamic–pituitary–adrenal axis, and experimental studies have shown that CRH can suppress the activity of GnRH neurons and that several forms of stress-induced impairment of reproductive function can be reversed by administering an antibody to CRH (i.e., footshock stress and inflammatory stresses). However, transgenic mice without expression of the CRH gene still show stress-induced suppression of reproductive hormone secretion in response to restraint stress and undernutrition. Thus, the activation of a particular neural system in response to stress does not necessarily indicate a causal role for that neurotransmitter in the etiology of stress-induced reproductive dysfunction. For many forms of stress, neural systems that are activated and inhibited are beginning to be mapped, but the role of these systems in mediating the suppression of GnRH neuronal activity, and how information regarding various modulatory factors (e.g., dominance status, perception of stress, and aggressiveness) interacts with these systems, awaits future research.

Glossary

amenorrhea A loss of ovarian cyclicity.
corticotropin-releasing hormone The hypothalamic neuropeptide that stimulates pituitary production and secretion of adrenocorticotropin, a hormone that regulates adrenal function.
functional hypothalamic amenorrhea A clinical state of subfertility in women resulting from stress exposure.
gonadotropin-releasing hormone The hypothalamic neuropeptide that stimulates pituitary production and secretion of gonadotropins.
gonadotropins Luteinizing hormone and follicle-stimulating hormone; hormones produced by the anterior pituitary gland that regulate ovarian and testicular function.
menarche The time of first menstrual bleeding.
stress An internal or external stimulus that causes a physiological challenge or evokes a state of anxiety.

See Also the Following Articles

Corticotropin-Releasing Hormone, Stress, and the Immune System • Eating Disorders • Endocrine Rhythms: Generation, Regulation, and Integration • Gonadotropin-Releasing Hormone (GnRH) • Sexual Differentiation, Molecular and Hormone Dependent Events in • Stress • Thyroid and Reproduction

Further Reading

Berga, S. L., Daniels, T. L., and Giles, D. E. (1997). Women with functional hypothalamic amenorrhea but not other forms of anovulation display amplified cortisol concentrations. *Fertil. Steril.* 67, 1024–1030.
Bronson, F. H. (1998). Energy balance and ovulation: Small cages versus natural habitats. *Reprod. Fertil. Dev.* 10, 127–137.
Cameron, J. L., Helmreich, D. L., and Schreihofer, D. A. (1993). Modulation of reproductive hormone secretion by nutritional intake: Stress signals versus metabolic signals. *Hum. Reprod.* 8(2), 162–167.
I'Anson, H., Manning, J. M., Herbosa, G. C., Pelt, J., Friedman, C. R., Wood, R. I., Bucholtz, D. C., and Foster, D. L. (2000). Central inhibition of gonadotropin-releasing hormone secretion in the growth-restricted hypogonadotropic female sheep. *Endocrinology* 141, 520–527.
Jeong, K. H., Jacobson, L., Widmaier, E. P., and Majzoub, J. A. (1999). Normal suppression of the reproductive axis following stress in corticotropin-releasing hormone-deficient mice. *Endocrinology* 140, 1702–1708.
Karsch, F. J., Battaglia, D. F., Breen, K. M., Debus, N., and Harris, T. G. (2002). Mechanisms for ovarian cycle disruption by immune/inflammatory stress. *Stress* 5, 101–112.
Marshall, J. C., and Kelch, R. P. (1979). Low dose pulsatile gonadotropin-releasing hormone in anorexia nervosa: A model for human pubertal development. *J. Clin. Endocrinol. Metab.* 49, 712–718.
McNeilly, A. S. (2001). Lactational control of reproduction. *Reprod. Fertil. Dev.* 13, 583–590.
Sapolsky, R. M. (1983). Endocrine aspects of social instability in the olive baboon (*Papio anubis*). *Am. J. Primatol.* 5, 365–379.
Tilbrook, A. J., Turner, A. I., and Clarke, I. J. (2002). Stress and reproduction: Central mechanisms and sex differences in nonrodent species. *Stress* 5, 83–100.
Warren, M. P., and Perlroth, N. E. (2001). The effects of intense exercise on the female reproductive system. *J. Endocrinol.* 170, 3–11.
Wood, J. W. (1994). Maternal nutrition and reproduction: Why demographers and physiologists disagree about a fundamental relationship. *Ann. N. Y. Acad. Sci.* 709, 101–116.
Xiao, E., and Ferin, M. (1997). Stress-related disturbances of the menstrual cycle. *Ann. Med.* 29, 215–219.

Systemins

CLARENCE A. RYAN AND GREGORY PEARCE
Washington State University

I. INTRODUCTION
II. TOMATO SYSTEMIN
III. TOMATO SYSTEMIN HOMOLOGUES
IV. TOBACCO SYSTEMIN
V. MODE OF ACTION
VI. SUMMARY

Systemin is an 18-amino-acid polypeptide hormone that is released in *Solanaceae* species from sites where there is tissue damage. Systemin activates genes throughout plant tissues for defense against predators and pathogens. The wound hormone is cleaved from a 200-amino-acid precursor called prosystemin that is synthesized in vascular bundle cells.

I. INTRODUCTION

Polypeptide hormones are common regulators of numerous physiological processes in eukaryotes. In 1922, the first polypeptide hormone discovered, insulin, was initially identified in the pancreatic secretions of dogs. Following the discovery of insulin, hundreds of polypeptide hormones that regulate a wide variety of physiological processes were isolated and characterized.

Polypeptide hormones in animals are nearly always produced as precursors that are proteolytically processed to their active forms. Many of the polypeptide hormones are derived from precursors that contain one copy of the hormone, but in many cases, the precursor contains more than one copy, and in other cases more than one type of hormone is produced from a single precursor.

Before 1991, polypeptides were not recognized as signaling molecules in plants; small organic molecules were thought to regulate the numerous physiological processes that govern growth and development. Evidence that supported a role for polypeptides as signaling molecules was not obvious. In 1991, an 18-amino-acid polypeptide called systemin was isolated and was found to regulate the expression of defensive genes in tomato leaves in response to insect attacks or severe mechanical wounding. Since then, five families and subfamilies of polypeptide signals that fulfill the definition of hormones have been identified in plants as regulators of various processes of defense and development.

II. TOMATO SYSTEMIN

Systemin, like animal polypeptide hormones, is derived proteolytically from the C-terminal region of a 200-amino-acid precursor protein called prosystemin (Fig. 1). The systemin precursor does not exhibit a signal sequence at its N-terminus, is not glycosylated or posttranslationally modified, is found in the cytoplasm, and is not known to be associated with any organelles. Alanine substitutions at each amino acid residue in systemin have variable effects on activity, with only a substitution of Thr to Ala at

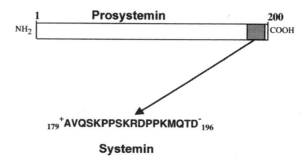

FIGURE 1 The location of the systemin sequence within its precursor, prosystemin.

position 17 totally eliminating activity. This analogue is a powerful antagonist of native systemin. Removal of the C-terminal Asp totally abolishes activity, and it too is a potent antagonist of native systemin. The N-terminal 14 amino acids are likely involved in receptor binding, whereas the C-terminal sequence [MQTD (using the one-letter amino acid code): M, methionine; Q, glutamine; T, threonine; and D, aspartic acid] appears to have a direct role in signaling.

The tertiary structure of systemin in solution has been analyzed by nuclear magnetic resonance (NMR) and circular dichroism spectroscopy; systemin exists as a mixture of random coils with β-sheet and β-turn motifs. The most interesting features of the systemin sequence are the prolines, at positions 6, 7, 12, and 13, which suggests that a poly(l-proline) II 3_1 helix secondary structure is present in the central region of the polypeptide. The polyproline II 3_1 helix may provide a signature kink in the systemin structure that is likely important to its recognition by the systemin receptor.

Prosystemin, generated in *Escherichia coli* or in a baculovirus/insect cell system, has been found to be as active as systemin. It has not been determined whether the intact prosystemin protein is active without being processed, or whether it is processed after being supplied to the plants. A prosystemin lacking the systemin sequence is totally inactive when supplied to excised tomato plants, indicating that the systemin sequence must be present for signaling to occur.

III. TOMATO SYSTEMIN HOMOLOGUES

Homologues of tomato prosystemin genes are found in other Solanaceae species, including potato, black nightshade, and bell pepper. The homologues are highly conserved among the species, with identities ranging from 73–88% and each encoding a systemin sequence that contains at most two to three amino acid replacements compared to tomato systemin

Tomato	AVQSKPPSKRDPPKMQTD
Potato-1	AVHSTPPSKRDPPKMQTD
Potato-2	AAHSTPPSKRDPPKMQTD
Nightshade	AVRSTPPPKRDPPKMQTD
Pepper	AVHSTPPSKRPPPKMQTD

FIGURE 2 Amino acid sequences of systemins from potato, nightshade, and pepper, compared to the sequence of tomato systemin. Conserved amino acids are in bold type.

(Fig. 2). No substitutions have been found among the seven residues at the C-terminus, and all prolines are conserved. Each systemin actively induces defense genes in tomato plants, with the exception that the nightshade systemin is about 10-fold less effective than the others.

IV. TOBACCO SYSTEMIN

A homologue of the tomato prosystemin gene has not been found in tobacco, a more distant relative of the tomato than nightshade, pepper, and potato. Additionally, tomato systemin does not induce defense gene expression in leaves of tobacco plants. A search for tobacco systemin in leaves of tobacco plants has resulted in the isolation of two tobacco 18-amino-acid hydroxyproline-rich, glycosylated polypeptides that are structurally dissimilar from tomato systemin, but that possess a strong defense gene induction in tobacco plants. All of the plant-derived polypeptides that activate defense genes are included under the general name of systemins. The two tobacco systemins, called Tob Sys I and Tob Sys II, are produced from a single gene that encodes a 150-amino-acid polyprotein precursor from which both systemins are processed, one systemin from the N-terminal region and one from the C-terminal region (Fig. 3).

Tobacco prosystemin bears no homology to tomato systemin, but the central regions of both of the tobacco systemins contain hydroxyproline-rich regions, which are similar to the proline-rich regions found in tomato systemin. These regions would likewise cause a kinking of the secondary structure and, like tomato systemin, are likely to be important in recognition of the polypeptides by their respective receptors.

V. MODE OF ACTION

A synthetic ^{14}C-labeled tomato systemin derivative has been shown to be mobile when applied to wounds,

and its movement in the phloem correlates with the movement of the systemic signal that is produced in response to wounding. Prosystemin synthesis is localized in the vascular bundles of the plants, and systemin signaling may be amplified in parenchyma cells as it moves through the phloem. This scenario is temporally compatible with the known rate of movement of the wound signal from a severe wound site to cells throughout the plants.

The functional role of systemin has been demonstrated by transforming tomato plants with an antisense prosystemin gene, driven by the constitutive 35S promoter. The transgenic antisense plants exhibit a severely reduced systemic induction of defense genes in response to wounding and are rapidly consumed by *Manduca sexta* larvae. However, supplying the plants with systemin through their cut stems results in a normal response. Additionally, tomato plants that are transformed with prosystemin cDNA in the sense orientation, driven by the 35S promoter, act as if they are in a permanently wounded state, synthesizing defense proteins constitutively. This phenotype is apparently caused by expression of the gene in cells in which it is not normally expressed, resulting in the release of systemin at a low but constitutive level, causing the plants to behave as if they are under attack by chewing insects. Grafting wild-type tomato scions to rootstocks overexpressing prosystemin also causes the wild-type scions to accumulate defense proteins as if they are wounded. This appears to be the result of the constitutive release of systemin in the rootstock. Wild-type plants grafted onto wild-type rootstocks do not exhibit this response. These experiments support the role of systemin as a mobile signal.

Systemin interacts with a 160-kDa membrane-bound receptor with a K_D of about 10^{-13} M and initiates a signal transduction cascade that activates over 20 defensive genes that help protect the plant from insect and pathogen attacks.

Two sets of genes are activated in response to wounding and systemin—signal pathway genes and defensive genes directly involved in deterring predators. Signal pathway genes are activated within 1–4 h after wounding and include the prosystemin gene and genes that code for some members of the octadecanoid pathway. The octadecanoid pathway is part of the signaling pathway that leads to synthesis of jasmonic acid, a second messenger for up-regulating the pathway as well as for signaling downstream activation of the defense response. The defensive genes are activated at about 4–8 h after wounding and they code for several proteinase inhibitor proteins that have specificities against all four classes of proteolytic

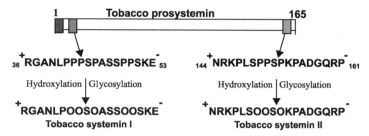

FIGURE 3 The origin of Tob Sys I and Tob Sys II from a common precursor. The precursor consists of 165 amino acids that contain a 16-amino-acid signal sequence (in black) that is lost during processing through the secretory pathway. Within the secretory pathway, the prolines are modified to hydroxyprolines and carbohydrate units are attached. The specific hydroxyprolines that are glycosylated have not been identified.

enzymes, and also for polyphenol oxidase. The proteinase inhibitor proteins can inhibit proteolytic digestive enzymes of attacking organisms, whereas the polyphenolase cross-links proteins in the digestive tracts of the predators, reducing the nutritional value of the proteins. The overall effect of the defense response is to facilitate systemic signaling and to reduce the ability of the predators to obtain nutrition from plant proteins, resulting in protein starvation.

VI. SUMMARY

Homologues of tomato systemin with a high percentage of amino acid similarities are found in potato, black nightshade, and pepper. Systemins have also been found in tobacco but are structurally different than tomato systemin and are cleaved from a polyprotein precursor. However, all systemins contain a central motif containing prolines or hydroxyprolines; this motif is likely involved in providing a structure that is recognized by cellular receptors. Although systemins have been isolated only from Solanaceae species, systemic signaling for defense is known to occur in over 100 plant families in which systemins may also play a hormonal role in signaling.

Glossary

octadecanoid pathway Signaling pathway in many plants; regulates a variety of cell-specific responses and is initiated by release of linolenic acid from membranes, in response to specific signals. Free linolenic acid is converted to jasmonic acid, a second messenger that activates genes, via several enzymes that cumulatively comprise this pathway.
polypeptide hormones Found ubiquitously in animals as two major classes: those synthesized in the endoplasmic reticulum, processed through the secretory pathway, stored in vesicles, and released in response to an appropriate signal, and those synthesized in the

secretory pathway, anchored to membranes with the hormone domain in the extracellular space, and released by proteolysis in response to an appropriate signal. Polypeptide hormones have been identified only recently in plants, and their mode of synthesis, storage, and release is poorly understood.
prohormone Precursor of an active hormone.
prohormone processing enzyme Enzyme that processes polypeptide prohormones to their active form.
prosystemin Precursor of a systemin.
systemins Polypeptide plant hormones that are released following attack (wounding) by insects and pathogens; regulate activation of defense-related genes.

See Also the Following Articles

Abscisic Acid • Auxin • Brassinosteroids • Cytokinins • Ethylene • Gibberellins • Jasmonates • Salicylic Acid

Further Reading

Pearce, K. G., Moura, D. S., Stratmann, J., and Ryan, C. A. (2001). Production of multiple plant hormones from a single polyprotein precursor. *Nature* **411**, 817–820.
Ryan, C. A. (1998). The discovery of systemin. *In* "Discoveries in Plant Biology," Vol. II. (S.-D. Kung and S.-F. Yang, eds.), pp. 175–188. World Scientific Press, Singapore.
Ryan, C. A. (2000). The systemin signaling pathway: Differential activation of plant defensive genes. *Biochim. Biophys. Acta* **1477**, 112–121.
Ryan, C. A., and Pearce, G. (1998). Systemin, a polypeptide signal for plant defense. *Annu. Rev. Cell Dev. Biol.* **14**, 1–17.
Ryan, C. A., and Pearce, G. (2001). Polypeptide signaling. *Plant Physiol.* **125**, 65–68.
Schaller, A. (1999). Oligopeptide signaling and the action of systemin. *Plant Mol. Biol.* **49**, 763–769.
Scheer, J. M., and Ryan, C. A. (1999). A 160-kD systemin receptor on the surface of *Lycopersicon peruvianum* suspension-cultured cells. *Plant Cell* **11**, 1525–1535.
Toumadje, A., and Johnson, W. C., Jr. (1995). Systemin has the characteristics of a poly(L-proline) II type helix. *J. Am. Chem. Soc.* **117**, 7023–7025.

Testis Descent, Hormonal Control of

Judith M. A. Emmen, J. Anton Grootegoed,
and Albert O. Brinkmann

Erasmus University Rotterdam, The Netherlands

In many species of mammals, during fetal development in males, the testes migrate out of the abdomen toward and into the scrotum; this process is called testis descent. Various mechanisms and factors are involved in the control of this process; this article examines the role that a number of hormones, including anti-Müllerian hormone, androgens, insulin-like factor 3, and estrogens, play in the control of testis descent.

I. DEVELOPMENT AND TESTIS DESCENT

In mammalian species, male sex is determined by a gene on the Y chromosome, encoding the protein SRY, which triggers the differentiation of the undifferentiated gonads to become testes. In the absence of expression of functional SRY, the gonads develop into ovaries. Following genetic sex determination at fertilization (formation of 46,XX or 46,XY zygotes in humans), gonadal sex determination is the next step in a series of events leading to male/female sex differentiation. In this process of sex differentiation, hormonal factors produced by the gonads during fetal and postnatal development appear to play very prominent roles. The major players are anti-Müllerian hormone (AMH), androgens, and estrogens. It was recently discovered that insulin-like growth factor 3 (INSL3) is also involved in sex differentiation, in particular with regard to establishing gonadal position.

The undifferentiated gonads develop in the abdomen close to the kidneys. Functional ovaries are found at this location throughout reproductive life. However, in male mouse and human, and in many other mammalian species, the testes migrate away from the kidneys during fetal life, to finally arrive at a position outside the abdomen, in the scrotum. In human, and also in several other mammalian species, the relatively low testis temperature that is attained at the scrotal position, some 2 °C below abdominal temperature, is essential for the production of spermatozoa (spermatogenesis). Many attempts have been made to explain why spermatogenesis in scrotal species would require the lower scrotal temperature, and hypotheses abound. However, a decisive answer cannot be given.

The migration of the testes toward and into the scrotum is called testis descent (or, for the plural, testes descent). The process of testis descent is generally subdivided into two phases. During the first or transabdominal phase, the testes move from their initial position to the bottom of the abdomen. During the second or inguino-scrotal phase, the testes leave the abdomen and move through the inguinal canal into the scrotum. The transabdominal movement of the testes appears to be dependent on the differential development of two paired structures, the cranial suspensory ligament (CSL) and the gubernaculum. At first, each ovary or testis is connected cranially to the diaphragm via the CSL and caudally to the bottom of the abdomen via the gubernaculum. In the male fetus, the gubernaculum further develops, whereas outgrowth of the CSL is lacking. This allows movement of the testes toward the bottom of the abdomen. In contrast, in the female fetus, gubernacular development is absent, and the CSL develops into a muscular cord-like structure, so that the ovaries remain located at the lower pole of the kidneys (Fig. 1).

With regard to the mechanisms and factors controlling testis descent, much evidence points to the respective roles of hormones, as will be described in this article. However, it should be taken into account that embryonic development of the body plan and the organ systems is based on highly complex gene expression networks. It is to be expected that many genes that control more general aspects of development are also involved in creating the structures that allow testis descent to occur.

II. ANTI-MÜLLERIAN HORMONE

A. AMH and the AMH Receptor

Anti-Müllerian hormone is also known as Müllerian inhibiting substance (MIS). This protein is a member of a family of growth and differentiation factors that

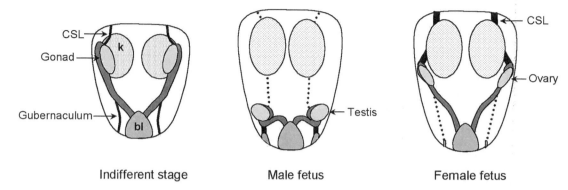

FIGURE 1 Sexually dimorphic development of the cranial suspensory ligament (CSL) and the gubernaculum. At the undifferentiated stage, before gonadal sex determination and differentiation have started, each gonad is located next to a kidney (k). The gonad and its associated duct system are attached to the abdominal body wall by two ligaments: the cranial suspensory ligament (CSL) and the gubernaculum. In the male fetus, the first phase of testis descent results the testis being positioned lateral to the bladder (bl), connected to the inguinal region via a developing gubernaculum; development of the CSL is lacking. In the female fetus, the ovary is found in a position lateral to the kidney, attached to a well-developed CSL; there is no further development of the gubernaculum. Based on Emmen, J. M., McLuskey, A., Adham, I. M., Engel, W., Grootegoed, J. A., and Brinkman, A. O. (2000). Hormonal control of gubernaculum development during testis descent: Gubernaculum outgrowth in vitro requires both insulin-like factor 3 and androgen. *Endocrinology* **141**, 4720–4727. Copyright owner, The Endocrine Society.

are related to, and include, transforming growth factor-β. The term hormone in the name AMH refers to its signaling role, rather than giving information about its position in the context of the endocrine and growth factor classification system. The action of AMH is mediated by a multimeric complex containing two related serine/threonine kinase receptors, a type I receptor and a type II receptor. The type II receptor for AMH (AMHR-II) has been identified, whereas ALK2 and ALK6 (BMPR-1B) are considered as candidate AMH type I receptors.

AMH is the first hormonal factor known to be produced by the testis, in the precursor Sertoli cells following embryonic testis determination. Later in life, these cells will develop into mature Sertoli cells, providing support to the germ cells during spermatogenesis. In addition to being the first testicular secreted hormonal factor, another hallmark of AMH production involves its testis specificity. The *AMH* gene is silent in embryonic ovaries and is also not transcribed in any other tissue.

B. AMH Action

Much is known about the role of AMH in embryonic/fetal sex differentiation. Evidence from studies on both humans and laboratory animals shows that AMH induces the regression of the Müllerian ducts in the male embryo. In the female, the Müllerian ducts develop into oviducts and uterus (and also the upper part of the vagina). Male *AMH* and *AMHRII* knockout mice, which are deficient for either AMH or AMHRII, retain Müllerian ducts that will develop. Also, female transgenic mice expressing AMH during fetal life lack oviducts and a uterus. There exists a rare syndrome in humans, called persistent Müllerian duct syndrome (PMDS), in which 46,XY individuals have Müllerian duct derivatives. PMDS in humans has been associated with mutations in either the *AMH* gene or the *AMHRII* gene. Patients with PMDS often have undescended testes. Additional research demonstrated that boys born with undescended testes often show a relatively low AMH level. Taken together, the available evidence indicates that incomplete regression of the Müllerian duct system in boys can lead to impairment of testis descent. However, this impairment is caused mainly by mechanical interference, due to the presence of female genital duct structures. Typically, the undescended testes are not seen in the mouse models. Male *AMH* knockout mice retain Müllerian ducts but their testes descend normally. In contrast to human females, which have a simple uterus, the uterus in rodents is bicornuate and highly movable, allowing the testes to reach the scrotum in a PMDS situation. Furthermore, female transgenic mice overexpressing AMH do not demonstrate ovarian descent or any difference in the position of the ovaries. The current view is that AMH is not a hormonal factor that is directly involved in the control of testis descent.

III. ANDROGENS

A. Androgens and the Androgen Receptor

Following the onset of AMH production by Sertoli cells, the next step in testis differentiation involves the formation of an interstitial population of Leydig cells situated in between the testicular tubules. Whereas the tubules are the spermatogenic compartment of the testis, the interstitial Leydig cells are responsible for steroid hormone production, or steroidogenesis, during fetal and postnatal life. The main steroid hormone to be produced is testosterone, formed by a series of enzymatic conversions from cholesterol. An important metabolite of testosterone is 5α-dihydrotestosterone. Each androgen has a quite specific role during male sexual differentiation; testosterone is directly involved in differentiation and development of the Wolffian duct-derived structures, including the epididymides, whereas 5α-dihydrotestosterone is the main active ligand in the differentiation and development of the prostate and male external genitalia.

The actions of testosterone and 5α-dihydrotestosterone are mediated by the androgen receptor, which is a member of the family of nuclear receptors. The available evidence indicates that there is only one gene encoding one type of androgen receptor. The *androgen receptor* (*AR*) gene is located on the X chromosome, in the human at Xq11–q12, and consists of eight coding exons, encoding a protein with a molecular mass of approximately 110 kDa. A polyglutamine stretch, encoded by a polymorphic $(CAG)_n CAA$ repeat, is present in the NH_2-terminal domain. Variation in length (9–33 glutamine residues) is observed in the human population, and the length of the repeat has been suggested to be negatively associated with a very mild modulation of androgen receptor activity. Whether subtle differences in $(CAG)_n CAA$ repeat lengths are important for modulation *in vivo* of androgen receptor activity is still a matter of debate, but could possibly play a role in later life, in relation to aging.

B. Androgen Insensitivity Syndrome

It is generally accepted that mutational defects in the androgen receptor can lead to impairment of the normal development of both internal and external male structures in 46,XY individuals. Detailed information about the DNA sequence of the human *AR* gene and the molecular structure of the AR protein has facilitated the study of mutational defects associated with androgen insensitivity. The end-organ resistance to androgens has been designated as androgen insensitivity syndrome (AIS). The main phenotypic characteristics of 46,XY individuals with the complete form of AIS are as follows: female external genitalia, a short and blind-ending vagina, the absence of Wolffian duct-derived structures (including epididymides) and the prostate, development of gynecomastia, the absence of pubic and axillary hair, and cryptorchidism. This cryptorchidism is not only related to the absence of male external genitalia, including a scrotum, but also is caused by marked disturbance of the early steps in the process of testis descent.

Mutations of the *AR* gene in AIS individuals are mostly single base mutations resulting in amino acid substitutions or premature stop codons, although complete or large deletions of the *AR* gene, and also intronic mutations in splice donor or acceptor sites, have been found.

Androgen insensitivity has also been noted in other mammalian species including the rat and the mouse. In the mouse, this condition also appeared to be X-linked and the locus was designated *Tfm* (testicular feminization). *Tfm* mice completely lack Wolffian duct-derived structures and show female external genitalia and cryptorchidism.

C. Androgens and Testis Descent

In male androgen-resistant *Tfm* mutant mice, development of the cranial suspensory ligament (CSL) is observed. This is of much interest, because outgrowth of this ligament is lacking in normal male mice, as opposed to its further development in normal female mice. The CSL is considered to be one of the main structures involved in determination of the gonadal position.

Several studies have supported the concept that development of the CSL is sex-dimorphic, which is probably relevant for the male-specific transabdominal phase of testis descent. When pregnant rats are treated with androgens to expose the fetuses to an increased level of androgens, this prevents the outgrowth of the CSL in the female fetuses, whereas males prenatally exposed to synthetic anti-androgens display CSL development. Furthermore, the AR is clearly expressed in primordial cells of the CSL, shortly before the onset of the first phase of testis descent, when this structure is highly sensitive to androgens. Interestingly, the sensitivity to androgens occurs within a small developmental time window and is lost after embryonic day 17 in the mouse, despite AR expression. The molecular mechanisms underlying the suppressive action of androgens on CSL development are largely unknown and remain to be elucidated. Thus far, no evidence that cell proliferation and cell death parameters of the CSL are different in female and male mouse fetuses has been obtained. The interactions between cells and their extracellular matrix, and the controlling actions of androgens and local signaling factors in the development of the CSL primordium, need to be studied in more detail.

A second important structure, which certainly plays a major role in testis descent and also is under androgenic control, is the mesenchymal layer of the gubernaculum. Initially, in both female and male fetuses, the gubernaculum expresses AR protein. Subsequently, when the sex differentiation mechanisms have started to come into play, AR expression decreases dramatically in the female gubernaculum, compared to maintenance of AR expression in the male gubernaculum. Most likely, this is an androgen-dependent process. *In vivo* and organ culture experiments have demonstrated that rat gubernaculum tissue shows cell proliferation under the influence of androgens. Given the fact that expression of the AR, which is a prerequisite for androgen action, is detected in the mesenchymal core of rodent gubernaculum, it is suggested that androgens act directly on the mesenchymal cells. These mesenchymal cells, in turn, may elicit a growth response of the myogenic cells through paracrine mechanisms. In several androgen-responsive tissues, including the prostate, androgens act via the AR expressed in the mesenchymal compartment.

It is concluded that androgens have a clear and unmistakable role in testis descent during the first phase, as demonstrated in mice and rats. This role involves the inhibition of CSL development and the stimulation of growth of the gubernaculum, probably through an indirect action, mediated by mesenchymal cells on the muscular component of the gubernaculum.

IV. INSULIN-LIKE GROWTH FACTOR 3

A. Insl3

For many years, it has been quite clear that testicular factors, in particular androgens, are involved in the control of testis descent. Yet, it also was clear that a piece of the puzzle was missing, and as discussed herein, this missing piece does not seem to be AMH. Several investigators have put much effort in trying to identify the factor, which was believed to be produced by the testis in addition to AMH and androgens. Descendin, a candidate protein, was not character-

ized in molecular detail. A very strong candidate for the unknown testicular factor was recently identified, by analysis of the phenotype of *Insl3* knockout mice. The *Insl3* gene is expressed in embryonic testis, by the early Leydig cell population. Like the expression of the *AMH* gene, this expression is specifically found in testis and not in ovaries or other embryonic tissues. The phenotype of the *Insl3* knockout mice showed a complete lack of testis descent.

Insl3 is a member of the insulin-like hormone family, which includes insulin, relaxin, and insulin-like growth factors I and II. Insl3, also called relaxin-like factor, is a single gene product, and is synthesized as a prepropeptide consisting of a signal peptide, a B-chain, a connecting C-peptide, and an A-chain. It is expected that bioactive Insl3 is formed after enzymatic removal of the C-peptide, as for insulin and relaxin. Insl3 probably mediates its action through binding to a specific receptor. However, no such receptor has been identified thus far.

With regard to transcriptional control of the *Insl3* gene, it is of interest to note that the transcriptional regulator steroidogenic factor 1 (SF1) might be involved. This factor plays a prominent role in the development of the gonads and steroidogenic tissues. Based on the identification of functional SF1 sites in the *Insl3* promoter, it can be suggested that SF1 may act as a co-mediator of *Insl3* gene expression during male sex differentiation. The production of Insl3 by the fetal Leydig cells is independent of gonadotropin stimulation. However, gonadotropins become essential for the maintenance of *Insl3* expression in the postnatal and adult testis, as supported by the observation that *hpg* mice, carrying a deletion in the *GnRH* gene, lack Insl3 expression in adulthood.

B. Insl3 Deficiency

Mice with a targeted deletion of the *Insl3* gene have been generated. Since no gross abnormalities are found in female Insl3-deficient mice, which are fertile and have normal-sized litters, it was initially assumed that Insl3 plays a redundant role in ovarian function. Recently, however, careful examination of female mutant mice showed that their estrous cycle was twice as long as that of wild-type littermates. In addition, the *Insl3* knockout ovary shows an acceleration of follicular atresia and luteolysis, indicating that Insl3 plays a role in normal ovarian function during reproductive life. Male mice deficient for Insl3 have a very clear phenotype: all have undescended testes in adulthood. This phenotype was unexpected but confirmed the previous proposed involvement of an additional testicular factor in testis descent. Analysis of male *Insl3* knockout mice revealed that gubernaculum development is severely affected. The action of both androgen and AMH appears not to be affected in these mutant mice, since they are completely virilized and no Müllerian duct remnants could be identified. The testis-specific expression of Insl3 during embryonic life is consistent with a role in gubernaculum development. It was demonstrated that impairment of spermatogenesis seen in Insl3-deficient mice is caused by the intra-abdominal position of the testis, rather than by a direct role of Insl3 in control of spermatogenesis. The molecular and cellular mechanism of Insl3 action on the gubernaculum remains to be studied.

C. Human INSL3 Gene

The human gene encoding INSL3 has been characterized and mapped to region p13.2–p12 of chromosome 19. Human serum contains a detectable level of INSL3, and the circulating INSL3 level in boys increases around puberty, resulting in a significantly higher level in postpubertal males than in females and prepubertal children. Similarly, the concentration of testosterone in plasma increases at puberty in normal boys. Since both testosterone and INSL3 are produced by testicular Leydig cells, such a correlation between testosterone and INSL3 levels might reflect coordinated control of their production.

Based on observations in mice, genetic analysis of cryptorchidism has recently been performed, by screening for *INSL3* gene mutations in cryptorchid boys. Several studies have been published, resulting in information about 350 individuals with (a history of) (one- or two-sided) cryptorchidism. Three mutations and several polymorphisms were found. Two heterozygous mutations are located in the connecting C-peptide and one mutation is found in the B-chain. No functional studies have been performed yet, so it remains to be determined whether these mutations are the underlying cause of the observed phenotypes.

It can be concluded that mutations in the *INSL3* gene appear not to be a frequent cause of cryptorchidism in human. One possible explanation might be that such a mutation will be effectively eliminated from the genetic pool, due to its adverse effect on fertility. There might also be a difference in the role of INSL3 among species. In human, mutations in the *INSL3* gene may lead to a phenotype possibly related to gonadal function but not resulting in a disturbance of testis descent.

It is to be expected that INSL3 acts through binding to a cell plasma membrane receptor. Recently, high-affinity INSL3-binding sites have been reported, although the binding molecules have not yet been identified. It would be of great interest to study the possible occurrence of INSL3 receptor mutations in the human population, in relation to the incidence of cryptorchidism.

V. ESTROGENS

Genes playing a role in the synthesis and biological action of estrogens have been identified, and mouse gene knockout models have been generated for the two genes encoding the two different estrogen receptors (ER-α and ER-β) and for the gene encoding aromatase, the enzyme that converts testosterone into estradiol. These mouse models indicate that there is no prominent direct role for estrogens in the development of the male reproductive tract, including the process of testis descent. In ER-α-deficient mice, quite excessive development of the cremaster muscle was observed, but there was no direct effect on the process of testis descent.

In contrast, exposure to an exogenous estrogenic agent before birth has been found to exert a clear adverse effect on male reproductive tract development. Urogenital tract abnormalities (including epididymal cysts, microphallus, testicular hypoplasia, and cryptorchidism) were found in male offspring of mothers taking the synthetic estrogenic compound DES (diethylstilbestrol) during pregnancy. The incidence of hypospadias, cryptorchidism, and testicular cancer in the general population has been reported to have increased over the past several decades. There is a general concern that chemicals with estrogenic activity that are present in the environment might act as endocrine disruptors and thereby contribute to the increasing incidence of male reproductive tract abnormalities, similar to that seen in DES-exposed males.

A possible mechanistic explanation for disruption of testis descent after fetal exposure to an exogenous estrogenic compound has become apparent during analysis of Insl3-deficient mice. The reproductive phenotype of Insl3-deficient mice is strikingly similar to a phenotype that can be induced by prenatal exposure of male mice to DES: an intra-abdominal position of the testes and a lack of gubernaculum development. It was hypothesized that this effect of DES might involve down-regulation of *Insl3* gene expression. Indeed, the expression of *Insl3* mRNA is markedly reduced in DES-exposed testes, compared to testes of control mice. Thus, the undescended testes

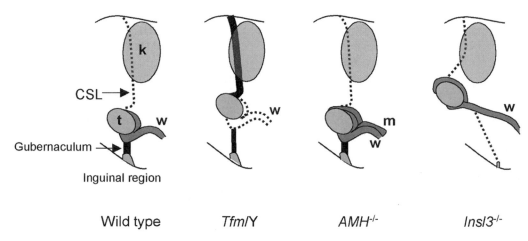

FIGURE 2 The first phase of testis descent in different genetic mouse models. In the normal (wild type) male fetus, the gubernaculum develops, whereas CSL development is lacking. When a functional androgen receptor is absent (*Tfm/*Y mouse), both the CSL and the gubernaculum develop, although shortening of the gubernaculum is less pronounced. The Wolffian duct system is not stabilized. In AMH-deficient male mice (*AMH* $^{-/-}$), both the Müllerian and Wolffian duct systems are maintained. CSL development is lacking, whereas the gubernaculum shows normal development. Finally, in Insl3-deficient male mice (*Insl3* $^{-/-}$), CSL development does not occur, and gubernaculum development is severely impaired. CSL, cranial suspensory ligament; k, kidney; m, Müllerian duct system; w, Wolffian duct system; t, testis.

observed in DES-exposed male mouse fetuses might be related to decreased Insl3 expression.

VI. CONCLUDING REMARKS

A clear picture has emerged with regard to the control of testis descent in the mouse, with androgens and Insl3 acting as principal factors (Fig. 2). However, the control of testis descent in the human male seems to involve additional factors, perhaps still unknown. It is of great importance to study this in more detail. The incidence of disturbed testis descent in the human male is very high—some type of problem is observed in at least 1% of all newborn males—and may be increasing due to environmental factors. Disturbed testis descent, resulting in unilateral or bilateral cryptorchidism, often can be completely repaired by surgical intervention. The surgical intervention might minimize the loss of fertility, as the scrotal location of the testis is needed to obtain normal spermatogenesis. Also, there is a correlation between testis maldescent and testicular cancer, which warrants the prevention and treatment of cryptorchidism, although it is not clear whether this correlation reflects a cause and effect relationship or whether a shared etiological factor is involved. By learning more about the mechanisms involved in testis descent and the factors that control this process, an understanding of other aspects of male reproductive health will be acquired.

Glossary

cranial suspensory ligament A ligament that connects the undifferentiated gonad to the upper wall of the abdominal cavity, in the early fetus. This ligament does not develop further in the male fetus, which is a prerequisite for testis descent. In adult females of most mammalian species, the cranial suspensory ligament (CSL) is a muscular cordlike structure that keeps the ovary and uterus in place, especially during pregnancy. The development and function of the human CSL are not completely understood.

cryptorchidism A disorder in which one testis or both testes do not descend into the scrotum, as detected at birth. This condition can originate from impairment at an early step or at later steps in testis descent. When cryptorchidism is not reversed spontaneously, surgical placement of the undescended testis into the scrotum is required to obtain normal spermatogenesis and fertility with the onset of adulthood.

gubernaculum A paired ligamentous cord present in both sexes that attaches to the gonad at the superior end and attaches to the bottom of the abdomen at the expanded inferior end (gubernacular bulb). Development and relative shortening of the gubernaculum, which occur only in the male, are essential for the first abdominal phase of testis descent. Later changes in the configuration of the gubernaculum are involved in passage of the testes through the inguinal canal into the scrotum.

insulin-like factor 3 A protein hormone that may be involved in the control of testis descent. During fetal development, insulin-like factor 3 (Insl3) is produced by the testis, in the interstitial Leydig cells, but not by the ovary. Inactivation of the gene encoding Insl3 in the mouse (*Insl3* knockout) results in complete blockade of testis descent.

See Also the Following Articles

Anti-Müllerian Hormone ● Dihydrotestosterone, Active Androgen Metabolites and Related Pathology ● Estrogen and Spermatogenesis ● Estrogen in the Male ● Insulin-like Growth Factor Signaling ● Male Hormonal Contraception ● Sexual Differentiation, Molecular and Hormone Dependent Events in ● Spermatogenesis, Hormonal Control of

Further Reading

Bartlett, J. E., Washburn, T., Eddy, E. M., Korach, K. S., Temelcos, C., and Hutson, J. M. (2001). Early development of the gubernaculum and cremaster sac in estrogen receptor knockout mice. *Urol. Res.* **29**, 163–167.

Brinkmann, A. O., and Trapman, J. (2000). Genetic analysis of androgen receptors in development and disease. *Adv. Pharmacol.* **47**, 317–341.

Emmen, J. M. A., McLuskey, A., Adham, I. M., Engel, W., Grootegoed, J. A., and Brinkmann, A. O. (2000a). Hormonal control of gubernaculum development during testis descent: Gubernaculum outgrowth *in vitro* requires both insulin-like factor and androgen. *Endocrinology.* **141**, 4720–4727.

Emmen, J. M. A., McLuskey, A., Adham, I. M., Engel, W., Verhoef-Post, M., Themmen, A. P., Grootegoed, J. A., and Brinkmann, A. O. (2000b). Involvement of insulin-like factor 3 (Insl3) in diethylstilbestrol-induced cryptorchidism. *Endocrinology.* **141**, 846–849.

Hutson, J. M., Hasthorpe, S., and Heyns, C. F. (1997). Anatomical and functional aspects of testicular descent and cryptorchidism. *Endocr. Rev.* **18**, 259–280.

Lim, H. N., Raipert-de Meyts, E., Skakkebaek, N. E., Hawkins, J. R., and Hughes, I. A. (2001). Genetic analysis of the INSL3 gene in patients with maldescent of the testis. *Eur. J. Endocrinol.* **144**, 129–137 and references therein.

MacLaughlin, D. T., Teixeira, J., and Donahoe, P. K. (2001). Perspective: Reproductive tract development—new discoveries and future directions. *Endocrinology.* **142**, 2167–2172.

Marin, P., Ferlin, A., Moro, E., Garolla, A., and Foresta, C. (2001). Different insulin-like 3 (INSL3) gene mutations not associated with human cryptorchidism. *J. Endocrinol. Invest.* **24**, RC13–RC15 and references therein.

Nef, S., Shipman, T., and Parada, L. F. (2000). A molecular basis for estrogen-induced crytorchidism. *Dev. Biol.* **224**, 354–361.

Toppari, J., and Skakkebaek, N. E. (1998). Sexual differentiation and environmental endocrine disruptors. *Bailliere's Clin. Endocrinol. Metab.* **12**, 143–156.

Zimmermann, S., Steding, G., Emmen, J. M. A., Brinkmann, A. O., Nayernia, K., Holstein, A. F., Engel, W., and Adham, I. M. (1999). Targeted disruption of the Insl3 gene causes bilateral cryptorchidism. *Mol. Endocrinol.* **13**, 681–691.

Thyroglobulin

GERALDO MEDEIROS-NETO

Hospital das Clinicas, University of São Paulo Medical School

Thyroglobulin (Tg) is a glycoprotein that is synthesized and secreted by thyroid cells; it is essential for the synthesis of thyroid hormone. In addition, large reserves of iodine and thyroid hormone are stored in the Tg molecule and are available for secretion when needed. Mutations in the Tg gene cause a structurally defective protein with a severely impaired ability to function. Defects in the synthesis of Tg have been described in both animals and humans, resulting in congenital goiter and reduced thyroid function.

I. INTRODUCTION

Thyroid hormone synthesis is intimately tied with thyroglobulin (Tg). Indeed, after the active transport of iodide into the thyroid cell, every subsequent step of triiodothyronine (T_3) and thyroxine (T_4) formation occurs within the Tg molecule. Thus, synthesis of T_3 and T_4 follows a metabolic pathway that depends on the integrity of the Tg structure. This large glycoprotein, a dimer of 660,000 Da, is synthesized and secreted by the thyroid cells into the lumen of the thyroid follicle (Fig. 1). Thyroglobulin serves two main purposes in the function of the thyroid gland. The first is related to the process of hormone production. Thus, Tg provides for the efficient coupling of the hormone precursors mono- and diiodotyrosine to form T_3 and T_4. The second function is that of a repository within the gland of a large supply of iodine and of hormone for secretion at a steady rate or upon demand. These two properties of Tg seem to permit the organism to operate in an

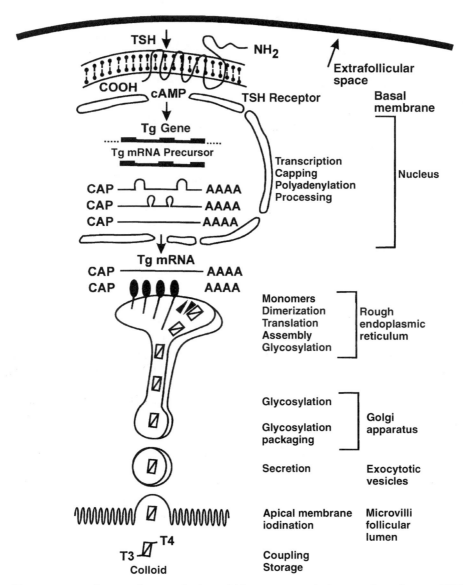

FIGURE 1 Tg gene expression, product synthesis, and Tg gene transcription are dependent on TSH stimulation through the interaction of TSH within the TSH receptor, via the cAMP pathway. The Tg gene (300 kb long) is transcribed into a Tg mRNA of 8448 bp and translated into a 2748-amino-acid (12S) Tg subunit. The mature protein is formed by joining two 12S subunits. After carbohydrate incorporation, the Tg is secreted into the follicular lumen via the Golgi apparatus. Modified from Medeiros-Neto, G., Targovnik, H. M., and Vassart, G. (1993). Defective thyroglobulin synthesis and secretion causing goiter and hypothyroidism. *Endocr. Rev.* **14**(2), 165–183, with permission from The Endocrine Society.

environment that is usually deficient in iodine and to accommodate wide variations in iodine supply. The efficiency of hormone synthesis of Tg depends on structural factors intrinsic to the protein matrix that favors the coupling reaction. It may be assumed that genetic mutations that would result in a structurally defective protein would severely impair the functional ability of Tg to serve as a matrix for the generation of T_3 and T_4.

II. THE STRUCTURE OF THYROGLOBULIN AND SYNTHESIS OF THYROID HORMONE

Thyroglobulin is synthesized on the endoplasmic reticulum as single polypeptide chains of approximately 300,000 Da. The nascent protein is transported to the Golgi, where the carbohydrate chains are completed. It then migrates to the apical membrane of the thyroid cell. Meanwhile, the iodide that has been trapped by the thyroid also accumulates at the apical cell border. Here, a complex series of reactions occurs, in which the iodide is oxidized through the action of a thyroidal peroxidase and hydrogen peroxide and is attached to tyrosyl residues within the Tg peptide chain. At this point, the Tg molecule contains iodinated tyrosines, monoiodotyrosine (MIT), and diiodotyrosine (DIT), but no thyroid hormone.

Through a further action of the peroxidase, two DIT residues, both in peptide linkage within Tg, couple to form T_4. This occurs by the formation of a diphenyl ether from the two DITs, leaving dehydro-alanine at the site formerly occupied by the DIT donating the outer ring of T_4. The other thyroid hormone (T_3) is formed by coupling one molecule of MIT with one molecule of DIT. Normally, approximately one-third of the iodine of Tg will be in the thyroid hormones T_4 and T_3, and the remainder will be in the inactive precursors DIT and MIT. By the time hormone synthesis is completed, two chains of 330,000 Da will associate to form the mature 660,000 Da Tg molecule. The two associating chains are probably identical. Thyroglobulin is stored extracellularly in the lumen of the thyroid follicle, where it is virtually the sole occupant (Fig. 1).

When the stored hormone is needed, Tg is retrieved by pinocytosis and ingested by the cell, where it fuses with lysosomes and is digested, and the hormone is released into the circulation. DIT and MIT are deiodinated and the iodine is returned to the intracellular iodide pool, where it is recycled. This is an important mechanism for iodine conservation.

The main metabolic steps of the biosynthesis of Tg appear in Fig. 1. Despite its huge size, Tg is not rich in tyrosine. Of more than 5000 amino acids in the 660,000 Da protein, only 4 to 8 are actually incorporated into hormone molecules. The synthesis of such an enormous molecule for this relatively small yield has perplexed many observers. The apparent wastefulness of this process may be explained in part by the storage function of Tg, through which large amounts of iodine are retained for long periods of time. This provides the thyroid with a constant reserve of iodine for hormone synthesis, even during periods when iodine is not immediately available from the environment.

Structural changes in the Tg molecule or its precursors, inability to couple iodotyrosines, defective glycosylation, or abnormal transport through the membrane system of the cell could impair or sub-stantially alter the synthesis of T_4 and T_3 and result in congenital goiter and various degrees of thyroid hypofunction.

III. THE TG GENE: STRUCTURE, EXPRESSION, AND REGULATION

The Tg gene, mapped to human chromosome 8q24.2–q24.3, covers at least 300 kb of genomic DNA and contains 8.5 kb of coding sequence divided over 48 exons separated by introns varying in size up to 64 kb. In 1987, the primary structure of human Tg was deduced from the sequence of its 8448-base messenger RNA and corresponding coding DNA (cDNA) sequence of 8304 bp. More recently, it was shown that the open reading frame of human Tg consists of 8307 bp, due to an extra nucleotide triplet (CAG) after position 2952. The frame encodes 2768 amino acid residues, including the signal peptide. The revised nucleotide positions resulted in the change of 12 amino acid residues and reduced the original number of tyrosine residues in the Tg monomer from 67 to 66.

The complete coding sequence of the 8307 nucleotides of the human Tg has been published with the encoded amino acid sequence (19-amino-acid signal peptide plus 2749 amino acids). To indicate the complexity of the Tg protein, other characteristics have been included such as the acceptor and donor tyrosine residues, the sites where thyroid hormones are synthesized, the N-glycosylation sites for the addition of carbohydrate molecules, the cysteine-rich repeated domains, the acetylcholinesterase homologous domain, and the most prominent antigenic epitopes. This work also described previously identified mutations and deletions found in human thyroid pathology and homologous positions in animals with hereditary thyroid disorders linked to a Tg defect (such as goats, Afrikander cattle, and cog/cog mice).

Four hormonogenic acceptor sites lie at positions 5, 1291, 2554, and 2747 in human Tg. Iodothyronine donor sites are at positions 130 and 1448. The acceptor sites map to the nonrepeated amino- and carboxy-terminal segments. The central portion of the molecule does not contain hormonogenic sites, yet it probably plays an important structural role in allowing the precise positioning of the hormonogenic tyrosines.

Two mechanisms for coupling are possible, one involving the free interaction of the donor and acceptor and the other assuming rigid juxtaposition of donor and acceptor. For this latter mechanism, a specific three-dimensional Tg structure is necessary.

The expression of the Tg gene is controlled at the level of transcription by TSH, the intracellular effects of which are mediated via cAMP. It is mimicked by forskolin, a universal activator of adenyl cyclase. No significant increase of Tg gene transcription was observed with chronic hyperstimulation of the rat thyroid gland with endogenous TSH. This indicates that the gene is close to being maximally expressed (at least in relative terms) under normal physiological conditions. In contrast, a dramatic decrease in Tg gene transcription was observed when endogenous TSH levels were suppressed. Injection of exogenous TSH in experimental animals restores transcriptional activity of the gene.

IV. ANIMAL MODELS OF DEFECTIVE Tg SYNTHESIS

Defects in Tg synthesis have been described in detail in sheep, cattle, bongo antelope, goats, and mice. Some of the animal studies are very informative. They serve as models for defective Tg synthesis in humans and provide important information about the molecular mechanisms of Tg defects.

A. Hereditary Goiter of the Afrikander Cattle

Congenital goiter with Tg deficiency has been described in a South African breed of cattle. Affected homozygotes were euthyroid despite huge goiters. The tissue contained iodoproteins, immunologically related to Tg but of abnormally low molecular weight. Iodoproteins with sedimentation coefficients of 4S, 9S, 12S, and 18S were isolated and purified into homogenous forms by gel chromatography and sucrose gradient ultracentrifugation.

In the Afrikander cattle thyroid, iodoalbumin constituted only 2.6% of the total soluble protein in the supernatant of the thyroid homogenate. In other examples of defective Tg biosynthesis, iodinated albumin frequently replaces Tg. The goiter of the homozygous animal contained a 7.3 kb Tg mRNA species in addition to the normal-sized 8.4 kb Tg mRNA. The mutation responsible for the disease is a cytosine to thymine transition, creating a stop codon at position 697 in exon 9. As a consequence, the goiter Tg mRNA encodes the shorter peptide of 75 kDa. The normal reading frame is conserved in the defective message, which is translatable into a potentially functional protein of approximately 2400 residues instead of the normal 2769 amino

acids. The euthyroid state of the affected animals is compatible with the fact that the major T_4 hormonogenic region of Tg near the amino-terminus is present on both the short and the long Tg-related peptides found in the goiter.

B. Hereditary Goiter of the Dutch Goats

A strain of hypothyroid goats with congenital goiter due to a defect in Tg synthesis has been extensively studied. The disease is inherited as an autosomal recessive. Only minute amounts of Tg were detected by radioimmunoassay (RIA). Ultracentrifugation, immunodiffuson, and immunoelectrophoresis demonstrated an absence of a normal 19S Tg in the goiter tissue.

Sequencing studies on goat complementary DNA were reported. A cytosine to guanine point mutation that caused a change from TAC (Tyr) to TAG (termination signal) at amino acid position 296 was found in exon 8. Chain termination in exon 8 will result in a Tg polypeptide chain with an estimated molecular weight of 39,000 that is similar in size to the *in vitro* translation product. The Tg fragment found in the goat's goiter containing the N-terminal hormonogenic site was able to produce T_4 *in vivo*. Administration of 1 mg iodide per day to a goitrous goat resulted in iodinated Tg with an iodotyrosine:iodothyronine ratio of 2.0:2.4. This is probably why the goitrous goats could be kept euthyroid by the administration of extra iodide.

C. Hereditary Goiter of the *cog/cog* Mice

A mouse mutation that in the homozygous state (*cog/cog*) causes primary hypothyroidism with goiter has been found. Young adult mutant mice are hypothyroid, as evidenced by significantly lower total serum concentrations of T_4 and T_3 and elevated serum levels of TSH. Studies of goitrous tissue showed marked deficiency in immunoreactive Tg. Further studies demonstrated linkage of goiter to the Tg gene on chromosome 15. A single amino acid change at position 2265 (leucine to proline) causes abnormal storage of the mutant thyroglobulin in the endoplasmic reticulum.

Ultracentrifugation procedures followed by RIA were used to determine the protein sedimentation properties. A small peak in the 3S to 8S area (13.7% of the total apparent immunologic activity) contained iodinated albumin. There were also broad, overlapping peaks at 12S, 19S, and 27S (86.3%). The sedimentation properties indicate that the formation of 19S Tg was not normal. There was an increase in unassociated 12S subunits and aggregated species larger than 19S.

V. HUMAN CONGENITAL GOITER WITH DEFECTIVE Tg SYNTHESIS

A. Clinical Features

Characteristically, the majority of patients have congenital goiter, with hypothyroidism or goiter appearing shortly after birth. Goiters are usually large and have a soft, elastic consistency. Many of these patients present as adults with nodular hyperplasia (Fig. 2). Symptoms of compression of the surrounding neck structures are quite common. Hypothyroidism may be partially compensated for by preferential T_3 secretion and normal serum T_3 levels. Therefore, many of these patients may attain near-normal stature and some are able to perform simple tasks and even to learn how to read and write. There is no impairment in hearing and the structure of the cochlea is normal in the few cases that have been examined by computerized tomography.

B. Genetics

A positive family history of goiter has been obtained in more than 50% of these patients. Both sexes are affected, but males are more frequently affected (38 females, 54 males). The parents were considered heterozygous and unaffected; frequently more than one sib was affected in a generation and the pattern of inheritance is autosomal recessive.

C. Laboratory Investigation and Diagnosis

In the early reports of defective Tg synthesis, it was found that the serum protein-bound iodine concentration (PBI) was higher than thyroxine iodine measured by RIA. This suggested the presence in serum of abnormal iodoproteins. These may be non-19S Tg subunits, iodoalbumin, iodohistidines, or iodogammaglobulin. The presence of abnormal iodoproteins is also frequently found in endemic goiter, sporadic goiter, and goitrous Hashimoto

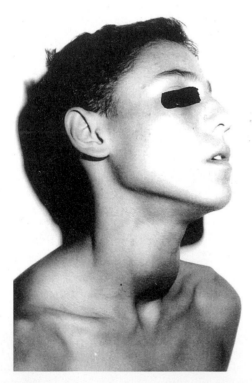 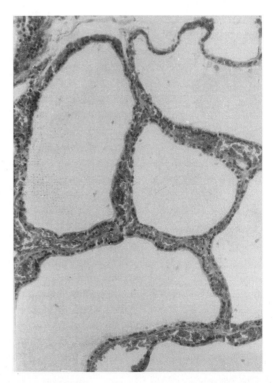

FIGURE 2   A 16-year-old male with congenital goiter with few signs of hypothyroidism treated with L-T4 since early childhood (left). Serum Tg was very low (1.8 ng/ml) and did not rise after 0.45 mg of human recombinant TSH (2.1 ng/ml) despite a large goiter (78 g). The pathological specimen was typical of a thyroglobulin defect with absent colloid (right). Immunochemistry was able to demonstrate immunoreactive Tg inside the follicular cells.

thyroiditis and should be considered as only indicative of a possible Tg defect.

With the increasing use of serum Tg determination by RIA, the presence of an abnormally low or borderline low serum Tg level in a goitrous individual became a good indicator of a Tg defect. The TSH stimulation test is used to differentiate the group of Tg defects from other possible types of dishormonogenesis. Subjects with Tg defects have relatively low or undetectable serum Tg values that do not increase 48 h after a single injection of bovine or, more recently, human recombinant TSH. By contrast, a fivefold increase in serum Tg values was obtained in goitrous patients with organification defects (low or absent thyroid peroxidase active). Therefore, goitrous patients with a suspected hereditary Tg defect may be differentiated from other congenital goitrous patients through the TSH stimulation test.

The radioiodide uptake is invariably elevated, indicating an activation of the iodine-concentrating mechanism, probably due to chronic TSH stimulation. As the thyroperoxidase system is also activated, there is an increased incorporation of iodine into protein. Since thyroglobulin is not available, albumin and other proteins are iodinated and secreted. Incorporation of iodine into proteins other than Tg generates iodotyrosines and iodohistidines. In situations in which the patient lives in an area where the supply of iodine is low, the loss of iodide may aggravate the functional deficiency of the dishormonogenetic gland. On the other hand, an adequate supply of iodide can lead to compensation for the relative lack of thyroidal Tg, as demonstrated in experimental animals.

The perchlorate discharge test is usually negative (less than 15% of the trapped iodide is released after an oral dose of 2.0 g of potassium perchlorate).

Thyroid images obtained by isotope scanning or by ultrasonography are not different from those seen in multinodular or hyperplastic goiters. Thus, although these procedures are routinely employed to estimate the thyroid volume and thyroid anatomy, they add little to the differential diagnosis.

D. Microscopic Examination

A number of reports include the histological examination of the thyroid, by both light microscopy and electron microscopy. The absence or pronounced scarcity of colloid and large follicular spaces lined by predominantly cuboidal cells with frequent atypical nuclei are indicative of a lack of Tg synthesis and chronic TSH stimulation (Fig. 2). In patients with impaired Tg export, electron microscopy has shown fragmented endoplasmic reticulum cisternae, with irregular contours that appeared overdistended. The Golgi complexes were numerous and had a large surface area. There were no colloid droplets inside the follicular cell and no immunofluorescence in the lumina after exposure to both anti-human Tg and anti-human serum albumin. Similarly, immunostaining with anti-human Tg using the immunoperoxidase method in two patients with a quantitative defect have shown Tg-related protein only inside the cytoplasm.

E. Biochemical Studies on Tissues with Defective Tg Synthesis

In patients with a defective synthesis of Tg, the normal Tg peak is usually absent in the filtration elution pattern and an abnormally large albumin peak preceding the hemoglobin peak is observed.

This pattern of absence of Tg can be confirmed by Tg radioimmunoassay. Normally, Tg is measurable in the thyroid-soluble protein fraction, ranging from 50 to 90 mg/g of tissue. In all patients with the quantitative Tg defect, the Tg content was less than 0.5 mg/g of tissue. Other methods for evaluating the presence of Tg in the thyroid extract are immunoelectrophoresis (using rabbit anti-human Tg) and sodium dodecyl sulfate-agarose gel electrophoresis. In both methods, the absence of Tg bands confirms the quantitative Tg defect.

F. Identified Defects in Human

Five different mutations in the Tg gene have been reported. All patients are homozygous for the mutations and fit the clinical description of a Tg synthesis defect, although the locations of the mutations and the corresponding defects at the protein level are strikingly dissimilar. The Tg disorders can be divided into three groups:

1. Structurally defective Tg that may not be functional or will yield thyroid hormones only at a very high intake of iodine.
2. The defective Tg molecule is not exported to the colloid (endoplasmic reticulum storage disease) as indicated in Fig. 3.
3. Defective glycosylation of Tg (low sialyc acid incorporation).

Approximately 113 patients from several families have been described in detail and molecular mechanisms have been determined in many of these patients. Two important deletions, of 68 amino acids from the

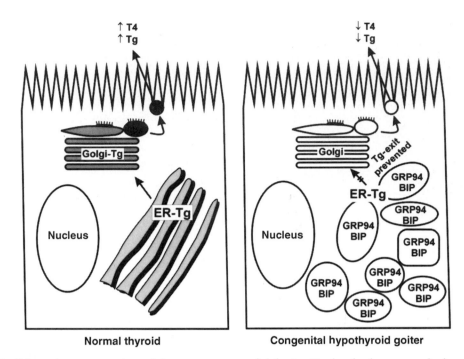

FIGURE 3 Schematic representation of the consequences of defective Tg that leads to an endoplasmic reticulum storage disease causing congenital hypothyroid goiter. In affected patients, the arrival of Tg in the Golgi complex and the subsequent secretion of Tg to form T4 are drastically inhibited. Instead, Tg accumulates in the ER, with accumulation of ER chaperones (GRP94, BIP) that assist the mutant Tg in migrating to the Golgi apparatus. The diminished synthesis of T4 triggers pituitary secretion of TSH, further stimulating the thyroid gland and contributing to goiter growth. Modified from Arvan *et al.* (1997). Intracellular protein transport to the thyrocyte plasma membrane: Potential implications for thyroid physiology. *Thyroid* 7(1), 89–105, with permission from Mary Ann Liebert Publishers.

N-terminal part of the Tg proteins and 46 amino acids of the middle of the protein, have been attributed to the in-frame deletion of exons 4 and 30, respectively.

A truncated Tg protein has been reported in a patient in whom exon 22 contains a premature stop codon that results in a very small Tg protein. The thyroid tissue also contains an alternative splice variant from which exon 22 was deleted.

In many patients, similar to the findings in *cog/cog* mice, the mutant Tg may not leave the endoplasmic reticulum, due to the quality control system of the cell. Therefore, very little Tg protein is actually stored in the colloid (Fig. 3).

VI. SERUM THYROGLOBULIN MEASUREMENTS IN THE MANAGEMENT OF THYROID CANCER

Thyroglobulin is a glycoprotein that is produced only by normal or neoplastic thyroid follicular cells. Most differentiated thyroid carcinomas secrete Tg. Patients with lung and bone metastases have the highest serum Tg concentrations, whereas those with metastases in lymph nodes may have only modest elevations of serum Tg. Medullary and anaplastic carcinomas do not secrete Tg, whereas Hürthle cell carcinoma, a variant of follicular carcinoma, secretes Tg but does not concentrate radioiodine.

Serum Tg should not be detectable in patients who have undergone total thyroidectomy followed by radioiodine ablation and its detection in such patients signifies the presence of persistent or recurrent disease.

Good thyroglobulin assays can detect concentrations as low as 1 ng/ml. The results, however, can be artifactually altered by the presence of serum anti-thyroglobulin antibodies, which are found in approximately 15% of patients with thyroid carcinoma. Tests for these antibodies should always be performed when serum thyroglobulin is measured, but the extent to which the presence of the antibodies alters the results of serum Tg assays depends on whether a radioimmunoassay (less affected) or an immunoradiometric assay (more affected) is performed.

The production of thyroglobulin in both normal and neoplastic thyroid tissue is in part dependent on TSH. Interpretation of the serum Tg concentrations should take into account the serum TSH value, as well as the presence or absence of thyroid remnants.

If the serum Tg level is detectable during L-T4 suppressive treatment, it will increase after the treatment is withdrawn, indicating that thyroid remnant or neoplastic tissue is actively producing and releasing thyroglobulin under the stimulation of endogenous TSH.

The serum thyroglobulin concentration is an excellent prognostic indicator. Patients with undetectable serum Tg concentrations after total thyroidectomy and radioiodine ablation and under L-T4 suppressive therapy are free of the disease (Fig. 4). Conversely, 80% of patients with serum thyroglobulin concentrations that are higher than 10 ng/ml during L-T4 treatment and higher than 40 ng/ml after withdrawal of L-T4 treatment have detectable foci of radioiodine uptake in the neck or bone/lung metastases (Fig. 4).

Patient 1, as shown in Fig. 4, developed a serum Tg that was close to 1 ng/ml by the end of the first postoperative year and subsequently had no recurrences during 15 years of follow-up. In contrast, patient 2 never had a serum Tg below 1 ng/ml despite a total thyroidectomy and radioiodine ablation. After approximately 5 years, this patient developed a clinically evident recurrence despite negative radioiodine scans and died of the disease 10 years later.

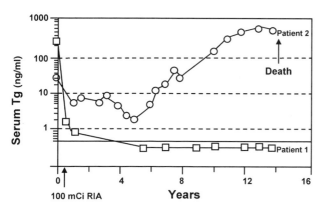

FIGURE 4 Serum Tg concentrations during L-T4 suppressive therapy in two patients. Patient 1 consistently had serum Tg levels below 1 ng/ml, whereas Patient 2 had elevated serum Tg values despite negative RAI scans. This patient developed clinically evident distant metastases. Modified from Spencer, C. A. (1998). Detection of residual and recurrent thyroid cancer by serum thyroglobulin measurement. American Thyroid Association 70th Annual Meeting, with permission.

In conclusion, it should be remembered that measurement of Tg in serum is technically challenging and it is difficult to compare serum Tg obtained by different methods. The clinical interpretation of serum Tg results should be made relative to two main factors that influence serum Tg concentrations: the mass of differentiated thyroid tissue present and the level of serum TSH and TSH receptor stimulation. Therefore, changes in the serum Tg levels during TSH suppression by L-T4 are a good indicative sign of the TSH sensitivity of the tumor and may indicate the potential efficiency of TSH suppression therapy.

Finally, the ability to stimulate serum Tg with recombinant human TSH during thyroxine suppression and to measure Tg mRNA from peripheral blood holds promise for improvement in the management of thyroid cancer patients over the next decade.

VII. SUMMARY

The integrity of the Tg protein structure is essential for adequate synthesis of thyroid hormone. Also, a large supply of iodine and of thyroid hormone is stored in the Tg molecule and is available for secretion on demand.

Mutations in the Tg gene or hyposialylated Tg due to defective sialyltransferase activity cause a structurally defective protein and severely impair the functional ability of Tg. Abnormalities in the synthesis of Tg have been described in both animals and human. Hereditary congenital goiter with or without hypothyroidism is the phenotypic major clinical finding in these species. Affected animals include sheep, cattle, bongo antelope, goats, and mice. The inheritance mode is autosomal recessive. In most animal studies, structurally abnormal Tg is present. The molecular basis for the defective Tg synthesis is attributable to a nonsense mutation in exon 9 (Afrikander cattle) and in exon 8 (Dutch goats).

In human, defective Tg synthesis has been reported in 113 patients and frequently more than one sibling is affected in a given generation. Characteristically, these patients exhibit hereditary congenital goiter with relatively low Tg levels that do not increase after stimulation with bovine TSH. High PBI concentrations with low serum T_4 values indicate the presence in serum of iodinated proteins (mainly iodoalbumin). Also, iodinated peptides are frequently excreted into the urine. Tissue studies confirm that there is no normal Tg peak on gel filtration and virtually no immunoassayable Tg in the tissue extracts.

The described mutations in the Tg gene include deletions of entire exons (exon 4 and exon 30) and point mutations with a premature stop codon generating a very truncated Tg protein. The mutant Tg protein may be functional (generating T_3 and T_4) in the constant presence of excess iodine. Many of the mutant Tg proteins are retained in the endoplasmic reticulum system of the cell and do not reach the follicular lumen (colloid).

Serum Tg measurements have greatly facilitated the clinical management of patients with differentiated thyroid cancer. The interpretation of any given Tg value requires the careful synthesis of all pertinent clinical and laboratory data available to the clinician. For instance, Tg autoantibodies remain a significant obstacle to the clinical use of Tg assays, although their presence may be indicative of persistent or residual metastatic disease. Finally, the ability to stimulate serum Tg with recombinant human TSH during L-T4 suppression and to measure Tg mRNA from peripheral blood holds promise for the management of thyroid cancer patients.

Glossary

allele Variant form of a gene at a specific locus.

autosomes A term for any chromosome other than the X or Y sex chromosome.

base pair Two nucleotides located on complementary strands of DNA and paired by hydrogen bonds.

cDNA (complementary DNA) DNA strand created *in vitro* by reverse transcription of a messenger RNA molecule.

chaperone A protein that assists in the correct folding (and assembly) of another protein.

codon Sequence of three nucleotides that encodes a particular amino acid or signals the initiation or termination of protein synthesis.

deletion Mutation that results in the removal of a sequence of DNA from a chromosome.

endocytosis Process by which extracellular material is transported into a cell, forming membrane-bound vesicles within the cytoplasm.

endonuclease Enzyme that cleaves a nucleotide chain.

endoplasmic reticulum Cellular organelle consisting of sheets of membranes; it functions in the synthesis of lipids and membrane proteins.

exon Portion of a gene that encodes a protein sequence or a specific part of a protein.

frameshift mutation Change in the DNA sequence that occurs by insertion or deletion of some number of nucleotides that is not a multiple of 3, thus altering the reading frame for protein translation.

gene Specific sequence of DNA at a particular chromosomal location; it codes for a specific protein.

heterozygote Organism with two different alleles at a particular locus.

homozygote Organism with the same alleles at a particular locus.

intron Noncoding segment of a gene that is transcribed into RNA but is spliced out before translation occurs.

linkage The association between two genes that are located near each other on the same chromosome and that as a result tend to be inherited together.

missense mutation Change in the DNA sequence that alters a codon so that it codes for a different amino acid.

mutation Change in the DNA sequence of a gene.

nonsense mutation Change in the DNA sequence that results in a codon that specifies an amino acid being replaced by a stop codon (codon that terminates protein synthesis).

oncogene Gene that can cause or contribute to cancerous growth or other unregulated cell proliferation.

PCR (polymerase chain reaction) Laboratory technique for exponentially amplifying the number of copies of a short segment of DNA.

point mutation Change in one nucleotide in a DNA molecule.

recessive allele Allele that is not expressed in the phenotype of a heterozygote, due to the presence of the dominant allele.

somatic mutation Change in the DNA sequence of any cell in an organism other than a germ cell; it cannot be inherited by the organism's offspring.

See Also the Following Articles

Environmental Disruptors of Thyroid Hormone Action • Iodine: Symporter and Oxidation, Thyroid Hormone Biosynthesis • Thyroid Hormone Receptor, TSH and TSH Receptor Mutations • Thyroid Stimulating Hormone (TSH) • Thyrotropin-Releasing Hormone (TRH)

Further Reading

Arvan, P., Kim, P. S., Kuhawat, R., Prabaran, D., Muresan, Z., Yoo, S. E., and Hossain, S. A. (1997). Intracellular protein transport to the thyrocyte plasma membrane: Potential implications for thyroid physiology. *Thyroid* 7(1), 89–105.

Kim, P. S., Kwon, O. Y., and Arvan, P. (1996). An endoplasmic reticulum storage disease causing congenital goiter with hypothyroidism. *J. Cell Biol.* **133**, 517–527.

Medeiros-Neto, G. (1994). Defects in Tg gene expression and Tg secretion. *In* "Inherited Disorders of the Thyroid System" (G. Medeiros-Neto and J. B. Stanbury, eds.), pp. 107–138. CRC Press, Boca Raton, FL.

Medeiros-Neto, G., Kim, P. S., Yoo, S. E., Vono, J., Camargo, R., Targovnik, H. M., Honain, S. A., and Arvan, P. (1996). Congenital hypothyroidism goiter with deficient thyroglobulin identification of an endoplasmic reticulum storage disease (ERSD) with induction of molecular chaperones. *J. Clin. Invest.* **98**, 2838–2844.

Medeiros-Neto, G., Targovnik, H. M., and Vassart, G. (1993). Defective thyroglobulin synthesis and secretion causing goiter and hypothyroidism. *Endocr. Rev.* **14**(2), 165–183.

Moya, C. M., Mendive, F. M., Rivolta, C. M., Vassart, G., and Targovnik, H. M. (2000). Genomic organization of the 5′

region of the human thyroglobulin gene. *Eur. J. Endocrinol.* **143**, 789–798.

Spencer, C. A. (1998). Detection of residual and recurrent thyroid cancer by serum thyroglobulin measurement. CMES Satellite Symposium, 70th Annual Meeting of the American Thyroid Association, Portland, OR.

Spencer, C. A., Takeuchi, M., Kazarosyan, M., Wang, C. C., Gruthler, R. B., Singer, P. A., Fatemi, S., LoPresti, J. S., and Nicoloff, J. T. (1998). Serum thyroglobulin auto-antibodies: Prevalence, influence on serum thyroglobulin measurements and prognostic significance in patients with differentiated thyroid carcinoma. *J. Clin. Endocrinol. Metab.* **83**, 1121–1127.

Targovnik, H. M., Rivolta, C. M., Mendive, F. M., Moya, C. M., Vono, J., and Medeiros-Neto, G. (2001). Congenital goiter with hypothyroidism caused by a $5'$ splice site mutation in the thyroglobulin gene. *Thyroid* **11**, 685–690.

Torrens, J. I., and Burch, H. B. (2001). Serum thyroglobulin measurement: Utility in clinical practice. *Endocrinol. Metab. Clin.* **30**(2), 429–465.

Van de Graaf, S. A. R., Ris-Stalpers, C., Pauws, E., Mendive, F. M., Targovnik, H. M., and DeViljder, J. J. M. (2001). Up to date with human thyroglobulin. *J. Endocrinol.* **170**, 307–321.

Van de Graaf, S. A. R., Ris-Stalpers, C., Veenboer, G. J. M., Cammenga, M., Santos, C. L. S., Targovnik, H. M., DeViljder, J. J. M., and Medeiros-Neto, G. (1999). A premature stop codon in thyroglobulin mRNA results in familial goiter and moderate hypothyroidism. *J. Clin. Endocrinol. Metab.* **84**, 2537–2542.

Thyroid and Reproduction

CHRISTOPHER LONGCOPE

University of Massachusetts Medical School

I. THYROID HORMONE ACTION ON THE GONADS
II. CLINICAL ASPECTS OF THYROID DYSFUNCTION
III. PREGNANCY

Thyroid hormones appear to have some effects on male and female reproductive capacities. Thyroid hormone receptors found on cells of reproductive tissues in both sexes are involved in activation of steroid hormones. Disorders of the thyroid gland are common in patient populations, and thus it is important to understand the impact thyroid dysfunction my have on sexual development and function.

I. THYROID HORMONE ACTION ON THE GONADS

Although much of the work on the effects of thyroid hormone at the tissue level has been carried out in animals, the results appear to be applicable to humans. The following discussions present the known effects of thyroid hormones on the reproductive axis in men and women.

A. Testis

Because the testis is stimulated by both luteinizing hormone (LH) and follicle-stimulating hormone (FSH), thyroid hormone effects on the pituitary, the source of LH and FSH, can result in changes in testicular function. In rats, both thyroid hormone administration and thyroidectomy result in decreases in concentrations of circulating LH and FSH. In the testis, thyroid hormone has been reported to increase LH receptors on Leydig cells initially, but with continued exposure there is a decrease in receptor number. Thyroid hormone appears to be active in the developing testis but to play a lesser role on the adult testis. Receptors for thyroid hormones, primarily TRα1 and TRα2, have been identified in prepubertal testes; primarily in the Sertoli and germ cells. Acting mainly through TRα1, thyroid hormone increases differentiation of the Sertoli cells and inhibits their proliferation. Similarly, thyroid hormone increases differentiation of Leydig cells from mesenchymal precursor cells. In adult testis, thyroid hormone has an acute effect, increasing steroid synthesis and enhancing steroidogenic acute regulatory protein (StAR) function. However, continued exposure to thyroid hormone results in decreases in both end points. Thyroid hormone also decreases aromatization in Sertoli cells. With maturation through puberty, both TRα1 and TRα2 decline in number; however, the decline appears to be much greater for TRα1 than TRα2, thus the ratio of TRα2/TRα1 increases. Because TRα2 may inhibit the action of TRα1, the fact that it is at a higher level than TRα1 may explain why thyroid hormone has less effect on the adult testis, compared to the prepubertal testis. However, male mice lacking both TRα1 and TRβ2 are fertile. Although some individuals with thyroid dysfunction may have problems related to reproduction, the presence of thyroid hormone does not appear to be absolutely necessary for male reproductive function.

B. Ovary

Thyroid hormone acts to decrease circulating levels of LH and to synergize with FSH to increase differentiation of granulosa cells. It is not clear that ovarian development is critically dependent on normal thyroid hormone levels. Thyroid hormone receptors TRα1 and TRβ1 are present in human and animal granulosa and stromal cells. Female mice lacking either TRα1 or TRβ are fertile, but those lacking both TRα1 and TRβ1 have markedly reduced fertility. Thus, it would appear that thyroid hormones are more important for reproduction processes in females, as opposed to males. A lack of thyroid hormone has been associated with the development of polycystic ovaries in rodents. Granulosa cell aromatase activity is inhibited by excess thyroid hormone, although progesterone synthesis is increased. Thyroid hormone not only has a direct effect on ovarian steroidogenesis but also augments action of gonadotropins in steroid synthesis. Thyroid hormones are important for normal ovulation and normal steroidogenesis.

Studies have indicated that triiodothyronine (T3) decreases estradiol secretion in both medium and large follicles but increases progesterone synthesis in medium follicles and decreases progesterone synthesis in large follicles. T3 also stimulates 3β-hydroxysteroid dehydrogenase activity in the pig corpus luteum. The development of hypothyroidism in prepubertal rats results in increased proliferation of granulosa cells but inhibition of differentiation. No copora lutea are noted in the ovaries of hypothyroid rats. Receptors for thyroid hormone have been noted in the endometrium and excess thyroid hormone in mice may cause a thickened endometrium. Thyroxine (T4) has been noted to decrease estradiol uptake by the rat uterus, but thyrotoxicosis in rats results in a decreased response to estrogen in the uterus.

II. CLINICAL ASPECTS OF THYROID DYSFUNCTION

A. Hypothyroidism

1. Males

Hypothyroidism during pregnancy may lead to the condition known as cretinism. Hypothyroidism does not appear to interfere with gonadal development in the male fetus, however, and cretins usually have a normal reproductive tract. As a reflection of the role of thyroid hormone in stimulating the differentiation of Sertoli cells, hypothyroidism in early life results in an increased number of Sertoli cells and an accordingly enlarged testis. Leydig cells may also be increased in number. Thus, hypothyroidism occurring in prepubertal boys may be associated with enlarged testis and precocious pseudopuberty. True puberty will occur in these individuals, however, and they will be capable of normal reproduction. Prepubertal hypothyroidism is more commonly associated with delayed sexual maturation.

Hypothyroidism in adults may be associated with defects in spermatogenesis and fertility, but this is not a universal phenomenon and many hypothyroid men will be fertile. In part, this is a manifestation of the degree of hypothyroidism. Hypothyroidism may alter the pituitary responsiveness to gonadotropin-releasing hormone (GnRH), resulting in lower levels of LH and a decrease in levels of circulating testosterone. In addition, hypothyroidism can be associated with hyperprolactinemia, which can be associated with hypogonadism.

2. Females

Perhaps because thyroid dysfunction is more common in women than in men, there have been more studies of hypothyroidism in females. Female cretins generally have normally developed reproductive tracts at birth. Hypothyroidism in prepubertal girls may cause precocious pseudopuberty with galactorrhea, caused by an increase in prolactin, and vaginal bleeding as a result of increased ovarian estrogen secretion, which stimulates the endometrium. The exact mechanisms are uncertain, but these conditions may be due to excess pituitary secretion of thyroid-stimulating hormone (TSH) and gonadotropins. A more common result of hypothyroidism in girls is delayed menarche and sexual maturation.

In postpubertal women, hypothyroidism is often associated with menstrual dysfunction, menometrorrhagia (irregular menstrual cycle) being the commonest. However, the incidence of menstrual irregularities appears to be less common now than previously. Earlier studies reported that 60–80% of hypothyroid women had menstrual abnormalities as compared to only 23% in more recent studies. The commonest symptom is menometrorrhagia in most studies. Anovulation is frequently present and endometrial biopsies often are out of phase. Paradoxically, hypothyroid women taking oral contraceptives may report an absence of withdrawal bleeding. LH and FSH levels are often low and, although this may be a direct result of low thyroid hormone levels, prolactin levels are often elevated and may result in hypogonadism.

B. Hyperthyroidism

1. Males

Excess thyroid hormone in prepubertal males may result in early maturation; a marked excess of thyroid hormone may cause a decrease in testis volume and an impairment of sexual development associated with low levels of LH.

In adults, increased levels of thyroid hormone result in an increase in circulating levels of sex hormone-binding globulin (SHBG) and an increase in circulating levels of testosterone and estradiol. Free testosterone levels generally remain within the normal range but bioavailability may be decreased. The increase in estrogen levels can be sufficient to cause gynecomastia. An increase in LH levels may occur; but this is not a universal finding. In males with thyrotoxicosis, fertility may be decreased because of low sperm counts and alterations in sperm motility. Receptors for T3 have been found in rat epididymis and these may play a role in the sperm abnormalities.

2. Females

In prepubertal women, thyrotoxicosis can result in delayed sexual maturity, but women with polycystic fibrous dysplasia (McCurre–Albright syndrome) may have associated precocious puberty and thyrotoxicosis. In adult women, menstrual abnormalities are frequently noted, with oligo- or amenorrhea being common. Gonadotropin levels are increased but the ovulatory peak of LH may be absent.

III. PREGNANCY

It has been proposed that hypothyroid women rarely became pregnant, but, despite the frequency of anovulation, pregnancy in untreated hypothyroid women is not uncommon. The course of pregnancy and its eventual outcome are influenced by thyroid function, and, in turn, pregnancy has an effect on thyroid function in euthyroid women.

Pregnancy in an untreated hypothyroid woman is associated with an increased risk of spontaneous abortion, gestational hypertension, low-birth-weight infants, and congenital fetal malformations. Subclinical hypothyroidism, i.e., elevated TSH levels with borderline low T4 and T3 levels, has been reported to be associated with an increased risk for these abnormalities. The frequency of these disorders is difficult to determine because of the scattered nature of the reports, many of which involve a questionable diagnosis of hypothyroidism or the institution of appropriate treatment at the time of diagnosis.

In a normal pregnancy, the high levels of human chorionic gonadotropin (hCG) stimulate the thyroid gland and there is a small increase in thyroxine and free T4 and T3. Elevations of thyroid hormone levels in turn suppress TSH levels. As hCG levels fall, the stimulus to the thyroid decreases and TSH levels start to rise.

Thyroid hormone has been shown to increase the concentration of SHBG, but the marked increase in thyroxine-binding globulin (TBG) and SHBG that occurs in pregnancy is secondary to the increase in estrogen levels. As TBG levels rise, the levels of T4 and T3 also increase and in most normal pregnancies will be above the upper limits for normal nonpregnant women. The free T4 and free T3 levels remain within the normal limits. However, in pregnant women being treated with replacement doses of thyroid hormone, the dose will need to be increased because of the increase in TBG.

Thyrotoxicosis in pregnant women is also associated with abnormalities, and there is an increased risk of low-birth-weight infants, congenital fetal malformations, pre-eclampsia, and premature delivery. Pregnant women with thyrotoxicosis are usually treated with an antithyroid drug, although in extreme cases surgery may be indicated. Antithyroid drugs cross the placenta and can act on the fetal thyroid, resulting in a fetal goiter. Thus, the dose of the antithyroid drug should be kept at the lowest dose needed to ameliorate the thyrotoxicosis, and in many instances can be discontinued in the third trimester.

In the postpartum period, thyroiditis may develop in association with hypothyroidism or hyperthyroidism. Either condition may be transient or prolonged.

Glossary

galactorrhea Production and secretion of milk from breast tissue.
granulosa cells Line the follicle in the ovary; take up and aromatize androgens to estrogens, primarily estradiol.
gynecomastia Enlargement of the breast; usually used in reference to the male breast.
Leydig cells Present in the interstitial space of the testes; stimulated by luteinizing hormone to synthesize steroids, primarily the androgen testosterone.
Sertoli cells Line the seminiferous tubules of the testes; necessary for spermatogenesis; respond to follicle-stimulating hormone.
sex hormone-binding globulin Protein made in the liver that binds certain steroids with high affinity, making them less available for uptake by tissues compared to albumin-bound or free (bioavailable) steroids. The binding affinity of SHBG is highest for dihydrotestosterone and testosterone but less for estradiol.

See Also the Following Articles

Environmental Disruptors of Thyroid Hormone Action • Follicle Stimulating Hormone (FSH) • Luteinizing Hormone (LH) • Sex Hormone-Binding Globulin (SHBG) • Stress and Reproduction • Thyroid Hormone Action on the Heart and Cardiovascular System ● Thyroid Hormone Action on the Skeleton and Growth ● Thyroid Hormone Receptor, TSH and TSH Receptor Mutations ● Thyroid Stimulating Hormone (TSH)

Further Reading

Ariyaratne, H. B. S., Mason, J. I., and Mendis-Handagama, S. M. L. C. (2000). Effects of thyroid and luteinizing hormones on the onset of precursor cell differentiation into Leydig progenitor cells in the prepubertal rat testis. *Biol. Reprod.* **63**, 898–904.

Buzzard, J. J., Morrison, J. R., OBryan, M. K., Song, Q., and Wreford, N. G. (2001). Developmental expression of thyroid hormone receptors in the rat testis. *Biol. Reprod.* **62**, 664–669.

Canale, D., Agostini, M., Giorgilli, G. *et al.* (2001). Thyroid hormone receptors in neonatal, prepubertal, and adult rat testis. *J. Androl.* **22**, 284–288.

Donnelly, P., and White, C. (2000). Testicular dysfunction in men with primary hypothyroidism; reversal of hypogonadotrophic hypogonadism with replacement thyroxine. *Clin. Endocrinol.* **52**, 197–201.

Doufas, A. G., and Mastorakos, G. (2000). The hypothalamic pituitary thyroid axis and the female reproductive system. *Ann. N.Y. Acad. Sci.* **900**, 65–76.

Fallah-Rad, A. H., Connor, M. L., and Del Vecchio, R. P. (2001). Effect of transient early hyperthyroidism on onset of puberty in Suffolk ram lambs. *Reproduction* **121**, 639–646.

Glinoer, D. (1999). What happens to the normal thyroid during pregnancy? *Thyroid* **9**, 631–635.

Glinoer, D. (2000). Thyroid disease during pregnancy. *In* "Werner & Ingbar's The Thyroid" (L. Braverman and R. D. Utiger, eds.), pp. 1014–1027. Lippincott, Williams & Wilkins, Philadelphia.

Jannini, E. A., Carosa, E., Rucci, N., Screponi, C. R., and D'Armiento, M. (1999). Ontogeny and regulation of ovarian thyroid hormone receptor isoforms in developing rat testis. *J. Endocrinol. Invest.* **22**, 843–848.

Krassas, G. E. (2000). Thyroid disease and female reproduction. *Fertil. Steril.* **74**, 1063–1070.

Krassas, G. E., Pontikides, N., Kaltsas, T. *et al.* (1999). Disturbances of menstruation in hypothyroidism. *Clin. Endocrinol.* **50**, 655–659.

Longcope, C. (2000). The male and female reproductive systems in hypothyroidism. *In* "Werner & Ingbar's The Thyroid" (L. E. Braverman and R. D. Utiger, eds.), pp. 824–827 Lippincott, Williams & Wilkins, Philadelphia.

Manna, P. R., Roy, P., Clark, B. J., Stocco, D. M., and Huhtaniemi, I. T. (2001). Interaction of thyroid hormone and steroidogenic acute regulatory (StAR) protein in the regulation of murine Leydig cell steroidogenesis. *J. Steroid Biochem. Mol. Biol.* **76**, 167–177.

Panidis, D. K., and Russo, D. H. (1999). Macro-orchidism in juvenile hypothyroidism. *Arch. Androl.* **42**, 85–87.

Trummer, H., Ramschak-Schwarzer, S., Haas, J., Habermann, H., Pummer, K., and Leb, G. (2001). Thyroid hormones and thyroid antibodies in infertile males. *Fertil. Steril.* **76**, 254–257.

Thyroid Hormone Action on the Heart and Cardiovascular System

Bernd R. Gloss

University of California, San Diego

I. INTRODUCTION
II. T3 TARGET GENES IN THE HEART
III. T3 EFFECTS ON MYOCYTE PHYSIOLOGY
IV. TARGET GENE PROMOTERS
V. T3 RECEPTOR EXPRESSION IN THE HEART
VI. SUMMARY

Both hyperthyroidism and hypothyroidism are associated with changes in cardiac function. A number of genes expressed in the heart are known to be regulated by thyroid hormone. This article examines the changes in cardiac performance that are associated with changes in thyroid hormone levels and discusses thyroid hormone regulation of target gene expression in the heart.

I. INTRODUCTION

In the late 1700s, a physician named Caleb Hillier Parry described an interesting correlation that he had observed during his medical career. He noted that an enlargement of the thyroid gland coincided with an enlargement of the heart.

Since these early descriptions of the correlation between thyroid disorders and cardiac function, many detailed studies have crystallized the concept that there must be genes in the heart that are regulated by thyroid hormone and that up- or down-regulation of such genes brings about the physiological effects in the heart that are observed in a particular thyroid condition. What are the changes in cardiac physiology that are associated with elevated or lowered thyroid hormone levels?

Hyperthyroidism is associated with an elevated heart rate (tachycardia) and to a significant degree also with cardiac arrhythmias. In addition, the speed and force of cardiac contraction are both elevated and there are hemodynamic changes largely caused by a decreased arterial tone and increased venous tone. Because most of the biological actions of thyroxine are mediated by its conversion to triiodothyronine (T3), in the hyperthyroid state T3 increases heart rate (chronotropic effects), increases the force and speed

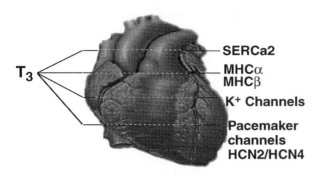

SERCa2
MHCα
MHCβ
K⁺ Channels
Pacemaker channels HCN2/HCN4

Phospholamban
β-Adrenergic receptor
Adenylyl cyclases
Guanine-nucleotide regulating protein
T3Rα1
Sodium-potassium ATPase
Sodium-calcium exchanger
Ryanodine receptor

FIGURE 1 Thyroid hormone in the form of T3 regulates the cardiac genes listed in this figure. The regulatory regions of the genes on the right have been studied extensively and in some the T3-response elements have been identified and characterized.

of systolic contraction (inotropic effect), and accelerates diastolic relaxation (lusitropic effect).

Hypothyroidism, in the long run, causes a lowering in heart rate (bradycardia) and often leads to an elevated blood pressure. It is the hemodynamic changes combined with the altered metabolic functions, for example, hypercholesterolemia, that eventually manifest in a failing heart, often in conjunction with coronary artery disease.

The T3-induced changes in hyper- and hypothyroidism in cardiac target genes are best studied in rodents and will be discussed in detail in Section II. Figure 1 illustrates schematically which target genes are described in this article and lists other genes known to be influenced by thyroid hormone but that are less well studied thus far.

II. T3 TARGET GENES IN THE HEART

A. The SERCa2 Gene

Thyroid hormone regulates the expression of sarcoplasmic–endoplasmic calcium ATPase type 2a (SERCa2) in myocytes. When rodents are injected with thyroxine at a dose of 1 mg per kilogram of body weight to make them hyperthyroid, both the mRNA for the SERCa2 gene and the protein levels are elevated. Figure 2 shows a Northern blot with total ventricular RNA of mice with different thyroid status. Conversely, when rodents are made hypothyroid by treatment with 5-propyl-2-thiouracil and a low-iodine

diet, the mRNA for SERCa2a as well as the protein levels are reduced by 20–30% (see Fig. 2). Interestingly, it has been noted that in heart failure patients and in rodents with failing hearts, the SERCa2 gene is down-regulated. Aortic constriction (banding) in mice and rats that leads to cardiac hypertrophy also reduces the transcription of the SERCa2 gene. Very recent findings indicated that in both the failing heart and the hypertrophied heart, the levels of thyroid hormone receptors, especially the T3Rα1 receptor, are reduced, which in turn could be the reason for the diminished transcription of the SERCa2 gene.

B. The Myosin Heavy Chain Genes

The gene for myosin heavy chain α (MHCα) encodes a large protein that is part of the thick filament in myocytes, facilitating contraction and relaxation. Transcription of the α isoform is regulated by thyroid hormone, as shown in Fig. 2, especially in mice, where hyperthyroidism leads to an elevation of

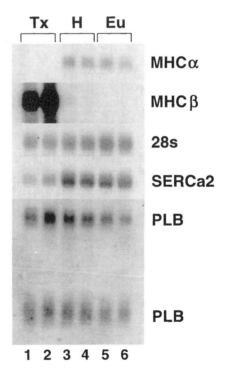

FIGURE 2 Northern blot with mouse heart total RNA. The mRNA levels in ventricles of hypothyroid (Tx, lanes 1 and 2), hyperthyroid (H, lanes 3 and 4), and euthyroid (Eu, lanes 5 and 6) animals were determined by probing the blot with radiolabeled oligonucleotides for myosin heavy chain α (MHCα), myosin heavy chain β (MHCβ), and 28S rRNA or with cDNA probes random-labeled for sarcoplasmic–endoplasmic reticulum calcium ATPase (SERCa2) and phospholamban (PLB).

transcripts and protein in cardiac myocytes. Particularly in the mouse heart, the up-regulation of MHCα expression is linked to the development of the neonatal myocyte into an adult myocyte and the onset of MHCα isoform expression coincides with an increase in circulating T3 and tetraiodothyronine levels during this developmental process.

The gene for the MHCβ isoform encodes a high-molecular-weight protein similar to MHCα and also localizes to the thick myosin filament. Transcription of the MHCβ gene is also regulated by thyroid hormone, and in mouse myocytes this T3 regulation is reversed compared with MHCα, which is nicely demonstrated in Fig. 2. In the adult mouse heart, there is very little MHCβ transcription when the animals are euthyroid; however, in hypothyroidism, the transcription of MHCβ is strongly induced, which points to a T3-dependent negative regulation of the promoter of this gene. This ligand-dependent repression of the MHCβ gene can be reestablished when the euthyroid status is restored.

It should be noted here that the expression of the myosins in general is very species specific although in mammals all members of the MHC gene family are regulated by T3. Surprisingly, however, whether T3 induces or represses the expression of a given MHC gene depends not only on the gene itself, but also on the muscle in which it is expressed. Indeed, the same gene can be induced by T3 in one muscle and repressed in another.

C. The K$^+$ Channel Genes

Some genes for the cardiac delayed inward rectifier potassium channels have been cloned in recent years. These channels are pores in the plasma membrane that are not always homogenous structures but are composed of two or more different proteins encoded by different genes. This makes it difficult to study the regulation of one particular gene and make a conclusion regarding the effect on a particular current that flows across the membrane using the channel pore that contains the gene product studied.

Nevertheless, a strong correlation was found between the prolonged relaxation times in hypothyroid papillary muscles of the mouse heart and reduced expression of genes that code for delayed inward rectifier channels, namely, Kv1.4, Kv4.2, and Kv4.3. Patch-clamping cardiac myocytes from hypothyroid hearts have indeed shown a reduced net current flow across the plasma membrane, which could explain the prolonged repolarization time and relaxation period observed in hypothyroid mouse papillary muscles.

Conversely, in hyperthyroid animals, the Kv4.3 gene was moderately up-regulated and the Kv1.4 gene was strongly up-regulated. This could lead to a faster repolarization of the myocyte to accommodate the more rapid action-potential cycles needed for the faster heartbeat that is observed in hyperthyroidism.

The Kv1.5 gene was also investigated for its regulation by thyroid hormone. In hypothyroid rat hearts, this gene was markedly down-regulated in contrast to the hyperthyroid status when the gene was expressed at a higher level. Interestingly, these thyroid hormone-induced changes in gene expression were not found in the mouse heart, which points toward a possible species-specific action of the thyroid hormone signaling pathway on this gene, similar to the species-specific regulation of the myosin genes by thyroid hormone.

The Long QT syndrome is a dominant autosomal disease, in some cases linked to congenital deafness. It can be linked to mutations in various ion channel genes, among them the KvLQT1 gene. In hypothyroid animals, the QT interval of the electrocardiogram (ECG) is significantly prolonged and the question of whether the KvLQT1 gene was down-regulated in hypothyroidism was examined. This was not the case, however, it was found that an associated protein encoded by the minK gene was actually up-regulated in hypothyroidism and down-regulated in hyperthyroidism. The increased expression of minK could potentially interfere with the gating properties of the pore formed by KvLQT1 and thereby contribute to the prolongation of the QT interval in the ECG.

D. Pacemaker Channels

Rapid rhythmic changes in membrane potentials are most prevalent in the cells of the brain and the heart. Rhythmic pacing of neuronal networks has been implicated with the encoding and controlling of information flow in the CNS. The involvement of a membrane current that was called I_h in the brain and I_f in the heart has been fairly well characterized. Recently, the HCN gene family whose gene products constitute the I_h or I_f channel was discovered. This article focuses on the two family members that are expressed in the heart, namely, HCN2 and HCN4. Both genes are highly homologous and their encoded proteins form the entire or at least the majority of the pore-forming units that presumably carry the I_f current. The I_f current acts at the very end of the action potential in cardiac myocytes just before the membrane rapidly depolarizes and the cell contracts. It is believed that the activation of the

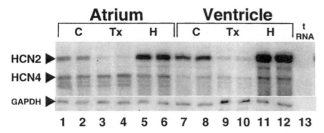

FIGURE 3 RNase protection, showing the mRNA levels for the pacemaker channels HCN2 and HCN4 in atria (lanes 1–6) and ventricles (lanes 7–12) of euthyroid (C), hypothyroid (Tx), and hyperthyroid (H) mice. In lane 13, a tRNA control was hybridized to all probes used and no specific protected signal was detected. A probe for the glyceraldehyde3-phosphate dehydrogenase (GAPDH) was used to confirm equal RNA input into each hybridization.

channel serves as a trigger for a new depolarization/repolarization cycle. These cycles are slower at a reduced heart rate and faster at an elevated heart rate. Because thyroid hormone modulates heart rate, the T3 responsiveness of the HCN2 and HCN4 genes has been investigated. Indeed, it could be demonstrated that mRNA levels for both genes are elevated in hyperthyroidism and diminished in hypothyroidism in mouse, rat, and rabbit hearts. Data from RNase protection experiments in mouse hearts are shown in Fig. 3. Because heart rate is controlled from the sinus node in the right atrium, the expression of HCN2 and HCN4 in atria and ventricles was studied and it was found that HCN2 is regulated by T3 in atria and ventricles; however, HCN4 responds to T3 only in ventricles and not in atria. The reason for this differential regulation of the pacemaker channels is currently unknown.

III. T3 EFFECTS ON MYOCYTE PHYSIOLOGY

When myocytes are isolated from adult or neonatal rat hearts and put in tissue culture, a spontaneous contraction can be observed. Addition of T3 to the culture medium increases this spontaneous beating, indicating an effect of T3 on the contractile physiology of these cells. Prolonged treatment of myocytes with T3 also increases the protein content of these cells, similar to what is seen in cardiac hypertrophy. Although not all of these T3 effects can be explained on the molecular level, the transcriptional stimulation of the SERCa2 gene by T3 and the concomitant decrease of phospholamban mRNA, as shown in Fig. 2, facilitate a more efficient shift of calcium from the cytoplasm into the sarcoplasm. The relocation of calcium to the cytoplasm to bring about a contraction

via the myosin/actin apparatus works through the ryanodine channel in the sarcoplasm; interestingly, the gene for this channel is also up-regulated by T3. In this way, T3 increases the calcium transients between the sarcoplasm and the cytoplasm, which provides for more rapid contraction/relaxation cycles. To coordinate the increased calcium cycling in the myocyte with an increased contractile capability, depolarizing and repolarizing must be accelerated as well. The depolarizing trigger could potentially be shifted toward a more positive voltage by modulating the I_f current that works just before the depolarization phase of the myocyte action potential. This is schematically indicated in Fig. 4, showing a ventricular myocyte action potential diagram. An increase of mRNA for HCN2 and HCN4 by T3 could potentially bring about the voltage shift in the I_f current. In the repolarization phase of the action potential, several delayed inward rectifier potassium channels control the flow of K^+ ions into the cytoplasm. Most of the genes that encode these potassium channels have been identified and it could be shown that Kv1.4, Kv1.5, Kv4.2, Kv4.3, and the minK gene are regulated by T3. This provides a basis for accelerated and decelerated depolarization and repolarization, indirectly evident in ECGs of hyper- and hypothyroid animals.

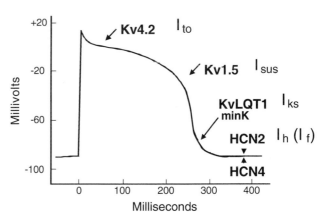

FIGURE 4 Ventricular action potential curve. During a single contraction of a ventricular myocyte, its membrane potential changes within 300 to 400 ms from a resting negative potential of 80–90 mV to a positive potential of approximately 20 mV. This is largely due to a rapid influx of sodium and calcium ions. The slow repolarization phase is characterized mainly by potassium efflux through channels that carry the I_{to}, I_{sus}, and I_{ks} currents. Pacemaker channels carry the I_h or I_f current with both sodium and potassium ions, triggering the rapid depolarization phase. I_{to}, transient outward potassium current; I_{sus}, sustained outward potassium current; I_{ks}, slow delayed rectifier potassium current.

Finally, the mechanical contraction apparatus within the cytoskeleton of the myocyte can be modified by T3. Especially in rodents, the myosin heavy chains (MHCα and MHCβ) that make up the thick filament of the contractile apparatus are thyroid hormone responsive. Transcription of MHCα is activated by T3, whereas transcription of MHCβ is repressed. In the mouse, this leads to an almost complete myosin isoform switch in hypo- and hyperthyroidism. Myosin V3 contains only MHCβ and myosin V1 is composed of two molecules of MHCα. In hypothyroidism, the V3 form, which hydrolyzes ATP slowly and therefore causes a slower contraction, dominates. In contrast, euthyroid and hyperthyroid mouse hearts contain the fast ATP-hydrolyzing V1 myosin that facilitates a rapid contraction.

Taken together, these findings indicate that thyroid hormone regulation of gene expression links the calcium pumps, ion channels, and myosins with one another for a coordinated faster performance or slower performance in the hyperthyroid heart and hypothyroid heart, respectively.

IV. TARGET GENE PROMOTERS

The most extensively studied promoters are those of the myosin heavy chain genes and the promoter of the rat SERCa2 gene. The MHCα promoter contains a complex arrangement of transcription factor-binding sites; these include the classical TATA-box and CAAT-box, a muscle enhancer factor 2 (MEF2)-binding site, a brain factor 2 (BF2) site, and a PNR (pannier gene encoded GATA transcription factor) element that binds two Ets factors as well as a thyroid hormone response element (TRE) with the consensus sequence 5'-AGGTGAcaggAGGACA-3'. Further upstream of the transcription start site at approximately −1.9 kb, a DNase I hypersensitive site that contained a conserved GATA-binding factor motif was found.

The rat and mouse MHCβ promoter is very strongly repressed by T3; a transferable negative regulatory element has not yet been found but several hexamer half-sites close to the transcription start site have been identified. It has also been hypothesized that the promoter could be T3 inhibited by a mechanism proposed for negative regulation by the glucocorticoid and retinoic acid receptors. In these models, the ligand-bound receptor molecules interact with positive-acting transcription factors (presumably off DNA), preventing them from transactivating their target gene. Among the factors proposed to bind to the MHCβ promoter within 300 bp upstream of the transcription start site are TFIID (TATA box binding

factor IID)-binding TATA-box, MyoD (muscle gene-transactivating helix-loop-helix factor), NFe (tissue specific nuclear factor), SP1 (Simian-virus 40 protein 1), M-CAT (muscle specific TEF), and AP5/GT-II (TEF-I binding element), as well as other binding sites that are shared between many muscle specific genes. Which of these factors could be inhibited by the ligand-bound T3 receptor is currently not known.

The rat SERCa2 promoter has been examined also. T3 responsiveness lies within 560 bp upstream of the transcription start site, and three TREs have been identified. All three TREs are needed for full activation or repression by non—ligand-bound T3R, but each TRE has a different half-site configuration. TRE1 is a direct repeat spaced by 4 nucleotides (DR + 4), TRE2 is an inverted palindrome spaced by 4 nucleotides (IP + 4), and TRE3 is configured as an IP + 6. Interestingly, a novel thyromimetic (GC-1) stimulates TRE1 but represses TRE2 and TRE3 when each TRE is isolated by pairwise mutation of the other two in the natural promoter context. The TREs of the rat SERCa2 promoter can potentially interact with the other transcription factors that bind to the promoter. One such interaction has been demonstrated with the MEF2a factor potentiating the T3 stimulation in a T3Rα isoform-specific manner. Other factors that could bind to the region within 560 bp upstream of the transcription start site are the TFIID-binding TATA-box, C/EBP (CCAAT/enhancer binding protein), SP1, and an E-box-binding helix-loop-helix protein.

Very recently, the promoters of the T3-regulated delayed inward rectifier potassium channel Kv4.2 and the pacemaker channels HCN2 and HCN4 were cloned. The Kv4.2 region linked to a CAT reporter gene responded significantly to T3 stimulation in neonatal rat myocyte transfections. The promoter regions of HCN2 and HCN4 have not been characterized fully and the HCN2 region failed to respond to T3 when linked to a reporter gene, which raises the possibility that other mechanisms besides transcriptional regulation may operate on this gene to elevate and diminish mRNA levels in hyper- and hypothyroidism, respectively.

V. T3 RECEPTOR EXPRESSION IN THE HEART

The above-described changes in nuclear gene regulation are likely to be mediated by the nuclear hormone receptors that bind T3. The ligand-binding isoforms that are found in the heart are the T3Rα1 and T3Rβ1 isoforms. Expression of T3Rα1 dominates in the heart with the mRNA levels of T3Rβ1 approximately 30% of those for T3Rα1. This is shown in an RNase protection experiment with total RNA from mouse hearts in Fig. 5. In the liver, for example, this ratio in inverted with the T3Rα1 mRNA levels approximately 10% of the T3Rβ1 mRNA levels. Which factors promote enhanced expression of the T3Rα gene in the heart and a lower ratio of expression of the T3Rβ gene is currently unknown.

Much has been learned from the knockout of the α or β isoforms of the thyroid hormone receptors in the mouse. Lack of T3Rα expression in the heart led to bradycardia and a "hypothyroid-like" gene expression profile. In contrast, lack of T3Rβ expression in the heart had virtually no phenotype when the animals were brought to a euthyroid status, except for the notion that T3Rα expression was reduced by nearly 40% in T3Rβ knockout animals (see Fig. 5). Interestingly, homozygous mutation of the ligand-binding domain of T3Rβ in the mouse to generate a dominant negative receptor significantly disturbed T3Rα action. This shows that T3Rβ is obviously expressed in the same cardiac cells as T3Rα. The question arises as to why T3Rβ cannot compensate for the lack of T3Rα expression. Do certain promoters of cardiac genes respond preferentially to T3Rα, and if so, what are the discriminating elements in such promoters? Further

studies are necessary to understand the contribution of each receptor isoform in the heart, for example, analyzing the cardiac phenotype and gene expression in receptor double-knockout mice. Rescue experiments of knockout mice with specific T3R isoforms in a cardiac gene therapy experiment will also reveal what each isoform can contribute to cardiac function. Finally, the temporal and spatial disruption of either T3R isoform in the heart will enable a refined analysis of the cardiac phenotype in inherently euthyroid animals.

VI. SUMMARY

Thyroid status in humans and in animals influences cardiac output. This article has attempted to describe the known molecular targets in the heart that T3 reaches to alter cardiac performance. The genes that are regulated by T3 contribute to the lusitropic effect, for example, the potassium channels Kv1.4, Kv1.5, Kv4.2, Kv4.3, and minK. Genes that contribute to the inotropic effect are, on the one hand, calcium pumps and channels like SERCa2a, phospholamban, ryanodine channel and the sodium–calcium exchanger and, on the other hand, the myosin heavy chains. The chronotropic effect of T3 probably has several components including the pacemaker channels that are up-regulated in hyperthyroid tachycardia and down-regulated in hypothyroid bradycardia. But there are also reports that the β-adrenergic receptor, adenylyl cyclase, and the T3Rα gene itself are regulated by T3, which may contribute to the chronotropic effect. Some of the target gene promoters have been characterized very well and contain distinct thyroid hormone-response elements, as well as muscle-specific elements. Other promoters still lack TREs and there may be other mechanisms by which T3 regulates the expression of those genes. Two isoforms of the thyroid hormone-binding nuclear receptors are expressed in the heart, T3Rα1 and T3Rβ1. Both seem to be present in the same myocytes but subserve distinct functions that are currently under intense investigation.

Glossary

K⁺ channels Multisubunit structures located in the plasma membrane that gate the flux of potassium into the cell. These include the so-called delayed inward rectifier channels that open to repolarize the cell after a contraction. Some of the genes for individual subunits are regulated by thyroid hormone.

myosins Proteins that are part of the contractile fibers found in myocytes. The genes for myosin heavy chain α

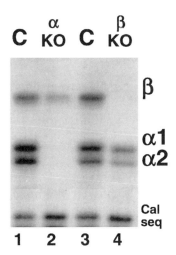

FIGURE 5 RNase protection, showing the mRNA levels for thyroid hormone receptors β (β1 and β2), α1 (α1), and α2 (α2) in mouse ventricles. Controls (C, lanes 1 and 3) were hybridized with RNA from isogenic wild-type animals of the respective mouse strain that was lacking either thyroid hormone receptor α (lane 2) or thyroid hormone receptor β (lane 4), designated αKO and βKO, respectively. To control for equal RNA input in each lane, a probe for calsequestrin (Calseq) was used.

(MHCα) and myosin heavy chain β (MHCβ) are regulated by thyroid hormone in some species. In rodents, MHCα is predominant in the adult heart and MHCβ can be strongly induced by hypothyroidism.

pacemaker channels The genes for these channels were only recently cloned and this article focuses on those that are expressed in the heart and regulated by thyroid hormone, namely, the HCN2 and HCN4 genes. A characteristic of the I_f conductance constituted by the gene products of HCN2 and HCN4 is that both sodium and potassium ions are conducted through the pore. Furthermore, gating is regulated by cyclic AMP and hyperpolarization of the cell membrane.

phospholamban A small 6 kDa protein that associates with SERCa2a and regulates the calcium pump activity dependent on the phospholamban phosphorylation status.

SERCa2a Sarcoplasmic-endoplasmic calcium ATPase type 2a is found primarily in the myocytes of the heart. The approximately 100 kDa protein is embedded in the sarcoplasmic membrane and transports calcium from the cytoplasm into the sarcoplasm while hydrolyzing ATP to ADP. The expression of the gene coding for SERCa2a is regulated by thyroid hormone.

See Also the Following Articles

Environmental Disruptors of Thyroid Hormone Action • Thyroid Hormone Action on the Skeleton and Growth • Thyroid Stimulating Hormone (TSH)

Further Reading

DiFrancesco, D. (1993). Pacemaker mechanisms in cardiac tissue. *Annu. Rev. Physiol.* 55, 455–472.

Dillmann, W. H. (1996). Thyroid hormone and the heart: Basic mechanistic and clinical issues. *Thyroid Today* 19, 1–11.

Gloss, B., Trost, S. U., Bluhm, W. F., Swanson, E. A., Clark, R., Winkfein, R., Janzen, K. M., Giles, W., Chassande, O., Samarut, J., and Dillmann, W. H. (2001). Cardiac ion channel expression and contractile function in mice with deletion of thyroid hormone receptor α or β. *Endocrinology* 142, 544–550.

Klein, I. (2001). Thyroid hormone—Targeting the heart. *Endocrinology* 142, 11–12. (Editorial).

Klein, I., and Ojamaa, K. (2001). Thyroid hormone and the cardiovascular system. *N. Engl. J. Med.* 344, 501–509.

Morkin, E. (2000). Control of cardiac myosin heavy chain gene expression. *Microsc. Res. Tech.* 50, 522–531.

Nadal-Ginard, B., and Mahdavi, V. (1993). Molecular mechanisms of cardiac gene expression. *Basic Res. Cardiol.* 88(Suppl. 1), 65–79.

Parry, C. H. (1825). Collections from the unpublished papers of the late Caleb Hillier Parry. *London* 2, 111.

Roden, D. M., and George, A. L., Jr. (1996). The cardiac ion channels: Relevance to management of arrhythmias. *Annu. Rev. Med.* 47, 135–148.

Rohrer, D. K., Hartong, R., and Dillmann, W. H. (1991). Influence of thyroid hormone and retinoic acid on slow sarcoplasmic

reticulum Ca^{2+} ATPase and myosin heavy chain alpha gene expression in cardiac myocytes: Delineation of cis-active DNA elements that confer responsiveness to thyroid hormone but not to retinoic acid. *J. Biol. Chem.* 266, 8638–8646.

Santoro, B., and Tibbs, G. R. (1999). The HCN gene family: Molecular basis of the hyperpolarization-activated pacemaker channels. *Ann. N. Y. Acad. Sci.* 868, 741–764.

Sussman, M. A. (2001). When the thyroid speaks, the heart listens. *Circ. Res.* 89, 557–559.

Zhang, J., and Lazar, M. (2000). The mechanism of action of thyroid hormones. *Annu. Rev. Physiol.* 62, 439–466.

Thyroid Hormone Action on the Skeleton and Growth

GRAHAM R. WILLIAMS

Imperial College London, Hammersmith Campus, London

I. CLINICAL AND EPIDEMIOLOGICAL OBSERVATIONS
II. THYROID HORMONE RECEPTORS
III. THE EPIPHYSEAL GROWTH PLATE
IV. THYROID HORMONE EFFECTS ON CHONDROCYTES AND GROWTH
V. GROWTH ABNORMALITIES IN TR NULL MICE
VI. THYROID HORMONE EFFECTS ON OSTEOBLASTS, OSTEOCLASTS, AND BONE TURNOVER

The skeleton is a specialized and complex organ that remodels its structure in response to systemic, local, and physical signals. It is highly vascularized, contains the hematopoietic bone marrow, and provides structural support and a reserve of calcium and phosphate ions for the maintenance of mineral homeostasis. Bone is formed either by direct transformation and ossification of condensed mesenchyme (intramembranous ossification) or by replacement of a cartilage scaffold with calcified bone (endochondral ossification). Development and growth of the skull and closure of its sutures result from intramembranous ossification. Linear growth, fracture repair, and bone remodeling, together with development of the remaining skeleton, result from endochondral ossification. A considerable number of clinical, epidemiological, and basic scientific studies indicate that thyroid hormones play a key role in skeletal development. They are essential for normal linear growth and are important regulators of bone turnover and the maintenance of bone mass.

I. CLINICAL AND EPIDEMIOLOGICAL OBSERVATIONS

Hypothyroidism in childhood causes growth arrest together with delayed bone age, epiphyseal dysgenesis, and immature body proportion. Furthermore, up to 50% of patients with the phenotypically variable syndrome of resistance to thyroid hormone (RTH), caused by mutant thyroid hormone receptor (TR) β proteins, suffer from growth retardation and developmental abnormalities of bone that may reflect tissue hypothyroidism. Thyroxine (T4) replacement therapy in hypothyroid children induces rapid catch-up growth that may be incomplete because bone age advances faster than height, leading to early epiphyseal growth plate fusion and speculation that skeletal responses to thyroid hormones are exaggerated in hypothyroidism. Accordingly, childhood thyrotoxicosis causes accelerated growth and advanced bone age, which may lead to premature growth plate closure and short stature. Advanced intramembranous ossification may also result in craniosynostosis in thyrotoxic children due to premature closure of the skull sutures. Indeed, stimulation of mineral apposition and osteogenesis, resulting in premature narrowing of the skull sutures, has been documented in a hyperthyroid rat model.

Thyrotoxicosis in adults results in increased bone turnover and net bone loss and causes osteopenia and fracture in patients with established disease. Thus, a series of studies has shown that thyrotoxicosis is associated with reduced bone density and an increased risk of osteoporotic hip fracture. Postmenopausal women are particularly at risk when confounding factors including age and sex are accounted for. Such findings have led to the contentious issue regarding whether treatment of hypothyroid or thyroid cancer patients with supraphysiological doses of T4 is also associated with osteoporosis and increased fracture risk. The current consensus suggests that overzealous treatment with T4, leading to suppression of circulating thyrotropin (TSH) concentrations, is probably associated with increased fracture risk, particularly in postmenopausal women and in those with a previous history of thyrotoxicosis.

II. THYROID HORMONE RECEPTORS

The complex actions of thyroid hormone (3,5,3'-L-triiodothyronine, T3) are mediated by TR proteins, which function as hormone-inducible transcription factors that regulate the expression of target genes and are members of the superfamily of hormone and orphan nuclear receptors. The TRα and TRβ genes are conserved in vertebrates. TRα encodes the widely expressed α1 and α2 C-terminal variants: TRα1 is a functional receptor that binds T3 and DNA, whereas TRα2 fails to bind T3 and is a weak antagonist *in vitro*, although its physiological role is unknown. A novel promoter in intron 7 of TRα generates the truncated Δα1 and Δα2 variants that act as repressors *in vitro* and have been implicated in intestinal development. TRβ encodes the functional β1, β2 isoforms and a new β3 N-terminal variant was recently identified in rat. TRβ2 expression is restricted to pituitary and hypothalamus, where it primarily regulates the activity of the hypothalamo–pituitary–thyroid feedback loop, but β1 and β3 are expressed widely. A truncated rat TRΔβ3 isoform is also expressed widely and acts as a potent antagonist in vitro, but its physiological significance is not yet known.

TRs are located at sites of intramembranous and endochondral bone formation in a variety of species; TRα1, TRα2, and TRβ1 mRNAs and proteins are expressed in osteoblasts and osteocytes and in reserve and proliferative zone epiphyseal growth plate chondrocytes. Functional TRs have also been identified in primary cultured osteoblasts and growth plate chondrocytes and in immortalized osteoblastic and chondrogenic cells from several species. Recent reports suggest that skeletal osteoblastic responses to T3 may vary according to anatomical site, although the mechanisms responsible for these findings are unknown. Thyroid hormones also stimulate osteoclastic bone resorption, but this effect is likely to be mediated by T3-responsive osteoblasts, as osteoclasts do not express functional TRs.

III. THE EPIPHYSEAL GROWTH PLATE

The epiphyses and metaphyses of long bones originate from independent ossification centers and are separated by a growth plate, which becomes ossified after puberty when epiphyseal fusion occurs (Fig. 1). In the normal growth plate, reserve zone progenitor cells lie immediately below the epiphysis and mature chondrocytes are located above the primary spongiosum, which communicates with the bone marrow. Immature reserve zone cells undergo clonal expansion to form organized columns in the proliferative zone, where they secrete a cartilage matrix containing type II collagen and proteoglycans. The largest proliferative cells differentiate to form hypertrophic chondrocytes, which secrete type X collagen, enlarge by five times their volume, and eventually undergo apoptosis to leave a cartilage scaffold. New blood

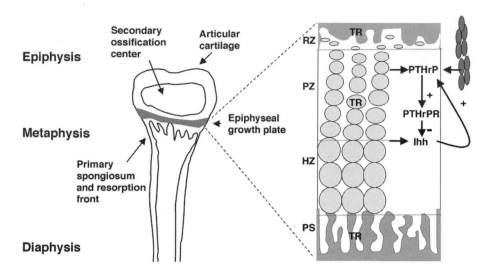

FIGURE 1 Long bone showing the location of the epiphyseal growth plate and an enlarged view to show the organization of chondrocytes, the localized expression of thyroid hormone receptors, and the feedback loop that controls the pace of chondrocyte proliferation. RZ, reserve zone; PZ, proliferative zone; HZ, hypertrophic zone; PS, primary spongiosum; TR, thyroid receptor; Ihh, Indian hedgehog; PTHrP, parathyroid hormone-related peptide; PTHrPR, PTHrP receptor.

vessels enter from the primary spongiosum and osteoblasts invade the growth plate to lay down trabecular bone on this cartilage template and complete the endochondral ossification process. Recent experiments have established that the pace of chondrocyte differentiation and bone formation is regulated by a negative feedback loop involving the paracrine factors Indian hedgehog (Ihh) and parathyroid hormone-related peptide (PTHrP). Ihh is secreted by pre-hypertrophic chondrocytes and stimulates PTHrP production from the peri-articular region of the epiphysis during bone development. PTHrP acts on PTHrP-receptor-expressing pre-hypertrophic chondrocytes to maintain cell proliferation, reduce Ihh production, and complete a feedback loop in which PTHrP exerts a negative signal that inhibits hypertrophic chondrocyte differentiation and delays bone formation (Fig. 1).

IV. THYROID HORMONE EFFECTS ON CHONDROCYTES AND GROWTH

Hypothyroidism results in gross abnormalities of growth plate structure with disorganized proliferating chondrocyte columns, abnormal cartilage matrix, reduced hypertrophic chondrocyte differentiation, and impaired vascular invasion of the growth plate at the primary spongiosum (Fig. 2). Alterations in PTHrP and PTHrP receptor mRNA expression in growth plate chondrocytes were identified in hypothyroid and thyrotoxic animals, suggesting that the setpoint of the critical Ihh/PTHrP feedback loop is sensitive to thyroid status. Whereas the majority of these effects probably result from direct actions of T3 in TR-expressing chondrocytes, other studies also indicate that the hypothyroid growth plate is relatively insensitive to the actions of growth hormone (GH) because of reduced local expression of insulin-like growth factor-I (IGF-I). Similar findings of delayed hypertrophic chondrocyte differentiation and impaired neovascularization of newly formed cartilage in fracture callus in hypothyroid rats reinforce the view that endochondral ossification during skeletal growth and repair requires thyroid hormones.

Until recently, the locations of T3 target cells within the growth plate were unknown. It has been shown that TRα1, TRα2, and TRβ1 proteins are expressed in reserve and proliferating zone chondrocytes but not in hypertrophic cells, suggesting that progenitor cells and proliferating chondrocytes are primary T3-target cells but that differentiated chondrocytes may lose the ability to express TRs and become unresponsive. A large body of data, in a variety of *in vitro* model systems using chondrocytes derived from several species, indicates that T3 regulates chondrocyte proliferation and the organization of proliferating chondrocyte columns, is required for terminal hypertrophic differentiation,

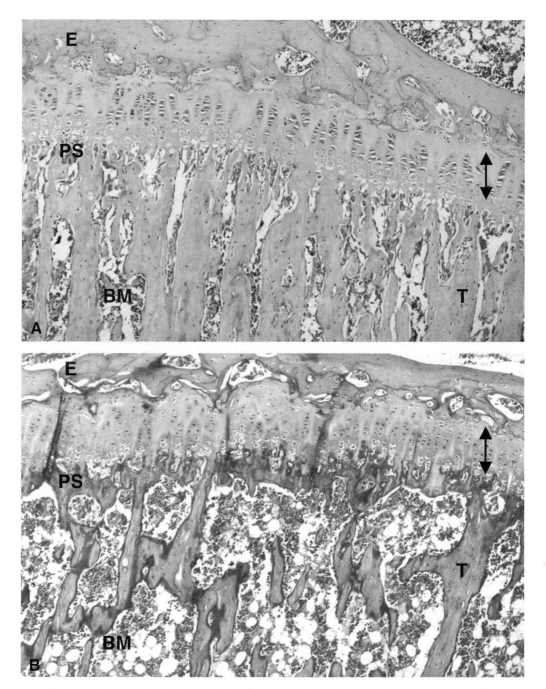

FIGURE 2 Sections of proximal tibial growth plate from 12-week-old euthyroid (A) and hypothyroid (B) rats stained with hematoxylin and eosin. The euthyroid growth plate contains organized columns of chondrocytes with neovascularization at the primary spongiosum. Longitudinal trabecular bone lies in continuity with proliferating and hypertrophic chondrocyte columns. The hypothyroid growth plate is disorganized and neovascularization is absent. Trabecular bone formation is diminished and disorganized relative to normal. E, epiphysis; PS, primary spongiosum; BM, bone marrow; T, trabecular bone; arrow delineates the growth plate.

and induces calcification of cartilage matrix. In other studies, rat tibial growth plate chondrocytes grown in primary suspension culture express TRs and maintain their differentiation potential. In this system, T3 directly inhibits clonal expansion and cell proliferation, while simultaneously promoting hypertrophic chondrocyte differentiation. Recent studies indicate that T3 might achieve this by induction of cyclin-dependent kinase inhibitors that may arrest cell cycle progression in proliferating chondrocytes and enable terminal hypertrophic differentiation to progress.

V. GROWTH ABNORMALITIES IN TR NULL MICE

The skeletal phenotypes of TR knockout mice reinforce the view that T3 acts directly in growth plate cartilage but reveal the complexity of thyroid hormone action in bone (Table 1). Deletion of the TRβ gene does not result in growth retardation or evidence of developmental abnormalities in bone and cartilage, indicating that TRβ is not essential for skeletal development. Nevertheless, the creation of distinct mouse models with different RTH mutations in TRβ has highlighted the phenotypic variability of the human RTH syndrome as only one mouse model, harboring the severe TRβ^{PV} mutation, suffers from impaired growth.

Several TRα knockouts have been produced, in which differing products of the TRα locus were deleted, with varying effects on the skeleton and on thyroid and GH/IGF-I status. TRα1$^{-/-}$ mice lack expression of TRα1 and Δα1, but TRα2, Δα2, and β are retained and skeletal development is normal. Combination of the TRα1$^{-/-}$ and β$^{-/-}$ mutations to produce a TRα1$^{-/-}$ β$^{-/-}$ double knockout results in growth retardation and delayed bone maturation. TRα1$^{-/-}$ β$^{-/-}$ mice are growth hormone and IGF-I deficient; GH replacement reverses some of the growth retardation but does not influence the defective

ossification, indicating that T3 exerts important direct effects on growth plate chondrocytes but mediates some of its effects on growth via GH and IGF-I.

In contrast, in TRα$^{-/-}$ mice there is growth arrest after weaning and disorganization of growth plate chondrocytes with delayed cartilage mineralization and bone formation. The TRα$^{-/-}$ mutation results in deletion of TRα1 and α2 but preservation of Δα1, Δα2, and TRβ. These animals become progressively hypothyroid in the postnatal period due to impaired thyroid hormone production and the skeletal phenotype can be rescued by T4 replacement, suggesting that TRβ can compensate for TRα in the growth plate in appropriate circumstances. Nevertheless, the delayed bone maturation seen in TRα$^{-/-}$ mice is not further modified in mice harboring a TRα$^{-/-}$ β$^{-/-}$ double gene deletion, suggesting that TRβ, in contrast to TRα, is dispensable in bone.

These studies have been interpreted to suggest that the non-T3-binding variants TRα2, Δα1, and Δα2 may play important roles in bone development. Thus, mice devoid of all TRα isoforms were generated. These TRα$^{0/0}$ mice display growth delay and retarded endochondral ossification with evidence of impaired hypertrophic chondrocyte differentiation and disorganized growth plate architecture. TRα$^{0/0}$ mice express TRβ and maintain normal TSH concentrations with slightly reduced T4 levels, indicating mildly increased thyroid hormone sensitivity and further suggesting that TRα is functionally predominant in bone. TRα$^{0/0}$β$^{-/-}$ double-mutant

---

TABLE 1   Genotypes and Growth Characteristics of Thyroid Hormone Receptor (TR) Null Mice

TR Knockout	Deleted TR mRNAs	Expressed TR mRNAs	Thyroid status	GH Status	Growth Retardation
α1$^{-/-}$	α1, Δα1	α2, Δα2, all β isoforms	Mildly hypothyroid	Normal	−
α$^{-/-}$	α1, α2	Δα1, Δα2, all β isoforms	Grossly hypothyroid	Normal	++
α$^{0/0}$	All α isoforms	All β isoforms	Euthyroid^a	Normal	+
β$^{-/-}$	All β isoforms	All α isoforms	RTH	Mildly deficient	−
β2$^{-/-}$	β2	All α isoforms, β1, β3, Δβ3	RTH	Mildly deficient	−
α1$^{-/-}$ β$^{-/-}$	α1, Δα1, all β isoforms	α2, Δα2	Severe RTH	GH/IGF-I^b deficient	++
α$^{-/-}$ β$^{-/-}$	α1, α2, all β isoforms	Δα1, Δα2	Severe RTH	Not determined	++
α$^{0/0}$β$^{-/-}$	All α isoforms, all β isoforms	None	Severe RTH	GH deficient	++

Note. GH, growth hormone; RTH, resistance to thyroid hormone; IGF-I, insulin-like growth factor-I, GH status was determined by comparison of pituitary GH mRNA expression in wild-type and mutant animals.

^{a}Dynamic testing demonstrated mild increased pituitary sensitivity to thyroid hormones.

^{b}GH and IFG-I serum concentrations and GH mRNA.

mice are viable and more severely growth retarded than their TRα$^{0/0}$ counterparts but less so than Pax8$^{-/-}$ mice in which congenital hypothyroidism results from thyroid follicular cell agenesis. Taken together, these findings indicate that differing consequences result from thyroid hormone deficiency, in which unoccupied receptors are present, compared to TR deficiency, and suggest a physiological role for unliganded TR or non-T3-binding TR variants in bone development. They also indicate that the TRα gene is essential for skeletal development and the timing of bone mineralization.

VI. THYROID HORMONE EFFECTS ON OSTEOBLASTS, OSTEOCLASTS, AND BONE TURNOVER

Thyroid hormones activate bone-forming osteoblasts and bone-resorbing osteoclasts, but in hyperthyroidism the normally tightly coupled activities of these two cell types are dissociated, resulting in bone loss. The bone remodeling cycle begins with activation of osteoclast lineage cells, which begin to resorb bone. Osteoblasts invade the area once a certain resorption depth is reached and lay down new matrix, which is mineralized to form new bone in areas of previous resorption. The activation–resorption–formation cycle normally lasts up to 200 days and occurs at discrete sites called bone-remodeling units. Bone remodeling occurs at differing rates in trabecular and cortical bone and in differing anatomical locations. The rate at which each site undergoes remodeling is known as the activation frequency and this is a major determinant of total bone turnover. Bone resorption, matrix deposition, and mineralization times are shortened in hyperthyroidism and the activation frequency is increased. These disproportionate changes uncouple osteoblasts and osteoclasts and lead to a net bone loss of approximately 10% per remodeling cycle in hyperthyroidism.

It is clear that osteoblasts express functional TRs, which have been identified at the mRNA and protein levels, by nuclear T3-binding activity and in transient transfection studies using T3-inducible reporter genes. Although osteoblasts in primary culture and several osteoblastic cell lines respond directly to T3 *in vitro*, the specific consequences of T3 stimulation vary considerably between studies. Such differences may occur between species and depend on the degree of cellular confluence, the stage of osteoblast differentiation, the cell type, passage number, and origin, and the dose and duration of T3 treatment. Furthermore, the response of osteoblastic cells to T3 has been reported to vary according to the anatomical site from which the cultured cells originate. Thus, T3 has been shown to stimulate, inhibit, or have no effect on osteoblastic cell proliferation. A general consensus, however, indicates that osteoblast activity is stimulated by T3. T3 increases production of osteocalcin and collagen type I matrix proteins, collagenase 3, gelatinase B, tissue inhibitor of metalloproteinase-1, alkaline phosphatase, IGF-I, IGF-binding proteins 2 and 4, fibroblast growth factor receptor 1, interleukin-6, and interleukin-8 in various osteoblastic cell culture systems. Furthermore, T3 may potentiate some of the osteoblast responses to PTH by modulating the expression of PTH/PTHrP receptor. Despite the many potential T3 target genes identified in osteoblasts, little information is available regarding mechanisms by which their expression is modulated and T3 regulation in many cases may be indirect and involve other signaling pathways. In contrast to effects on the activity of mature osteoblasts, osteoblast progenitor cell differentiation is inhibited by thyroid hormones, although the effects in vitro are complex and dose-related and involve interactions with other factors including IGF-I, steroid hormones, vitamin D, cytokines, and other growth factors.

Bone resorption is stimulated by T3 in bone organ cultures by mechanisms that are unclear but certainly complex and likely to involve other systemic hormones and locally acting cytokines. There is controversy regarding whether osteoclasts express TRs, although most studies indicate they do not and coculture experiments have revealed that osteoclastic bone resorption is stimulated by T3 only in the presence of osteoblastic cells. These findings suggest that the resorptive effects of T3 in bone are mediated via direct stimulation of TR-expressing osteoblasts, which may induce the recruitment and differentiation of osteoclast progenitor cells or increase the activity of mature osteoclasts.

Glossary

cortical bone Dense surface layer of mature compact bone.
endochondral ossification Bone formation by replacement of a preformed cartilage scaffold that occurs during skeletal development and fracture repair.
epiphyseal growth plate Specialized strip of cartilage located at the ends of long bones, in which programmed proliferation and maturation of chondrocytes result in the production of cartilage to form a template for new bone formation during linear growth.

intramembranous ossification Bone formation by direct transformation and ossification of condensed mesenchyme that occurs during development of flat bones, including the skull, mandible, scapula, and ileum.

osteoporosis A progressive systemic skeletal disease characterized by low bone mass and microarchitectural deterioration of bone tissue with a consequent increase in bone fragility and susceptibility to fracture.

primary spongiosum Region of trabecular bone forming the interface between the growth plate and bone marrow and the site for neovascularization and osteoblast invasion during endochondral ossification.

trabecular bone Interior network of organized calcified spongy bone, the space between which contains bone marrow and communicates with the marrow cavity.

See Also the Following Articles

Bone Morphogenetic Proteins • Environmental Disruptors of Thyroid Hormone Action • Osteogenic Proteins • Osteoporosis: Hormonal Treatment • Osteoporosis: Pathophysiology • Thyroid Hormone Action on the Heart and Cardiovascular System • Thyroid Hormone Receptor Isoforms • Thyroid Stimulating Hormone (TSH)

Further Reading

Ballock, R. T., Zhou, X., Mink, L. M., Chen, H. C., Mita, B. C., and Stewart, M. C. (2000). Expression of cyclin-dependent kinase inhibitors in epiphyseal chondrocytes induced to terminally differentiate with thyroid hormone. *Endocrinology* 141, 4552–4557.

Bauer, D. C., Ettinger, B., Nevitt, M. C., and Stone, K. L. (2001). Risk for fracture in women with low serum levels of thyroid-stimulating hormone. *Ann. Intern. Med.* 134, 561–568.

Bland, R. (2000). Steroid hormone receptor expression and action in bone. *Clin. Sci.* 98, 217–240.

Chung, U.-I., Schipani, E., McMahon, A. P., and Kronenberg, H. M. (2001). Indian hedgehog couples chondrogenesis to osteogenesis in endochondral bone development. *J. Clin. Invest.* 107, 295–304.

Gauthier, K., Plateroti, M., Harvey, C. B., Williams, G. R., Weiss, R. E., Refetoff, S., Willott, J. E., Sundin, V., Roux, J.-P., Malaval, L., Hara, M., Samarut, J., and Chassande, O. (2001). Genetic analysis reveals different functions for the products of the thyroid hormone receptor α locus. *Mol. Cell. Biol.* 21, 4748–4760.

Gothe, S., Wang, Z., Ng, L., Kindblom, J. M., Campos-Barros, A., Ohlsson, C., Vennstrom, B., and Forrest, D. (1999). Mice devoid of all known thyroid hormone receptors are viable but exhibit disorders of the pituitary–thyroid axis, growth, and bone maturation. *Genes Dev.* 13, 1329–1341.

Robson, H., Siebler, T., Stevens, D. A., Shalet, S. M., and Williams, G. R. (2000). Thyroid hormone acts directly on growth plate chondrocytes to promote hypertrophic differentiation and inhibit clonal expansion and cell proliferation. *Endocrinology* 141, 3887–3897.

Ross, D. S. (1998). Bone disease in hyperthyroidism. *In* "Metabolic Bone Disease and Clinically Related Disorders" (L. V. Avioli and S. M. Krane, eds.), 3rd ed., pp. 531–544. Academic Press, San Diego, CA.

Stern, P. H. (1996). Thyroid hormone and bone. *In* "Principles of Bone Biology, Part I, Basic Principles" (J. P. Bilezikian, L. G. Raisz and G. A. Rodan, eds.), pp. 521–531. Academic Press, San Diego, CA.

Stevens, D. A., Hasserjian, R. P., Robson, H., Siebler, T., Shalet, S. M., and Williams, G. R. (2000). Thyroid hormones regulate hypertrophic chondrocyte differentiation and expression of parathyroid hormone-related peptide and its receptor during endochondral bone formation. *J. Bone Miner. Res.* 15, 2431–2442.

Uzzan, B., Campos, J., Cucherat, M., Nony, P., Boissel, J. P., and Perret, G. Y. (1996). Effects on bone mass of long term treatment with thyroid hormones: A meta-analysis. *J. Clin. Endocrinol. Metab.* 81, 4278–4289.

Vortkamp, A., Lee, K., Lanske, B., Segre, G. V., Kronenberg, H. M., and Tabin, C. J. (1996). Regulation of rate of cartilage differentiation by Indian hedgehog and PTH-related protein. *Science* 273, 613–622.

Weiss, R. E., and Refetoff, S. (1996). Effect of thyroid hormone on growth: Lessons from the syndrome of resistance to thyroid hormone. *Endocrinol. Metab. Clin.* 25, 719–730.

Williams, G. R. (2000). Cloning and characterization of two novel thyroid hormone receptor β isoforms. *Mol. Cell. Biol.* 20, 8329–8342.

Williams, G. R., Robson, H., and Shalet, S. M. (1998). Thyroid hormone actions on cartilage and bone: Interactions with other hormones at the epiphyseal plate and effects on linear growth. *J. Endocrinol.* 157, 391–403.

Thyroid Hormone Receptor Isoforms

PAUL M. YEN

National Institute of Diabetes and Digestive and Kidney Diseases, National Institutes of Health, Maryland

I. TR ISOFORMS AND RELATED GENE PRODUCTS
II. TISSUE EXPRESSION OF TR ISOFORMS
III. HORMONAL REGULATION OF TR ISOFORMS
IV. ISOFORM-SPECIFIC REGULATION OF TARGET GENES
V. TR KNOCKOUT MODELS OF TR ISOFORMS
VI. CONCLUSION

Multiple isoforms of thyroid hormone receptors are expressed in a variety of tissues. Serving as transcription factors, these receptors play isoform-specific roles in regulation of hormonal activity and target gene expression. Genetic studies of the isoforms as well as their tissue expression, hormone regulation, and isoform-specific functions with respect to phenotype and transcription of target genes provide insights into mechanisms of disorders related to thyroid hormones.

I. TR ISOFORMS AND RELATED GENE PRODUCTS

Thyroid hormone receptors (TRs) are ligand-dependent transcription factors that belong to the nuclear hormone receptor superfamily. TRs and other nuclear hormone receptor family members share a similar domain organization in that they contain a central DNA-binding domain with two zinc fingers, a carboxy-terminal ligand-binding domain, and multiple transactivation domains (Fig. 1). They also bind to thyroid hormone response elements (TREs) composed of two or more hexamer sequences arranged as direct repeats or inverted repeats (separated by four and six nucleotides, respectively), typically located in the promoter region of target genes.

There are two major TR isoforms, TRα and TRβ, encoded on separate genes located on human chromosomes 17 and 3, respectively. The multiple TR isoforms have been found in tissues of amphibia, chicks, mice, rats, and humans. In mammalian species, TRα and TRβ vary from 400 to slightly over 500 amino acids in size and contain highly homologous DNA-binding and ligand-binding domains (Fig. 2). Both TR isoforms bind triiodothyronine (T3) with high affinity and mediate thyroid hormone-regulated gene expression. In positively regulated target genes, liganded TR recruits co-activators such as the steroid-related co-activator (SRC) family members and other cofactors that lead to increased histone acetylation of chromatin in the promoter of target genes (Fig. 3). This may then be followed by recruitment of another complex that contains components of the RNA polymerase II complex, which, in turn, leads to recruitment and stabilization of RNA polymerase II and enhanced transcription. In contrast, unliganded TRs bind to TREs and recruit corepressors, including the silencing mediator of retinoic acid and thyroid hormone (SMRT) receptors and the nuclear receptor corepressor (N-CoR), with histones deacetylases, which cause decreased acetylation of local chromatin and repression of transcription.

In addition to the TRs encoded by the two TR genes, TR isoforms can be produced by alternative splicing. Alternative splicing of the initial RNA transcript of the TRα gene generates two mature mRNAs, each encoding two proteins, TRα-1 and c-erbAα-2. In the rat, these proteins are identical from amino acid residue 1 to residue 370, but their respective sequences diverge markedly afterward. As a consequence of the replacement of the carboxy terminus with a 122-amino-acid sequence, c-erbAα-2 does not bind T3. Additionally, c-erbAα-2 binds TREs weakly but cannot transactivate thyroid hormone-responsive genes. It also may block TH action on certain target genes by binding to TREs and preventing TRs from regulating transcription.

The TRα gene also encodes another gene product, rev-erbA, on the opposite strand. The rev-erbA mRNA contains a 269-nucleotide stretch that is complementary to the c-erbAα-2 mRNA due to its transcription from the DNA strand opposite of that used to generate TRα-1 and c-erbAα-2. The protein product also belongs to the nuclear hormone receptor superfamily, is expressed in adipocytes and muscle cells, and can bind to TREs and retinoic acid response elements (RAREs) and repress gene transcription. However, rev-erbA should be considered an orphan receptor because its cognate ligand and function are not known. The rev-erbA receptor may be involved in regulating the splicing that generates c-erbAα-2 because increased levels of rev-erbA mRNA correlate with increased TRα-1 mRNA relative to c-erbAα-2. The rev-erbA receptor also may be involved in adipocyte differentiation.

The TRβ gene also generates two isoforms, TRβ-1 and TRβ-2. This gene contains two promoter regions that regulate the transcription of an mRNA encoding TRβ-1 or TRβ-2. One or both of the coding mRNAs are generated by selective promoter choice. The amino acid sequences of the DNA-binding, hinge region, and ligand-binding domains of these two TRβ isoforms are identical; however, the amino-terminal regions share no sequence homology. Both are bona

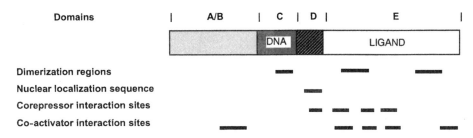

FIGURE 1   General organization of major thyroid hormone receptor domains and functional subregions.

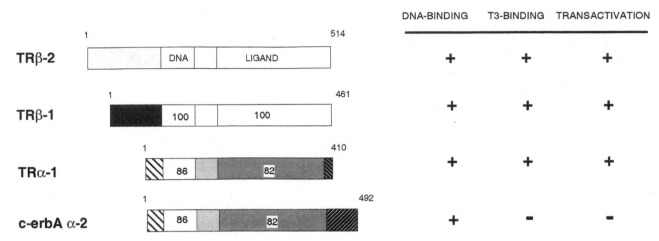

FIGURE 2 Comparison of amino acid homologies and their functional properties among thyroid hormone receptor isoforms; length of each receptor is indicated by numbers just above receptor diagrams; amino acid homology (%) with TRβ-2 is indicated by numbers in the receptor diagrams.

fide receptors in that they bind TREs and TH with high affinity and specificity and mediate TH-dependent transcription. Expression of the two TRβ isoforms may be regulated by pituitary-specific transcription factors such as Pit-1.

II. TISSUE EXPRESSION OF TR ISOFORMS

TRα-1 and TRβ-1 mRNAs and proteins are ubiquitously expressed in rat and human tissues. However, TRα-1 mRNA has highest expression in rat skeletal muscle and brown fat whereas TRβ-1 mRNA has highest expression in brain, liver, and kidney. TRβ-2 mRNA and protein have a restricted tissue expression in the anterior pituitary, hypothalamus, and developing brain and inner ear. In chicks and mice, TRβ-2 mRNA also is expressed in the developing retina. Last, a number of short forms of TRα and TRβ generated by alternative splicing of mRNA or by use of intrinsic promoters have been found in embryonic stem cells and in fetal bone cells, and may have biological significance. In particular, some of these short forms have dominant negative activity on TH-mediated transcription and may also affect intestine and bone development.

III. HORMONAL REGULATION OF TR ISOFORMS

TR mRNA regulation varies among the different isoforms. In the intact rat anterior pituitary, T3 decreases TRβ-2 mRNA, modestly decreases TRα-1 mRNA, and slightly increases rat TRβ-1 mRNA. Despite these countervailing effects, the total T3

binding decreases by 30% in the T3-treated rat pituitary. In other tissues, T3 slightly decreases TRα-1 and c-erbAα-2 mRNA, with the exception of the brain, where c-erbAα-2 levels are not changed. TRβ-1 mRNA is minimally affected in nonpituitary tissues. The hypothalamic tripeptide, thyrotropin-releasing hormone (TRH), also regulates TR mRNA expression because it decreases TRβ-2 mRNA, slightly decreases TRα-1 mRNA, and minimally affects TRβ-1 mRNA in cultured rat pituitary cells. Retinoic acid blunts the negative regulation by T3 in these cells. Additionally, in patients with nonthyroidal illness who have decreased circulating serum free T3 and tetraiodothyronine (T4) levels, TRα and TRβ mRNAs are increased in peripheral mononuclear cells and liver biopsy specimens. Thus, increased TR expression may potentially compensate for decreased circulating thyroid hormone levels in these patients.

IV. ISOFORM-SPECIFIC REGULATION OF TARGET GENES

The amino acids of each of the TR isoforms are highly homologous across mammalian species. This conservation suggests that there may be important specialized functions for each TR isoform. Recent studies have suggested that TRβ-1 may exhibit isoform-specific regulation of the TRH and myelin basic protein genes, and TRβ-2 may play important roles in the regulation of the growth hormone and thyroid-stimulating hormone β (TSHβ) gene expression in the pituitary. The differential expression of TR isoforms in various tissues (e.g., TRβ-1 is the

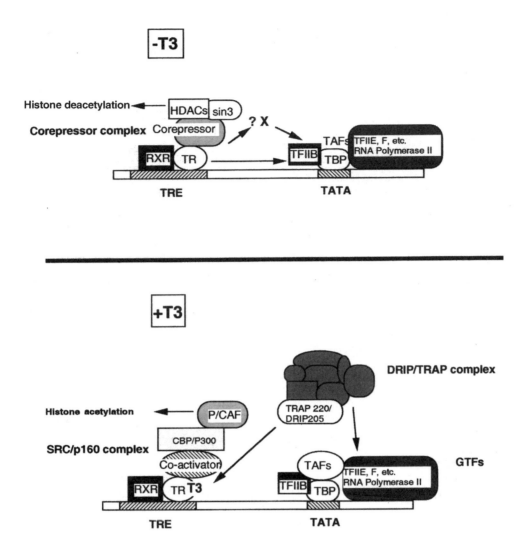

FIGURE 3 Molecular model for basal repression in the absence of triiodothyronine (T3) and transcriptional activation in the presence of T3. Possible additional cofactors (X) remain to be identified. HDAC, Histone deacetylase; RXR, retinoid acid X receptor; TR, thyroid hormone receptor; TAFs, TBP-associated factors; SRC, steroid receptor co-activator; CBP, cAMP response element binding protein; P/CAF, p300/CBP-associated factor; DRIP, vitamin D-interacting protein; TRAP, thyroid hormone receptor-associated protein; TBP, TATA-binding protein. See text for additional details.

predominant isoform expressed in liver whereas TRα-1 is the major isoform expressed in heart) has fostered attempts to develop TRβ-specific thyroid hormone analogues that may have cholesterol-lowering effects but minimal cardiac toxicity.

V. TR KNOCKOUT MODELS OF TR ISOFORMS

The selective ablation of TR isoforms in mice by homologous recombination has provided insight on the roles of TR isoforms in the development and function of various tissues. Two different groups have generated TRα knockout mice that have different phenotypes. The structure of the TRα gene is complex

because it encodes TRα-1, c-erbAα-2 (which cannot bind T3), and rev-erbA (generated from the opposite strand encoding TRα); thus, the locus of homologous recombination will determine which isoforms will be knocked out. Transgenic mice in which both TRα-1 and c-erbAα-2 have been deleted (TRα − /−) have a more severe phenotype, involving hypothyroidism, intestinal malformation, growth retardation, and early death shortly after weaning. The early death can be partially rescued by T3 injection of pups. Transgenic mice that lack only TRα-1 (TRα-1 − /−) have a milder phenotype compared to TRα − /− mice because they have decreased body temperature and heart rate and a prolonged electrocardiogram ventricular depolarization/repolarization (QT) interval. These findings suggest that TRα-1 plays an important role in regulating cardiac function. The differences in the two knockout phenotypes could be due to specific functions of c-erbAα-2; however, specific knockout of c-erbAα-2 does not affect the survival of pups. Short TRα isoforms can be generated from an internal promoter within the seventh intron, which then have dominant negative activity on wild-type TR function. It thus is likely that these short TR isoforms may be responsible for the more severe phenotype of the TRα − /− knockout mice. In this regard, a TRα knockout mouse that lacks both TRα-1 and c-erbA α-2, and does not express the short TRα isoforms (TRα$_{o/o}$), has a milder phenotype compared to TRα $_{-/-}$.

TRβ knockout mice (TRβ$_{-/-}$) display modest phenotypic changes, including elevated TSH and T4, thyroid hyperplasia, and hearing and retinal defects. These abnormalities in the hypothalamic–pituitary–thyroid (HPT) axis are similar to those seen in patients with the syndrome of resistance to thyroid hormone. Additionally, these findings suggest a critical role for TRβ in the development of the auditory and visual systems. Interestingly, ligand-independent elevation of TSH is normal in hypothyroid TRβ − /− mice, but the suppression of TSH by TH is impaired. Recently, TRβ-2 has been selectively knocked out. The mice had elevated levels of TH and TSH, implicating TRβ-2 as the major TR isoform regulating TSH production. Interestingly, the mice did not have any hearing defects, suggesting that TRβ-2 may not be required for auditory development or that its function can be compensated by TRβ-1.

Because the TRα-1 and TRβ knockout mice have relatively mild phenotypes, it is likely that the TR isoforms may have redundant transcriptional activity and can compensate for each other in most target genes. To examine the effects of abolishing all TR isoforms, TRα-1 − /− TRβ − /− double knockouts have been generated and, surprisingly, these mice are still viable. These mice have markedly elevated T4, T3, and TSH levels and large goiters. The mice also have growth retardation and decreased fertility, as well as impaired bone development and reduced bone mineral content. Furthermore, the mice have reduced heart rate and impaired control of body temperature, similar to the TRα-1 − /− mice. It is noteworthy that the effects on peripheral tissues generally are milder in the double-knockout mice compare to those seen in congenital hypothyroidism. It is possible that nongenomic effects of TH may be involved in double-knockout mice but not in mice with congenital hypothyroidism. It also is possible that lack of TRs is less deleterious than the presence of TRs during hypothyroidism. Because unliganded TRs bind to TREs and recruit corepressors to repress basal transcription of some positively regulated target genes, it is possible that critical target genes may be shut down in the hypothyroid mice whereas basal transcription is maintained in the double-knockout mice.

VI. CONCLUSION

Tissue-restricted expression and knockout mice studies suggest that the multiple TR isoforms may have specialized roles, although cotransfection studies suggest that most of the known target genes can be coregulated. Future studies with microarrays, proteomics, and isoform-specific ligands, perhaps in conjunction with knockout mice, should help identify isoform-specific roles in the transcription of specific genes.

Glossary

basal repression Target gene transcription repression by unliganded thyroid hormone receptor and its recruitment of corepressors.

dominant negative activity Blockade of thyroid hormone receptor transcriptional activity by a transcription factor or mutant receptor, typically by competitive binding to the thyroid hormone response element.

nuclear hormone receptor superfamily Nuclear receptor family that includes the steroid, vitamin D, retinoic acid, and thyroid hormone receptors.

thyroid hormone response elements Discrete enhancer sequences in the promoters of target genes to which thyroid hormones bind and regulate transcription.

thyroid hormones Triiodothyronine (T3) and thyroxine (T4); secreted by the thyroid gland and converted by peripheral deiodination.

transactivation Ligand-dependent transcription of target genes mediated by a thyroid hormone receptor and its recruitment of co-activators.

See Also the Following Articles

Co-activators and Corepressors for the Nuclear Receptor Superfamily • Estrogen Receptor Biology and Lessons from Knockout Mice • Thyroglobulin • Thyroid Hormone Receptor, TSH and TSH Receptor Mutations • Thyroid Stimulating Hormone (TSH)

Further Reading

Abel, E. D., Boers, M. E., Pazos-Moura, C., Moura, E., Kaulbach, H., Zakaria, M., Lowell, B., Radovick, S., Liberman, M. C., and Wondisford, F. (1999). Divergent roles for thyroid hormone receptor beta isoforms in the endocrine axis and auditory system. *J. Clin. Invest.* **104**, 291–300.

Chassande, O., Fraichard, A., Gauthier, K., Flamant, F., Legrand, C., Savatier, P., Laudet, V., and Samarut, J. (1997). Identification of transcripts initiated from an internal promoter in the c-erbA alpha locus that encode inhibitors of retinoic acid receptor-alpha and triiodothyronine receptor activities. *Mol. Endocrinol.* **11**, 1278–1290.

Davis, P. J., and Davis, F. B. (1996). Nongenomic actions of thyroid hormone. *Thyroid* **6**, 497–504.

Forrest, D., and Vennstrom, B. (2000). Functions of thyroid hormone receptors in mice. *Thyroid* **10**, 41–52.

Gothe, S., Wang, Z., Ng, L., Kindblom, J. M., Barros, A. C., Ohlsson, C., Vennstrom, B., and Forrest, D. (1999). Mice devoid of all known thyroid hormone receptors are viable but exhibit disorders of the pituitary–thyroid axis, growth, and bone maturation. *Genes Dev.* **13**, 1329–1341.

Hodin, R. A., Lazar, M. A., and Chin, W. W. (1990). Differential and tissue-specific regulation of the multiple rat c-erbA mRNA species by thyroid hormone. *J. Clin. Invest.* **85**, 101–105.

Lazar, M. A. (1993). Thyroid hormone receptors: Multiple forms, multiple possibilities. *Endocr. Rev.* **14**, 348–399.

Refetoff, S., Weiss, R. A., and Usala, S. J. (1993). The syndromes of resistance to thyroid hormone. *Endocr. Rev.* **14**, 348–399.

Trost, S. U., Swanson, E., Gloss, B., Wang-Iverson, D. B., Zhang, H., Volodarsky, T., Grover, G. J., Baxter, J. D., Chiellini, G., Scanlan, T. S., and Dillmann, W. H. (2000). The thyroid hormone receptor-beta-selective agonist GC-1 differentially affects plasma lipids and cardiac activity. *Endocrinology* **141**, 3057–3064.

Williams, G. R., Franklyn, J. A., Neuberger, J. M., and Sheppard, M. C. (1989). Thyroid hormone receptor expression in the "sick euthyroid" syndrome. *Lancet* **2**, 1477–1481.

Wood, W. M., Dowding, J. M., Bright, T. M., McDermott, M. T., Haugen, B. R., Gordon, D. F., and Ridgway, E. C. (1996). Thyroid hormone receptor beta2 promoter activity in pituitary cells is regulated by Pit-1. *J. Biol. Chem.* **271**, 24213–24220.

Yen, P. M. (2001). Physiological and molecular basis of thyroid hormone action. *Physiol. Rev.* **81**, 1097–1142.

Zhang, J., and Lazar, M. A. (2000). The mechanism of action of thyroid hormones. *Annu. Rev. Physiol.* **62**, 439–466.

Thyroid Hormone Receptor, TSH and TSH Receptor Mutations

Roy E. Weiss and Peter M. Sadow
University of Chicago

The thyroid hormone receptor interacts with the thyroid hormone triiodothyronine, which is secreted from the thyroid following interaction of thyroid-stimulating hormone and its receptor. Mutations in any of the genes regulating the production and function of these molecules lead to pathological conditions. In addition to the importance of these mutations as a cause of human disease, such errors of nature allow for an understanding of the structure and function of these molecules in normal physiology.

I. INTRODUCTION

At each juncture in the hypothalamic–pituitary–thyroid axis, there is an interaction between hormone and receptor that produces a specific biologic effect. Thyrotropin-releasing hormone (TRH), secreted from the hypothalamus, interacts with TRH receptors on the thyrotroph cell surface. This results in production and release of thyroid-stimulating hormone (TSH) from the pituitary. TSH, in turn, interacts with thyroid follicular cell surface receptors, resulting in synthesis and release of thyroid hormones (THs) from the thyroid gland. Finally, TH binds to nuclear TH receptors in target tissues for TH action. All of this is controlled by a series of negative feedback loops at the level of the hypothalamus and pituitary involving primarily TH. The focus of this article is on what has been learned from mutations in these hormones and their receptors in humans, how the mutations relate to human disease, and the structure and function of these molecules in normal physiology.

Abnormalities in either the hormone or the receptor can result in altered states of hormone sensitivity, such as resistance (loss of function) or hypersensitivity (gain of function). In the human thyroid axis, there are examples of both types of mutations. Resistance is defined as a condition of reduced or absent target tissue responsiveness to the hormone. Resistance manifests as higher than normal levels of the hormone without the expected biological effect. Resistance may be due to any of the following reasons: (1) a mutation in the hormone, resulting in altered biologic activity; (2) production of a substance, such as an antibody, that interferes with hormonal action; (3) an abnormal receptor due to a loss-of-function mutation, resulting in failure to bind the hormone or failure to activate the appropriate postreceptor response cascade; (4) an abnormality in any of the multiple cofactors involved in the process of hormone action; or (5) any postreceptor defect, such as abnormal G-protein, that could also result in hormone resistance. "Pseudoresistance" refers to lab assay results indicating excessive amounts of hormone when, in fact, the results are false, due to an interfering substance.

Hormone hypersensitivity is a condition of exaggerated effects of a hormone in the presence of normal to low levels of the hormone. Theoretically, this may be due to an increase in biological activity, as in a "superhormone," or to an abnormal constitutively activated receptor. Additionally, hypersensitivity can be due to a substance other than the hormone which stimulates the receptor.

II. TH RECEPTOR MUTATIONS AND RESISTANCE TO TH

A. Summary of TH Action

Thyroid hormone penetrates all body tissues and is believed to enter cells by a process of concentration-dependent passive diffusion after its dissociation from the serum hormone-binding proteins. Triiodothyronine (T3), the biologically active form of the hormone in blood, or generated from tetraiodothyronine (T4, thyroxine) within the cell, reaches its site of action, the cell nucleus. There it binds with DNA-bound specific molecules known as TH receptors (TRs). Hormone-bound TRs then interact with various cofactors that modify the receptor–ligand complex and allow it to regulate gene transcription.

B. General Introduction to Nuclear Receptors

Thyroid hormone receptors belong to the nuclear hormone receptor superfamily, which includes receptors for the sex hormones, testosterone and estrogen, as well as for vitamin D, retinoic acid, and the peroxisome proliferation receptor. These receptors are characterized by a carboxy-terminal ligand-binding domain (LBD) and a more proximal DNA-binding domain (DBD). These receptors act as nuclear transcription factors by binding to specific sequences of DNA located in target genes. In the case of TH, these sequences are TH response elements (TREs). Some regions of the receptor are involved in interacting with a variety of cofactors that modify the receptor–hormone complex on the TRE, thus modulating transcriptional activity.

C. The TR and Mode of Action

Mutations have been described that result in a failure to initiate TH-responsive transcription. Either the LBD is altered, preventing the recognition of the hormone, or the DBD or the hinge region is altered, inactivating the hormone–receptor complex. Mutations in TRs may result in the syndrome of resistance to TH. In a subject heterozygous for an abnormal TR allele, a dominant negative interaction occurs whereby the abnormal allele interferes with function of the normal allele, resulting in the phenotype of resistance.

D. Clinical Aspects of Resistance to TH

Resistance to TH (RTH) is an inherited syndrome (usually autosomal dominant) of reduced target tissue responsiveness to TH. More than 700 cases in 250 families have been described that fit this definition. It is suggested that the incidence is 1:50,000. With the exception of a single family, inheritance is autosomal dominant. In practice, patients with autosomal dominant RTH are identified by a persistent elevation of serum free 3,5,3',5'-tetraiodothyronine and free 3,5,3'-triiodothyronine levels without TSH suppression. In these RTH patients, this combination of abnormal laboratory test results occurs in the absence of intercurrent illness, drugs, or alterations of TH transport proteins in serum. More importantly, administration of supraphysiological doses of TH fails to produce the expected suppressive effect on the secretion of pituitary TSH and the anticipated metabolic responses in peripheral tissues.

The common features of RTH are (1) elevated serum levels of free T4 and free T3, (2) normal or slightly increased concentrations of serum TSH that responds to TRH stimulation, (3) absence of typical symptoms and metabolic consequences of TH excess, and (4) goiter.

E. Molecular Basis of RTH: TRβ Mutations

Mutations in the gene encoding thyroid hormone receptor β (TRβ) have been described in the majority of families with RTH. All mutations affect the LBD or adjacent hinge region of the TRβ molecule and are distributed in three clusters (Fig. 1). In the *TRβ* gene, 43 mutations in 86 families have been found in cluster 1 (corresponding to amino acids 429–460), 49 mutations in 113 families have been found in cluster 2 (amino acids 309–383), and 16 mutations in 31 families have been found in cluster 3 (amino acids 234–282). A complete *TRβ* gene deletion has been reported in one family. Mutations have been identified in 64 codons of the *TRβ* gene, with 30 of these codons altered by more than one mutation. Of the 109 identified *TRβ* gene mutations, 71 are unique in

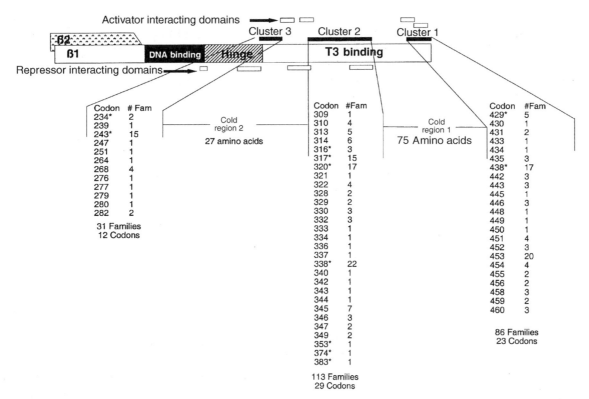

FIGURE 1 Functional domains of the thyroid hormone receptor β-subunit and reported mutations in the *TRβ* gene. The mutated codon is listed along with the number of families known to have mutations in that particular codon. There may be more than one mutation in a particular codon. In several codons, identical mutations have been found in multiple families. The mutations are present in three clusters, separated by two regions in which natural mutations have not been reported. *TRβ1* and *TRβ2* have different ATG start sites and differ only in the amino terminus. Asterisks indicate a CpG dinucleotide.

that they occur in only one family, and 38 occur in multiple unrelated families. Using the single-letter amino acid code to describe the protein mutations, the five most frequent mutations in the *TRβ* gene correspond to R338W (19 families); A317T (14 families); R438H (11 families); R243Q (10 families), and P453T (9 families). Of the mutations described, 95 (87.2%) are due to a single-base-pair substitution resulting in a single-amino-acid substitution (92) or a premature stop codon (3). The remaining mutations are due to dinucleotide substitution (1), complete deletion (1), single-base-pair deletion (1), three-base-pair deletion (5), single-base-pair insertion (4), three-base-pair insertion (1), and seven-base-pair duplication (1). Of 109 mutations, 17 occur in CpG dinucleotides and these account for 43% of the families with *TRβ* gene mutations. In 37 of 236 families with RTH, the *TRβ* mutation has occurred *de novo* and the mutant allele can be traced to the normal progenitor of one of the two parents. In contrast to syndromes of vitamin D and androgen

resistance, mutations in the DNA-binding region are not found in RTH.

No mutations have been reported in the *TRα* gene. Mice with deletion of TRα1 and TRα2 isotypes have hypersensitivity to TH. Therefore, the phenotype of a mutant TRα is unlikely to manifest as RTH and may explain the lack of observed mutations in this protein.

Normal TRβ is found in 10% of RTH patients. Patients with non-TRβ RTH and patients with TRβ mutations have identical phenotypes. Whereas the majority of patients with glucocorticoid resistance syndromes usually have mutations in the glucocorticoid receptor (GR), similar to RTH, some patients have been described with non-GR glucocorticoid resistance. Based on the observation of RTH in mice deficient in steroid receptor co-activator-1 (SRC-1), it is logical to postulate that abnormalities of co-activators or corepressors, known to be involved in hormone action, may also cause hormonal resistance.

III. TSH MUTATIONS

Thyroid-stimulating hormone is a 30-kDa glyco-protein secreted by the thyrotroph; it is encoded on human chromosome 1. Similar to other glycoprotein hormones secreted by the anterior pituitary, TSH is composed of a common α-subunit noncovalently bound to a specific β-subunit. The CAGYC (C, cysteine; A, alanine; G, glycine; Y, tyrosine) region of the protein forms the "seat belt" part of the TSH β-subunit, which allows for interaction with the α-subunit. It is the unique β-subunit that confers the hormonal specificity. In some instances, as in a molar pregnancy, a condition in which there are very high levels of chorionic gonadotropin (CG), stimulation of the TSH receptor by CG α-subunit can cause hyperthyroidism. All reported mutations in the *TSHβ* gene result in significant hypothyroidism. The patients present with typical findings of central hypothyroidism, namely, low levels of T3 and T4 with inappropriately very low or absent concentrations of serum TSH. The low serum TSH concentrations can be understood based on the observation that TSHβ is degraded intracellularly. TSHβ degradation occurs when TSHβ is not bound to the α-subunit, and the mutation prevents this binding. Therefore, any abnormality of the protein in the CAGYC region would result in undetectable TSH. Whereas most cases of central hypothyroidism are associated with disruptions in other components in the pathways of the pituitary hormone axis, such as adrenocorticotropic hormone (ACTH)/cortisol or luteinizing hormone (LH)/follicle-stimulating hormone (FSH)/sex hormone, TSHβ mutations present as isolated central hypothyroidism. Attempts to stimulate pituitary secretion by thyrotropin-releasing hormone results in prolactin release but fails to result in TSH stimulation in patients with TSHβ mutations.

The first reported cases of TSHβ mutations were found in three (possibly related) Japanese families homozygous for a G to A substitution encoded in codon 29 of the *TSHβ* gene; the substitution results in a conversion of glycine to an arginine (G29R). The second abnormal TSHβ was found in two Greek families in which a G to T substitution encoded in codon 12 results in a premature stop codon and leads to the deletion of amino acid residues 12–118. A third variant described in four families is a 1-bp deletion in codon 105 that produces a frameshift. This causes Cys-105 to be converted to valine and the addition of eight nonsense amino acids. The fourth variant was described in a consanguineous Turkish family whose members were homozygous for a C to T transition at nucleotide 654 of the region encoding the TSH β-subunit, resulting in Gln-49 becoming a stop codon and premature termination of the protein. This removes the region necessary for α-subunit heterodimerization and no TSH is secreted by the thyrotrophs (Fig. 2).

IV. TSH RECEPTOR MUTATIONS

The TSH receptor (TSHR) belongs to the superfamily of G-protein-coupled receptors, which are characterized by serpentine-like looping through the membrane, with seven-transmembrane segments. The molecule can be divided into three domains: extracellular, intramembranous, and intracellular. The extracellular domain consists of the 398-residue amino-terminal segment and three extracellular loops; the membranous domain consists of seven α-helices; and the intracellular domain consists of the carboxy-terminal amino acids of the molecule, with three intracellular loops. The specificity of the receptor for the ligand is encoded in the amino-terminal segment, which is responsible for ligand recognition. The carboxy-terminal segment contains the sites that interact with the cascade of G-proteins, leading to the generation of cyclic adenosine monophosphate (cAMP). The cAMP pathway, when stimulated, results in thyroid cell growth and TH secretion. The intramembranous domain is also coupled to the activation of the phospholipase C cascade. The latter requires TSH concentrations 5–10 times higher than are required for the cAMP pathway. The phospholipase C stimulation of diacylglycerol and inositol

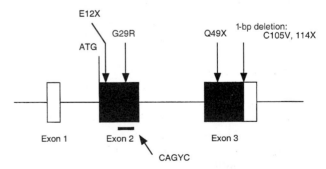

FIGURE 2 Thyroid-stimulating hormone gene mutations; organization of the *TSHβ* gene and reported mutations. The region encoding CAGYC (see text for discussion) is important for noncovalent interaction between the TSH β- and α-subunits.

phospholipase is mainly involved in the control of iodination and TH synthesis.

Abnormalities in the TSHR can result in either activation of the G-proteins in the absence of TSH, known as "gain-of-function" mutations, or reduced or absent activation of the G-proteins, known as "loss-of-function" mutations. Gain-of-function mutations in the TSHR usually result in hyperthyroidism and goiter through constitutive activity of the TSHR. This is due to a mutation activating the TSHR. Excessive amounts of TH released by the thyroid gland cause the symptoms associated with an overactive thyroid, including rapid heart beat (tachycardia), weight loss, jitteriness, fatigue, and goiter. Loss-of-function mutations in the TSHR usually cause hypothyroidism, manifesting as weight gain, tiredness, and dry skin. The hypothyroidism is caused by the resistance of the TSHR, resulting in failure of the thyroid gland to respond to TSH, despite high circulating levels of TSH. Gain-of-function and loss-of-function mutations have also been described for other glycoprotein hormone receptors, including LH, FSH, and parathyroid hormone.

To date, 39 gain-of-function mutations have been reported in the TSHR (Fig. 3). Only one of these mutations occurs in the 398-residue amino terminus; the rest occur in the third cytoplasmic loop or in the adjacent sixth transmembrane segment of the receptor. This observed clustering of mutations underlines the importance of this portion of the molecule. Of the mutations, 23 are found only as somatic mutations, 9 are found only as germ-line mutations, and 8 have been described as somatic in some families and germ-line in other families. The most common setting to observe these gain-of-function mutations is in patients with "toxic adenomas." These are nodules of the thyroid gland that autonomously secrete TH. In some series of studies, up to 80% of toxic adenomas have TSHR mutations, but other populations have a lower incidence, perhaps related to levels of environmental iodine. One TSHR mutation (L677V) was also associated with thyroid carcinoma.

A mutation of the TSHR has been determined to be the cause of familial gestational hyperthyroidism in one family whose members experienced hyperthyroidism only when pregnant. Investigation of this

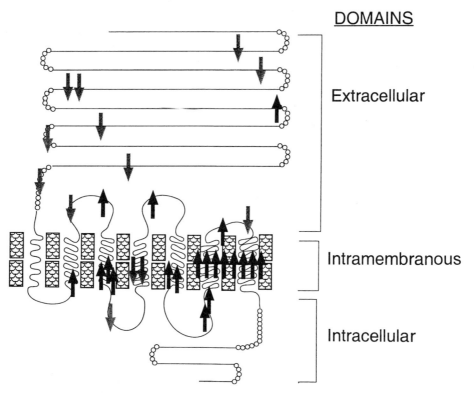

DOMAINS

Extracellular

Intramembranous

Intracellular

FIGURE 3 Organization of the thyroid-stimulating hormone receptor and reported mutations. Black arrows pointing up indicate gain-of-function mutations; gray arrows pointing down indicate loss-of-function mutations. Note that a majority of the gain-of-function mutations are in the intramembranous domains, whereas the loss-of-function mutations are in the extracellular domains.

family revealed a heterozygous mutation (K183R) located in the extracellular domain of the TSHR, causing chorionic gonadotropin to bind with higher affinity than TSH. However, the receptor also maintained normal responsiveness to TSH. Therefore, when the CG levels increased dramatically during pregnancy, the TSHR was activated, causing hyperthyroidism that resolved spontaneously when the CG levels decreased following delivery. This shows that some mutations can produce a promiscuous TSHR that responds to other hormones.

Cases involving 16 loss-of-function mutations in the TSHR have been described. In contrast to the gain-of-function mutations, a majority of the loss of function mutations are located in the amino-terminal extracellular domain, with the remainder in the extracellular loops of the and fourth intramembranous region. These mutations can result in either partial or complete resistance to TSH (RTSH). In all instances, TSH is elevated but does not cause goiter. In partial RTSH, there is a compensatory increase in TSH, stimulating the thyroid to produce just the needed amount of TH. In complete RTSH, the thyroid gland is completely insensitive to TSH and the patients are severely hypothyroid. Administration of TH to these patients appropriately suppresses their elevated TSH and they become euthyroid. This supports the notion that the defect in RTSH is in responding to TSH and that TH acts normally. Loss of function implies that both alleles are abnormal. Of the 14 families described, 8 were euthyroid and 6 were hypothyroid; RTSH occurred in 6 families homozygous for the TSHR mutations and 8 families were compound heterozygous.

Acknowledgments

Supported in part by NIH Grant DK-58258 and funds from the Seymour J. Abrams Thyroid Research Center.

Glossary

co-activators Molecules that modulate gene transcription, usually through bound receptor; generally have histone acetyl transferase activity, which allows for unraveling of DNA and initiation of transcription.

corepressors Proteins that modulate gene transcription in the presence of receptor; generally stabilize the receptor complex on the response element of the target gene, recruiting histone deacetylase. When ligand is present, corepressor binding is unfavorable and the corepressor dissociates from the receptor–ligand–DNA complex, allowing for the recruitment of a co-activator.

gain-of-function mutations Gene alterations that render a receptor constitutively active, in the absence of hormone. In the thyroid-stimulating hormone receptor, such mutations usually result in hyperthyroidism.

germ-line mutations Gene alterations that are present in germ cells (ova or sperm) and are thus transmitted to the progeny.

goiter Enlargement of the thyroid gland; occurs in hypothyroid states, when thyroid cells are under TSH stimulation to produce more hormone, or in hyperthyroid states, when stimulating substances, usually antibodies, bind to the TSH receptor and stimulate thyroid function.

hyperthyroidism Condition of thyroid hormone excess; commonly associated with weight loss, tachycardia, excessive sweating, heat intolerance, moist skin, and fatigue; usually due to excessive thyroid gland production of thyroid hormone.

hypothyroidism Condition of thyroid hormone deficit; commonly associated with weight gain, slow mentation, decreased energy, cold intolerance, edema, and dry skin; usually due to failure of the thyroid gland to synthesize and release thyroid hormone.

loss-of-function mutations Gene alterations that reduce or abolish receptor activity; result in impaired ligand–receptor interaction. Such mutations in thyroid-stimulating hormone receptor produce resistance to TSH, which, when severe, causes hypothyroidism. Such mutations in thyroid hormone receptor produce resistance to thyroid hormone.

resistance to thyroid hormone Inherited syndrome of reduced target tissue responsiveness to thyroid hormone. Diagnostic criteria are elevated serum levels of free thyroid hormone, nonsuppressed TSH, and absence of classic signs and symptoms of thyrotoxicosis.

resistance to thyrotropin Inherited syndrome of reduced responsiveness of the thyroid gland to TSH. All patients have elevated serum levels of TSH with serum thyroid hormone concentrations that are normal (in compensated forms) or low (in noncompensated forms).

somatic mutation Gene alteration that occurs in any cell that is not destined to become a germ cell.

thyroid hormone receptor Nuclear receptor for triiodothyronine (T3, the active form of thyroid hormone). The two thyroid hormone receptor genes, α and β, are located on human chromosomes 17 (q21–q22) and 3 (p22–p24.1), respectively. Various splicing arrangements of these genes result in several isoforms of both α and β.

See Also the Following Articles

Co-activators and Corepressors for the Nuclear Receptor Superfamily • Parathyroid Hormone • Thyroid Hormone Receptor Isoforms • Thyroid Stimulating Hormone (TSH) • Thyrotropin Receptor Signaling • Thyrotropin-Releasing Hormone (TRH) • Thyrotropin-Releasing Hormone Receptor Signaling

Further Reading

Corvilain, B., Van Sande, J., Dumont, J. E., and Vassart, G. (2001). Somatic and germline mutations of the TSH receptor and thyroid diseases. *Clin. Endocrinol.* 55, 143–158.

Kopp, P. (2001). The TSH receptor and its role in thyroid disease. *Cell. Mol. Life Sci.* 58, 1301–1322.

Matzuk, M. M., Kornmeier, C. M., Whitfield, G. K., Kourides, I. A., and Boime, I. (1988). The glycoprotein alpha-subunit is critical for secretion and stability of the human thyrotropin β-subunit. *Mol. Endocrinol.* 2, 95–100.

Refetoff, S., Dumont, J. E., and Vassart, G. (2001). Thyroid disorders. *In* "The Metabolic and Molecular Bases of Inherited Disease" (C. R. Scriver, A. L. Beaudet, W. S. Sly and D. Vale, eds.), pp. 4029–4076. McGraw Hill, New York.

Refetoff, S., and Weiss, R. E. (1997). Resistance to thyroid hormone. *In* "Molecular Genetics of Endocrine Disorders" (T. V. Thakker, ed.), pp. 85–122. Chapman & Hill, London.

Refetoff, S., Weiss, R. E., and Usala, S. J. (1993). The syndromes of resistance to thyroid hormone. *Endocr. Rev.* 14, 348–399.

Rodien, P., Bremont, C., Sanson, M. L., Parma, J., Van Sande, J., Costagliola, S., Luton, J. P., Vassart, G., and Duprez, L. (1998). Familial gestational hyperthyroidism caused by a mutant thyrotropin receptor hypersensitive to human chorionic gonadotropin. *N. Engl. J. Med.* 339, 1823–1826.

Sunthornthepvarakul, T., Gottschalk, M. E., Hayashi, Y., and Refetoff, S. (1995). Resistance to thyrotropin caused by mutations in the thyrotropin-receptor gene. *N. Engl. J. Med.* 332, 155–160.

Vuissoz, J.-M., Deladoey, J., Buyukgebiz, A., Cemeroglu, P., Gex, G., Gallati, S., and Mullis, P. E. (2001). New autosomal recessive mutation of the TSH-β subunit gene causing central isolated hypothyroidism. *J. Clin. Endocrinol. Metab.* 86, 4468–4471.

Weiss, R. E., and Refetoff, S. (2000). Resistance to thyroid hormone. *Rev. Endocr. Metab. Disord.* 1, 97–108.

Yen, P. M. (2001). Physiological and molecular basis of thyroid hormone action. *Physiol. Rev.* 81, 1097–1142.

Thyroid Hormone Transport Proteins: Thyroxine-Binding Globulin, Transthyretin, and Albumin

SAMUEL REFETOFF

The University of Chicago

Thyroid hormones are transported in blood bound to serum proteins. They are in equilibrium with a minute fraction of free hormones immediately available to tissues. Acquired abnormalities and inherited defects of transport proteins can have a profound effect on the serum concentration of the hormones but little or no consequences on their metabolic effects. Recognition of such defects prevents unnecessary and often harmful therapeutic interventions.

I. INTRODUCTION

Thyroxine (T_4)-binding globulin (TBG) is the principal thyroid hormone transport protein; the other two are transthyretin (TTR) and human serum albumin (HSA). TBG transports 75% of serum T_4 and TTR and HAS carry 20 and 5%, respectively. TBG also transports 75% of serum triiodothyronine (T_3). The benefit of thyroid hormone associating with proteins is unknown since the absence or inherited loss of binding function of the proteins does not result in a demonstrable disadvantage. However, it has been speculated that thyroid hormone-binding proteins may (1) safeguard the body from the effects of abrupt fluctuations in hormone secretion; (2) protect against iodine wastage by imparting macromolecular properties to the small thyroid hormone molecules and thus reducing their loss in urine; (3) facilitate the uniform cellular distribution of T_4; and (4) target the hormone to sites of inflammation through its release through TBG cleavage by neutrophil-derived elastase.

Important changes in TBG, either quantitative or qualitative, result in profound alterations in the total thyroid hormone level in serum without disturbing the free hormone concentration. Thyroid function tests in these circumstances may be misinterpreted as indicative of hyper- or hypothyroidism and could result in unnecessary treatment. Many physiologic, pathologic, and genetic conditions, as well as certain drugs, can alter the concentration of TBG (see below). In addition, drugs can compete with the binding of iodothyronine ligands.

II. STRUCTURAL, PHYSICAL, AND BIOLOGICAL PROPERTIES

A. TBG

TBG is a 54 kDa acidic glycoprotein synthesized by the liver (see Table 1). It is composed of a single polypeptide chain of 395 amino acids and four heterosaccharide units with five to nine terminal sialic acids. The carbohydrate chains are not necess-

TABLE 1   Properties of the Principal Thyroid Hormone-Binding Proteins in Serum

	TBG	TTR	HSA
Molecular weight (kDa)	54[a]	55	66.5
Structure	Monomer	Tetramer	Monomer
Carbohydrate content (%)	20		
Number of binding sites for T_4 and T_3	1	2	Several
Association constant K_a (M^{-1})			
For T_4	1×10^{10}	2×10^{8b}	1.5×10^{6b}
For T_3	1×10^9	1×10^6	2×10^5
Concentration in serum (mean normal, mg/liter)	16	250	40,000
Relative distribution of T_4 and T_3 in serum (%)			
T_4	75	20	5
T_3	75	<5	20
In vivo survival			
Half-life (days)	5[c]	2	15
Degradation rate (mg/day)	15	650	17,000

[a]Apparent molecular weight on acrylamide gel electrophoresis is 60 kDa.
[b]Value given is for the high-affinity binding site only.
[c]Longer half-life under the influence of estrogen.

ary for hormone binding but are required for the correct posttranslational folding and secretion of the molecule. However, secreted TBG that has been properly folded can be deglycosylated without loss of its hormone-binding and immunologic properties.

Serum TBG is stable at room temperature but undergoes rapid denaturation and loses its binding activity at temperatures above 55 °C and pH below 4. The half-life of TBG *in vivo* is approximately 5 days but that of asialo TBG is only 15 min.

TBG has a single iodothyronine-binding site with higher affinity for T_4 than T_3 (Table 1). In the euthyroid state, approximately one-third of TBG molecules carry thyroid hormone, mainly T_4. When fully saturated, TBG carries ~20 mg of T_4 per deciliter of serum. Normal serum concentration in adults ranges from 1.1 to 2.1 mg/dl. TBG is detected in the 12-week-old fetus, and in newborns and in children up to the age of 2–3 years, its concentration is 1.5-fold that in adults. Denatured TBG does not bind iodothyronines but can be detected with antibodies that recognize the primary structure of the molecule.

B. TTR

TTR is a 55 kDa, highly acidic tetramer devoid of carbohydrate. It forms a complex with retinol-binding protein (RBP) and thus plays a role in the transport of vitamin A.

TTR is present in blood as a stable tetramer of identical subunits, each containing 127 amino acids. Together they form a symmetrical structure with a double-barreled hydrophobic channel forming the two iodothyronine-binding sites. Yet, TTR usually binds only one T_4 molecule because the binding affinity of the second site is greatly reduced through a negative cooperative effect. The presence of RBP does not interfere with T_4 binding and vice versa.

Despite the 20-fold higher concentration of TTR in serum relative to that of TBG, it plays a lesser role in iodothyronine transport. The first T_4 molecule binds to TTR with a K_a that is approximately 100-fold higher than that for HSA and approximately 100-fold less than that for TBG. Relative to T_4, T_3 has lower affinity and tetraiodoacetic acid has higher affinity for TTR. Among the drugs that compete with T_4 binding to TTR are ethacrynic acid, salicylates, 2,4-dinitrophenol, and penicillin.

The average concentration of TTR in serum is 25 mg/dl and corresponds to a maximal binding capacity of 300 μg T_4. Changes in TTR concentration have relatively little effect on the concentration of serum iodothyronines. Only 0.5% of the circulating TTR is occupied by T_4. TTR has a relatively rapid turnover ($t_{1/2} = 2$ days). Hence, acute diminution in the rate of synthesis is accompanied by a rapid decrease of its concentration in serum.

C. HSA

HSA is a 66.5 kDa protein synthesized by the liver. It comprises 585 amino acids, has a high cysteine content, and has a high proportion of charged amino acids but contains no carbohydrate. The three domains of the molecule can be depicted in a model as three tennis balls packaged in a cylindrical case.

HSA associates with a wide variety of substances including hormones and drugs possessing a hydrophobic region, and thus the association of thyroid hormone with HSA can be viewed as being nonspecific. Fatty acids and chloride ions decrease the binding of iodothyronine to HSA.

The biological $t_{1/2}$ of HSA is longer than that of TBG and TTR. HSA constitutes more than half of the total protein content in serum and it is thus the principal contributor to the maintenance of colloid osmotic pressure. Despite the high iodothyronine-binding capacity, the low affinity is responsible for the minor contribution of HSA to thyroid hormone transport. Thus, even the most marked fluctuations in HSA concentration, including analbuminemia, have no significant effect on thyroid hormone levels.

III. GENE STRUCTURE AND TRANSCRIPTIONAL REGULATION

A. TBG

TBG is encoded by a single-copy gene located on the long arm of the human X chromosome (Xq22.2) (see Fig. 1). The gene consists of five exons and has two polyadenylation sites giving rise to mRNAs of different sizes. The gene organization and amino acid sequences are similar to those of other members of the serine protease inhibitor family, which includes cortisol-binding globulin, α_1-anti-trypsin, and α_1-anti-chymotrypsin. An upstream sequence of 218 bp contains liver-specific enhancer elements and is required for the transcription of the TBG gene. The promoter has no estrogen receptor-binding sites and estradiol does not appear to have a direct effect on TBG gene transcription.

B. TTR

TTR is encoded by a single-copy gene located on chromosome 18 (18q11.2–q12.1). The gene consists of four exons spanning 6.8 kb. Knowledge about the transcriptional regulation of the human TTR gene comes from studies of the mouse gene structural and sequence homology, which extends to the promoter region. In both species, a TATAA-box and binding sites for hepatocyte nuclear factor-1 (HNF-1), HNF-3, and HNF-4 are located within 150 bp of the transcription start site.

Although TTR in serum originates from the liver, TTR mRNA is also found in kidney cells, the choroid plexus, and pancreatic islet cells. TTR constitutes up

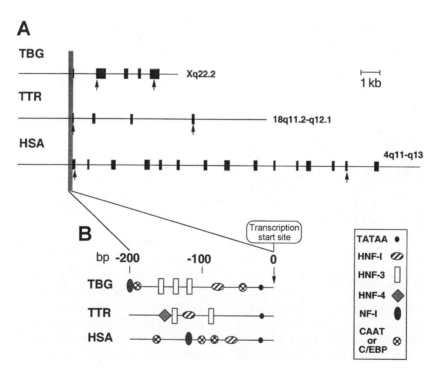

FIGURE 1 Genomic organization and chromosomal localization of thyroid hormone serum-binding proteins. (A) Filled boxes represent exons. Locations of initiation codons and termination codons are indicated by arrows. (B) Structure of promoter regions with the location of *cis*-acting transcriptional regulatory elements.

to 25% of the total protein present in ventricular cerebrospinal fluid.

C. HSA

HSA is encoded by a single-copy gene located on human chromosome 4 (4q11–q13). The gene contains 15 exons. The promoter region contains binding sites for hepatocyte-enriched nuclear proteins, such as HNF-1, CCAAT/enhancer-binding protein, and D-site binding protein, a member of the C/EBP family.

IV. ACQUIRED DEFECTS

A. TBG

Altered synthesis, degradation, or both are responsible for the majority of acquired TBG abnormalities. Severe terminal illness is undoubtedly the most common cause of an acquired decrease in TBG concentration. Interleukin-6 is a likely candidate for mediation of this effect. Altered rates of degradation are responsible for the decrease and increase of serum TBG concentration in thyrotoxicosis and hypothyroidism, respectively.

Partially desialylated TBG may be present in relatively higher proportion than intact TBG in the serum of some patients with severe liver disease and in a variety of nonthyroidal illnesses. Patients with carbohydrate-deficient glycoprotein syndrome show a characteristic cathodal shift in the relative proportion of TBG isoforms compatible with diminished sialic acid content.

Estrogen excess from an endogenous (hydatidiform mole, estrogen-producing tumors, etc.) or exogenous source is the most common cause of increased serum TBG concentrations. The levels of several other serum proteins such as corticosteroid-binding globulin and sex hormone-binding globulin are also increased. This effect of estrogen is mediated through an increase in the complexity of the oligosaccharide residues in TBG, prolonging its biological half-life.

B. TTR

The reduction of serum TTR concentration surpasses that of TBG in major illness and protein-calorie malnutrition. This is caused by either a decrease in the rate of synthesis or an increase in the rate of degradation. Increased serum TTR concentration can occur in some patients with islet cell carcinoma.

V. INHERITED DEFECTS

A. TBG

With a single exception, the inheritance of TBG abnormalities, including TBG deficiency and TBG excess, follows an X-linked pattern. Clinically, patients present with euthyroid hyper- or hypothyroxinemia. TBG deficiency can present as partial deficiency (TBG-PD) or complete deficiency (TBG-CD), depending on the serum TBG level in hemizygotes. In addition, TBG variants can be characterized by their properties that include (1) immunologic identity; (2) isoelectric focusing (IEF) pattern; (3) rate of inactivation at various temperatures or pH; and (4) affinity for ligands. More precise characterization of TBG defects requires sequencing of the TBG gene.

1. Complete Deficiency

TBG-CD is defined as an undetectable TBG concentration in hemizygotes (XY males or XO females) who express only the mutant allele. Obligatory carriers (mother or daughters of affected hemizygotes) have on the average a TBG concentration that is half that of normal individuals. On occasion, selective X-chromosome inactivation can cause a female heterozygote to manifest the hemizygous phenotype of TBG-CD. The prevalence of TBG-CD is approximately 1:15,000 newborn males.

Fifteen distinct mutations have been identified in subjects with TBG-CD (Fig. 2). Thirteen have truncated molecules due to an early stop codon. In 2 of these (TBG-K and TBG-Ja), nucleotide substitutions in introns caused abnormal splicing. In 2 other mutations, TBG-CD was caused by a missense mutations. The substitution of the normal Leu-227 with a Pro, in TBG-CD5, prevented secretion of the variant molecule due to aberrant posttranslational processing.

No mutations were found in the coding sequences or in the promoter regions of the TBG gene in two families with X-linked TBG-CD. The cause of TBG deficiency in these families remains unknown.

2. Partial Deficiency

With a prevalence of 1:4000 newborns, partial deficiency is the most common inherited TBG defect. Yet, the precise genetic error has been identified in only a few families. The serum level of TBG in hemizygotes is detectable but reduced and levels in heterozygous females often overlap the normal range. This invalidates the assignment of genotype based solely on serum TBG concentration.

Seven variants manifesting as TBG-PD have been identified. Two of these, TBG-S and TBG-A, are

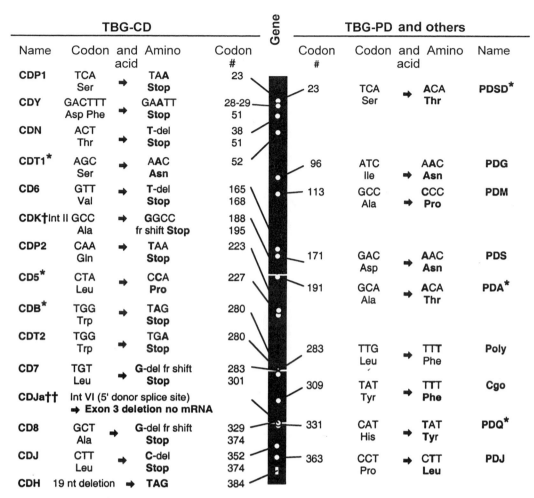

FIGURE 2 Mutations in the TBG gene and their locations. The TBG variants, in order of location, are as follows: SD, San Diego; CDP1, complete deficiency Portuguese 1; CDY, complete deficiency Yonago; CDN, complete deficiency Negev, formerly Bedouin (SDBe); CDT1, complete deficiency Taiwan 1; G, Gary; M, Montreal, CD6, complete deficiency 6; S, slow; CDK, complete deficiency Kankakee; A, Aborigine; CDP2, complete deficiency Portuguese 2; CD5, complete deficiency 5; CDB, complete deficiency Buffalo; CDT2, complete deficiency Taiwan 2; CD7, complete deficiency 7; Poly, polymorphic; Cgo, Chicago; CDJa, complete deficiency; CD8, complete deficiency 8, Quebec; CDJ, complete deficiency Japan; PDJ, partial deficiency Japan; CDH, Hatwichport. Asterisks indicate the coexistence of TBG-Poly. Dagger indicates a mutation in the acceptor splice site of intron II.

present in high frequency in some populations. TBG-S has a frequency of 5–16% in Black Africans. It has a characteristic cathodal shift on IEF due to loss of negative charge, caused by substitution of the normal Asp-171 with Asn. TBG-A was found in 40% of Australian Aborigines. It has a normal IEF pattern but is more heat-labile than the common type TBG (TBG-C). It was also found to have reduced affinity for T_4 (54%) and T_3 (30%), reducing the total T_4 and T_3 concentrations in serum out of proportion to that of TBG.

TBG-SD has a normal IEF pattern but is more -heat-labile and the affinities to T_4 and T_3 are reduced

by ~50%. The mean TBG concentration in hemizygotes can be low or overlap the normal range. TBG variants that have normal serum concentrations but reduced affinity for T_4 produce erroneous values for the estimated free thyroxine index (FT_4I).

Three of the seven TBG-PD variants are characterized by decreased stability at 37 °C and hence increased levels of denatured TBG in serum that correlated inversely with the native TBG concentration. These are TBG-Q, TBG-M, and TBG-G. TBG-Q and TBG-M were found in French Canadians. Expression of TBG-G in COS-1 cells showed impaired secretion of the variant molecule, leading to excessive intracellular degradation. This is caused by improper folding of the molecule due to the presence of an additional carbohydrate chain at a new N-linked glycosylation site.

TBG-PDJ (Japan) has only a mild reduction in heat stability, suggesting that impaired secretion is responsible for the low TBG level.

Recently, a Japanese family with partial TBG deficiency, transmitted in an autosomal dominant pattern, was described. The sequences of the proband's TBG gene and promoter region were normal. An abnormality in a transcription factor that is important for TBG gene expression is a distinct possibility.

3. TBG Variants Present in Normal Concentrations

Four TBG variants with minimal or no alterations in serum concentrations have been identified. TBG-Poly with a silent polymorphism was found in 16% of French Canadians and 20% of Japanese. TBG-Cgo is heat- and acid-resistant. The substitution of the normal Tyr-309 with a Phe ties the internal α-helixes to the molecule, stabilizing its tertiary structure.

4. TBG Excess

Inherited TBG excess is a relatively rare cause of increased TBG. The prevalence of inherited TBG excess is estimated to be 1:25,000. TBG levels in hemizygous affected subjects range from 2.5 to 5 times the normal mean value. TBGs of several unrelated families were shown to have normal properties and no abnormalities were found in the coding sequence or promoter regions of the gene. Gene dosing studies revealed that gene duplication and triplication were the causes of TBG excess in two families. The latter was proven by fluorescence *in situ* hybridization. More recently, a double TBG gene dose was found in two individuals with TBG excess, whose mothers were normal, suggesting *de novo* gene duplication occurring in gametes during meiosis.

B. TTR

Some of the TTR variants are responsible for the dominantly inherited familial amyloidotic polyneuropathy. TTR variants with reduced affinity for T_4 have little effect on the concentration of serum T_4. Only variant TTRs with a substantially increased affinity for iodothyronines produce significant elevations in serum T_4 and reverse T_3 concentrations. They account for 2% of subjects with euthyroid hyperthyroxinemia. The inheritance pattern is autosomal dominant.

A single family with elevated total T_4 concentration due to the replacement of the normal Ala-109 with a Thr has been described. The mutation increases its affinity for T_4, rT_3, tetraiodothyroacetic acid, and to a lesser extent T_3 and triiodothyroacetic acid. Crystallographic analysis of this variant TTR revealed an alteration in the size of the T_4-binding pocket. Another TTR gene mutation involving the same codon with a Val-109 has an increased affinity for T_4 that is of similar magnitude.

A more common defect found in subjects with TTR-associated hyperthyroxinemia is a point mutation in the TTR gene replacing the normal Thr-119 with Met. Despite an increase in the fraction of T_4 and rT_3 associated with this variant TTR, only a few subjects have serum T_4 levels above the upper limit of normal. Several TTR variants that do not alter the properties of the molecule and that are thus of no clinical significance have been found.

C. HSA

1. Familial Dysalbuminemic Hyperthyroxinemia

Another form of dominantly inherited euthyroid hyperthyroxinemia, later to be linked to the albumin gene, is known as familial dysalbuminemic hyperthyroxinemia (FDH). It is the most common cause of an inherited T_4 increase in the Caucasian population, producing on the average a twofold increase in the serum total T_4 concentration. The prevalence varies from 0.01 to 1.8%, depending on ethnic origin, with the highest prevalence occurring among Hispanics. This form of FDH has not been reported in subjects of African or Asian origin. Falsely elevated free T_4 values, when estimated by standard clinical laboratory techniques, have often resulted in inappropriate treatments.

FDH is suspected when serum total T_4 concentration is increased without a proportional elevation in total T_3 level and nonsuppressed serum TSH. Half of affected subjects have also rT_3 values above the normal range (Table 2). Since the same combination of test results is found in subjects with the Thr-109 TTR variant, the diagnosis of FDH should be confirmed by the demonstration of an increased proportion of the total serum T_4 migrating with HSA. This form of FDH is caused by a missense mutation in codon 218 of the HSA gene replacing the normal Arg with a His. Its association with a SacI$^+$ polymorphism suggests a founder effect and is compatible with ethnic predilection of FDH.

TABLE 2 Serum Iodothyronines in FDH

| Variant | Serum concentration (fold of the normal mean) | | | Binding affinity (K_a) of the variant albumins as fold of the normal mean | |
	T_4 (µg/dl)	T_3 (ng/dl)	rT_3 (ng/dl)	T_4	T_3
R218H	16.0 (2)	147 (1.2)	29 (1.4)	10–15	4
R218P	146 (18.2)	253 (2.3)	135 (6.1)	11–13[a]	1.1[a]
L66P	8.7 (1.1)	320 (3.3)	22.3 (1)	1.5	40

[a]Determined at saturation. Affinities are higher at the concentration of T_4 and T_3 found in serum.

Two other mutations of the HSA gene that increased the affinity of the molecule for iodothyronines have been recently identified. One is also located in codon 218 but the mutant amino acid is Pro. This variant HSA has a 90-fold increase in the affinity to T_4, resulting in serum total T_4 concentrations that are 22-fold the mean normal and the highest observed in any physiological or pathological circumstances. Corresponding increases of rT_4 and T_3 are on the average 5- and 2-fold the normal mean (Table 2). The other mutation, a replacement of the normal Leu-66 with a Pro, produces a 40-fold increase in the affinity for T_3 but only a 0.5-fold increase in the affinity for T_4. As a consequence, patients have hypertriiodothyroninemia but not hyperthyroxinemia. It should be noted that serum T_3 concentrations are falsely low, or even undetectable, when measured using an analogue of T_3 as a tracer rather than a radioisotope.

2. Bisalbuminemia and Analbuminemia

Variant HSAs, with altered electrophoretic mobility, produce "bisalbuminemia" in heterozygotes. T_4 binding has been studied in subjects from unrelated families with a slow HSA variant. In one study, only the slow-moving HSA bound T_4, while in another study, both did. The differential binding of T_4 to one of the components of bisalbumin may be due to enhanced binding to the variant component with a charged amino acid sequence.

Analbuminemia is extremely rare. T_4 transport has been studied in only two subjects with this homozygous condition. The virtual absence of HSA had no clear effect on the concentration of serum iodothyronines as judged by determination of protein-bound iodine, despite an increased binding capacity of TBG and TTR. TBG and TTR become normalized when serum HSA was restored to normal by multiple transfusions.

Acknowledgments

A great part of the information provided in this article represents the contributions of the following investigators who have worked in the author's laboratory (in alphabetical order): Kenneth B. Ain, Piamsook Angkeow, Richard B. Bertenshaw, Jr., Gisah Amaral de Carvalho, Alexandra Dumitrescu, Yoshitaka Hayashi, Onno E. Janssen, Peizhi Li, Paolo E. Macchia, Ventzislav Marinow, Yuichi Mori, Yoshiharu Murata, Silvana Pannain, Joachim Pohlenz, Theodore N. Pullman, David H. Sarne, Neal H. Scherberg, Hisao Seo, Piotr Sobieszczyk, Sylwester Sobieszczyk, Junta Takamatsu, Kyoko Takeda, Margaret Waltz, and Roy E. Weiss. This work was supported in part by Grants RR 00055 and DK 15070 from the National Institutes of Health and in part by the Blum-Kovler Fund.

Glossary

ligand A functional group, atom, or molecule that is attached to the central atom of a coordination compound, particularly a nonmetallic substance that combines with another substance in solution to form a coordination compound.

polyadenylation A process by which a sequence of adenylic acid residues is added to the 3'-end of many eukaryotic mRNA molecules immediately after transcription.

tetramer A polymer that is assembled from four identical monomers.

transcription The formation of a nucleic acid molecule using another molecule as a template, particularly the synthesis of an RNA using a DNA template.

See Also the Following Articles

Environmental Disruptors of Thyroid Hormone Action • Iodine: Symporter and Oxidation, Thyroid Hormone Biosynthesis • Thyroglobulin • Thyroid Hormone Receptor Isoforms • Thyroid Hormone Receptor, TSH and TSH Receptor Mutations • Thyroid Stimulating Hormone (TSH) • Thyrotropin-Releasing Hormone (TRH)

Further Reading

Ain, K. B., and Refetoff, S. (1988). Relationship of oligosaccharide modification to the cause of serum thyroxine-binding globulin excess. *J. Clin. Endocrinol. Metab.* **66**, 1037–1043.

Burr, W. A., Ramsden, D. B., and Hoffenberg, R. (1980). Hereditary abnormalities of thyroxine-binding globulin concentration. *Q. J. Med.* **49**, 295–313.

Cody, V. (1980). Thyroid hormone interactions: Molecular conformation, protein binding and hormone action. *Endocr. Rev.* **1**, 140–166.

Flink, I. L., Bailey, T. J., Gustefson, T. A., Markham, B. E., and Morkin, E. (1986). Complete amino acid sequence of human thyroxine-binding globulin deduced from cloned DNA: Close homology to the serine antiproteases. *Proc. Natl. Acad. Sci. USA* **83**, 7708–7712.

Hayashi, Y., Mori, Y., Janssen, O. E., Sunthornthepvarakul, T., Weiss, R. E., Takeda, K., Weinberg, M., Seo, H., Bell, G. I., and Refetoff, S. (1993). Human thyroxine-binding globulin gene: Complete sequence and transcriptional regulation. *Mol. Endocrinol.* **7**, 1049–1060.

Mori, Y., Miura, Y., Takeuchi, H., Igarashi, Y., Sugiura, J., and Oiso, Y. (1995). Gene amplification as a cause for inherited thyroxine-binding globulin excess in two Japanese families. *J. Clin. Endocrinol. Metab.* **80**, 3758–3762.

Peters, T., Jr (1985). Serum albumin. *Adv. Protein Chem.* **37**, 161–245.

Petersen, C. E., Ha, C.-E., Jameson, D. M., and Bhagavan, N. V. (1996). Mutations in a specific human serum albumin thyroxine binding site define the structural basis of familial dysalbuminemic hyperthyroxinemia. *J. Biol. Chem.* **271**, 19110–19117.

Refetoff, S. (1984). Inherited thyroxine-binding globulin (TBG) abnormalities in man. *Endocr. Rev.* **10**, 275–293.

Refetoff, S., Fang, V. S., and Marshall, J. S. (1975). Studies on human thyroxine-binding globulin (TBG). IX. Some physical, chemical and biological properties of radioiodinated TBG and partially desialylated TBG (STBG). *J. Clin. Invest.* **56**, 177–187.

Refetoff, S., Murata, Y., Vassart, G., Chandramouli, V., Marshall, J. S. (1984). Radioimmunoassays specific for the tertiary and primary structures of thyroxine-binding globulin (TBG): Measurement of denatured TBG in serum. *J. Clin. Endocrinol. Metab.* **59**, 269–277.

Rosen, H. N., Moses, A. C., Murrell, J. R., Liepnieks, J. J., and Benson, M. D. (1993). Thyroxine interactions with transthyretin: A comparison of 10 naturally occurring human transthyretin variants. *J. Clin. Endocrinol. Metab.* **77**, 370–374.

Sunthornthepvarakul, T., Angkeow, P., Weiss, R. E., Hayashi, Y., and Refetoff, S. (1994). A missense mutation in the albumin gene produces familial disalbuminemic hyperthyroxinemia in 8 unrelated families. *Biochem. Biophys. Res. Commun.* **202**, 781–787.

Sunthornthepvarakul, T., Likitmaskul, S., Ngowngarmratana, S., Angsusingha, K., Sureerat, K., Scherberg, N. H., and Refetoff, S. (1998). Familial dysalbuminemic hypertriiodothyroninemia: A new dominantly inherited albumin defect. *J. Clin. Endocrinol. Metab.* **83**, 1448–1454.

Tsuzuki, T., Mita, S., Maeda, S., Araki, S., and Shimada, K. (1985). Structure of human prealbumin gene. *J. Biol. Chem.* **260**, 12224–12227.

Thyroid-Stimulating Hormone (TSH)

H. MIRCESCU, J. C. GOFFART, AND J. E. DUMONT
Université Libre de Bruxelles

I. PHYSIOLOGICAL EFFECTS OF THYROID-STIMULATING HORMONE
II. BIOCHEMISTRY OF TSH ACTION: THE THYROTROPIN RECEPTOR
III. BIOCHEMISTRY OF TSH ACTION: TSH RECEPTOR-ACTIVATED CASCADES
IV. THYROTROPIN CONTROL OF THYROID GROWTH
V. THYROTROPIN ACTION IN DISEASE

The subject of this article is the action of thyroid-stimulating hormone (TSH) on the thyroid gland. The main function of the thyroid gland is the synthesis and secretion of thyroid hormones. These hormones are necessary for body and brain development in the fetus and in the child. Throughout the lifetime of an individual, they set the level of metabolism of the body and its various organs. Thyroid gland function and growth are essentially controlled by two major physiological systems: TSH from the hypophysis and iodide from the diet. The first system functions as a thermostat maintaining the serum levels of thyroid hormones at a constant level by negative feedback regulation. Thyroid hormones negatively control the synthesis and secretion of TSH by specialized cells of the anterior pituitary lobe: the thyrotrophs. TSH stimulates the function and growth of the thyroid. Serum iodide, the main precursor of thyroid hormones, negatively controls the thyroid, ensuring that the gland becomes more efficient when the supply of its substrate in the diet declines. TSH stimulates by various mechanisms all steps of iodine metabolism and thyroid hormone synthesis and secretion by the gland. On a chronic basis, it exerts trophic control of the gland, maintaining or increasing its size, i.e., the number of cells it contains in relation to the long-term level of serum thyroid hormones.

I. PHYSIOLOGICAL EFFECTS OF THYROID-STIMULATING HORMONE

Thyroid-stimulating hormone (TSH) exerts two types of effects on the thyroid gland (see Fig. 1). When

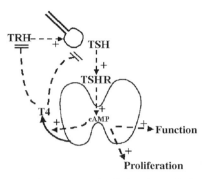

FIGURE 1 Pituitary control of the thyroid through TSH. TSHR, TSH receptor; TRH, TSH-releasing hormone; cAMP, 3′-5′ cyclic AMP.

administered acutely, it stimulates within minutes or hours thyroid hormone synthesis and secretion; in addition, its tonic level controls the growth and proliferation of the thyrocytes (see Fig. 2). The synthesis of thyroid hormones takes place at the apex of the thyrocyte, which faces a closed lumen: the follicular lumen. Synthesis requires (1) at the base of the cell, the trapping of iodide from the extracellular fluid by the Na^+/I^- symporter (NIS); (2) at the apex of the cell, the export of iodide from the cell to the lumen through specialized channels; (3) the synthesis of a very large protein, thyroglobulin (MW 680,000), which will serve as a matrix for the synthesis of thyroid hormones; (4) the export by exocytosis of thyroglobulin in the lumen; (5) the generation of H_2O_2 by a specialized enzyme, THOX (thyroid H_2O_2-generating system); (6) the oxidation of iodide and its covalent linkage to the tyrosines of thyroglobulin by thyroperoxidase using H_2O_2 as oxidizing cofactor; (7) the coupling in iodothyronines [thyroxine (T4), triiodothyronine (T3)] of iodotyrosyls of thyroglobulin by thyroperoxidase. Iodide channels, THOX, and thyroperoxidase are all located in the apical membrane of the cell.

Secretion also takes place at the apex of the cell. It involves the endocytosis of lumenal thyroglobulin, its hydrolysis in secondary lysosomes, and the secretion by an unknown mechanism of the iodothyronines released from thyroglobulin. Endocytosis may involve the bulk endocytosis of thyroglobulin by macropinocytosis or micropinocytosis with selective binding of thyroglobulin by protein acceptors, such as megalin and asialoglycoprotein, and its subsequent uptake (Fig. 3).

TSH stimulates within minutes several steps of synthesis and secretion: iodide efflux in the follicular lumen, H_2O_2 generation and thyroglobulin iodination, iodotyrosine coupling, and the uptake of thyroglobulin by macropinocytosis and therefore secretion. Iodide transport at the base of the cell is regulated by the level of the transporter NIS: its synthesis in significant amounts in response to TSH requires an effect at the level of gene transcription and therefore requires several hours.

Other effects on transcription supplement the acute effects of TSH: thus, TSH enhances the synthesis of thyroperoxidase and, in some species, of THOX and thyroglobulin. The latter effects represent the functional counterpart of the differentiating effects of TSH in thyroid cell cultures. In such cultures, stimulation of the cells by growth factors such as EGF (epidermal growth factor), hepatocyte growth factor, or phorbol esters induces proliferation and the loss of thyroid-specific gene expression, i.e., of differentiation. TSH re-induces such expression; it has a differentiating action. Such effects, involving changes in the pattern of transcription, require several hours.

In vivo or *in vitro*, if administered for at least 24 h and at a high enough level, TSH also induces thyroid cell proliferation and consequently thyroid growth. Due to the negative feedback regulation of thyroid hormones on TSH secretion, any treatment decreasing thyroid hormone secretion by inhibiting its synthesis, such as anti-thyroid drugs or iodine deficiency, will thus lead to thyroid enlargement, i.e., goiter.

Although it promotes the growth and differentiation of thyrocytes, TSH is not necessary for these developments in the fetus. Decapitated fetuses or fetuses lacking TSH develop a normal thyroid, although the growth of this thyroid will be slowed in the second part of pregnancy. By far, the most important effect of TSH in the fetus is the induction of NIS and therefore of iodide transport.

II. BIOCHEMISTRY OF TSH ACTION: THE THYROTROPIN RECEPTOR

Thyrotropin (7000 MW) is a heterodimer of an α-subunit, common to follicle-stimulating hormone,

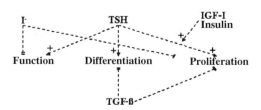

FIGURE 2 Effects of extracellular signals on human thyroid follicular cells.

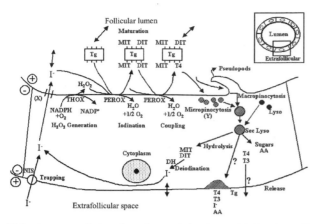

FIGURE 3 Cellular physiology of the thyroid follicular cell. AA, amino acids; DH, iodotyrosine dehalogenase; DIT, diiodotyrosine; MIT, monoiodotyrosine; NIS, Na^+/I^- symporter; PEROX, thyroid peroxidase; Tg, thyroglobulin; T4, thyroxine; THOX, thyroid H_2O_2-generating system; X, iodide apical channel; Y, acceptor involved in thyroglobulin uptake.

luteinizing hormone, and TSH, and a β-subunit specific to TSH. This glycoprotein is synthesized and secreted by the pituitary thyrotrophs. It is specifically recognized by a seven-transmembrane receptor expressed only in thyrocytes and, in some species, in some preadipocytes and adipocytes. The TSH receptor links the thyroid with its controlling system; i.e., it is its connection with the physiology of the cell. The TSH receptor is a classical seven-transmembrane receptor. It is a linear sequence of 764 amino acids from the exterior N-terminal to the interior C-terminal. Its external part contains 419 amino acids. Its doughnut-shaped structure recognizes and accommodates TSH. The membrane part of the receptor contains seven transmembrane α-helical segments, three extracellular loops, and three intracellular loops. The intracellular loops, especially the third loop, but also the second loop and the intercellular C-terminal, presumably interact with their GTP-binding protein effectors. The binding of TSH to the extracellular N-terminal induced a conformational change of the intramembrane part— a shift in the position of the α-helices—thus opening the intracellular loops for the effector GTP-binding proteins. The extracellular part of the receptor acts as an inhibitory domain, switching when bound to TSH from a negative to a positive regulator on GTP-binding proteins G_s, G_q, and G_i (Fig. 4).

The TSH receptor activates at least three effectors: the GTP-binding proteins G_s, G_q, and G_i. G_s itself activates adenylate cyclases, which generate cyclic AMP from ATP. G_q activates phospholipase C β,

which generates from phosphatidylinositol 3,5-phosphate the intracellular signals inositol 1,5-phosphate and diacylglycerol. G_i inhibits adenylate cyclases and through its βγ-subunits may affect other signal transduction proteins. Although the TSH receptor is able to activate both G_s and G_q, in some species such as dog it effectively activates only G_s. In human thyroid cells, it stimulates G_s and G_q and therefore stimulates two regulatory cascades: the cyclic AMP and the phospholipase C pathways.

III. BIOCHEMISTRY OF TSH ACTION: TSH RECEPTOR-ACTIVATED CASCADES

Like other hormones, the TSH receptor exerts its effects through two biochemical cascades: the cyclic AMP pathway and the phospholipase C inositol–1,4,5-phosphate and diacylglycerol pathway.

The human thyroid cell generates cyclic AMP through adenylate cyclases III, VI, and IX. cAMP then binds to and activates at least two effector proteins: the two isoforms of protein kinase A (cyclic AMP-dependent protein kinase), which modulate the activity of target proteins through phosphorylation, and EPAC protein, a guanyl nucleotide exchanger protein that activates the small G-proteins Rap1 and Rap2, which modulate other proteins themselves. Until recently, only protein kinase A was considered, although only a few substrates have been identified in thyroid. One of these, CREB (Ca^{2+}/cAMP-response element-binding protein), is a transcription factor that is activated by phosphorylation, which might account for some transcriptional effects of cAMP. The role of the Rap activator is still unknown. Although most effects of TSH and its mediator of cAMP are currently ascribed to the action of PKA, it is surprising that, in fact, as the availability of more or less specific PKA inhibitors has followed the study of cAMP effects, such a role of PKA has only rarely been investigated.

In the human thyroid, TSH activates phospholipase C β and thus releases two intracellular signal molecules: diacylglycerol and inositol 1,4,5-trisphosphate (IP_3). This effect requires higher concentrations of TSH than the stimulation of adenylate cyclase. The role of diacylglycerol is to stimulate protein kinase C (PKC). This role can be inferred from the effects of phorbol esters, which behave as nonhydrolyzable analogues of diacylglycerol. Thus, the activation of PKC leads to the stimulation of H_2O_2 generation, protein iodination, and thyroid hormone synthesis. IP_3, on the other hand, presumably, as in other cells activates the release of Ca^{2+} stored in the endoplasmic

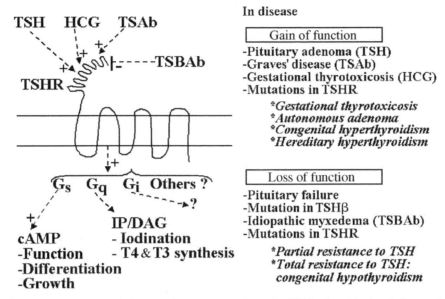

FIGURE 4 The TSH receptor. HCG, human chorionic gonadotropin; TSAb, thyroid-stimulating antibodies; TSBAb, thyroid stimulation-blocking antibodies; G_s, G_q, G_i, GTP-binding proteins mediating the activation (G_s) or inhibition (G_i) of adenylate cyclase and the activation of phospholipase (G_q).

reticulum, leading to an increased influx of extracellular calcium in the cell. Such effects of IP$_3$ would account for the known effects of TSH on thyrocyte calcium metabolism. Free intracellular calcium in its turn, presumably mainly through calmodulin, activates a variety of enzymes in cascade. The main physiological effect of this cascade is the activation of H_2O_2 generation and consequently of protein iodination and iodothyronine synthesis. Thus, through both arms of the phospholipase C cascade, TSH stimulates these processes; cyclic AMP, in contrast, inhibits them. These effects take place within minutes.

TSH stimulates to various extents the expression of the genes corresponding to specific thyroid proteins. These effects are mediated mostly by cyclic AMP and presumably by protein kinase A phosphorylation of various transcription factors of the CREB, cAMP response element modulator (CREM), and activator protein-1 families. Thyroid-specific transcription factors (Pax8, paired box gene 8; TTF1 and TTF2, thyroid transcription factors 1 and 2) are necessary for these syntheses but their function is not regulated directly by TSH or cyclic AMP. The induction of thyroglobulin and NIS mRNA expression requires an intermediary protein synthesis, but the induction of thyroperoxidase does not. Although the expression of NIS and TPO is greatly enhanced by TSH, that of thyroglobulin is not, but it is decreased in the absence of normal TSH levels. Of course, in time, *in vivo*, the synthesis of most proteins is increased, reflecting the growth of the cell. General protein synthesis is increased in thyroid cells by insulin and insulin-like growth factor-I (IGF-I) acting mostly through the IGF-I receptor. The synthesis of most thyroid-specific proteins is decreased by growth factors such as EGF, reflecting the dedifferentiating action of these factors.

IV. THYROTROPIN CONTROL OF THYROID GROWTH

Thyrotropin exerts a positive control on thyroid growth *in vivo*. In its absence, either because of a pituitary disease or because of a treatment with thyroid hormone, the gland becomes hypoplastic, with a decrease in the number and the size of the thyrocytes. Conversely, excess thyrotropin causes the hypertrophy of the thyroid, i.e., goiter. Inactivating or activating mutations of the TSH receptor similarly lead to thyroid atrophy or goiter. Antibodies blocking or activating the receptor have similar effects. The mechanism of the growth effect of thyrotropin has been studied *in vitro*. It corresponds to a DNA-synthesizing and mitogenic activity. It is mediated by cyclic AMP and can be mimicked by agents increasing intracellular cyclic AMP levels such as forskolin. It requires the activation of protein kinase A but this activation is not sufficient to trigger it. The role of EPAC and Rap in this action is under study. The effect of thyrotropin requires the action of IGF-I on its receptor. The respective roles of TSH and IGF-I can be summarized as follows: IGF-I provides the necessary cyclins for the cyclin–cyclin-dependent kinase complexes, which relieve the inhibition by retinoblastoma (RB) proteins of DNA synthesis; TSH, through cyclic AMP, activates these complexes.

Although thyrotropin growth-promoting action is the main controlling factor of thyroid size after birth, it is not required for thyroid differentiation and development in early fetal life. The thyroid differentiates, migrates to its normal location, and develops, albeit to a lesser extent, in the absence of the hypophysis or when the TSH receptor is inactivated.

V. THYROTROPIN ACTION IN DISEASE

Different diseases cause abnormalities in thyrotropin action. Lack of thyrotropin action through decreased thyrotropin synthesis or secretion occurs in various pituitary diseases through congenital hypopituitarism, a defect in TSH synthesis, or pituitary destruction by an adenoma. Inactivating defects of the TSH receptor have similar effects. In all of these cases, the thyroid becomes inactive, thus causing a decrease in thyroid hormone secretion and hypothyroidism and causing atrophy of the thyroid.

Conversely, hyperstimulation of the TSH by excessive pituitary secretion, by stimulating antibodies, or by congenital activating mutations of the TSH receptor causes hyperthyroidism and goiter.

Somatic activating mutations of the TSH receptor generate a hyperactive adenoma that, because of its excessive thyroid hormone secretion, will depress TSH blood levels and induce the quiescence of the unaffected thyroid cells.

Antibodies to the TSH receptor, depending on whether their action is stimulatory or inhibitory, will cause similar diseases: Graves' disease and hyperthyroidism with the thyroid-stimulating antibodies and hypothyroidism with the thyroid stimulation-blocking antibodies.

Glossary

NIS Na$^+$/I$^-$ symporter that actively transports three Na$^+$ ions for two iodide ions.

See Also the Following Articles

Environmental Disruptors of Thyroid Hormone Action • Iodine: Symporter and Oxidation, Thyroid Hormone Biosynthesis • Parathyroid Hormone • Thyroid and Reproduction • Thyroid Hormone Action on the Heart and Cardiovascular System • Thyroid Hormone Action on the Skeleton and Growth • Thyroid Hormone Receptor Isoforms • Thyroid Hormone Receptor, TSH and TSH Receptor Mutations • Thyrotropin-Releasing Hormone (TRH) • Thyroid Hormone Transport Proteins

Further Reading

Dremier, S., Coppee, F., Delange, F., Vassart, G., Dumont, J. E., and Van Sande, J. (1996). Clinical review 84. Thyroid autonomy: Mechanism and clinical effects. *J. Clin. Endocrinol. Metab.* **81**, 4187–4193.

Dumont, J. E., Lamy, F., Roger, P., and Maenhaut, C. (1992). Physiological and pathological regulation of thyroid cell proliferation and differentiation by thyrotropin and other factors. *Physiol. Rev.* **72**, 667–697.

Dumont, J. E. (2002). Ontogeny, Anatomy, Metabolism and Physiology. Available at www.Thyroidmanager.org (L. DeGroot, ed.). Endocrine Education, South Dartmouth, MA.

Dumont, J. E., Vassart, G., and Refetoff, S. (1989). Thyroid disorders. In "The Metabolic Basis of Inherited Disease" (C. R. Scriver, A. L. Beaudet, W. S. Sly, and D. Valle, eds.), 7th ed., Vol. II, Chap. 73, pp. 1843–1879.

Kimura, T., Van keymeulen, A., Golstein, J., Fusco, A., Dumont, J. E., and Roger, P. P. (2001). Regulation of thyroid cell proliferation by TSH and other factors: A critical evaluation of in vitro models. *Endocr. Rev.* Oct. **22**(5), 631–656.

Van Sande, J., Parma, J., Tonacchera, M., Swillens, S., Dumont, J., and Vassart, G. (1995). Genetic basis of endocrine disease. Somatic and germline mutations of the TSH receptor gene in thyroid diseases. *J. Clin. Endocrinol. Metab.* **80**, 2577–2585.

Vassart, G. (2002). Diseases Caused by Defects in TSH Receptors. Available at www.Thyroidmanager.org (L. DeGroot, ed.). Endocrine Education, South Dartmouth, MA.

Vassart, G., and Dumont, J. E. (1992). The thyrotropin receptor and the regulation of thyrocyte function and growth. *Endocr. Rev.* **13**, 596–611.

Thyrotropin Receptor Signaling

LEONARD D. KOHN[*] AND MINHO SHONG[†]

[*]*Edison Biotechnology Institute and Ohio University* • [†]*Chungnam National University, Korea*

I. INTRODUCTION
II. THE TSH RECEPTOR—STARTING POINT OF SIGNAL GENERATION
III. THE SIGNALS THEMSELVES
IV. TSHR SIGNALING AND TRANSCRIPTIONAL CONTROL OF GENE EXPRESSION
V. FEEDBACK CONTROL OF TSHR SIGNALING

The functional role of the thyroid is to synthesize and secrete the thyroid hormones necessary for the normal metabolic homeostasis of every cell

in the human body. This process is under the primary control of the pituitary glycoprotein hormone, thyrotropin (TSH), but requires the coordination of multiple genes and the activities of multiple gene products. This article explains the interaction of TSH with its receptor to govern thyroid gland growth and function.

I. INTRODUCTION

In addition to stimulating the synthesis and secretion of thyroid hormones, thyroid-stimulating hormone (TSH) regulates thyroid cell function and growth. TSH acts via a single molecular entity on the surface of the cell, the TSH receptor (TSHR). TSH interacting with this receptor accomplishes its complex array of duties by using a multiplicity of signals that are coordinated with the signals of other receptors, in particular, the insulin/insulin-like growth factor-I (IGF-I) signal system.

The thyroid is composed of a multiplicity of follicles, wherein thyrocytes surround a central lumen. Each follicle is surrounded by a vascular network that imports and exports raw materials or product from the thyrocyte and follicle. The primary function of the thyroid is to synthesize thyroglobulin (TG), the thyroid hormone precursor; the TSHR signal transduction system is devoted to its synthesis, storage, iodination, and degradation.

Humans ingest iodide, the key component of thyroid hormones, in episodic bursts. TSH/TSHR, by its control of the sodium iodide symporter (NIS), regulates the ability of ingested iodide to be scavenged from the bloodstream and concentrated within the thyrocytes surrounding the follicular lumen. TSH/ TSHR is involved in iodide transport and secretion into the follicular lumen; Pendrin is one porter now known to be important for this process. TG, to which the iodide is coupled and on which iodotyrosine residues are converted to thyroid hormones, is synthesized, glycosylated, phosphorylated, and vectorially transported to the follicular lumen. Thyroid peroxidase (TPO), which is necessary to iodinate the TG and couple iodotyrosine residues to form thyroid hormones, is synthesized, inserted into the apical membrane facing the follicular lumen, and coupled to a system to generate the hydrogen peroxide necessary for the TPO-dependent iodination process. The iodinated TG is stored and then transported to the lysosome where it is degraded to form thyroid hormones. The thyroid hormones are finally secreted into the bloodstream both to maintain a steady-state level necessary to achieve normal homeostasis and to respond in stress situations. These processes are not synchronized, since the thyroid follicles are functionally heterogeneous. The TSHR and its signaling process control and coordinate all of these steps by regulating gene expression, by posttranslational activation of genes, and by inducing morphologic changes in the cell important for TG degradation and thyroid hormone release.

The TSHR also controls the growth of the thyrocytes. In this case, it is now clear that TSH/ TSHR signaling is a preconditioning prelude for insulin, IGF-I, and possibly other growth factors to cause cell cycle progression. Moreover, TSH/TSHR signaling exerts a negative control on major histocompatibility (MHC) and intracellular adhesion molecule 1 gene expression to preserve self-tolerance. This is necessary to avoid an autoimmune response when TSHR-induced positive regulatory signals increase the multiplicity of genes and gene products needed for growth and function.

The concept that all of this is accomplished by a single signal transduction system, the adenylate cyclase system, and a single signaling molecule, cyclic AMP (cAMP), has been eliminated. Although some clinicians may still consider this signal the sole cause of Graves' hyperthyroidism and goiter. Graves' disease is caused by autoantibodies to the TSHR that cause its signal generation system to function excessively.

II. THE TSH RECEPTOR—STARTING POINT OF SIGNAL GENERATION

The TSH receptor is a member of the G-protein-coupled family of receptors with seven transmembrane domains. The receptor has two parts (Fig. 1), a long hydrophilic region that binds TSH followed by a region with seven hydrophobic, membrane-spanning domains, similar in sequence to other G-protein-coupled receptors and its sister receptors, the lutropin/chorionic gonadotropin receptor (LH/CGR) and follicle-stimulating hormone receptor (FSHR). Unlike many receptors in this family that couple to a single G-proteins, i.e., the α- or β-adrenergic receptors, TSHR, LH/CGR, and FSHR couple to more than one G-protein, thereby activating both the phosphatidylinositol 4,5-biphosphate (PIP$_2$) and cAMP cascades (Fig. 1).

The TSHR hydrophilic extracellular domain is longer than that of the LH/CGR or FSHR by approximately 60 residues (Fig. 1). These are located in a long ≥ 50-residue insert in the region of residues 300–400 of the TSHR and a short insert involving

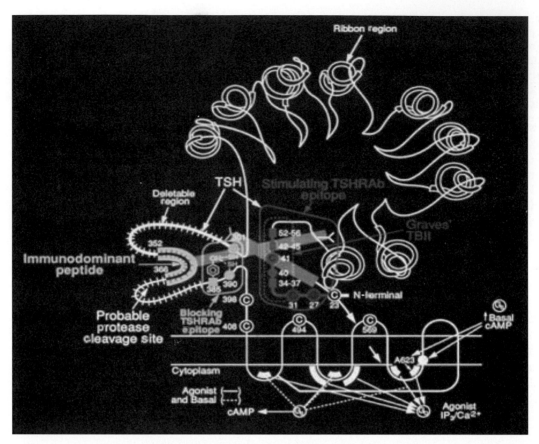

FIGURE 1 Putative model of TSHR. Determinants for blocking TSHR Abs and stimulating TSHR Abs are approximated to make up the TSH site. The former are implicated in high-affinity TSH binding and in the expression of disease by patients with idiopathic myxedema and hypothyroidism. The latter are implicated in patients with Graves' disease and hyperthyroidism. The loop between residues 303 and 382 is separated from the remainder of the external domain, since residues within it can be deleted with no loss in receptor function. This loop includes residues 352–366, which constitute the immunogenic peptide used to produce a specific antibody to the receptor. The hatched lines denote the regions of the receptor in close approximation based on antibody-peptide inhibition studies and by studies of TSHR relationships with the LH/CGR. The first, second, and third intracytoplasmic loops, particularly Ala-623 and the N- and C-terminal 5 residues of the third loop, are identified as the critical link for hormone and TSHR Ab coupling to G_q and the PIP_2 cascade. All loops interact with G_s to regulate constitutive or basal cAMP levels. The middle of the second cytoplasmic loop is coupled to agonist-increased cAMP signaling via G_s.

residues 38–47 (Fig. 1). The former region can be deleted with little loss of TSHR signaling; modification of the latter causes a loss in signal generation. TSH binds to multiple parts of this extracellular domain; however, the high-affinity binding site has important residues between residues 280 and 400. Binding to the extracellular domain perturbs the transmembrane domain where the signal is generated and induces a conformational change that converts the receptor to its agonist state.

TSHR residues 8–165 can be replaced by the equivalent N-terminal portion of the LH/CGR with no significant loss of TSHR signal generation; in contrast, stimulating TSHR autoantibodies from patients with Graves' disease largely lose their ability to increase cAMP levels or activate the $PIP_2/Ca^{2+}/$ arachidonate signal system. The residues in this region that are important for coupling to the cAMP and $PIP_2/Ca^{2+}/$arachidonate signals appear to be different; critical sites linked to cAMP signaling lie predominantly between residues 90 and 165, whereas several residues important for the $PIP_2/Ca^{2+}/$ arachidonate signal lie in the region between residues 30 and 90. The probability is that the two regions on the N-terminus, residues 30–60 and 90–165, act together in a conformational epitope, approximating helices and creating the agonist face of the TSH-binding site (Fig. 1).

Like adrenergic receptors (ARs), mutation of each of the extracellular loops of the transmembrane domain results in a loss of TSH-stimulated and TSHR autoantibody activities as a result of a conformational change rather than abnormal receptor synthesis, processing, or incorporation into the bilayer. The short cytoplasmic peptides of the transmembrane domain of the TSHR differ in length, are relatively nonhomologous among receptor types, contain one or more potential phosphorylation sites, and couple to G_q, which signals the PIP_2 cascade, as well G_s, which initiates the cAMP cascade.

Residues in the first, second, and third cytoplasmic loops are important for TSH and Graves' immunoglobulin G (IgG) induction of the PIP_2 signal, but also control constitutive cAMP levels (Fig. 1). Thus, all the first, second, and third cytoplasmic loop mutations affecting agonist-induced signaling also have decreased basal or constitutive cAMP levels and in some cases are hot spots that result in constitutively high basal cAMP signaling, i.e., in a receptor conformation that will bind and activate a G-protein in the absence of ligand. The latter mutations have been associated with functioning adenomas in patients; similar mutations in the LH/CGR are associated with precocious puberty. The middle region of the second cytoplasmic loop, particularly residues 525–527, is involved in agonist-induced G_s coupling, whereas the entire loop is important for agonist-induced G_q coupling.

The amino acid sequence in the second cytoplasmic loop, as an example, is identical in rat, human, and dog TSHR, suggesting that interactions and signals are likely to be applicable to all species of TSHR. The number of residues in the second cytoplasmic loop of TSH and LH/CGR is the same; further, the sequences of LH/CGR or FSHR are 60% identical and most differences are conservative substitutions. This suggests that the second cytoplasmic loop will share common signal transduction/G-protein interactions among the family of receptors. In the second cytoplasmic loop, the number of residues in the TSH, gonadotropin, and adrenergic receptors is the same, but the conformations of TSHR and ARs are very different with respect to helix, extended coil, or β-turn. This may contribute to the ability of the TSHR to couple to both G_s and G_q, whereas AR or muscarinic receptors couple to only one type of G-protein.

Since it is unlikely that G_q and G_s couple simultaneously and since TSHR transfections result in an increased basal cAMP level, it is possible that TSHR transmembrane domains are in a partial agonist conformation in the absence of ligand. Alternatively, there are several TSHR forms, precoupled to G_s, to G_q, or to neither one, and an equilibrium exists among them. Mutations might influence this equilibrium by allowing interactions not usually evident in the absence of ligand; they might also alter the affinity of each for G_s or G_q. This might explain curvilinear TSH-binding isotherms, i.e., high- and low-affinity binding sites, with low and high capacities, respectively. This also might explain why different concentrations of TSH are necessary to induce the cAMP and PIP_2 signals *in vitro*; i.e., the cAMP signal is linked to a high-affinity G_s-coupled TSHR form, whereas the PIP_2 signal is linked to a low-affinity G_q-coupled form.

The P_1 purinergic receptor regulates TSH and Graves' IgG induction of the cAMP and PIP_2 signals; P_1 purinergic agonists (phenylisopropyladenosine, PIA) inhibit TSHR-induced cAMP production but enhance inositol phosphate formation, despite the fact that they have little direct effect on either signal. The effect of PIA is mediated by a pertussis toxin-sensitive G-protein (G_i). The ability of TSH to modulate the cAMP signal system has also been related to pertussis toxin-sensitive ADP ribosylation of a G_i family member.

III. THE SIGNALS THEMSELVES

A. Adenylate Cyclase–cAMP Signal

A close correlation exists between TSH binding and stimulation of the adenylate cyclase/cAMP signal. It induces TG, TPO, and NIS gene expression and is important in their posttranslational activation. This dual role is exemplified by NIS, where there is a clear-cut dichotomy between gene induction (RNA levels), protein, and iodide uptake (function). Little is still known about the mechanism by which TSH activates Pax-8, the critical transcription factor that regulates NIS gene expression, or about the mechanism by which TSH activates the NIS protein. Pax-8 is the homeoprotein encoded by the PAX-8 gene, a member of the HOX network of transcription factors. Recent work suggests that cAMP modulation of redox potential is important for the activation of Pax-8 and that cAMP-modulated protein phosphorylation is important for protein activation.

The increase in cAMP activates protein kinase A. More than one form of protein kinase A exists. These differ in their regulatory subunits and in thyrocytes from different species, perhaps contributing to signal differences. Despite overwhelming evidence that kinase A mediates cAMP activity and despite the identification of a multiplicity of phosphorylated proteins resulting from the TSH/TSHR/cAMP signal, a cohesive view remains an enigma.

TSH-increased cAMP has been linked to thyroid cell growth, and cAMP is a necessary but insufficient signal. Thus, in the absence of insulin/IGF-I, TSH increases cAMP perfectly well but does not induce growth. TSH was found to be a preconditioner for insulin/IGF-I regulation of cell cycle progression; the insulin/IGF-I effect is, at the least, related to the action of Akt or PKB, a downstream kinase of the insulin signaling system.

TSH/TSHR and cAMP, together with insulin/IGF-I, increase 3-hydroxy-3-methylglutaryl coenzyme A (HMG-CoA) reductase, thereby increasing the formation of gerranylgerranyl phosphate. This eliminates p27Kip1 by accelerating its degradation; cyclin-dependent kinase 2 is activated, causing the cyclin cascade to proceed, and S6 kinase 1 (S6K1) is activated. Rho proteins necessary for S-phase development are also gerranylated and translocated to membranes during $G_{1/S}$ progression. The effect of gerranylgerranyl pyrophosphate is abolished with botulinum C3 exoenzyme, which specifically ADP ribosylates Rho proteins. The connection of TSHR/cAMP signaling to phosphatidylinositol 3-kinase (PI3K), phosphoinositide-dependent kinase 1 (PDK1), and insulin/IGF-I-coordinated actions to increase S6 kinase activity is increasingly clear (Fig. 2).

TSH/TSHR/cAMP signaling causes morphologic changes in cells. The signals induce pseudopod and microvilli formation on the apical membrane adjacent to the follicular lumen and initiate the fluid pinocytosis process whereby colloid containing TG is engulfed and taken into the cell to lysosomes for degradation. They initiate the secretion process as lysosomes that had moved to the apical membrane to fuse with the pinocytotic vesicles return toward the basal membrane while digesting the TG and converting it to amino acids. Contractile and cytoskeleton proteins are altered during this process. Increased membrane fluidity needed for these processes may derive from TSHR/cAMP signaling inducing HMG CoA reductase to produce cholesterol, not simply gerranylgerranyl phosphate.

B. PIP_2/Ca^{2+}/Arachidonate Signaling

TSH stimulates the hydrolysis of PIP_2 by phospholipase C. The best characterized functional effect of this signal is on iodide efflux from the apical membrane and H_2O_2 generation important for TPO activity, iodination of TG, and iodotyrosine coupling.

The importance of this pathway in thyrocyte growth is recognized clinically. Thus, two populations of TSHR antibody (Ab)-stimulating autoantibodies exist, one increasing cAMP levels and the second increasing PIP_2/Ca^{2+}/arachidonate signaling. The two together maximally increase growth and are associated with the largest goiters.

Only approximately 50% of TSH-increased cytosolic Ca^{2+} levels is phospholipase C-dependent; the remaining 50% is linked to phospholipase A2 activation. Phospholipase A2 produces arachidonic acid; cyclooxygenase-, lipoxegenase-, and expoxygenase-derived metabolites of arachidonic acid are important end products regulating cell activity, i.e., prostaglandins and leukotrienes.

Currently, the importance of this pathway focuses on TSH-regulated hydrolysis of phosphatidylinositol 3,4-bisphosphate and phosphatidylinositol 3,4,5-trisphosphate and phosphatidylinositol 3,4-biophosphate and phosphatidylinositol 3,4,5-triphosphate. The complexity of the effects of TSH action and its connection to insulin/IGF-I regulated Akt (PKB) is illustrated in a report by Rameh and Cantley (1999).

C. PI3K Signaling

Recently, pituitary glycoprotein hormone receptors, including the TSHR, have been shown to activate PI3K-dependent signaling pathways to regulate the growth of target endocrine glands. Signaling in thyrocytes is TSHR-specific, is mediated by the cAMP signal, and involves the p85 subunit of PI3K that is bound to the TSHR as well as G_s (Fig. 2). PDK1 is a major regulator for transmitting PI3K-dependent signaling pathways to downstream kinases, such as Akt/PKB and S6K1, in response to TSH and insulin/IGF-I in thyroid cells (Fig. 2). TSH preferentially activates S6K1 signaling pathways compared to Akt/PKB in thyroid cells (Fig. 2). However, insulin independently activates two PDK1 downstream signaling pathways, Akt/PKB and S6K1, thus exhibiting synergistic actions with TSH on S6K1 activation (Fig. 2). The inhibition of S6K1 by rapamycin results in inhibition of $G_{1/S}$ cell cycle progression by TSH/insulin *in vitro*. S6K1 is also involved in the regulation of thyroid follicle activity, for example, uptake of colloid, which is regulated by endogenous TSH *in vivo*.

D. Other Signals

TSH/TSHR-increased ADP ribosylation is not mediated by cAMP and has been related to modulation of G_s. Thus, the cholera toxin subunit has an intrinsic ADP-ribosyltransferase activity that

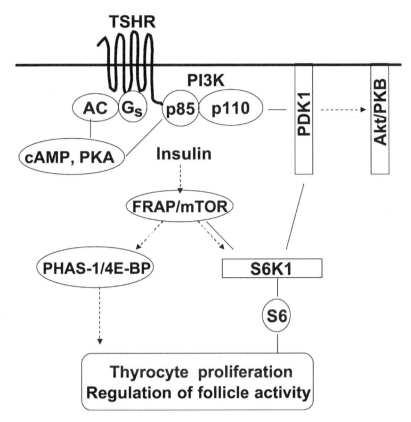

FIGURE 2 TSHR and PI3K signaling: involvement of PDK1 and link to insulin/Akt. TSHR is associated with the p85 regulatory subunit of PI3K and its PI3K activity is induced by TSH and cAMP. TSH is able to translocate PDK1 into the plasma membrane and PDK1 preferentially phosphorylates S6K1, but not Akt/PKB. However, insulin phosphorylates Akt/ PKB and PHAS-1/4E-BP1 in a PI3K- and FRAP/mTOR-dependent manner. Rapamycin inhibits the cooperative actions of PHAS-1/4E-BP1 and S6K1 and results in the inhibition of TSH-mediated follicle proliferation and activity. The solid lines represent the pathways preferentially activated by TSH and the dashed lines represent pathways activated by insulin but not by TSH in thyroid cells. PHAS-1, the small, heat- and acid-stable protein 4E-BPI; FRAP, flouride-resistant acid phosphates; mTOR, mammalian target of rapamycin.

ADP-ribosylates G_s, altering ATP/ATP hydrolysis and binding, and shifting G_s to a "permanently activated" state. TSH activates a membrane ADP-ribosyltransferase imputed to act similarly and activates a deribosylating enzyme. Little is known about the significance of this potential signal. TSH/TSHR can regulate the membrane electrical potential and pH gradient via a non-cAMP mechanism. It does not seem to involve ion flux mechanisms exhibited by prototypical seven-transmembrane domain receptors such as rhodopsin.

E. Signaling Crosstalk

Phorbol esters mimic or potentiate TSHR effects. There is clear feedback regulation between the cAMP and PIP_2 signal systems in FRTL-5 cells and transgenic animals. Catecholamines and β_1-adrenergic agents modulate TSHR signal transduction via cAMP. However, perhaps the least recognized yet most important receptor signal system able to regulate TSHR signaling is the transforming growth factor-β (TGF-β) signal.

TGF-β up-regulates upstream stimulatory factors (USF). As will be noted below, USF transcription factor sites are directly competitive with Pax-8 sites and reverse TSHR/ cAMP signal transduction by competing for Pax-8 binding, most notably on the NIS promoter. However, USF sites exist on TG, TPO, and the TSHR. TGF-β-induced Smad signaling can regulate TTF-1 action. Smad/TTF-1 complexes up-regulate Pendrin gene expression.

Basic fibroblast growth factor (bFGF) decreases TSHR mRNA levels, cAMP signal generation, and cAMP signal action. Despite this, bFGF increases thyrocyte thymidine incorporation and cell growth.

This appears to be explained by the ability of bFGF to activate the PIP$_2$ signal system, the Ca^{2+} signal, and a novel tyrosine kinase activity that is able to activate the insulin/c-*ras* pathway. It mimics the crosstalk between the TSHR-induced PIP$_2$ and cAMP signal systems.

IV. TSHR SIGNALING AND TRANSCRIPTIONAL CONTROL OF GENE EXPRESSION

A. TG, TPO, and NIS

A fundamental advance in TSHR signaling is dependent on the work of DiLauro and colleagues, who described the importance of tissue-specific thyroid transcription factors in the function of thyrocytes: thyroid transcription factor-1, (TTF-1), TTF-2, and Pax-8 (Fig. 3). TG synthesis is controlled by TTF-1, TTF-2, and Pax-8. Thus, there are three TTF-1 sites within the minimal promoter, A to C, from 5′ to 3′; the C site also binds Pax-8. TSH/TSHR/cAMP decreases TTF-1 gene expression and binding to the three TTF-1 sites but increases Pax-8 expression, phosphorylation, redox potential, and binding. This allows TG synthesis to persist or increase, despite decreases in TSHR, which is controlled by TTF-1 alone. TTF-2 is a forkhead protein controlled by insulin/IGF-I. This allows TG synthesis in the absence

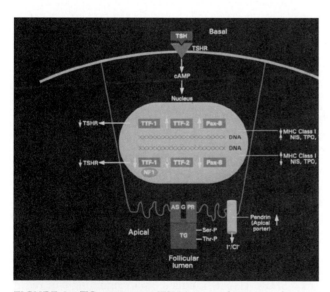

FIGURE 3 TG counteracts TSH-increased Pax-8 and TTF-2 and is additive in suppressing TTF-1. Both TSH and TG therefore decrease TSHR. TSH increases NIS, TPO, and TG, whereas TG suppresses them. TSH decreases MHC class I, whereas TG increases class I as well as the Pendrin gene product. TG activity is mediated by binding to the ASGPR; TG activity is regulated by serine and threonine phosphorylation.

and in the presence of TSH, so TG can accumulate in the follicular lumen to act as an iodide trap.

TPO gene expression is similarly controlled by TSHR/cAMP signaling, TTF-1, TTF-2, and Pax-8. NIS gene expression is predominantly up-regulated by Pax-8, but not TTF-1 or TTF-2. The Pax-8 site contains within it a consensus USF-binding site termed an E-box. USFs are up-regulated and phosphorylated by TGF-β; these compete for Pax-8 binding and down-regulate NIS gene expression, counteracting TSHR/cAMP signals. USF sites also exist in the TPO B site for TTF-1, the TG TTF-1/Pax-8 site, and the downstream but not upstream TSHR TTF-1 site. USF thus plays a role in controlling the TSH/TSHR/cAMP-signaled synthesis of genes important for triiodothyronine (T3) or tetraiodothyronine (T4) formation.

B. TSHR

Signaling by TSHR/TSH/cAMP autoregulates TSHR gene expression. Thus, these signals decrease TSHR gene expression rather than up-regulate it, like TG, TPO, or NIS, because the TSHR has only a TTF-1 site and TSH/TSHR/cAMP decreases TTF-1 gene expression. Thus, gene expression of TSHR is decreased, whereas gene expression of NIS, TPO, and TG is increased because Pax-8 can replace the TTF-1. This may be an important feedback control for TSHR signaling. It is hypothesized that TSH/TSHR/ cAMP decreased TSHR gene expression is important for cell cycle progression; functional genes are expressed followed by growth signals.

C. MHC Genes

MHC class I genes are negatively regulated by the TSHR-mediated cAMP signal. Insulin and IGF-I also are negative regulators of MHC class I gene expression in the thyroid. In the thyroid, hormonal suppression of class I genes appears to be a means of preserving self-tolerance in the face of hormone action to increase the expression of tissue-specific genes such as TG, TPO, and the TSHR. TG, TPO, and the TSHR are the autoantigens associated with autoimmune disease. Inappropriate class I expression in the thyroid, i.e., if induced by interferon, viruses, or some as yet unknown agent, is hypothesized to contribute to the generation of autoimmune disease by the loss of negative regulation.

This hypothesis has been supported by studies showing that TSHR, MHC class I, and MHC class II have common *cis* elements that are regulated by the same transcription factors. Moreover, MHC class I knockouts result in a loss in the ability to induce several autoimmune diseases. Finally, the thesis has been supported by the development of a mouse model of Graves' disease, the Shimojo model, wherein Graves' disease is induced by immunizing mice that have normal immune systems with fibroblasts over-expressing MHC class II and TSHR.

The model suggests that Graves' disease is initiated by an insult to the thyrocyte in an individual with a normal immune system. The insult, infectious or otherwise, causes double-stranded DNA or RNA to enter the cytoplasm of the cell. This causes abnormal expression of MHC class I as a dominant feature, but also aberrant expression of MHC class II, as well as changes in genes or gene products needed for the thyrocyte to become an antigen-presenting cell. A critical factor in these changes is the loss of normal TSHR/cAMP-induced negative regulation of MHC class I, MHC class II, and TSHR gene expression, which is necessary to maintain self-tolerance during TSHR-signaled increases in genes involved in growth and function. Self-tolerance of the TSHR is maintained in normals because there is a population of CD8$^+$ cells that normally suppresses a population of CD4$^+$ cells that can interact with the TSHR. This is a host self-defense mechanism that probably leads to autoimmune disease in persons with a specific viral infection or perhaps a genetic predisposition. The model is suggested to be important in explaining the development of other autoimmune diseases including systemic lupus and diabetes.

As noted above, TSHR/cAMP-induced inhibition of constitutive MHC class I gene expression requires the expression of several transcription factors. In addition, TSHR/cAMP inhibits upstream interferon-γ (IFN-γ) signaling pathways, in particular Janus kinase 1 (JAK1). TSH/TSHR-mediated inhibition of JAK1 is caused by TSH-induced suppressor of cytokine signaling-1 (SOCS-1) and SOCS-3. TSH/TSHR-induced SOCSs are negative regulators of IFN-γ-mediated signal transducer and activator of transcription 1 activation in thyroid cells. This TSH/TSHR-induced inhibitory cross talk of IFN-γ may also participate in thyrocyte survival in an autoimmune environment.

V. FEEDBACK CONTROL OF TSHR SIGNALING

As noted above, the synthesis of TG is the primary function of the thyrocyte, since this is the scaffold upon which thyroid hormones are formed. TG is now recognized not to be simply an inert scaffold for T3/T4 formation; it is an important transcriptional regulator of thyroid function and T3/T4 formation (Fig. 3). TG stored in the follicular lumen is a feedback suppressor, counterregulating the actions of TSH, insulin, and IGF-I to up-regulate TG, TPO, NIS, and TSHR gene expression by specific down-regulation of the thyroid-specific transcription factors, TTF-1, TTF-2, and Pax-8. It simultaneously up-regulates the synthesis of the Pendrin gene product, thus maximizing TG iodination in the follicular lumen even in the suppressed state. TG suppression involves binding to the asialoglycoprotein receptor (ASGPR) on the apical membrane of the thyrocyte, which faces the follicular lumen. TG suppresses TTF-1 by decreasing nuclear factor 1 binding to two sites within 200 bp of the transcriptional start site. The feedback regulation process is an important determinant of follicular heterogeneity and up-regulates the MHC class I gene. This has been related to autoimmune phenomena associated with goiters where poorly iodinated TG accumulates.

In vivo evidence supporting these data includes findings that TG binding to the apical surface of thyrocytes facing the follicular lumen suppresses iodide uptake by NIS. TG also suppresses vascular endothelial growth factor (VEGF) gene expression, decreasing vascular permeability and further decreasing iodide uptake.

In a follicle rich in follicular TG, TG would suppress NIS and VEGF/VPF (vascular permeability factor) gene expression, as well as TG and TPO expression and synthesis. In this follicle, TSH would act predominantly to cause resorption and degradation of follicular TG and the secretion of thyroid hormones into the bloodstream. Because TSH-induced resorption/degradation of TG exceeds the rate of TSH-increased synthesis and replacement of TG in the colloid, the TG concentration in the lumen of this follicle will decrease. The decrease in follicular TG releases transcriptional suppression and reinitiates TSH-increased NIS, VEGF/VPF, TG, and TPO gene expression. Pendrin gene expression is maximally induced by a low concentration of TG. The increased vascular permeability, NIS, and Pendrin gene expression will increase iodide uptake; increased TG and TPO will contribute to the synthesis and storage of T3 and T4 most efficiently. When the accumulation of follicular TG reaches a certain level, TG suppression of gene expression would again dominate TSH-stimulated gene expression and the whole process would be repeated.

Glossary

Akt (PKB) Insulin-regulated downstream serine/threonine kinase important in thyroid-stimulating hormone receptor-regulated signaling of growth and function.

Graves' disease Disorder caused by overexpression of thyroid-stimulating hormone receptor (TSHR) signaling, which is induced by TSHR autoantibodies.

major histocompatibility genes Expression in thyroid is regulated by thyroid-stimulating hormone receptor signaling and is important for preserving self-tolerance, i.e., preventing autoimmunity.

Pendrin (PDS gene product) An apical membrane iodide porter controlling iodide export from the thyrocyte into the follicular lumen.

thyroglobulin The primary protein synthesized by thyrocytes; it is both the precursor of thyroid hormone formation and a feedback regulator controlling thyroid-stimulating hormone receptor signaling.

thyroid follicle Structural component of the thyroid, composed of thyrocytes that surround a central lumen and whose function and growth are controlled by thyroid-stimulating hormone receptor signaling.

thyroid peroxidase The enzyme catalyzing the iodination of thyroglobulin and catalyzing the coupling of iodotyrosine residues to form thyroid hormones, whose activity is controlled by thyroid-stimulating hormone receptor signaling.

thyroid transcription factor-1 Thyroid-restricted transcription factor controlling thyroid-specific gene expression, whose levels and activity are controlled by thyroid-stimulating hormone receptor signaling.

thyroid transcription factor-2 Thyroid-restricted transcription factor controlling thyroid-specific gene expression, whose levels and activity are controlled by insulin signaling but which influences thyroid-stimulating hormone receptor signaling.

See Also the Following Articles

Thyroglobulin ● Thyroid Hormone Receptor, TSH and TSH Receptor Mutations ● Thyrotropin-Releasing Hormone (TRH) ● Thyrotropin-Releasing Hormone Receptor Signaling ● Thyroid Stimulating Hormone (TSH)

Further Reading

Chung, J., *et al.* (2000). Thyrotropin modulates interferon-gamma-mediated intercellular adhesion molecule-1 gene expression by inhibiting Janus kinase-1 and signal transducer and activator of transcription-1 activation in thyroid cells. *Endocrinology* **141**, 2090–2097.

Czech, M. (2000). PIP2 and PIP3: Complex roles at the cell surface. *Cell* **100**, 603–606.

Damante, G., and Di Lauro, R. (1994). Thyroid-specific gene expression. *Biochim. Biophys. Acta* **1218**, 255–266.

Dremier, S., *et al.* (2002). The role of cyclic AMP and its effect on protein kinase A in the mitogenic action of thyrotropin on the thyroid cell. *Ann. N. Y. Acad. Sci.* **968**, 106–121.

Dumont, J. E., *et al.* (1990). Transducing systems in the control of human thyroid cell function, proliferation, and differentiation. *In* "Control of the Thyroid: Regulation of Its Normal Growth and Function" (R. Ekholm, L. D. Kohn, S. Wollman, eds.), pp. 357–372. Plenum Press, New York.

Kohn, L. D. (1990). Receptors of the thyroid gland: The thyrotropin receptor is only the first violinist of a symphony orchestra. *In* "Control of the Thyroid: Regulation of Its Normal Growth and Function" (R. Ekholm, L. D. Kohn, and S. Wollman, eds.), pp. 151–210. Plenum Press, New York.

Kohn, L. D. (1995). Antireceptor immunity. *In* "Thyroid Autoimmunity" (D. Rayner and B. Champion, eds.), pp. 115–170. R. G. Landes, Austin/Georgetown, TX.

Kohn, L. D., *et al.* (1995). The Thyrotropin Receptor. *Vitam. Horm.* **50**, 287–384.

Kohn, L. D., *et al.* (2000). Graves' disease: A host defense mechanism gone awry. *Int. Rev. Immunol.* **19**, 633–644.

Park, E. S., *et al.* (2000). Involvement of JAK/STAT (Janus kinase/signal transducer and activator of transcription) in the thyrotropin signaling pathway. *Mol. Endocrinol.* **14**, 440–448.

Rameh, L. E., and Cantley, L. C. (1999). The role of phosphoinositide 3-kinase lipid products in cell function. *J. Biol. Chem.* **274**, 8347–8350.

Suzuki, K., *et al.* (2000). Thyroglobulin autoregulation of thyroid-specific gene expression and follicular function. *In* "Reviews in Endocrine and Metabolic Disorders," (D. Le Roith, ed.), Vol. 1, pp. 217–224. Kluwer Academic, Boston.

Shimojo, N., *et al.* (2000). A novel mouse model of Graves' disease: Implications for a role in aberrant MHC class II expression in its pathogenesis. *Int. Rev. Immunol.* **19**, 619–631.

Suzuki, K., *et al.* (1998). Autoregulation of thyroid-specific gene transcription by thyroglobulin. *Proc. Natl. Acad. Sci. USA* **95**, 8251–8256.

Tomer, Y., and Davies, T. (1993). Infection, thyroid disease, and autoimmunity. *Endocr. Rev.* **14**, 107–121.

Thyrotropin-Releasing Hormone Receptor Signaling

MARVIN C. GERSHENGORN

National Institute of Diabetes and Digestive and Kidney Diseases of the National Institutes of Health, Maryland

  I. INTRODUCTION
  II. THREE-DIMENSIONAL STRUCTURE OF TRH-Rs
 III. TRH-Rs AND G-PROTEINS
 IV. TRH-R AND SIGNAL TRANSDUCTION PATHWAYS
  V. CONSTITUTIVE SIGNALING BY TRH-Rs
 VI. TRH DESENSITIZATION
VII. TRH-R INTERNALIZATION
VIII. SUMMARY

Thyrotropin-releasing hormone signaling occurs primarily, if not exclusively, by binding of the hormone to one of two hormone-specific

receptor subtypes, TRH-R1 and TRH-R2, members of the large superfamily of G-protein-coupled receptors. The primary pathway of signal transduction is mediated by activation of G_q or G_{11} proteins; this, in turn, activates a series of further enzymatic reactions, leading to an increase in $[Ca^{2+}]_i$. The increase in $[Ca^{2+}]_i$ activates Ca^{2+}/calmodulin protein kinase and is further augmented by activation of cell surface membrane channels that allow influx of extracellular Ca^{2+}. One end result of all of these activities is stimulation of hormone secretion and gene transcription in the anterior pituitary.

I. INTRODUCTION

Thyrotropin-releasing hormone (TRH; thyroliberin) is a tripeptide (pyro-glutamyl-histidyl-proline-amide; pyro-Glu-His-Pro-NH₂) that functions as a hormone, a paracrine regulatory factor, and a neurotransmitter/neuromodulator. TRH initiates some, if not all, of these effects by interacting with receptors on cell surfaces. A complementary DNA (cDNA) for a TRH receptor (TRH-R) was initially cloned from mouse pituitary tissue. Using nucleotide sequence information derived from the mouse pituitary receptor, cDNA clones of rat, human, bovine, and chicken TRH-Rs were isolated. There is very high sequence homology in the protein-coding regions of these TRH-Rs. A second subtype of TRH-R was subsequently cloned from rat and then mouse tissue. The two subtypes of TRH-Rs are now referred to as TRH-R1 and TRH-R2. The primary amino acid sequences and the putative two-dimensional topologies of the two mouse TRH-Rs are illustrated in Fig. 1. The two-dimensional topology is based on hydropathy analyses of the receptor proteins and, because TRH-Rs couple primarily to G-proteins (see Section III), on the consensus two-dimensional structure of all G-protein-coupled receptors (GPCRs). The two TRH-Rs are most similar in the transmembrane regions and differ significantly within the extracellular amino terminus and within the intracellular carboxyl terminus (see Section II).

The roles of TRH-Rs in normal physiology are only partly understood. Within the central nervous system, the two TRH-R subtypes exhibit distinct patterns of expression, signaling properties, and regulation, but similar ligand-binding characteristics, thus it is likely that they serve different physiological roles. TRH-R1 is the predominant receptor in the anterior pituitary gland and has a major regulatory role in stimulating thyrotropin (thyroid-stimulating hormone; TSH) synthesis and secretion and, thereby,

plays a central role in thyroid hormone homeostasis. A role for TRH-R1 in regulation of prolactin secretion from the anterior pituitary is less clear. In the central nervous system, in which there is widespread but discrete expression of the two TRH-R subtypes, a number of pharmacological experiments have been performed in which effects of inhibiting or stimulating the TRH/TRH-R systems have been observed. Nevertheless, the physiologic roles of TRH-R1 and TRH-R2 in the central nervous system have not been clearly elucidated.

The emphasis here is on the molecular aspects of cellular signaling by TRH-Rs. The following issues are addressed: TRH-R structure, how TRH binds to TRH-Rs, which coupling proteins initiate TRH-R signaling, which transduction pathways mediate signaling, and what cellular mechanisms regulate TRH-R signaling.

II. THREE-DIMENSIONAL STRUCTURE OF TRH-Rs

To understand the relationship between the three-dimensional structure of a receptor protein at an atomic level of detail and function is a major goal of receptor research. TRH-Rs, like all GPCRs, contain an extracellular amino terminus, three extracellular loops (ECLs), seven transmembrane-spanning helices (TMHs), three intracellular loops (ICLs), and an intracellular carboxyl terminus. A major advance in understanding the structure–function relationships of all GPCRs was made with the resolution of the structure of the inactive state of bovine rhodopsin by X-ray crystallography. Three-dimensional models of mouse TRH-R1 have been constructed based on data from molecular genetic experimental analyses, computer simulations, and the structure of rhodopsin. The model of TRH-R1 in the unliganded (unbound) state attempts to depict the overall structure of the receptor, including the intramolecular atomic interactions that constrain TRH-R in an inactive conformation. The model of TRH-bound TRH-R1 tries to illustrate the interactions between TRH and TRH-R1 that allow for high-affinity binding and, by comparison with the unliganded model, the changes in conformation that the receptor underwent on assuming the active state. These models are used, therefore, to generate hypotheses regarding TRH binding and the mechanism of TRH-R activation.

TRH-R1 is a cylindrical protein that traverses the cell surface membrane seven times, with the amino terminus and three loops outside of the cell membrane, facing the extracellular environment

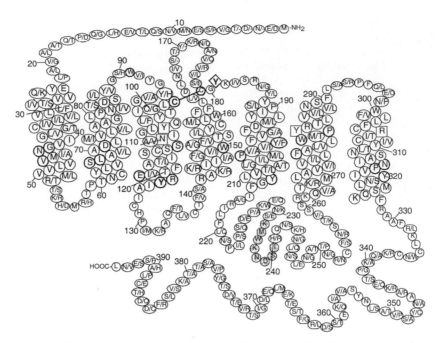

FIGURE 1 Putative two-dimensional topologies of murine TRH-R1 and TRH-R2 sequences. The amino acids are numbered beginning with the first putative residue at the amino terminus. The amino terminus and three extracellular loops are at the top and the three intracellular loops and the carboxyl terminus are at the bottom. The sequences for both receptors (TRH-R1/TRH-R2) are represented by giving within each circle the specific single-letter amino acid symbols for each position; when the amino acid at any position is the same in both receptors, the symbol is given once, and when TRH-R2 does not have a corresponding residue, a hyphen is used (X/-). Residues that are important for binding TRH (see text) are presented within squares.

[i.e., ECL-1-ECL-3: connecting TMHs 2 and 3 (ECL-1), 4 and 5 (ECL-2), and 6 and 7 (ECL-3)], and three loops within the cell [i.e., ICL-1-ICL-3: connecting TMHs 1 and 2 (ICL-1), 3 and 4 (ICL-2), and 5 and 6 (ICL-3)] (Fig. 2). The "core" of the cylinder, which does not form a channel, has projecting into it hydrophilic and hydrophobic residues that form interhelical interactions, which hold the protein in its native conformation. The side chains of specific residues that are found in the core interact directly with TRH. In contrast, positioned on the surface of the cylinder there are principally hydrophobic residues that allow interaction with the lipid environment of the cell surface membrane.

Like binding pockets for small ligands in other GPCRs, the pocket for TRH is within the upper third of the TMH core of the receptor. A computer simulation of TRH-R predicts that there is water in the core of the unliganded receptor. It is noteworthy that evidence has been presented that TRH binds initially to residues in the ECLs of TRH-Rs and then moves through a "channel" formed by the ECLs to gain access to the binding pocket within the TMHs. (The waters that are present in the "channel" are shown in Fig. 2 as the lighter gray spheres.) A number of critical interactions between TRH and residues within the TMH core of the receptor are responsible for high-affinity binding (Fig. 3). These include the hydrogen bond (H-bond) between the C—O of the *pyro*-Glu moiety of TRH and the OH group of Tyr-106 in TMH-3 of TRH-R1; the H-bond between the NH of *pyro*-Glu and the C—O of Asn-110, which is one helical turn below Tyr-106 in TMH-3; the imidazole of the His residue of TRH, in close proximity to Tyr-282 in TMH-6, forming a stacking or hydrophobic interaction; the C—O group of the Pro-NH$_2$, which forms the H-bond with Arg-306 in TMH-7; and the guanidino group of Arg-306, which also forms an H-bond with the backbone C—O of *pyro*-Glu. All of these interactions are important for TRH binding because mutation of any of these residues within the receptor or change by chemical synthesis of any moiety of TRH leads to decreases in binding affinity. It is noteworthy in this regard that of literally hundreds of analogues of TRH that have been synthesized, only one, *pyro*-Glu-[*methyl*]His-Pro-NH$_2$, exhibits a higher affinity for TRH-Rs than does native TRH.

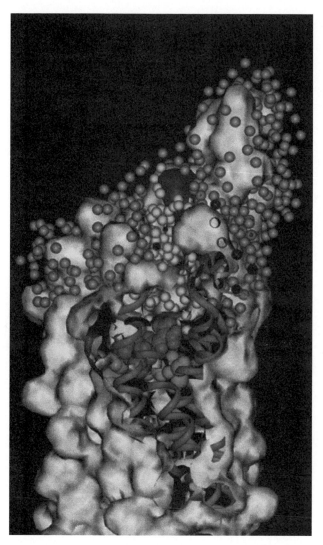

FIGURE 2 Computer-simulated three-dimensional model of mouse TRH-R1. The model was constructed by computational techniques that include the extracellular loops obtained in primary hydration cell simulations (constructed by Avia Rosenhouse-Dantzker and Roman Osman, Mount Sinai School of Medicine). The model is surrounded by a surface to illustrate the path from the initial anchoring site at Tyr-181 into the transmembrane binding pocket defined by Arg-306, Tyr-282, and Tyr-106. The waters used in the primary hydration shell simulations are displayed as dark spheres. The waters that define the path from Tyr-181 into the transmembrane binding pocket are the lighter spheres.

Although TRH-R1 and TRH-R2 differ at approximately 30% of amino acid residues within the most conserved domains of the TMHs, all of the residues just described that appear to interact directly with TRH are present at the same positions within both receptor subtypes. It is, therefore, not surprising that a series of TRH analogues that differ from one another at all three amino acids of the tripeptide have been shown to bind to both receptors with similar hierarchies of affinities.

The conformational changes within the receptor that constitute activation of TRH-Rs are not known. Because the TRH binding pocket appears to be present in the extracellular third of the TMH bundle, it is assumed that the conformational changes in the TMHs that occur on agonist binding secondarily affect the G-protein-coupling domains on the cytoplasmic surface of the receptor protein. It is probable that the unoccupied receptor is restrained in an inactive state in the absence of TRH and that TRH binding releases these restraints. Interactions between residues in different TMHs have been suggested to fulfill this function because mutation of TMH residues that are predicted to dissociate these interactions leads to receptors that are active in the absence of agonist. For example, in the model of the unliganded state of TRH-R1, there is a hydrophobic stacking interaction between Phe-199 in TMH-5 and Trp-279 in TMH-6 that holds TMH-5 and TMH-6 close to one another. In the model of TRH-bound TRH-R1, this interaction is disrupted and helices 5 and 6 are further apart. Experiments in which either Phe-199 or Trp-279 is mutated to Ala lead to receptors that are constitutively active, and models for this demonstrate positioning of TMH-5 and TMH-6 further apart than in the unoccupied receptor model due to lack of interaction of the residues in positions 199 and 279. Thus, work providing initial insights into the changes that constitute TRH-R activation caused by binding of TRH is underway.

III. TRH-Rs AND G-PROTEINS

The proposed structure of TRH-R1 is similar to that of all GPCRs and it is therefore likely that TRH-Rs couple to a heterotrimeric, signal-transducing G-protein(s) composed of α-, β-, and γ-subunits. Specific G-proteins that interact with TRH-R have been identified. TRH-Rs couple primarily to G_q and G_{11}, which are pertussis-toxin-insensitive G-proteins (see later) that activate phosphoinositide-specific phospholipase C (PPI-PLC). One of the most important observations supporting this conclusion was the demonstration that antibodies directed toward the common carboxyl terminus of these two G-protein α-subunits inhibit TRH stimulation of this enzyme activity. Several lines of evidence have been presented that support the idea that TRH-Rs couple to other G-proteins in addition to G_q and G_{11}. Bacterial toxins

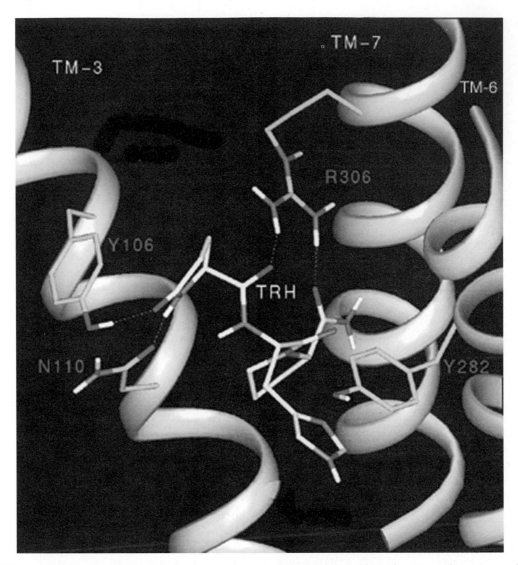

FIGURE 3 Computer-simulated three-dimensional model of the binding pocket of a mouse thyrotropin-releasing hormone receptor subtype (TRH-R1). A close-up view of TRH (light gray bond representations) in the binding pocket, showing the proposed interactions with Tyr-106 and Asn-110 in transmembrane-spanning helix 3 (TM-3), Tyr-282 in TM-6, and Arg-306 in TM-7 (dark gray). The ribbons represent the backbones of the α-helices, which are the part of the receptor that spans the cell surface membrane.

that covalently modify certain G-proteins (pertussis toxin modifies proteins of the G_i class and cholera toxin modifies proteins of the G_s class), have provided evidence in studies of model systems that G_{i2} and G_{i3} can mediate TRH stimulation of voltage-sensitive calcium channels and that TRH-Rs can couple to G_o, which is a pertussis-toxin-sensitive G-protein that is found at high levels in the brain. The most controversial aspect of TRH-R/G-protein coupling involves G_s or a G_s-like protein; G_s is known to activate adenylyl cyclase and calcium channels and to inhibit sodium channels in different cell types.

Evidence has been presented that both supports and refutes coupling of TRH-Rs to G_s or G_s-like proteins. Thus, it appears that under specific conditions in model systems, TRH-Rs couple to G_q, G_{11}, G_{i2}, and G_{i3}, and, perhaps, to a G_s-like protein that does not activate adenylyl cyclase. Because the principal pathway for TRH-R signaling appears to be through the cascade initiated by phosphoinositide hydrolysis, it appears that coupling of TRH-R to G_q and G_{11} is of primary importance.

The regions of TRH-Rs that are involved in coupling to G-proteins include ICL-3 and the carboxyl-terminal tail. In both ICL-3 and the carboxyl tail, it is the regions just underneath the cell surface membrane that are important for coupling. For example, a large part of the middle portion of ICL-3 and a large part of the distal aspect of the carboxyl tail of TRH-R1 can be deleted without any effect on $G_{q/11}$ activation. Thus, TRH-Rs behave like most GPCRs and couple selectively to a limited number of G-proteins that are members of several G-protein families.

IV. TRH-R AND SIGNAL TRANSDUCTION PATHWAYS

TRH-Rs predominantly utilize a ubiquitous second-messenger system that is initiated by the hydrolysis of phosphoinositides, which are phospholipids that contain the sugar *myo*-inositol as the polar head group, for signal transduction. When TRH binds to TRH-Rs, G_q/G_{11} proteins are activated; in turn, a PPI-PLC that is activated primarily hydrolyzes phosphatidylinositol 4,5-bisphosphate (PIP_2) to generate two molecules that serve as second messengers, i.e., inositol 1,4,5-trisphosphate ($InsP_3$) and 1,2-diacylglycerol (1,2-DAG). $InsP_3$, which is water soluble, is released into the cytoplasm and diffuses away from the membrane whereas 1,2-DAG remains membrane bound. $InsP_3$ leads to release of intracellular stores of Ca^{2+} into the cytoplasm and elevates the cytoplasmic free Ca^{2+} concentration ($[Ca^{2+}]_i$), and 1,2-DAG activates protein kinase C (PKC). These two second messengers then induce signal transduction via two parallel pathways.

A central aspect of Ca^{2+} signaling stimulated by TRH is that increases in $[Ca^{2+}]_i$ are translated into changes in cellular function through a number of specific, Ca^{2+}-binding regulatory proteins or protein subunits. On binding Ca^{2+}, these proteins undergo conformational changes that regulate their activity. For example, calmodulin is a ubiquitous Ca^{2+}-binding protein that, on binding Ca^{2+}, binds to and activates several enzymes, including Ca^{2+}/calmodulin-dependent multifunctional protein kinases, which phosphorylate a broad array of proteins and may mediate regulation of gene transcription, protein synthesis, and secretion.

TRH-R stimulation of PIP_2 hydrolysis leads to formation of $InsP_3$, which causes an elevation of $[Ca^{2+}]_i$ within seconds. $InsP_3$ rapidly diffuses in the cytoplasm away from the cell surface membrane to bind to receptors on the endoplasmic reticulum. $InsP_3$ receptors are Ca^{2+} channels that "open" on binding $InsP_3$, allowing the flow of previously sequestered

Ca^{2+} from the lumen of the endoplasmic reticulum into the cytoplasm and thereby elevating $[Ca^{2+}]_i$. This component of elevation of $[Ca^{2+}]_i$ is rapid and transient. Within seconds of TRH activation of TRH-Rs in excitable cells, such as those in the anterior pituitary and nervous system, Ca^{2+} channels within the cell surface membrane are activated by a mechanism that is incompletely understood. When "opened," these channels allow rapid influx of Ca^{2+} down the electrochemical gradient from the extracellular space to the cytoplasmic compartment, thus also elevating $[Ca^{2+}]_i$. The increase in $[Ca^{2+}]_i$ secondary to stimulated Ca^{2+} influx is more prolonged. TRH-stimulated increases in $[Ca^{2+}]_i$ can occur as a rapid but transient increase followed by a plateau phase, as increases in the frequency of oscillations ("spikes"), or as a combination of a transient increase followed by a plateau with superimposed oscillations (Fig. 4). Ca^{2+} influx across the cell surface membrane is also increased when Ca^{2+} stores in the endoplasmic reticulum are depleted during TRH stimulation. This has been termed "capacitative Ca^{2+} entry" and may be more important in "nonexcitable" cells than in excitable cells. Thus, several different processes that lead to elevations in $[Ca^{2+}]_I$ or replenishment of intracellular Ca^{2+} stores, or both, are initiated rapidly after TRH-R activation.

The other limb of the PPI pathway activated after TRH stimulation of PIP_2 hydrolysis is mediated by 1,2-DAG. 1,2-DAG, in combination with phosphatidylserine (PS) and, depending on the isoenzyme subtype, with or without a requirement for an elevation of $[Ca^{2+}]_i$, activates phospholipid-dependent PKC. PKC enzymes are a family of serine and threonine kinase isoenzymes that phosphorylate many proteins involved in regulating downstream cellular responses. In unstimulated cells, the level of 1,2-DAG in membranes is very low, but 1,2-DAG accumulates in response to TRH, causing within seconds a transient translocation of some isoforms of PKC to the plasma membrane. An important proximate effect of activation of PKC is one of negative feedback to inhibit PPI signaling, which may be mediated by phosphorylation of TRH-Rs (see Section VI). The more distal effects of activation of PKC by TRH signaling include stimulation of hormone secretion and gene transcription in the anterior pituitary.

Other protein kinases are also activated after TRH-R activation. The elevation of $[Ca^{2+}]_i$ caused by TRH stimulation leads to activation of multifunctional Ca^{2+}/calmodulin-dependent protein kinase II. Evidence has been provided that this kinase has a role

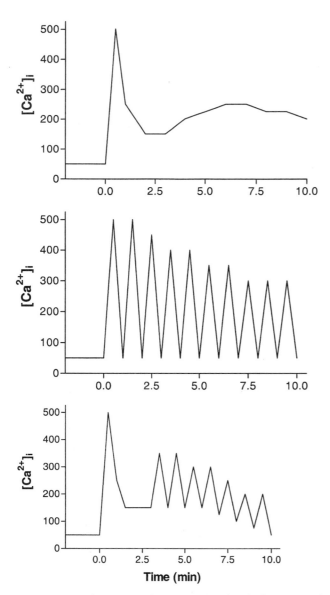

FIGURE 4 Three ways that TRH-stimulated elevations of $[Ca^{2+}]_i$ occur in pituitary cells. TRH was added to cells in tissue culture at time zero. See text for discussion.

in regulation of gene transcription in pituitary cells. TRH activates mitogen-activated protein kinases (MAPKs), a family of differentially regulated serine/threonine kinases, which also appears to lead to regulation of gene transcription. Activation of MAPK is in part secondary to PKC activation and is enhanced via the βγ subunit dimer of heterotrimeric G-proteins. The set of genes regulated by these protein kinases after TRH stimulation has only begun to be delineated. Although a number of signal transduction pathways initiated by TRH-R activation have been identified, cellular responses other than

stimulation of hormone synthesis and secretion by the anterior pituitary are poorly understood.

V. CONSTITUTIVE SIGNALING BY TRH-Rs

Constitutive (basal; i.e., agonist-independent) signaling is a well-documented characteristic of some native receptors and of receptors that are mutated and cause human disease. Both TRH-R subtypes, at least when they are expressed at high levels in cells in tissue culture, exhibit constitutive signaling. However, the level of basal signaling exhibited by TRH-R2 is much greater than that of TRH-R1. Indeed, in some assays in certain cell types, basal signaling by TRH-R1 cannot be measured. As with most native GPCRs, whether basal signaling occurs *in situ* under normal conditions and whether it has an important physiological role is not known for TRH-Rs. It is noteworthy that some drugs (for example, benzodiazepines) are able to bind to TRH-Rs and inhibit their basal signaling activities. Ligands that inhibit basal signaling are termed inverse agonists (or negative antagonists). Inverse agonists may be used in future studies to determine whether basal signaling by TRH-Rs is physiologically relevant.

VI. TRH DESENSITIZATION

Persistent stimulation by a constant level of TRH, as with many agonists that act at GPCRs, leads to a diminished response over time. This phenomenon of TRH-induced desensitization is an important regulatory mechanism that may be mediated at several steps in the signal transduction pathway. Perhaps the most important mechanisms of desensitization involve effects on the receptor. These include receptor phosphorylation, which decreases G-protein coupling, and receptor down-regulation, which is a decrease in the number of receptors on the cell surface. These two types of desensitization can often be dissociated because uncoupling of receptors from G-proteins occurs rapidly, within seconds to minutes, whereas receptor down-regulation is usually slower, requiring several hours.

TRH stimulation of InsP$_3$ formation rapidly causes desensitization. (TRH-induced elevation of $[Ca^{2+}]_i$ is also rapidly desensitized, but this may be due in part to depletion of Ca^{2+} stores.) Although not proved, rapid TRH desensitization likely involves receptor phosphorylation, which may be caused by the action of PKC or by a member of the family of GPCR-specific kinases. The Ser or Thr residues that are likely to be phosphorylated are within ICL-2 and ICL-3 and in the carboxyl tail of TRH-R. These proposals are based on observations that pharmacologic activation of PKC (for example, by phorbol myristate acetate) and overexpression of GPCR kinases inhibit TRH stimulation of $InsP_3$ generation. TRH-induced TRH-R down-regulation can be observed after approximately 1 h of initiation of signaling. Down-regulation of TRH-Rs leads to diminished TRH responsiveness because the magnitude of the TRH response is usually directly related to the number of TRH-Rs expressed on the cell surfaces. TRH-R down-regulation may be caused by a number of extracellular regulatory factors, including TRH, thyroid hormones, and vasoactive intestinal polypeptide acting in pituitary cells. The number of TRH-Rs can be decreased by decreasing their rate of synthesis or by increasing their rate of degradation, or both. Changes in the rate of TRH-R protein degradation have not been studied.

Modulation of the rate of TRH-R synthesis secondary to decreases in the level of TRH-R mRNA has been shown by monitoring gene transcription and mRNA degradation. These studies were of TRH-R1 but may apply to TRH-R2 as well. Decreases in the levels of TRH-R mRNA can occur by decreasing the rate of TRH-R gene transcription or by increasing TRH-R mRNA degradation, or both. TRH causes a decrease in the level of endogenous TRH-R mRNA by increasing the rate of TRH-R mRNA degradation. This effect of TRH appears to involve activation of PKC and elevation of $[Ca^{2+}]_i$. Thus, it appears that TRH increases TRH-R mRNA degradation through its well-characterized signal transduction pathway, which is initiated by hydrolysis of PIP_2. TRH also decreases TRH-R mRNA levels by inhibiting TRH-R gene transcription; however, the signaling pathway that mediates this effect has not been demonstrated. In conclusion, down-regulation of the TRH-R number by a mechanisms that involves modulation of TRH-R protein turnover, although likely, has not been studied directly, whereas regulation of TRH-R synthesis is well documented and involves several distinct mechanisms that are initiated by different regulatory factors.

VII. TRH-R INTERNALIZATION

Internalization (or endocytosis) of TRH-Rs occurs rapidly after TRH binds. This process serves to bring TRH and receptors into the cell, where either or both can be recycled to the cell surface or sorted to lysosomes for degradation. Although it has not been specifically shown with TRH-Rs, GPCR recycling allows for receptor resensitization because protein phosphatases associated with recycling vesicles can dephosphorylate receptors that have been acutely desensitized by phosphorylation. Unoccupied TRH-Rs are almost exclusively present on the cell surface. TRH/TRH-R complexes are internalized via clathrin-coated vesicles by a mechanism that involves arrestin and perhaps dynamin. The majority of TRH and TRH-Rs recycle to the cell surface membrane under most conditions studied. On binding TRH, TRH-R2 internalizes at a much faster rate than does TRH-R1. The reason for this difference is not clear. It is thought that proteins that reside in the cell surface membrane and undergo internalization contain a "signal" that directs them to plasma membrane clathrin-coated pits, from which coated vesicles pinch off during the initial steps in internalization. Evidence has shown that two distinct domains within the carboxyl terminus of TRH-R1 are necessary for TRH-stimulated TRH-R internalization. Although it has been suggested that coupling to G-proteins is necessary for internalization, it is not clear whether there is coupling to proteins of the internalization machinery in the absence of coupling to G-proteins.

VIII. SUMMARY

The primary pathway of TRH signal transduction is mediated by activation of G_q or G_{11} proteins; activation of PPI-PLC follows, leading to formation of $InsP_3$ and 1,2-DAG. $InsP_3$ elevates $[Ca^{2+}]_i$ by releasing Ca^{2+} from the endoplasmic reticulum and 1,2-DAG activates PKC. The increase in $[Ca^{2+}]_i$ is further augmented by activation of cell surface membrane channels, allowing influx of extracellular Ca^{2+}. The elevation of $[Ca^{2+}]_i$ activates $Ca^{2+}/$ calmodulin protein kinase. Although increases in $[Ca^{2+}]_i$ and activation of these protein kinases are known to result in stimulation of anterior pituitary hormone secretion and gene transcription, the effects in the central nervous system are still poorly understood.

Glossary

agonist Ligand that activates a receptor.

Ca^{2+}/calmodulin-dependent protein kinase Family of serine/threonine protein kinases; activated by Ca^{2+} and calmodulin.

constitutive signaling Receptor signaling that occurs in the absence of agonist binding; also termed basal or agonist-independent signaling.

1,2-diacylglycerol Lipid product of phospholipase C-mediated hydrolysis of phospholipids; a neutral lipid with fatty acyl chains at positions 1 and 2; activates protein kinase C.

G-proteins Family of signal-transducing (or coupling) proteins made up of three subunits (α, β, and γ); activated by members of the largest family of receptors and, in turn, activate ion channels and a number of effector molecules, including enzymes such as adenylyl cyclase and phospholipase C.

G-protein-coupled receptors Seven-transmembrane-spanning (heptahelical, or serpentine) cell surface receptors that bind extracellular regulatory molecules such as hormones, neurotransmitters, and growth factors, and bind and activate G proteins.

inositol 1,4,5-trisphosphate Sugar product of phospholipase C-mediated hydrolysis of phosphatidylinositol 4,5-bisphosphate; a hexahydroxy, cyclic sugar with phosphate groups at the 1, 4, and 5 positions; activates channels in the endoplasmic reticulum to release previously sequestered Ca^{2+}.

ligand Any molecule, such as a hormone, neurotransmitter, growth factor, or drug, that binds to a receptor.

phospholipase C Lipid-hydrolyzing enzyme that cleaves phospholipids at the 3 position to form two products— the head group, such as $InsP_3$, and 1,2-diacylglycerol.

protein kinase C Serine/threonine protein kinase that is activated by 1,2-diacylglycerol, phospholipids, and/or Ca^{2+} downstream of activation of certain receptors.

See Also the Following Articles

Calmodulin • GPCR (G-Protein-Coupled Receptor) Structure • Heterotrimeric G-Proteins • Inositol Phosphate Signaling • Thyrotropin Receptor Signaling • Thyroid Hormone Receptor, TSH and TSH Receptor Mutations • Thyrotropin-Releasing Hormone (TRH)

Further Reading

Arvanitakis, L., Geras-Raaka, E., and Gershengorn, M. C. (1998). Constitutively signaling G protein-coupled receptors and human disease. *Trends Endocrinol. Metab.* **9**, 27–31.

Ashworth, R., Yu, R., Nelson, E. J., Dermer, S., Gershengorn, M. C., and Hinkle, P. M. (1995). Visualization of the thyrotropin-releasing hormone receptor and its ligand during endocytosis and recycling. *Proc. Natl. Acad. Sci. U.S.A.* **92**, 512–516.

Faick-Pedersen, E., Heinflink, M., Alvira, M., Nussenzveig, D. R., and Gershengorn, M. C. (1994). Expression of thyrotropin-releasing hormone receptors by adenovirus-mediated gene transfer reveals that thyrotropin- releasing hormone desensitization is cell specific. *Mol. Pharmacol.* **45**, 684–689.

Gershengorn, M. C., and Hinkle, P. M. (2001). Second messenger signaling pathways: phospholipids and calcium. *In* "Endocrinology" (L. J. DeGroot and J. L. Jameson, eds.), pp. 89–98. W.B. Saunders Company, Philadelphia.

Gershengorn, M. C., and Osman, R. (2001). Minireview: Insights into G protein-coupled receptor function using molecular models. *Endocrinology* **142**, 2–10.

Osman, R., Colson, A.-O., Perlman, J. H., Laakkonen, L. J., and Gershengorn, M. C. (1999). Mapping binding sites for peptide G protein-coupled receptors: The receptor for thyrotropin-releasing hormone. *In* "Structure/Function of G-Protein Coupled Receptors" (J. Wess, ed.), pp. 59–84. John Wiley and Sons, Inc., New York.

Palczewski, K., Kumasaka, T., Hori, T., Behnke, C. A., Motoshima, H., Fox, B. A., Le Trong, I., Teller, D. C., Okada, T., Stenkamp, R. E., Yamamoto, M., and Miyano, M. (2000). Crystal structure of rhodopsin: A G protein-coupled receptor. *Science* **289**, 739–745.

Perlman, J. H., Colson, A.-O., Jain, R., Czyzewski, B., Cohen, L. A., Osman, R., and Gershengorn, M. C. (1997). Role of the extracellular loops of the thyrotropin-releasing hormone receptor: Evidence for an initial interaction with thyrotropin-releasing hormone. *Biochemistry* **36**, 15670–15676.

Pitcher, J. A., Freedman, N. J., and Lefkowitz, R. J. (1998). G protein-coupled receptor kinases. *Annu. Rev. Biochem.* **67**, 653–692.

Wess, J. (1999). "Structure/Function Analysis of G-Protein Coupled Receptors." John Wiley and Sons, Inc., New York.

Thyrotropin-Releasing Hormone (TRH)

RONALD M. LECHAN[*] AND ANTHONY HOLLENBERG[†]

*Tufts–New England Medical Center and Tufts University School of Medicine • †Harvard Medical School

I. INTRODUCTION
II. BIOSYNTHESIS AND PROCESSING OF TRH
III. TRH GENE AND PROMOTER REGULATION
IV. ANATOMY OF THE HYPOTHALAMIC TRH TUBEROINFUNDIBULAR SYSTEM
V. FEEDBACK REGULATION OF HYPOPHYSIOTROPIC TRH BY THYROID HORMONE
VI. REGULATION OF HYPOPHYSIOTROPIC TRH BY COLD EXPOSURE AND SUCKLING
VII. REGULATION OF HYPOPHYSIOTROPIC TRH BY FASTING AND INFECTION (NONTHYROIDAL ILLNESS SYNDROME)
VIII. EXTRAHYPOTHALAMIC FUNCTIONS OF TRH

Thyrotropin-releasing hormone (TRH) arises from posttranslational processing of a large precursor protein but it is only one of several other potentially biologically active peptides derived from the same precursor. The biosynthesis of TRH is dependent on feedback regulation of thyroid hormone, mediated by its interaction with the β2 thyroid hormone receptor and negative thyroid hormone-responsive elements in the TRH gene. Whereas TRH originating in neurons of the hypothalamic paraventricular nucleus contributes to the hypothalamic tuberoinfundibular system and regulates anterior pituitary secretion, the TRH gene is expressed in many other regions of the brain and in peripheral tissues where TRH and other proTRH-derived peptides are expressed in a region- and tissue-specific manner to exert a variety of biologic actions.

I. INTRODUCTION

The maintenance of thyroid function is dependent on a complex interplay between the hypothalamus, anterior pituitary, and thyroid gland, as well as other factors that influence the function of these organ systems. This function is critical in achieving a constant level of free thyroid hormone in the bloodstream to support peripheral tissues by affecting protein synthesis and/or altering the metabolic activity of cells, as well as for brain development during fetal growth and early infancy. The hypothalamic peptide primarily responsible for this action by stimulating the biosynthesis and release of thyrotropin (TSH) from the anterior pituitary gland is thyrotropin-releasing hormone (TRH). TSH then stimulates the release of the thyroid hormones thyroxine (T4) and tri-iodothyronine (T3) from the thyroid gland into the circulation; T4 and T3 in turn feed back on the hypothalamic TRH neurons and anterior pituitary thyrotropes, completing what is recognized as a classic example of a negative feedback loop system (Fig. 1). Elucidation of the normal anatomy and connectivity of the TRH neurons responsible for the secretion of TSH and characterization of the TRH gene has vastly improved the understanding of the normal physiology of hypophysiotropic TRH and the mechanisms by which the thyroid axis is modified under adverse conditions such as fasting, infection, and cold exposure.

TRH should not be considered to have an exclusive action on the secretion of TSH as its name suggests, however, as it also subserves a wide range of other biologic functions both within the central nervous system and in some peripheral tissues. The recognition that posttranslational products of the TRH prohormone include not only TRH but also other cryptic peptides that may have biologic activity further expands the diversity of the actions of the products of proTRH and raises the possibility that in some tissues, the primary product of posttranslational processing may not be TRH.

II. BIOSYNTHESIS AND PROCESSING OF TRH

TRH (pyroGlu-His-ProNH$_2$, MW 362) arises by a mRNA-directed ribosomal mechanism and posttranslational processing of a larger precursor prohormone. The complete sequence of the TRH precursor,

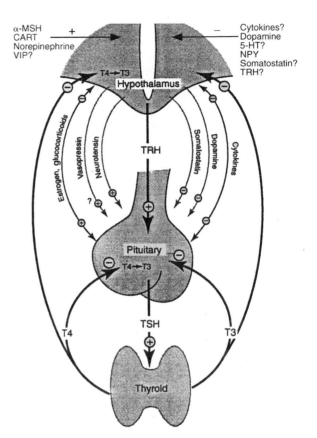

FIGURE 1 Neuroregulatory control systems involved in the secretion of thyroid hormone. Boldface lines denote the negative feedback loop of thyroid hormone on TRH secretion from the hypothalamus and TSH secretion from the anterior pituitary. Both the hypothalamic TRH neurons and the anterior pituitary thyrotropes are impinged upon by numerous other potential regulatory influences that are activated under specific physiological or pathological conditions.

deduced from its cDNA, has been elucidated for frog, rat, mouse, and human and is schematically illustrated in Fig. 2. Common to each prohormone are multiple copies of a progenitor sequence for TRH, Gln-His-Pro-Gly, flanked on either side by paired basic amino acids, Lys-Arg or Arg-Arg, that are processing signals for carboxypeptidase B-like enzymes. The C-terminal glycine functions as a substrate for α-amidating enzymes that convert TRH-Gly to TRH and the N-terminal glutaminyl is modified by glutaminyl cyclase to result in the fully mature and biologically active TRH.

Rat preproTRH contains 255 amino acids and five copies of the TRH progenitor sequence and is approximately 88% homologous to the mouse preproTRH, which contains 256 amino acids and also gives rise to five copies of TRH by proteolytic

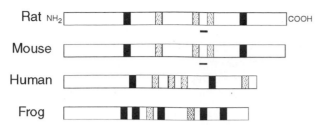

FIGURE 2 Schematic representation of rat, mouse, frog, and human preproTRH. Each sequence contains multiple copies of a TRH progenitor sequence (Gln-His-Pro) preceded by Lys-Arg and followed by Lys-Arg or Arg-Arg. Unique to the frog is one TRH progenitor sequence that is preceded by Arg-Arg and followed by Lys-Arg. The cryptic peptides preproTRH$_{160-169}$ and preproTRH$_{178-199}$ are located between the third and the fourth progenitor TRH sequences and between the fourth and the fifth progenitor TRH sequences, respectively.

processing. The human preproTRH contains 242 amino acids and six copies of the progenitor sequence for TRH. Frog brain has at least three different TRH preprohormones ranging between 224 and 227 amino acids and contains seven copies of the TRH progenitor sequence. Common to all species are the repeating progenitor sequences of TRH in the prohormone, presumably important in magnifying the response to signals that trigger TRH secretion.

In addition to the sequences that give rise to TRH, the TRH precursor contains several cryptic peptides between the TRH progenitor sequences and the N- and C-terminal flanking peptides that may be biologically active. At least one peptide, preproTRH$_{160-169}$, a decapeptide containing the amino acid sequence Ser-Phe-Pro-Trp-Met-Glu-Ser-Asp-Val-Thr that follows the third TRH sequence in the rat prohormone, is also present in mouse preproTRH and has been isolated from bovine hypothalamus. This peptide is released from the medial hypothalamus into the system of veins that conveys releasing hormones to the anterior pituitary, the portal capillary system, and specific binding sites for the decapeptide have been identified in the anterior pituitary as well as in other regions in the brain. PreproTRH$_{160-169}$ has little effect on anterior pituitary secretion by itself, but in the presence of TRH, it potentiates the secretion of TSH by increasing TSHβ mRNA in thyrotropes. The action of preproTRH$_{160-169}$ is probably not directly on thyrotropes, however, as receptors have been identified only in folliculostellate cells, a specialized glial cell of anterior pituitary origin that is not known to secrete TSH. Presumably, therefore, the effect of preproTRH$_{160-169}$ to potentiate the action of TRH

on TSH secretion is indirect via paracrine interactions between the processes of folliculostellate cells and anterior pituitary thyrotropes.

In addition to TSH secretion, preproTRH$_{160-169}$ enhances both the synthesis and the secretion of prolactin and possibly growth hormone release. PreproTRH$_{160-169}$ also potentiates the effect of TRH to induce gastric acid secretion when the two peptides are simultaneously microinjected into the dorsal motor nucleus of the vagus.

PreproTRH$_{178-199}$, which separates the fourth and fifth progenitor TRH sequences, is also released from the rat median eminence but as yet, no receptors for this peptide have been identified. Claims for biologic activity of preproTRH$_{178-199}$ were based on its ability to act as a corticotropin-inhibiting factor, blocking both ACTH release and proopiomelanocortin (POMC) mRNA transcription, but these claims are still controversial. PreproTRH$_{178-199}$ may also have a number of other potential actions including inhibition of growth hormone secretion and neuro-endocrine responses to stress, antidepressant activity, and neuroprotection against cerebral ischemia. PreproTRH$_{178-184}$ and preproTRH$_{186-199}$, posttranslational products of preproTRH$_{178-199}$, may have prolactin-releasing activity.

Despite the potential for the above rodent proTRH-derived peptides to have biologic activity, most of these sequences are not present in the human or frog preproTRH, raising questions as to their importance across animal species. Hydropathy profiles of the rat, human, and frog preproTRH sequences, however, do show a peak hydrophobicity over the region corresponding to the C-terminal flanking peptide. In particular, this region has remarkable resemblance over a 47- to 50-amino-acid span in the rat, mouse, and human prohormone. In the human, this sequence contains within it the sixth progenitor TRH that may have arisen from evolutionary changes between the fifth TRH coding sequence and the stop codon. No data that establish a definite biologic action of the C-terminal flanking peptide have been reported, however. Several preproTRH sequences have been identified in extracts of human hypothalamus including preproTRH$_{141-149}$, preproTRH$_{158-183}$, and preproTRH$_{192-224}$. PreproTRH$_{141-149}$ (referred to as human thyrotropin-releasing hormone-associated peptide 3 or hTAP-3) is also present in human serum and corresponds in position to the intervening sequence preproTRH$_{160-169}$ in the rat prohormone.

Processing of proTRH to its final products is region specific and dependent on the type of processing enzymes in the cell. In the hypothalamus, preproTRH is fully processed to yield all five copies of TRH and each of the spacer peptides. In contrast, in the olfactory lobes, C-terminal extended forms of TRH, preproTRH$_{154-169}$, and preproTRH$_{172-199}$ are the predominant end products, suggesting incomplete processing at Arg-Arg residues. Furthermore, in the midbrain periaqueductal gray, the N-terminal cryptic peptide preproTRH$_{83-106}$ is selectively increased during opiate withdrawal while TRH and the C-terminal peptide are reduced.

Two enzymes that are critical for the processing of proTRH are the proconvertase enzymes, PC1 and PC2. These enzymes cleave at the C-terminal end of single or paired basic amino acid residues and the remaining basic amino acids are removed by carboxypeptidases. PC1 appears to be capable of processing the entire proTRH precursor to mature TRH, whereas PC2 processes only specific regions of the prohormone. Along these lines, it is of interest that both PC1 and PC2 are present in the majority of TRH neurons in the paraventricular nucleus (PVN), whereas primarily PC2 is expressed in the olfactory lobes and periaqueductal gray. Accordingly, differences in the expression of PC1 and PC2 in different regions of the brain may be responsible for the differential processing of proTRH observed in these regions.

A schema for the processing of proTRH is shown in Fig. 3. In this model, the 26 kDa prohormone is cleaved at one of two sites to generate either 15 and 10 kDa fragments (preproTRH$_{25-151}$ and preproTRH$_{160-255}$) or 9.5 and 16.5 kDa fragments (preproTRH$_{25-112}$ and preproTRH$_{115-255}$), respectively. This initial cleavage occurs in the Golgi apparatus. Subsequently, the 15 kDa N-terminal fragment is processed in vesicles to a 6 kDa intermediate (preproTRH$_{25-74}$) and a 3.8 kDa peptide (preproTRH$_{77-106}$), and the 10 kDa fragment produces a 5.6 kDa intermediate (preproTRH$_{160-199}$) and a 5.4 kDa intermediate corresponding to the C-terminal peptide, preproTRH$_{208-255}$. The 5.6 kDa fragment is then further processed to preproTRH$_{160-169}$ and preproTRH$_{178-199}$. PreproTRH$_{178-199}$ can then be further processed to the smaller peptides, preproTRH$_{178-184}$ and preproTRH$_{186-199}$, mediated by the action of PC2. Alternatively, processing of the 9.5 kDa N-terminal fragment is proposed to yield preproTRH$_{25-50}$, preproTRH$_{53-74}$, and preproTRH$_{83-106}$, and the 16.5 kDa C-terminal fragment is proposed to yield preproTRH$_{160-199}$ and preproTRH$_{208-255}$. Following cleavage at all paired basic residues, the mature TRH (pGlu-His-Pro-NH$_2$)

is generated by amidating the C-terminal end of the tripeptide using the glycine residue in the immediate precursor to TRH, TRH-Gly, as a substrate for the α-amidating enzyme, PAM, and cyclization of the N-terminal glutaminyl to pGlu by glutaminyl cyclase.

III. TRH GENE AND PROMOTER REGULATION

The murine, rat, and human TRH genomic structures are identical, with each structure containing three exons and two introns (Fig. 4); exon 1 encodes the 5′-untranslated region, whereas exon 2 and 3 contain the sequence that encodes the preproTRH message. The DNA sequences of the exons are well conserved across species, but the sequences of the introns are poorly conserved. The promoter region of the TRH gene is located immediately 5′ to exon 1 and presumably is the major locus where regulation of the gene takes place. In vivo studies in transgenic mice using TRH promoter fragments linked to a luciferase reporter gene suggest that sequences within the proximal promoter as well as the first exon are critical for TRH expression in the hypothalamus. It remains unclear, however, which regions of the TRH gene allow for its expression in other tissues, such as the pituitary, pancreas, or heart.

The TRH promoter region is heralded by the presence of a conserved TATAA-box, allowing for transcriptional initiation by RNA polymerase II. Just proximal to the TATAA-box is an important regulatory element, termed Site 4 (TGACCTCA), that is conserved in the mouse, rat, and human promoters (Fig. 4). This sequence is important for basal expression of the TRH promoter in many different mammalian cell lines when assessed using transfection studies. In addition, Site 4 serves as a multifunctional binding site for the transcription factor cyclic AMP-response element-binding protein (CREB) and thyroid hormone receptors (TRs), including TR homodimers and heterodimers of TR and the retinoic acid X receptor (RXR). It appears that Site 4 cooperates with a second weak TR-binding site 11 bp 3′ to Site 4 that binds both TR homodimers and TR/RXR heterodimers. Taken together, Site 4 appears to be a critical sequence within the TRH promoter that is preserved across species and controls both basal and regulated expression of the TRH gene.

The importance of Site 4 in the regulation of TRH expression was first demonstrated in functional studies in mammalian cell lines that showed that it was required for down-regulation of TRH promoter constructs by T3 in the presence of the TR. T3

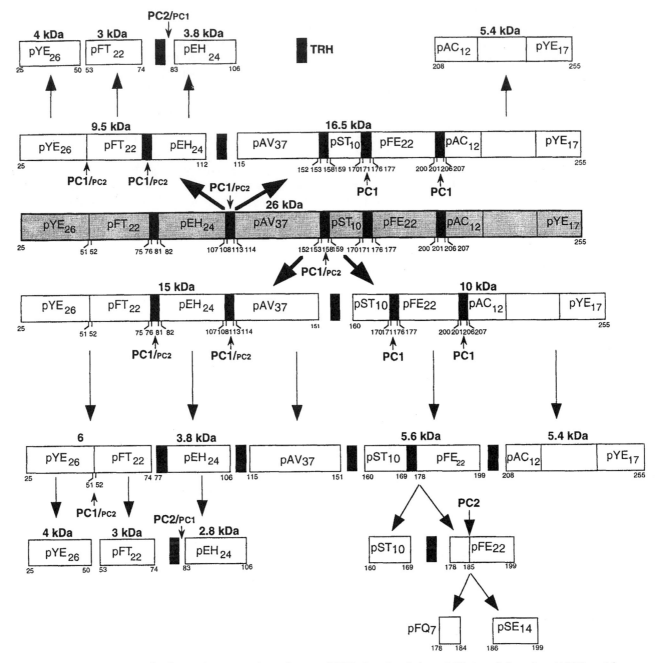

FIGURE 3 Proposed schema for processing of preproTRH. Reprinted from Nillni and Sevarino (1999), with permission from The Endocrine Society.

mediates its effects on gene expression via the three TR isoforms (TRα₁, TRβ₁, and TRβ₂). TRα₁ is expressed in many tissues but plays only a small role in negative regulation by T3. Its actions are critical for the effects of T3 in the heart, bone, and small intestine. The TRβ isoforms are products of a single gene and differ only in their amino-terminal regions. TRβ₁ mediates the effect of T3 in the inner ear, liver,

and kidney, and recent genetic studies have confirmed that TRβ₂ is critical for negative regulation of the TRH, TSHα subunit, and TSHβ subunit genes by T3. The molecular mechanism governing negative regulation of the TRH promoter by T3 has not been firmly established. Site 4 and its surrounding region can bind TRβ₂, which appears to be necessary for negative regulation. However, it is not clear which co-factors

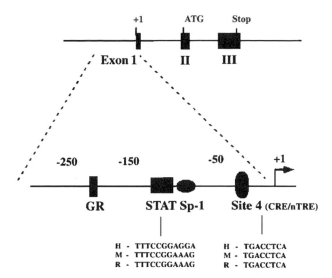

FIGURE 4 Genomic and promoter structure of TRH. The murine, rat, and human TRH genes are composed of three exons and two introns. The coding sequence for the precursor protein is present on exons 2 and 3. As depicted, the TRH promoter region precedes the transcription start site in exon 1. The proximal 250 bp sequences of the human, mouse, and rat promoters are similar and share the indicated transcription factor-binding sites. The sequences of the STAT element and Site 4 across species are indicated.

are involved. On genes positively regulated by T3, the TR isoforms are bound constitutively to thyroid hormone-response elements (TREs). In the absence of T3, they recruit the nuclear co-repressors (nuclear receptor co-repressor and silencing mediator for retinoid and thyroid hormone receptor) that repress transcription of target genes. The presence of T3 causes the release of co-repressors and the recruitment of co-activators such as SRC-1, which lead to transcriptional activation. The role of co-repressors and co-activators in the negative regulation of the TRH gene remains less clear, given that the recruitment of co-activators by TRβ2 in the presence of T3 would be expected to activate rather than repress TRH expression. However, they also appear to be important because mutations in TRs that prevent binding of either co-repressors or co-activators without altering DNA binding are unable to mediate negative regulation. In addition to Site 4, a second region within the TRH gene present within the first 55 bp of exon 1 may be important in mediating the effects of T3. This region interacts with TRβ monomers and its removal in functional studies causes a loss of negative regulation by T3.

Site 4 can also be bound by CREB. CREB binding and TR binding appear to be mutually exclusive and

there is no evidence that they interact on Site 4. Thus, it is possible that they in fact compete for Site 4. CREB is bound constitutively to target promoters, usually as a homodimer or as a heterodimer with other members of the ATF-1 family. When phosphorylated by protein kinase A after activation of the cAMP signaling cascade by activators such as forskolin, PCREB recruits the co-activator CREB-binding protein (CBP), which allows for transcriptional activation of the TRH gene. CBP functions as a histone acetyl transferase, allowing modification of surrounding histones to enhance transcription. Mutation or deletion of Site 4 prevents the activation of TRH promoter constructs by forskolin. The phosphorylation of CREB, therefore, is likely a key mechanism for positive regulation of TRH gene expression, and by competing with PCREB for Site 4, TRβ2 could prevent activation of the TRH promoter. Binding of PCREB to Site 4 also has an important role in mediating the effects of melanocortin signaling on the TRH gene (see below).

Activation of the TRH gene also occurs via a canonical signal transducer and activator of transcription (STAT)-binding site in the murine and rat promoter 5′ to Site 4. A similar site in the human promoter located between −150 and −125 has also been identified, suggesting the importance of this sequence across animal species (Fig. 4). A number of STAT isoforms (STAT1, STAT3, and STAT5) have been identified and appear to be ubiquitously expressed. In the inactivated state, STAT proteins are present in the cytoplasm. Activation occurs after a cell surface receptor (usually a member of the cytokine receptor family) is bound by its ligand. This leads to a cascade that results in recruitment and activation of Janus tyrosine kinase (JAK), which in turn leads to recruitment and phosphorylation of the STAT isoforms. Tyrosine phosphorylation allows phospho-STAT to dimerize and enter the nucleus to bind to its target regulatory elements such as that found in the TRH promoter. STAT activates transcription by recruiting co-activators such as CBP. The leptin receptor also activates transcription via the JAK/STAT signaling pathway and is able to significantly enhance TRH promoter activity in transfection experiments in mammalian cells. This direct action of leptin on the TRH promoter is the best example to date of a downstream transcriptional target of the leptin signaling pathway. The presence of such a STAT site also suggests that the TRH promoter is poised to respond to other cytokine signaling pathways that could engage TRH neurons in the paraventricular nucleus (PVN) or elsewhere.

The TRH promoter also contains binding sites for the glucocorticoid receptor (GR) and Sp-1. The glucocorticoid receptor is also a member of the nuclear receptor family, and Sp-1 is a widely expressed transcription factor that binds to GC-rich motifs in target promoters. Their role in its regulation are less well understood. The GR-response element is located just upstream of the STAT element and appears to be functional in the pituitary, where glucocorticoids enhance TRH gene expression (Fig. 4). However, glucocorticoids appear to be inhibitory to TRH gene expression in the PVN. There are multiple potential Sp-1 sites within the promoter. One is located adjacent to the STAT site and is required for full induction by leptin.

IV. ANATOMY OF THE HYPOTHALAMIC TRH TUBEROINFUNDIBULAR SYSTEM

The origin of TRH-containing neurons that regulate anterior pituitary TSH secretion is the hypothalamic PVN, a triangular, midline nuclear group symmetrically located on either side of the dorsal portion of the third ventricle (Fig. 5A). The PVN is composed of two major parts: magnocellular neurons located in more lateral portions of the nucleus and parvocellular neurons located in more medial portions of the nucleus. The magnocellular component gives rise to the hypothalamic neurohypophyseal tract that carries vasopressin and oxytocin to the posterior pituitary. The parvocellular component has a number of subcompartments including anterior, medial, periventricular, ventral, dorsal, and lateral parvocellular subdivisions. TRH-synthesizing neurons are found primarily in the anterior, medial, and periventricular parvocellular subdivisions (Fig. 5B) and to a lesser extent in the dorsal and lateral subnuclei. However, only TRH neurons in medial and periventricular parvocellular subdivisions project to the median eminence (often referred to as hypophysiotropic neurons because they are involved in regulation of the anterior pituitary) and thereby are functionally distinct from the TRH neurons in the anterior parvocellular subdivision. Further support for the anatomical diversity of medial and periventricular parvocellular subdivision TRH neurons is the presence of the peptide cocaine- and amphetamine-regulated transcript (CART) in hypophysiotropic TRH neurons but not in other TRH neuronal populations.

Axons from hypophysiotropic TRH neurons in the PVN project to the median eminence, one of five so-called "circumventricular organs" in the mammalian brain that lie outside of the blood–brain barrier.

Here, they terminate in the external zone of the median eminence where they have access to the fenestrated capillaries of the portal system (Fig. 5C). Some fibers also descend in the pituitary stalk to terminate in the posterior pituitary and may provide an alternative pathway by which TRH can regulate anterior pituitary secretion through the vascular channels (short portal veins) that connect the posterior pituitary to the anterior pituitary.

By residing in the PVN, TRH-producing neurons are situated in a region highly enriched by afferent inputs from other regions in the brain. These inputs are important to establish the setpoint for feedback regulation of hypophysiotropic TRH by thyroid hormone under basal conditions and during times when it is necessary to increase or decrease circulating levels of thyroid hormone (described below). Synaptic contacts between axon terminals and both the perikarya and the dendrites of TRH-producing neurons have been observed by ultrastructural analysis, including both the symmetric type, suggesting inhibitory control, and the asymmetric type, suggesting excitatory control. Symmetric synapses containing small and large electron-lucent vesicles tend to predominate on TRH perikarya, whereas both symmetric and asymmetric contacts containing small, round and oval, clear vesicles predominate on TRH dendrites. Central modulation of hypophysiotropic TRH neurons through afferent projections may also occur in the external zone of the median eminence, which could influence tuberoinfundibular TRH release by axo-axonal associations, but true axo-axonic synapses have only rarely been recognized in the mammalian median eminence.

Although several regions of the brain project to the PVN, at least two regions provide the major input to hypophysiotropic TRH neurons, brainstem catecholamine neurons and the hypothalamic arcuate nucleus (Fig. 6A). Axon terminals containing catecholamines give one of the most conspicuous innervations to TRH neurons in the PVN arising primarily from C1/A1 groups in the medulla, contributing approximately 20% of all synapses on these cells. These axons establish mostly asymmetric synapses with both perikarya and dendrites of TRH neurons, suggesting an excitatory function. Noradrenergic axon terminals have also been identified in close apposition to TRH axons in the external layer of the rat median eminence, indicating that catecholamine inputs may influence TRH hypophysiotropic neurons not only through direct effects on their perikarya and dendrites but also on their axon terminals. The trajectory of catecholamine-contain-

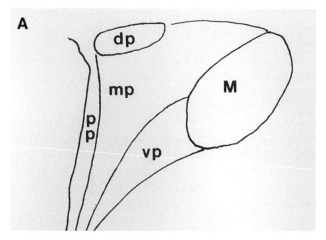

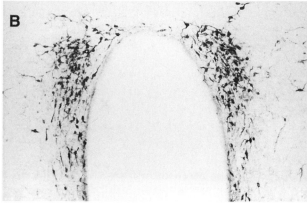

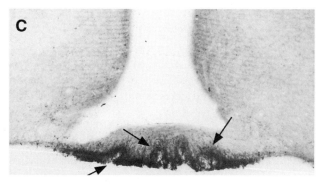

FIGURE 5 (A) Location of the major subdivisions in the PVN showing its major subdivisions. pp, periventricular parvocellular subdivision; mp, medial parvocellular subdivision; dp, dorsal parvocellular subdivision; vp, ventral parvocellular subdivision; M, magnocellular division. (B) TRH neurons originate in the medial and periventricular parvocellular subdivisions of the PVN and (C) terminate in the external zone of the median eminence in contact with capillaries of the portal vascular system (arrows).

ing axons from the brainstem is to course rostrally in the dorsal and ventral noradrenergic bundles to ultimately enter the median forebrain bundle in the hypothalamus before terminating in the PVN

(Fig. 6B). Transection of the noradrenergic bundle at the level of the midbrain results in marked depletion of the catecholamine input to the PVN, in keeping with their origin from the brainstem.

At least four different peptides of arcuate nucleus origin, α-melanocortin-stimulating hormone (α-MSH), CART, neuropeptide Y (NPY), and agouti-related peptide (AGRP), are contained in axon terminals in synaptic contact with TRH hypophysiotropic neurons (Fig. 6A,C). Neurons of the arcuato-PVN pathway project their axons primarily ipsilateral to the PVN and, like the catecholamine axon trajectory from the brainstem, course through the medial forebrain bundle prior to entering the PVN. In the rat, α-MSH and CART arise from the same neurons located in lateral portions of the arcuate nucleus, whereas NPY and AGRP are both contained in a distinct population located in more medial portions of the nucleus. A similar organization is also present in the human brain, suggesting the evolutionary importance of this neuroregulatory control system. Indeed, in the rat and mouse, pharmacologic ablation of the arcuate nucleus not only results in profound reduction in the number of axons contacting TRH neurons in the PVN that contain these neuropeptides, but also reduces circulating levels of TSH and thyroid hormone.

Similar to the catecholamine innervation, asymmetric specializations between axons containing α-MSH/CART and TRH neurons in the PVN are observed, suggesting an excitatory function, whereas axon terminals containing NPY and AGRP establish primarily symmetric synaptic specializations, suggesting an inhibitory function. The latter associations are sometimes so dense as to completely envelop the perikarya and first-order dendrites of TRH neurons. In addition to the arcuate nucleus, however, which constitutes more than 80% of the NPY innervation to TRH neurons in the PVN and 100% of the AGRP innervation, brainstem catecholaminergic neurons may also contribute to the NPY innervation of hypophysiotropic TRH neurons in a minor way, particularly to their distal dendrites. Nevertheless, a major NPY projection pathway from the brainstem to the PVN does exist, but is primarily targeted to CRH neurons in the PVN. This target-specific innervation of the PVN by axons containing NPY originating from at least two discrete sources in the brain may be a mechanism by which a single peptide can exert independent actions on discrete populations of neurons under different physiologic conditions.

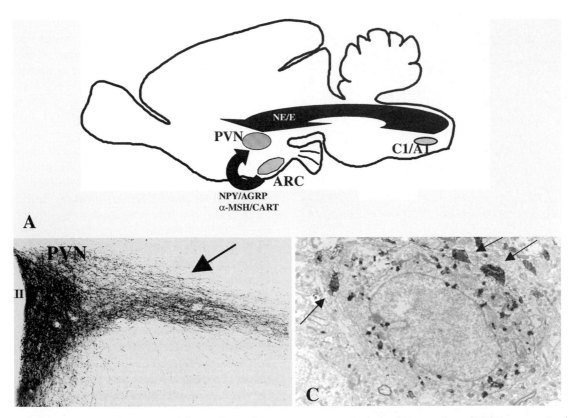

FIGURE 6 (A) Sagittal drawing of the rat brain showing two major sources of innervation of TRH neurons in the hypothalamic PVN: the hypothalamic arcuate nucleus (ARC) that carries the neuropeptides NPY, AGRP, α-MSH, and CART to the PVN and brainstem C1/A1 cell groups that carry the catecholamines norepinephrine (NE) and epinephrine (E) to the PVN. (B) Neurons arising in the arcuate nucleus and brainstem innervate the PVN by traversing the medial forebrain bundle (arrow). (C) Electron micrograph showing that these axons (arrows) establish synaptic contacts with the cell body and dendrites of TRH neurons.

V. FEEDBACK REGULATION OF HYPOPHYSIOTROPIC TRH BY THYROID HORMONE

The anatomical specificity of the TRH neuronal population in the medial and periventricular parvocellular subdivisions of the PVN is associated with a functional specificity of these cells with respect to feedback regulation by thyroid hormone. When circulating levels of thyroid hormone fall below normal values, perikaryal size and the content of proTRH and proTRH mRNA increases in these neurons, but not other TRH neurons in the forebrain (Figs. 7A and 7B). This increase is accompanied by a decline in the content of TRH in the median eminence due to an increase in the secretion of TRH into the portal blood for conveyance to the anterior pituitary. Conversely, increased circulating levels of T4 cause marked suppression of proTRH mRNA in the PVN and a reduction in the secretion of TRH into the portal plexus, establishing an inverse relationship between thyroid hormone and the biosynthesis and secretion of hypophysiotropic TRH.

The increase or decrease in the amount of hypophysiotropic TRH secreted into the portal system for conveyance to the anterior pituitary as dictated by variations in circulating levels of thyroid hormones is important in establishing the setpoint for feedback regulation by thyroid hormone on anterior pituitary TSH secretion. When portal blood TRH concentrations are low, TSH can be suppressed by less T4 circulating in the bloodstream (reduced setpoint), whereas high portal blood TRH concentrations raise the setpoint for feedback regulation by thyroid hormone. Thus, thyroidectomized animals with lesions of the hypothalamus that include the PVN can suppress TSH with smaller doses of T4 than animals with an intact hypothalamus, whereas chronic intrathecal infusion of TRH can elevate TSH and circulating free and total thyroid hormones.

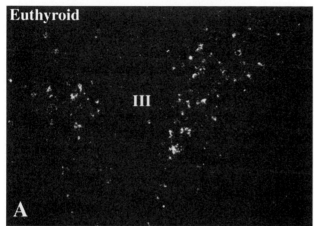

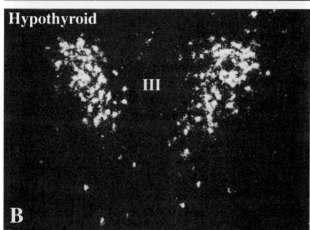

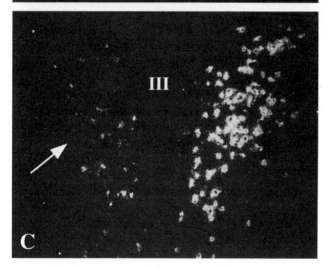

FIGURE 7 *In situ* hybridization autoradiographs of proTRH mRNA in the PVN of (A) euthyroid and (B) hypothyroid animals. Note the marked increase in hybridization signal in (B). (C) Effect of stereotaxic placement of thyroid hormone adjacent to one side of the PVN in a hypothyroid animal. Marked asymmetry of hybridization signal is apparent with diminished signal on the side of the implant (arrow).

The selectivity of TRH neurons in the medial and periventricular parvocellular subdivisions of the PVN to negative feedback regulation by thyroid hormone is an intrinsic property of these cells, mediated by the presence of thyroid hormone receptors in these neurons and the high vascular flow to the PVN. Stereotaxic implantation of microcrystals of T3 adjacent to one side of the PVN in hypothyroid animals, therefore, leads to marked inhibition of proTRH mRNA on that side, but not on the opposite side (Fig. 7C). Although TRH neurons in the PVN contain all of the known thyroid hormone receptors in their nucleus, TRα1 and TRβ2 are the most highly expressed in these cells. However, TRβ2 is the most important thyroid hormone receptor isoform responsible for thyroid hormone-mediated negative feedback regulation of TRH gene expression in hypophysiotropic neurons. Thus, mice with targeted deletion of TRβ2 alone show no significant increase in proTRH mRNA concentration in response to PTU-induced hypothyroidism or a decrease in proTRH mRNA concentration in response to the exogenous administration of T3.

The source of nuclear T3 responsible for feedback regulation of TRH neurons in the PVN differs from the source of T3 in other regions of the central nervous system (CNS) such as the cerebral cortex and anterior pituitary, where the majority of T3 arises from the intracellular monodeiodination of T4 to T3 by type II iodothyronine 5′-monodeiodinase (D2). This is because the PVN contains little, if any, D2 activity or D2 mRNA, indicating that cells in this region are not capable of intracellular conversion of T4 to biologically active T3. Thus, hypophysiotropic TRH neurons in the PVN must receive T3 from an exogenous source, directly from the bloodstream, from the cerebrospinal fluid, from adjacent glia, or by transneuronal transport. The possibility that feedback regulation by thyroid hormone on TRH neurons in the PVN is mediated exclusively by circulating levels of T3 alone is unlikely since the systemic infusion of graded doses of T3 to hypothyroid animals that restore plasma levels of T3 to normal do not suppress proTRH mRNA levels in the PVN to euthyroid levels. Only after constant infusion with higher concentrations of T3 that raise plasma T3 into the supranormal range is there an apparent reduction in hybridization signal for proTRH mRNA to euthyroid levels. Thus, the calculated plasma level of T3 required to suppress proTRH mRNA to normal in the absence of T4 is approximately 1.6 times euthyroid levels, suggesting that like other regions of the brain, feedback regulation of thyroid hormone on

TRH neurons in the PVN is partially dependent on circulating T4.

One potential source of T4 to T3 conversion is the base of the third ventricle where contained among the ependymal cells are specialized glial cells or tanycytes, which contain one of the highest concentrations of D2 mRNA in any region of the brain. Tanycytes extend apical blebs into the CSF and cytoplasmic extensions into the neuropil that envelop the portal capillaries in the median eminence and blood vessels in the hypothalamic arcuate nucleus. Thus, tanycytes may provide a cytoplasmic conduit between the bloodstream and the CSF, allowing bidirectional movement of substances between the vascular and CSF compartments. "D2 tanycytes," therefore, may have an important role in the conversion of T4 to T3 either by the uptake of T4 from the CSF or from vascular compartments in the median eminence/arcuate nucleus and then the delivery of T3 to the CSF. By volume transmission, T3 would have access to extracellular spaces in the brain, such as the hypothalamic PVN, where it could mediate actions directly on hypophysiotropic TRH neurons. Alternatively, tanycytes may release T3 directly into the arcuate nucleus through tanycyte–neuronal interactions, where it could influence the activity of arcuate nucleus neurons that have known projections to TRH neurons in the PVN.

VI. REGULATION OF HYPOPHYSIOTROPIC TRH BY COLD EXPOSURE AND SUCKLING

Thyroid hormone levels and TSH are acutely elevated by cold exposure in several animal species due to the increased secretion of TRH in the median eminence. This response is accompanied by a rapid increase in proTRH mRNA in the PVN, peaking within 30 to 60 min of the stimulus, suggesting that the response is mediated at least in part at the level of TRH gene transcription. A particularly intriguing finding regarding the acute cold-induced stimulation of the thyroid axis is that proTRH mRNA is increased at a time when circulating levels of thyroid hormone are high. This is in contrast to the mechanism of inverse feedback regulation by thyroid hormone as discussed above where proTRH mRNA would be expected to be inhibited. Thus, cold exposure may override the normal mechanism for feedback regulation by altering the setpoint for inhibition of TRH gene expression by T3.

The mechanism whereby the setpoint for feedback inhibition by thyroid hormone changes with cold exposure and suckling is still uncertain but there is strong evidence to suggest a role of catecholamines. Norepinephrine stimulates the release of TRH from hypothalamic preparations in culture, and depletion of catecholamines with inhibitors of catecholamine biosynthesis, such as α-methyl-para-tyrosine, or selective catecholamine neurotoxins, such as 6-hydroxydopamine, abolishes the response of the hypothalamic–pituitary–thyroid axis to cold exposure. In addition, the TSH response to acute cold exposure does not occur within the first 10 days after birth in the rat when the hypothalamic norepinephrine innervation is still immature. As noted previously, the PVN receives dense, afferent input from catecholamine-containing neurons in the brainstem that form asymmetric-type synaptic interactions on the cell body and dendrites of TRH neurons, suggesting an excitatory role. Norepinephrine may also stimulate TRH secretion by interacting with α-1 receptors directly in the median eminence.

Suckling increases proTRH mRNA in the PVN within 30 to 60 min of the response but for the primary purpose of increasing prolactin secretion from the anterior pituitary. TSH and thyroid hormone levels do not increase, perhaps due to the simultaneous release of oxytocin, which can attenuate TRH-induced TSH secretion. Although serotonergic afferents from the midbrain raphe may mediate this response, the mechanism for the increase in TRH gene expression remains elusive.

VII. REGULATION OF HYPOPHYSIOTROPIC TRH BY FASTING AND INFECTION (NONTHYROIDAL ILLNESS SYNDROME)

Infection and fasting also alter the normal mechanisms of feedback regulation by circulating levels of thyroid hormone on hypophysiotropic TRH. In these circumstances, however, there is a fall in thyroid hormone levels but a seemingly paradoxical reduction of proTRH mRNA in the PVN, reduced secretion of TRH into the portal blood, and low or inappropriately normal plasma TSH levels rather than the anticipated increase in all of these parameters as seen in primary hypothyroidism. Thus, these conditions override the normal feedback mechanism described above and induce a state of central hypothyroidism, commonly referred to as "nonthyroidal illness" or the "sick euthyroid syndrome" in human. By reducing thyroid thermogenesis and preserving nitrogen stores, this mechanism is an important adaptive response to reduce energy expenditure until the adverse stimulus has been removed.

The state of central hypothyroidism induced by fasting is orchestrated by a circulating cytokine of white adipose tissue origin, leptin, which declines with fasting and is restored to normal levels by refeeding. Thus, if leptin is administered exogenously to fasting animals, the reduction in circulating levels of thyroid hormone, TSH, and hypophysiotropic proTRH mRNA in the PVN is prevented (Fig. 8). The primary action of leptin on the hypothalamic–pituitary–thyroid (HPT) axis is mediated primarily by the hypothalamic arcuate nucleus via the arcuato-PVN pathway. If the arcuate nucleus is destroyed, not only is the response of the thyroid axis to fasting abolished, its response to the exogenous administration of leptin is lost as well. The arcuate nucleus, therefore, serves as a critical locus to mediate the effects of leptin on the HPT axis and in so doing presumably establishes the setpoint for feedback sensitivity of proTRH-producing neurons in the PVN to thyroid hormone, lowering the setpoint when leptin levels are suppressed during fasting.

At least two anatomically distinct populations of neurons in the arcuate nucleus with opposing functions, the α-MSH-producing neurons that co-express CART and the NPY-producing neurons that co-express AGRP, are responsible for the actions of leptin on hypophysiotropic TRH. When leptin levels are suppressed during fasting, expression of the genes encoding POMC, the precursor protein of α-MSH, and CART are reduced simultaneously with a marked increase in the genes encoding NPY and AGRP. As suggested by the appearance of the synaptic specializations between axons containing α-MSH and CART and TRH neurons, both peptides, when administered intracerebroventricularly to fasting animals, activate proTRH gene expression and each can increase the suppressed levels of proTRH mRNA in hypophysiotropic neurons induced by fasting. Suppression of α-MSH and CART by fasting, therefore, is an important component of the effect of fasting on the thyroid axis, and their increase with refeeding may partly explain the recovery of the thyroid axis to normal. Since the TRH gene contains a multifunctional cAMP-response element that is activated by the phosphorylated form of CREB (PCREB) and inhibited by thyroid hormone bound to its receptor, and all melanocortin receptors couple to stimulatory G-proteins, an increase in cAMP generation may have the effect of decreasing the sensitivity of the TRH gene to feedback inhibition by thyroid hormone by increasing PCREB. Nevertheless, in contrast to the systemic administration of leptin, which restores the thyroid axis to normal in fasting animals, α-MSH is capable of only partly restoring circulating thyroid hormone levels and TSH, and CART has no effect on these hormones, suggesting that other central regulatory mechanisms also participate in this response.

It is likely that NPY has an important role in resetting the hypothalamic–pituitary–thyroid axis during fasting since fasting up-regulates NPY gene expression simultaneously with a decrease in POMC/CART gene expression and NPY receptors couple to inhibitory G-proteins that reduce cAMP. An inhibitory effect of NPY is suggested by the morphologic specializations between NPY-containing axon term-

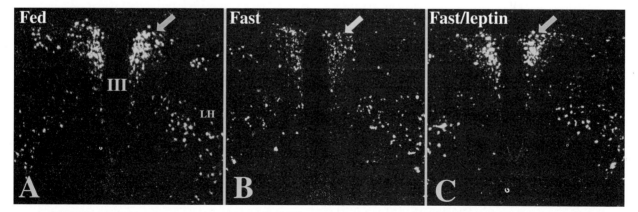

FIGURE 8 *In situ* hybridization autoradiographs of proTRH mRNA in the PVN (arrow) of (A) normal fed and (B) fasting animals. Note the marked reduction in hybridization signal by fasting. (C) ProTRH mRNA levels are restored to normal in fasting animals administered leptin.

inals and TRH neurons in the PVN. Indeed, the exogenous administration of NPY to normal, fed rats reduces circulating thyroid hormone and TSH levels and induces a greater than 50% reduction in proTRH mRNA in PVN neurons. The inhibitory action of NPY is mediated primarily by NPY Y1 and NPY Y5 receptors, with little or no effect of NPY Y2 receptors. NPY may also antagonize the activating effect of α-MSH on hypophysiotropic TRH neurons at a postreceptor level by preventing the phosphorylation of CREB.

Since the NPY-deficient transgenic mouse retains typical homeostatic responses to fasting, including a fall in thyroid hormone levels, it is likely that inhibitory factors other than NPY also contribute to the regulatory responses of fasting on the HPT axis. A likely candidate is AGRP, which is co-expressed in the same arcuate nucleus neurons and axon terminals that innervate TRH neurons in the PVN and which is also a potent inhibitor of proTRH mRNA when administered exogenously to fed animals. As AGRP is an endogenous antagonist at melanocortin receptors, its primary role may be to prevent the stimulatory effects of α-MSH on the TRH gene. Not all TRH neurons in the PVN receive contacts by α-MSH-containing axon terminals, however, indicating that AGRP may also function as an inverse agonist to constitutively active melanocortin receptors that may be uniformly expressed in hypophysiotropic TRH neurons or at a separate, as yet unknown receptor.

Although a decrease in POMC and CART gene expression contributes to fasting-induced suppression of the HPT axis, this mechanism does not appear to participate in other causes of nonthyroidal illness syndromes such as infection. In fact, following the administration of endotoxin, both POMC mRNA and CART mRNA increase in the arcuate nucleus despite suppression of proTRH mRNA in the PVN, and circulating levels of leptin are increased. Presumably, therefore, a set of regulatory controls over the hypothalamic–pituitary–thyroid axis that is different than that observed during fasting must be utilized under these conditions, superceding the stimulatory action of these substances on hypophysiotropic TRH.

The inhibitory effect of infection on hypophysiotropic TRH neurons is likely multifactorial and may involve direct and indirect effects of cytokines other than leptin such as interleukin-1, interleukin-6, tumor necrosis factor, and interferon. Supporting a direct action of cytokines on hypophysiotropic TRH neurons is the presence of a STAT-binding site in the promoter of the TRH gene. The potential contribution of cytokine-inducible inhibitors of signaling such as the SOCS (suppressor of cytokine signaling) proteins that prevent activation of the JAK/STAT pathway should also be considered. Glucocorticoids, which rise dramatically following endotoxin administration, may also contribute to the abnormal feedback responses to thyroid hormone. Both the normal circadian variation and the pulsatile secretion of TSH can be abolished by glucocorticoids, and glucocorticoids can reduce proTRH mRNA in the PVN, although the mechanism is unclear.

VIII. EXTRAHYPOTHALAMIC FUNCTIONS OF TRH

Not all populations of TRH neurons subserve a hypophysiotropic function. As noted above, even within the PVN itself, TRH neurons in the anterior and dorsal parvocellular subdivisions do not project to the median eminence and instead are probably involved in the regulation of autonomic function and behavior. There are many TRH-rich regions in the brain including such diverse groups as the lateral hypothalamus, preoptic region, olfactory lobes, periaqueductal gray, dorsal motor nucleus of the vagus, and spinal cord, to name only a few. Rather than influence anterior pituitary TSH secretion, these neurons have a number of independent functions (depending upon their location), as described in Table 1. The spinal cord, for example, contains one of the highest concentrations of TRH in the CNS, exceeding even that in the hypothalamus. Here, TRH is located in axon terminals in the intermediolateral column and ventral horn (Fig. 9), originating from a large population of neurons in the brainstem medullary raphe. The dense concentration of TRH

TABLE 1 Nonhypophysiotropic Effects of TRH/TRH-Derived Peptides

Analgesia	Increased gastric acid secretion
Anticonvulsant activity	Increased gastrointestinal motility
Arousal	Increased glucagon secretion
Cerebral vasodilation	Increased locomotor activity
Diaphoresis	Increased respiration
Facilitation of memory	Inhibition of food intake
Facilitation of motoneuron excitability	Neurotropic effects on spinal cord motoneurons
Hypertension	Peripheral vasoconstriction
Improved memory	Reduced pancreatic exocrine secretion
Increased blood pressure	Tachycardia
Increased body temperature	Tremor

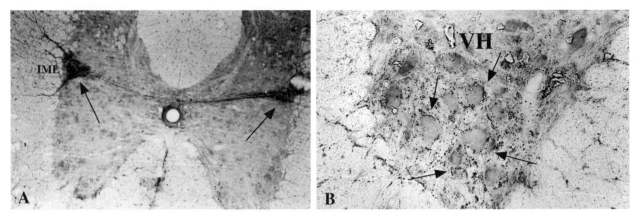

FIGURE 9 TRH terminal fields in the spinal cord (A) intermediolateral column (IML) [arrows in (A)], and (B) ventral horn (VH). Arrows in (B) show dense terminal fields in association with α-motoneurons.

in the intermediolateral column mediates some of the autonomic effects of TRH including cardiovascular function. Ventral horn TRH may act as a facilitatory (excitatory) modulator of lower motoneuron function but could also have a tropic role, stimulating the outgrowth of motoneurons and promoting recovery following traumatic or ischemic spinal injuries. The effect of TRH on gut motility and gastric acid secretion is mediated by neurons in the dorsal motor nucleus of the vagus. TRH in the hippocampus exerts an anticonvulsant action, whereas TRH in the lateral hypothalamus and septum is involved in arousal and locomotor activity. Of particular interest are regions in the brain such as the midbrain periaqueductal gray, reticular nucleus of thalamus, and olfactory bulbs, where products of the TRH prohormone other than TRH itself may be the primary end products of proTRH processing. In the periaqueductal gray, for example, opiate withdrawal results in preferential accumulation of preproTRH$_{83-106}$ and may be involved in nociception or recovery from the physical manifestations of opiate withdrawal.

TRH (and/or TRH mRNA) has also been identified in anterior pituitary somatotropes, where it may contribute to basal secretion of TSH by a paracrine mechanism, and in many peripheral tissues including the retina, thyroid (parafollicular cells), heart, adrenal medulla, epididymis, testis (Leydig cells), placenta (syncytiotrophoblast cells), ovary, spleen, gastrointestinal tract, and pancreas (beta cells). The demonstration that mice with targeted deletion of the TRH gene develop diabetes has implicated TRH or products of proTRH in islet cell development and/or glucose homeostasis.

Glossary

cyclic AMP-response element-binding protein A nuclear transcription factor mediating intracellular signaling systems that activate cyclic AMP.

deiodinase One of three different enzymes (D1, D2, and D3) responsible for removal of iodine from tyrosine residues to activate or inactivate thyroid hormone.

hypophysiotropic That pertaining to regulation of anterior pituitary secretion.

paraventricular nucleus A collection of small (parvocellular) and large (magnocellular) neurons in the hypothalamus that contain the neurons of origin of the thyrotropin-releasing hormone tuberoinfundibular system.

proconvertase enzymes Proteolytic enzymes of the subtilisin/kexin-like family that participate in the conversion of peptide precursors to their final biologically active forms by cleaving at the C-terminal basic amino acids.

promoter The region of a gene that directs regulation of transcription of its specific mRNA.

retinoid acid X receptor A member of the nuclear receptor family capable of forming heterodimers with thyroid hormone receptors.

signal transducers and activators of transcription A family of transcription factors mediating the effects of cytokines.

tuberoinfundibular system The collection of neurons in the brain and their axon trajectory that terminate in the neural–hemal contact zone of the hypothalamic median eminence.

See Also the Following Articles

Parathyroid Hormone • Thyroglobulin • Thyroid Hormone Receptor Isoforms • Thyroid Stimulating Hormone (TSH) • Thyrotropin Receptor Signaling • Thyrotropin-Releasing Hormone Receptor Signaling

Further Reading

Abel, E. D., Ahima, R. S., Boers, M.-E., Elmquist, J. K., and Wondisford, F. E. (2001). Critical role for thyroid hormone receptor β2 in the regulation of paraventricular thyrotropin-releasing hormone neurons. *J. Clin. Invest.* **107**, 1017–1023.

Arancibia, S., Rage, F. L., Astier, H., and Tapia-Arancibia, L. (1996). Neuroendocrine and autonomous mechanisms underlying thermoregulation in cold environment. *Neuroendocrinology* **6**, 257–267.

Fekete, C., Kelly, J., Mihaly, E., Sarkar, S., Rand, W. M., Legradi, G., Emerson, C. H., and Lechan, R. M. (2001). Neuropeptide Y has a central inhibitory action on the hypothalamic–pituitary–thyroid axis. *Endocrinology* **142**, 2606–2613.

Fekete, C., Legradi, G., Mihaly, E., Huang, Q.-H., Tatro, J. B., Rand, W. M., Emerson, C. H., and Lechan, R. M. (2000). α-Melanocyte-stimulating hormone is contained in nerve terminals innervating thyrotropin-releasing hormone-synthesizing neurons in the hypothalamic paraventricular nucleus and prevents fasting-induced suppression of prothyrotropin-releasing hormone gene expression. *J. Neurosci.* **20**, 1550–1558.

Fekete, C., Mihaly, E., Luo, L.-G., Kelly, J., Clausen, J. T., Mao, Q. F., Rand, W. M., Moss, L. G., Kuhar, M., Emerson, C. H., Jackson, I. M. D., and Lechan, R. M. (2000). Association of cocaine- and amphetamine-regulated transcript-immunoreactive elements with thyrotropin-releasing hormone-synthesizing neurons in the hypothalamic paraventricular nucleus and its role in the regulation of the hypothalamic–pituitary–thyroid axis during fasting. *J. Neurosci.* **20**, 9224–9234.

Flier, J. S., Harris, M., and Hollenberg, A. N. (2000). Leptin, nutrition, and the thyroid: The why, the wherefore, and the wiring. *J. Clin. Invest.* **105**, 859–861.

Harris, M., Aschkenasi, C., Elias, C. F., Chadfrankunnel, A., Nillni, E. A., Bjorbaek, C., Wlmquist, J. K., Flier, J. S., and Hollenberg, A. N. (2000). Transcriptional regulation of the thyrotropin-releasing hormone gene by leptin and melanocortin signaling. *J. Clin. Invest.* **107**, 111–120.

Hollenberg, A. N., Monden, T., Flynn, T. R., Boers, M.-E., Cohen, O., and Wondisford, F. E. (1995). The human thyrotropin-releasing hormone gene is regulated by thyroid hormone through two distinct classes of negative thyroid hormone response elements. *Mol. Endocrinol.* **9**, 540–550.

Lechan, R. M., and Toni, R. (2002). Thyroid Hormones in Normal Tissue. "Hormones, Brain and Behavior" (D. Pfaff, ed.), Vol. 2, 157–238. Academic Press, San Diego, CA.

Legradi, G., Emerson, C. H., Ahima, R. S., Flier, J. S., and Lechan, R. M. (1997). Leptin prevents fasting-induced suppression of prothyrotropin-releasing hormone messenger ribonucleic acid in neurons of the hypothalamic paraventricular nucleus. *Endocrinology* **138**, 2569–2576.

Legradi, G., Emerson, C. H., Ahima, R. S., Rand, W. M., Flier, J. S., and Lechan, R. M. (1998). Arcuate nucleus ablation prevents fasting-induced suppression of proTRH mRNA in the hypothalamic paraventricular nucleus. *Neuroendocrinology* **68**, 89–97.

Legradi, G., and Lechan, R. M. (1998). The arcuate nucleus is the major source of neuropeptide Y-innervation of thyrotropin-releasing hormone neurons in the hypothalamic paraventricular nucleus. *Endocrinology* **139**, 3262–3270.

Mihaly, E., Fekete, C. S., Tatro, J. B., Liposits, Z. S., Stopa, E. G., and Lechan, R. M. (2000). Hypophysiotropic thyrotropin-releasing hormone-synthesizing neurons in the human hypo-

thalamus are innervated by neuropeptide Y, agouti-related protein, and α-melanocyte-stimulating hormone. *J. Clin. Endocrinol. Metab.* **85**, 2596–2603.

Nillni, E. A., and Sevarino, K. A. (1999). The biology of pro-thyrotropin-releasing hormone-derived peptides. *Endocr. Rev.* **20**, 599–648.

Yamada, M., Saga, Y., Shibusawa, N., Hirato, J., Murakami, M., Iwasaki, T., Hashimoto, K., Satoh, T., Wakabayashi, K., and Taketo, M. M. (1997). Tertiary hypothyroidism and hyperglycemia in mice with targeted disruption of the thyrotropin-releasing hormone gene. *Proc. Natl. Acad. Sci. USA* **94**, 10862–10867.

TNF

See *Tumor Necrosis Factor*

Transcortin and Blood-Binding Proteins of Glucocorticoids and Mineralocorticoids

AGNÈS EMPTOZ-BONNETON, CATHERINE GRENOT, AND MICHEL PUGEAT
INSERM ERM 03 22

I. INTRODUCTION
II. STRUCTURE, BIOCHEMISTRY, AND BIOSYNTHESIS OF CBG
III. CBG GENE
IV. PHYSIOLOGICAL VARIATIONS
V. PATHOLOGY AND FAMILIAL CBG DEFICIENCY
VI. ROLE OF CBG

Transcortin or corticosteroid-binding globulin (CBG) is the specific plasma transport protein that binds glucocorticoid hormones and regulates their biological disposal to target cells. Analysis of its primary structure, gene organization, and chromosomal location shows a close relationship with α1-anti-trypsin as well as other serine protease inhibitors. During acute inflammatory stress, the fall in circulating CBG levels enhances the bioavailability of cortisol and further amplifies the acute stimulation of adrenal function. In addition to its role as a steroid transport protein, there are indications of a possible role played by CBG in the release of glucocorticoids at inflammation sites and in steroid hormone targeting through the binding of CBG–steroid complexes to cell membranes.

I. INTRODUCTION

In blood, hydrophobic steroid hormones circulate while bound to proteins. Albumin binding is the nonspecific, high-capacity transport system that is generally nonsaturated in normal physiological circumstances, whereas corticosteroid-binding globulin (CBG), also referred to as transcortin, represents a specific high-affinity but low-capacity transport system for cortisol, the main glucocorticoid hormone secreted by adrenal glands in humans. No specific binding protein for aldosterone, which is the main mineralocorticoid hormone secreted by the adrenals, has been identified thus far.

Most vertebrate species examined have circulating CBG with varying serum concentrations and steroid-binding specificities. In each species, the binding specificity of CBG is correlated with the biological activity of glucocorticoids. In humans, CBG-binding affinity is much higher for glucocorticoids (cortisol, corticosterone, and deoxycortisol) and progesterone than for mineralocorticoids (aldosterone and deoxycorticosterone) (Table 1). The binding capacity of CBG is close to the highest physiological cortisol concentration, and more than 90% of circulating cortisol is bound to CBG. Thus, according to the free hormone hypothesis, CBG, by limiting cortisol access to target cells, regulates cortisol biodisposal.

II. STRUCTURE, BIOCHEMISTRY, AND BIOSYNTHESIS OF CBG

Human CBG is a monomeric glycoprotein of 50–55 kDa, as estimated by polyacrylamide gel electrophoresis under denaturing conditions, with one steroid-binding site per molecule. The mature protein is a 383-amino-acid polypeptide, derived from a 405-residue precursor polypeptide.

TABLE I   Affinity (K_a) of Adrenal Steroids for CBG at 37°C

	K_a (liter·mol^{-1})
Cortisol	76×10^6
Corticosterone	76×10^6
Deoxycortisol	76×10^6
Cortisone	7.8×10^6
Aldosterone	1.9×10^6
Deoxycorticosterone	45×10^6

CBG comprises five N-linked oligosaccharide chains per molecule, of which three are biantennary and two triantennary. A pregnancy-specific variant containing only triantennary oligosaccharide chains has been described, but does not affect steroid-binding activity. These carbohydrate chains potentially influence the biological half-life of the protein and may play a role in the interaction of CBG with the membrane receptors that are reported to be present at the surface of some target cells.

CBG is a member of the serine protease inhibitor (SERPIN) superfamily and shares a high degree of sequence homology with α1-anti-trypsin (α1AT), α1-anti-chymotrypsin (AACT), and another plasma transport protein, thyroxin-binding globulin (TBG). The role of α1AT (structurally and genetically the closest to CBG) is to protect tissue from hydrolysis by elastase, released by activated neutrophils during inflammation. CBG is specifically cleaved in vitro by neutrophil elastase at a single site in the neighborhood of the steroid-binding site. This cleavage induces a conformational change in the molecule, resulting in a 10-fold decrease in cortisol-binding affinity and the subsequent release of cortisol from its steroid-binding site.

Circulating CBG is synthesized by the liver. However, small amounts of CBG are also present in tissues such as pituitary corticotrophs, lung, kidney, uterus, and testis. It is not yet clear whether the presence of CBG at these sites is due to local synthesis or to sequestration from blood circulation. The physiological significance of this extrahepatic production of CBG, which probably has no influence on the plasma CBG concentration but could alter the local bioavailability of steroids that bind to CBG, has also not yet been established.

III. CBG GENE

Human CBG is encoded by a single gene located on the long arm of chromosome 14, at position 32.1 (14q32.1). This region, the SERPIN gene cluster, includes five other SERPIN genes: α1AT, AACT, kallistatin, protein C inhibitor, and ATR, an anti-trypsin-related sequence.

The human CBG gene (Cbg) comprises five exons distributed over approximately 19 kb, with the complete coding sequence for CBG spanning exons 2 to 5 (Fig. 1). Cis-acting sequence elements identified in rat Cbg promoter (pCbg) and highly conserved in the human pCbg indicate that hepatocyte nuclear factor-1β and hepatocyte nuclear factor-3α (HNF-1β and HNF-3α), CCAAT-binding protein, D-site-bind-

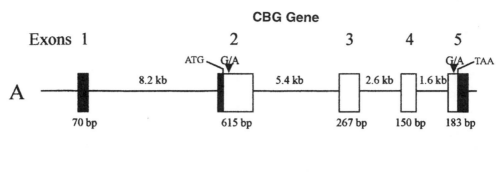

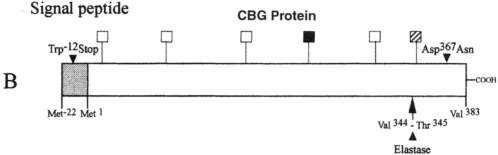

FIGURE 1 Schematic representation of the human CBG gene and CBG protein. (A) The human CBG gene comprises five exons (boxes), numbered 1–5; the black areas correspond to 5'- and 3'-untranslated regions; the size of the exons [in base pairs (bp)] is indicated at the bottom; the size of the introns [in kilobases (kb)] is indicated at the top. The start codon (ATG) and stop codon (TAA) are indicated at the top. The two known mutations inducing CBG deficiency are indicated by arrows (CBG null, c.121G → A in exon 2; and CBG Lyon, c.1254G → A in exon 5). (B) Human CBG and its signal peptide (shaded area). The consensus sites for N-linked carbohydrate chains are indicated by squares; the evolutionarily highly conserved site, essential for the production of CBG with steroid-binding activity, is shown as a black square, and the site that appears to be partially utilized is shown as a diagonally striped square. The position of the elastase cleavage site is indicated by an arrow. The amino acid substitutions corresponding to the mutations in the CBG gene are indicated by arrowheads (CBG null, Trp^{-12}Stop; and CBG Lyon, Asp^{367}Asn).

ing protein, and interleukin-6 (IL-6) can contribute to the regulation of *Cbg*. It has also been demonstrated recently that HNF-1α and HNF-4 control both the chromatin structure and the gene activity of the entire α1AT/CBG gene locus within the SERPIN gene cluster at 14q32.1.

IV. PHYSIOLOGICAL VARIATIONS

In mammals, CBG biosynthesis varies considerably during development, independently of maternal hepatic CBG biosynthesis. Fetal hepatic CBG mRNA and plasma CBG levels increase during mid to late gestation and decrease shortly before birth (rabbit, rat, and mouse) or immediately postnatally (sheep). Thereafter, the production of CBG by the liver increases during the first weeks of postnatal life. This decrease in hepatic CBG biosynthesis around the time of birth may control the amount of glucocorticoids available to tissues, especially to the lungs, the

glucocorticoid-dependent maturation of which is critical to neonate survival at birth.

In humans, CBG levels are low in cord blood, rise rapidly during the first week of life, and then rise steadily during infancy (Fig. 2). Maximum plasma CBG levels are observed at 4 to 6 years of life. A decrease of 30% is observed before puberty (between 6 and 12 years), and then the level of plasma CBG decreases gradually from 12 to 18 years and remains remarkably stable throughout adult life, except in women during pregnancy. CBG levels rise from the 9th week to the 24th week of pregnancy, reach values two or three times as high as basal levels, and return to nonpregnant levels 1 week after delivery. By analogy to animal models, in which CBG variations during pregnancy reflect changes in CBG mRNA levels, this increment has been said to be associated with the inducing effect of estrogens on CBG biosynthesis rather than to a decreased clearance rate.

Gender differences in CBG levels have been reported: CBG values have a bimodal distribution in

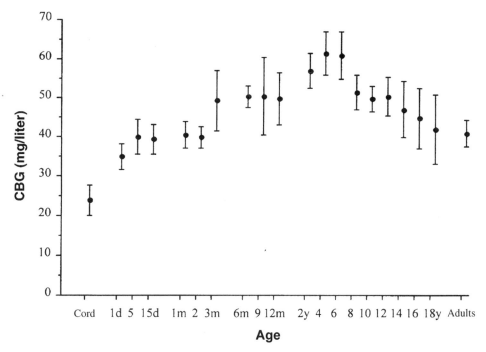

FIGURE 2 Plasma CBG levels (± SEM) according to age from birth to adulthood (cord, cord blood; d, days; m, months; y, years).

men but not in women. No diurnal fluctuation in plasma CBG levels is observed in humans, in contrast to diurnal variations in plasma glucocorticoid levels, and the level of CBG remains unchanged with aging.

V. PATHOLOGY AND FAMILIAL CBG DEFICIENCY

A. Acute Inflammation

Acute inflammation (documented in sepsis, burn injury, and cardiac surgery) induces a rapid and prolonged decrease in plasma CBG concentration. This two-step decrease can be explained by (1) an increased CBG clearance rate after proteolytic cleavage by neutrophil elastase and (2) IL-6 repression of hepatic CBG biosynthesis, as suggested by *in vitro* and *in vivo* experiments (Fig. 3). During inflammation, CBG depletion enhances the bioavailability of cortisol and further amplifies the acute stimulation of adrenal function escaping the normal cortisol negative feedback regulation.

B. Glucocorticoid Excess

Glucocorticoid excess (Cushing's syndrome or glucocorticoid treatment) is associated with low CBG levels, most likely by reduced CBG gene transcription rate, as demonstrated in adult rats. In contrast, the increased cortisol levels observed during depressive syndrome or anorexia nervosa are not associated with any significant decrease in CBG levels.

C. Insulin-Dependent Diabetes Mellitus

In insulin-dependent diabetes mellitus, CBG levels tend to be elevated and return to normal after insulin treatment. Obese subjects with glucose intolerance have higher CBG levels than do lean or normally glucose-tolerant obese subjects, and CBG levels are negatively correlated with the insulin response to intravenous glucose. These results are in line with evidence that insulin is a potent inhibitor of hepatic CBG production, as demonstrated on a human hepatoma (HepG2) cell line (Fig. 3).

D. Thyroid Disease

In thyroid diseases, CBG levels have a tendency to be negatively correlated with free thyroid-hormone levels; patients with thyroxin excess have low CBG plasma concentrations and, conversely, hypothyroid patients have high CBG levels. Treatment of hyper- or hypothyroidism normalizes CBG concentrations. The relationship between CBG and thyroid function is unclear.

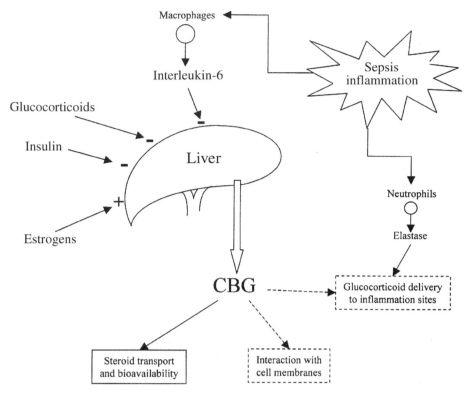

FIGURE 3 Schematic representation of CBG biosynthesis regulation and of the roles played by CBG (dashed lines indicate hypothetical roles).

E. Diseases Involving Protein Metabolism

In diseases involving protein metabolism alterations, such as liver cirrhosis and nephrotic syndrome, the CBG plasma concentration is decreased proportionally to the decrease in albumin concentration.

F. Familial CBG Deficiency

Familial CBG deficiency is a rare occurrence. Recently, two independent mutations (one in exon 2 and one in exon 5) have been described in patients with unexplained fatigue, obesity, low blood pressure, and abnormally low basal and adrenocorticotropic hormone (ACTH)-stimulated cortisol concentrations despite normal free urinary cortisol and ACTH levels. The low cortisol concentrations in CBG-deficient patients illustrate the crucial effect of CBG on the metabolic clearance rate of cortisol, whereas the normal functioning of the hypothalamo–pituitary–adrenal axis indicates that negative cortisol feedback on ACTH secretion is exerted by the free cortisol fraction, which is in the normal range in these patients. Interestingly, obesity is a common clinical feature in CBG-deficient subjects and may be explained by enhanced cortisol activity on adipose tissue, since it

has recently been shown that these patients have low CBG mRNA expression in preadipocytes.

VI. ROLE OF CBG

A. Steroid Transport and Bioavailability

The main circulating cortisol fraction is bound to CBG (90 to 95%), suggesting that CBG may provide a buffer reservoir of cortisol in the vascular compartment that can become rapidly available to the free and active hormone pool by simple dissociation from CBG-binding sites. During pregnancy, increased CBG levels may optimize this cortisol reservoir function of CBG.

CBG protects cortisol from peripheral metabolism and thus reduces the rate of synthesis required by the adrenal to maintain a given level of unbound or biologically active hormone.

B. Glucocorticoid Delivery to Inflammation Sites

As a member of the SERPIN family, CBG is specifically cleaved by elastase released at the surface of activated neutrophils. It is unlikely that elastase cleavage of CBG occurs in the general circulation because of the large surplus of α1AT (the main inhibitor of elastase). Nevertheless, at inflammation sites, CBG cleavage can occur at the surface of activated neutrophils that produce superoxide anions inactivating α1AT. Thus, large amounts of glucocorticoid could be released directly to inflammatory cells.

C. CBG Interaction with Cell Membranes

Although the intracellular presence of CBG can be attributed to *de novo* synthesis in some cases, it can only be explained by sequestration from blood circulation in many other instances, and this may involve a process of cellular internalization. In support of this notion, a specific interaction has been demonstrated between CBG and binding sites on the plasma membrane of various cell types, and the binding is influenced by the conformation of CBG and by the structure of its carbohydrate chains. Furthermore, a CBG–receptor complex has been characterized on placental plasma membranes. It has also been shown that CBG binding to trophoblast cells increases intracellular cyclic AMP levels. Taken together, these findings suggest that CBG could be involved in the guided transport of steroid hormones to target cells and transmembrane transfer of hormones and/or hormonal signals.

Glossary

free hormone hypothesis Plasma-specific binding proteins sequester circulating hormones and therefore only the non-protein-bound fraction (= free) of hormones is available for movement out of capillaries and for cell biodisposal, where it may either initiate a biological response or be metabolized and cleared from the circulation.

interleukin-6 (IL-6) One of the major cytokines secreted by macrophages. IL-6 induces the synthesis of hepatic acute-phase proteins and activates the hypothalamic–pituitary–adrenal axis during inflammation.

serine protease inhibitors (SERPIN) Superfamily of proteins that undergo a relaxed/stressed transition state on binding with serine protease to form an inactive complex. The subgroup including corticosteroid-binding globulin, α1-anti-trypsin, and α1-anti-chymotrypsin derives from a common ancestral gene by gene duplication.

See Also the Following Articles

Glucocorticoid Biosynthesis • Glucocorticoid Effects on Physiology and Gene Expression • Glucocorticoid Receptor, Natural Mutations of • Glucocorticoid Resistance • Heterodimerization of Glucocorticoid and Mineralocorticoid Receptors • Interleukin-6 • Mineralocorticoid Biosynthesis • Mineralocorticoid Effects on Physiology and Gene Expression • Mineralocorticoid Receptor, Natural Mutations of

Further Reading

Abou-Samra, A. B., Pugeat, M., Déchaud, H., Nachury, L., Bouchareb, R., Fèvre-Montange, M., and Tourniaire, J. (1984). Increased plasma concentration of N-terminal beta-lipotrophin and unbound cortisol during pregnancy. *Clin. Endocrinol.* 20, 221–228.

Bernier, J., Jobin, N., Emptoz-Bonneton, A., Pugeat, M., and Garrel, D. (1998). Decreased corticosteroid-binding globulin in burn patients: Relationship with interleukin-6 and fat in nutritional support. *Crit. Care Med.* 26, 452–460.

De Moor, P., Meulepas, E., Hendrikx, A., Heynes, W., and Vandenschrieck, H. G. (1967). Cortisol-binding capacity of plasma transcortin: A sex-linked trait? *J. Clin. Endocrinol. Metab.* 27, 959–965.

Dunn, J. F., Nisula, B. C., and Rodbard, D. (1981). Transport of steroid hormones: Binding of 21 endogenous steroids to both testosterone-binding globulin and corticosteroid-binding globulin in human plasma. *J. Clin. Endocrinol. Metab.* 53, 58–67.

Emptoz-Bonneton, A., Cousin, P., Seguchi, K., Avvakumov, G. V., Bully, C., Hammond, G. L., and Pugeat, M. (2000). Novel human corticosteroid-binding globulin (CBG) variant with low cortisol-binding affinity. *J. Clin. Endocrinol. Metab.* 85, 361–367.

Emptoz-Bonneton, A., Crave, J. C., Lejeune, H., Brébant, C., and Pugeat, M. (1997). Corticosteroid-binding globulin synthesis regulation by cytokines and glucocorticoids in human hepatoblastoma-derived (HepG2) cells. *J. Clin. Endocrinol. Metab.* 82, 3758–3762.

Fernandez-Real, J. M., Grasa, M., Casamitjana, R., Pugeat, M., Barret, C., and Ricart, W. (1999). Plasma total and glycosylated corticosteroid-binding globulin levels are associated with insulin secretion. *J. Clin. Endocrinol. Metab.* 84, 3192–3196.

Forest, M. G., Bonneton, A., Lecoq, A., Brébant, C., and Pugeat, M. (1986). Ontogeny of corticosteroid binding globulin (CBG) and sex steroid binding protein (SBP) in primates: Physiological variations and study in various biological fluids. *In* "Binding Proteins of Steroid Hormones" (M. G. Forest and M. Pugeat, eds.), pp. 263–291. John Libbey Eurotext, London/Paris.

Grenot, C., Blachère, T., Rolland de Ravel, M., Mappus, E., and Cuilleron, C. Y. (1994). Identification of Trp-371 as the main site of specific photoaffinity labelling of corticosteroid-binding globulin using Δ6 derivatives of cortisol, corticosterone, progesterone as unsubstituted photoreagents. *Biochemistry* 33, 8969–8981.

Hammond, G. L. (1995). Potential functions of plasma steroid-binding proteins. *Trends Endocrinol. Metab.* 6, 298–304.

Hammond, G. L., Smith, C. L., Gopping, I., Underhill, D. A., Harley, M. J., Reventos, J., Musto, N. A., Gunsalus, G. L., and Bardin, C. W. (1987). Primary structure of human corticosteroid-binding globulin, deduced from hepatic and pulmonary cDNAs, exhibits homology with serine protease inhibitors. *Proc. Natl. Acad. Sci. USA* 84, 5153–5157.

Pemberton, P. A., Stein, P. E., Pepys, M. B., Potter, J. M., and Carrell, R. W. (1988). Hormone binding globulin undergoes serpin conformation change in inflammation. *Nature* **336,** 257–258.

Rollini, P., and Fournier, R. E. K. (1999). The HNF-4/HNF-1α transactivation cascade regulates gene activity and chromatin structure of the human serine protease inhibitor gene cluster at 14q32.1. *Proc. Natl. Acad. Sci. USA* **96,** 10308–10313.

Rosner, W. (1990). The functions of corticosteroid-binding globulin and sex hormone-binding globulin: Recent advances. *Endocr. Rev.* **11,** 80–91.

Torpy, D. J., Bachmann, A. W., Grice, J. E., Fitzgerald, S. P., Phillips, P. J., Whitworth, J. A., and Jackson, R. V. (2001). Familial corticosteroid-binding deficiency due to a novel null mutation: Association with fatigue and relative hypotension. *J. Clin. Endocrinol. Metab.* **86,** 3692–3700.

TRH

See *Thyrotropin-Releasing Hormone*

TSH

See *Thyroid Stimulating Hormone*

Thymic Stromal Lymphopoietin (TSLP)

STEVEN D. LEVIN[*‡], DAVID J. RAWLINGS[*],
STEVEN F. ZIEGLER[†], AND ANDREW G. FARR[*]

[*]*University of Washington ● *[†]*Virginia Mason Research Center, Seattle, Washington ● *[‡]*ZymoGenetics, Inc., Seattle*

I. CLONING AND CHARACTERIZATION OF TSLP
II. CHARACTERIZATION OF THE TSLP RECEPTOR COMPLEX
III. SIGNAL TRANSDUCTION THROUGH THE TSLP RECEPTOR
IV. FUNCTION OF TSLP *IN VITRO*
V. BIOLOGY OF TSLP *IN VIVO*
VI. CONCLUSIONS

Thymic stromal lymphopoietin was first identified as an activity in supernatants from the thymic stromal cell line, Z210R.1. This cell line was derived from medullary thymic epithelium from an adult Balb/C mouse. Specifically, conditioned media from Z210R.1 cells supported the outgrowth of B lymphocytes from fetal liver precursors, and this activity was determined to be distinct from IL-7 and other known cytokines.

I. CLONING AND CHARACTERIZATION OF TSLP

Using a cDNA library from Z210R.1 cells and a transient expression strategy, Sims *et al.* isolated a cDNA clone whose product supported the growth of the fetal liver-derived pre-B-cell line NAG8/7 in a bioassay. The cDNA encoded a protein of 140 amino acids, including the 19-amino-acid leader sequence. The mature polypeptide contained seven cysteine residues and three potential N-linked glycosylation sites. Further examination showed that the protein was predicted to fold into the canonical four-helix bundle structure common to members of the cytokine family. Expression studies have shown that thymic stromal lymphopoietin (TSLP) mRNA is most highly expressed in thymus and lung, with lower levels found in a wide variety of tissues. The *Tslp* gene was localized to mouse chromosome 18.

Recently, a cDNA clone encoding human TSLP was isolated using database search methods. The predicted amino acid sequence of the cDNA showed 43% identity with the mouse TSLP sequence and was also predicted to form a four-helix bundle structure. For both mouse and human TSLP, the most closely related member of the cytokine family was interluekin-7 (IL-7), consistent with the similarities in the biological properties of these cytokines (see below).

II. CHARACTERIZATION OF THE TSLP RECEPTOR COMPLEX

Using radiolabeled TSLP, Park and colleagues identified two classes of TSLP-binding sites, high affinity (ranging from $7 \times 10^9 \, M^{-1}$ to $1.0 \times 10^{10} \, M^{-1}$) and low affinity ($< 4 \times 10^8 \, M^{-1}$). All of the cell lines that were capable of binding TSLP were of hematopoietic origin, including those derived from the B-cell, T-cell, and monocyte lineages. No binding of the mouse protein was found on any human cell line tested, suggesting that TSLP binding was species-specific. Interestingly, all cell lines found to bind TSLP were also capable of binding IL-7. A direct expression cloning strategy was used to isolate cDNA clones that encode a protein capable of binding TSLP. Using either database searching or a signal-sequence trap, three other groups also isolated cDNA clones shown to encode the mouse TSLP receptor (TSLPR). In all three cases, the cDNA clones were predicted to encode a 359-amino-acid polypeptide with a resemblance to members of the cytokine receptor family. Homology studies showed that the common cytokine receptor γ-chain (γc) was most closely related to the

TSLPR. However, the primary sequence of the TSLPR differed from that of other members of the cytokine receptor family in several important ways. First, the second of four conserved cysteine residues in the extracellular domain was missing. Second, the hallmark WSXWS sequence found in all other members of the family was missing, with the sequences PSEWT or WTAVT present instead. The significance of these changes remains unclear. In the cytoplasmic domain, the TSLPR had a sequence that corresponded to the "Box 1" motif found in members of the cytokine receptor family, but it lacked the linked "Box 2" motif. These sequences have been shown to be important in initiating signal transduction cascades following receptor engagement through binding of members of the Janus family of protein tyrosine kinases. The final structural feature of note in the TSLPR cytoplasmic domain is a single tyrosine residue, 4 amino acids from the carboxy-terminus.

As discussed above, only cells of the hematopoietic lineage were found to bind TSLP. However, using RNA analyses, Pandey et al. found TSLPR mRNA in a wide variety of tissues, with the highest levels in liver, lung, and testis. Message was also found in thymus, spleen, brain, and heart. Fujio et al. found a similar expression profile. One possible explanation for the widespread expression of TSLPR mRNA comes from Hiroyama et al., who found that myeloid cells displayed the highest levels of TSLPR expression. The expression of TSLPR mRNA in nonhematopoietic tissue may reflect the presence of resident cells of the myeloid lineage in those tissues. Support for this hypothesis comes from expression studies of the human TSLPR. Like the mouse gene, the human TSLPR gene was found to be expressed predominantly in myeloid cells, with the highest levels seen in myeloid-derived dendritic cells. The fact that these cells are known to be present throughout the body may help to explain the broad expression profile of the TSLPR gene.

As described above, two affinity classes of TSLP-binding sites were found, suggesting the possibility of multiple subunits in a functional TSLP receptor complex. In support of this model, when the TSLP-binding properties of the TSLPR were examined by Scatchard analysis, only the low-affinity binding site was seen. Clues as to the identity of this second receptor subunit were suggested by the similarities between the biological responses generated by TSLP and those generated by IL-7 (see below) and by the observation that anti-IL-7 receptor α (IL-7Rα) chain antibodies inhibited responses to TSLP. Hence, experiments were performed to test whether the IL-7Rα chain contributed to TSLP-binding affinity. Binding studies using cells transiently transfected with cDNAs encoding TSLPR, IL-7Rα, or both showed that only those cells expressing both chains displayed high-affinity TSLP binding and only cell lines expressing both receptors responded to TSLP. The absolute requirement for IL-7Rα in delivering TSLP signals was further supported by the observation that chimeric receptors containing the TSLPR cytoplasmic domain and an extracellular domain capable of homodimerization failed to generate intracellular signals when expressed in cell lines. However, responses could be stimulated when chimeric molecules including the cytoplasmic domains of the TSLPR and IL-7Rα were induced to heterodimerize. Taken as a whole, these data demonstrate that the low-affinity binding of TSLP to the TSLPR does not generate responses and that a functional TSLP receptor complex consists of the TSLPR and IL-7Rα (Fig. 1).

III. SIGNAL TRANSDUCTION THROUGH THE TSLP RECEPTOR

The inclusion of IL-7Rα in both the TSLP and IL-7 receptor complexes suggested that TSLP and IL-7 may generate similar biochemical signals. Generally speaking, cytokine binding by members of the cytokine receptor family activates a similar signaling pathway, the Janus kinase/signal transducers and activators of transcription (JAK/STAT) pathway. Following receptor engagement, one or more members of the Janus family of protein tyrosine kinases are phosphorylated, associate with the receptor at the Box 1 and Box 2 motifs, and become activated. In turn, these activated kinases phosphorylate a member of STAT family of transcription factors, leading to their dimerization, localization to the nucleus, and induced transcription of specific target genes. For example, engagement of the IL-7 receptor activates JAK1 and JAK3, leading to the tyrosine phosphorylation and subsequent activation of STAT5 (Fig. 1).

TSLP signaling studies have taken advantage of the ability of the fetal liver-derived pre-B-cell line NAG8/7 to respond to either TSLP or IL-7, allowing a comparison of the signaling properties of each receptor complex. As expected, treatment of NAG8/7 cells with IL-7 led to the tyrosine phosphorylation of JAK1, JAK3, and STAT5. Likewise, TSLP treatment of these cells led to the tyrosine phosphorylation of STAT5, but not of JAK1 or JAK3 (Fig. 1). In fact, TSLP was unable to activate any of the known JAK family members. This is in contrast to data from Fujio

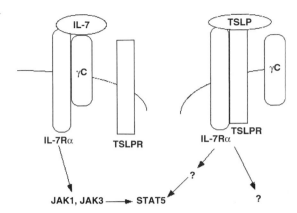

FIGURE 1 The TSLP–receptor complex utilizes the IL-7Rα chain and the TSLPR chain, but not γc. Whereas the IL-7–receptor complex utilizes the IL-7Rα chain and γc, the TSLP–receptor complex uses the IL-7Rα chain and the TSLPR complex. This leads to a number of downstream signaling differences, the most notable of which is JAK-independent activation of the STAT5 transcription factor in response to TSLP. IL-7 also activates STAT5, but does so through the more conventional pathway of activating JAKs (specifically, JAK1 and JAK3).

et al., who found that substituting the membrane-proximal region of the erythropoietin receptor with that of the TSLPR did lead to tyrosine phosphorylation of JAK2. Similarly, Hiroyama and colleagues found JAK2 constitutively associated with a chimeric receptor consisting of the extracellular domain of CD8 and the TSLPR cytoplasmic domain. One possible explanation for the different results may be that the chimeric receptors, by virtue of being homodimers, may adopt a confirmation that allows JAK2 to associate. In addition, it now appears that there is a fundamental difference in the signaling properties of the mouse and human TSLP receptors. The human receptor can recruit and activate JAK2, whereas the mouse receptor cannot. This difference may in part account for some of the unique biological properties of human and mouse TSLP (see below).

Support for the lack of JAK activation by engagement of at least the mouse TSLP receptor comes from receptor reconstitution experiments. Isaksen *et al.* used transient transfection of the hepatoma cell line HepG2 to demonstrate that TSLP signaling required STAT5 uniquely and that activation of STAT5 was independent of JAK. Treatment of cells that were co-transfected with cDNAs encoding the TSLPR, IL-7Rα, and a STAT-responsive reporter plasmid did not lead to reporter activation. However, addition of a STAT5 cDNA did lead to activation. As these cells express STAT1 and

STAT3, these data showed that STAT5, but not STAT1 or STAT3, could be activated by TSLP. In addition, dominant-negative forms of JAK1 and JAK2 did not affect reporter activity driven by TSLP treatment, although responses to IL-7 were inhibited by dominant-negative JAK1. Other experiments have demonstrated that JAK3 also has no effect on TSLP-mediated responses. Collectively, these data support the notion of JAK-independent STAT5 activation. Notably however, a cDNA encoding dominant-negative Tec partially inhibited TSLP-mediated STAT5 activation, suggesting a role for Tec family kinases in TSLP signal transduction.

IV. FUNCTION OF TSLP *IN VITRO*

Three cell types have been shown to respond to TSLP *in vitro*. First, thymocytes and peripheral T cells exposed to suboptimal antigen receptor stimulation can be co-stimulated by the addition of TSLP. The magnitude of the augmentation of proliferation mediated by TSLP supplementation is similar to the co-stimulatory effect of IL-7 on the same populations. However, IL-7 alone will induce a low level of proliferation in these cells as well, whereas TSLP by itself does not promote DNA replication at all. Consistent with what is known about the TSLP receptor complex, antibody blocking experiments have shown that TSLP co-stimulation is dependent on the IL-7Rα chain and the TSLPR but is independent of γc.

Second, TSLP has been shown to influence the development of B lymphocytes in *in vitro* culture systems. B-cell development from both bone marrow and fetal liver cultures is enhanced in the presence of TSLP. However, although IL-7 will also promote B lymphopoiesis in the same culture systems, there are several differences in the effects of IL-7 and TSLP. First, the vast majority of cells that develop in IL-7-supplemented bone marrow or fetal liver cultures fail to express surface immunoglobulin M (IgM). This is due to the fact that although many of these cells have rearranged heavy chain alleles, they have not yet rearranged their light chain loci. On the other hand, most of the cells that develop in cultures supplemented with TSLP express surface IgM, indicating that these cells have successfully rearranged one or more light chain loci. However, it should also be noted that TSLP imparts a less dramatic proliferative effect than IL-7, although the absolute number of IgM[+] cells produced in TSLP-treated cultures is still generally greater than what is obtained from IL-7-treated cultures.

Similar results have been obtained evaluating the contribution of TSLP to human B-cell development using an *in vitro* culture system. Specifically, human TSLP (huTSLP) promoted the development of CD19$^+$/VpreB$^+$ pre-B cells from CD34$^+$ cord blood progenitors. However, TSLP induced only a modest increase in total cell numbers with a concomitant increase in the percentage of CD19$^+$/Vpre-B$^+$ cells. In contrast, IL-7 induced a prominent expansion in cell numbers, but a proportional decrease in the CD19$^+$/Vpre-B$^+$ cells. Moreover, addition of TSLP to CD19$^+$ cells derived from established cultures resulted in a marked increase in the number of CD19$^+$/IgM$^+$ cells in the absence of stroma. These events were associated with an increase in kappa light chain transcripts, suggesting that TSLP may promote light chain rearrangement, perhaps by altering locus accessibility or the expression of germ-line transcripts. These effects were not observed in cultures treated with other B-cell lineage cytokines, including IL-7. The similar influence of TSLP on B-cell development in both the mouse and human systems strongly suggests that a unique function of TSLP may be to promote the development of IgM$^+$ B cells.

Finally, it has recently been established that human TSLP will stimulate the maturation and survival of CD11c$^+$ dendritic cells (DCs) and induce the production of a number of chemokines that promote the recruitment of T lymphocytes. This information collectively suggests the possibility that the enhanced proliferation of T cells and thymocytes induced by TSLP after suboptimal antigen receptor stimulation could be the consequence of the maturation and up-regulation of co-stimulatory molecules on antigen-presenting cells in these cultures. However, despite these clear effects of huTSLP on human DCs, mouse TSLP does not have similar effects on mouse DCs. This species-specific difference is somewhat surprising given that, as discussed above, the mouse receptor complex is expressed at high levels on cells from the myeloid lineage.

V. BIOLOGY OF TSLP *IN VIVO*

An interesting aspect of the biology of TSLP centers around the observations that mice that are genetically deficient in the gene encoding IL-7Rα have more severe defects in the development of B and T lymphocytes than those lacking the IL-7 gene. When this observation was initially made, it was suggested that perhaps the ability of another IL-7Rα-chain-utilizing cytokine accounted for the differences. Hence, it is possible that the action of TSLP

ameliorates some of the effects of IL-7 deficiency but that this is also eliminated in IL-7Rα-deficient mice. The specific differences in the developmental defects support this possibility. For example, B-cell precursors in IL-7Rα-chain knockout mice generally progress poorly beyond the pro-B-cell Hardy fraction A/B stage, which leads to dramatic reductions in mature B cells. B-cell development in IL-7-deficient mice generally proceeds to the pre-B-cell or Hardy fraction C stage, but the cells subsequently fail to expand, leading to reduced numbers of mature B cells. This is consistent with the *in vitro* activity of these two cytokines since IL-7 treatment of bone marrow or fetal liver precursors *in vitro* supports considerable expansion. TSLP, on the other hand, is less able to support expansion, but does promote maturation to later stages and some pre-B-cell expansion. Hence, it seems likely that either TSLP is responsible for the transition from the pro-B- to pre-B-cell stage normally or it can adequately serve the function of IL-7 in its absence at this stage. In any case, in the mouse, it is clear that TSLP cannot completely replace the need for IL-7 in expanding the numbers of pre-B cells *in vivo* or *in vitro*.

A possible role for TSLP in T-cell development has been suggested by the fact that the thymus was one of the areas of highest expression and by the observation that TSLP co-stimulates thymocytes and mature T cells. Moreover, observed differences in thymocyte maturation in IL-7Rα-chain- and IL-7-deficient mice also suggest this possibility. However, results regarding this hypothesis have been inconsistent. Specifically, IL-7-deficient mice have smaller thymi (approximately 10% of the normal cell numbers) and reduced numbers of T lymphocytes, although subset distributions appear grossly normal. Mice lacking IL-7Rα had an interesting dichotomy in their thymic phenotype, with some mice grossly resembling the IL-7-deficient mice and others showing more dramatic perturbations. This second group had thymocyte numbers approximately 1% of normal and they failed to develop CD4$^+$/CD8$^+$ double-positive thymocytes. Again, a potential role for TSLP in mediating these different phenotypes was suggested, although it is less clear why TSLP might partially rescue thymocyte development in some mice and not others. One possibility might be a difference in TSLP expression in these two subsets of mice in the thymus, with more severely affected individuals expressing less TSLP than the IL-7 knockout "look-a-likes." However, this is only speculation and has not been investigated.

A knockout of the *Tslp* gene has not yet been reported, but the gene encoding the receptor has recently been disrupted. However, no discernible phenotype involving the development of either B or T lymphocytes has been noted in mice that lack the receptor. It is possible that this reflects an ability of IL-7 to completely substitute for TSLP or that the subtlety of the defect has thus far escaped detection.

Perhaps the most intriguing clues as to the function of TSLP come from the study of mice that overexpress TSLP as a transgene. Notably, mice that express the TSLP protein in immature thymocytes develop an autoimmune disease that is characterized by the development of skin lesions, splenomegaly, lymphadenopathy, and mixed leukocytic infiltrates in multiple tissues including the skin, lungs, and liver. This autoimmune disease exhibited an earlier onset with greater severity in female mice, which intriguingly is also observed in many human autoimmune diseases as well. In addition, there was considerable evidence for an accumulation of polyclonal immunoglobulins precipitating from serum samples at low temperature. Accumulation of such "cryoglobulins" is characteristic of a type III cryoglobulinonemia, which is observed in certain types of infections (e.g., hepatitis C) and in various human autoimmune diseases. Apart from the skin lesions, the nature of this autoimmune disease is considerably different than what is observed when other cytokines including IL-7 are overexpressed in transgenic mice. In addition, the phenotype of mice overexpressing TSLP under the control of the Lck proximal promoter was very similar to that of mice expressing the cytokine under control of the keratin-14 promoter. The similarity in phenotype of transgenic mice expressing the same cytokine under a different type of transcriptional regulation suggests that these soluble proteins are systemically distributed and produce similar effects regardless of their point of origin. The same was true of IL-7 transgenic mice in which different promoters drove expression of the cytokine. Hence, it seems likely that the abnormalities observed in mice overexpressing these cytokines reflect perturbations of cell populations that they normally affect and that the development and character of this autoimmune disease in TSLP-transgenic mice reveals something important about its function in the regulation of the mouse immune system.

As discussed above, there is some evidence that both IL-7 and TSLP serve different functions in mice and humans. Most notably, as discussed above, deficiencies in the mouse IL-7 or IL-7 receptor gene result in severe defects in both B- and T-cell development. However, humans deficient in the IL-7 receptor have defects in T-cell development, but normal B-cell compartments. This indicates that neither IL-7 nor TSLP signaling is an obligate requirement for B-cell development in humans. Moreover, expression of the human TSLP receptor is highest in cells of the myeloid lineage and human TSLP triggers the release of T-cell-attracting chemokines in both monocytes and dendritic cells. In addition, TSLP treatment triggers the maturation of CD11c$^+$ dendritic cells, which enhances their ability to co-stimulate T cells. This suggests a possible mechanism whereby TSLP overexpression could mediate the lymphocytic infiltrates and autoimmune disease discussed above in transgenic mice. However, it has been reported that mouse TSLP does not have the same effects on mouse monocytes and dendritic cells despite the fact that monocytes at least express both the IL-7 and the TSLP receptors.

These effects on myeloid cells have now been shown to have profound consequences on the development of allergic inflammatory responses in humans. Soumelis and co-workers have recently demonstrated that TSLP triggers the maturation of CD11c$^+$ DCs. These mature DCs promote CD4$^+$ T-cell expansion, recruit T_H2-phenotype T cells, and promote the development of T_H2 cells from naive T cells. This turns out to be physiologically important because it was also shown that epithelial cells isolated from sites of acute atopic dermatitis expressed high levels of TSLP, whereas expression was undetectable in normal skin. Collectively, these data suggest a model whereby affected skin produces TSLP and promotes the recruitment, maturation, and survival of DCs to the site and the subsequent recruitment and development of allergy-promoting T_H2 T cells.

VI. CONCLUSIONS

The initial characterization of TSLP and its biological effects suggested that it may be simply a "lesser" version of IL-7—it does everything IL-7 does, but simply not as well. The study of TSLP is still in its infancy and the availability of reagents and systems to facilitate understanding of this unique cytokine suggest that the next few years will produce a vast expansion in information regarding TSLP. At this point, it is known that TSLP can influence the development of B lymphocytes in both mice and humans. In addition, findings in TSLP transgenic mice strongly suggest that this cytokine influences immune system homeostasis at some level and can contribute to the development of autoimmune disease. Such a role is also suggested by the recent demonstration that TSLP plays a major role in allergic inflammatory responses in humans. Collectively, available information suggests that TSLP is much more than just a "poor man's IL-7."

Glossary

common cytokine receptor γ-chain (γc) A transmembrane protein that was first identified for its contribution to interleukin-2 (IL-2) binding and signaling. It has subsequently been shown to be involved in binding and signaling from a number of other cytokines, which are collectively known as the γc-utilizing cytokines. These include IL-2, IL-4, IL-7, IL-9, IL-15, and IL-21.

interleukin-7 A cytokine that promotes the growth of pre-B cells and co-stimulates thymocytes and mature T cells.

interleukin-7 receptor α-chain A transmembrane protein that was first identified for its capacity to bind interleukin-7 (IL-7). Subsequent research revealed that it binds IL-7 in conjunction with another transmembrane protein termed the common cytokine receptor γ-chain.

Janus family kinases (Jaks) A family of protein tyrosine kinases that are activated by cytokines binding to their receptors. Their best-characterized substrates are members of the signal transducers and activators of transcription family.

signal transducers and activators of transcription (Stats) A family of transcription factors that are induced to dimerize and translocate to the nucleus after being tyrosine phosphorylated in response to cytokine stimulation. This phosphorylation is most commonly carried out by members of the Janus kinase family.

See Also the Following Article

Interleukin-7

Further Reading

Fujio, K., Nosaka, T., Kojima, T., Kawashima, T., Yahata, T., Copeland, N. G., Gilbert, D. J., Jenkins, N. A., Yamamoto, K., Nishimura, T., and Kitamura, T. (2000). Molecular cloning of a novel type 1 cytokine receptor similar to the common gamma chain. *Blood* 95(7), 2204–2210.

Hiroyama, T., Iwama, A., Morita, Y., Nakamura, Y., Shibuya, A., and Nakauchi, H. (2000). Molecular cloning and characterization of CRLM-2, a novel type I cytokine receptor preferentially expressed in hematopoietic cells. *Biochem. Biophys. Res. Commun.* 272(1), 224–229.

Ihle, J. N., Witthuhn, B. A., Quelle, F. W., Yamamoto, K., and Silvennoinen, O. (1995). Signaling through the hematopoietic cytokine receptors. *Annu. Rev. Immunol.* 13, 369–398.

Isaksen, D. E., Baumann, H., Trobridge, P. A., Farr, A. G., Levin, S. D., and Ziegler, S. F. (1999). Requirement for Stat5 in thymic stromal lymphopoietin-mediated signal transduction. *J. Immunol.* 163(11), 5971–5977.

Isaksen, D. E., Baumann, H., Zhou, B., Nivollet, S., Farr, A. G., Levin, S. D., and Ziegler, S. F. (2002). Uncoupling of proliferation and Stat5 activation in thymic stromal lympho-poietin-mediated signal transduction. *J. Immunol.* 168(7), 3288–3294.

Levin, S. D., Koelling, R. M., Friend, S. L., Isaksen, D. E., Ziegler, S. F., Perlmutter, R. M., and Farr, A. G. (1999). Thymic stromal lymphopoietin: A cytokine that promotes the development of IgM$^+$ B cells *in vitro* and signals via a novel mechanism. *J. Immunol.* 162(2), 677–683.

Pandey, A., Ozaki, K., Baumann, H., Levin, S. D., Puel, A., Farr, A. G., Ziegler, S. F., Leonard, W. J., and Lodish, H. F. (2000). Cloning of a receptor subunit required for signaling by thymic stromal lymphopoietin. *Nat. Immunol.* 1(1), 59–64.

Park, L. S., Martin, U., Garka, K., Gliniak, B., Di Santo, J. P., Muller, W., Largaespada, D. A., Copeland, N. G., Jenkins, N. A., Farr, A. G., Ziegler, S. F., Morrissey, P. J., Paxton, R., and Sims, J. E. (2000). Cloning of the murine thymic stromal lymphopoietin (TSLP) receptor: Formation of a functional heteromeric complex requires interleukin 7 receptor. *J. Exp. Med.* 192(5), 659–670.

Peschon, J. J., Morrissey, P. J., Grabstein, K. H., Ramsdell, F. J., Maraskovsky, E., Gliniak, B. C., Park, L. S., Ziegler, S. F., Williams, D. E., Ware, C. B., Meyer, J. D., and Davison, B. L. (1994). Early lymphocyte expansion is severely impaired in interleukin 7 receptor-deficient mice. *J. Exp. Med.* 180, 1955–1960.

Puel, A., Ziegler, S. F., Buckley, R. H., and Leonard, W. J. (1998). Defective IL7R expression in T$^-$B$^+$NK$^+$ severe combined immunodeficiency. *Nat. Genet.* 20(4), 394–397.

Quentmeier, H., Drexler, H. G., Fleckenstein, D., Zaborski, M., Armstrong, A., Sims, J. E., and Lyman, S. D. (2001). Cloning of human thymic stromal lymphopoietin (TSLP) and signaling mechanisms leading to proliferation. *Leukemia* 15(8), 1286–1292.

Reche, P. A., Soumelis, V., Gorman, D. M., Clifford, T., Liu, M.-R., Travis, M., Zurawski, S. M., Johnston, J., Liu, Y.-J., Spits, H., de Waal Malefyt, R., Kastelein, R. A., and Bazan, J. F. (2001). Human thymic stromal lymphopoietin preferentially stimulates myeloid cells. *J. Immunol.* 167(1), 336–343.

Rich, B. E., Campos-Torres, J., Tepper, R. I., Moreadith, R. W., and Leder, P. (1993). Cutaneous lymphoproliferation and lymphomas in interleukin 7 transgenic mice. *J. Exp. Med.* 177, 305–316.

Sims, J. E., Williams, D. E., Morrissey, P. J., Garka, K., Foxworthe, D., Price, V., Friend, S. L., Farr, A., Bedell, M. A., Jenkins, N. A., Copeland, N. G., Grabstein, K., and Paxton, R. J. (2000). Molecular cloning and biological characterization of a novel murine lymphoid growth factor. *J. Exp. Med.* 192(5), 671–680.

Soumelis, V., Reche, P. A., Kanzler, H., Yuan, W., Edward, G., Homey, B., Gilliet, M., Ho, S., Antonenko, S., Lauerma, A., Smith, K., Gorman, D. M., Zurawski, S. M., Abrams, J., Menon, S., McClanahan, T., de Waal Malefyt, R., Bazan, J. F., Kastelein, R. A., Liu, Y.-J., and Zurawski, S. M. (2002). Human epithelial cells trigger dendritic cell-mediated allergic inflammation by producing TSLP. *Nat. Immunol.* 3(7), 673–680.

Taneda, S., Segerer, S., Hudkins, K. L., Cui, Y., Wen, M., Segerer, M., Wener, M. H., Khairallah, C. G., Farr, A. G., and Alpers, C. E. (2001). Cryoglobulinemic glomerulonephritis in thymic stromal lymphopoietin transgenic mice. *Am. J. Pathol.* 159(6), 2355–2369.

Tumor Necrosis Factor (TNF)

BRUCE BEUTLER

The Scripps Research Institute, La Jolla, California

Tumor necrosis factor was originally defined as the principal cause of hemorrhagic necrosis of transplantable tumors in mice and cytolytic destruction of cultured tumor cells *in vitro*. This cytokine, produced primarily by macrophages, and another factor, lymphotoxin, produced by lymphocytes, have identical biological activities. Both cytokines, through interactions with their receptors, are important mediators of normal immune responses and immune diseases.

I. BACKGROUND AND IMPORTANCE

The tumor necrosis factor (TNF) that was originally defined as causing hemorrhagic necrosis of murine transplantable tumors and cytolytic destruction of cultured tumor cells *in vitro* is now also referred to as TNFα. Induced by lipopolysaccharide (LPS) and other substances of microbial origin, TNFα is produced chiefly by macrophages, but also by other cells under certain conditions. Its biological activity is identical to that of what was initially known as lymphotoxin (LT, or LTα), although this protein is induced in response to different stimuli and is produced by lymphocytes. Lymphotoxin is now often referred to as TNFβ.

In the early 1980s, TNFα and TNFβ were purified to homogeneity, sequenced partially (or entirely, in the case of TNFβ) at the protein level, and cloned from cDNA libraries. Independent of these efforts, an LPS-induced macrophage factor termed "cachectin" was defined by its ability to suppress lipoprotein lipase synthesis in cultured preadipocytes (3T3-L1 cells). Cachectin was purified to homogeneity, partially sequenced, and found to represent the murine orthologue of human TNF. The central premise that cachectin is responsible for cachexia in chronic disease remains unsubstantiated, and TNF (or TNFα) is now the standard appellation for this cytokine mediator.

TNF is produced in abundance in response to LPS and is a central mediator of LPS-induced shock. As such, its inherent toxicity precludes its effective use as an antineoplastic drug. At the same time, TNF is considered an essential effector component of the host innate immune system, and animals that lack TNF or are subjected to TNF blockade fare poorly when infected with a variety of pathogens, particularly intracellular bacteria. Because TNF production is one of the most important end points of cellular LPS activation, positional cloning of the mammalian LPS sensor, Toll-like receptor 4 (TLR4), was pursued and achieved by monitoring the LPS-induced TNF response. This has led to an understanding of the sensing mechanism utilized by the innate immune system.

Judicious blockade of TNF activity *in vivo* is now routinely applied as a means of treating Crohn's disease and rheumatoid arthritis, diseases in which the cytokine plays an important though ill-understood etiologic role. Blockade is enforced using chimeric, soluble versions of the TNF receptor, or anti-TNF antibodies. Recent evidence suggests that anti-TNF therapy may also be useful in ankylosing spondylitis.

II. CONTROL OF BIOSYNTHESIS

TNF is primarily an effector molecule of the innate immune system and it is produced in copious quantities in response to microbial "signature" molecules that herald infection of the host. LPS is the best studied stimulus for TNF production. It activates synthesis via TLR4, one member of a paralogous family of receptors that collectively serve in the recognition of molecules produced by microbes. The activation signal proceeds through recruitment of MyD88, which is a signaling adapter containing a Toll/interleukin-1 receptor (TIR), and MyD88 adapter-like (MAL)/TIR domain-containing adapter protein (TIRAP) molecules; these, in turn, stimulate the activation of interleukin-1 receptor-associated kinase (IRAK) and IRAK4, both of which are serine kinases, and secondarily, members of the mitogen-activated protein kinase (MAPK) family, including p38. Downstream from IRAK4, TGFβ-activating kinase (TAK-1) is activated, leading to the activation of the inhibitor of κB (IκB) and its dissociation from nuclear factor κB (NF-κB). This augments transcription of the TNF gene. Separate events, involving p38, lead to enhanced translation of the TNF mRNA, which is subject to repressive control that depends on a UA-rich element in the 3′ untranslated region. Tristetraproline (TTP), an RNA-binding factor, seems to be involved in repression, and targeted deletion of the TTP gene or deletion of the UA-rich element causes TNF-dependent systemic inflammatory disease.

Probably all of the TLRs, when activated, stimulate TNF production in some measure. Other stimuli, including physical stimuli such as ultraviolet light, can also activate TNF production, albeit in far lower quantities. Other cytokines may also activate TNF synthesis under some conditions. However, TNF occupies a position near the apex of the cytokine cascade that occurs following macrophage activation, and it has a greater propensity to induce the synthesis of other cytokines than to be induced. The proximal cause of TNF production in diseases such as rheumatoid arthritis and Crohn's disease is not known.

III. STRUCTURE

TNF, a homotrimer, is synthesized as a transmembrane protein but is efficiently released from membrane anchorage by the action of a matrix metalloproteinase, TNFα-converting enzyme (TACE), concurrent with synthesis, or, in some instances, at the cell surface. A trimeric quaternary structure is essential for biological activity, insofar as the protein must stimulate a conformational response in a dimeric receptor, which engages two of three identical active sites on the ligand surface. Bivalent inhibitors of TNF activity are highly effective because they occupy two of the three binding sites, leaving only one site available for receptor binding.

Paralogous proteins in the TNF superfamily are also trimeric, although some are heteromers [e.g., lymphotoxinβ (LTβ)], and most remain stably attached to the cell membrane. In this regard, the sole exception is lymphotoxinα (LTα), which is entirely secreted. The three-dimensional structure of TNFα and LTα have been solved crystallographically. Likewise, the liganded and unliganded p55 TNF receptor ectodomain structure has been solved. These studies contribute to a model of receptor activation events.

IV. RECEPTORS AND SIGNAL TRANSDUCTION

The TNF protein binds to two receptors, both of which have elongated extracellular domains with four cysteine-rich repeat motifs. Different numbers of these repeats are observed in paralogous members of the TNF receptor family, and, indeed, define the family. The type I (p55) TNF receptor is distinguished from the type II (p75) TNF receptor by the presence of a "death domain" motif in the cytoplasmic domain of the former. The death domain

permits heterotypic interaction with signaling molecules such as Fas-associated death domain (FADD), TNF receptor-associated death domain (TRADD), and receptor-interacting protein (RIP), which have similar domains of their own.

Death domains ultimately elicit cell death by means of caspase recruitment and activation. FADD, in particular, is known to activate caspase-8, with ensuing activation of more distal cell apoptotic machinery. Among the critical targets for caspase cleavage is polyadenosine diphosphate (polyADP)-ribose polymerase (PARP), which is believed to kill cells when activated by consuming cellular nicotinamide adenine dinucleotide (NAD). Other targets, yet unknown, may also participate in cell killing.

The TNF signal transduction pathway is complex and, in part, is mimicked by the imd (immunodeficient) pathway in Drosophila melanogaster, which is responsible for sensing gram-negative bacterial infection. The Drosophila genome does not encode orthologues of TNF or either TNF receptor, but the imd gene encodes a facsimile of RIP, one of the transducers of TNF signals in mammals, and mutations of imd render flies susceptible to infection. RIP and Drosophila FADD signal a Drosophila death effector domain-like domain (DREDD), a homologue of caspase-8, Drosophila TAK-1, and kenny, a homologue of IκB kinase γ (IKKγ), to activate Relish, a homologue of NF-κB. Galere, a gene encoding a homologue of Tab2, also affects signaling through the pathway, and at the apex, a sensing protein similar to mammalian peptidoglycan recognition proteins (PGRPs) is required to transduce bacterial signals across the membrane.

In mammals, TRADD and RIP engage the strongly proapoptotic p55 TNF receptor and signal to activate proteins of the caspase cascade, as well as NF-κB. FADD, which serves the Fas receptor, is activated by interaction with TRADD. The p75 TNF receptor can, under some circumstances, mediate cell death as well, although the mechanism by which it does so is unclear. It is best known to engage members of the (TNF receptor-associated factor (TRAF) family, which leads to the activation of NF-κB. In mice, p75 stimulates lymphoid proliferation, although it also contributes to the net toxic effect of TNF.

Some of the proinflammatory effects of TNF are undoubtedly mediated by both receptors. Gene knockout work, however, has established that the preponderance of the toxicity of TNF is mediated through the p55 receptor, as is the tumoricidal effect. Receptor-selective TNF mutants have been fashioned and used to dissociate cytotoxic from growth-stimulatory effects of the two receptor subtypes.

V. BIOLOGICAL EFFECTS

Shock and inflammation are caused by TNF, which to a large extent mediates the effects of microbial toxins such as LPS. At the same time, TNF offers protection against a wide array of pathogens, including viruses (some of which have fashioned systems for TNF inhibition), gram-positive bacteria, mycobacteria, and protozoa. It is quite clear that this immunoprotective, innate immune function is the central raison d'être of TNF.

Some chronic inflammatory and autoimmune disorders are clearly orchestrated by TNF, insofar as TNF blockade has ameliorative effects, and biologically significant amounts of TNF can be found within involved tissues or in biological fluids that surround them. Both the toxic and beneficial effects of TNF are mediated by its proinflammatory actions, which include neutrophil activation, a procoagulant effect on the vascular endothelium, stimulation of proteolytic enzyme synthesis, and enhancement of microbicidal activity (including enhancement of oxidative radical production) within various cells. Hence, both the benefits and liabilities of inflammation are embodied within this single molecule and the signals that it initiates.

A developmental role for the TNF type I receptor is seen in its requirement for normal development of germinal centers and follicular dendritic cell clusters in the spleen and other peripheral lymphoid organs. LTα signaling as a part of the LTα/LTβ heteromer via the LTβ receptor has an even more pronounced role in this regard, acting to organize lymphoid tissue throughout the body. The tumorolytic effect that gave TNF its name is now seen as the combined result of the procoagulant activity that TNF exerts with disproportionate efficacy in tumor vasculature, and the apoptotic effect that it exerts on sensitive tumor cells. It is apparently something of a curiosity in a biological sense, insofar as mice lacking TNF do not seem to be more susceptible to the *in vivo* development of tumors.

VI. THERAPEUTIC MEASURES THAT INVOLVE TNF

Once regarded primarily as an antineoplastic drug—biotechnology's premiere reply to cancer—TNF proved to be far too toxic in humans to permit routine use for induction of remissions in patients with metastatic neoplasia. Isolated limb perfusion with TNF has been used with some success to treat localized tumors, such as melanomas that have not yet produced visible metastases. The greatest therapeutic success has been witnessed in the arena of TNF inhibition. Although TNF blockade has not shown significant efficacy as a means of treating septic shock, it has been highly effective in the management of selected chronic inflammatory diseases, including rheumatoid arthritis, Crohn's disease, and ankylosing spondylitis. Psoriatic arthritis has also been approached with TNF blockade, with promising results. Inhibition of TNF activity is generally not considered to be effective therapy for multiple sclerosis, ulcerative colitis, osteoarthritis, heart failure, or systemic lupus erythematosus. Indeed, TNF blockade appears to induce signs and symptoms of SLE in a small proportion of patients. This observation, taken together with the fact that several autoimmune diseases involve defects in cell death pathways, suggests that TNF-mediated apoptosis is normally required for the removal of cells that cause certain types of autoimmunity.

Although macromolecules with high specificity have been used as the most effective means of blocking TNF activity, other approaches aimed at preventing TNF signaling or preventing TNF synthesis have also been entertained. A number of small molecular antagonists of LPS signaling have been described, and some of them may also block TNF production under other circumstances. Among these, thalidomide, pentoxifylline, p38 MAPK inhibitors, and glucocorticosteroids have been studied extensively. Each class of agents displays numerous side effects, however, and in some cases, poor efficacy. Specific inhibitors of TNF or TNF receptor processing have not yet been used for clinical effect.

VII. GENETIC VARIABILITY AT THE TNF LOCUS

Although no major coding variants of the TNF gene have been reported, mutations affecting promoter sequences have been identified and exist at fairly high (polymorphic) frequency in the normal population. Numerous attempts have been made to link these polymorphisms to human disease phenotypes and, in particular, to infectious disease susceptibility or outcome. The results have been conflicting; to date, no solid proof of any relationship between a given TNF isoform and any specific phenotype has ever been made. In all events, it is possible to explain associations by linkage disequilibrium; in the most rigorous analyses, no difference in gene expression has been shown to result from mutational differences within the promoter region.

VIII. PRESENT CHALLENGES IN TNF RESEARCH

The TNF field has reached a high degree of maturity. Nonetheless, there remains much uncertainty about fine details of the TNF signaling pathways, and there are inviting possibilities that bear on the selective exploitation of these pathways. Small molecular TNF mimetic drugs might yet see a role in cancer chemotherapy, provided that their effects are channeled so as to split the proapoptotic effect of the cytokine from the proinflammatory effects. In addition, approximately 30 paralogous genes encode all of the members of the TNF receptor and ligand families in mammals. To some extent, cooperativity and receptor "sharing" occur, so that a higher degree of complexity is observed in specific target cell populations. Considerable work must still be devoted to deciphering the pathways that are involved.

Glossary

apoptosis Programmed cell death.
Crohn's disease Form of inflammatory bowel disease in which TNF is inappropriately produced and contributes to disease.
death domain Signature motif of the type I TNF receptor, responsible for inducing programmed cell death. Also found in other members of the TNF receptor superfamily.
endotoxic shock Severe, acute disorder caused by gram-negative infection; excess TNF is produced in response to bacterial lipopolysaccharide as a result of signaling via Toll-like receptor 4. Marked by fever, hypotension, and inadequate tissue perfusion.
lipopolysaccharide Principal glycolipid (also called endotoxin) of the outer membrane of gram-negative bacteria. The most potent known inducer of TNF synthesis.
lymphotoxin The closest paralogue of TNFα, but produced by different cells; also referred to as LTα and as TNFβ; also important for normal immune development and function.
rheumatoid arthritis Autoimmune inflammatory disorder, affecting joints and other tissues, in which TNF is inappropriately produced and contributes to disease.
Toll-like receptors Primary sensors of the innate immune system; named after the *Toll* gene found in *Drosophila*, provide essential signals for TNF production under conditions of infection.
tumor necrosis factor Proinflammatory cytokine mediator essential for normal immune development and function; the factor first discovered to be produced primarily by macrophages, also referred to as TNFα and as TNF.

See Also the Following Articles

Apoptosis • Anti-Inflammatory Actions of Glucocorticoids • CC, C, and CX$_3$C Chemokines • CXC Chemokines • Defensins • Flt3 Ligand • Glucocorticoids and Autoimmune Diseases • Interferons: α, β, ω, and τ • Interleukin-1 (IL-1) • Osteoporosis: Pathophysiology • Pro-Inflammatory Cytokines and Steroids

Further Reading

Bazzoni, F., and Beutler, B. (1996). The tumor necrosis factor ligand and receptor families. *N. Engl. J. Med.* **334**, 1717–1725.

Beutler, B., Greenwald, D., Hulmes, J. D., Chang, M., Pan, Y.-C. E., Mathison, J., Ulevitch, R., and Cerami, A. (1985). Identity of tumour necrosis factor and the macrophage-secreted factor cachectin. *Nature* **316**, 552–554.

Beutler, B., Milsark, I. W., and Cerami, A. (1985). Passive immunization against cachectin/tumor necrosis factor (TNF) protects mice from the lethal effect of endotoxin. *Science* **229**, 869–871.

Carswell, E. A., Old, L. J., Kassel, R. L., Green, S., Fiore, N., and Williamson, B. (1975). An endotoxin-induced serum factor that causes necrosis of tumors. *Proc. Natl. Acad. Sci. U.S.A.* **72**, 3666–3670.

Chaplin, D. D., and Fu, Y. (1998). Cytokine regulation of secondary lymphoid organ development. *Curr. Opin. Immunol.* **10**, 289–297.

Feldmann, M. (2002). Development of anti-TNF therapy for rheumatoid arthritis. *Nat. Rev. Immunol.* **2**, 364–371.

Havell, E. A. (1989). Evidence that tumor necrosis factor has an important role in antibacterial resistance. *J. Immunol.* **143**, 2894–2899.

Hoffmann, J. A., and Reichhart, J. M. (2002). *Drosophila* innate immunity: An evolutionary perspective. *Nat. Immunol.* **3**, 121–126.

Jones, E. Y., Stuart, D. I., and Walker, N. P. C. (1989). Structure of tumour necrosis factor. *Nature* **338**, 225–228.

Loetscher, H., Pan, Y.-C. E., Lahm, H.-W., Gentz, R., Brockhaus, M., Tabuchi, H., and Lesslauer, W. (1990). Molecular cloning and expression of the human 55 kd tumor necrosis factor receptor. *Cell* **61**, 351–359.

Pennica, D., Nedwin, G. E., Hayflick, J. S., Seeburg, P. H., Derynck, R., Palladino, M. A., Kohr, W. J., Aggarwal, B. B., and Goeddel, D. V. (1984). Human tumor necrosis factor: Precursor structure, expression and homology to lymphotoxin. *Nature* **312**, 724–729.

Peppel, K., Crawford, D., and Beutler, B. (1991). A tumor necrosis factor (TNF) receptor-IgG heavy chain chimeric protein as a bivalent antagonist of TNF activity. *J. Exp. Med.* **174**, 1483–1489.

Poltorak, A., He, X., Smirnova, I., Liu, M.-Y., Van Huffel, C., Du, X., Birdwell, D., Alejos, E., Silva, M., Galanos, C., Freudenberg, M. A., Ricciardi-Castagnoli, P., Layton, B., and Beutler, B. (1998). Defective LPS signaling in C3H/HeJ and C57BL/10ScCr mice: Mutations in *Tlr4* gene. *Science* **282**, 2085–2088.

Smith, C. A., Davis, T., Anderson, D., Solam, L., Beckmann, M. P., Jerzy, R., Dower, S. K., Cosman, D., and Goodwin, R. G. (1990). A receptor for tumor necrosis factor defines an unusual family of cellular and viral proteins. *Science* **248**, 1019–1023.

Uterine Contractility

Satoshi Obayashi and R. Ann. Word

University of Texas Southwestern Medical Center

The preponderance of biochemical evidence indicates that Ca^{2+}-dependent myosin phosphorylation serves an obligatory role in the regulation of uterine contraction, although additional mechanisms for regulation are not entirely excluded. This article examines the mechanisms by which uterine smooth muscle contraction is regulated. There remain a number of unresolved aspects of regulation specific to the uterus including the mechanisms by which the processes are regulated during pregnancy and parturition.

I. OVERALL CELLULAR BASIS FOR UTERINE SMOOTH MUSCLE CONTRACTION AND RELAXATION

A. Activation of Contraction

Interactions between actin and myosin provide the molecular basis for muscle contraction. Whereas Ca^{2+} regulates this interaction in all muscle types, mechanisms of regulation are fundamentally different for smooth muscle compared with skeletal or cardiac muscle. The discoveries that phosphorylation of smooth muscle myosin results in marked stimulation of actin-activated myosin Mg^{2+} ATPase activity and that myosin light chain kinase (MLCK), the enzyme responsible for myosin phosphorylation, requires Ca^{2+} and calmodulin (CaM) for activity led to the evolution of an overall system for the regulation of smooth muscle contraction. These regulatory mechanisms include the central role of Ca^{2+}-dependent phosphorylation of myosin regulatory light chain in the initiation of smooth muscle contraction (Fig. 1). Activators of contraction lead to increases in intracellular Ca^{2+} concentrations ($[Ca^{2+}]_i$) and the formation of Ca^{2+}/calmodulin complexes that bind to and activate the enzyme MLCK. Activated MLCK catalyzes the phosphorylation of myosin regulatory light chain. The resulting dramatic increases in actin-activated Mg^{2+} ATPase activity of smooth muscle myosin initiate cross-bridge cycling and generation of contractile force. Increases in Ca^{2+} may occur by influx of Ca^{2+} through Ca^{2+} channels in the plasma membrane, by Ca^{2+}-induced Ca^{2+} release, or by release of Ca^{2+} from the sarcoplasmic reticulum (SR). According to this simplified scheme, smooth muscle contraction is regulated by the relative activities of MLCK and myosin phosphatase and Ca^{2+} homeostasis exerts predominant control over the MLCK:myosin phosphatase ratio. In recent years, the discoveries of additional regulatory mechanisms that modulate the kinase:phosphatase ratio emphasize the increasing complexity of contractile mechanisms in smooth muscle. These regulatory mechanisms include alterations in the Ca^{2+} sensitivity of regulatory light chain phosphorylation and the dependence of contractile force on regulatory light chain phosphorylation (Fig. 2).

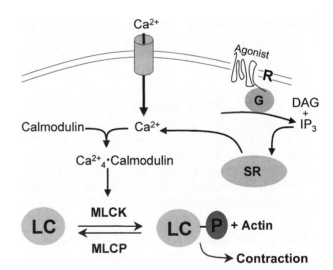

FIGURE 1 Scheme for initiation of smooth muscle contraction via myosin light chain phosphorylation. Increases in intracellular $[Ca^{2+}]$ occur by receptor-activated phosphatidylinositol hydrolysis, inositol 1,4,5-trisphosphate (IP_3) formation, and release of Ca^{2+} from IP_3-sensitive stores and/or by influx of extracellular Ca^{2+} via plasma membrane Ca^{2+} channels. This increase in cytoplasmic $[Ca^{2+}]$ is the primary event that initiates the activation of smooth muscle contractile elements by Ca^{2+}/calmodulin/myosin light chain kinase (MLCK)-dependent phosphorylation of myosin regulatory light chain (LC⁻Op). Phosphorylated myosin undergoes ATP-dependent cyclic interactions with actin to produce contraction. MLCP, myosin light chain phosphatase.

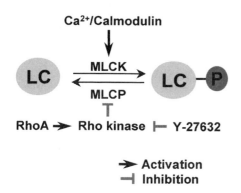

Activation
Inhibition

FIGURE 2 The ratio of activities of myosin light chain kinase (MLCK) and myosin light chain phosphatase (MLCP) affects contraction and relaxation in smooth muscle. Increased intracellular Ca^{2+} concentration ($[Ca^{2+}]_i$) activates calmodulin/MLCK, resulting in increased light chain (LC) phosphorylation and contraction. Inhibition of MLCP by Rho kinase linked to receptor activation sensitizes myosin light chain phosphorylation to $[Ca^{2+}]_i$.

The intracellular Ca^{2+} concentration remains the mainstay for control of myometrial contraction. In the uterus, in the absence of extracellular Ca^{2+} the force of contraction is $< 5\%$ of that obtained in the presence of extracellular Ca^{2+}. Thus, in myometrium, it appears that influx of Ca^{2+} through voltage-dependent Ca^{2+} channels in the sarcolemma is the main source of activating Ca^{2+} for initiation of contraction. However, the intimate relationship between the release of Ca^{2+} from the sarcoplasmic reticulum and the influx of Ca^{2+} through Ca^{2+}-induced Ca^{2+}-release mechanisms confounds the precise localization of activating Ca^{2+} sources. In addition, the release of Ca^{2+} from inositol trisphosphate (IP_3)-dependent Ca^{2+} stores provides additional layers of Ca^{2+} regulation. Particular pathways of excitation–contraction coupling differentially affect Ca^{2+} homeostasis. Elevation of $[Ca^{2+}]_i$ sets in motion the activation of the contractile elements by Ca^{2+}/calmodulin-dependent phosphorylation of myosin. Alterations in the Ca^{2+} sensitivity of force may arise from effects on regulatory light chain phosphorylation or other contractile proteins.

In myometrial tissues, electrical depolarization results in rapid and synchronous depolarization of smooth muscle cells, influx of extracellular Ca^{2+}, and force development. Increases in $[Ca^{2+}]_i$ precede light chain phosphorylation and force development with immediate increases in $[Ca^{2+}]_i$ after electrical stimulation. After a period of latency (200 ms), significant increases in regulatory light chain phosphorylation and force occur, and these values decrease as a function of time despite maintenance of force. In uterine smooth muscle, maintenance of force in the presence of declining levels of light chain phosphorylation is not sustained for long periods of time. Nevertheless, the recruitment of nonphosphorylated cross-bridges into force-bearing structures may be an important mechanism for force generation in uterine smooth muscle during pregnancy.

B. Activation of Contraction in Uterine Smooth Muscle During Pregnancy

In myometrium from nonpregnant women, spontaneous contractions (~ 10 per hour) are associated with cyclic increases in $[Ca^{2+}]_i$ and phosphorylation/dephosphorylation of myosin. Myosin light chain phosphorylation increases from 0.10 to 0.49 mol phosphate per mole of light chain within 10% of the time required to develop the maximal force of spontaneous contraction. During the declining phase of the contraction, force and light chain phosphorylation dissociate. Experiments from a number of laboratories indicate that, although myosin light chain phosphorylation plays an important role in the initiation of uterine contraction, other cellular mechanisms are involved in the regulation of contraction and relaxation, particularly during pregnancy. In most mammalian species, maximal force generation capacity is increased in myometrial tissues during pregnancy. In myometrium from pregnant women, similar levels of force per cross-sectional area develop in nonpregnant and pregnant women. However, the rate and extent of light chain phosphorylation during contraction are significantly diminished in tissues from pregnant women. The extent of myosin light chain phosphorylation in contracting myometrial tissues from pregnant women is very low. Modifications in $[Ca^{2+}]_i$ may be responsible for these observations because they are not due to changes in the amounts of contractile proteins or the activities of myosin light chain kinase or phosphatase. Other signal transduction pathways may be involved.

C. Mechanisms of Uterine Smooth Muscle Relaxation

Decreases in $[Ca^{2+}]_i$, brought about by Ca^{2+} extrusion or uptake into the SR, result in inactivation of MLCK, regulatory light chain dephosphorylation by myosin phosphatase, and muscle relaxation. Decreases in $[Ca^{2+}]_i$ are mediated predominantly by decreases in membrane potential and extrusion of cytoplasmic Ca^{2+} by plasma membrane Ca^{2+} pumps or uptake of

Ca^{2+} into the sarcoplasmic reticulum by SR Ca^{2+} ATPases.

Recently, the search for mediators of uterine relaxation that maintain uterine quiescence during pregnancy has been intense. For many years, cyclic AMP (cAMP) was identified as a mediator of uterine smooth muscle relaxation, and the mechanism of relaxation has been shown to occur primarily through a lowering of $[Ca^{2+}]_i$. In addition, activation of soluble guanylate cyclase by nitric oxide leading to increased tissue levels of cyclic GMP (cGMP) has been identified as a major mechanism of cGMP-induced vasorelaxation through activation of cGMP-dependent protein kinase. Activation of cGMP-dependent protein kinase also results in decreased free intracellular Ca^{2+} and increased myosin phosphatase activity in vascular smooth muscle. Although evidence supporting a role for this signaling pathway in maintenance of uterine quiescence during pregnancy has been published, experimental evidence from other studies conducted both *in vivo* and *in vitro* indicates that mechanisms other than cGMP-induced activation of cGMP-dependent protein kinase regulate myometrial relaxation during pregnancy.

D. Role of Other Thin Filament-Associated Proteins

Two thin filament-associated proteins, h-caldesmon and calponin, are believed to modify contractility by inhibiting actin-activated myosin ATPase activity and, in the case of caldesmon, by tethering actin to myosin and inhibiting the velocity of actin/tropomyosin filaments in the presence of nonphosphorylated myosin. Caldesmon is a basic protein associated with actin filaments. In uterine smooth muscle cells, caldesmon is the most abundant calmodulin-binding protein. Calponin is a smooth muscle-specific, thin-filament protein with biochemical properties very similar to those of caldesmon. However, the subcellular distribution of these two proteins differs in smooth muscle cells. The total amounts of caldesmon are increased four- to fivefold in pregnant myometrium. Although the total amount of calponin does not increase in pregnant myometrium, calponin is redistributed in pregnant myometrium with increased amounts in the cytoplasmic fraction and decreased amounts in the myofilaments, suggesting a lower affinity for cytoskeletal and myofilament proteins during pregnancy. At this time, it is not clear whether these changes in thin filament proteins are involved in the regulation of uterine contractility during pregnancy.

E. Anatomic and Cellular Considerations of Uterine Contractility

Myometrium belongs to the broad classification of smooth muscles termed phasic smooth muscle. Phasic smooth muscle is characterized by transient increases in force generation in response to K^+, initiation of force by action potentials inherent in the muscle cell, and differential expression patterns of contractile proteins. In general, phasic contractile activity of the myometrium (either spontaneous contractions or in response to K^+) is a response to the underlying electrical activity of the muscle cells. As such, contraction and relaxation of myometrium result from the cyclic depolarization and repolarization of muscle cell membranes, and the driving force for contractility is extracellular Ca^{2+}. The action potentials (voltage- and time-dependent changes in membrane ionic permeabilities) are characterized by depolarization and repolarization phases. The depolarization phase is due to an inward current carried predominantly by Ca^{2+} ions and Na^+ ions. The outward current (repolarization) is carried by K^+ ions consisting of fast voltage-dependent and slow Ca^{2+}-activated components. Thus, the frequency and intensity of myometrial contractions are proportionate to the consistency and duration of action potentials in each muscle cell and the total number of cells that are active. The number of cells activated in response to the action potential is thereby determined by the propagation of the electrical impulses in myometrial cells, i.e., low-resistance pathways for current spread. Intercellular channels specified as gap junctions link cells by allowing the passage of inorganic ions and small molecules from one cell to another. Uterine contractions are thereby controlled by intracellular signal transduction mechanisms and by intercellular communications involving the synthesis, organization, size, and gating of gap junctions.

II. REGULATION OF CA^{2+} SENSITIVITY OF THE CONTRACTILE ELEMENTS

A. Ca^{2+} Sensitivity of Myosin Light Chain Phosphorylation

1. Regulation of Myosin Light Chain Phosphorylation by Phosphorylation of Myosin Light Chain Kinase

The sensitivity of MLCK to activation by Ca^{2+}/ calmodulin is diminished upon phosphorylation at a regulatory site A. As predicted, phosphorylation of MLCK has been shown to desensitize light chain phosphorylation to $[Ca^{2+}]_i$. Initial investigations on the phosphorylation-dependent desensitization of MLCK focused on the possibility that phosphorylation of MLCK by cAMP may be a potential mechanism whereby increases in cAMP and activation of protein kinase A lead to the relaxation of smooth muscle. In human myometrium and other smooth muscles, however, cAMP does not cause relaxation via phosphorylation of MLCK. Nevertheless, MLCK is phosphorylated at site A by calmodulin kinase II, resulting in desensitization of the contractile elements to elevated levels of intracellular Ca^{2+}. During the initiation of contraction and rapid phase of light chain phosphorylation (between 0.5 and 2 s in electrically stimulated tissues), there are no changes in MLCK activation properties. Thereafter, MLCK is phosphorylated and the Ca^{2+} sensitivity of light chain phosphorylation is diminished.

2. Regulation of Myosin Light Chain Phosphorylation by Myosin Phosphatase Activity

The Ca^{2+} sensitivity of myosin regulatory light chain phosphorylation is affected by myosin phosphatase activity. Protein serine/threonine phosphatases are regulated by protein–protein interactions with formation of oligomeric complexes that direct phosphatase catalytic subunits toward specific substrates by association with regulatory proteins. In addition, phosphatase subunits and their inhibitor proteins are regulated by phosphorylation. Smooth muscle myosin light chain phosphatase is a holoenzyme consisting of three subunits: a 38 kDa catalytic subunit (PP1C), a myosin-targeting subunit (MYPT, 110–133 kDa), and a small 20 kDa subunit. The small subunit has no established function and is not required for either catalytic activity or activation of the catalytic subunit.

Two well-described myosin phosphatase inhibitory pathways may result in increased levels of myosin phosphorylation and force in response to contractile agonists. Although most of the work in this area has been conducted in other muscles, recent studies suggest that these pathways may be involved in the regulation of myometrial contractions as well. The first is through the small GTPase RhoA, in which GTP-bound RhoA translocates to the membrane and activates Rho kinase. Activation of Rho kinase results in inhibition of myosin phosphatase activity either through direct phosphorylation of the myosin-bind-

ing subunit or through other indirect mechanisms. Dissociation of $PP1_C$ from the M complex occurs by phosphorylation of MYPT. Dissociation of the catalytic subunit from the myosin-targeting subunit results in the inhibition of phosphatase activity. The second signaling pathway, present in only some smooth muscles, involves phosphorylation of a phosphatase inhibitor, CPI-17 (PKC-potentiated phosphatase inhibitor protein-17 kDa), CPI-17 phosphorylation inhibits the catalytic subunit of myosin phosphatase. Currently, there is no information regarding the role of CPI-17 in uterine smooth muscle.

In myometrium, the expression of RhoA protein does not change during pregnancy. Expression of Rho kinase, however, increases in the uterus during pregnancy. The potential role of the RhoA/Rho kinase pathway in oxytocin-induced uterine contraction has been reported. A Rho-kinase inhibitor, Y-27632, inhibits oxytocin-induced rat uterine contraction on day 21 of pregnancy in a concentration-dependent manner. In rat myometrium, Y-27632 has no effect on oxytocin-induced increases in intracellular Ca^{2+}; yet, it is reported that oxytocin-induced increases in light chain phosphorylation are attenuated. Oxytocin increases the phosphorylation of MYPT, and the Rho-kinase inhibitor Y-27632 reduces phosphorylation of the phosphatase subunit by oxytocin. These results indicate that agonist-induced contractions involving G-protein-coupled receptors in the uterus may involve Ca^{2+} sensitization through Rho-kinase-associated inhibition of myosin phosphatase. In addition to the well-described up-regulation of oxytocin receptors during pregnancy, up-regulation of Rho kinase in the myometrium during pregnancy may augment responsiveness to oxytocin.

B. Myosin Light Chain Phosphorylation/Force Relationship

Conditions in which small increases in light chain phosphorylation result in large increases in force have been most frequently reported when smooth muscles are stimulated with activators of protein kinase C (PKC). In human myometrium, it appears that PKC augments agonist-induced contractions. In some smooth muscles, activators of PKC act to cause a slow, forceful contraction, but light chain phosphorylation is not increased. In rat myometrium, phorbol esters inhibit contraction by inhibiting increases in $[Ca^{2+}]_i$. It should be noted that PKC activators may also stimulate contractions with concomitant increases in $[Ca^{2+}]_i$ and phosphorylation of myosin light chain in some smooth muscles from some species.

Several laboratories working with a variety of smooth muscle types have reported that force may be desensitized (rather than sensitized) to increases in light chain phosphorylation. For example, both arterial and uterine muscles are relaxed upon addition of high external Mg^{2+} without reduction in myosin light chain phosphorylation, and high concentrations of sodium nitroprusside have been shown to relax arterial smooth muscle without decreases in light chain phosphorylation. It has been proposed that complex interactions of the contractile proteins with thin filament regulatory proteins may alter the myosin light chain phosphorylation/force relationship, particularly in myometrium during pregnancy.

III. MODULATION OF UTERINE CONTRACTILITY BY STEROID HORMONES AND PREGNANCY

A. Estrogen and Progesterone

It has been suggested that the contractile phenotype of uterine smooth muscle is increased by estradiol treatment and decreased by progesterone. The concept that estrogen promotes a "contractile" state and progesterone gives rise to "quiescence" suggests that the tissue functions as one or the other of these physiological states depending on the hormonal milieu. In general, procontractile mechanisms are expressed and function under estrogen domination, and prorelaxant mechanisms act under the influence of progesterone. Many examples in the literature suggest that this paradigm may be operative in myometrial cells. Estrogen results in increased expression of oxytocin receptors, connexin-43, and smooth muscle myosin. Estrogen also acts to increase smooth muscle-specific expression of cGMP-dependent protein kinase, and this protein is involved in smooth muscle relaxation. Progesterone opposes the effect of estrogen on many, but not all, estrogen-regulated myometrial proteins. Thus, in most species at term, progesterone withdrawal, together with increasing levels of estrogen, leads to increased expression of oxytocin receptors, cervical collagenase, and formation of gap junctions, thereby providing effective contractions of labor and cervical ripening.

In ovariectomized animals, estrogen increases the expression of oxytocin receptor mRNA, even if combined with progesterone. Importantly, however, progesterone inhibits estrogen-induced increases in oxytocin-binding sites. It has been shown that progesterone inhibits oxytocin receptor binding and oxytocin-induced increases in the generation of intracellular second messengers though nongenomic mechanisms. The precise mechanisms of steroid-induced modulation of G-protein-linked receptor signaling remain to be determined.

B. Pregnancy

This article has alluded to the effects of pregnancy on the contractile machinery of uterine smooth muscle. Although beyond the scope of this article, it should be noted that the uterus, like other smooth muscles, is regulated by the expression of a number of G-protein-coupled receptors. The best characterized of uterine G-protein-coupled receptors is the high-affinity oxytocin receptor.

Unlike the closely related vasopressin receptors, oxytocin receptor expression is highly regulated in a tissue-specific manner. Specifically, prior to parturition, uterine oxytocin receptors are increased up to 100-fold. Although, in the human, increases in oxytocin receptor are less dramatic than in many other species (approximately 2-fold), virtually every mammalian species exhibits changes in the expression of uterine oxytocin receptors before or during parturition. Moreover, expression of the receptor decreases dramatically within 24 h of parturition. Temporal expression patterns in the uterus are unique compared with patterns in the brain, mammary gland, and kidney. In addition, uterine stretch seems to be required for dramatic parturition-associated changes in uterine oxytocin receptor gene expression. These findings suggest that myometrial cell-specific transcriptional factors regulate oxytocin receptor gene expression.

IV. SUMMARY

There have been major advances in the understanding of the regulation and physiological functions of contractile proteins in myometrium in recent years. Phosphorylation of the regulatory light chain of myosin by Ca^{2+}/CaM-dependent MLCK plays a pivotal role in activation. The simple view that contractile force in smooth muscle is proportionate to $[Ca^{2+}]_i$ and myosin light chain phosphorylation has been modified as additional experiments have provided insights into the mechanisms of regulation of the contractile elements. It is apparent that, although $[Ca^{2+}]_i$ is undoubtedly the master mediator of regulation, additional pathways act to modulate the regulatory components, particularly during pregnancy. The sensitivity of myosin light chain phosphorylation to $[Ca^{2+}]_i$ can be shifted by second messengers modulating the activities of MLCK and myosin phosphatase. MLCK is phosphorylated, which desensitizes its activation by Ca^{2+}/CaM; protein phosphatase activity toward myosin is also regulated by phosphorylation and dephosphorylation of regulatory subunits or cytosolic inhibitors. The dependence of force on myosin phosphorylation is established in the steady state of tonic contractions; however, in uterine smooth muscle, transient increases and decreases in light chain phosphorylation parallel cyclic increases in contractile force. Pregnancy can shift the relationship between regulatory light chain phosphorylation and force development, indicating that the number of cross-bridges can be altered independent of myosin light chain phosphorylation. The physiologic importance and relative contributions of other regulatory components for uterine smooth muscle function *in vivo* are not entirely clear. Moreover, the role of these mechanisms in various hormonal states and pregnancy remains to be defined. The uterus exhibits physiologic properties unique from other smooth muscle types characterized by unique ligand receptors, electrical properties, and Ca^{2+} homeostatic mechanisms. In addition, there is growing appreciation for differences in contractile protein contents and differing patterns of expressed contractile protein isoforms in the uterus during pregnancy. The future holds exciting new information that will increase understanding of the regulatory processes in uterine contractility.

Acknowledgments

This work was supported by National Institutes of Health Grant HD11149.

Glossary

G-protein Any of a class of guanine nucleotide-binding proteins associated with the cytoplasmic face of the plasma membrane of mammalian cells; proteins involved in transmitting signals from certain types of hormone and neurotransmitter receptors to intracellular pathways.

protein kinase An enzyme that phosphorylates proteins, specifically phosphorylating the amino acids serine, threonine, and tyrosine.

sarcoplasmic reticulum A membranous organelle system of muscle cells, composed of vesicular and tubular components, that stores calcium ions involved in muscle contraction.

See Also the Following Articles

Oxytocin/Vasopressin Receptor Signaling ● Placental Development ● Progesterone Action in the Female Reproductive Tract

Further Reading

Cornwell, T. L., Li, J., Sellak, H., Miller, R. T., and Word, R. A. (2001). Reorganization of myofilament proteins and decreased cGMP-dependent protein kinase in the human uterus during pregnancy. *J. Clin. Endocrinol. Metab.* 86, 3981–3988.

Kimura, K., Ito, M., Amano, M., Chihara, K., Fukata, Y., Nakafuku, M., Yamamori, B., Feng, J., Nakano, T., Okawa, K., Iwamatsu, A., and Kaibuchi, K. (1996). Regulation of myosin phosphatase by Rho and Rho-associated kinase (Rho-kinase) [see comments]. *Science* 273, 245–248.

Longbottom, E. R., Luckas, M. J., Kupittayanant, S., Badrick, E., Shmigol, T., and Wray, S. (2000). The effects of inhibiting myosin light chain kinase on contraction and calcium signalling in human and rat myometrium. *Pflug. Arch. Eur. J. Physiol.* 440, 315–321.

Sanborn, B. M. (2000). Relationship of ion channel activity to control of myometrial calcium. *J. Soc. Gynecol. Invest.* 7, 4–11.

Somlyo, A. P., and Somlyo, A. V. (1998). From pharmacomechanical coupling to G-proteins and myosin phosphatase. *Acta Physiol. Scand.* 164, 437–448.

Tahara, M., Morishige, K., Sawada, K., Ikebuchi, Y., Kawagishi, R., Tasaka, K., and Murata, Y. (2002). RhoA/Rho-kinase cascade is involved in oxytocin-induced rat uterine contraction. *Endocrinology* 143, 920–929.

Word, R. A., Stull, J. T., Casey, M. L., and Kamm, K. E. (1993). Contractile elements and myosin light chain phosphorylation in myometrial tissue from nonpregnant and pregnant women. *J. Clin. Invest.* 92, 29–37.

Word, R. A., Tang, D. C., and Kamm, K. E. (1994). Activation properties of myosin light chain kinase during contraction/relaxation cycles of tonic and phasic smooth muscles. *J. Biol. Chem.* 269, 21596–21602.

Wray, S. (1993). Uterine contraction and physiological mechanisms of modulation. *Am. J. Physiol.* 264, C1–18.

Zingg, H. H., Grazzini, E., Breton, C., Larcher, A., Rozen, F., Russo, C., Guillon, G., and Mouillac, B. (1998). Genomic and non-genomic mechanisms of oxytocin receptor regulation. *Adv. Exp. Med. Biol.* 449, 287–295.

Vagal Regulation of Gastric Functions by Brain Neuropeptides

YVETTE TACHÉ AND HONG YANG

VA Greater Los Angeles Healthcare System and University of California, Los Angeles

The vagal innervation of the stomach plays a role in the parasympathetic regulation of digestive function through interaction with the myenteric nervous system. This article outlines novel neuroanatomical aspects of vagal innervation of the stomach and focuses on selective brain neuropeptides known to stimulate or inhibit gastric secretory and motor function and to alter the resistance of gastric mucosa to withstand damaging agents through vagal pathways.

I. INTRODUCTION

The vagus was recognized to play a primary role in the cephalic control of gastric functions at the beginning of the 20th century after Pavlov's original observations made in dogs with vagally denervated pouch. However, the identification of transmitters in the central nervous system regulating gastric vagal efferent activity lagged behind. During the past two decades, the characterization of several neuropeptides and advances in combined neuroanatomical, electrophysiological, and pharmacological techniques have expanded our understanding of the central vagal regulation of gastric function.

II. PARASYMPATHETIC CONTROL OF GASTRIC FUNCTIONS: NEUROANATOMICAL BASIS

A. Vagal Innervation of the Stomach

The parasympathetic innervation to the stomach is derived exclusively from the vagus nerve, which is composed of a majority of vagal afferent fibers (80%) and a smaller proportion of vagal efferent fibers (20%). The vagal efferent fibers provide neural connections from the brain to the stomach and afferent fibers convey sensory information from the gut to the brain. The vagal efferent fibers originate from cell bodies located in the dorsal motor nucleus of the vagus (DMN) and the gastric vagal afferent fibers have their cell bodies located in the nodose ganglia. The two cervical vagi (right and left) emerge from the brain medulla at the jugular foramen, extend via the nodose ganglia into the neck, and course along the esophagus; then the cervical vagus enters the diaphragm as the anterior and posterior vagal trunks that divide into five branches, two gastric, two celiac, and one hepatic (Fig. 1). The anterior gastric branch of the vagus innervates the ventral part of the stomach and the pyloric sphincter, and the posterior gastric branch innervates the dorsal part of the stomach. The common hepatic branch contains a gastroduodenal/pyloric branch, which contributes additional innervation to the antrum and pylorus (Fig. 1).

B. Organization and Characteristics of DMN Neurons with Axonal Projections to the Stomach

Tracing studies by Powley and Berthoud revealed that the vagal preganglionic cell bodies in the DMN exhibit a viscerotopic organization with a distinctive rostrocaudally symmetrical pair of longitudinal columns contributing to the vagal innervation of the gut (Fig. 1). The anterior and posterior gastric vagal branches originate from ipsilateral projections of DMN neurons located in the medial column of the left and right DMN nuclei, respectively. Morphological and electrophysiological studies revealed that the columnar organization of DMN neurons shows quantitative and regional differences. In particular, preganglionic vagal motor neurons in the medial column innervating the stomach are small in size and large in number. Consistent with the "size principle" whereby neurons with the smallest cell bodies have

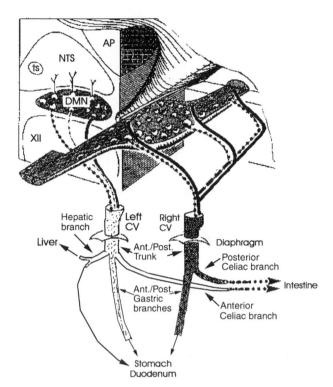

FIGURE 1 Rostrocaudal schematic representation of DMN neurons providing vagal innervation of the stomach through the gastric and hepatic branches. Dendritic projections of DMN motoneurons into the nucleus tractus solitarius are also shown. AP, area postrema; CV, cervical vagus; NTS, nucleus tractus solitarius. Reprinted with permission from Powley, T. L., Berthoud, H.-R., Prechtl, J. C. and Fox, A. E. (1991). Fibers of the vagus regulating gastrointestinal function. *In* "Brain–Gut Interactions" (Y. Taché and D. Wingate, eds.), pp. 73–82. Copyright CRC Press, Boca Raton, Florida.

the lowest threshold for synaptic activation, DMN neurons projecting to the fundus have smaller and shorter after-hyperpolarization and a higher frequency of action potential firing than neurons projecting to the cecum through the vagal celiac branch. Within the medial column, there is also a site-specific organization of neurons. Those projecting to the fundus are more laterally located and those innervating the antrum/pylorus are more medially positioned.

Neurons in the DMN also display dendritic fields that are spread in the horizontal plane with each column harboring spatial separation. Of particular significance are the dendrites of DMN neurons that extend to the overlying nucleus tractus solitarius (NTS) with the highest density in the subnucleus gelatinosus of the dorsal medial NTS, just rostral to the obex where gastric vagal afferent fibers project. This wiring provides the anatomic basis for gastric

vago-vagal reflexes whereby signaling from gastric vagal afferent endings in the dorsal medial NTS feed back onto DMN neurons to modulate vagal outflow to the stomach and thereby regulate gastric functions.

Immunohistochemistry combined with retrograde tracing studies revealed that the neurochemical phenotypes of DMN neurons projecting to the stomach are mainly cholinergic. In addition, nitric oxide (NO), a recognized neuronal messenger molecule detected by NO synthase (NOS), is present in 12% of medial neurons of the caudal DMN projecting to the fundus. Nitric oxide innervation may play an important role in vagally mediated gastric reflex relaxation.

C. Projections to the DMN from Brain Nuclei Involved in Regulating Gastric Functions

DMN neurons receive direct neural input from many brain nuclei. Tracing studies revealed that the parvocellular part of the paraventricular nucleus of the hypothalamus (PVN), the central amygdala, the locus coeruleus, and the bed nucleus stria terminalis are an interconnected continuum of "prevagal neurons" that send direct projections to influence DMN neurons. In the medulla, the DMN receives direct projections from a number of NTS neurons as well as from specific nuclei located in the ventral regions, namely, the raphe pallidus (Rpa), the raphe obscurus (Rob), and the parapyramidal regions (PPR). The biochemical coding of identified neurons projecting from the PVN to the dorsal vagal complex (DVC) includes a large number of peptides such as bombesin-like peptide, somatostatin, enkephalins, corticotropin-releasing factor (CRF), neuropeptide Y, vasopressin, and oxytocin.

Consistent with these anatomical circuits for regulatory process, the activation of these specific hypothalamic, limbic, pontine, and medullary neurons influences the neuronal activity of DVC neurons and results in the vagal-dependent alterations of gastric motor and secretory function. In addition, peptides shown to project from the PVN to the DVC, such as bombesin, CRF, and somatostatin, when applied directly into the DVC alter gastric function through vagal pathways.

D. Vagal Efferent Innervation of the Stomach

The vagal preganglionic projections originating from DMN neurons end in the enteric nervous system, predominantly in the myenteric plexus located between the circular and the longitudinal muscular layers. The prevailing concept is that, due to their small number, vagal efferent fibers provide parasympathetic input to the gut through projections to selected "mother cells/command enteric neurons." However, this concept has been recently challenged. There is now convincing evidence that vagal efferent terminals encircle or make putative contacts with all the ganglia in the myenteric plexus and, to a lesser extent, in the submucosal plexus of the stomach. Electrophysiological probing is also consistent with the notion that a high percentage of gastric myenteric neurons receive direct synaptic fast excitatory postsynaptic potential input from the vagus nerve. Therefore, the current understanding of an interface between vagal efferent fibers and myenteric neurons supports the existence of a dense network of direct interactions between the extrinsic and the enteric nervous systems.

The neurochemical phenotypes of gastric myenteric neurons receiving vagal efferent input encompass serotonin (5-HT)-, vasoactive intestinal peptide (VIP)-, NOS-, gastrin-releasing peptide (GRP)-, and GRP/VIP-containing neurons. Moreover, 60–70% of myenteric neurons in the stomach are cholinergic and surrounded by cholinergic positive fibers, showing the importance of vagal efferent cholinergic/nicotonic input to postganglionic cholinergic myenteric neurons innervating the muscular and mucosal layers of the stomach.

III. BRAIN MEDULLARY THYROTROPIN-RELEASING HORMONE AND VAGAL REGULATION OF GASTRIC FUNCTIONS

The combined use of neuroanatomical, electrophysiological, and pharmacological techniques provided increasingly detailed understanding on the role of medullary thyrotropin-releasing hormone (TRH) in the vagal regulation of gastric function. These studies greatly expanded initial observations from the 1980s that injection of TRH into the cerebrospinal fluid (CSF) at the level of the cisterna magna induced a vagal-dependent stimulation of gastric acid secretion in rats. Currently, TRH-containing projections to the DVC are the only brain peptidergic circuit known to have physiological relevance in the central vagal stimulation of gastric function.

A. Neuroanatomical and Electrophysiological Evidence

Tracing studies revealed that neurons in the Rpa, Rob, and PPR are the exclusive source of the TRH fibers innervating the DVC. Immunoelectron microscopy showed that TRH immunoreactive fibers make direct synaptic contacts with dendrites of DMN neurons projecting to the stomach. Likewise, in humans, TRH immunoreactive fibers represent the most prominent neuronal network compared with that of 12 other neuropeptides investigated. In addition, there is a strong anatomical relationship between TRH nerve terminals in the DVC and the localization of TRH receptors. Earlier studies pointed out that the highest concentration of TRH-binding sites occurs within the medial DMN where gastric preganglionic motor neurons are located and in the subnucleus gelatinosus of the NTS where gastric vagal afferents project. This was further confirmed by the mapping of TRH receptor gene distribution after the cloning of TRH receptor subtype 1 and subtype 2 (TRH_1 and TRH_2). TRH_1 mRNA, but not TRH_2 mRNA, is highly expressed in DMN and NTS neurons. Electrophysiological reports demonstrated that TRH directly stimulates the firing rates of DMN neurons by increasing the inward cationic current and reducing the calcium-dependent after-hyperpolarizing current. TRH also indirectly activates DMN neurons by inhibiting the activity of the NTS neurons that are responsive to gastric distention. Indeed, electrophysiological evidence shows that distention of the stomach and/or duodenum increased the firing rate of the majority of NTS neurons and decreased the firing rate of most DMN neurons, suggesting suppressive input onto DMN neurons from gastric distention-responsive NTS neurons. The activation of DMN neurons by central injection of TRH stimulates vagal efferent outflow to the stomach as monitored electrophysiologically in the cervical vagus as well as in the gastric vagal branch. It also induces a widespread activation of myenteric neurons in the gastric corpus and antrum as shown by Fos expression, a marker of neuronal activation.

B. Gastric Responses to Central TRH-Induced Vagal Stimulation

TRH injected into the CSF of the cisterna magna or brain ventricle or directly into the DMN results in a vagal-dependent and atropine-sensitive stimulation of gastric secretions (acid, pepsin, mucus, histamine, prostaglandin, NO, serotonin, and gastrin), gastric motor function (motility, transit), and gastric mucosal blood flow. The gastric acid secretion in response to central TRH results from the activation of cholinergic postganglionic neurons, which directly stimulate parietal cell secretion through interaction with muscarinic receptors localized on these cells. In addition, the vagally mediated increase of gastric histamine release also stimulates the parietal cells. The gastric hyperemia in response to a maximally effective dose of TRH injected intracisternally is mediated by the cholinergic activation of peripheral NO pathways. This increase in blood flow is independent of the release of established vasoactive substances, such as histamine, calcitonin gene-related peptide (CGRP), VIP, and prostaglandins (Fig. 2).

By contrast, under conditions of submaximal increase of vagal efferent activity, induced by low doses of TRH injected into the cisterna magna, the gastric acid response is largely blunted or abolished. This is related to the action of vagally released anti-acid secretory transmitters, namely, prostaglandins, CGRP, and 5-HT. However, despite this minimal acid response, there is a robust gastric hyperemia resulting from the vagal cholinergic-dependent activation of capsaicin-sensitive CGRP/NO vasodilatory pathways without the involvement of prostaglandins. These observations support the notion that various transmitters are released in the stomach by central vagal cholinergic stimulation. Their interplay varies with

the degree of vagal activation and contributes to the differential patterns of gastric responses elicited by low or high levels of vagal efferent drive (Fig. 2).

C. Roles of Endogenous Medullary TRH in the Vagal Regulation of Gastric Functions

The use of specific TRH antibody and TRH_1 receptor antisense oligodeoxynucleotides as well as the monitoring of changes in medullary TRH gene expression provided valuable approaches to examine the physiological role of endogenous medullary TRH in the absence of selective TRH receptor antagonists. There is now convincing evidence that this peptide participates in the central vagal stimulation of gastric function during the digestive process, specific stress conditions, and thyroid-related endocrine alterations.

The cephalic phase of gastric acid secretion is mediated by centrally driven vagal-dependent pathways as initially demonstrated by Pavlov's pioneering studies in dogs. Medullary TRH plays an important role in the cephalic phase of gastric acid secretion as shown by the dampening of the gastric acid response to sham feeding by pretreatment into the cisterna

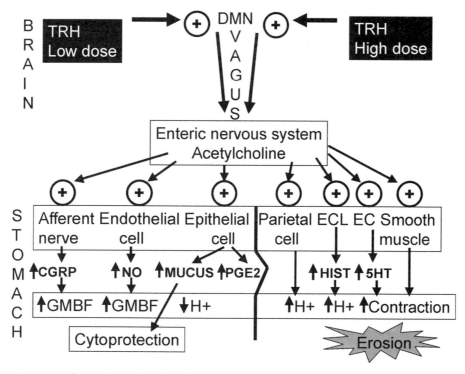

FIGURE 2 Summary of experimental studies showing the gastroprotective and ulcerogenic actions of central vagal stimulation induced by low and high doses of TRH, respectively, and related transmitters involved in the dual gastric responses. CGRP, calcitonin gene-related peptide; EC, enterochromaffin cells; ECL, enterochromaffin-like cells; GMBF, gastric mucosal blood flow; HIST, histamine; NO, nitric oxide.

magna with antisense oligodeoxynucleotides targeted to the TRH_1 receptor. Another established role of the vagus was in the modulation of the gastric mucosa to withstand damaging agents such as strong acid or ethanol. Low doses of TRH injected into the cisterna magna or DVC confer gastric protection against ethanol-induced mucosal lesions. The gastric protection is brought about by medullary TRH inducing a vagal cholinergic-dependent release of gastric prostaglandins and NO, as well as the activation of a local effector function of capsaicin-sensitive splanchnic afferents containing CGRP and related gastric hyperemia (Fig. 2). Likewise, the endogenous release of TRH in the DVC induced by the activation of TRH cell bodies in the Rpa is also gastroprotective. Other phenomena, such as the vagal-dependent adaptive gastric protection whereby a mild gastric irritant reduced the damaging effect of a strong irritant, are also mediated by TRH in the brain medulla. In view of these findings, the cephalic phase of gastric secretion, which results in a mild vagal stimulation, may have beneficial effects on the gastric mucosa by triggering these mucosal protective mechanisms. Conversely, a deficient cephalic phase (nongustatory appreciation) may facilitate the damaging effect of ulcerogenic stimuli due to the reduction or absence of vagally recruited protective mechanisms.

By contrast, a high and sustained level of vagal activation is known to cause gastric hemorrhagic erosions. There is now evidence that intracisternal injection of a maximal acid secretory dose of TRH and maximal chemical stimulation of TRH-synthesizing neurons in the Rpa also result in the development of gastric erosions through the activation of vagal cholinergic pathways. Moreover, this gastric erosive response is potentiated when gastric prostaglandins, also released under these conditions of vagal stimulation, are blocked by an inhibitor of prostaglandin synthesis. Acute exposure of fasted rats to cold (an experimental model known since the 1960s to reliably induce vagal-dependent stimulation of gastric acid secretion, motility, and gastric lesions) is now clearly linked with the activation of medullary TRH pathways. Acute cold exposure increased TRH gene expression in the medullar nuclei selectively in the Rpa, Rob, and the PPR along with Fos expression, which is indicative of cell activation and gene transcription. TRH antibody injected into the cisterna magna reduced cold exposure-induced vagal-dependent gastric acid secretion and mucosal lesion formation. Antisense oligodeoxynucleotides targeted to the TRH_1 receptor, given centrally, prevented acute cold exposure-induced vagal cholinergic acceleration

of gastric emptying. Collectively, these findings highlighted the dual role of medullary TRH, which, depending upon the differential level of activity, confers to the gastric mucosa a vagal cholinergic-mediated prevalence of protective or erosive mechanisms.

Another important role of medullary TRH is related to the alterations of autonomic activity linked with diseased thyroid states. Indeed, the synthesis of TRH gene expression in the Rpa, Rob, and PPR neurons is regulated by the feedback inhibition of thyroid hormones as established for TRH neurons located in the PVN. There is recent evidence that hypothyroidism significantly increased Fos expression in TRH-synthesizing neurons as well as TRH mRNA expression in the Rpa, Rob, and PPR neurons. Conversely, hyperthyroidism reduced TRH gene expression in these neurons. The localization of thyroid hormone receptors in these medullary nuclei indicates that the feedback regulation of TRH gene expression is mediated by a direct action of thyroid hormone on TRH neurons. The alterations of TRH neuroanatomical circuitry by hypo/hyperthyroidism along with the established effects of TRH to stimulate vagal outflow provide new insight into the understanding of autonomic disorders associated with altered thyroid states. Functional studies support the notion that hypothyroidism associated with increased TRH gene expression in raphe neurons is also linked with increased vagal drive to the viscera.

D. Modulation of Medullary TRH Action by Other Brain Peptides

There is growing evidence that TRH excitatory action on DMN neurons occurs in concert with other modulatory influences exerted by other neuropeptides or neurotransmitters innervating the DVC. Neuroanatomical support for this interaction came with the co-localization of TRH with substance P (SP) and 5-HT immunoreactivity in neurons of the Rpa, Rob, and PPR projecting to the DVC. These substances modulate the activities of the vagal preganglionic motor neurons as they are co-released with TRH in the DVC. In particular, SP immunoreactive fibers innervate the entire lengths of the DMN and the NTS in rats and humans. Retrograde labeling studies identified DMN neurons projecting to the stomach located at the rostral level of the obex that are in contact with terminals containing SP fibers. In addition, gastric-projecting preganglionic vagal motor neurons expressed neurokinin-1 (NK_1) receptor. The biological consequence of activation of NK_1 receptors in the DMN is the reduction of the gastric secretory and motor responses to exogenous or endogenous TRH. Therefore, co-released SP with TRH in the DVC dampens the excitatory action of TRH in the DMN. By contrast, 5-HT, which is also co-localized with TRH in medullary raphe nuclei and PPR projecting into the DVC, potentiates TRH stimulatory action through 5-HT$_2$ receptors within the DVC. A number of brain peptides co-injected with TRH into the DMN have been reported to inhibit the vagal-dependent stimulation of gastric function by TRH. These include interleukin-1, opioid peptides, adrenomedulin, CGRP, bombesin, and calcitonin, providing pharmacological evidence of their central action to influence vagal outflow to the gut.

IV. BRAIN BOMBESIN-LIKE PEPTIDES AND VAGAL INHIBITION OF GASTRIC FUNCTIONS

Thirty years ago, Erspamer *et al.* isolated the 14-amino-acid peptide bombesin from extracts prepared from the skin of the European frog, *Bombina bombina*. Earlier studies showed that bombesin-like immunoreactivity (-LI) was widely distributed in the brain and that central injection of bombesin exerted potent centrally mediated actions on thermoregulation, glucoregulation, and gastric function in rats. In addition, other reports showed the presence of bombesin-LI in the gut of rodents that fostered research to identify a mammalian bombesin counterpart. This resulted in the late 1970s in the characterization of a 27-amino-acid peptide displaying strong homology with the carboxyl-terminus of bombesin and potent gastrin-releasing activity and was accordingly named gastrin-releasing peptide. With these observations, bombesin/GRP was added to the list of peptides co-existing and acting both in the brain and in the gut, giving support to the emerging concept of the peptidergic brain–gut axis.

A. Neuroanatomical Evidence

The neuroanatomical substrate role for the bombesin-LI terminal fields in the modulation of vagal outflow to the stomach came from the identification by retrograde tracing of bombesin-LI in cell bodies within the medial parvocellular part of the PVN projecting to the DVC. These projections constitute an important source of bombesin-LI terminals in the DVC with the strongest labeling in the medial NTS. A similar distribution of bombesin-LI in the rat DVC was confirmed with an N-terminal antibody selective for GRP and bombesin gene expression by *in situ*

hybridization. Ultrastructural analysis identified a large number of bombesin-LI-labeled nerve terminals making mostly axo-dendritic synaptic contact on medium and small dendrites in the DMN and medial NTS. These data indicated that bombesin action was directly exerted on postsynaptyic neurons. Autoradiographic studies also revealed a high to moderate density of binding sites for ^{125}I-[Tyr^4]bombesin in the caudal NTS.

B. Biological Role

Bombesin was the first peptide shown to act in the brain to inhibit gastric function. The peptide administered into the cisterna magna induced a potent, dose-related, and long-lasting inhibition of acid secretion in several mammalian species including the rabbit, cat, dog, and rodents. The specificity and potency of bombesin action were established as 30 unrelated natural neuropeptides tested under the same conditions in rats and dogs were found to be inactive or less potent.

Consistent with bombesin action being mediated by altering vagal outflow to the stomach, bombesin-responsive hindbrain nuclei include the DVC. When microinjected at low doses (0.6–6.2 pmol), bombesin inhibited the gastric acid and contractile responses to the TRH analogue RX 77368 co-injected into the DVC. In addition, the delayed gastric emptying induced by central injection of bombesin was completely prevented by ganglionic blockade and vagotomy but not adrenalectomy in rats and dogs. The dose ranges at which central injection of bombesin delayed gastric emptying also correlated well with those inhibiting vagal outflow as monitored by electrophysiological recording of gastric vagal efferent discharges.

The biological actions of bombesin-like peptides are mediated by their binding to high-affinity receptors. Four members of the bombesin receptor family have been cloned: the mammalian neuromedin B-preferring receptor (neuromedin B receptor), the GRP-preferring receptor (GRP receptor), the bombesin subtype 3 (bombesin-3), and the amphibian bombesin subtype 4 (bombesin-4) receptors. The receptor subtype involved in bombesin anti-secretory action is unlikely to involve the neuromedin B receptor since neuromedin B injected into the CSF did not influence gastric acid secretion. The pharmacological characterization of bombesin-3 receptor showed that litorin, ranatensin, and bombesin have a low affinity and that [Phe^{13}]bombesin has no affinity for this subtype. Since these peptides also act centrally to inhibit acid secretion, this rules out a possible mediation through bombesin-3 receptor. Therefore, it is likely that the GRP receptor is involved in bombesin action. The bombesin/GRP receptor antagonist N-acetyl-GRP$_{20-26}$–O–CH$_3$ injected at a 52:1 antagonist:agonist ratio blocked intracisternal bombesin-induced anti-secretory action.

Taken together, these neuroanatomical and functional studies support an inhibitory action of bombesin-LI peptides in the DVC to regulate gastric function through vagal pathways. Additional actions of bombesin are also exerted at sites influencing sympathetic activity and the activation of this pathway contributes to the potent centrally mediated anti-secretory effect of bombesin injected intracisternally or into the rostroventral medulla. The elucidation of the physiological importance of bombesin-like peptide-induced regulation of gastric function through vagal pathways will be forthcoming with the development of more selective and specific GRP receptor antagonists and/or the use of GRP receptor subtype gene knockout mice.

V. BRAIN CRF RECEPTORS AND VAGAL INHIBITION OF GASTRIC MOTOR RESPONSE TO STRESS

The characterization of the 41-amino-acid peptide CRF in the 1980s and, more recently, of the CRF-related family members urocortin, urocortin II, and urocortin III, as well as the cloning of CRF receptor subtypes 1 (CRF$_1$) and 2 (CRF$_2$) and the development of specific CRF$_1$/CRF$_2$ receptor antagonists provided key tools to unravel the neurochemical basis of the stress response. Evidence has emerged that the activation of brain CRF receptors triggers almost the entire repertoire of behavioral, neuroendocrine, autonomic, immunological, and visceral responses characteristic of stress in rodents and primates. In particular, the activation of brain CRF receptors modulates autonomic outflow and plays a role in stress-related autonomic alterations of gut function.

A. Activation of Brain CRF Receptors and Vagal Inhibition of Gastric Motor Function

Several reports consistently established that CRF and related peptides injected into the CSF act in the brain to inhibit gastric emptying of a solid or liquid meal and gastric contractility in rats and dogs. CRF and related peptides also act in the brain to inhibit gastric

acid secretion and somatostatin release. These actions are mediated through modulation of vagal pathways. Brain sites responsive to CRF to inhibit gastric motor function are located in nuclei established to influence parasympathetic outflow to the viscera, namely, the PVN and DVC. In particular, CRF microinjected into the DVC blocked exogenous or endogenous TRH-induced vagal stimulation of gastric function. Functional mapping of brain neuronal activity using Fos expression also showed that central injection of CRF inhibits cold exposure-induced activation of DMN neurons and increases NTS neuronal activity. Moreover, direct electrophysiological recording of gastric vagal efferent discharges showed that intracisternal injection of CRF and related peptides inhibits gastric vagal efferent discharges. Finally, vagotomy prevented intracisternal CRF-induced inhibition of gastric motor function.

CRF actions in the medulla to decrease vagal outflow to the stomach may be primarily mediated by the CRF$_2$ receptor. This is supported by functional studies showing that selective CRF$_2$ receptor antagonists blocked central CRF- or urocortin-induced inhibition of gastric motor function. In addition, mapping studies of the distribution of CRF receptor gene expression in the medulla showed the presence of CRF$_2$ receptors particularly in the NTS. The network of CRF immunoreactive fibers in the NTS suggests that CRF may act through activation of NTS inhibitory input to the DMN preganglionic neurons.

B. Role of Brain CRF Receptors in Stress-Related Alterations of Gastric Motor Function

Activation of brain CRF receptors plays a role in the vagally mediated alterations of gastric function evoked by stress. Delayed gastric emptying is a common pattern of response to exposure to various acute stressors such as operant avoidance, water avoidance, radiation, handling, acoustic stimulation, hemorrhage, abdominal or cranial surgery, tail shock, trunk clamping, wrap restraint at room temperature, swimming, and anesthetic exposure in experimental animals (mice, rats, guinea pigs, dogs, and/or monkeys). Likewise, in healthy subjects, anger, fear, labyrinthine stimulation, painful stimuli, preoperative anxiety, or intense exercise results in a slowing of gastric transit.

Various CRF receptor antagonists injected into the CSF or the PVN at doses preventing the biological actions of centrally injected CRF blocked the delayed gastric emptying resulting from exposure to various forms of acute stress. These include those elicited by immunological agents (intravenous or intracisternal injection of interleukin-1β), physico-psychological factors (partial restraint, forced swimming), exogenous chemical stimulation (short anesthetic), and body injury (abdominal or cranial surgery or peritoneal irritation). These findings provide new venues for understanding brain pathways contributing to gastric stasis in response to an acute stress including the underlying mechanisms of postoperative ileus. It is also noteworthy that the intercommunications between the immune and hypothalamic CRF systems impact the central regulation of gastric motor function.

VI. VAGAL INHIBITION OF GASTRIC FUNCTION BY POSTPRANDIAL RELEASE OF THE GUT PEPTIDE, PEPTIDE YY

Peripherally originating gut peptides can enter the brain and act in specific brain nuclei outside the blood–brain barrier to regulate gastric functions. Recent studies have established that peptide YY (PYY) is a representative peptide with this mechanism of action. PYY is a 36-amino-acid hormone that was originally isolated from the pig intestine and localized in the open-ended L-type endocrine cells of the terminal ileum and colon in the rat, dog, and human. PYY is released postprandially via extramural neural or endocrine mechanisms that originate in the foregut and by intralumenal nutrients. However, the basal release of PYY seems to be partly regulated by tonic vagal activity. PYY_{1-36} and PYY_{3-36} are the two molecular forms of PYY that are abundant in the blood. Circulating PYY displays a profound inhibitory action on gastric emptying and acid secretion. Recent studies have revealed two important mechanisms involved in the inhibitory action of PYY on gastric acid secretion, one of which is its central action on vagally mediated regulation of gastric functions.

A. Peripheral PYY Is a Potent Inhibitor of Vagally Mediated Gastric Acid Secretion

Intravenous infusion of PYY at doses reproducing circulating levels induced by food ingestion inhibits gastric acid secretion in several experimental animals and in humans irrespective of acid secretion being stimulated by peripheral (pentagastrin and liver extract) or central vagal (insulin, baclofen, and TRH) mechanisms. However, earlier observations indicated that PYY was more potent at inhibiting gastric acid secretion induced by central–vagal

secretagogues than peripheral secretagogues. It was first speculated that PYY acts by inhibiting acetylcholine release from vagal nerve fibers rather than by inhibiting the action of acetylcholine on the parietal cell. This viewpoint was further supported by studies in rats showing that administration of PYY had no effect on bethanechol-induced acid output, but inhibited baclofen-induced acid output. Baclofen is a γ-aminobutyric acid receptor agonist that stimulates gastric acid output through atropine-sensitive and vagally mediated pathways. The demonstration that vagotomy markedly impaired the anti-secretory potency of peripherally infused PYY indicated that PYY inhibitory action on gastric acid secretion required the integrity of vagal innervation.

B. Neuroanatomical Basis for PYY Action in the DVC

Recent studies revealed that PYY acts in the medullary DVC particularly at the level of the area postrema (AP) located close to the surface of the fourth ventricle (Fig. 1) and portions of the NTS are defined as circumventricular organs where the blood–brain barrier is incomplete. These regions can therefore act as portals of entry for circulating peptide hormones. PYY-binding sites are present in the AP and DVC. Specific binding sites for both ^{125}I-[Leu^{31}Pro^{34}]PYY (Y$_1$ agonist) and ^{125}I-PYY$_{3-36}$ (Y$_2$ agonist) have been detected in the NTS and AP. A recent study revealed that Y$_1$, Y$_2$, and Y$_4$ receptor subtype mRNAs are located in the AP, NTS, and the DMN with a high level of expression in the AP and DMN. Labeled PYY, injected intravenously at doses that produce a blood concentration of PYY within the range observed after a meal is consumed, binds specifically to the region of the rat brainstem containing the DVC. Likewise, peripheral injection of PYY activates NTS and AP cells as shown by Fos expression. Collectively these data provide neuroanatomical evidence supporting a receptor-mediated action of PYY in the brain medulla.

C. Central Action of Peripheral PYY in Inhibiting Gastric Function

The centrally mediated action of peripheral PYY in inhibiting vagally stimulated gastric acid secretion was observed in studies using immunoneutralization with a PYY polyclonal antibody. PYY infused intravenously inhibited in a dose-dependent manner the acid response to TRH analogue injected intracisternally. PYY or the Y$_2$ agonist PYY$_{3-36}$ injected intracisternally reproduced the anti-secretory effect observed after peripheral administration of the peptides. In addition, intravenous injection of PYY antibody that shows a 35% cross reaction with PYY_{3-36} by radioimmunoassay completely prevented the inhibitory effect of intravenous infusion of PYY. When injected intracisternally, the PYY antibody reversed not only the inhibition of gastric acid secretion induced by centrally administered PYY but also the inhibition elicited by PYY infused peripherally. These results strongly indicated that peripheral PYY acts within the area of the AP/NTS outside of the blood–brain barrier to inhibit central-vagally stimulated gastric acid secretion. The role of Y_2 receptors in mediating the anti-secretory action of PYY is further supported by the strong expression of Y_2 receptor mRNA in the AP and NTS. The central action of circulating PYY released postprandially to suppress vagally stimulated gastric response induced by TRH may have relevance in the dampening of the cephalic phase of gastric secretion in response to a meal.

VII. SUMMARY

Brain medullary TRH is a physiologically important stimulant of vagal efferent discharges to the stomach and thereby stimulates gastric secretory and motor functions and blood flow. Medullary TRH also regulates the gastric mucosal resistance against injury with a dual action, protective or ulcerogenic in relation to the intensity of the vagal activity. The central action of this peptide is to function in the course of normal physiological digestive activities, in particular during the cephalic phase of the gastric response to a meal. Impaired thyroid levels feed back on the regulation of medullary TRH gene expression and impact on autonomic regulation of the viscera through TRH–vagal pathway. Within the brain, several selective nuclei send inputs to the DVC neurons and modulate the action of TRH through the release of peptides and transmitters. There is evidence that TRH action is modulated by inhibitory actions of medullary SP and PVN–DVC projections containing bombesin-LI, whereas medullary 5-HT potentiates TRH excitatory action in the DVC. In addition, postprandially released gut peptides, such as PYY, may impact on the cephalic phase of gastric secretion through a direct action on the medullary area outside of the blood–brain barrier.

New information is emerging about the stress-related inhibition of gastric motor function through the activation of brain CRF receptors, which suppressed vagal outflow to the stomach. The brain–gut peptidergic interaction is part of the mechanisms through which digestive function is coordinated and adjusted in response to internal and external environmental changes.

Acknowledgments

The authors' work was supported by the National Institute of Diabetes and Digestive and Kidney Disease Grants DK 30110 (Y. T.), DK 41301 (Y. T.), DK 33061 (Y. T.), and DK 50255 (H. Y.). Thanks are extended to Paul Kirsh for his help in the preparation of the manuscript.

Glossary

dorsal vagal complex Association of two medullary nuclei: the dorsal motor nucleus of the vagus and the nucleus tractus solitarius. The dorsal motor nucleus contains cell bodies with axons that form the vagal innervation of the gut. The nucleus tractus solitarius contains cell bodies of interneurons and of neurons projecting to other brain areas as well as terminal fibers of vagal afferents originating from cell bodies in the nodose ganglia; fibers from cell bodies located in the other parts of the brain (central amygdala, hypothalamus) are also present in the nucleus tractus solitarius.

enteric nervous system Network of neuronal cells and fibers embedded within the gut wall that serve as a relay for signals to and from the brain or spinal cord. This network can respond to stimuli from various sensory receptors and generate changes in neuronal activity independent of the central nervous system.

hypothalamus A region in the forebrain that contains control centers for homeostatic regulation of pituitary hormone secretions, behavior, and visceral functions.

peptides Molecules composed of small numbers of amino acids (fewer than 100).

thyrotropin-releasing hormone (TRH) A tripeptide amide originally isolated from the hypothalamus and expressed in many extrahypothalamic brain nuclei, especially the medulla. Hypothalamic TRH regulates thyroid function by releasing pituitary thyrotropin hormone, whereas medullary TRH regulates autonomic function by acting as an excitatory neurotransmitter on autonomic regulatory neurons.

vagus nerve The 10th cranial nerve that emerges from the brainstem and passes through the neck and thorax to the abdomen, innervating visceral organs including the heart, lungs, and digestive organs; it plays a major role in the parasympathetic regulation of gut functions.

See Also the Following Articles

Appetite Regulation, Neuronal Control • Bombesin-like Peptides • Cholecystokinin (CCK) • Gastrointestinal Hormone-Releasing Peptides • Motilin • Peptide YY

● Thyrotropin-Releasing Hormone (TRH) ● Vasoactive Intestinal Peptide (VIP)

Further Reading

Browning, K. N., Renehan, W. E., and Travagli, R. A. (1999). Electrophysiological and morphological heterogeneity of rat dorsal vagal neurons which project to specific areas of the gastrointestinal tract. *J. Physiol.* **517**(Pt. 2), 521–532.

Habib, K. E., Weld, K. P., Rice, K. C., Pushkas, J., Champoux, M., Listwak, S., Webster, E. L., Atkinson, A. J., Schulkin, J., Contoreggi, C., Chrousos, G. P., McCann, S. M., Suomi, S. J., Higley, J. D., and Gold, P. W. (2000). Oral administration of a corticotropin-releasing hormone receptor antagonist significantly attenuates behavioral, neuroendocrine, and autonomic responses to stress in primates. *Proc. Natl Acad. Sci. USA* **97**, 6079–6084.

Holst, M. C., Kelly, J. B., and Powley, T. L. (1997). Vagal preganglionic projections to the enteric nervous system characterized with *Phaseolus vulgaris*-leucoagglutinin. *J. Comp. Neurol.* **381**, 81–100.

Martinez, V., and Taché, Y. (2000). Bombesin and the brain–gut axis. *Peptides* **21**, 1617–1625.

Miampamba, M., Yang, H., Sharkey, K. A., and Taché, Y. (2001). Intracisternal TRH analog induces Fos expression in gastric myenteric neurons and glia in conscious rats. *Am. J. Physiol. Gastrointest. Liver Physiol.* **280**, G979–G991.

Miselis, R. R., Rinaman, L., Altschuler, S. M., Bao, X., and Lynn, R. B. (1991). Medullary viscerotopic representation of the alimentary canal innervation in the rat. *In* "Brain–Gut Interactions" (Y. Taché and D. Wingate, eds.), pp. 3–21. CRC Press, Boca Raton, FL.

Sawchenko, P. E., Li, H. Y., and Ericsson, A. (2000). Circuits and mechanisms governing hypothalamic responses to stress: A tale of two paradigms. *Prog. Brain. Res.* **122**, 61–78.

Taché, Y. (2002). The parasympathetic nervous system in the pathophysiology of the gastrointestinal tract. *In* "Handbook of Autonomic Nervous System in Health and Disease" (C. L. Bolis, J. Licinio and S. Govoni, eds.), pp. 453–503. Dekker, New York.

Taché, Y., Kaneko, H., Kawakubo, K., Kato, K., Kiraly, A., and Yang, H. (1998). Central and peripheral mechanisms involved in gastric protection against ethanol injury. *J. Gastroenterol. Hepatol.* **13**(Suppl.), S214–S220.

Taché, Y., Martinez, V., Million, M., and Wang, L. (2001). Stress and the gastrointestinal tract III. Stress-related alterations of gut motor function: Role of brain corticotropin-releasing factor receptors. *Am. J. Physiol.* **280**, G173–G177.

Taché, Y., Yang, H., and Kaneko, H. (1995). Caudal raphe–dorsal vagal complex peptidergic projections: Role in gastric vagal control. *Peptides* **16**, 431–435.

Yang, H. (2002). Central and peripheral regulation of gastric acid secretion by peptide YY. *Peptides* **23**, 349–358.

Yang, H., Yuan, P., Wu, V., and Taché, Y. (1999). Feedback regulation of thyrotropin-releasing hormone gene expression by thyroid hormone in the caudal raphe nuclei in rats. *Endocrinology* **140**, 43–49.

Zhang, X., Fogel, R., and Renehan, W. E. (1999). Stimulation of the paraventricular nucleus modulates the activity of gut-sensitive neurons in the vagal complex. *Am. J. Physiol.* **277**, G79–G90.

Vascular Endothelial Growth Factor B (VEGF-B)

ULF ERIKSSON AND XURI LI

Ludwig Institute for Cancer Research, Stockholm

I. DISCOVERY
II. PROTEIN STRUCTURE
III. GENE STRUCTURE AND REGULATION
IV. TISSUE DISTRIBUTION
V. RECEPTORS
VI. BIOLOGICAL ACTIVITIES AND PATHOLOGY
VII. FUTURE DIRECTIONS

Vascular endothelial growth factor (VEGF)-B was found serendipitously as a partial mouse cDNA clone encoding a VEGF-related peptide. The partial cDNA was then used to isolate full-length mouse and human cDNA clones from mouse and human cDNA libraries.

I. DISCOVERY

A full-length cDNA that encoded a homologue of vascular endothelial growth factor (VEGF) was discovered, and in analogy with the nomenclature of the related platelet-derived growth factors (PDGFs), the new protein was denoted VEGF-B. Independently, other researchers found the same gene when attempting to identify the locus involved in multiple endocrine neoplasia type 1 (MEN1). The protein encoded by this gene was designated VEGF-related factor and was later excluded from being involved in MEN1.

II. PROTEIN STRUCTURE

Two isoforms of mouse and human VEGF-B have been identified. Both isoforms are secreted proteins and have 167 (VEGF-B$_{167}$) and 186 (VEGF-B$_{186}$) amino acid residues, respectively. The isoforms have an identical amino-terminal domain of 115 amino acid residues, excluding the signal sequence, whereas the two different carboxyl-terminal domains are not related to each other. The highly conserved pattern of eight cysteine residues found in VEGFs and PDGFs, involved in intra- and intermolecular disulfide bonding, was present in the common amino-terminal domain. Both human and mouse VEGF-B isoforms lack the consensus sequence for N-linked glycosylation (-Asn-Xxx-Thr/Ser-), unlike the structurally related factors of the PDGF/VEGF family. However, VEGF-B$_{186}$ is O-glycosylated in the unique carboxyl-terminal domain, which is rich in serine and threonine residues. Pairwise comparisons of the amino acid sequences showed that mouse VEGF-B$_{167}$ is $\approx 43\%$ identical to mouse VEGF$_{164}$, $\approx 30\%$ identical to human placenta growth factor (PlGF), and $\approx 20\%$ identical to mouse PDGF-A and PDGF-B.

The two VEGF-B isoforms are produced as disulfide-linked homodimers and under reducing conditions the molecular mass of secreted VEGF-B$_{167}$ is 21 kDa. The secreted O-glycosylated VEGF-B$_{186}$ isoform has an apparent molecular mass of 32 kDa, and the unmodified intracellular form of VEGF-B$_{186}$ has a molecular mass of 26 kDa.

The different carboxyl-terminal domains of the two isoforms of VEGF-B affect their biochemical and cell biological properties. The highly hydrophilic carboxyl-terminal domain of VEGF-B$_{167}$ is related to the corresponding region in several isoforms of VEGF, with several conserved cysteine residues and stretches of basic amino acid residues. VEGF-B$_{167}$ will remain cell-associated upon secretion by binding to pericellular heparan sulfate proteoglycans. The cell association is likely to occur via its unique basic carboxyl-terminal region, as noted for the highly basic splice variants of VEGF.

The carboxyl-terminal domain of the VEGF-B$_{186}$ isoform is rather hydrophobic with several conserved alanine, proline, serine, and threonine amino acid residues, and its characteristics contrast with those of the hydrophilic and basic carboxyl-terminal domain in VEGF-B$_{167}$. The amino acid sequence of the carboxyl-terminus of this isoform has no significant similarity with other known amino acid sequences. On secretion, VEGF-B$_{186}$ does not remain cell-associated. Instead, it is proteolytically processed, and the processing regulates the biological properties of the growth factor.

Both isoforms of VEGF-B form disulfide-linked heterodimers with VEGF when co-expressed in transfected cells, but it has not been established whether naturally occurring VEGF·VEGF-B heterodimers exist. It is known that VEGF forms naturally occurring heterodimers with PlGF, and such heterodimers display functional properties distinct from those of both VEGF and PlGF homodimers. Similarly, VEGF·VEGF-B heterodimers may have unique functional properties.

Heterodimers of VEGF-B$_{167}$·VEGF remain cell-associated, whereas homodimers of VEGF$_{165}$ are secreted from cells in a soluble form. In contrast, heterodimers of VEGF-B$_{186}$ and VEGF are freely secreted. Thus, VEGF-B$_{167}$ determines the release of heterodimers from cells, and heterodimerization of VEGF with either of the two isoforms of VEGF-B might therefore control the release and bioavailability of VEGF·VEGF-B heterodimers. Whether the VEGF-B polypeptides act as homodimers, as heterodimers with VEGF, or as both is not known.

The ability of VEGF-B isoforms to affect the release of VEGF·VEGF-B heterodimers from the producing cells is intriguing since the two factors are co-expressed in many tissues, most prominently in heart and muscle.

III. GENE STRUCTURE AND REGULATION

The human VEGF-B gene is localized to chromosome 11q13, close to the MEN1 locus. The mouse and human genes for VEGF-B are almost identical and both span approximately 4 kb of DNA. The genes are composed of seven exons and their exon–intron organization is similar to that of the VEGF and PlGF genes. The common amino-terminal domain in the two isoforms of VEGF-B is encoded by exons 1–5, and differential use of the remaining three exons gives rise to the two isoforms. The transcript for VEGF-B$_{167}$ is generated by exons 1–5, exon 6b, and exon 7. In contrast, the transcript encoding VEGF-B$_{186}$ is generated by the use of an alternative splice acceptor site in exon 6, leading to an insertion of 101 bp (exon 6a) that introduces a frameshift mutation and termination of the coding region in exon 6b (Fig. 1). In VEGF and PlGF, several isoforms are encoded by the use of alternative splice acceptor sites and different combinations of exons in the 3'-regions of the genes, but the corresponding transcripts are translated using the same reading frame. The use of partially overlapping but different reading frames is rare among higher eukaryotes, but is frequently used by different viruses.

The expression of the two isoforms of VEGF-B appears to be strictly regulated. In most adult and embryonic tissues, the transcript encoding VEGF-B$_{167}$ accounts for more than 80% of the total level of expression of VEGF-B. However, in several primary tumors and tumor cell lines, the expression of transcripts encoding VEGF-B$_{186}$ is up-regulated. The differential expression of VEGF-B isoforms would contribute to a genetically controlled mechanism involved in the release of VEGF·VEGF-B heterodimers in co-expressing tissues.

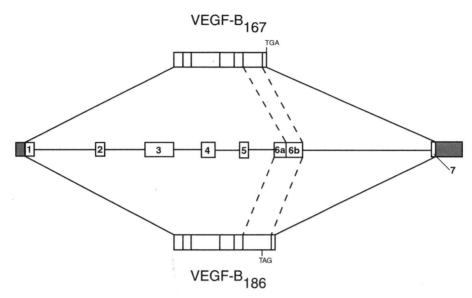

FIGURE 1 Schematic structure of the gene encoding VEGF-B. The genomic region harboring the seven coding exons spans approximately 4 kb. Alternative use of the splice acceptor site in exon 6 generates the transcripts for the two VEGF-B isoforms. Translation terminates in exon 7 in VEF-B$_{167}$ and in exon 6b in VEGF-B$_{186}$.

The gene for VEGF-B does not contain binding sites for hypoxia-inducible factors, and accordingly, VEGF-B mRNA expression is not regulated by hypoxia, unlike VEGF expression. Instead, the expression levels of VEGF-B are remarkably stable and not influenced by a variety of other stimuli including several growth factors and cytokines.

IV. TISSUE DISTRIBUTION

In adult mouse and human tissues, VEGF-B is abundantly expressed as a 1.4 kb mRNA in heart, brain, skeletal muscle, and kidney, and lower levels are present in most other tissues. VEGF-B and VEGF mRNAs are co-expressed in many tissues, such as heart, skeletal muscle, pancreas, and prostate, generating the possibility that VEGF-VEGF-B heterodimers may occur *in vivo*.

VEGF-B is expressed during embryonic development and is widely distributed. It is prominently expressed in the developing cardiac myocytes and less abundantly expressed in several other tissues, including developing muscle, bone, pancreas, adrenal, and the smooth muscle cell layer of several larger vessels. On embryonic day (E) 11.5–12.5, VEGF-B was strongly expressed in the developing heart. Later, on E14, VEGF-B was expressed in most tissues of the embryo, although most prominently in heart, spinal cord, and cerebral cortex. On E17, VEGF-B expression was concentrated in the heart, brown fat, and spinal cord. Throughout embryonic

development, no expression of VEGF-B was detected in endothelial cells. Based on the expression pattern, VEGF-B was suggested to have a role in vascularization of the heart, skeletal muscles, and other tissues and act via paracrine interactions between endothelial cells and surrounding tissue cells.

V. RECEPTORS

Two receptors have been identified for the two isoforms of VEGF-B, the vascular endothelial growth factor receptor (VEGFR)-1 and the co-receptor neuropilin-1 (NP-1). VEGFR-1 is a cell surface receptor tyrosine kinase containing seven immunoglobulin-like domains in the extracellular portion and an intracellular tyrosine kinase domain. In addition to VEGF-B, VEGFR-1 is a receptor for VEGF and PlGF. VEGF-B and PlGF form a subgroup of VEGFR-1-specific ligands since VEGF also binds to VEGFR-2, the main mitogenic VEGF receptor. The first three immunoglobulin-like domains are sufficient for VEGF-B binding, and the binding site is identical to, or at least overlaps, the binding site for VEGF and PlGF. VEGFR-1 binds to the common growth factor domains present in both VEGF-B isoforms. The receptor is expressed on the endothelium of blood vessels during embryonic development and in adult tissues, and it is also expressed by monocytes, macrophages, and certain stem cell populations. Targeted deletion of VEGFR-1 has shown that it is crucial for vascular development during embryogenesis.

Embryos homozygous for VEGFR-1 deletion die at E9–11 due to extensive accumulation of endothelial cells in the developing vessels. In contrast, embryos with a deletion of the intracellular tyrosine kinase domain of VEGFR-1 are viable. These data suggest that the extracellular ligand-binding portion of the receptor is sufficient to support normal development of the vasculature.

NP-1, the second receptor for VEGF-B, is also an isoform-specific co-receptor for some isoforms of VEGF and PlGF and is a receptor for semaphorins/collapsins involved in axonal guidance. In addition to its neuronal expression, NP-1 is present in the endothelial cells of blood vessels and in mesenchymal cells surrounding the blood vessels during embryonic development, as well as in certain other nonneuronal tissues. Embryos with targeted deletion of NP-1 die of cardiovascular failure at E10.5–12.5, and overexpression of NP-1 under the β-actin promoter is lethal due to severe anomalies of both the nervous system and the cardiovascular system.

NP-1 binds to both VEGF-B isoforms via the carboxy-terminal domains. In VEGF-B$_{167}$, the interaction is mediated by the heparin-binding exon 6B-encoded domain, which is homologous to the NP-1-binding domain of VEGF$_{165}$. VEGF-B$_{186}$, the non-heparin-binding isoform, binds to NP-1 following proteolytic cleavage of the unique carboxy-terminal domain that unmasks the binding epitope. The binding epitope has been mapped to the first 12 amino acid residues of the carboxy-terminal domain.

VI. BIOLOGICAL ACTIVITIES AND PATHOLOGY

VEGF-B is poorly, if at all, mitogenic for endothelial cells. This property accompanies the weak ligand-induced activation of VEGFR-1. Initially, it was reported that conditioned medium from cells transfected with an expression vector generating VEGF-B$_{167}$ stimulated DNA synthesis in primary cultures of endothelial cells. However, at least part of this mitogenic activity is probably contributed by the formation of VEGF·VEGF-B heterodimers as most *in vitro* grown cell lines express VEGF endogenously.

The poor mitogenic effect of VEGF-B on endothelial cells seen *in vitro* is also reflected in *in vivo* studies. Transgenic mice overexpressing VEGF-B under strong promoters show no obvious vascular phenotypes, and mice carrying a targeted deletion in the VEGF-B gene develop normally. No gross abnormalities can be seen in such mice, even in organs in which normal expression of VEGF-B is high, such as heart, muscle, and kidney. These results have shown that VEGF-B is not required for embryonic angiogenesis. Similar results have been shown in mice deficient in PlGF, the functional homologue of VEGF-B, suggesting that neither VEGFR-1-specific ligand is a critical regulator of embryonic vessel development. This is in contrast to the essential role of VEGF in vasculogenesis and angiogenesis.

VEGF-B is expressed in most tumors and tumor-derived cell lines analyzed. Given its poor mitogenic capacity on endothelial cells, VEGF-B is unlikely to directly control the growth of the tumor vasculature like VEGF. Instead, the effects of VEGF-B may be indirect and related to the recruitment of stem cells, progenitor cells, and inflammatory cells to the tumors (see below).

Recent results have suggested that the receptor for VEGF-B, VEGFR-1, is important in the recruitment and mobilization of hematopoietic stem cells and endothelial progenitors from the bone marrow. Such cells are likely to have important functions in therapeutic angiogenesis whereby new vessels are generated or existing vessels are remodeled in ischemic tissues to allow increased blood flow. Furthermore, these cells also contribute to pathological vessel growth in several diseases, including cancer and retinopathies, and contribute to inflammatory conditions, such as atherosclerosis and arthritis. VEGF-B is also able to induce an endothelial cell phenotype of mesenchymal stem cells from the bone marrow. Given that expression of VEGF-B is widespread, and rather abundant in some tissues, a role of VEGF-B in stem cell biology and inflammation is likely.

VII. FUTURE DIRECTIONS

The exciting finding that VEGFR-1 and its ligands control the recruitment and mobilization of hematopoietic stem cells and endothelial progenitor cells and the differentiation of mesenchymal stem cells suggests that they provide important tools for the therapeutic modulation of vessel growth in cardiovascular disease, cancer, retinopathies, inflammation, atherosclerosis, and hematopoiesis. Clearly, more extensive studies of these molecules, and particularly VEGF-B, in various experimental models are warranted.

Glossary

angiogenesis Sprouting and growth of blood vessels from preexisting blood vessels.

stem cells Primitive cells that have an unlimited capacity to divide and that can differentiate into different functional cell types.

vasculogenesis *De novo* formation of blood vessels from mesodermal precursors.

See Also the Following Articles

Angiogenesis • Cancer Cells and Progrowth/Prosurvival Signaling • Corpus Luteum: Regression and Rescue • Epidermal Growth Factor (EGF) Family • Estrogen Receptor (ER) Actions through Other Transcription Factor Sites • Heparin-Binding Epidermal Growth Factor-like Growth Factor (HB-EGF) • HGF (Hepatocyte Growth Factor)/MET System • Platelet-Derived Growth Factor (PDGF) • Vascular Endothelial Growth Factor D (VEGF-D)

Further Reading

Aase, K., Lymboussaki, A., Kaipainen, A., Olofsson, B., Alitalo, K., and Eriksson, U. (1999). Localization of VEGF-B in the mouse embryo suggests a paracrine role of the growth factor in the developing vasculature. *Dev. Dyn.* **215**, 12–25.

Aase, K., von Euler, G., Li, X., Pontén, A., Thorén, P., Cao, R., Cao, Y., Olofsson, B., Gebre-Medhin, S., Pekny, M., Alitalo, K., Betsholtz, C., and Eriksson, U. (2001). Vascular endothelial growth factor-B-deficient mice display an atrial conduction defect. *Circulation* **104**, 358–364.

Hattori, K., Heissig, B., Wu, Y., Hicklin, D., Zhu, Z., Bohlen, P., Witte, L., Ferris, B., Dias, S., Hendriks, J., Hacket, N. R., Crystal, R. G., Moore, M. A. S., Werb, Z., Lyden, D., and Raffi, S. (2002). Placental growth factor reconstitutes hematopoiesis by recruiting VEGFR1[+] stem cells from bone marrow microenvironment. *Nat. Med.* **8**, 841–849.

Li, X., Aase, K., Li, H., von Euler, G., and Eriksson, U. (2001). Isoform-specific expression of VEGF-B in normal tissues and tumors. *Growth Factors* **19**, 49–59.

Luttun, A., Tjwa, M., Moons, L., Wu, Y., Angelillo-Scherrer, A., Liao, F., Nagy, J. A., Hooper, A., Priller, J., De Klerck, B., Compernolle, V., Daci, E., Bohlen, P., Dewerchin, M., Herbert, J.-M., Fava, R., Mattys, P., Carmeliet, G., Collen, D., Dvorak, H. F., Hicklin, D., and Carmeliet, P. (2002). Revascularization of ischemic tissues by PlGF treatment and inhibition of tumor angiogenesis, arthritis and atherosclerosis by anti-Flt-1 antibody. *Nat. Med.* **8**, 831–840.

Olofsson, B., Korpeleinen, E., Pepper, M. S., Mandriota, S., Aase, K., Gunji, Y., Jeltsch, M. M., Shibuya, M., Alitalo, K., and Eriksson, U. (1998). VEGF-B binds to VEGFR-1 and regulates plasminogen activator activity in endothelial cells. *Proc. Natl. Acad. Sci. USA* **95**, 11709–11714.

Olofsson, B., Pajusola, K., Kaipainen, A., von Euler, G., Joukov, V., Saksela, O., Orpana, O., Pettersson, R., Alitalo, K., and Eriksson, U. (1996). Vascular endothelial growth factor B, a novel growth factor for endothelial cells. *Proc. Natl. Acad. Sci. USA* **93**, 2576–2581.

Olofsson, B., Pajusola, K., von Euler, G., Chilov, D., Alitalo, K., and Eriksson, U. (1996). Genomic organization of the mouse and human genes for vascular endothelial growth factor B (VEGF-B) and characterization of a second splice isoform. *J. Biol. Chem.* **271**, 19310–19317.

Vascular Endothelial Growth Factor D (VEGF-D)

MARC G. ACHEN AND STEVEN A. STACKER
Ludwig Institute for Cancer Research, Melbourne

I. DISCOVERY AND ALTERNATIVE NAMES
II. PROTEIN STRUCTURE
III. BIOSYNTHESIS
IV. RECEPTORS
V. BIOLOGICAL ACTIVITIES
VI. GENE STRUCTURE AND REGULATION
VII. TISSUE DISTRIBUTION
VIII. PATHOLOGY
IX. FUTURE DIRECTIONS

Vascular endothelial growth factor D (VEGF-D) is a member of the VEGF family of growth factors. These growth factors are secreted glycoproteins that contain a cysteine knot motif. Human VEGF-D is mitogenic for vascular endothelial cells *in vitro* and can induce the growth of both blood vessels and lymphatic vessels *in vivo*. VEGF-D is expressed at many sites in the developing embryo including lung and kidney mesenchyme, skin, liver, heart, and limb buds, likely playing a role in inducing the growth of blood and lymphatic vessels in these regions. In adult tissues, VEGF-D is expressed in the vascular smooth muscle of blood vessels, where it may play a role in the repair of blood vessels after vascular damage.

I. DISCOVERY AND ALTERNATIVE NAMES

Vascular endothelial growth factor D (VEGF-D) is the most recently discovered mammalian member of the VEGF family of growth factors, which consists of the secreted glycoproteins VEGF (VEGF-A), VEGF-B, VEGF-C, VEGF-D, placenta growth factor, and VEGF-like molecules encoded by viruses and present in snake venoms. VEGF family members form part of a structural superfamily of growth factors containing a cysteine knot motif in which six conserved cysteine residues contribute to a three-dimensional fold involving an unusual clustering of three cysteine bridges intertwined to resemble a knot. VEGF-D was originally reported as c-*fos*-induced growth factor because it was identified as a protein that was downregulated in fibroblasts deficient in c-*fos*. Subsequently, the protein was renamed VEGF-D when its capacity to bind and activate VEGF receptors was demonstrated. VEGF-D is most closely related to VEGF-C (these proteins share 48% amino acid identity throughout the entire molecule and 61% identity within the central VEGF homology domain); similarities in the structure, proteolytic processing, and receptor binding of these two growth factors indicate that they form a subfamily within the VEGF family.

II. PROTEIN STRUCTURE

Human VEGF-D and mouse VEGF-D are 354 and 358 amino acids in length, respectively (including the signal sequence for protein secretion), are 87% identical in amino acid sequence, and contain three potential N-linked glycosylation sites. VEGF-D is initially synthesized as a precursor protein containing N- and C-terminal propeptides in addition to a central VEGF homology domain (VHD) (Fig. 1). The VHD contains the known receptor-binding regions and shares homology with all VEGF family members. The free N-terminal propeptide has an apparent molecular weight of approximately 10 kDa as assessed by sodium dodecyl sulfate–polyacrylamide gel electrophoresis (SDS–PAGE) under reducing conditions, whereas the VHD is approximately 21 kDa and the C-terminal propeptide is approximately 29 kDa. The C-terminal propeptide contains numerous cysteine residues, many of which are arranged in motifs resembling those of the Balbiani ring 3 protein (BR3P) ($CysX_{10}CysXCysXCys$).

Approximately 50 of these motifs are found in BR3P, a cysteine-rich protein synthesized in the larval salivary glands of the midge *Chironomus tentans*. It has been speculated that the cysteine residues in the C-terminal propeptide of VEGF-D may have a role in intermolecular interactions (as is the case for the BR3P motifs), possibly modulating the bioavailability, localization, or biological half-life of the growth factor.

Two distinct isoforms of mouse VEGF-D, VEGF-D_{358} and VEGF-D_{326}, which differ in the structure of the C-terminal propeptide, have been reported. Alternative use of an RNA splice donor site in exon 6 of the mouse *VEGF-D* gene produces the two different protein isoforms. The two isoforms are both expressed in a wide range of adult mouse tissues and embryonic stages of development. Both isoforms are proteolytically processed in a fashion similar to human VEGF-D to generate a range of secreted derivatives (Section III). The isoforms are differently glycosylated when expressed *in vitro*. Hence, RNA splicing, protein glycosylation, and proteolysis are mechanisms for generating structural diversity of mouse VEGF-D. Multiple isoforms of human VEGF-D, generated by alternative RNA splicing, have not been reported.

III. BIOSYNTHESIS

Studies carried out with VEGF-D *in vitro* demonstrated that the N- and C-terminal propeptides are proteolytically cleaved from the VHD in a step-wise

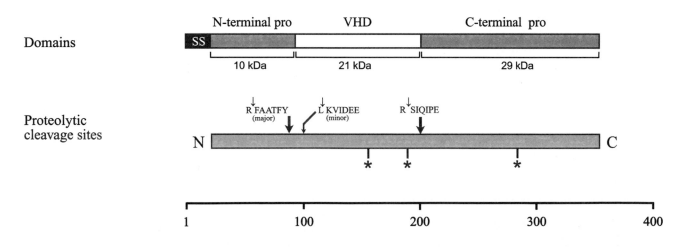

FIGURE 1 Schematic representation of the domain structure of human VEGF-D. SS denotes signal sequence for protein secretion and pro denotes propeptide. Proteolytic cleavage sites are indicated by arrows and potential N-linked glycosylation sites by asterisks. Apparent molecular weights, indicated under the domains, were determined by SDS–PAGE under reducing conditions.

fashion after secretion from the cell to ultimately generate a mature form consisting of dimers of the VHD (Fig. 2A). The VHD dimers are assumed to be anti-parallel in nature based on the three-dimensional structure of VEGF, and the association between them is predominantly noncovalent. Proteolytic processing at the N-terminus of the VHD occurs at multiple sites in a region that appears to be prone to proteolysis, whereas cleavage at the C-terminus occurs at a unique site (Fig. 1) that is located at the same position in VEGF-C. Expression of VEGF-D in mammalian cells *in vitro* leads to the production of a mixture of unprocessed, partially processed, and fully processed forms that accumulate in the cell culture medium. Predominant forms observed by SDS–PAGE are the free N-terminal propeptide (~ 10 kDa), the free C-terminal propeptide (~ 29 kDa), the free VHD (~ 21 kDa), the VHD linked to the N-terminal propeptide (~ 31 kDa), and full-length material (~ 58 kDa). Analysis of VEGF-D purified from

mouse lung demonstrated that this growth factor is proteolytically processed *in vivo*.

IV. RECEPTORS

The receptors for human VEGF-D identified thus far are VEGFR-2 (also known as KDR in human and Flk1 in mouse) and VEGFR-3 (also known as Flt4) (Fig. 2B). These are cell surface receptor tyrosine kinases that are closely related in structure, contain seven Ig-like domains in their extracellular regions, and are bound, cross-linked, and activated by VEGF-D. VEGFR-2 is localized on the endothelium of blood vessels during embryonic development but is generally down-regulated in adult tissues. In contrast, VEGFR-3 is localized on lymphatic endothelium in adult tissues. During embryogenesis, VEGFR-3 is initially expressed on a wide range of vessels but subsequently becomes restricted to developing veins and then to the lymphatics. An extensive range of

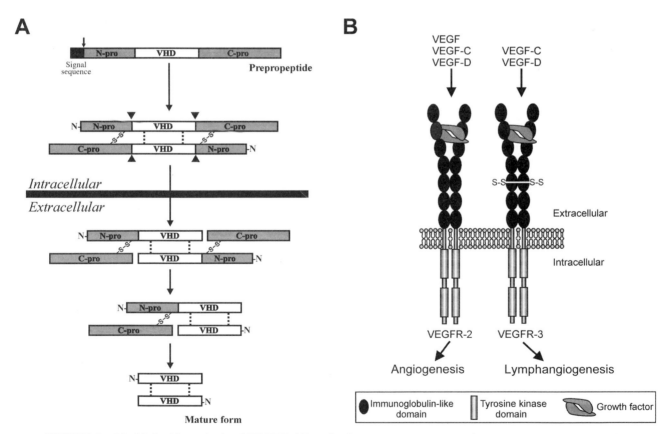

FIGURE 2 Model for biosynthesis of VEGF-D (A) and schematic representation of receptor interactions (B). (A) Stepwise proteolytic processing gives rise to a mature form consisting of dimers of the VHD. Arrowheads indicate sites of proteolytic cleavage; -S-S-, disulfide bridges; N-Pro, the N-terminal propeptide; C-pro, the C-terminal propeptide; dotted lines, noncovalent interactions. (B) Mammalian VEGF family members dimerize VEGFR-2 and VEGFR-3 to induce angiogenesis and lymphangiogenesis, respectively.

in vivo studies have indicated that VEGFR-2 signals for angiogenesis, whereas VEGFR-3 signals for lymphangiogenesis.

Both VEGFR-2 and VEGFR-3 are crucial for vascular development during embryogenesis. Embryos homozygous for *VEGFR-2* gene inactivation, which die at approximately 9 days post coitum (dpc), lack both hematopoietic precursor cells and endothelial cells, indicating that this receptor plays a crucial role in early vasculogenesis. In contrast, VEGFR-3 is not required for vasculogenesis as mouse embryos lacking this receptor have both hematopoietic and endothelial cells; however, large vessels become abnormally organized with defective lumens, leading to fluid accumulation in the pericardial cavity and cardiovascular failure at 9.5 dpc. On the basis of these findings, it has been proposed that VEGFR-3 is required for the maturation of primary vascular networks into larger blood vessels. As the *VEGFR-3* mutant mice die before the lymphatic vessels emerge, it may be necessary to generate conditional knockout *VEGFR-3* mice in order to test the role of VEGFR-3 in the development of the lymphatic vasculature.

Unexpectedly, mouse VEGF-D, in contrast to human VEGF-D, fails to bind mouse VEGFR-2 but activates VEGFR-3. Mutation of amino acids in mouse VEGF-D to those in the human homologue indicated that residues important for the VEGFR-2 interaction are clustered at, or are near, the receptor-binding surface predicted from the structure of VEGF. The different receptor-binding specificities of mouse and human VEGF-D indicate that this growth factor may have different biological functions in mouse and human.

Analyses of the interaction of human VEGF-D with immobilized receptor extracellular domains revealed that proteolytic processing modulates VEGF-D function as the mature form of human VEGF-D binds VEGF-2 and VEGFR-3 with 290- and 40-fold greater affinity, respectively, than does unprocessed VEGF-D. Therefore, proteolytic processing is essential for generation of VEGF-D, which binds these receptors with high affinity. VEGF-D activates both VEGFR-2 and VEGFR-3 as the treatment of cells expressing these receptors with VEGF-D induces the phosphorylation of tyrosine residues on these receptors.

V. BIOLOGICAL ACTIVITIES

Human VEGF-D is mitogenic for vascular endothelial cells *in vitro* and can induce both angiogenesis and lymphangiogenesis *in vivo*, although the predominant response to this growth factor depends on the timing and location of its application. For example, VEGF-D was demonstrated to be angiogenic in the adult rabbit cornea and in a mouse tumor model. When expressed during embryonic development in the epidermis of mouse skin, under the control of the *keratin-14* gene promoter, VEGF-D induced lymphatic hyperplasia/lymphangiogenesis, but not angiogenesis, in the underlying dermis. The biological response induced by VEGF-D, be it angiogenesis or lymphangiogenesis, most likely depends on the proximity of blood vessels and lymphatic vessels expressing VEGFR-2 and/or VEGFR-3 to the site of application of the growth factor. VEGF-D also induced lymphangiogenesis in a mouse tumor model. Importantly, the tumor lymphangiogenesis induced by VEGF-D promoted metastatic spread via the lymphatics, suggesting that the route of metastatic spread of a tumor is dependent on the capacity of tumor-derived growth factors to induce angiogenesis and/or lymphangiogenesis.

Some members of the VEGF family, such as VEGF and VEGF-C, potently induce a rapid and transient increase in the permeability of microvessels to macromolecules. However, the mature form of human VEGF-D did not exhibit any activity in the Miles vascular permeability assay. This suggests that VEGF-D is unlikely to induce edema in a therapeutic setting and that activation of VEGFR-2 alone may not be sufficient to induce vascular permeability.

VI. GENE STRUCTURE AND REGULATION

The gene encoding human VEGF-D consists of seven exons, is approximately 50 kb in size, and is located on the X chromosome at position Xp22.1. The mouse *VEGF-D* gene is similar in structure and is also located on the X chromosome. The *VEGF-D* gene is highly homologous to that for VEGF-C, further illustrating the relatedness of these two growth factors. It is clear that the genes for VEGF-D and VEGF-C arose from duplication of a common ancestor gene. Although it is known that c-*fos* induces *VEGF-D* gene expression, few studies have addressed the regulation of this gene. VEGF-D gene expression is induced by cell–cell contact mediated by cadherin-11, but unlike VEGF-C, VEGF-D is not up-regulated by interleukin-1β, tumor necrosis factor α, or serum. Distinct mechanisms of gene regulation occur among VEGF family members to enable independent expression during blood and lymphatic vessel growth and development.

The mechanism by which the transcripts for mouse VEGF-D$_{358}$ and VEGF-D$_{326}$ are generated can be explained by the structure of exon 6 of the mouse *VEGF-D* gene. The VEGF-D$_{358}$ transcript is generated by a splice event from within exon 6 to the beginning of exon 7. In contrast, the transcript for VEGF-D$_{326}$ arises when this splice event does not occur. Therefore, the 3' region of exon 6 is represented in the VEGF-D$_{326}$ transcript but not in the VEGF-D$_{358}$ transcript. Such alternative splicing events have not been reported for the human *VEGF-D* gene.

VII. TISSUE DISTRIBUTION

VEGF-D is expressed at many sites in the developing embryo including lung and kidney mesenchyme, skin, liver, heart, and limb buds. As this growth factor can induce both angiogenesis and lymphangiogenesis, it is likely that it plays a role in attracting the growth of blood and lymphatic vessels into these regions of the embryo during development. In adult tissues, VEGF-D is localized in the vascular smooth muscle of blood vessels. Although VEGFR-2 is not strongly expressed on the endothelium of blood vessels in adult tissues, it can be up-regulated in response to various forms of vascular stress or damage. As VEGF-D is an activating ligand for VEGFR-2, the VEGF-D produced by vascular smooth muscle may play a role in repair of blood vessels after vascular damage.

VIII. PATHOLOGY

VEGF-D is expressed in a range of human tumors including malignant melanoma, glioma, and breast and lung carcinomas. In non-small-cell lung carcinoma, VEGF-D was detected in tumor cells and the endothelium of nearby vessels. Furthermore, mRNA for VEGF-D was detected in the tumor cells but not in the endothelium, indicating that VEGF-D is produced by tumor cells and accumulates in nearby endothelium due to receptor-mediated uptake. These findings suggest a paracrine model by which VEGF-D derived from tumor cells promotes tumor angiogenesis and lymphangiogenesis. Direct demonstration of such a role was established by studies of VEGF-D action in a mouse tumor model that indicated that this growth factor can induce tumor angiogenesis, lymphangiogenesis, and metastatic spread via lymphatic vessels. Therefore, VEGF-D may be a useful target for anti-cancer therapy designed to block metastatic spread via the lymphatics.

IX. FUTURE DIRECTIONS

Recent studies of VEGF-D action in tumor models suggest that inhibition of VEGF-D may be of use to block metastatic spread. Neutralizing monoclonal antibodies, peptidomimetic inhibitors of receptor binding, and small-molecule inhibitors of the catalytic domains of VEGFR-2 and VEGFR-3 must be carefully tested in animal models of tumor development to establish the utility of targeting the signaling pathways in which VEGF-D is involved. Other possible clinical utilities for VEGF-D include induction of endothelial cell mitogenesis for prevention of restenosis, induction of collateral vessel formation for treatment of diseases involving ischemia, and induction of lymphangiogenesis/lymphatic hyperplasia for treatment of primary and secondary lymphedema. Testing the utility of VEGF-D in these clinical contexts is a matter of high priority.

Glossary

angiogenesis Growth of blood vessels.
lymphangiogenesis Growth of lymphatic vessels.
lymphatic system An open-ended network of vessels that collect fluid from tissue spaces and ultimately drain it into the venous system.
lymphedema Swelling of tissue due to accumulation of lymphatic fluid.
vasculogenesis *De novo* formation of blood vessels from mesodermal precursors.

See Also the Following Articles

Angiogenesis ● Cancer Cells and Progrowth/Prosurvival Signaling ● Corpus Luteum: Regression and Rescue ● Epidermal Growth Factor (EGF) Family ● Estrogen Receptor (ER) Actions through Other Transcription Factor Sites ● Heparin-Binding Epidermal Growth Factor-like Growth Factor (HB-EGF) ● HGF (Hepatocyte Growth Factor)/MET System ● Platelet-Derived Growth Factor (PDGF) ● Vascular Endothelial Growth Factor B (VEGF-B)

Further Reading

Achen, M. G., and Stacker, S. A. (1998). The vascular endothelial growth factor family: Proteins which guide the development of the vasculature. *Int. J. Exp. Pathol.* **79**, 255–265.

Achen, M. G., Jeltsch, M., Kukk, E., Makinen, T., Vitali, A., Wilks, A. F., Alitalo, K., and Stacker, S. A. (1998). Vascular endothelial growth factor-D (VEGF-D) is a ligand for the tyrosine kinases VEGF receptor-2 (Flk1) and VEGF receptor-3 (Flt4). *Proc. Natl. Acad. Sci. USA* **95**, 548–553.

Achen, M. G., Williams, R. A., Minekus, M. P., Thornton, G. E., Stenvers, K., Rogers, P. A. W., Lederman, F., Roufail, S., and

Stacker, S. A. (2001). Localization of vascular endothelial growth factor-D in malignant melanoma suggests a role in tumour angiogenesis. *J. Pathol.* **193**, 147–154.

Baldwin, M. E., Catimel, B., Nice, E. C., Roufail, S., Hall, N. E., Stenvers, K. L., Karkkainen, M. J., Alitalo, K., Stacker, S. A., and Achen, M. G. (2001). The specificity of receptor binding by vascular endothelial growth factor-D is different in mouse and man. *J. Biol. Chem.* **276**, 19166–19171.

Jenkins, N. A., Woollatt, E., Crawford, J., Gilbert, D. J., Baldwin, M., Sutherland, G. R., Copeland, N. G., and Achen, M. G. (1997). Mapping of the gene for vascular endothelial growth factor-D in mouse and man to the X chromosome. *Chromosome Res.* **5**, 502–505.

Stacker, S. A., and Achen, M. G. (1999). The vascular endothelial growth factor (VEGF) family: Signaling for vascular development. *Growth Factors* **17**, 1–11.

Stacker, S. A., Caesar, C., Baldwin, M. E., Thornton, G. E., Williams, R. A., Prevo, R., Jackson, D. G., Nishikawa, S.-I., Kubo, H., and Achen, M. G. (2001). VEGF-D promotes the metastatic spread of tumor cells via the lymphatics. *Nat. Med.* **7**, 186–191.

Stacker, S. A., Stenvers, K., Caesar, C., Vitali, A., Domagala, T., Nice, E., Roufail, S., Simpson, R. J., Moritz, R., Karpanen, T., Alitalo, K., and Achen, M. G. (1999). Biosynthesis of vascular endothelial growth factor-D involves proteolytic processing which generates non-covalent homodimers. *J. Biol. Chem.* **274**, 32127–32136.

Vasoactive Intestinal Peptide (VIP)

BAHRİ KARAÇAY AND M. SUE O'DORISIO
University of Iowa College of Medicine

I. VASOACTIVE INTESTINAL PEPTIDE
II. VIP EXPRESSION DURING DEVELOPMENT
III. VIP RECEPTORS
IV. MECHANISM OF VIP ACTION (SIGNAL TRANSDUCTION PATHWAY)
V. BIOLOGICAL EFFECTS OF VIP
VI. CONCLUSION AND PERSPECTIVES

Vasoactive intestinal peptide is a 28-amino-acid hormone belonging to the secretin/glucagon superfamily of peptides. Through receptor-specific interactions, vasoactive intestinal peptide activates signal transduction pathways that confer vasodilatory effects throughout the body. In its roles as neurotransmitter, hormone, and cytokine, this peptide also plays a role in oncologic disease; further studies may lead to important therapeutic applications.

I. VASOACTIVE INTESTINAL PEPTIDE

A. Discovery of VIP

Vasoactive intestinal peptide (VIP), first discovered in porcine duodenum, was initially considered to be a gastrointestinal hormone. The peptide was named for its profound and long-lasting vasodilatory effects in laboratory animals. This initial identification, however, belies a much broader function of VIP in the central and peripheral nervous systems as well as in the immune system. Today we know that VIP functions as a neurotransmitter, a hormone, and a cytokine through neuroendocrine and neuroimmune axes. VIP regulates intestinal water and electrolyte secretion; vaginal fluid secretion; pituitary hormone, neuronal growth factor, and lymphocyte cytokine release; and glycogenolysis in the liver and cerebral cortex. Through its vasodilatory effect, VIP modulates the vascular reactivity for penile erection, influences cervical and vaginal blood flow, and induces bronchodilation. One or more of these functions is essential to the role of VIP in oocyte maturation, neurogenesis, neuroprotection, and immune homeostasis.

B. Structure of the Peptide

VIP is a 28-amino-acid peptide with structural similarity to other gastrointestinal hormones, including secretin, glucagon, pituitary adenylate cyclase-activating polypeptides (PACAP-37 and PACAP-38), gastric inhibitory peptide (GIP), growth hormone-releasing hormone (GHRH), peptide histidine isoleucine (PHI; in pigs and rodents), and peptide histidine methionine (PHM; in humans) (Fig. 1). Thus, VIP belongs to the secretin/glucagon superfamily of peptides. The sequence is identical in human, porcine, bovine, sheep, goat, rabbit, rat, and mouse VIP, suggesting strict amino acid conservation during evolution.

C. Structure of the VIP Gene

The approximately 9-kb gene encoding human VIP is located on chromosome 6q24. The VIP gene consists of six introns and seven exons. Exon sizes vary from 89 to 165 bp. Isolation and sequence determination of the cDNA for human VIP reveal that the messenger RNA encodes a second peptide, PHM (PHI in rodents). PHM is encoded by exon four and VIP is encoded by exon five (Fig. 2). The prepro-VIP consists of 170 amino acids; during proteolytic

```
VIP       H-S-D-A-V-F-T-D-N-Y-T-R-L-R-K-Q-M-A-V-K-K-Y-L-N-S-I-L-N
PACAP-27  H-S-D-G-I-F-T-D-S-Y-S-R-Y-R-K-Q-M-A-V-K-K-Y-L-A-A-V-L
PHM       H-A-D-G-V-F-T-S-D-F-S-K-L-L-G-Q-L-S-A-K-K-Y-L-E-S-L-M
SECRETIN  H-S-D-G-T-F-T-S-E-L-S-R-L-R-D-S-A-R-L-Q-R-L-L-Q-G-L-V
GLUCAGON  H-S-Q-G-T-F-T-S-D-Y-S-K-Y-L-D-S-R-R-A-Q-D-F-V-Q-W-L-M-N-T
```

FIGURE 1 Structures of the secretin/glucagon family of peptides. VIP, Vasoactive intestinal peptide; PACAP, pituitary adenylate cyclase-activating peptide; PHM, peptide histidine methionine. Areas of amino acid sequence homologies with VIP are shaded. PACAP-27, PHM, secretin, and glucagon share 68, 44, 37, and 20% amino acid homology with VIP, respectively.

cleavage, five peptides are formed: prepro-VIP(22–79) (N-terminal flanking peptide), peptide histidine isoleucine/methionine (PHI/PHM)(81–107), prepro-VIP (111–122) (bridging peptide), VIP(125–152), and prepro-VIP(156–170) (C-terminal flanking peptide). Alternative splicing generates a C-terminally extended PHM, a peptide designated as PHV-42 that has been shown to be a potent smooth muscle relaxer (Fig. 2). The amino acid homology between VIP and PHM (37%) is less than the degree of similarity between VIP and PACAP (68%). The evolutionary process leading to the generation of different precursors for secretin/glucagon superfamily members probably includes serial gene duplication accompanied by exon loss events. The fact that two different peptides (VIP and PHM) are encoded by the same messenger RNA suggests cosynthesis of the two peptides in the same tissue. However, colocalization is not always found in the same cells in the brain.

The differential regulation of these two peptides may be due to differences at translational or posttranslational levels.

D. Regulation of Gene Expression

Cell-type-specific expression of the human VIP gene requires several cis-acting sequences located at the 5′ flanking region of VIP. Among these, a 425-bp tissue-specifier element (TSE) located between −4.6 and −4.0 kb and a region with multiple positive- and negative-acting elements, along with a cyclic adenosine monophosphate (cAMP) response element located between −1.55 kb and −904 bp, play important roles in regulation of VIP gene expression (Fig. 2). The ubiquitously expressed POU-homeodomain proteins Oct-1 and Oct-2 as well as AP-2/Ets transcription factors physically interact with the TSE and play a central role in regulation of VIP gene expression. Accurate spatial expression of the

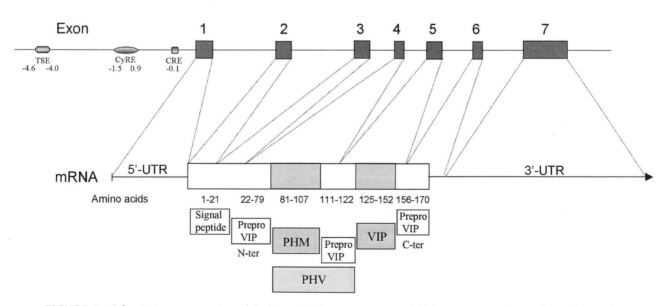

FIGURE 2 Schematic representation of the human VIP gene structure, mRNA transcript, and peptide products. The VIP gene is approximately 9 kb in size and is located on human chromosome 6q24. Exon sizes vary from 89 to 165 bp. PHM, Peptide histidine methionine; PHV, peptide histidine valine; VIP, vasoactive intestinal peptide; TSE, tissue-specifier element; CyRE, cytokine response element; CRE, cyclic AMP response element; UTR, untranslated region.

VIP gene requires combinatorial effects of the cis-elements within the TSE and the proximal 1.55-kb 5′ flanking sequence. The proximal promoter region contains cis-acting elements such as E-boxes, MEF-2-like motifs, and a cytokine-responsive element. Interactions between the TSE and proximal promoter elements lead to either transcriptional repression or activation of VIP gene expression in different cell lineages, resulting in varying levels of VIP message in different cell types.

The spatial expression pattern of VIP is remarkably well conserved between rodents and human genes. Consistent with this, analysis of 5′ flanking regions of mouse and human VIP genes demonstrates a high level of conservation (80%) immediately upstream of the transcription initiation site that also includes the cAMP response element (Fig. 2). A higher level of conservation (91%) has been found between human and mouse genes within a 210-bp fragment located more than 1.1 kb upstream from the transcription start site; this sequence contains cis-acting elements such as PEA-3 and NGF–IL-6. Studies aimed at determining whether 5′ flanking sequences of the VIP gene could recapitulate the endogenous gene expression have demonstrated that a 5.2-kb promoter region of the human VIP gene is able to direct reporter gene expression to the small intestine of transgenic mice. In a later study, a 2-kb promoter fragment was shown to direct the expression of a reporter gene to tissues in a pattern similar to the endogenous VIP gene expression profile. However, the transgene expression was also detected in smooth muscle and Schwann cells, in which endogenous VIP mRNA is rare. When a 16.5-kb upstream sequence of the mouse VIP gene was fused to β-galactosidase, reporter gene expression was targeted to neurons in the esophagus, stomach, small intestine, and colon, where endogenous VIP is present. However, this reporter gene was not expressed in brain, including the regions that contain high levels of VIP such as the cerebral cortex, thalamus, hippocampus, amygdala, and suprachiasmatic nucleus. These results demonstrate that gene regulation at the level of transcription is of fundamental importance for VIP gene expression, but the results also suggest that additional studies are necessary to provide a better understanding of *in vivo* regulation of VIP gene expression. Recent studies demonstrate that VIP gene expression is also regulated at the posttranscriptional level; elements that regulate RNA stability are localized at the 3′ untranslated region of the VIP message. The presence of different sizes of VIP mRNA with varied half-lives, along with competition studies employing heterologous RNA stability elements, suggest an important role for tissue-specific posttranscriptional regulation of VIP levels (Fig. 2). The multiple levels of control of VIP gene expression provide a highly specific spatial expression pattern.

II. VIP EXPRESSION DURING DEVELOPMENT

Developmental regulation of the VIP gene has not been studied in great detail. Although samples from different species have been used, most of the data regarding VIP expression have been obtained from rats. Early studies demonstrated no VIP expression in the central nervous system (CNS) of rats until birth, when a rapid increase in expression is observed. However, later studies employing *in situ* hybridization and histochemistry detected VIP message as early as embryonic day 14 (E14) in the hindbrain of a mouse. This may be due to the increased sensitivity of the method used, or to the interspecies differences between mice and rats. After birth, rat VIP mRNA increases in most brain regions until the level and distribution reach the expression profile of the adult. In the cortex, however, VIP message level increases until postnatal day 14 but decreases after postnatal day 21 until it reaches adult levels, suggesting that VIP may be involved in the development of the cortex. VIP is expressed earlier in the peripheral nervous system than in the CNS. *In situ* hybridization detects VIP message in the embryonic body in E14 rat embryos. By E16, VIP message is detectable in the sphenopalatine ganglion, aorta, and intestine. Contrary to late appearance of VIP message in the CNS during development, binding sites for VIP appear earlier (E13 in rats and E9 in mice). VIP binding sites are particularly abundant in brain regions where rapid cell division takes place, such as neuroepithelial regions of the brain or the intermediate medial thalamus. The observation that maternal VIP levels peak during midgestation raises the possibility that maternal VIP may be involved in early embryonic development, when embryonic VIP binding sites are apparent but embryonic VIP is still undetectable.

In the adult central nervous system, VIP is expressed in the cerebral cortex, hypothalamus, amygdala, hippocampus, and corpus striatum at high levels. Potentiation of cAMP levels in the cortex results in promotion of glycogenolysis. Localization of binding sites for VIP in cortex by *in vitro* autoradiography suggests that VIP may function in the energy metabolism of the cortex. Processes of some VIP-containing neurons penetrate the cortical surface, enter the pial membranes, and make contacts with cerebral blood vessels. VIP binding sites are abundant throughout the cortex, with the highest binding in layers of the cortex exhibiting greatest dendritic arborization of VIP neurons (layers I, II, IV, and VI). *In situ* hybridization reveals vasoactive intestinal peptide receptor 1 (VPAC1) message in the cortex of rat, suggesting that VPAC1 may mediate the effects of VIP in cerebral cortex. VIP neurons are also present in the hippocampal formation and send their axons to nearby pyramidal and granule cells, where VIP receptors are expressed. These neurons receive input from the γ-aminobutyric acid (GABA)-ergic septohippocampal pathway and diagonal band. *In vitro* binding studies localize VIP binding throughout the hippocampal formation, with higher levels in the molecular layer of the dentate gyrus. Thus, VIP may play a role in the regulation of electrical activity in the hippocampal formation.

Within the hypothalamus, the suprachiasmatic nucleus (SCN) has the highest density of VIP neurons and VIP binding sites. Both VIP peptide and message levels vary over the day/night cycle, with peak levels occurring at night. Microinjection of VIP or PACAP into the rodent SCN shifts the circadian pace maker whereas VIP antagonists and oligonucleotides disrupt the circadian cycle. Overexpression of VPAC2 in the SCN alters the circadian phenotype of mice, leading to a quicker resynchronization in transgenic mice compared to wild-type animals. VPAC2-overexpressing mice also exhibit a shorter circadian period in constant darkness. Some early studies focused on VIP regulation of prolactin release from the anterior pituitary. Subsequent studies have reported a role for VIP as an important modulator of other pituitary

hormones, such as adrenocorticotropic hormone (ACTH), growth hormone, and luteinizing hormone (LH). VIP may also regulate anterior pituitary GABA concentrations.

III. VIP RECEPTORS

A. Receptor Subtypes

VIP binds with high affinity to specific G-protein-coupled receptors with seven transmembrane domains. Two receptor subtypes with different affinities for VIP have been isolated and designated as vasoactive intestinal peptide receptors 1 and 2 (VPAC1 and VPAC2) (Table 1). VPAC1 was first isolated from rat lung. The human homologue has also been cloned and expressed in different cell lines. VPAC1 consists of 457 amino acids with an estimated molecular mass of 52 kDa. Murine VPAC1 has 93 and 83% identity with previously cloned rat and human counterparts, respectively. The powerful fluorometric quantitative polymerase chain reaction (PCR) assay has demonstrated that expression of VPAC1 is highest in the small intestine and colon of the mouse, followed by the liver and the brain. VPAC1 message was also detected in thymus, spleen, lung, kidney, gonads, adrenal gland, spinal cord, and heart. Human, mouse, and rat VPAC1 genes map to syntenic regions of human chromosome 3p21.33–p21.31; the distal region of mouse chromosome 9, and to rat chromosome 8q32.

A second high-affinity VIP receptor has been cloned from rat olfactory bulb and designated as VPAC2. VPAC2 has 438 amino acids with an estimated molecular mass of 47 kDa. The VPAC2 gene

TABLE 1 Receptor-Specific Agonists and Antagonists for VPAC1 and VPAC2

Ligand	IC$_{50}$		Activity
	VPAC1	VPAC2	
VIP	1 nM^a	3–4 nM^a	VPAC1 agonist, VPAC2 agonist
[Lys^{15}, Arg^{16}, Leu^{27}]VIP$_{(1-7)}$GRF$_{(8-27)}$-NH$_2$	1 nM	—	VPAC1 agonist
[Arg^{16}]chicken secretin	2 nM	—	VPAC1 agonist
[Acetyl-His^1, D-Phe^2, lys^{15}, Arg^{16}]VIP$_{(3-7)}$GRF$_{(8-27)}$-NH$_2$	1–10 nM	3 μM	VPAC1 antagonist
RO25-1392	—	10 nM	VPAC2 agonist
RO25-1553	—	1 nM	VPAC2 agonist
PACAP-27	1 nM	10 nM	VPAC1 agonist, VPAC2 agonist
PACAP-38	30 nM	2 nM	VPAC1 agonist, VPAC2 agonist
Secretin	1.5 μM	—	VPAC1 agonist
GRF	—	5–30 μM	VPAC2 agonist
VIPhyb	0.5 μM	—	VPAC1 agonist
VIP$_{(10-28)}$	1 μM	—	VPAC1 antagonist

^{a}Value is K_d instead of IC$_{50}$.

was mapped to human chromosome 7q36.3. Northern blot analysis shows that the rat VPAC2 gene is expressed in lung, stomach, and intestine, with lower levels in telencephalon, diencephalon, brain stem, cerebellum, and olfactory bulb. VPAC2 message is also detected in rat thymus, spleen, pancreas, adrenal gland, heart, placenta, and pituitary. The two receptors have similar affinities for VIP (Table 1) when expressed in cell lines, with an IC_{50} of 1 and 3 nM for VPAC1 and VPAC2, respectively. Both receptors also recognize the related peptide PACAP. VPAC1 has similar affinity for PACAP-27 and PACAP-38 (IC_{50}, 1 nM), but VPAC2 has different affinities for PACAP-27 and PACAP-38 (IC_{50}, 10 and 2 nM, respectively). A PACAP-selective receptor (PAC1) has been isolated, cloned, and shown to have a strong affinity for both PACAP-27 and PACAP-38 (IC_{50}, 1 nM), but has 1000-fold less affinity for VIP (IC_{50}, 1 μM).

B. Receptor Pharmacology

Long-term goals to use VIP analogues for the treatment of cancer, immune disorders, nerve degeneration, and impotence have been hampered by a lack of receptor-specific agonists and antagonists. Similarly, basic research into understanding the biological functions of VIP and its receptors would be facilitated by the availability of specific agonists and antagonists. However, few synthetic VPAC1- and VPAC2-specific agonist or antagonists have yet been designed. Molecular cloning of VIP receptors has facilitated functional testing of several newly developed compounds. These potential peptide agonists and antagonists have been examined for their ability to mimic or inhibit the physiological actions of VIP (Table 1).

Stearyl-Nle-VIP (SNV) is a VIP analogue designed by the addition of a fatty acid moiety to VIP; this enables penetration of the analogue through membranes while maintaining binding and functional activity. SNV also contains a norleucine at position 17, which increases the stability of the molecule against oxidation and increases its lipophilicity. SNV is 100-fold more potent than VIP in providing neuroprotection to cerebellar granule neurons. SNV binds both VPAC1 and VPAC2 with similar affinities as compared to VIP (Table 1). This peptide has also been shown to be effective in potentiation of sexual performance in a variety of impotence models in rats. Toxicological studies in animals indicate that SNV is safe, making it a possible candidate for clinical studies.

Two VPAC1-specific agonists have been described. The VIP/GRF hybrid [Lys[15],Arg[16], Leu[27]]-VIP$_{(1-7)}$GRF$_{(8-27)}$-NH$_2$ has an IC_{50} value of 1 nM for VPAC1 but does not bind to the GRF receptor. [Arg[16]]chicken secretin is an agonist at both VPAC1 and secretin receptors, but can be used as a highly selective VPAC1 agonist in tissues, such as brain, that do not express the secretin receptor. [Acetyl-His[1], D-Phe[2],lys[15],Arg[16]]VIP$_{(3-7)}$GRF$_{(8-27)}$-NH$_2$ acts as a selective VPAC1 antagonist (IC_{50}, 1–10 nM). IC_{50} values of ^{125}I-labeled VIP binding inhibition by this antagonist, also known as PG 97-269, were 10 and 2 nM for rat and human VPAC1, compared to 2 and 3 μM for rat and human VPAC2.

RO25-1553, a VPAC2-specific agonist, was designed with a lactam ring that is introduced within the VIP peptide between positions 21 and 25. It exhibits a high potency and long duration of action. It is a selective agonist for VPAC2, having an affinity for this receptor (IC_{50}, 1 nM) that is 1000-fold higher than for the VPAC1 receptor (IC_{50}, 1 μM). It exhibits anti-inflammatory effects using the VPAC2 signal transduction pathway in lipopolysaccharide (LPS)-stimulated human monocytes, leading to inhibition of tumor necrosis factor α (TNFα) and interleukin-12 (IL-12) synthesis.

A VIP cyclic analogue RO25-1392 is also highly potent and specific for VPAC2 (300-fold greater affinity than for VPAC1). It increases the intracellular concentration of calcium and cAMP. It also down-regulates VPAC2 expression when tested on Chinese hamster ovary cells stably expressing recombinant human VPAC1 or VPAC2. Several VIP antagonists have also been developed using VIP or a peptide from the same family as part of their structure, including [4-Cl-D-Phe[6],Leu[7]]VIP, VIP$_{(10-28)}$, neurotensin$_{(6-11)}$-VIP$_{(7-28)}$ (also designated VHA), stearyl-Nle[17]-hybrid antagonist (SNH), and [Ac-Tyr[1], D-Phe[2]]-growth hormone-releasing factor(1–29) amide. VHA inhibits VIP-mediated cAMP formation or VIP-associated maintenance of neuronal survival in spinal cord cultures. A new derivative of this antagonist yields the stearyl-VIP-hybrid antagonist, stearyl-Nle[17]-neurotensin$_{(6-11)}$-VIP$_{(7-28)}$; it has been shown to be 100-fold more potent in producing neuronal death than the parent VHA molecule and also a growth inhibitor in lung cancer. Although several candidate compounds have been developed within the past few years, the need for specific agonists and antagonists for each VIP receptor remains unfulfilled.

Despite the lack of extensive studies, endogenous peptide fragments of natural VIP, such as VIP$_{(4-28)}$ or

VIP$_{(10-28)}$, may play roles as agonist or antagonist, providing another level of regulation for the VIP–VPAC signal transduction pathway.

IV. MECHANISM OF VIP ACTION (SIGNAL TRANSDUCTION PATHWAY)

An increase in the intracellular concentrations of cyclic 3', 5'-adenosine monophosphate is generated by activation of a membrane-associated enzyme, adenylate cyclase, that is stimulated on binding of VIP to either VPAC1 or VPAC2 (Fig. 3). VIP binding to its receptors has been shown to elevate cellular cAMP levels through a guanosine triphosphate (GTP)-regulated coupling of the receptor to a stimulatory guanine nucleotide-binding (G$_s$) protein. In turn, cAMP binds cooperatively to two sites on the regulatory subunit of protein kinase A (PKA). This binding results in release of the active catalytic subunit that phosphorylates its substrate (the serine in the context X-Arg-Arg-X-Ser-X), present in a number of cytoplasmic and nuclear proteins such as cAMP response element binding (CREB) protein or CREMτ. Activated PKA modulates the function of transcription factors that bind to cis-acting elements present in the promoter regions of cAMP-induced

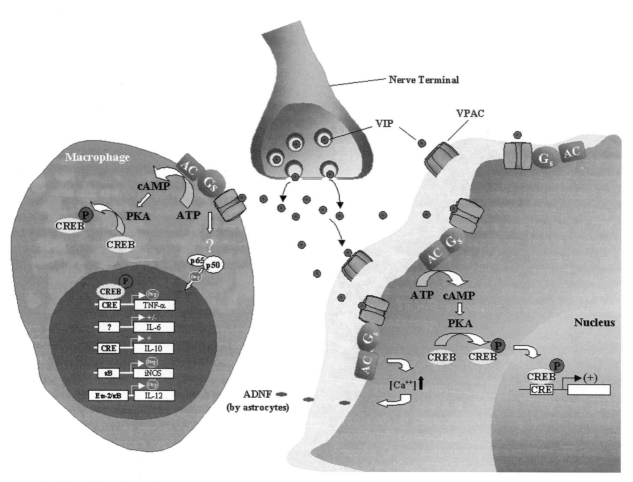

FIGURE 3 Signal transduction pathway activated by vasoactive intestinal peptide (VIP) binding to receptor VPAC1 or VPAC2. Binding of VIP initiates VPAC1 or VPAC2 association with membrane-bound G-protein (G$_s$), activating adenylate cyclase (AC) and generating cAMP, which, in turn, binds to a regulatory subunit in protein kinase A (PKA). The active catalytic subunit of PKA is then released to phosphorylate its substrate, cAMP response element (CRE) binding protein (CREB). Phospho-CREB binds to cis-acting elements present in the promoter regions of cAMP-induced genes. Through this signal transduction pathway, VIP stimulates synthesis and secretion of neuroprotective molecules such as the cytokine interleukin-1α (IL-1α), activity-dependent neurotropic factor (ADNF), and activity-dependent neuroprotective protein (ADNP) from astrocytes. In macrophages, VIP inhibits the production of proinflammatory factors tumor necrosis factor α (TNFα), IL-6, IL-12, and nitric oxide (iNO) and stimulates the production of the anti-inflammatory cytokine IL-10. A cAMP-independent pathway of VIP is involved in the nuclear factor κB (NF-κB; p65/p50), the inactivation of which affects the transcription of the TNFα, IL-12, and iNOS genes.

genes. Most of the cAMP-responsive genes have one or more copies of cAMP response elements (CREs) within their promoters. The consensus CRE is constituted by the palindromic sequence TGACGTCA (Fig. 3). CRE binding protein, a member of the basic region/leucine zipper (bZip) transcription factor family and the first to be cloned, also binds to CRE. CREB cloning has been followed by cloning of many other proteins that have the characteristic bZip domains. Although heterodimerization is possible among the members, some specific combinations are more common than others. Certain CRE binding factors, such as ATF-2, ATF-3, and ATF-4, can heterodimerize with the bZip oncogenes Fos and Jun, allowing the cAMP/PKA pathway to interact with the diacylglycerol/protein kinase C pathways. Depending on the CRE binding factors, this pathway may result in the activation or repression of the expression of downstream genes.

In some neuronal preparations, inositol phosphate production and protein kinase C activation has been observed, suggesting that VIP signal transduction may follow alternative pathways in addition to adenylate cyclase. After VIP binds to its receptor, the peptide is rapidly internalized by receptor-mediated endocytosis. Most of the receptors are recycled and move back to the cell surface, although some are degraded in lysosomes. VIP peptide is cleaved and inactivated by tissue neutral endopeptidase 24.11, which is widely distributed in the peripheral circulation. VIP is also susceptible to trypsin and plasma-catalyzed cleavage.

V. BIOLOGICAL EFFECTS OF VIP

A. VIP in the Nervous System

VIP acts as a neurotransmitter in the nervous system; its presence and synthesis in neurons, its release from the nerve terminals in response to electrical stimulation, its target tissue response after neuronal stimulation, and its enzymatic degradation after binding to VPAC1 or VPAC2 are all characteristics of a true neurotransmitter. Furthermore, electrophysiological studies demonstrate that VIP can affect membrane potential and can act in concert with other neurotransmitters to modulate electrical responses. The effects of VIP on electrical activity can be either excitatory or inhibitory in the same brain region, suggesting that VIP modulates effects of other neuroactive substances. In early studies carried out on isolated spinal cords, VIP led to depolarization of the dorsal root terminals and motoneurons. However,

VIP had both inhibitory and excitatory actions on neurons from preoptic, septal, and midbrain regions. VIP enhanced both the inhibitory effects of GABA and excitatory responses to acetylcholine. Although VIP binding to VPAC1 or VPAC2 has been shown to increase the cAMP levels in many cell types, the slow depolarization and decreased membrane resistance of retinal horizontal neurons on VIP treatment are not replicated by analogues of cAMP or forskolin (a lipophilic agent that causes an increase in intracellular cAMP levels). These results suggest that effects of VIP can be mediated through other signal transduction pathways or, alternatively, may be indirect. VIP shares some of the functional characteristics of neurotropins, which play fundamental roles in the nervous system, including neuroprotective neurotropins that are expressed after neural injury. VIP modulates cell proliferation, differentiation, neurite outgrowth, and neuronal survival. Early studies on the ability of VIP to prevent cell death associated with tetrodotoxin demonstrated that VIP stimulates secretion of neuroprotective molecules such as cytokine IL-1α, a serine protease inhibitor (protease nexin I), and an extracellular stress protein, activity-dependent neurotropic factor (ADNF), from astrocytes (Fig. 3). Hence, many of the neurotropic and neuroprotective effects of the VIP have been attributed to the secretagogue action of the peptide. The survival-promoting action of VIP is mediated indirectly through nonneuronal astroglia via induction of glial cell neuroprotective proteins. Stimulation of high-affinity VIP receptors on astroglia results in the release of several neurotropic substances, including cytokines, protease nexin I, ADNF, and activity-dependent neuroprotective protein (ADNP). The active sites of ADNF and ADNP (ADNF-9 and NAP, respectively) have been shown to be effective in femtomolar concentrations. The neurotropic action of VIP occurs at very low peptide concentrations (0.1 nM) and appears to be correlated with mobilization of calcium and the translocation of specific isoenzymes of protein kinase C. On the other hand, cAMP increases are associated with neurotropic effects in developing sympathetic nervous system.

B. VIP in Immunomodulation

The endocrine and immune systems are linked through a communication system that utilizes cytokines and neuropeptides. Studies employing immunohistochemistry and flow cytometry demonstrate that VIP is present in all lymphoid organs and in several lymphocyte subpopulations, including T and

B lymphocytes, and splenic lymphocytes. VIP is released by peptidergic nerve fibers that innervate primary and secondary lymphoid organs in mammalian species. VPAC1 and VPAC2 receptors have been detected in rodent and human immune systems by autoradiography. These receptors have been also detected in established cell lines of immune origin. Studies in rodents and humans demonstrate that VPAC1 and VPAC2 genes are differentially distributed and regulated in the immune system. Murine VPAC1 is expressed in stimulated and unstimulated thymocytes and in splenic CD4 and CD8 T cells. In contrast, VPAC2 is expressed on splenic T-cell subpopulations only following stimulation. Resting and LPS-stimulated murine B cells do not express either VIP receptor. VPAC1 is constitutively expressed in resting human T cells and monocytes. VPAC2 is expressed at very low levels in resting human T cells but is not detectable in resting monocytes. *In vitro* stimulation of T cells with soluble anti-CD3 plus phorbol myristic acid (PMA) induces a T-cell activation-dependent down-regulation of VPAC1.

In vitro studies have demonstrated that secretion of VIP is enhanced in mitogen-stimulated cell suspensions from different murine lymphoid organs. VIP secretion is also stimulated by corticosteroids and proinflammatory cytokines (IL-1, IL-6, and TNFα) produced by activated murine macrophages. VIP plays a role in modulation of the immune response through its effect on the expression of various key cytokines. VIP inhibits the production of proinflammatory factors TNFα, IL-6, IL-12, and nitric oxide and stimulates the production of anti-inflammatory cytokine IL-10 (Fig. 3). VIP may have inhibitory (inflammatory or endotoxemia models) or stimulatory (unstimulated macrophages or after low LPS doses) effects on IL-6 production, depending on the conditions. These results support the role of VIP as an immune homeostasis mediator. VIP has been shown to suppress collagen-induced arthritis in mice and to correct the associated cytokine imbalance. T_H1 and T_H2 cells are responsible for phagocyte-mediated host defense and phagocyte-independent host defense, respectively, and have relatively restricted cytokine production profile and effector functions. Enhancement of T_H2 function and suppression of T_H1 cells have been proposed as a therapeutic approach for rheumatoid arthritis. VIP suppresses T_H1 cell function and differentiation but enhances T_H2 function, as revealed by decreased interferon γ (IFNγ) and increased IL-4 production, respectively. VPAC1 was shown to be the major mediator of the anti-inflammatory effect of VIP.

VIP message is also detected within granulomas of murine schistosomiasis and expression is localized to granuloma T cells. In murine schistosomiasis, VIP invokes IL-5 release from granuloma T cells. Furthermore, VIP suppresses mitogen- and antigen-induced T-cell proliferation, possibly by inhibiting IL-2 production. The granuloma T cells express both VPAC1 and VPAC2 receptors. VIP also inhibits activation-induced cell death (AICD) *in vivo* and *in vitro* in peripheral T cells and T-cell hybridomas. The effect is dose dependent and is mediated through VPAC1 and VPAC2 receptors. A functional study has demonstrated that inhibition of AICD is achieved through inhibition of activation-induced FasL expression at protein and mRNA levels. VIP has also been shown to increase the survival of thymocytes against glucocorticoid-induced apoptosis, and this action of VIP is mediated by VPAC1. Phenotypic analysis shows that VIP, PACAP-27, and PACAP-38 protect predominantly CD4 + CD8 + thymocytes from glucocorticoid-induced apoptosis.

C. VIP in Pulmonary and Cardiac Systems

Many systemic and pulmonary blood vessels are innervated by VIP immunoreactive nerve fibers that cause vascular smooth muscle dilation. VIP activation of adenylate cyclase has been observed in cerebral, heart, and coronary vessels and in the portal vein, aorta, mesenteric artery, and ovarian artery of mice. The vasodilatory effect of VIP in different species and tissues is not only due to increased cAMP but also to activation of lipoxygenase, nitric oxide synthase, or the guanylate cyclase and cyclooxygenase pathways. In some species, VIP effects may involve hyperpolarization of the vascular smooth muscle membrane, which reduces calcium influx and intracellular Ca^{2+} concentration. The relative contribution of these various mediators to the vasodilatory effects of VIP is not known; however, interaction between different mediators may modulate VIP action. A possible example of this interaction is seen in gastrointestinal smooth muscle, in which relaxation is stimulated by both cAMP- and cGMP-dependent pathways. The effects of VIP on coronary arteries have been studied in isolated vascular tissue, in intact hearts, and *in vivo* in rodents as well as humans; VIP is shown to have a significant dilatory effect in each species. VIP has a stronger vasodilatory effect on arteries than on veins, possibly due to higher receptor density on the arteries. In ventricular myocytes, VIP binding to its receptor results in increased levels of cAMP, which can stimulate protein kinase A activity. This, in turn, enhances calcium channel phosphorylation and L-type calcium currents, leading to increased intracellular calcium concentration. As a result, cardiac myocyte tension rate and extent of contraction are enhanced. An increase in cAMP can also lead to sequestration of intracellular calcium via decreased troponin affinity for calcium, which subsequently enhances the rate and extent of myocyte relaxation. In this manner, VIP can increase cardiac myocyte contraction and relaxation. *In vivo* studies have also demonstrated that both administered and endogenous VIP can increase coronary blood flow. The vasodilatory effect of VIP is not limited to coronary arteries; similar effects have been observed in cerebral arteries as well as vessels of the eyes, thyroid, and pancreas. A vasodilatory effect of VIP was also confirmed by using a monoclonal anti-VIP antibody that significantly attenuated VIP-induced vasodilation in the *in situ* hamster cheek pouch.

VIP is present in nerves innervating the airway smooth muscles and pulmonary and nasal vessels. VIP produces prolonged relaxation of airway smooth muscles and mimics the electrophysiological changes produced by noncholinergic, nonadrenergic nerve stimulation. VIP has been shown to prevent lung injury and to improve survival in different experimental models of acute respiratory distress syndrome. Protective effects of VIP include inhibition of transcription factor nuclear factor κB (NF-κB) activation (Fig. 3) and inhibition of caspase activity coupled with an increase in antiapoptotic Bcl-2 protein. Both receptor subtypes, VPAC1 and VPAC2, are expressed by several lung cell lines. VPAC2 is expressed in airway epithelial, glandular, and immune cells of the lung but not in airway and vascular smooth muscles. The absence of VPAC2 mRNA in vascular and airway smooth muscle myocytes along with presence of high-affinity VIP binding in the lung suggest that the effects of VIP on vasodilation and bronchodilation are mediated by VPAC1 in the lung.

D. VIP in the Gastrointestinal System

VIP nerves have been demonstrated in the esophageal wall, mostly in the circular muscle layer. More VIP-containing neurons are located near the sphincter region. Both *in vitro* and *in vivo* studies show that VIP has a relaxing affect on the lower esophageal sphincter, the sphincter of Oddi, and the anal sphincter. In the stomach as well as the small and large intestines, VIP is involved in relaxation of smooth muscles. VIP is a major peptide with relaxant

activity and is considered a transmitter of inhibitory motor neurons of the gut. The relaxation-inducing effect of VIP has also been demonstrated using VIP antiserum, which blocks this effect. VIP stimulates the secretion of ductal pancreatic and biliary bicarbonate and water and simultaneously inhibits gastric acid and pepsinogen secretion as well as absorption from the intestinal lumen. VIP also stimulates enzyme secretion from pancreatic acinar cells and regulates chloride secretion. All layers of the gut contain VIP fibers. VIP nerve fibers are most dense in the lamina propria, where they associate with blood vessels and come into contact with the surface epithelium. VIP acts on neurons and muscle cells to regenerate nitric oxide (NO). VIP inhibits the growth of certain colonic adenocarcinoma cell lines and both VIP and VPAC1 expression are elevated during the enterocytic differentiation of a colonic adenocarcinoma cell line *in vitro*.

E. VIP in Oncology

In 1958, Verner and Morrison described a clinical syndrome that included the triad of pancreatic islet cell tumors, severe watery diarrhea, and hypokalemia. In 1973, Bloom and colleagues made the association between Verner–Morrison syndrome and vasoactive intestinal peptide. They reported that patients with this syndrome also had elevated plasma levels of VIP. These VIP-secreting tumors of the pancreas are also known as VIPomas, watery diarrhea/hypokalemia/hypochlorhydria syndrome, or pancreatic cholera syndrome. VIP is the major mediator of the diarrhea, as demonstrated by a rapid fall in VIP levels and cessation of diarrhea after tumor removal as well as the demonstration that intravenous injection of VIP in normal subjects can induce diarrhea. Some patients develop hypotension resulting from peripheral vasodilation, and severe hypertension may develop after tumor removal; hypotension is also induced by intravenous administration of VIP. These features are compatible with the known cardiovascular effect of VIP. A recent 15-year retrospective review of patients with VIPoma showed that VIP-secreting tumors are usually metastatic at the time of diagnosis. However, survival of the patients with VIPoma has improved due to supportive treatment and the use of chemotherapy.

In approximately 20% of the VIPoma cases, the tumor is too small to localize with computerized tomography (CT) scanning. However, all of these patients receive symptomatic relief of the watery diarrhea. However, in a recent Verner–Morrison syndrome case study, octreotide, an analog of somatostatin, was shown to be effective in reducing the serum VIP level of the patient and in decreasing water loss, but both CT scan and octreoscan failed to detect the tumor. The tumor was detectable in the pancreatic tail using ^{123}I-labeled VIP scintigraphy. Surgical resection of the tumor resulted in complete remission of the syndrome. Recent data also indicate that ^{123}I-labeled VIP receptor scintigraphy is clinically useful for the *in vivo* localization of adenocarcinomas, liver metastases, and certain endocrine tumors of the gastrointestinal tract. Although ^{123}I-labeled VIP receptor scintigraphy is a highly promising method for imaging, the high uptake of the peptide by the lung does not allow therapeutic use of VIP labeled with isotopes such as ^{131}I or [90]Y. Thus, related compounds with different binding profiles, such as ^{99m}Tc-labeled VIP conjugates, have been developed and currently are undergoing testing for clinical use. Further scintigraphic studies with patients need to be carried out using newly designed VIP-based radioligands with high specific activity.

In a study to evaluate whether VIP can be used as a tumor marker, serum levels of VIP were evaluated in a total of 135 patients; 45 patients had metastatic colorectal cancer, 45 suffered from metastatic pancreatic cancer, and 45 healthy volunteers served as controls. As opposed to pancreatic cancer and healthy controls, patients with metastatic colorectal cancer had elevated serum VIP levels that were statistically significant ($p < 0.0001$). Several pediatric tumors, including neuroblastoma, primitive neuroectodermal tumors (PNET), and tumors of the Ewing's sarcoma/peripheral PNET family, express either VIP or VIP receptors. High levels of expression of VIP and VIP receptors are a favorable prognostic factor in neuroblastoma, a tumor of neuroectodermal origin. Patients with high levels of VIP and associated diarrhea have a more favorable prognosis. VIP can also slow the rate of proliferation and induce *in vitro* differentiation of neuroblastoma cells. Both medulloblastoma (infratentorial PNET) and supratentorial PNET (tumors derived from neuroepithelial precursors) express VIP receptors as demonstrated by reverse transcriptase (RT) and PCR, high-affinity binding of ^{125}I-labeled VIP on quantitative autoradiography, and in competitive binding assays. VIP also inhibits tumor cell proliferation in a dose-dependent manner in PNET cell lines.

VIP inhibits proliferation of small-cell lung carcinoma cells (SCLCs) in culture and dramatically suppresses the growth of SCLC tumor cell implants in athymic nude mice. The effect of VIP is mediated by a cAMP-dependent mechanism. High-affinity VIP binding sites are also detected in several breast cancer cell lines as well as breast cancer biopsy specimens as revealed by ^{125}I-labeled VIP. Several breast cancer cell lines make and secrete immunoreactive VIP; cAMP levels are elevated in these cell lines following VIP treatment. Furthermore, VIPhyb, a VIP antagonist, inhibits breast cancer growth *in vitro* and *in vivo*. Retinoic acid treatment of breast carcinoma cell lines leads to the down-regulation of the VPAC1 receptor.

VI. CONCLUSION AND PERSPECTIVES

The previously unknown role and contribution of VIP to certain biological processes have been discovered within the past few years. During the preparation of this article, for example, a possible role for VIP in autism was reported. In the first study, in which neuropeptide and neurotropin concentrations were determined, plasma concentrations of VIP were found to be higher at birth in children with autism or mental retardation without autism than in healthy control children. The roles of VIP in brain development and its functions as neurotransmitter and neuromodulator warrant more research on its role in autism.

Anti-inflammatory effects of VIP in the immune system have also recently been documented. These studies have led to the use of VIP in the treatment of inflammatory collagen-induced arthritis in mice, suggesting a new therapeutic approach for rheumatoid arthritis. VIP inhibits the production of proinflammatory factors TNFα IL-6, IL-12, and nitric oxide, and stimulates the production of anti-inflammatory cytokine IL-10.

Receptor targeting with radiolabeled peptides is rapidly developing in nuclear oncology. These naturally occurring peptides are clinically useful diagnostic imaging agents and have future implications for the treatment of tumors expressing target receptors. Radiolabeled VIP and VIP analogues are being developed and evaluated for clinical application because of observations that most human carcinomas express VIP receptors as measured by *in vitro* receptor autoradiography. The application of radiolabeled VIP (^{123}I-labeled VIP) is generally safe and scintigraphy results can be obtained within 2–4 h after injection of the peptide.

Availability of genomic and cDNA sequences for VIP peptide and its receptors will facilitate the disruption of corresponding genes in mice using homologous recombination techniques, thus uncovering the biological processes in which VIP is involved as well as the relative contributions of each receptor for VIP action. Together with the development of receptor-specific analogues, these studies should lead to development of alternative therapies that will take advantage of manipulating VIP-initiated signal transduction pathways. Although use of native VIP as a drug is limited due to its susceptibility to endopeptidases and its limited passage across biological membranes, several VIP analogues have been developed to overcome this problem and are under investigation for their possible use.

Vasoactive intestinal peptide clearly functions in multiple ways, including neurotransmission; neuromodulation, immunomodulation, bronchodilation, vasodilation, smooth muscle relaxation, and modulation of reproduction. One peptide that can fulfill multiple roles as a cytokine, neurotransmitter, and hormone must be a physiologic VIP, a "very important peptide."

Glossary

agonist Peptide, hormone, or drug that binds to a specific receptor and activates its signal transduction cascade.

antagonist Peptide, hormone, or drug that binds to a specific receptor and blocks its signal transduction cascade.

autoradiography Visualization of radioactively labeled molecules on X-ray film.

complementary DNA Nucleic acid synthesized by reverse transcription of RNA; cDNA is complementary to the RNA template.

G-proteins Guanine nucleotide-binding trimeric proteins that reside in the plasma membrane and transduce a signal from a receptor–ligand complex to the signal transduction cascade.

IC$_{50}$ Concentration of ligand that inhibits by 50% the binding of a homologous radiolabeled ligand to a specific receptor.

K_d Concentration of ligand that inhibits by 50% the binding of an identical radiolabeled ligand to a specific receptor.

signal transduction Process by which a ligand–receptor interaction activates a cascade of biochemical reactions, leading to a change in cellular activity.

T$_H$1 A T helper lymphocyte that makes interleukin-2 and interferon γ, promoting a cellular immune response.

T$_H$2 A T helper lymphocyte that makes interleukin-4, -5, -9, and -10, promoting humoral or allergic responses.

transfection Introduction of new genetic material into a cell.

transgenic Describes animals that are generated by insertion of new DNA into the germ line via DNA microinjection into the one-cell-stage embryo.

See Also the Following Articles

Gastrin ● Gastrointestinal Hormone-Releasing Peptides ● Glucagon Action ● Growth Hormone-Releasing Hormone (GHRH) ● Oocyte Development and Maturation ● Peptide YY ● Pituitary Adenylate Cyclase-Activating Polypeptide (PACAP) and Its Receptor ● Secretin ● Vagal Regulation of Gastric Functions by Brain Neuropeptides

Further Reading

Albers, A. R., O'Dorisio, M. S., Balster, D. A., Caprara, M., Gosh, P., Chen, F., Hoeger, C., Rivier, J., Wenger, G. D., O'Dorisio, T. M., and Qualman, S. J. (2000). Somatostatin receptor gene expression in neuroblastoma. Regul. Pept. 82, 61–73.

Delgado, M., Abad, C., Martinez, C., Leceta, J., and Gomariz, R. P. (2001). Vasoactive intestinal peptide prevents experimental arthritis by downregulating both autoimmune and inflammatory components of the disease. Nat. Med. 7, 563–568.

Fahrenkrug J., and Said S. I., ed., (2000). "VIP, PACAP, Glucagon, and Related Peptides," Vol. 9. New York Academy of Science, New York.

Frühwald, M. C., O'Dorisio, M. S., Fleitz, J., Summers, M. A., Pietsch, T., and Reubi, J.-C. (1999). Vasoactive intestinal peptide (VIP) receptors: Gene expression and growth modulation in medulloblastoma and other central primitive neuroectodermal tumors of childhood. Int. J. Cancer 81, 165–173.

Gomariz, R. P., Martinez, C., Abad, C., Leceta, J., and Delgado, M. (2001). Immunology of VIP: A review and therapeutical perspectives. Curr. Pharm. Des. 7, 89–111.

Gozes, I., and Brenneman, D. E. (2000). A new concept in the pharmacology of neuroprotection. J. Mol. Neurosci. 14, 61–68.

Gressens, P., Besse, L., Robberecht, P., Gozes, I., Fridkin, M., and Evrard, P. (1999). Neuroprotection of the developing brain by systemic administration of vasoactive intestinal peptide derivatives. J. Pharmacol. Exp. Ther. 288, 1207–1213.

Harmar, A. J., Arimura, A., Gozes, I., Journot, L., Laburthe, M., Pisegna, J. R., Rawlings, S. R., Robberecht, P., Said, S. I., Sreedharan, S. P., Wank, S. A., and Waschek, J. A. (1998). International Union of Pharmacology. XVIII. Nomenclature of receptors for vasoactive intestinal peptide and pituitary adenylate cyclase-activating polypeptide. Pharmacol. Rev. 50, 265–270.

Henning, R. J., and Sawmiller, D. R. (2001). Vasoactive intestinal peptide: Cardiovascular effects. Cardiovasc. Res. 49, 27–37.

Metwali, A., Blum, A. M., Li, J., Elliott, D. E., and Weinstock, J. V. (2000). IL-4 regulates VIP receptor subtype 2 mRNA (VPAC2) expression in T cells in murine schistosomiasis. FASEB J. 14, 948–954.

Pozo, D., Delgado, M., Martinez, M., Guerrero, J. M., Leceta, J., Gomariz, R. P., and Calvo, J. R. (2000). Immunobiology of vasoactive intestinal peptide (VIP). Immunol. Today 21, 7–11.

Raderer, M., Kurtaran, A., Leimer, M., Angelberger, P., Niederle, B., Vierhapper, H., Vorbeck, F., Hejna, M. H., Scheithauer, W., Pidlich, J., and Virgolini, I. (2000). Value of peptide receptor scintigraphy using (123)I-vasoactive intestinal peptide and (111)In-DTPA-D-Phe1-octreotide in 194 carcinoid patients: Vienna University Experience, 1993 to 1998. J. Clin. Oncol. 18, 1331–1336.

Said, S. I., and Dickman, K. G. (2000). Pathways of inflammation and cell death in the lung: Modulation by vasoactive intestinal peptide. *Regul. Pept.* **93**, 21–29.

Smith, S. L., Branton, S. A., Avino, A. J., Martin, J. K., Klingler, P. J., Thompson, G. B., Grant, C. S., and van Heerden, J. A. (1998). Vasoactive intestinal polypeptide secreting islet cell tumors: A 15-year experience and review of the literature. *Surgery* **124**, 1050–1055.

Vasopressin (AVP)

WILLIAM E. ARMSTRONG

University of Tennessee College of Medicine

I. INTRODUCTION
II. NEUROANATOMICAL LOCALIZATION AND CONNECTIONS OF AVP NEURONS
III. AVP ACTIONS AND RECEPTORS
IV. STIMULI FOR AVP RELEASE
V. ELECTROPHYSIOLOGY OF AVP NEURONS
VI. SUMMARY

Vasopressin, also called antidiuretic hormone because of its actions on the kidney, is formed with an arginine at position 8 in all mammals but pigs. Arginine vasopressin is a 9-amino-acid polypeptide hormone that is synthesized in and released from mammalian hypothalamic neurosecretory cells. It functions in blood pressure regulation and water reabsorption by the kidneys.

I. INTRODUCTION

Arginine vasopressin (AVP) and the closely related peptide oxytocin (OT) were the first pituitary hormones for which the amino acid structures were characterized (Fig. 1). Each hormone consists of 9 amino acids with an NH_2 terminus; the amino acids form a ring via disulfide bonds at the two cysteine residues. These hormones are similar to peptides serving related functions in fishes, birds, and amphibians. In pigs, vasopressin is formed with a lysine substituted for arginine at position 8.

The production of neurohypophyseal hormones in brain tissue first was established by Ernst Bargmann and the Scharrers, who utilized Gomori-positive histochemistry (which reveals sulfide-rich elements) to demonstrate the axonal pathway from the hypothalamus to the neurohypophysis. These early studies have been confirmed and expanded with

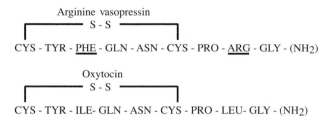

FIGURE 1 The amino acid sequences for arginine vasopressin and oxytocin. The nonapeptides share all but two amino acids, with substitutions at positions 3 and 8. Note the cysteine ring formed by disulfide bonds.

more advanced biochemical and immunohistochemical studies. AVP is synthesized in neurons of the supraoptic nuclei (SON) and paraventricular hypothalamic nuclei (PVN) of the central nervous system (CNS) (Fig. 2). Synthesis begins with a preprohormone complex containing a signal peptide; the latter is cleaved and the remaining protein is glycosylated to a prohormone in the Golgi apparatus. The prohormone is packaged into large (150–200 nm) neurosecretory vesicles, which are axonally transported to the neural lobe of the pituitary gland for release into the general circulation. The prohormone contains AVP, a large protein called neurophysin, and a 39-amino-acid glycopeptide (absent in the OT complex). These products are separated by several enzymes within the neurosecretory granules during axonal transport and are released as separate products. There is no generally accepted peripheral function for neurophysin or the glycopeptide, although each may have some biological activity. A natural "knockout" for the AVP gene, the Brattleboro rat, is characterized by a single base deletion. The Brattleboro rat has extreme polydipsia and polyuria and has been a model for diabetes insipidus.

Although in most situations AVP and OT are found in separate cells, many neurons can synthesize both peptides, as shown by extensive colocalization of mRNA when amplification procedures are employed. During enhanced hormone release, the amount of colocalization may be increased for OT and AVP as well as for other peptides, although in lesser quantities (e.g., neuropeptide Y), found in the same neurons. Synthesis is at least partly regulated by the stimuli that evoke AVP release. For example, osmotic stimulation increases transcription of AVP and mRNA abundance and increases the length of the RNA poly(A) tail. Transcription of AVP mRNA appears to be regulated in part by immediate-early genes such as c-*fos*, but other regulators, such as the cAMP response element binding protein, are

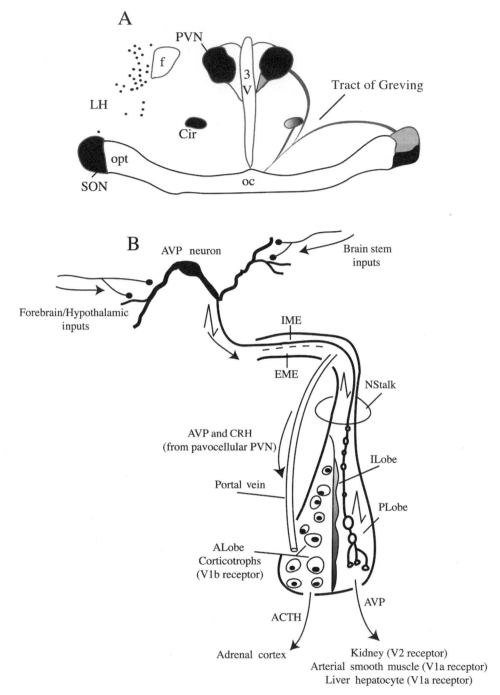

FIGURE 2 Anatomical location and connectivity of arginine vasopressin (AVP) neurons. (A) Drawing of a coronal section through the rat hypothalamus, illustrating the location of AVP and oxytocin neurons and schematizing their projection toward the pituitary. On the left, paraventricular hypothalamic nuclei (PVN) and supraoptic nuclei (SON) fiber tracts are named. On the right, AVP neuronal clusters are shown in black and oxytocin clusters are in gray. In addition to the PVN and SON, accessory neurosecretory nuclei are shown. At this plane, there are scattered neurons in the lateral hypothalamus (LH), and a cluster called the nucleus circularis (Cir). The axons from all nuclei collect in the tract of Greving, which eventually leads to the internal layer of the median eminence before projecting into the posterior (neural) lobe of pituitary. Abbreviations: f, fornix; oc, optic chiasm; opt, optic tract; 3V, third ventricle. (B) Schematic representation of an AVP neuron and its axonal projection to the posterior lobe of the pituitary. The neuron has a sparse dendritic tree but receives important brain stem synapses that relay vascular reflex signals; from the forebrain and rostral hypothalamus, synapses relay osmotic, vascular, and other stimuli. The single axon projects into the internal layer of

involved. These factors can be activated by neurotransmitter actions and/or increases in intracellular ($[Ca^{2+}]_i$).

II. NEUROANATOMICAL LOCALIZATION AND CONNECTIONS OF AVP NEURONS

For neurohypophyseal release, the neurons synthesizing AVP are located in the SON, PVN, and a few accessory magnocellular nuclei (Fig. 2). Neurons in these regions send axons arching through the lateral hypothalamus (tract of Greving) to collect along the midline of the ventral hypothalamus in the internal lamina of the median eminence. These axons lead into the neural stalk and terminate in the posterior (or neural) lobe of the pituitary gland in varicosities, largely $1-2$ μm in diameter, near fenestrated capillaries. Larger swellings ($5-15$ μm) called Herring bodies are more visible with histochemical stains but typically do not form endings per se. Herring bodies serve to store hormone but can also release it with prolonged stimulation. In addition to axon terminals and a dense capillary bed, the neural lobe contains a large number of modified astrocytes, called pituicytes, which have an intimate morphological relationship with the terminals. Pituicyte processes normally separate terminals from capillaries and can engulf terminals. The processes recede during periods of great hormone demand.

Magnocellular PVN and SON neurons have a relatively simple morphology (Fig. 2). A typical neuron has an egg-shaped somata $25-30$ μm in diameter, two to three short dendrites with few branches, and a single axon arising from the soma or primary dendrite. A few axons may branch and form local connections (not shown in Fig. 2). This simple morphology computes to a relatively small surface area and, electrically speaking, a large input resistance. Thus, even distal synaptic inputs may reach the soma and exert significant control over the membrane potential and spike initiation. The dendrites are varicose, moderately spinous, and also contain AVP.

Varicosities dot the axons along their course and form the classic "string of pearls" described in original Gomori-positive material.

Within the SON and PVN, AVP and OT neurons cluster into separate regions. In many species, a large cluster of AVP neurons characterizes the lateral wing of the PVN. Although all mammals, including humans, have a mix of OT and VP neurons in both the PVN and SON, the distribution and proportions vary widely across species. SON and PVN somata and dendrites receive a variety of synaptic inputs. Quantitatively, the most numerous synaptic terminals contain the excitatory amino acid glutamate or the inhibitory amino acid γ-aminobutyric acid (GABA). All of the sources of these two transmitters are not known, but two important contributors are the median preoptic nucleus and organum vasculosum of the lamina terminalis (OVLT), two areas known to participate in osmoregulation. Another strong forebrain input comes from the subfornical nucleus, also involved in water regulation. Although accounting for a minority of synapses, noradrenergic and other inputs arising from the ventrolateral medulla and nucleus of the solitary tract have great importance for cardiovascular functions. Additional inputs to the SON and/or the PVN include the locus coeruleus, the parabrachial nucleus, the bed nucleus of the stria terminalis, adjacent hypothalamic nuclei, and midbrain and/or hypothalamic dopaminergic neurons. Neurochemically, AVP neurons receive a rich variety of peptidergic and other neuromodulators, many of which colocalize with glutamate or GABA.

AVP also is found in other CNS neurons and synaptic terminals. Within the PVN, a parvocellular group of neurons synthesizes both AVP and corticotropin-releasing hormone (CRH). These neurons control the release of adrenocorticotropic hormone (ACTH) from the anterior pituitary via projections to the portal vascular plexus of the external layer of the median eminence (Fig. 2). The suprachiasmatic nucleus contains AVP neurons involved in circadian rhythms. The bed nucleus of the stria terminalis and

the median eminence and into the neural stalk before arborizing in the posterior lobe. AVP-containing vesicles are present in the many varicosities along the axon, the largest of which are called Herring bodies. The axons terminate near fenestrated capillaries, where released hormone enters the bloodstream. Action potentials from the neuron drive release at the terminals. The external layer of the median eminence also contains AVP terminals from axons of parvocellular PVN neurons that colocalize with corticotropin-releasing hormone (not shown). These neurons release these two hormones into the external layer of the median eminence, where portal veins carry the products into the anterior lobe of the pituitary. Abbreviations: ALobe, anterior lobe (adenohypophysis) of the pituitary; ACTH, adrenocorticotropic hormone; EME, external layer of the median eminence; ILobe, intermediate lobe of the pituitary; IME, internal layer of the median eminence; NStalk, neural stalk; PLobe, posterior (neural) lobe of the pituitary gland.

medial amygdaloid nucleus have widespread outputs; AVP neurons in these nuclei are highly responsive to gonadal steroids. The central effects of AVP on a variety of neuronal functions are well documented.

III. AVP ACTIONS AND RECEPTORS

The pressor effects of AVP were discovered over 100 years ago. Shortly thereafter, the antidiuretic effects of AVP in kidney were appreciated, and, more recently, effects of AVP in liver, brain, anterior pituitary, and testis have been demonstrated. The receptors for AVP, now cloned, fall into three main classes: V1a, V1b, and V2 receptors. Along with the OT receptor, all are part of the G-protein-coupled superfamily. V1a receptors are coupled to G-proteins ($G_{q/11}$, G_i). Activation leads to increased phospholipases, production of inositol 1,4,5-trisphosphate and diacylglycerol, the activation protein kinase C, and the mobilization of intracellular calcium. V1a receptors also can increase $[Ca^{2+}]_i$ via extracellular influx by coupling to voltage-gated Ca^{2+} channels (primarily L type). For vascular smooth muscle, V1a activation results in contraction and an increase in arterial blood pressure, and activation has a mitogenic effect as well. Because of the wide vascular distribution, V1a receptors can be found in most tissues, including the medullary vessels in the kidney. In the liver, AVP activation of V1a receptors on hepatocytes leads to gluconeogenesis and glycogenolysis. In the brain, V1a receptors are found on a variety of neurons, including autoreceptors on AVP cells, and on the pituicytes of the neural lobe. Although sensitivity to AVP can vary, even across vascular beds, AVP typically activates V1a receptors with K_d values in the low nanomolar or high picomolar range. Occupation of a divalent binding site on the receptor, preferentially by Mg^{2+}, increases the affinity of AVP for the receptor.

The V1b receptor population is dense on corticotrophs of the anterior pituitary. Like V1a activation, yet with distinct intracellular pathways, V1b occupation leads to increased $[Ca^{2+}]_i$. Although the details of these messaging signaling differences are not fully known (e.g., cAMP may be increased with strong V1b activation), V1b receptors have a different pharmacological profile compared to V1a receptors, with a lower affinity for various V1a antagonists. V1b activation on corticotrophs leads to release of ACTH. AVP expression is low (even undetectable) in parvocellular PVN neurons but increases during stress or in the absence of negative glucocorticoid feedback (as with adrenalectomy). Because of the potency differences, AVP may normally serve as a

cofactor augmenting the response of colocalized CRH. Like the V1a receptors, V1b receptors are found on neurons as well as in other tissues.

V2 receptors are the classic renal receptors and are concentrated on the collecting ducts and distal tubules of the kidney medulla. Activation of V2 receptors leads to a G-protein (G_s) stimulation of adenylyl cyclase, an increase in cyclic adenosine monophosphate (cAMP), activation of protein kinase A, and insertion of new water (aquaporin-2) channels. These new channels enhance reabsorption of water in the collecting ducts and tubules, producing concentrated urine. The affinity of AVP for the V2 receptor is in the low picomolar range.

IV. STIMULI FOR AVP RELEASE

Increased plasma osmolality, decreased blood volume, and hypotension are the most effective and well-studied stimuli for the release of AVP. A low release threshold and the exquisite sensitivity of the kidney suggest that small osmolality perturbations near basal levels (~ 285 mOsm/kg H_2O) are finely controlled by AVP release (Fig. 3). The osmotic threshold for release is 1–3% in a well-hydrated subject, which can lead to an antidiuresis from the release of just a few picomoles of AVP. Suprathreshold stimulation results in a linear relationship between plasma osmolality of AVP release. Although a purely osmotic stimulus is apparently sufficient for AVP release, Na^+ is the most abundant and effective physiological osmotic particle, and brain Na^+ detection is a part of the normal response to hypertonicity. Release of AVP is triggered locally with the SON and PVN by these same stimuli. Locally released AVP can feed back on the neurons to modulate their electrical activity (see later).

The hypothesis first proffered by Verney some 60 years ago, that brain osmoreceptors were located near the SON, has been confirmed in a variety of studies and species. Indeed, the SON neurons are osmoreceptive. The mechanism is demonstrated to be a volume-dependent modulation of stretch-inactivated, nonselective cationic channels (SICs). Membrane stretching associated with hypotonic cell swelling decreases SIC channel openings. Cell shrinkage increases them, provoking membrane depolarization. Furthermore, extracellular Na^+ increases the permeability of SIC channels, and prolonged hypertonicity has been shown to increase Na^+ channel density in SON neurons. However, the intrinsic osmoreceptivity of the AVP neuron is insufficient to account for the full activation of SON neurons and

A

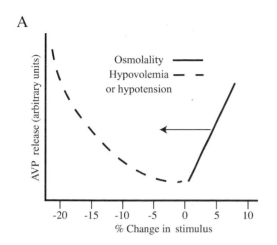

B

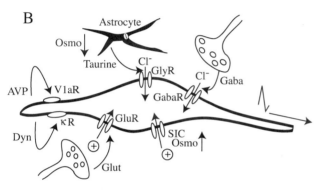

FIGURE 3 Integration of vascular and osmotic signals by arginine vasopressin (AVP) neurons. (A) Schematic diagram illustrating the responsiveness of AVP neurons to both vascular (dashed line) and osmotic (solid line) stimuli. AVP release is linearly related to changes in osmotic pressure above threshold and is more sensitive to this than to vascular stimuli. Vascular stimuli are exponentially related to release, but ultimately can cause release of larger quantities of AVP compared to hypertonicity. The arrow shows that the osmotic curve is displaced to the left in the presence of hypovolemia/hypotension, such that release in response to osmotic stimuli is enhanced. (B) Neural, glial, and osmotic signals are integrated by AVP neurons and lead to changes in action potential activity. Osmotic stimuli have two effects: first, increased osmolality (Osmo)/Na$^+$ concentration opens stretch-inactivated cation (SIC) channels directly on the AVP cell, depolarizing it; second, decreases in osmolality increase the release of taurine from astrocytes in the supraoptic nuclei. Taurine increases Cl$^-$ influx through glycine receptors (GlyR). Thus, during hypertonicity, the neuron is released from this inhibitory stimulus in addition to being depolarized directly. Excitatory and inhibitory transmitters (and many modulators not shown) impinge on the AVP neuron. Some carry information from cardiovascular receptors, transducing blood volume and pressure signals, others carry information from additional osmoreceptive neurons. Increased activity is associated with increased somato-dendritic release of AVP and the colocalized peptide, dynorphin (Dyn). AVP acts on V1a receptors to increase intracellular [Ca^{2+}] and to modulate neuronal activity. Dynorphin acts on κ receptors (κR), but the exact second

AVP release. Additional osmosensitive elements are located along the lamina terminalis of the hypothalamus, in the OVLT and median preoptic nucleus. Direct osmoreceptivity has been demonstrated in excitatory OVLT neurons projecting to the SON. Activation of these neurons increases the frequency of glutamate-mediated excitatory postsynaptic potentials and contributes strongly to SON activation. Indeed, damage to the ventral wall of the lamina terminalis strongly impairs osmoregulation and can be associated with chronic hypernatremia in humans. Astrocytes invested within the SON are also osmosensitive and release the inhibitory amino acid taurine during hypotonicity. Thus, intrinsic SON and glial cell osmoreceptivity, as well as the activity of osmosensitivity afferent inputs, all participate in the fully integrated response of AVP neurons (Fig. 3).

Dehydration incurs hypovolemia and hypertonicity. Plasma volume deficits as low as 5%, induced with hemorrhage or isotonic fluid withdrawal, stimulate AVP release in the absence of any change in osmolality (Fig. 3). For AVP release, purely volemic stimuli are transduced in the thoracic vasculature, primarily by atrial stretch receptors. Unloading these receptors results in strong neuronal activation of the SON via brain stem nuclei such as the nucleus of the solitary tract, the ventrolateral medulla, and the parabrachial nucleus. Osmotic and volemic signals clearly interact, because small changes in blood volume result in a stronger osmotic response. Conversely, osmotic dilution will blunt the response to hypovolemia. The integration of these signals likely occurs in the hypothalamus, if not the SON. Hypovolemia also triggers the release of renin, which leads to a pressor response from angiotensin II (AII). By stimulating AII receptors in the subfornical organ, AII can augment AVP release via a strong projection from this organ to the SON.

Hypotension often accompanies hypovolemia and it can be difficult to separate the stimuli. Hypotensive stimuli are primarily transduced by arterial receptors in the carotid sinus and aortic arch and reach the SON via related, but not identical, brain stem neurons, as for hypovolemia. In some animal models,

messengers and/or channels modulated are not known. However, dynorphin decreases the depolarizing afterpotential and inhibits burst length. Abbreviations: Gaba, γ-aminobutyric acid; GabaR, γ-aminobutyric acid receptor; Glut, glutamate; GluR, glutamate receptor; V1aR, V1a subclass of AVP receptor.

hypovolemia induces AVP release only when there is an associated drop in arterial pressure, and this response is dependent on nerve activity from sino-aortic receptors. Nevertheless, considerable data suggest that volume and pressure signals are separately transduced, if often integrated. In humans, the release of 1–2 pmol of AVP can be triggered by a reduction in arterial pressure by ~5%, and further reductions are exponentially related to AVP release, resulting in a large release (~100 pmol) with reductions near 40%. Receptor activation need not depend on total blood or water loss, however, because shifts in regional blood pools induced by temperature or body position are effective at altering AVP release. Like volume stimuli, hypotension also enhances the response to increased osmolality (Fig. 3).

Although V1a receptors with high affinity are densely distributed on hepatocytes, the physiological role of AVP in the regulation of blood glucose is questionable. Pronounced hypoglycemia is a trigger for AVP release, but the levels of AVP required to increase plasma glucose are thought to be high for day-to-day regulation.

V. ELECTROPHYSIOLOGY OF AVP NEURONS

The pioneering studies of Harris and Douglas showed clearly that Ca^{2+}-dependent stimulus-secretion coupling, much like that observed at the neuromuscular junction, characterizes neurohypophyseal hormone release. It is now widely appreciated that release of AVP from the neural lobe is a function of both the pattern and the rate of action potential activity originating in SON and PVN neurons. Action potentials depolarize the axon terminals and increase Ca^{2+} influx, which triggers the exocytosis of AVP-containing vesicles.

Hypotension, hypovolemia, and hyperosmolality all trigger a stereotypic electrical response from AVP neurons. This response consists of a phasic, bursting pattern of activity (Fig. 4). In normal animals, very few neurons exhibit this pattern. With even moderate dehydration, the majority of AVP neurons adopt this pattern. Stimulation of phasic neurons increases the firing rate within bursts and can increase burst length. Phasic activity is clearly the most efficient means of releasing AVP (Fig. 5). Studies directly using the action potential distribution of bursts to stimulate the axons electrically in the neural lobe have shown that this pattern is superior to continuous trains of stimuli at the same mean frequency for releasing AVP. The maximally efficient frequency is ~13 Hz. Efficiency is related both to the high frequency of discharge at the beginning of each burst (facilitation) and to the recovery from fatigue during interburst intervals. Recovery during these silent intervals maximizes Ca^{2+} uptake into the terminals for successive bursts.

Although phasic activity is instigated and controlled by the peripheral stimuli known to release AVP, the mechanisms for this activity are intrinsic properties of the AVP neuron and can be observed in synaptically uncoupled neurons. Phasic activity is voltage dependent, with a threshold from −60 to −50 mV. Thus, peripheral stimuli must depolarize the neuron to this range before the activity can commence, regardless of whether isolated action potentials occur. With depolarization, action potentials open voltage-gated Ca^{2+} channels and induce a Ca^{2+}-dependent depolarizing afterpotential (DAP) (Fig. 4). The DAP summates with repetitive firing and forms a plateau potential on which a long (10- to 60-s) discharge is maintained. The current underlying the DAP appears to result from the reduction in a resting K^+ conductance, although inward cationic currents participate. SON neurons contain many other conductances that could shape the activity of the burst, the best studied of which are low- and high-threshold Ca^{2+} currents, a Ca^{2+}-dependent K^+ current that gates the firing rate, voltage-gated K^+ currents that influence the firing rate and spike width, and voltage-gated, nonselective cation currents, such as I_H.

Recent data of great interest concern an auto-inhibitory feedback mechanism controlling burst length. AVP neurons also synthesize the opiate peptide dynorphin and package it within AVP dense core vesicles. Both dynorphin and AVP are released locally during neuronal activity. Dynorphin acts on κ opioid receptors on AVP neurons and serves to inhibit phasic bursting. At least one mechanism for this inhibitory effect is a direct inhibition of the DAP. Thus, accumulative release of dynorphin during spike activity may eventually terminate the burst.

The V1a (and possibly V1b or related variant) receptors are located on the membrane of AVP neurons, just as OT receptors have been found on OT neurons. Activation of these receptors increases $[Ca^{2+}]_i$ and also modulates AVP neuronal activity. The precise effect (i.e., inhibitory or excitatory) varies with the ongoing level of activity, so as to reinforce the most efficient firing rate for AVP release.

VI. SUMMARY

Arginine vasopressin released from the posterior pituitary is synthesized within a preprohormone complex by large neurons in SON and PVN of the

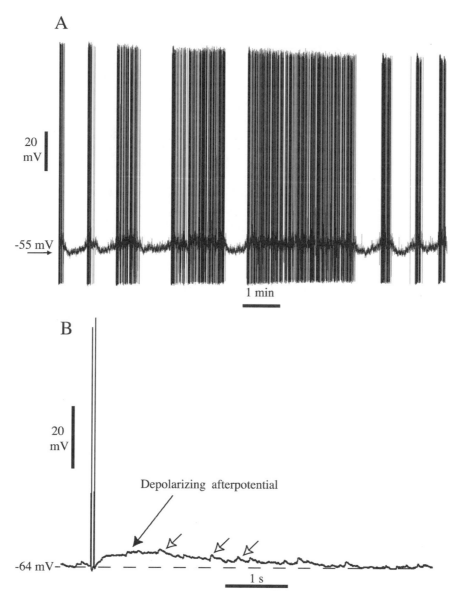

FIGURE 4 (A) Example of a phasically bursting AVP neuron from a whole-cell recording in a hypothalamic slice from an adult rat. Note the periods of action potential activity associated with membrane depolarizations, interrupted by silent periods when the membrane is hyperpolarized. (Recording courtesy of Chunyan Li). (B) The depolarizing afterpotential implicated in phasic activity is shown following two action potentials evoked with current injection. At this more hyperpolarized potential, a depolarizing afterpotential can be evoked, but the resulting depolarization does not reach spike threshold. Note the excitatory synaptic potentials (open arrowheads).

mammalian hypothalamus. After axonal transport to the neurohypophysis, the hormone is released into the peripheral circulation by stimuli such as dehydration, hypovolemia, and hypotension. At least three cloned AVP receptors are present. V1a receptors are found primarily on vascular smooth muscle and act to transduce muscle contraction. V1b receptors are found on pituitary corticotrophs and their activation leads to ACTH release. V2 receptors are found in the kidney, where they mediate antidiuresis. AVP neurons are osmoreceptive.

Glossary

anterior pituitary lobe Also called the adenohypophysis, this region contains numerous hormone-secreting cells under humoral control from hypothalamic inhibitory and excitatory factors.

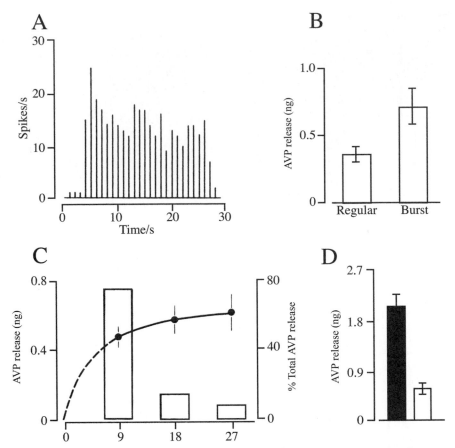

FIGURE 5 The relationship between phasic bursting activity and arginine vasopressin (AVP) release in isolated neural lobes. (A) Rate meter of a burst recorded in an AVP neuron. This burst was used to program the electrical stimulation of isolated neural lobes. The burst contained 348 spikes, lasted 26.7 s, and had a mean firing rate of 13 Hz. Note that firing rate is higher at the beginning of the burst. (B) Total AVP release evoked in isolated neural lobes is much greater with the burst as compared to when lobes are stimulated at the same frequency, with the same number of pulses, in a regular manner (i.e., the interpulse interval was constant). (C) Groups of neural lobes were stimulated with the AVP burst for the first 9 s, the first 18 s, or the complete burst. The black circles show the AVP release from each group. The bars show the amount of AVP attributable to each 9-s period as a percentage of the total amount released. Release is high in the beginning of the burst, when frequency is higher, and low in the final 18 s of the burst. The efficiency is likewise highest in the first 9 s, when each pulse evoked an average of 3.3 pg AVP, compared with 0.7 and 0.6 pg AVP, respectively, in the second and third 9-s periods. (D) Neural lobes were stimulated with four successive bursts that were either separated by 21-s silent intervals (filled bar) or were administered without silent periods (open bar). Release is higher when recovery from fatigue is allowed during the silent periods. Modified from Cazalis *et al.* (1985).

median eminence Collection of neurosecretory axons along middle, ventral, and posterior portions of the hypothalamus; connects the brain with the pituitary gland.

neurohypophysis Posterior (neural) and intermediate lobes of the mammalian pituitary gland.

oxytocin Polypeptide hormone closely related to vasopressin. Composed of 9 amino acids, oxytocin is synthesized in and released from neurosecretory cells in the hypothalamus of mammals; promotes uterine contractions, salt excretion, and milk ejection.

posterior (neural) pituitary lobe Houses vasopressin- and oxytocin-containing axon terminals, fenestrated capillaries, and a large population of astrocyte-like cells, the pituicytes.

supraoptic and paraventricular nuclei Clusters of neurons in the mammalian hypothalamus with axons that project to the neurohypophysis; synthesize vasopressin and oxytocin.

vasopressin Polypeptide hormone composed of 9 amino acids. Synthesized and released from neurosecretory cells in the hypothalamus of mammals, vasopressin increases blood pressure and promotes water reabsorption from the kidneys.

See Also the Following Articles

Adrenocorticotropic Hormone (ACTH) and Other Proopiomelanocortin (POMC) Peptides • **Neuropeptides**

and Control of the Anterior Pituitary • Oxytocin
• Oxytocin/Vasopressin Receptor Signaling

Further Reading

Acher, R., Chauvet, J., and Rouille, Y. (2002). Dynamic processing of neuropeptides: Sequential conformation shaping of neuro-hypophysial preprohormones during intraneuronal secretory transport. *J. Mol. Neurosci.* 18, 223–228.

Armstrong, W. E. (1995). Morphological and electrophysiological classification of hypothalamic supraoptic neurons. *Prog. Neurobiol.* 47, 291–339.

Baylis, P. H. (1987). Osmoregulation and control of vasopressin secretion in healthy humans. *Am. J. Physiol.* 253, R671–R678.

Brown, C. H., Ludwig, M., and Leng, G. (1998). Kappa-opioid regulation of neuronal activity in the rat supraoptic nucleus in vivo. *J. Neurosci.* 18, 9480–9488.

Cazalis, M., Dayanithi, G., and Nordmann, J. J. (1985). The role of patterned burst and interburst interval on the excitation-coupling mechanism in the isolated rat neural lobe. *J. Physiol.* 369, 45–60.

Dayanithi, G., Widmer, H., and Richard, P. (1996). Vasopressin-induced intracellular Ca^{2+} increase in isolated rat supraoptic cells. *J. Physiol.* 490, 713–727.

Dunn, F. L., Brennan, T. J., Nelson, A. E., and Robertson, G. L. (1973). The role of blood osmolality and volume in regulating vasopressin secretion in the rat. *J. Clin. Invest.* 52, 3212–3219.

Gouzenes, L., Desarmenien, M. G., Hussy, N., Richard, P., and Moos, F. C. (1998). Vasopressin regularizes the phasic firing pattern of rat hypothalamic magnocellular vasopressin neurons. *J. Neurosci.* 18, 1879–1885.

Hatton, G. I. (1997). Function-related plasticity in hypothalamus. *Annu. Rev. Neurosci.* 20, 375–397.

Hussy, N., Deleuze, C., Bres, V., and Moos, F. C. (2000). New role of taurine as an osmomediator between glial cells and neurons in the rat supraoptic nucleus. *Adv. Exp. Med. Biol.* 483, 227–237.

North, W. G. (1987). Biosynthesis of vasopressin and neurophysins. In "Vasopressin: Principles and Properties" (D. M. Gash and G. J. Boer, eds.), pp. 175–209. Plenum, New York and London.

Poulain, D. A., and Wakerley, J. B. (1982). Electrophysiology of hypothalamic magnocellular neurones secreting oxytocin and vasopressin. *Neuroscience* 7, 773–808.

Sladek, C. D. (1999). Antidiuretic hormone: Synthesis and release. In "Handbook of Physiology, Section 7: Endocrinology Volume III: Hormonal Regulation of Water and Electrolyte Balance" (John C. S. Fray, ed.), pp. 436–495. Oxford University Press, Oxford, U.K.

Thibonnier, M., Berti-Mattera, L. N., Dulin, N., Conarty, D. M., and Mattera, R. (1998). Signal transduction pathways of the human V1-vascular, V2-renal, V3-pituitary vasopressin and oxytocin receptors. *Prog. Brain Res.* 119, 147–161.

Voisin, D. L., and Bourque, C. W. (2002). Integration of sodium and osmosensory signals in vasopressin neurons. *Trends Neurosci.* 25, 199–205.

Xi, D., Kusano, K., and Gainer, H. (1999). Quantitative analysis of oxytocin and vasopressin messenger ribonucleic acids in single magnocellular neurons isolated from supraoptic nucleus of rat hypothalamus. *Endocrinology* 140, 4677–4682.

VEGF

See *Vascular Endothelial Growth Factor*

VIP

See *Vasoactive Intestinal Peptide*

Vitamin D

ANTHONY W. NORMAN

University of California, Riverside

I. VITAMIN OR HORMONE?
II. CHEMISTRY
III. PHOTOBIOLOGY
IV. VITAMIN D ENDOCRINE SYSTEM
V. NUTRITIONAL REQUIREMENTS
VI. DISEASE STATES
VII. SUMMARY

Vitamin D is essential for life in higher animals. Classically, vitamin D has been shown to be one of the most important biological regulators of calcium homeostasis. This important biological effect is only achieved as a consequence of the conversion of vitamin D into a family of daughter metabolites, including the two key kidney-produced metabolites $1\alpha,25(OH)_2$-vitamin D_3 [$1\alpha,25(OH)_2D_3$] and $24R,25(OH)_2$-vitamin D_3 [$24R,25(OH)_2D_3$]. $1\alpha,25(OH)_2D_3$, is a steroid hormone and there is increasing evidence that $24R,25(OH)_2D_3$ is also a steroid hormone.

I. VITAMIN OR HORMONE?

The first scientific description of the bone disease rickets, which is the hallmark of vitamin D deficiency, was provided in written scientific treatises as early as 1645. The major breakthrough in understanding the causative factors of rickets was the development of nutrition as an experimental science and the appreciation of the existence of vitamins. Considering the fact that the biologically active form of vitamin D is now known to be a steroid hormone, it is somewhat ironic that vitamin D, through a historical accident, became classified as a vitamin. In 1919–1920, Sir Edward Mellanby, while working with dogs raised exclusively indoors (in the absence of sunlight or ultraviolet light), devised a diet that allowed him to unequivocally establish that rickets was caused by a deficiency of a trace lipid component present in the dog's diet. In 1921, he wrote, "The action of fats in rickets is due to a vitamin or accessory food factor which they contain, probably identical with the fat-soluble vitamin." Furthermore, he established that cod liver oil was an excellent anti-rachitic agent. This ultimately led to the anti-rachitic factor being classified as a vitamin or as an essential dietary trace component that prevents rickets. However, in 1924 it was discovered that a precursor of vitamin D that could be converted into vitamin D by exposure to sunlight or ultraviolet light was present in skin. Thus, the substance known as vitamin D is correctly termed "a vitamin" only when there is a deficiency of sunlight exposure.

The modern era of vitamin D began in 1965–1970 with the discovery and chemical characterization of a metabolite of vitamin D, namely, $1\alpha,25(OH)_2$-vitamin D_3 [$1\alpha,25(OH)_2D_3$] and its nuclear receptor, VDR. It is now accepted that vitamin D is a precursor of $1\alpha,25(OH)_2D_3$, which generates biological responses as a steroid hormone.

II. CHEMISTRY

Vitamin D_3 is the naturally occurring form of vitamin D and is produced from 7-dehydro-cholesterol. Vitamin D_2 is a synthetic form of vitamin D that is produced by irradiation of the yeast steroid, ergosterol. The structures of vitamin D_3 (cholecalciferol) and its provitamin 7-dehydrocholesterol are presented in Fig. 1. Vitamin D is a generic term and indicates a molecule of the general structure shown for rings A, B, C, and D with differing side chain structures. The A-, B-, C-, and D-ring structure is derived from the cyclopentanoperhydrophenanthrene ring structure for steroids. Technically, the steroid vitamin D is classified as a seco-steroid. Seco-steroids are those in which one of the rings has been broken; in vitamin D, the 9,10 carbon–carbon bond of ring B is broken, and it is indicated by the inclusion of "9,10-seco" in the official nomenclature. Vitamin D (synonym calciferol) is named according to the revised rules of the International Union of Pure and Applied Chemists (IUPAC). Because vitamin D is derived from a steroid, the structure retains its numbering from the parent compound cholesterol

(see Fig. 1). Asymmetric centers are designated by using the R,S notation; the configuration of the double bonds is indicated as E for "eingang" or *trans* and Z for "zuzammen" or *cis*. Thus, the official name of vitamin D_3 is 9,10-seco(5Z,7E)-5,7,10(19)cholestatriene-3β-ol. Vitamin D_3 is currently the form of calciferol that is used for food supplementation, particularly of milk, in the United States. Vitamin D_2 differs from D_3 by virtue of the presence of a 22-ene and 24-methyl group in the side chain. Historically, vitamin D_2 was used in the years 1940–1960 as a food supplement to supply vitamin D activity. The official name of vitamin D_2 is 9,10-seco(5Z,7E)-5,7,10(19),22-ergostatetraene-3β-ol.

III. PHOTOBIOLOGY

Vitamin D_3 can be produced photochemically by the action of sunlight or ultraviolet light on the precursor sterol 7-dehydrocholesterol, which is present in the epidermis or skin of most higher animals (see Fig. 2). The chief structural prerequisite of a provitamin D is that it be a sterol with a Δ5-7 diene double bond system in ring B (see Fig. 1). The conjugated double bond system in this specific location of the molecule allows the absorption of light quanta (energy) at certain wavelengths in the ultraviolet (uv) range; this can readily be provided in most geographical locations by natural sunlight. This initiates a complex series of transformations (partially summarized in Fig. 2) that ultimately results in the transformation into vitamin D_3. Thus, it is important to appreciate that vitamin D_3 can be endogenously produced and that as long as the animal (or human) has access on a regular basis to sunlight there is no dietary requirement for this vitamin.

IV. VITAMIN D ENDOCRINE SYSTEM

Vitamin D_3 is not known to have any intrinsic biological activity itself. It is only after vitamin D_3 is metabolized, first into 25(OH)-vitamin D_3 [25-(OH)D_3] in the liver and then into $1\alpha,25(OH)_2D_3$ and $24R,25(OH)_2D_3$ by the kidney, that biologically active molecules are produced. *In toto*, some 37 vitamin D_3 metabolites have been isolated and chemically characterized. Fig. 3 illustrates the concept of the vitamin D endocrine system. The elements of the vitamin D endocrine system include the following: (1) in the skin, photoconversion of 7-dehydrocholesterol to vitamin D_3 or dietary intake of vitamin D_3; (2) conversion vitamin D_3 by the liver to 25(OH)D_3, which is the major form of vitamin D

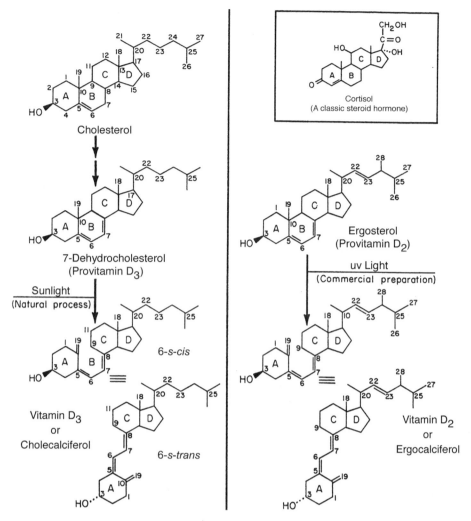

FIGURE 1 Structural relationship of vitamin D_3 (cholecalciferol) and vitamin D_2 (ergocalciferol) with their respective provitamins (7-dehydrocholesterol and ergosterol), cholesterol, and a classic steroid hormone, cortisol (see inset box). The two structural representations presented at the bottom for both vitamin D_3 and vitamin D_2 result from the conformational flexibility in the B ring that allows 180° rotation about the 6,7 single carbon bond. This rotation generates a population of conformers that are represented by the 6-*s-cis* and the 6-*s-trans* orientations indicated in the figure. Vitamin D_3 is the naturally occurring form of the vitamin; it is produced from 7-dehydrocholesterol, which is present in the skin, by the action of sunlight or ultraviolet light. Vitamin D_2 is produced commercially by the irradiation of the sterol ergosterol with ultraviolet light.

circulating in the blood compartment; (3) conversion of $25(OH)D_3$ by the kidney (functioning as an endocrine gland) to produce the two principal dihydroxylated metabolites, $1\alpha,25(OH)_2D_3$ and $24R,25(OH)_2D_3$; (4) systemic transport of the dihydroxylated metabolites $24R,25(OH)_2D_3$ and $1\alpha,25(OH)_2D_3$ to distal target organs; (5) binding of the steroid hormone $1,25(OH)_2D_3$ to either a nuclear receptor or a membrane receptor at the target organs followed by the subsequent generation of appropriate biological responses. An additional key component in the operation of the vitamin D

endocrine system is the plasma vitamin D-binding protein (DBP), which carries vitamin D_3 and all its metabolites to their various target organs.

The three enzymes responsible for the conversion of vitamin D_3 into its two key daughter metabolites include the hepatic vitamin D_3-25-hydroxylase and the two kidney enzymes, $25(OH)D_3$-1α-hydroxylase and $25(OH)D_3$-24R-hydroxylase. All three enzymes have been demonstrated to be cytochrome P450 mixed-function oxidases. Both renal enzymes are localized in mitochondria of the proximal tubules of the kidney. The $25(OH)D_3$-1α-hydroxylase has been

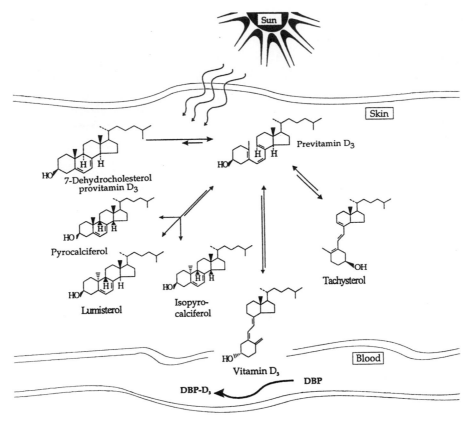

FIGURE 2 Photochemical pathway of production of vitamin D_3 (calciferol) from 7-dehydrocholesterol. The starting point is the irradiation of a provitamin D, which contains the mandatory $\Delta^{5,7}$-conjugated double bonds; in the skin, this is 7-dehydrocholesterol. After absorption of a quantum of light from sunlight (ultraviolet B), the activated molecule can return to the ground state and generate at least six distinct products. The four steroids that do not have a broken 9,10 carbon bond (provitamin D, lumisterol, pyrocalciferol, and isopyrocalciferol) represent the four diastereomers with either an α- or a β-orientation of the methyl group on carbon 10 and the hydrogen on carbon 9. The three seco-steroid products, vitamin D_3, previtamin D, and tachysterol, have the three conjugated double bonds at different positions. In the skin, the principal product is previtamin D, which then undergoes a 1,7-sigmatropic hydrogen transfer from C-19 to C-9, yielding the final vitamin D. Vitamin D can be drawn as either a *6-s-trans* representation (this figure) or a *6-s-cis* representation (Fig. 1), depending upon the state of rotation about the 6,7 single bond. The resulting vitamin D_3, which is formed in the skin, is removed by binding to the plasma transport protein, the vitamin D-binding protein (DBP), present in the capillary bed of the dermis. The DBP-D_3 then enters the general circulatory system.

cloned and the specific site of mutations that result in the appearance in patients of vitamin D-resistant rickets type I (VDRR-I) has been identified. These patients lack the ability to produce $1\alpha,25(OH)_2D_3$ and thus express the phenotype of vitamin D deficiency. In addition, $25(OH)D_3$-24R-hydrodroxylase and vitamin D_3-25-hydroxylase have been cloned.

The most important point of regulation of the vitamin D endocrine system occurs through the stringent control of the activity of the renal $25(OH)D_3$-1α-hydroxylase. In this way, the production of the hormone $1\alpha,25(OH)_2D_3$ can be modulated according to the calcium needs and other endocrine needs of the organism. The chief regulatory factors are $1\alpha,25(OH)_2D_3$ itself, parathyroid hormone (PTH), and the serum concentrations of calcium and phosphate. The secretion of PTH is inversely proportional to the serum Ca^{2+} concentration and increased secretion of PTH will result in stimulation of the renal $25(OH)D_3$-1α-hydroxylase and a concomitant increase in the serum concentration of $1\alpha,25(OH)_2D_3$. Probably the most important determinant of 1α-hydroxylase is the vitamin D status of the animal. When the circulating concentration of $1\alpha,25(OH)_2D_3$ is low, a lowered serum Ca^{2+} results and production of $1\alpha,25(OH)_2D_3$ by the kidney is high; when the circulating concentration of $1\alpha,25(OH)_2D_3$ is high, the output of $1\alpha,25(OH)_2D_3$ by the kidney is sharply reduced.

A. Mode of Action of 1α,25(OH)₂

1α,25(OH)₂D₃ produces a wide spectrum of biological responses through interaction with both its nuclear receptor to regulate gene transcription and a second receptor associated with the cellular membrane that mediates the generation of a variety of rapid signal transduction processes (see Fig. 2).

1. Genomic Responses of 1α,25(OH)₂D₃

The genomic responses to $1\alpha,25(OH)_2D_3$ are a consequence of the stereospecific interaction of this steroid hormone with its nuclear vitamin D receptor, the VDR. The VDR is a protein of 50 kDa that binds $1\alpha,25(OH)_2D_3$ with high affinity; the $K_d \approx 0.5$ nM. The VDR is not able to bind the parent vitamin D, whereas $25(OH)D_3$ and $1\alpha (OH)D_3$ only bind 0.1–0.3% as well as $1\alpha,25(OH)_2D_3$. The primary amino acid sequence of the VDR, like all nuclear receptors for steroid hormones, is divided into five functional domains: these include regions (from the N-terminal to the COOH-terminal) involved in nuclear localization, DNA binding, heterodimerization with other nuclear proteins, ligand binding, and transcriptional activation.

The process of nuclear receptor-mediated regulation of gene transcription is exquisitely dependent upon the complementary relationship between the unoccupied receptor and its cognate ligand. Thus, the unoccupied receptor is largely unable to engage in a productive fashion with the transcriptional machinery to effect meaningful regulation of gene transcription. It is only after the ligand-receptor complex has formed, resulting in conformational changes in the receptor protein, that a functional receptor protein is generated. Thus, acquisition of a detailed understanding of the complementarity of the ligand shape with that of the interior surface of the nuclear VDR receptor ligand-binding domain is believed to be the key to understanding not only the structural basis of receptor action and its formation of heterodimers and interactions with co-activators, but also to designing new drug forms of the various hormones, including $1\alpha,25(OH)_2D_3$.

The protein receptors for all steroid hormones (estrogen, progesterone, testosterone, cortisol, and aldosterone) and the protein receptors for $1\alpha,25(OH)_2D_3$, retinoic acid, and thyroid hormone are all members of the same gene superfamily; accordingly, there is a high level of conservation in their amino acid sequences, particularly in their DNA- and ligand-binding domains. The X-ray crystallographic structures of the ligand-binding domains (LBDs) of the thyroid hormone receptor, the retinoic acid receptor, the estrogen receptor, and the progesterone receptor have all been determined with their respective ligands bound. Also, the crystal structure of the nuclear receptor for vitamin D bound to its natural ligand $1\alpha,25(OH)_2D_3$ has been determined at a 1.8 Å resolution. The VDR LBD structure, as well as that of the other nuclear receptors, consists of 12 α-helices that are arranged to create a three-layer sandwich that completely encompasses the ligand $1\alpha,25(OH)_2D_3$ in a hydrophobic core. The secondary and tertiary structural features of this family of receptor proteins were found to be remarkably similar.

An animal model in which the gene for the VDR has been deleted (termed a gene knockout or KO) has been engineered by targeted disruption of both the first and the second zinc-fingers of the DNA-binding domain of the VDR. This VDR KO displays the phenotype of vitamin D-dependent rickets type II (VDDR-II). Despite the widespread tissue distribution of the VDR (see Fig. 2), the resultant animals were phenotypically normal at birth, indicating that there is biological redundancy with respect to most of the functions of this receptor. The most surprising observation was that all of the VDR KO mice developed alopecia (hair loss) by 7 weeks. In addition, the male and female VDR KO mice were infertile.

2. Rapid Responses of 1α,25(OH)₂D₃

The "rapid" responses mediated by $1\alpha,25(OH)_2D_3$ (see Fig. 3) are postulated to be mediated through interaction of $1\alpha,25(OH)_2D_3$ with a second protein receptor located on the external membrane of the cell. Rapid responses stimulated by $1\alpha,25(OH)_2D_3$ include the following: transcaltachia [the rapid stimulation by $1\alpha,25(OH)_2D_3$ of intestinal Ca^{2+} absorption], the opening of voltage-gated Ca^{2+} and Cl^- channels, rapid uptake of $^{45}Ca^{2+}$ into (ROS, rat osteosarcoma 17/2.8) osteoblast cells, enhancement of the concentration of phospholipid second messengers in the intestine, activation of protein kinase C, tyrosine kinases, and mitogen-activated protein kinase.

3. 24R,25(OH)₂D₃ Biological Properties

In comparison to $1\alpha,25(OH)_2D_3$, the biological actions of $24R,25(OH)_2D_3$ have been relatively less studied. One key question that has attracted attention is whether $1\alpha,25(OH)_2D_3$ acting alone can generate *all* the biological responses that are attributed to the parent vitamin D_3 or whether a second vitamin D_3 metabolite may be required for some responses.

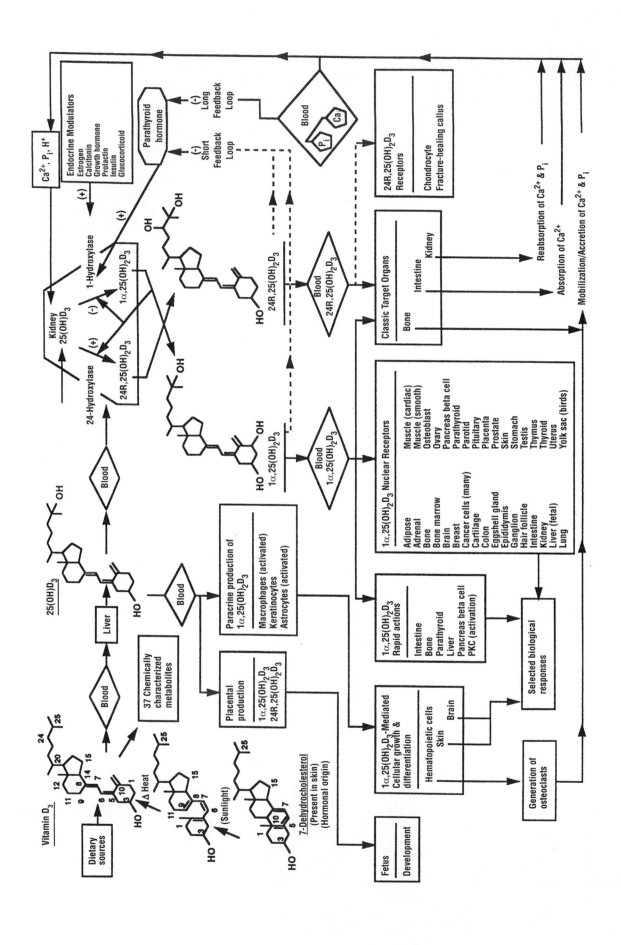

Evidence supports the view that the combined presence of both $1\alpha,25(OH)_2D_3$ and $24R,25(OH)_2D_3$ is necessary to generate the complete spectrum of biological responses attributable to the parent vitamin D_3. Current research on $24R,25(OH)_2D_3$ focuses on elucidating its actions in cartilage and bone cells.

V. NUTRITIONAL REQUIREMENTS

A. Recommended Dietary Allowance (RDA)

The World Health Organization has responsibility for defining the "International Unit" of vitamin D_3. Their most recent definition, provided in 1950, stated that "the International Unit of vitamin D recommended for adoption is the vitamin D activity of 0.025 μg of the international standard preparation of crystalline vitamin D_3." Thus, 1.0 IU of vitamin D_3 is 0.025 μg, which is equivalent to 65.0 pmol. With the discovery of the conversion of vitamin D_3 to other active seco-steroids, particularly $1\alpha,25(OH)_2D_3$, it was recommended that 1.0 Unit of $1\alpha,25(OH)_2D_3$ be set equivalent in molar terms to that of the parent vitamin D_3. Thus, 1.0 Unit of $1\alpha,25(OH)_2D_3$ has been operationally defined to be equivalent to 65 pmol.

The vitamin D requirement for healthy adults has never been precisely defined. Since vitamin D_3 is produced in the skin after exposure to sunlight, the human does not have a requirement for vitamin D when sufficient sunlight is available. The tendencies of humans to wear clothes, to live in cities where tall buildings block adequate sunlight from reaching the ground, to live indoors, to use synthetic sunscreens that block ultraviolet rays, and to live in geographical regions of the world that do not receive adequate sunlight all contribute to the inability of the skin to biosynthesize sufficient amounts of vitamin D_3. Thus, vitamin D does become an important essential nutritional factor in the absence of sunlight. It is known that a substantial proportion of the U.S. population is exposed to suboptimal levels of sunlight. This is particularly true during the winter months. Under these conditions, vitamin D becomes a true vitamin, which dictates that it must be supplied in the diet on a regular basis.

The current "adequate intake" allowance of vitamin D recommended in 1998 by the United States Food and Nutrition Board of the Institute of Medicine is 200 IU/day (5 μg/day) for infants, children, and adult males and females up to age 51. For adults ages 51–70, the adequate indicated level is set at 400 IU/day (10 μg/day). For adults >70 years of age, the adequate indicated level is set at 600 IU (15 μg/day). The adequate allowance for pregnancy and lactation is set at 200 IU/day (5 μg/day). These recommendations are all summarized in a 1998 publication from the Food and Nutrition Board of the Institute of Medicine.

In the United States, adequate amounts of vitamin D can readily be obtained from the diet and/or from casual exposure to sunlight. The uv exposure can be as little as three times per week exposure of the face and hands to ambient sunlight for 20 min. However, in some parts of the world where food is not routinely fortified and sunlight is often limited during some periods of the year, obtaining adequate amounts of vitamin D becomes more of a problem. As a result, the incidence of the bone disease rickets in these countries is higher than in the United States.

1. Food Sources of Vitamin D

Animal products constitute the bulk source of vitamin D that occurs naturally in unfortified foods. Salt water fish, such as herring, salmon, and sardines, and fish liver oils are good sources of vitamin D_3. Small quantities of vitamin D_3 are also derived from eggs, veal, beef, butter, and vegetable oils, whereas plants, fruits, and nuts are extremely poor sources of vitamin D. In the United States, fortification of foods such as milk (both fresh and evaporated), margarine and butter, cereals, and chocolate mixes help in meeting the RDA recommendations. Because only fluid milk is fortified with vitamin D, other dairy products (cheese, yogurt, etc.) do not provide the vitamin.

B. Excess and Toxicity

1. Vitamin D

Excessive amounts of vitamin D are not normally available from usual dietary sources and thus reports

---

FIGURE 3 Summary of the vitamin D endocrine system. The kidney is the principal endocrine gland that produces in a regulated fashion small amounts of both $1\alpha,25(OH)_2D_3$ and $24R,25(OH)_2D_3$. During pregnancy, these same two metabolites are also produced by the placenta. Target organs for the steroid hormone $1\alpha,25(OH)_2D_3$ by definition contain the nuclear receptor $1\alpha,25(OH)_2D_3$ (VDR). Also, $1\alpha,25(OH)_2D_3$ produces selected biological responses via a rapid signal transduction process. The biological roles of $24R,25(OH)_2D_3$ are believed to occur in the bone and cartilage.

of vitamin D intoxication are rare. However, there is always the possibility that vitamin D intoxication may occur in individuals who are taking excessive amounts of supplemental vitamins. In 1993, there was one report of vitamin D intoxication occurring from drinking milk that had been fortified with inappropriately high levels of vitamin D_3. Symptoms of vitamin D intoxication include hypercalcemia, hypercalciuria, anorexia, nausea, vomiting, thirst, polyuria, muscular weakness, joint pains, diffuse demineralization of bones, and general disorientation. If allowed to go unchecked, death will eventually occur. The extent of toxicity has been shown in some instances to be related to the level of dietary intake of calcium.

The biological basis for intoxication resulting from the inappropriate intake of the parent vitamin D_3 is believed to occur from the unrestrained conversion by the liver of the vitamin D_3 to $25(OH)D_3$; this is a largely unregulated metabolic step. The vitamin D intoxication is thought to occur as a result of high plasma levels of $25(OH)D$ rather than high plasma levels of $1\alpha,25(OH)_2D_3$. Patients suffering from hypervitaminosis D have been shown to exhibit a 15-fold increase in plasma $25(OH)D$ concentration compared to normal individuals; however, their $1\alpha,25(OH)_2D$ levels are not substantially altered. It has also been shown that large concentrations of $25(OH)D_3$ can mimic the actions of $1\alpha,25(OH)_2D_3$ at the level of the VDR, which can lead to a massive stimulation of intestinal Ca^{2+} absorption and bone Ca^{2+} resorption and ultimately

the occurrence of soft tissue calcification and kidney stones. The use of pamidronate, a bisphosphonate inhibitor of bone resorption, has been proposed to reduce the hypercalcemia secondary to acute vitamin D intoxication.

VI. DISEASE STATES

Figure 4 describes human disease states related to vitamin D and the vitamin D endocrine system. Conceptually, human clinical disorders related to vitamin D can be considered as those arising because of the following: (1) altered availability of vitamin D; (2) altered conversion of vitamin D_3 to $25(OH)D_3$; (3) altered conversion of $25(OH)D_3$ to $1\alpha,25(OH)_2D_3$ and/or $24R,25(OH)_2D_3$; (4) variations in end organ responsiveness to $1\alpha,25(OH)_2D_3$ or possibly $24R,25(OH)_2D_3$; and (5) other conditions of uncertain relation to vitamin D. Thus, the clinician/nutritionist/biochemist is faced with a problem, in a diagnostic sense, of identifying parameters of hypersensitivity, antagonism, or resistance (including genetic aberrations) to vitamin D or one of the other of its metabolites as well as identifying perturbations of metabolism that result in problems in production and/or delivery of the hormonally active form, $1\alpha,25(OH)_2D_3$.

A. Vitamin D Deficiency and Rickets

The classic deficiency state resulting from a dietary absence of vitamin D or lack of ultraviolet (sunlight)

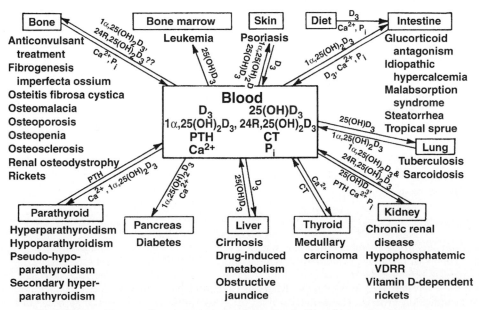

FIGURE 4 Human disease states related to vitamin D and its endocrine system.

exposure is the bone disease rickets (in children) or osteomalacia (in adults). The clinical features of rickets and osteolmalacia depend on the age of onset. The classical skeletal disorder of rickets includes deformity of the bones, especially the knees, wrists, and ankles, as well as associated changes in the costochondrial joint functions, which have been termed by some as the rachitic rosary. If rickets develops in the first 6 months, infants may suffer from convulsions or develop tetany due to a low blood calcium level (usually <7 mg/100 ml; normal blood calcium levels are 9–10.5 mg/100 ml) but may have only minor skeletal changes. After 6 months, bone pain as well as tetany is likely to be present. Since osteomalacia occurs after growth and development of the skeleton are complete (i.e., the adult stage of life), its main symptoms are muscular weakness and bone pain with little bone deformity.

A characteristic feature of bone osteomalacia and rickets is the failure of the organic matrix of bone (osteoid) to calcify. This leads to the appearance of excessive quantities of uncalcified osteoid. In addition, there is often a high serum level of alkaline phosphatase, a fact that is often used to assist in the clinical diagnosis of osteomalacia. Also, low serum levels of 25(OH)D$_3$ have been found to be diagnostic for the presence of rickets or osteomalacia. The normal serum level of 25(OH)D$_3$ is 25–35 ng/ml. When the serum 25(OH)D$_3$ level is below 5 ng/ml, the individual is classified as being vitamin D-deficient. When the serum 25(OH)D$_3$ level is below 10 ng/ml, the individual is "at risk" for development of vitamin D deficiency.

The nutritional availability of vitamin D is particularly important both in the newborn and young child and in the elderly. Thus, circumstances of deprivation of sunlight through seasonal variation (winter) or skin pigmentation in Africans or African Americans or certain cultural groups, including Muslims, associated with clothing that covers the entire body and face, can lead to the onset of clinical rickets or osteomalacia, characterized by low serum 25(OH)D$_3$ levels. Accordingly, the nursing infant can be at risk for rickets if her/his mother is vitamin D-deficient.

VII. SUMMARY

Current evidence substantiates the concept that the classical biological actions of the nutritionally important fat-soluble vitamin D in mediating calcium homeostasis are supported by a complex vitamin D endocrine system that coordinates the conversion of vitamin D$_3$ into 1α,25(OH)$_2$D$_3$ and 24R,25(OH)$_2$D$_3$. It is now clear that the vitamin D endocrine system embraces many more target tissues than simply the intestine, bone, and kidney. Notable additions to this list include the pancreas, pituitary, breast tissue, placenta, hematopoietic cells, skin, and cancer cells of various origins. Key advances in understanding the mode of action of 1α,25(OH)$_2$D$_3$ have been made by a thorough study of nuclear receptors as well as emerging studies describing a membrane receptor for this steroid hormone. Integral to these observations are efforts to define the signal transduction systems that are subservient to the nuclear and membrane receptors for 1α,25(OH)$_2$D$_3$ and to obtain a thorough study of the tissue distribution and subcellular localization of the gene products induced by this steroid hormone. There are clinical applications for 1α,25(OH)$_2$D$_3$ or related analogues for treatment of the bone diseases of renal osteodystrophy and osteoporosis, psoriasis, and hypoparathyroidism. Other clinical targets for 1α,25(OH)$_2$D$_3$ currently under investigation include its use in leukemia and breast, prostate, and colon cancer as well as its use as an immunosuppressive agent.

Glossary

endocrine system The integrated interaction between an endocrine gland (source of a hormone) and target cells (location of the hormone's receptor) to generate in a regulated fashion the selective biological responses for that system.

hormone Any of several chemical classes of compounds produced in regulated quantities by an endocrine gland that acts as a chemical messenger, usually delivered through the circulatory system to a target cell, which by definition possesses a receptor for that hormone so that a specific biological response may be generated.

photochemical reaction A chemical reaction mediated or enhanced by some wavelength of light.

receptor A protein molecule that binds very specifically to its cognate hormone to generate a receptor–hormone complex that initiates a cellular signal transduction process resulting in a biological response.

Recommended Dietary Allowance (RDA) Recommendations for the amounts of various dietary nutrients (e.g., vitamins and minerals) required to maintain human health.

rickets A bone disease in infants and children characterized by a reduction of bone calcium content that results from a dietary deficiency of vitamin D or lack of adequate exposure to sunlight.

steroid A member of the lipid class of compounds that is composed of a four-ring structure, the cyclopentano-perhydro-phenanthrene nucleus, and is the basic structural component of steroid hormone families such as estrogens, progestogens, androgens, mineralocorticoids, and glucocorticoids.

vitamin Any of a group of essential organic substances provided in trace amounts in food components to effect the normal function of a cellular metabolic process.

See Also the Following Articles

Steroid Nomenclature ● Vitamin D and Cartilage ● Vitamin D and Human Nutrition ● Vitamin D: Biological Effects of 1,25(OH)$_2$D$_3$ in Bone ● Vitamin D Deficiency, Rickets and Osteomalacia ● Vitamin D: 24,25-Dihydroxyvitamin D ● Vitamin D Metabolism ● Vitamin D: Nuclear Receptor for 1,25(OH)$_2$D$_3$

Further Reading

Bouillon, R., Okamura, W. H., and Norman, A. W. (1995). Structure–function relationships in the vitamin D endocrine system. *Endocr. Rev.* **16**, 200–257.

Feldman, D., Glorieux, F. H., Pike, J. W. (eds.) (1997). "Vitamin D," pp. 1–1285. Academic Press, San Diego, CA.

Food and Nutrition Board (1998). "Dietary Reference Intakes: A Risk Assessment Model for Establishing Upper Intake Levels for Nutrients." National Academy Press, Institute of Medicine, Washington, DC.

Haddad, J. G. (1995). Plasma vitamin D-binding protein (Gc-globulin): Multiple tasks. *J. Steroid Biochem. Mol. Biol.* **53**, 579–582.

Haussler, M. R., Whitfield, G. K., Haussler, C. A., Hsieh, J. C., Thompson, P. D., Selznick, S. H., Dominguez, C. E., and Jurutka, P. W. (1998). The nuclear vitamin D receptor: Biological and molecular regulatory properties revealed. *J. Bone Miner. Res.* **13**, 325–349.

Malloy, P. J., Pike, J. W., Feldman, D., and Ryaby, J. T. (1999). The vitamin D receptor and the syndrome of hereditary 1,25-dihydroxyvitamin D-resistant rickets. *Endocr. Rev.* **20**, 156–188.

Norman, A. W. (2001). Vitamin D. *In* "Present Knowledge in Nutrition" (B. Bowman and R. Russell, eds.), pp. 134–143. International Life Sciences Institute, Washington, DC.

Norman, A. W., Bouillon, R., Thomasset, M., 2000. Vitamin D endocrine system: Structural, biological, genetic and clinical aspects. *In* Proceedings of the 11th Workshop on Vitamin D, pp. 1–1014. University of California, Riverside.

Reichel, H., Koeffler, H. P., and Norman, A. W. (1989). The role of the vitamin D endocrine system in health and disease. *N. Engl. J. Med.* **320**, 980–991.

Rochel, N., Wurtz, J. M., Mitschler, A., Klaholz, B., and Moras, D. (2000). The crystal structure of the nuclear receptor for vitamin D bound to its natural ligand. *Mol. Cell* **5**, 173–179.

Verstuyf, A., Verlinden, L., van Etten, E., Shi, L., Wu, Y., D'Halleweyn, C., Van Haver, D., Zhu, G.-D., Chen, Y.-J., Zhou, X., Haussler, M. R., De Clercq, P., Vandewalle, M., Van Baelen, H., Mathieu, C., and Bouillon, R. (2000). Biological activity of CD-ring modified 1α,25-dihydroxyvitamin D

analogues: C-ring and five membered D-ring analogues. *J. Bone Miner. Res.* **15**, 237–252.

Webb, A. R., and Holick, M. F. (1988). The role of sunlight in the cutaneous production of vitamin D$_3$. *Annu. Rev. Nutr.* **8**, 375–399.

Vitamin D and Cartilage

BARBARA D. BOYAN[*,**], VICTOR L. SYLVIA[*], DAVID D. DEAN[*], AND ZVI SCHWARTZ[*,**,†]

[*]*University of Texas Health Science Center at San Antonio* ● [**]*Georgia Institute of Technology and Emory University, Atlanta* ● [†]*Hebrew University Hadassah, Jerusalem*

I. INTRODUCTION
II. ROLE OF 1α,25(OH)$_2$D$_3$
III. ROLE OF 24R,25(OH)$_2$D$_3$
IV. METABOLISM OF 25(OH)D$_3$
V. MEMBRANE-MEDIATED ACTIONS
VI. SUMMARY

Two metabolites of vitamin D, 1α,25-dihydroxy vitamin D$_3$ (1α,25(OH)$_2$D$_3$) and 24R,25-dihydroxy vitamin D$_3$ (24R,25(OH)$_2$D$_3$) regulate growth plate physiology. The effects of each metabolite are limited to different subsets of cells in specific zones of the growth plate; different mechanisms of action are used by the metabolites to exert their effects in their target cells.

I. INTRODUCTION

Cartilage is one of the primary target tissues for vitamin D action. During embryonic development, a cartilage anlage provides the form of the skeleton. Mineralization of the cartilage must occur before it can serve as a structural support for bone formation, ultimately being replaced by bone marrow. At the ends of the long bones of the skeleton, at cranial sutures, at the scapula, and at the mandibular condyle, the embryonic cartilage forms a specialized tissue called the growth plate. This tissue remains in postfetal life and provides the mechanism for continued bone growth.

Cartilage cells in the growth plate proceed through a lineage cascade that culminates in the calcification of the tissue (Fig. 1). Chondrocytes in the resting zone, also called the reserve zone, of the growth plate are surrounded by an extracellular matrix that is rich in type II collagen and sulfated

Cell zone

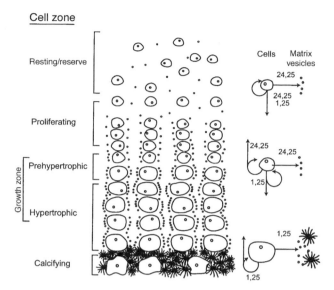

FIGURE 1 Growth plate cartilage. Cells progress through their lineage in a linear fashion in time and space. Vitamin D metabolites 1,25(OH)$_2$D$_3$ (1,25) and 24,25(OH)$_2$D$_3$ (24,25) produced by the chondrocytes act back on the cells in an autocrine manner or on adjacent chondrocytes in a paracrine manner. In addition, they act on matrix vesicles in the extracellular matrix.

glycosaminoglycans in the form of proteoglycan aggregates. This region of the growth plate cushions the tissue from mechanical load. Upon signals that are not yet understood, chondrocytes at the base of the resting zone align in columns and undergo a set number of divisions. Once proliferation is complete, the phenotype of the cartilage cells is altered. The cells are described as being in the zone of maturation or the prehypertrophic cell zone. There are many features of this zone that are not well understood but it appears to be a staging ground for the rapid increase in cell size that characterizes the zone of hypertrophy. This increase in size is primarily in the longitudinal direction and is accompanied by rapid turnover of extracellular matrix, particularly the breakdown of type II collagen and proteoglycan aggregate. In addition, the cells produce increased numbers of extracellular matrix vesicles that contain matrix-processing enzymes and serve as focal points for initial calcification of the tissue. Many of the chondrocytes in this zone are apoptotic. At the base of the hypertrophic cell zone, calcification of the cartilage is complete. This is accompanied by vascular invasion and migration of mesenchymal cells that ultimately differentiate into osteoblasts and marrow stromal cells, resulting in bone and bone marrow

formation. A similar sequence of events is recapitulated during fracture repair and during the process of osteoinduction.

In the absence of vitamin D, mineralization of the growth plate fails to occur. As a consequence, the hypertrophic cell zone increases in length since proliferation continues at its normal rate. Because the hypertrophic zone is weak structurally, it cannot withstand weight-bearing loads. As a result, a condition known as rickets develops, in which there is characteristic bowing of the long bones.

In experimental animals, rickets can be cured rapidly by injection with either 25-hydroxy vitasmin D$_3$ (25(OH)D$_3$) or metabolites of vitamin D that are hydroxylated on the 1-carbon, such as 1α,25(OH)$_2$D$_3$. This effect is due to the rapid release of Ca^{2+} into the extracellular matrix of the cells. Other studies have shown that rickets in rats that are deficient in vitamin D as well as phosphate can be cured by systemic injection of 24R,25(OH)$_2$D$_3$ or local injection of this metabolite into the bone. Since this metabolite is not associated with Ca^{2+} transport, these observations suggest either that the 24R,25(OH)$_2$D$_3$ is further metabolized to 1,24,25-trihydroxy vitamin D$_3$ (1,24,25(OH)$_3$D$_3$) in the tissue or that 24R,25(OH)$_2$D$_3$ also regulates growth plate chondrocytes directly, affecting other aspects of cell physiology that contribute to the development of the rachitic syndrome.

Vitamin D is also an important regulator of growth plate physiology in vitamin D replete animals. When vitamin D replete adolescent rats are given radiolabeled 25(OH)D$_3$, both 1,25(OH)$_2$D$_3$ and 24,25(OH)$_2$D$_3$ are concentrated in the growth plate to a greater extent than in kidney or serum. This supports the hypothesis that these vitamin D metabolites have functions in the growth plate in addition to calcium ion transport. There are numerous studies that indicate this to be the case and these are reviewed below.

The sensitivity of growth plate cartilage to vitamin D and the fact that this tissue contains a single cell type that transits its lineage cascade in a linear manner that can be visualized under a dissecting microscope have made this tissue an excellent model for studying the mechanisms of action of this hormone. The development of techniques for the culture of growth plate chondrocytes has enabled investigators to identify specific subpopulations of cells that respond to 24R,25(OH)$_2$D$_3$ and 1α,25(OH)$_2$D$_3$. These studies have also led to rapid advances in our understanding of the mechanisms involved.

II. ROLE OF 1α,25(OH)$_2$D$_3$

Growth plate chondrocytes contain nuclear receptors for 1α,25(OH)$_2$D$_3$ and respond to this vitamin D metabolite via traditional nuclear receptor-mediated mechanisms. In addition to the rapid release of Ca^{2+} ions after treatment with 1α,25(OH)$_2$D$_3$, there are a number of other changes that occur in the growth plate in response to this metabolite. 1α,25(OH)$_2$D$_3$ causes an increase in alkaline phosphatase activity in the hypertrophic zone of the growth plate, as well as an increase in phospholipase A$_2$ activity. This results in the increased production of lysophospholipids. Other aspects of phospholipid metabolism are affected as well, including the specific breakdown of phospholipids not associated with the nucleation of hydroxyapatite crystals in the extracellular matrix. Moreover, the activity of various matrix-processing enzymes is increased. These observations indicate that the primary functions of 1α,25(OH)$_2$D$_3$ are to prepare the matrix for calcification and to ensure that the mineral ions necessary for calcium phosphate formation are present in sufficient quantity. This hypothesis is supported by the fact that many of the effects described above involve matrix vesicles, which are extracellular organelles produced by the chondrocytes that contain matrix-processing enzymes and serve as foci for initial mineral formation.

Studies examining the effects of 1α,25(OH)$_2$D$_3$ on growth plate chondrocytes in culture show that this metabolite inhibits the proliferation of both resting zone and growth zone (prehypertrophic and upper hypertrophic cell zones) cells. However, the effects of this metabolite on differentiation are limited to cells from the growth zone. In confluent cultures of rat costochondral growth plate chondrocytes grown in the presence of serum, 1α,25(OH)$_2$D$_3$ increases the production of prostaglandin E1 (PGE1) and PGE2, stimulates the activity of matrix vesicle alkaline phosphatase and phospholipase A$_2$, and increases the activity of matrix metalloproteinases in these extracellular organelles. In contrast, cultures of chick epiphyseal growth plate chondrocytes grown under serum-free conditions respond to 1α,25(OH)$_2$D$_3$ with a decrease in cellular alkaline phosphatase activity. Whether these differences are due to the species, the presence of serum, or the tissue from which the cells were derived, cells versus matrix vesicles, or the experimental design is not known.

1α,25(OH)$_2$D$_3$ also modulates growth plate physiology indirectly by regulating the storage and activation of transforming growth factor-β (TGF-β) in the extracellular matrix of prehypertrophic and hypertrophic chondrocytes (Fig. 2). Synthesis of latent TGF-β-binding protein by growth zone chondrocytes is regulated by 1α,25(OH)$_2$D$_3$ both in vivo and in vitro. 1α,25(OH)$_2$D$_3$ also acts directly on matrix vesicle membranes, increasing phospholipase A$_2$ activity and releasing enzymes that can activate latent TGF-β1. It is now known that 1α,25(OH)$_2$D$_3$ is involved in the release of active stromelysin-1, also called matrix metalloproteinase-3, from matrix vesicles and that this enzyme is responsible for the release of latent TGF-β1 from the matrix and its subsequent activation. Interestingly, TGF-β1 regulates the metabolism of 25(OH)D$_3$ in the growth plate, thereby completing the regulatory feedback loop.

III. ROLE OF 24R,25(OH)$_2$D$_3$

A role for 24R,25(OH)$_2$D$_3$ in the growth plate has been controversial. Rickets can be treated by direct injection of this metabolite into the growth plate, but the possibility exists that this is due to conversion of 24R,25(OH)$_2$D$_3$ to 1,24,25(OH)$_3$D$_3$. In experiments using difluorinated analogues of 24,25(OH)$_2$D$_3$ that prevented further metabolism to 1,24,25(OH)$_3$D$_3$, rapid healing of rickets did not occur, leading to the assumption that 24R,25(OH)$_2$D$_3$ had no active function in the tissue. However, there were a number of studies using rat mandibular condyle organ cultures as an experimental model that argued to the contrary. In addition, the effects of systemically administered 24R,25(OH)$_2$D$_3$ on matrix-processing enzymes in rachitic rat epiphyseal growth plates are very different from the effects of 1α,25(OH)$_2$D$_3$, supporting the contention that they are not due to further metabolism of the metabolite on the 1-carbon. Moreover, specific binding of radiolabeled 24,25(OH)$_2$D$_3$ was found in the growth plate by autoradiography, indicating that receptors for this metabolite are present. Although a nuclear receptor for this vitamin D metabolite has not been purified to homogeneity, recent studies indicate that membrane receptors specific for 24R,25(OH)$_2$D$_3$ exist.

Cell culture studies confirm that 24R,25(OH)$_2$D$_3$ directly affects rat costochondral growth plate chondrocytes, but the response to this metabolite is primarily seen in cells from the resting zone. 24R,25(OH)$_2$D$_3$ stimulates matrix vesicle alkaline phosphatase activity, but it inhibits phospholipase A$_2$ activity and decreases the production of PGE1 and PGE2. The activity of matrix-processing enzymes in matrix vesicles is also decreased. 24R,25(OH)$_2$D$_3$ stimulates the synthesis of latent TGF-β-binding protein by resting zone cells both in vivo and in vitro,

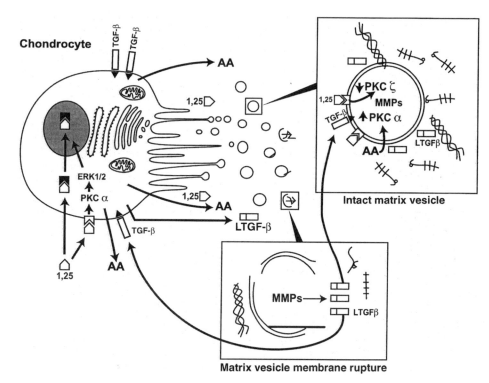

FIGURE 2 Growth plate chondrocytes secrete 1,25(OH)$_2$D$_3$ (1,25) into the extracellular matrix, where it acts directly on matrix vesicles via membrane-associated receptors (1,25-mVDR), decreasing protein kinase C ζ (PKC ζ) activity. Alkaline phosphatase and phospholipase A$_2$ activities are also increased, leading to increased local phosphate concentration, calcium phosphate crystal formation (line on inner surface of matrix vesicle membrane), and destabilization of the membrane. The mineral within the matrix vesicle provides calcification initiation sites. Matrix-processing enzymes are released into the matrix, causing proteoglycan degradation and facilitating further calcification. Matrix vesicle stromelysin-1 releases and activates latent TGF-β1 stored in the matrix. TGF-β1 can then act back on the cell. Secreted 1,25(OH)$_2$D$_3$ also binds to the 1,25-mVDR on the cell membrane, causing activation of PKC and MAP kinase, ultimately leading to new gene expression. 1,25(OH)$_2$D$_3$ binds to the 1,25-nVDR as well, also contributing to genomic regulation of the cells. Phospholipase A$_2$ is activated by 1,25(OH)$_2$D$_3$, releasing arachidonic acid, which can participate in the cell response and act on matrix vesicle PKC as well.

but this metabolite is not involved in the activation of latent TGF-β. These observations all suggest that 24R,25(OH)$_2$D$_3$ modulates the differentiation of the cells, but down-regulates matrix turnover that leads to calcification of the matrix. This is supported by the fact that 24R,25(OH)$_2$D$_3$ causes uptake rather than release of Ca^{2+}.

However, these results do not explain how injection of 24R,25(OH)$_2$D$_3$ into a rachitic growth plate can lead to repair of a rachitic lesion. It is now known that 24R,25(OH)$_2$D$_3$ induces resting zone cells to acquire a growth zone phenotype. Short-term exposure to 24R,25(OH)$_2$D$_3$ increases the proliferation of resting zone cells, and this is accompanied by an increase in the levels of stathmin. Prolonged exposure to 24R,25(OH)$_2$D$_3$ causes a decrease in proliferation. Responsiveness to the metabolite is also reduced, and the cells become responsive to

1α,25(OH)$_2$D$_3$. In addition, 24R,25(OH)$_2$D$_3$ regulates the expression and activity of 1-hydroxylase, leading to production of 1,25(OH)$_2$D$_3$ and potentially to production of 1,24,25(OH)$_3$D$_3$.

IV. METABOLISM OF 25(OH)D$_3$

The fact that growth plate cartilage has the ability to metabolize 25(OH)D$_3$ has been known for some time. Recent studies using the rat costochondral cartilage cell model have enabled us to examine the mechanisms involved. Resting zone and growth zone chondrocytes constitutively produce 1,25(OH)$_2$D$_3$ and 24,25(OH)$_2$D$_3$ at levels that are comparable to kidney cells, with production of 1,25(OH)$_2$D$_3$ being greater than production of 24,25(OH)$_2$D$_3$. This correlates with mRNA levels for 1-hydroxylase

(Cyp27B1) and 24-hydroxylase (Cyp24), as well as with constitutive activities of these enzymes. The metabolism of $25(OH)D_3$ is regulated in a cell-specific manner. In resting zone cells, the production of $1,25(OH)_2D_3$ is regulated by TGF-β1 within 1 h and by dexamethasone within 24 h. Production of $24,25(OH)_2D_3$ is regulated by TGF-β1 within 24 h, suggesting that it may be due to the earlier increase in $1,25(OH)_2D_3$. This is in fact the case. TGF-β1 stimulates an increase in 24-hydroxylase gene expression and activity, whereas expression of 1-hydroxylase is decreased. In contrast to its effects on $25(OH)D_3$ metabolism in resting zone cells, TGF-β1 has no effect on the production of either $1,25(OH)_2D_3$ or $24,25(OH)_2D_3$ in growth zone cell cultures. $24R,25(OH)_2D_3$ decreases 24-hydroxylase and 1-hydroxylase activity in resting zone cells, but affects neither hydroxylase in growth zone cells. $1\alpha,25(OH)_2D_3$ increases 24-hydroxylase activity and $24,25(OH)_2D_3$ production in growth zone cells but has no effect on 1-hydroxylase activity.

These complex interrelationships indicate that the secreted hormones can act back on the cells that produce them. The 24-hydroxylase gene Cyp24 has a $1\alpha,25(OH)_2D_3$-response element in its promoter, but to date there have been no reports of a $1\alpha,25(OH)_2D_3$-response element in the promoter of the Cyp27B1 gene. Recent studies indicate that both promoters contain activator protein 1 (AP-1) sites, and AP-1 is sensitive to mitogen-activated protein (MAP) kinase, which is activated by $24R,25(OH)_2D_3$ in resting zone cells and by $1\alpha,25(OH)_2D_3$ in growth zone cells. These observations suggest that the secreted metabolites may modulate their own metabolism through mechanisms that are independent of the nuclear vitamin D receptor (1,25-nVDR) or that augment the actions of the 1,25-nVDR.

V. MEMBRANE-MEDIATED ACTIONS

Rat costochondral growth plate chondrocytes produce $1,25(OH)_2D_3$ and $24,25(OH)_2D_3$ at levels that correspond to those at which biological effects are observed in cell culture, 10^{-8} and 10^{-7} M, respectively. This also corresponds to the amount of radiolabeled $1,25(OH)_2D_3$ and $24,25(OH)_2D_3$ found in the growth plates of vitamin D replete rats treated with radiolabeled $25(OH)D_3$. These observations indicate that locally produced metabolites are important in the physiology of the cells and suggest that they act in an autocrine or paracrine manner. In fact, $1\alpha,25(OH)_2D_3$ and $24R,25(OH)_2D_3$ act directly

on the cells via mechanisms involving activation of protein kinase C α (PKC α) by specific membrane-associated receptors (1,25-mVDR; 24, 25-mVDR). Both resting zone cells and growth zone cells possess both types of membrane receptors, yet the effects of $1\alpha,25(OH)_2D_3$ are limited to growth zone cells and the effects of $24R,25(OH)_2D_3$ are limited to resting zone cells. It is now known that distinctly different mechanisms are responsible for the action of the metabolites in their target cells.

$1\alpha,25(OH)_2D_3$ causes a rapid increase in arachidonic acid release via cytosolic phospholipase A_2. The arachidonic acid acts as a co-factor, activating PKC α directly. It also serves as a substrate for constitutive cyclooxygenase 1 (COX-1), resulting in increased prostaglandin production. Inhibition of COX-1 inhibits the action of $1\alpha,25(OH)_2D_3$ on PKC as well as the membrane-mediated effects of $1\alpha,25(OH)_2D_3$ on the physiology of the cell. PGE2 produced as a consequence of $1\alpha,25(OH)_2D_3$ action on growth zone cells acts on its own prostaglandin E type 1 (EP1) receptors, increasing PKC through a protein kinase A-dependent mechanism. $1\alpha,25(OH)_2D_3$ also activates phosphatidylinositol-specific phospholipase C-β, leading to the formation of diacylglycerol and inositol 1,4,5-trisphosphate (IP_3). Diacylglycerol binds to cytosolic PKC α and activates the translocation of the enzyme to the plasma membrane, thereby increasing the plasma membrane enzyme activity. The released IP_3 activates the release of Ca^{2+} from the endoplasmic reticulum, which is also a co-factor for PKC α. These effects of $1\alpha,25(OH)_2D_3$ on PKC are mediated by the 1,25-mVDR.

$24R,25(OH)_2D_3$ also activates PKC α, but it can do so only in resting zone cells. $24R,25(OH)_2D_3$ causes a rapid decrease in arachidonic acid release, followed by an increase in release after 15 min. Production of prostaglandin is also reduced. The action of PGE2 on its EP1 receptor inhibits PKC activity in these cells, so reduction of PGE2 has the effect of reducing the inhibition, in essence contributing to the stimulatory effect of $24R,25(OH)_2D_3$ on the enzyme. $24R,25(OH)_2D_3$ also causes an increase in diacylglycerol production but there is no corresponding increase in IP_3. Instead, the diacylglycerol is a result of the activation of phospholipase D. Moreover, translocation of PKC α to the plasma membrane does not occur.

Many of the physiological effects of $1\alpha,25(OH)_2D_3$ on growth zone cells and of $24R,25(OH)_2D_3$ on resting zone cells are mediated, at least in part, by the activation of PKC α. Some of these effects do not require new gene expression, but other effects clearly have a genomic component. For $1\alpha,25(OH)_2D_3$, the 1,25-nVDR is likely to play a role. However, an equivalent receptor for $24R,25(OH)_2D_3$ has not been isolated, raising the possibility that any genomic response may be mediated through other mechanisms, such as the 24,25-mVDR. In other systems, MAP kinase has been shown to mediate the downstream effects of the PKC α-dependent signaling pathway. This appears to be the case in cartilage as well. $1\alpha,25(OH)_2D_3$ activates the extracellular signal-related kinase 1/2 (ERK1/2) family of MAP kinases at the same time that peak activation of PKC α is observed. Similarly, $24R,25(OH)_2D_3$ activates ERK1/2 MAP kinase at the time that peak increases in PKC α occur in resting zone cells.

These experiments explain how $1\alpha,25(OH)_2D_3$ and $24R,25(OH)_2D_3$ exert their membrane-mediated effects in the chondrocytes but they do not explain how secreted metabolites can elicit one set of responses in the cells but another set of responses in matrix vesicles. Matrix vesicles are produced by resting zone and growth zone chondrocytes under genetic control. $1\alpha,25(OH)_2D_3$ increases PKC activity in matrix vesicles produced by growth zone cells by increasing the synthesis of protein kinase ζ (PKC ζ). Similarly, $24R,25(OH)_2D_3$ increases PKC activity in matrix vesicles produced by resting zone cells by increasing the synthesis of PKC ζ. Thus, one mechanism for discriminating the effects of the vitamin D metabolites on matrix vesicles versus cells is by differential segregation of PKC isoforms; PKC α predominates in the cell and PKC ζ predominates in the matrix vesicle. In addition, when matrix vesicles are incubated directly with the vitamin D metabolites, the responsive isoform is PKC ζ rather than PKC α, and activity is decreased rather than increased. These effects are mediated by the membrane receptors for each metabolite and are by definition nongenomic because matrix vesicles lack DNA and RNA. In addition to the direct regulation of PKC ζ by $1\alpha,25(OH)_2D_3$ and $24R,25(OH)_2D_3$, matrix vesicle PKC is regulated by arachidonic acid, causing an increase in enzyme activity. Since arachidonic acid is a co-factor for PKC α, which is also present in the matrix vesicles, it is likely that this is the affected isoform. Arachidonic acid is released by growth zone chondrocytes as a consequence of the action of $1\alpha,25(OH)_2D_3$ on phospholipase A_2, providing another membrane-mediated mechanism by which the cell can transmit signals to the extracellular organelles and regulate their activity nongenomically.

VI. SUMMARY

This article has described how two metabolites of vitamin D, $1\alpha,25(OH)_2D_3$ and $24R,25(OH)_2D_3$, regulate the physiology of growth plate cartilage. Each metabolite exerts its effects primarily on a subset of the cells as the chondrocytes mature through the endochondral lineage cascade. Some of the responses are mediated through traditional 1,25-nVDR mechanisms, resulting in new gene expression and protein synthesis. Other responses involve the action of membrane-associated receptors for each metabolite, and these too can result in gene expression through the PKC α signaling pathway and MAP kinase activation. $1\alpha,25(OH)_2D_3$ and $24R,25(OH)_2D_3$ also exert direct effects on extracellular organelles via their respective membrane receptors, thereby modulating matrix maturation, growth factor activation, and calcification.

Glossary

chondrocyte Cartilage cell.
matrix vesicles Extracellular organelles produced by chondrocytes that are sites for initiation of calcification and also contain matrix-processing enzymes.
1,25-nVDR Nuclear receptor for $1\alpha,25(OH)_2D_3$.
1,25-mVDR Membrane-associated receptor for $1\alpha,25(OH)_2D_3$.
24,25-mVDR Membrane-associated receptor for $24R,25(OH)_2D_3$.

See Also the Following Articles

Vitamin D • Vitamin D and Human Nutrition • Vitamin D-Binding Protein • Vitamin D: Biological Effects of $1,25(OH)_2D_3$ in Bone • Vitamin D Deficiency, Rickets and Osteomalacia • Vitamin D: 24,25-Dihydroxyvitamin D • Vitamin D Metabolism

Further Reading

Balmain, N., Hauchecorne, M., Pike, J. W., Cuisinier-Gleizes, P., and Matlieu, H. (1993). Distribution and subcellular immunolocalization of 1,25-dihydroxyvitamin D3 receptors in rat epiphyseal cartilage. Cell. Mol. Biol. 39, 339–350.
Boyan, B. D., Dean, D. D., Sylvia, V. L., and Schwartz, Z. (1997). Cartilage and vitamin D: Genomic and nongenomic regulation by 1,25-(OH)2D3 and 24,25-(OH)2D3. In "Vitamin D" (D. Feldman, F. H. Glorieux and J. W. Pike, eds.), pp. 395–421. Academic Press, San Diego, CA.
Boyan, B. D., Sylvia, V. L., Dean, D. D., Del Toro, F., and Schwartz, Z. (2002). Differential regulation of growth plate chondrocytes by 1,25-(OH)2D3 and 24,25-(OH)2D3 involves cell maturation specific membrane receptor activated phospholipid metabolism. Crit. Rev. Oral Biol. Med. 13, 143–154.
Dean, D. D., Schwartz, Z., Muniz, O. E., Carreno, M. R., Maeda, S., Howell, D. S., and Boyan, B. D. (2001). Effect of 1α,

$25(OH)_2D_3$ and $24R,25(OH)_2D_3$ on metalloproteinase activity and cell maturation in growth plate cartilage in vivo. *Endocrine* **14**, 311–323.

Kato, S. (1999). Genetic mutation in the human 25-hydroxyvitamin D_3 1α-hydroxylase gene causes vitamin D-dependent rickets type I. *Mol. Cell. Endocrinol.* **156**, 7–12.

Maeda, S., Dean, D. D., Gay, I., Schwartz, Z., and Boyan, B. D. (2001). Activation of latent transforming growth factor-β1 by stromelysin 1 in extracts of growth plate chondrocyte-derived matrix vesicles. *J. Bone Miner. Res.* **16**, 1281–1290.

Nemere, I., Schwartz, Z., Pedrozo, H., Sylvia, V. L., Dean, D. D., and Boyan, B. D. (1998). Identification of a membrane receptor for 1,25-dihydroxy vitamin D_3 which mediates rapid activation of protein kinase C. *J. Bone Miner. Res.* **13**, 1353–1359.

Ohyama, Y., Ozono, K., Uchida, M., Shinki, T., Kato, S., Suda, T., Yamamoto, O., Noshiro, M., and Kato, Y. (1994). Identification of a vitamin D-responsive element in the 5′-flanking region of the rat 25-hydroxyvitamin D_3 24-hydroxylase gene. *J. Biol. Chem.* **269**, 10545–10550.

Pedrozo, H. A., Boyan, B. D., Mazock, J., Dean, D. D., Gomez, R., and Schwartz, Z. (1999). TGF-β1 regulates 25-hydroxyvitamin D_3 1α- and 24-hydroxylase activity in cultured growth plate chondrocytes in a maturation-dependent manner. *Calcif. Tissue Int.* **64**, 50–56.

Pedrozo, H. A., Schwartz, Z., Mokeyev, T., Ornoy, A., Xin-Sheng, W., Bonewald, L. F., Dean, D. D., and Boyan, B. D. (1999). Vitamin D_3 metabolites regulate LTBP1 and latent TGF-β1 expression and latent TGF-β1 incorporation in the extracellular matrix of chondrocytes. *J. Cell. Biochem.* **72**, 151–165.

Pedrozo, H. A., Schwartz, Z., Rimes, S., Sylvia, V. L., Nemere, I., Posner, G. H., Dean, D. D., and Boyan, B. D. (1999). Physiological importance of the $1,25\text{-}(OH)_2D_3$ membrane receptor and evidence for a membrane receptor specific for 24, $25\text{-}(OH)_2D_3$. *J. Bone Miner. Res.* **14**, 856–867.

Schwartz, Z., Dean, D. D., Walton, J. K., Brooks, B. P., and Boyan, B. D. (1995). Treatment of resting zone chondrocytes with 24, 25-dihydroxyvitamin D_3 $[24,25\text{-}(OH)_2D_3]$ induces differentiation into a $1,25\text{-}(OH)_2D_3$-responsive phenotype characteristic of growth zone chondrocytes. *Endocrinology* **136**, 402–411.

Schwartz, Z., Pedrozo, H. A., Sylvia, V. L., Gomez, R., Dean, D. D., and Boyan, B. D. (2001). $1α,25\text{-}(OH)_2D_3$ regulates 25-hydroxyvitamin D_3 24R-hydroxylase activity in growth zone costochondral growth plate chondrocytes via protein kinase C. *Calcif. Tissue Int.* **69**, 365–372.

Schwartz, Z., Sylvia, V. L., Del Toro, F., Hardin, R. R., Dean, D. D., and Boyan, B. D. (2000). $24R,25\text{-}(OH)_2D_3$ mediates its membrane receptor-dependent effects on protein kinase C and alkaline phosphatase via phospholipase A_2 and cyclooxygenase-1 (Cox-1) but not Cox-2 in growth plate chondrocytes. *J. Cell. Physiol.* **182**, 390–401.

Seo, E. G., Schwartz, Z., Dean, D. D., Norman, A. W., and Boyan, B. D. (1996). Preferential accumulation in vivo of 24R,25-dihydroxyvitamin D_3 in growth plate cartilage of rats. *Endocrine* **5**, 147–155.

Sylvia, V. L., Schwartz, Z., Del Toro, F., DeVeau, P., Whetstone, R., Dean, D. D., and Boyan, B. D. (2001). $24R,25\text{-}(OH)_2D_3$ regulates phospholipase D2 (PLD2) activity of costochondral chondrocytes in a metabolite specific and cell maturation dependent manner. *Biochim. Biophys. Acta* **1499**, 209–221.

Vitamin D and Human Nutrition

NORMAN H. BELL

Medical University of South Carolina

I. INTRODUCTION
II. RICKETS
III. OSTEOMALACIA
IV. OSTEOPOROSIS
V. TREATMENT
VI. SUMMARY

Vitamin D is an essential fat-soluble vitamin that is acquired from dietary sources or by dermal synthesis in response to exposure to sunlight. Nutritional deficiency of vitamin D causes rickets in infants and children and osteomalacia in adults; it may also be a contributing factor in the development of osteoporosis and fractures in the elderly. Treatment with vitamin D can correct and prevent these bone diseases.

I. INTRODUCTION

Vitamin D, an essential fat-soluble vitamin, is derived from the diet as vitamin D_2 (irradiated ergosterol) or by dermal synthesis from 7-dehydrocholesterol as vitamin D_3 in response to solar ultraviolet light and body heat. Vitamin D itself is biologically inactive and must undergo hydroxylation in the liver to form 25-hydroxyvitamin D [25(OH)D] and in the kidney to form 1,25-dihydroxyvitamin D $[1,25(OH)_2D]$, by vitamin D 25-hydroxylase and 25(OH)D-1α-hydroxylase, respectively. The metabolites of vitamin D_2 and D_3 have similar biologic activity, although those of vitamin D_2 are less toxic. 24-Hydroxylase is the rate-limiting enzyme for degradation of 25(OH)D and $1,25(OH)_2D$ and is genomically induced by $1,25(OH)_2D$.

Nutritional deficiency of vitamin D leads to rickets in infants and children and to osteomalacia in adults and can be a contributing factor to the development of osteoporosis and fractures in older adults. These bone diseases can be corrected and prevented by treatment with vitamin D. Dark-skinned individuals who reside in areas of limited sunlight exposure are at particular risk for developing vitamin D deficiency and its consequences. This occurs because melanin pigment in skin absorbs the photons of light energy and prevents activation of 7-dehydrocholesterol to eventually form vitamin D_3. Vitamin D deficiency is prevalent worldwide, especially in underdeveloped countries where foods are not fortified.

II. RICKETS

Deficiency of vitamin D is the major cause of rickets in infants and children and results from inadequate exposure to sunlight or intake of dietary vitamin D. Except for oily fishes and fortified foods, the normal diet provides little in the way of vitamin D so that adequate dermal exposure to sunlight or supplementation of vitamin D is essential to prevent rickets. In human milk, the concentrations of vitamin D and 25(OH)D are not adequate to meet daily requirements. Thus, rickets occurs in breast-fed infants who are not given vitamin D supplements, in infants before they are able to walk and be outdoors, in children living at extremes of latitude, and in children who have diminished exposure of skin as a consequence of excess clothing and lack of exposure to sunlight. African American infants with dark skin are at particular risk. In underdeveloped countries in the Middle East, for example, vitamin D deficiency is prevalent in Arab adults and children who reside near the equator because of avoidance of sunlight, wearing of clothes and veils that cover the body, lack of vitamin D supplements, and consumption of nonfortified foods and diets that are low in calcium or high in inhibitors of calcium absorption. Vitamin D deficiency also occurs in vegetarians and those who consume macrobiotic diets, regardless of where they live.

Deficiency of vitamin D leads to decrease in serum 25(OH)D and 1,25(OH)$_2$D and the intestinal absorption of calcium that in turn causes hypocalcemia, secondary hyperparathyroidism, and hypophosphatemia and results in diminished mineralization of the skeleton (Fig. 1). A decrease in serum 25(OH)D is the hallmark of vitamin D deficiency.

Children with rickets may have muscle weakness, stridor (a harsh, high-pitched respiratory sound), a waddling gait, impaired growth, and fractures and may have cataracts, seizures, tetany sometimes associated with carpopedal spasm, and a positive Chvostek sign as a consequence of hypocalcemia and tetany. Dental problems include delayed tooth eruption, defects in tooth structure, and increased incidence of caries. Patients are prone to develop pneumonia. It is not clear whether this is caused by immune deficiency as a consequence of vitamin D

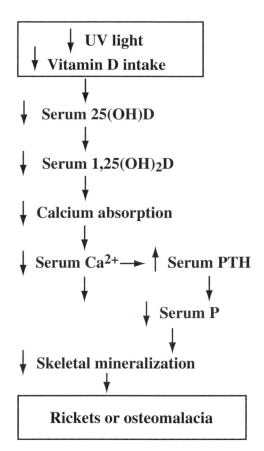

FIGURE 1   Pathogenesis of rickets and osteomalacia.

deficiency or myopathy resulting in poor clearing of bronchopulmonary secretions. Myopathy may include left ventricular myocardial dysfunction. These abnormalities are all corrected by vitamin D and adequate calcium intake.

The rate of growth of different bones varies with age. Since skeletal deformities develop at sites of rapid growth, skeletal changes of rickets vary with age and may indicate the age of onset of the disease. With rapid growth in neonates, the skull is particularly affected. Softening of the cranium or craniotabes may occur with parietal flattening, frontal bossing, and widened sutures. Rapid growth of the arms and rib cage in early childhood is associated with widening of the forearm at the wrist and thickening of the costochondral junctions that results in the rachitic rosary. There may be forward projection of the breastbone or "pigeon chest" and scoliosis or kyphosis of the spine. Indentations of the lower ribs at the site of attachment of the diaphragm may occur and are called Harrison's groove. With rapid growth of long bones, bowing of the lower extremities, genu varus (bowleg) or valgus (knock-knee), may result because of weight-bearing. Deformities of the pelvis may also occur and may severely compromise weight-bearing. Secondary hyperparathyroidism may cause resorption of the phalanges and distal ends of long bones, such as the clavicles and humeri.

Biochemical findings include low serum 25(OH)D, calcium, and phosphorus and elevated serum immunoreactive parathyroid hormone (PTH) and alkaline phosphatase. Serum 1,25(OH)$_2$D may be low, normal, or increased depending on the degree of 25(OH)D deficiency and secondary hyperparathyroidism. When present, increases in serum 1,25(OH)$_2$D induce 24-hydroxylase, enhance degradation of 25(OH)D and 1,25(OH)$_2$D, and hasten the development of vitamin D deficiency.

III. OSTEOMALACIA

Osteomalacia caused by nutritional deficiency of vitamin D occurs primarily in Asian Indians and Pakistanis, more commonly in those who live far from the equator and have limited exposure to sunlight. Inadequate intake of vitamin D, increased skin pigmentation, practice of purdah by women in which veils are worn during pregnancy, parturition, and lactation, and consumption of a vegetarian diet are contributing factors.

Patients with osteomalacia may be asymptomatic or have muscle weakness and diffuse skeletal pain in the lower back, hip, or sites of fractures. Decreased skeletal density is the most common X-ray finding. Looser zones or pseudo-fractures may occur and are typically bilateral and symmetrical. Common sites are axillary margins of the scapulae, lower ribs, superior and inferior pubic rami, inner margins and neck of the proximal femora, and posterior margins of the proximal ulnae. Bone resorption caused by secondary hyperparathyroidism is sometimes the most prominent radiographic finding.

In patients with osteomalacia, bone density determined by dual-photon absorptiometry is reduced and bone scans show increased uptake of technetium-99m pyrophosphate by long bones and wrists and prominence of the calvaria and mandible. Beading of the costochondral junctions may occur and increased tracer uptake by the sternum and its margins produces the so-called "tie sternum." Pseudo-fractures appear as hot spots.

IV. OSTEOPOROSIS

Vitamin D deficiency is often present in older men and women. Decreased dermal production of 7-dehydrocholesterol, the precursor of vitamin D$_3$, decreased

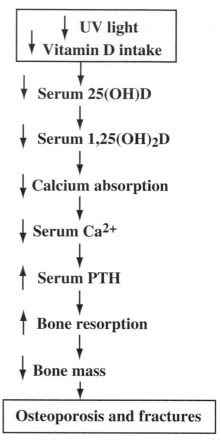

FIGURE 2   Pathogenesis of osteoporosis.

exposure intake of vitamin D, decreased exposure to sunlight, down-regulation of the vitamin D receptor in the small intestine, and decreased production of 25(OH)D and 1,25(OH)$_2$D are contributing factors. Older individuals may be house-bound as well. In addition to vitamin D, calcium intake is often inadequate in older men and women.

Deficiency of vitamin D leads to decrease in serum 25(OH)D and 1,25(OH)$_2$D, the intestinal absorption of calcium that in turn causes hypocalcemia, secondary hyperparathyroidism, increased bone resorption, bone loss, osteoporosis, and fractures (Fig. 2).

V. TREATMENT

The most recent recommended daily intakes of vitamin D and calcium by the National Academy of Science are listed in Table 1; values for vitamin D range from 200 IU per day in children to 600 IU per day in older individuals. The normal range for serum 25(OH)D is between 10 and 60 ng/ml. However, an increase in circulating PTH is the most sensitive

TABLE I Recommendations for Daily Intake of Calcium and Vitamin D

Age (years)	Calcium (mg)	Vitamin D (IU)[a]
4–8	800	200
9–18	1300	200
19–50	1000	200
51–65	1200	400
>65	1200	600

[a]1 IU equals 15 ng.

indicator of vitamin D deficiency, and the lowest value for serum 25(OH)D at which there is a plateau of circulating immunoreactive PTH ranges from approximately 30 to 40 ng/ml. In a recent study, serum 25(OH)D (28 to 50 ng/ml) and serum and urinary calcium remained in the normal range in normal men and women given 4000 IU per day for 2 to 5 months. Furthermore, a comprehensive review of the literature indicated that serum 25(OH)D does not begin to increase abnormally and cause hypercalcemia until a daily dose of more than 10,000 IU is administered. Thus, there is a wide margin of safety between therapeutic and toxic doses of vitamin D.

In patients with rickets or osteomalacia, the goals of treatment are to correct and prevent the effects of hypocalcemia, cataracts, seizures, and skeletal effects of secondary hyperparathyroidism, to prevent and correct the skeletal deformities of rickets and osteomalacia, to prevent hypercalcemia, hypercalciuria, and their consequences, and to produce normal growth and development of the skeleton in children.

Vitamin D deficiency is treated with vitamin D. Although 400 IU per day of the vitamin is an adequate maintenance dose, the initial dose should be larger, perhaps 1200 IU per day.

Stoss therapy with an intramuscular dose of 150,000 IU of vitamin D or more is recommended by some. Excess vitamin D produces intoxication that is associated with hypercalcemia and hypercalciuria; it is caused by increased circulating 25(OH)D and is produced by daily doses in excess of 10,000 IU. Serum 1,25(OH)$_2$D is usually in the normal range. Available evidence indicates that hypercalcemia does not occur at doses of 10,000 IU per day of vitamin D or less. Vitamin D intoxication is treated by discontinuing the vitamin D, by forcing fluids, and, if necessary, by treatment with dexamethasone or hydrocortisone.

Although it is well documented that elderly subjects may be deficient in vitamin D, that vitamin D deficiency can lead to secondary hyperparathyroidism, increased bone resorption, and increased bone loss, and that the incidence of fractures can be reduced by treatment with vitamin D and calcium, results of studies in which 25(OH)D$_3$ and calcium were given separately to men and women show that calcium is more effective than 25(OH)D$_3$ at increasing bone mineral density. The recommended intake for calcium in individuals over the age of 65 years is 1200 mg per day.

VI. SUMMARY

Vitamin D deficiency is prevalent especially in underdeveloped countries where foods are not fortified with vitamin D. Breast-fed infants, particularly African American infants, are at risk for rickets if they are not given vitamin D or exposed to sunlight. Asian Indians and Pakistanis are at risk for developing rickets and osteomalacia especially when they have limited access to sunlight and vitamin D. Aging men and women are prone to vitamin D deficiency, osteoporosis, and fractures and can be treated with calcium and vitamin D. Recent evidence indicates that daily doses of vitamin D as high as 4000 IU are well tolerated and do not increase serum 25(OH)D or serum or urinary calcium abnormally.

Glossary

carpopedal spasm Spasm of the wrist and foot produced by hypocalcemia and tetany.

Chvostek's sign A spasm of the facial muscles in response to tapping of the facial nerve that is caused by hypocalcemia and tetany.

craniotabes Caused by softening of the cranium and associated with parietal flattening of the sides of the skull, frontal bossing or exaggeration of the curvature of the forehead, and widened sutures or sites of attachment of bones to one another.

kyphosis Enhanced curvature of the spine as seen from the side, or hunchback.

osteomalacia A bone disease that occurs in adults as a result of vitamin D deficiency and that is caused by abnormal mineralization of the skeleton and weak bone that is prone to bend and fracture.

osteoporosis A bone disease that is characterized by decreased bone mass and alterations in microarchitecture, resulting in increased skeletal fragility and risk of fracture.

pigeon chest The forward projection of the breastbone that occurs with rickets.

pseudo-fracture A thickening of periosteum or bone surface and formation of new bone over what appears to be a fracture on X ray. It is usually found at the site of a pulsating artery and may result from softening of bone and arterial pulsation.

rachitic rosary Caused by thickening of the costochondral junctions of the ribs.

rickets A bone disease that occurs in children as a result of vitamin D deficiency and is caused by abnormal mineralization of the skeleton and weak bone that is prone to bend and fracture. Rapid growth of the arms and rib cage in early childhood is associated with widening of the forearm at the wrist and scoliosis or kyphosis of the spine. Indentations of the lower ribs at the site of attachment of the diaphragm may occur and are called Harrison's groove.

scoliosis A lateral curvature of the spine.

See Also the Following Articles

Osteoporosis: Hormonal Treatment • Osteoporosis: Pathophysiology • Vitamin D • Vitamin D and Cartilage • Vitamin D: Biological Effects of 1,25(OH)₂D₃ in Bone • Vitamin D: Biological Effects of 1,25(OH)₂D₃ in the Intestine and Kidney • Vitamin D Deficiency, Rickets and Osteomalacia • Vitamin D Metabolism

Further Reading

Awumey, E. M. K., Mitra, D. A., Hollis, B. W., Kumar, R., and Bell, N. H. (1998). Vitamin D metabolism is altered in Asian Indians in the southern United States: A Clinical Research Center Study. *J. Clin. Endocrinol. Metab.* **83**, 169–173.

Bell, N. H. (2001). Osteomalacia and rickets. *In* "Principles and Practice of Endocrinology and Metabolism" (K. Becker, K. L. Bilezikian, W. J. Bremner, W. Hung, C. R. Kahn, L. D. Loriaux, E. S. Nylen, R. W. Rebar, G. L. Robertson, R. H. Snider, Jr., L. Wartofsky, eds.), 3rd ed., pp. 615–623. Lippincott Williams & Wilkins, Philadelphia.

Chapuy, M.-C., and Meunier, P. J. (1997). Vitamin D insufficiency in adults and the elderly. *In* "Vitamin D" (D. Feldman, F. H. Glorieux, and J. W. Pike, eds.), pp. 679–693. Academic Press, San Diego, CA.

Chesney, R. W. (2001). Vitamin D deficiency and rickets. *Rev. Endocrinol. Metab. Dis.* **2**, 145–151.

Fuleihan, G. E.-H., Nabulsi, M., Choucair, M., Salamoun, M., Shahine, C. H., Kizirian, A., and Tannous, R. (2001). Hypovitaminosis D in healthy schoolchildren. *Pediatrics* **107**, E53–E59.

Gannage-Yared, M. H., Chemalii, R., Yaacoub, N., and Halaby, G. (2000). Hypovitaminosis D in a sunny country: Relation to lifestyle and bone markers. *J. Bone Miner. Res.* **15**, 1856–1862.

Kreiter, S. R., Schwartz, R. P., Kirkman, H. N., Jr., Charlton, P. A., Calikoglu, A. S., and Davenport, M. L. (2000). Nutritional rickets in African American breast-fed infants. *J. Pediatr.* **137**, 153–157.

Lips, P., Duong, T., Oleksik, A., Black, D., Cummings, S., Cox, D., and Nickelsen, T. (2001). A global study of vitamin D status and parathyroid function in postmenopausal women with osteoporosis: Baseline data from the multiple outcomes of raloxifene evaluation clinical trial. *J. Clin. Endocrinol. Metab.* **86**, 1212–1221.

Mitra, D., and Bell, N. H. (1997). Racial, geographic, genetic, and body habitus effects on vitamin D metabolism. *In* "Vitamin D" (D. Feldman, F. H. Glorieux, and J. W. Pike, eds.), pp. 521–532. Academic Press, San Diego, CA.

Peacock, M., Liu, G., Carey, M., McClintock, R., Ambrosius, W., Hui, S., and Johnston, C. C. (2000). Effect of calcium or 25(OH)vitamin D₃ dietary supplementation on bone loss at the hip in men and women over the age of 60. *J. Clin. Endocrinol. Metab.* **85**, 3011–3019.

Pettifor, J. M., and Daniel, E. D. (1997). Vitamin D deficiency and nutritional rickets in children. *In* "Vitamin D" (D. Feldman, F. H. Glorieux, and J. W. Pike, eds.), pp. 663–678. Academic Press, San Diego, CA.

Uysal, S., Kalayci, A. G. J., and Baysal, K. (1999). Cardiac functions in children with vitamin D deficiency rickets. *Pediatr. Cardiol.* **20**, 283–286.

Vieth, R. (1999). Vitamin D supplementation, 25-hydroxyvitamin D concentrations, and safety. *Am. J. Clin. Nutr.* **69**, 842–856.

Vieth, R., Chan, P.-C. R., and MacFarlane, G. D. (2001). Efficacy and safety of vitamin D3 intake exceeding the lowest observed adverse effect level. *Am. J. Clin. Nutr.* **73**, 288–294.

Vitamin D-Binding Protein

IVY HURWITZ AND NANCY E. COOKE
University of Pennsylvania

I. INTRODUCTION
II. REGULATION AND EXPRESSION OF DBP
III. DBP POLYMORPHISMS
IV. DBP FUNCTIONS
V. SUMMARY

Vitamin D-binding protein (DBP) plays a major role in the binding, solubilization, and serum transport of the principal vitamin D metabolites 25-hydroxyvitamin D₃, the major circulating metabolite, and 1,25-dihydroxyvitamin D₃, the more biologically active metabolite. However, circulating DBP concentrations are approximately 20-fold higher than that of total vitamin D metabolites. This large excess is unusual among other serum carrier proteins, suggesting other roles for this protein.

I. INTRODUCTION

Vitamin D-binding protein (DBP), also referred to as group-specific component of serum or Gc-globulin, was initially identified by its polymorphic migration pattern on serum electrophoresis. Although its function remained relatively unknown at that time, its highly polymorphic nature allowed DBP to play a major role in population genetics and forensic medicine. The multifunctionality of DBP has now been recognized. In addition to transporting vitamin D metabolites, DBP is proposed to be involved in the transport of fatty acids, to function as a plasma actin scavenger following tissue damage, and to play a role in complement C5a-mediated chemotaxis, and DBP may be involved in the activation of macrophages.

II. REGULATION AND EXPRESSION OF DBP

DBP is a member of the albumin (ALB), α-fetoprotein (AFP), and α-albumin/afamin (AFM) gene family that is encoded on human chromosome 4. Initial studies have sublocalized the DBP gene to 4q11–q13, and refined mapping of this region has demonstrated that these four related genes are linked in the following order: centromere–3′-DBP-5′–5′-ALB-3′–5′-AFP-3′–5′-AFM-3′–telomere. Despite this linkage and the high degree of sequence and structural similarities among DBP, ALB, AFP, and AFM, the multifunctionality of DBP is a unique characteristic.

The human DBP gene itself is composed of 13 exons and spans over 42 kb from the transcription initiation site to the polyadenylation site. The cDNA structure of DBP was initially reported for humans and was subsequently determined for rat, mouse, rabbit, turtle, and chicken. Turtle DBP occupies a unique niche because it also binds thyroxine. Thus far, DBP appears to be limited to vertebrate species; a search of the *Drosophila melanogaster* genome database revealed no sequence homologues to DBP.

Human DBP mRNA encodes a 458-amino-acid secreted protein following cleavage of its 16-amino-acid signal sequence. DBP is a monomeric protein, migrating at approximately 58 kDa (Table 1). Its exact size is dependent on its glycosylation state. Like other members of the ALB family, DBP is cysteine rich. In the case of DBP, all 28 cysteine residues are present in the disulfide form and define a signature modular structure of three internally repeated peptide domains. Biochemical binding studies initially identified a vitamin D sterol-binding domain near the amino-terminus and an actin-binding domain closer to the carboxyl-terminus. The X-ray crystallographic details of DBP structure including its vitamin D- and actin-binding domains have recently become available. DBP has significant similarity to the α-helical structure of ALB, but the overall three-dimensional orientation of DBP's three internal peptide domains is quite dissimilar and is responsible for its binding properties. The helices of domain I in the N-terminus form an open vitamin D-binding cleft, accessible to

TABLE I Features of DBP

General properties	
Size	58 kDa
Plasma concentration	4–8 μM
Plasma half-life	2.5–3 days
Daily production rate	∼10 mg/kg
Vitamin D-binding abilities	
Plasma capacity	2.4 mg/liter
Affinity	
25(OH)D$_3$	$K_a = 5 \times 10^8$ M^{-1}
1,25(OH)$_2$D$_3$	$K_a = 4 \times 10^7$ M^{-1}
Actin-binding abilities	
Plasma capacity	270 mg/liter
Affinity	$K_a = 2 \times 10^9$ M^{-1}
Macrophage and osteoclast activation abilities	
DBP "activation"	By β-galactosidase and sialidase
Macrophage effects	Increased superoxide production, increased phagocytic activities
Osteoclast effects	Increased osteoclastogenesis
Chemotactic abilities	
C5a enhancement	Binding of DBP to leukocytes
DBP leukocyte-binding site	Chondroitin sulfate proteoglycans
Affinity	Low affinity, nonselective

solvent and lined with hydrophobic residues. Such a cleft cannot be formed in ALB, and this binding cleft is dissimilar to the internal and closed vitamin D-binding pocket in the nuclear vitamin D receptor molecule. The unique organization of DBP's three internal domains compared to ALB is central to its unique ability to bind G-actin. DBP clamps onto G-actin by narrowing the distance between domain I on one side and domains II and III on the other side, by virtue of a hinge at glycine 227. Thus, a very large binding interface is formed by the overall fold of DBP; this may account for the high-affinity association between DBP and actin. Human DBP expression is detected by the end of the first trimester and reaches normal adult circulation levels (4–8 μM) by term. Estimations from kinetic studies suggest that the daily production rate of DBP is approximately 10 mg/kg. The plasma half-life of DBP is 2.5 to 3 days, whereupon it is recycled by megalin or degraded completely in various tissues. The expression of DBP appears to undergo hormonal and growth factor regulation. Modest increases in DBP expression have been reported during pregnancy and in subjects receiving estrogen. In the Hep3B hepatoma cell line, interleukin-6 and dexamethasone were shown to increase DBP mRNA by approximately twofold and transforming growth factor-β decreased DBP mRNA in a dose-dependent fashion by up to fivefold. Decreased DBP titers have also been reported in plasma from patients with advanced liver or kidney disease.

DBP is expressed at low levels in a variety of tissues, but most serum DBP is derived from the liver. Tissue-specific regulation of DBP has been postulated to be dependent on the relative abundance of two transcription factors, hepatocyte nuclear factor 1α (HNF1α) and HNF1β. These two closely related homeodomain-containing transcription factors bind to DNA as either homodimers or heterodimers. The DBP proximal promoter has three functional HNF1-binding sites. In this model, HNF1α homodimers stimulate a high level of DBP expression in the liver. In the kidney, the increased expression of HNF1β, and therefore formation of heterodimers, results in reduced DBP expression. In this situation, HNF1β functions as a *trans*-dominant inhibitor of HNF1α-mediated enhancing activity. The unique role of HNF1 in DBP expression is supported by the observation that DBP expression is reduced by 50% in the livers of HNF1 null mice. These observations would suggest that the net expression of the DBP gene reflects a balance between the two major HNF1 isoforms. Recently, mutations in human HNF1α and HNF1β have been identified to be the cause of some cases of maturity onset diabetes of the young (MODY). Whether or not DBP expression is affected in individuals with these MODY mutations remains undetermined.

III. DBP POLYMORPHISMS

The 3 most common allelic variants of DBP differ based on four single-nucleotide polymorphisms at codons 152, 311, 416, and 420. These protein variants are known as Gc*1F, Gc*1S, or Gc*2, where F and S refers to relative fast or slow migration rate following gel electrophoresis. The gene products of each variant allele differ from one another by amino acid substitution and/or by polysaccharide attachment. In addition to these 3 common alleles, there are over 124 rare variant alleles described to date, thus making DBP one of the most polymorphic proteins known. The geographical occurrences of some of these variants have been correlated with patterns of human migration and are therefore of anthropological interest. The affinities for vitamin D metabolites by several of these DBP isoforms have been determined, and for the most part, it was found that variants with higher isoelectric points have slightly lower ligand affinity. Any biological impli-

cations of these minor changes in binding affinity remain to be identified.

In the late 1980s, there was much controversy linking the expression of different DBP variants with susceptibility to human immunodeficiency virus infection. These initial reports were later proven to be erroneous by many investigators. Multiple studies have also been conducted over the years in an attempt to link the DBP variants to susceptibility or resistance to a variety of diseases such as multiple sclerosis, chronic obstructive pulmonary disease, pulmonary tuberculosis, and even schizophrenia. To date, no conclusive correlation has been reported in any of these cases. More recently, several attempts have been made to link DBP with the occurrence of diabetes. A higher prevalence of the Gc*1S-Gc*2 genotype was observed in type 2 diabetes in Japan. This genotype was also associated with higher fasting insulin levels and a higher index of insulin resistance in nondiabetic Japanese. In this population and in Dogrib Indians, the lowest fasting insulin levels were seen in individuals harboring the Gc*1F-Gc*1F genotype. Interestingly, a difference in response to the oral glucose tolerance test was also observed in nondiabetic Pima Indians with this genotype, suggesting a link between the prediabetic state and DBP genotype. Conversely, in a mixed population study of nondiabetic Hispanic Americans and Caucasians, this Gc*1F-Gc*1F genotype was associated with high fasting glucose levels. Studies in Caucasian populations would suggest that there is no association between DBP genetic variants and disease. These conflicting data may reflect the ethnic diversity in the populations sampled. Nonetheless, it is most unlikely that polymorphisms within the DBP gene are directly related to the diabetic trait.

IV. DBP FUNCTIONS

A. Sterol Binding

Under normal physiological conditions, most circulating vitamin D metabolites are protein bound. DBP binds 88% of serum 25-dihydroxyvitamin D_3 [25(OH)D_3] ($K_a = 5 \times 10^8$ M^{-1}) and 85% of serum 1,25-dihydroxyvitamin D_3 [1,25(OH)$_2$D$_3$] ($K_a = 4 \times 10^7$ M^1), leaving 0.40% "free" and the remainder associated with other serum proteins. Because DBP is in significant molar excess over vitamin D, only approximately 5% of the total circulating DBP actually carries vitamin D metabolites. This large molar excess of serum DBP has been hypothesized to play a role in protecting against vitamin D intoxication by buffering the levels of free vitamin D metabolites. But work using a DBP-deficient (Dbp-null) mouse model had challenged the validity of this idea. Dbp-null mice were generated at the expected Mendelian frequency from intercrosses of Dbp heterozygous animals. These animals are of normal size and appearance. There is no evidence for impairment of fertility in either males or females because intercrosses between Dbp-null animals resulted in normal-sized litters. This conclusion was surprising because extensive population studies had failed to identify a human DBP-null allele. The successful generation of the Dbp-null mice clearly demonstrated that DBP is not essential for viability.

The major role of DBP appears to be in sterol transport. *Dbp*-null mice on normal diets demonstrate only a modest decrease in serum levels of $25(OH)D_3$ and $1,25(OH)_2D_3$, and show no evidence of biological vitamin D deficiency, clearly indicating that free hormone levels are still physiologically adequate. However, when subjected to a vitamin D-deficient diet for 4 to 6 weeks, end-organ effects of vitamin D deficiency become apparent in these animals, suggesting that normal DBP levels offer a degree of protection against short-term, dietary-induced vitamin D deficiency.

To test the buffering capacity of DBP *in vivo*, sublethal doses of vitamin D were administered to *Dbp*-null and wildtype animals. Vitamin D toxicity is manifested by hypercalcemia, bone resorption, and calcification of soft tissues. Surprisingly, *Dbp*-null mice were less susceptible to hypercalcemia and the secondary soft-tissue calcifications of vitamin D toxicity than the wild-type controls. This protection may have arisen secondary to an accelerated clearance of $25(OH)D_3$ from serum and a rapid urinary excretion in the absence of DBP. A partial explanation for this paradoxical phenomenon was provided by the recent hypothesis that megalin in the proximal renal tubule may function to recycle DBP and $25(OH)D_3$.

Megalin/gp330 is a transmembrane protein with a large extracellular domain, a single transmembrane domain, and a short cytoplasmic tail. This protein belongs to the low-density lipoprotein (LDL) receptor family. Megalin is expressed in the proximal brush border surfaces of the kidney epithelium where it appears to function as an endocytic DBP receptor for the reabsorption of apo–DBP and DBP–$25(OH)D_3$ complexes from the glomerular filtrate into the proximal tubular cells (Fig. 1). Here, $25(OH)D_3$ is metabolized to the physiologically active $1,25(OH)_2D_3$. In the absence of DBP, renal uptake and activation of $25(OH)D_3$ via the megalin endocytic recycling pathway would also be absent, thereby resulting in increased $25(OH)D_3$ excretion in

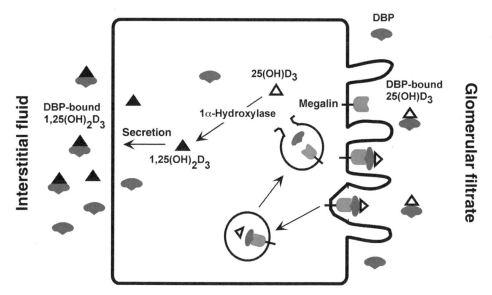

FIGURE 1 Receptor-mediated endocytosis and activation of $25(OH)D_3$ by megalin. DBP-bound $25(OH)D_3$ interacts with megalin located at the brush border surface of the proximal tubule. This complex enters the cell by endocytosis and $25(OH)D_3$ is released and undergoes metabolic activation by 1α-hydroxylase. This active form of vitamin D, $1,25(OH)_2D_3$, is secreted back into the interstitial fluid, where it is rebound by DBP and delivered to target organs. Adapted from White *et al.* (2000). The multifunctional properties and characteristics of vitamin D-binding protein, *Trends in Endocrinology and Metabolism*, **11**, 320–327, with permission from Elsevier Science.

the urine and contributing to the observed resistance to vitamin D toxicity in the *Dbp*-null mice.

Like other members of the LDL receptor family, megalin exhibits broad ligand specificity. Megalin has been demonstrated to bind apolipoproteins, amino-glycosides, receptor-associated protein, and a variety of growth factors as well as DBP. A megalin-deficient mouse model has been generated to further elucidate the significance of this protein. A large percentage of megalin-deficient mice die perinatally from holosprosencephaly. Animals that do survive to adulthood demonstrate severe growth retardation, bone formation defects, and reduced bone density with scalloped bone surfaces. These animals also demonstrate tubular resorption deficiencies and excrete low-molecular-weight plasma proteins in their urine including DBP and albumin, reminiscent of patients with Fanconi syndrome. The loss of plasma carrier proteins such as DBP is concomitant with the loss of 25(OH)D$_3$. The disturbances in bone metabolism in the megalin knockout animals as a consequence of vitamin D deficiency have therefore been attributed to the urinary wasting of DBP–25(OH)D$_3$ complexes. These studies may overemphasize the physiological role of megalin-mediated 25(OH)D$_3$ in reclamation from the urine. Unlike the megalin knockout mice, *Dbp*-null mice are physiologically normal and show no evidence of biological vitamin D deficiency. This clearly indicates that in the absence of DBP, uptake and activation of 25(OH)D$_3$ occur via a pathway that is independent of the proposed DBP–megalin endocytic recycling route. Thus, the role of megalin in vitamin D metabolism and its linkage to DBP recycling remains unclear.

B. Actin Scavenger Activity

DBP is part of an "actin scavenger system" that functions by sequestering G-actin from the circulation for subsequent disposal (Fig. 2). DBP binds monomeric actin (G-actin) with very high affinity ($K_a = 2 \times 10^9 \, M^{-1}$). This interaction occurs independent of sterol binding, and all three common polymorphic forms of DBP appear to have equal avidity for binding to G-actin.

The function of DBP in actin scavenging appears to be interrelated with the function of the protein gelsolin (GSN). Serum GSN functions mainly as a nonenzymatic fibrous actin (F-actin) severing molecule but has been demonstrated to also bind G-actin in the absence of DBP. As the G-actin monomers dissociate from the pointed ends of the severed actin

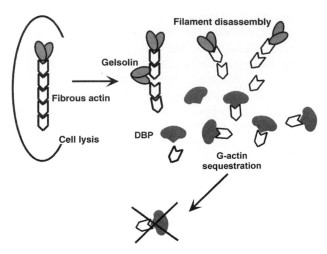

FIGURE 2 DBP and serum gelsolin (GSN) act in concert to prevent actin toxicity following tissue injury. When released from the cell, fibrous actin is disassembled by GSN. Monomeric actin released by this reaction is sequestered by DBP and to some extent by GSN. The bound actin is subsequently cleared from the circulation.

polymer, they are rapidly bound by DBP and cleared from the circulation by Küpffer cells in the liver. The coordinated action of DBP and GSN has been demonstrated to inhibit actin-stimulated platelet aggregation. It is hypothesized that these two serum proteins function in concert to clear free actin from the circulation, thereby preventing the consequences of actin toxicity in the host. For example, G-actin is released into the circulation following tissue injury. If left unattended, G-actin will rapidly polymerize into F-actin, resulting in microemboli that may further damage the microvasculature. DBP–actin and GSN–actin complexes have been reported in the circulation of patients with a wide range of serious illnesses including hepatitis, acute lung injury, septic shock, severe trauma, and pregnancy. The levels of these complexes are also increased following tissue ischemia, inflammation, or injury. Clinical studies have recently described DBP as an acute-phase reactant after major surgery. Studies of rats injected with increasing concentrations of G-actin demonstrate progressive binding followed by saturation of DBP by G-actin. Saturation is then followed by the observation of new F-actin polymers and the appearance of emboli in the microcirculation of the lungs and hearts of these animals, resulting in death. In humans, marked decreases in total DBP followed by increased levels of DBP–actin complexes were reported in patients suffering from multiple organ failure and trauma. Saturation of the DBP–actin scavenger system has been correlated with poor patient survival rates. Although decreases in hepatic DBP production may be due to initial liver damage, the increase in DBP–actin complexes is likely the result of the sequestration of the free actin released from the failing or damaged organs by circulating DBP. Depletion of the circulating pool of DBP often precedes death in these settings.

C. Macrophage Activation and Osteoclastogenesis

Studies suggest that during inflammation DBP is transformed by sequential deglycosylation by two membrane-bound galactosidases into a potent macrophage-activating factor known as DBP–MAF. Increases in superoxide production and phagocytotic activities have been reported in macrophages activated by DBP–MAF *ex vivo*. These activated macrophages have been reported to successfully eradicate Ehrlich ascites tumors in mice. DBP–MAF has also been demonstrated to be an osteoclast activator in rat studies. Because osteoclast progenitor cells are blood-borne cells of the monocyte–macrophage lineage, this connection between macrophage activation and osteoclastogenesis is not totally surprising.

The structural requirements of DBP that relate to its bone resorbing activities were recently examined. It was demonstrated that DBP–MAF activates osteoclasts *ex vivo* in a dose-dependent manner. This activation occurs in the presence or absence of sterol binding to DBP. Furthermore, the study demonstrated that glycosylation of DBP is imperative for its ostesoclast-activating activities. Unglycosylated *Escherichia coli*-expressed recombinant DBP failed to activate osteoclasts, whereas glycosylated DBP expressed in a baculovirus system demonstrated significant osteoclast-activating function. Although it was not demonstrated in this study, it is likely that initial DBP glycosylation is also critical for macrophage activation by the scheme described previously.

The abnormal macrophages of several osteopetrotic mice and rats have been studied in detail. These animal models generally exhibit varying degrees of immunological as well as bone disorders. Analysis of B cells from two different strains of osteopetrotic mice (*mi/mi* and *op/op*) and one osteopetrotic rat (*op*) demonstrated that they lack β-galactosidase activities. This galactosidase has been shown to work in concert with sialidase, found on T cells, to deglyco-sylate DBP to its purported DBP–MAF active form. Treatment of the *op* rat from birth with DBP–MAF resulted in the reversal of the macrophage defect and partially ameliorated bony abnormalities. These results indicated a role for DBP in osteoclastogenesis. However, *Dbp*-null mice do not display bony defects and do not show a defect in macrophage recruitment or activation or in mounting an immune response to microorganisms requiring activated macrophages as the first line of defense. These observations would suggest that DBP–MAF generation is nonessential *in vivo* and that alternative pathways must exist for each of the activities attributed to DBP–MAF.

In vitro experiments demonstrated that whereas the Gc*1 human DBP protein requires sequential treatment by β-galactosidase (B cells) and sialidase (T cells) for activation to DBP–MAF, the Gc*2 DBP protein is predicted to be activated by β-galactosidase alone. A site located between amino acids 416 and 420 in domain III of DBP is thought to be the O-linked glycosylation site for *N*-acetylagalactosamine (GalNAc). Galactose and sialic acid residues are attached to this sugar molecule in the Gc*1 DBP proteins, creating a branched structure. Early work on human DBP has in fact demonstrated that a contributing factor to the difference in electrophoretic mobility between the Gc*1F and the Gc*1S DBP isoforms is related to the number of sialic acid residues attached to this sugar moiety. Treatment of Gc*1F with sialidase results in its migration to the position of GC*1S. Upon activation, the terminal structure of the DBP–MAF derived from the Gc*1 proteins appears to be GalNAc-threonine. The situation for Gc*2 human DBP is unclear. It is proposed that the polysaccharide chain for this isoform of DBP is linear in that it lacks sialic acid. Removal of the terminal galactose by β-galactoside would result in a DBP–MAF structure as described above. However, only a very small percentage of Gc*2 human DBP appears to be O-glycosylated, suggesting that the glycosylation site might be at amino acid 420. A single nucleotide polymorphism (A to C) at this codon results in an amino acid change from threonine (Gc*1) to lysine (Gc*2). The lysine residue cannot be glycosylated. If this were the case, then Gc*2 homozygous individuals would be incapable of utilizing the macrophage activation pathway. Recently, threonine 418 was suggested to be the putative Gc*2 glycosylation site. Evidence supporting this idea, however, is lacking. Further biochemical studies in this area are clearly required.

D. Chemotaxis Enhancing Activity

DBP has been demonstrated to interact with a variety of different cell types. When bound to the surface of leukocytes, DBP plays an essential role in augmenting the chemotactic effect of complement factor C5a for neutrophils, monocytes, and fibroblasts *ex vivo*. DBP has been isolated from bronchoalveolar lavage fluid from patients with chronic obstructive pulmonary disease and adult respiratory distress syndrome, suggesting that it may indeed be a critical player in the inflammatory and chemotactic response to lung injury.

The chemotactic activity of DBP is dependent on its binding to chondroitin sulfate proteoglycans on the cell surface of neutrophils. Unlike DBP's interaction with vitamin D and actin, binding to these cell surface molecules is nonselective and of rather low affinity. Recently, it was reported that binding of DBP to neutrophils plateaus with time, possibly reflecting a steady state between binding and shedding of DBP on the plasma membrane. Inhibition of serine proteases with phenylmethylsulfonyl fluoride appears to disrupt this balance and allows for the accumulation of DBP on the plasma membrane of these cells. By a process of elimination, it was discovered that only inhibitors of neutrophil elastase prevented the loss of membrane-bound DBP-binding activity. A decrease in C5a chemotactic activities was correlated with the loss of DBP from the cell surfaces. Taken together, these results would suggest that neutrophil elastase plays a regulatory role in DBP-mediated C5a chemotactic activities. The exact mechanism by which DBP mediates its co-chemotactic response to C5a remains to be elucidated.

V. SUMMARY

DBP is a multifunctional protein that plays a critical role in regulating the bioavailability of $25(OH)D_3$. New data implicate DBP as a ligand for the endocytic recycling receptor, megalin. The folding of DBP's three internal structural domains results in a large, high-affinity G-actin-binding interface. Serum DBP's actin-binding function is postulated to work in concert with serum gelsolin as part of an actin scavenger system that prevents actin toxicity in the host following tissue injury. From an immunological standpoint, DBP is a co-factor for C5a-mediated chemotaxis and appears to be involved in macrophage and osteoclast activation in *ex vivo* experiments. Many of the mechanisms underlying the different roles played by DBP remain obscure.

Future studies using the *Dbp*-null mouse model may provide long-awaited answers.

Glossary

F-actin (filamentous actin) Protein that results from the self-assembly of G-actin into head-to-tail polymers. This assembly is regulated by a large class of actin-binding proteins.

G-actin (globular actin) The major protein of the microfilament system in eukaryotic cells.

gelsolin A calcium- and polyphosphoinositide-regulated F-actin severing and capping protein found in both cytosol and serum.

megalin A multifunctional, transmembrane clearance receptor of the low-density lipoprotein family that mediates the uptake and lysosomal degradation of numerous ligands, particularly in renal proximal tubular cells.

vitamin D-binding protein An abundant serum protein of the albumin family that functions to bind and solubilize vitamin D sterols for transport to target tissues and for storage; it is also an extracellular G-actin-binding and sequestration protein.

See Also the Following Articles

Vitamin D ● Vitamin D and Cartilage ● Vitamin D and Human Nutrition ● Vitamin D: Biological Effects of $1,25(OH)_2D_3$ in Bone ● Vitamin D: Biological Effects of $1,25(OH)_2D_3$ in the Intestine and the Kidney ● Vitamin D Deficiency, Rickets and Osteomalacia ● Vitamin D: 24,25-Dihydroxyvitamin D ● Vitamin D Metabolism ● Vitamin D: Nuclear Receptor for $1,25(OH)_2D_3$

Further Reading

Bogaerts, I., Verboven, C. C., Rabijns, A., Van Baelen, H., Bouillon, R., and De Ranter, C. (2000). Crystallization and preliminary X-ray investigation of the human vitamin D-binding protein in complex with 25-hydroxyvitamin D3. *In* "Vitamin D Endocrine System: Structural, Biological, Genetic and Clinical Aspects" (A. W. Norman, R. Bouillon, and M. Thomasset, eds.), pp. 117–120. University of California, Riverside.

Cooke, N. E., and Haddad, J. G. (1997). Vitamin D binding protein. *In* "Vitamin D" (D. Feldman, F. H. Glorieux, and J. W. Pike, eds.), pp. 87–100. Academic Press, San Diego, CA.

DiMartino, S. J., and Kew, R. R. (1999). Initial characterization of the vitamin D binding protein (Gc-globulin) binding site on the neutrophil plasma membrane: Evidence for a chondroitin sulfate proteoglycan. *J. Immunol.* **163**, 2135–2142.

DiMartino, S. J., Shah, A. B., Trujillo, G., and Kew, R. R. (2001). Elastase controls the binding of the vitamin D-binding protein (Gc-globulin) to neutrophils: A potential role in the regulation of C5a co-chemotactic activity. *J. Immunol.* **166**, 2688–2694.

Haddad, J. G., Harper, K. D., Guoth, M., Pietra, G. G., and Sanger, J. W. (1990). Angiopathic consequences of saturating the plasma scavenger system for actin. *Proc. Natl. Acad. Sci. USA* **87**, 1381–1385.

Haddad, J. G., Hu, Y. Z., Kowalski, M. A., Laramore, C., Ray, K., Robzyk, P., and Cooke, N. E. (1992). Identification of the sterol- and actin-binding domains of plasma vitamin D binding protein (Gc-globulin). *Biochemistry* 31, 7174–7181.

Head, J. F., Swamy, N., and Ray, R. (2002). Crystal structure of the complex between actin and human vitamin D-binding protein at 2.5 Å resolution. *Biochemistry* 41, 9015–9020.

Lee, W. M., and Galbraith, R. M. (1992). The extracellular actin-scavenger system and actin toxicity. *N. Engl. J. Med.* 326, 1335–1341.

Norman, A. W., Ishizuka, S., and Okamura, W. H. (2001). Ligands for the vitamin D endocrine system: Different shapes function as agonists and antagonists for genomic and rapid response receptors or as a ligand for the plasma vitamin D binding protein. *J. Steroid Biochem. Mol. Biol.* 76, 49–59.

Nykjaer, A., Dragun, D., Walther, D., Vorum, H., Jacobsen, C., Herz, J., Melsen, F., Christensen, E. I., and Willnow, T. E. (1999). An endocytic pathway essential for renal uptake and activation of the steroid 25-(OH) vitamin D3. *Cell* 96, 507–515.

Otterbein, L. R., Cosio, C., Graceffa, P., and Dominguez, R. (2002). Crystal structure of the vitamin D-binding protein and its complex with actin: Structural basis of the actin-scavenger system. *Proc. Natl. Acad. Sci. USA* 99, 8003–8008.

Safadi, F. F., Thornton, P., Magiera, H., Hollis, B. W., Gentile, M., Haddad, J. G., Liebhaber, S. A., and Cooke, N. E. (1999). Osteopathy and resistance to vitamin D toxicity in mice null for vitamin D binding protein. *J. Clin. Invest.* 103, 239–251.

Song, Y. H., Naumova, A. K., Liebhaber, S. A., and Cooke, N. E. (1999). Physical and meiotic mapping of the region of human chromosome 4q11–q13 encompassing the vitamin D binding protein DBP/Gc-globulin and albumin multigene cluster. *Genome Res.* 9, 581–587.

Song, Y. H., Ray, K., Liebhaber, S. A., and Cooke, N. E. (1998). Vitamin D-binding protein gene transcription is regulated by the relative abundance of hepatocyte nuclear factors 1α and 1β. *J. Biol. Chem.* 273, 28408–28418.

Verboven, C., Rabijns, A., De Maeyer, M., Van Baelen, H., Bouillon, R., and De Ranter, C. (2002). A structural basis for the unique binding features of the human vitamin D-binding protein. *Nat. Struct. Biol.* 9, 131–136.

Vitamin D: Biological Effects of 1α,25(OH)₂D₃ in Bone

TATSUO SUDA

Saitama Medical School, Japan

I. INTRODUCTION
II. DISCOVERY OF BONE MINERAL MOBILIZATION ACTIVITY OF VITAMIN D
III. ESTABLISHMENT OF A MOUSE CO-CULTURE SYSTEM TO EXAMINE OSTEOCLASTOGENESIS
IV. MOLECULAR MECHANISM OF OSTEOCLASTOGENESIS
V. ROLE OF 1α,25(OH)₂D₃ IN MAINTAINING SERUM CALCIUM HOMEOSTASIS
VI. SUMMARY

Vitamin D, in concert with parathyroid hormone and calcitonin, plays a critical role in regulating serum calcium homeostasis. A metabolite of vitamin D₃, 1α,25(OH)₂D₃, stimulates osteoblastic bone formation and mineralization at least in an indirect manner, by stimulating the intestinal absorption of calcium. 1α,25(OH)₂D₃ also stimulates osteoclastic bone resorption by inducing osteoclast differentiation factor (ODF) receptor activator of NF-κB ligand (RANKL) in osteoblasts.

I. INTRODUCTION

It is well known that, in healthy animals and humans, serum calcium levels are tightly regulated and are maintained at 9 to 10 mg/dl. Intestine, bone, and kidney are the three major organs involved in calcium homeostasis. Vitamin D plays a major role in regulating serum calcium homeostasis in concert with parathyroid hormone (PTH) and calcitonin. Most of the biological effects generated by vitamin D are produced by its metabolite 1α,25-dihydroxyvitamin D₃ [1α,25(OH)₂D₃]. Vitamin D receptors (VDRs), which bind 1α,25(OH)₂D₃, have been reported to be present in these three organs. In bone, VDRs are located preferentially in osteoblasts. In addition, vitamin D-deficient animals and humans exhibit severe rickets and osteomalacia. From these results, it was postulated that vitamin D directly stimulates bone formation, in particular, bone mineralization.

In 1997, Kato and his associates in Japan succeeded in generating mice deficient in VDR by gene targeting. They showed that in VDR null mutant mice [VDR (−/−)], no appreciable defects in development and growth were observed before weaning, irrespective of the reduced expression of vitamin D target genes. After weaning, however, mutant mice failed to thrive, and alopecia, hypocalcemia, and infertility resulted (Fig. 1a). Both bone formation and mineralization were severely impaired as a typical feature of type II vitamin D-dependent rickets. Most of the null mutant mice died within 15 to 25 weeks after birth due to severe hypocalcemia (Fig. 1b). Unexpectedly, when these null mutant mice were fed a rescue diet containing high levels of calcium, they developed normally even at 50 weeks, but severe alopecia remained (Fig. 1, inset). Bone formation and mineralization in the null mutant mice maintained on

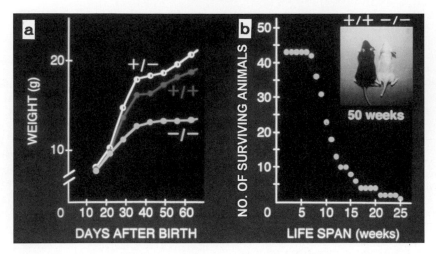

FIGURE 1   Representative growth curves of wild-type (+/+), heterozygous (+/−), and homozygous (−/−) littermates of VDR gene knockout mice (a) and the survival rate of 43 VDR (−/−) mice (b). The inset shows VDR (+/+) mice and VDR (−/−) mice fed a rescue diet containing high levels of calcium for 50 weeks. Reprinted from Yoshizawa *et al.* (1997), *Nature Genetics* **16**, 391–396 with permission.

a high-calcium diet were completely reestablished. From these results, it can be concluded that the stimulating effect of 1α,25(OH)₂D₃ on bone formation and mineralization is indirect, occurring through the stimulation of intestinal absorption of calcium by vitamin D.

II. DISCOVERY OF BONE MINERAL MOBILIZATION ACTIVITY OF VITAMIN D

It appears to be paradoxical, but vitamin D functions in the process of calcium mobilization from calcified bone, making calcium available to the extracellular fluid upon demand by the calcium homeostatic system. This important observation was first reported by Carlsson in 1952. He showed that when hypocalcemic rats fed a vitamin D-deficient, low-calcium diet were orally given 100 IU (2.5 μg) of vitamin D₃, their serum calcium was increased from 5 to 8 mg/dl 3 days after administration (Fig. 2a). Parathyroidectomy (PTX) 2 h prior to vitamin D₃ administration abolished the increase in serum calcium levels (Fig. 2a). Since the diet did not contain any appreciable amounts of calcium, he concluded that vitamin D stimulates mineral mobilization from calcified bone to blood in concert with PTH.

The metabolite of vitamin D₃ responsible for bone mobilization is 1α,25(OH)₂D₃. Using an *in vitro* organ culture system, in 1972 Raisz *et al.* reported that 1α,25(OH)₂D₃ and 25(OH)D₃ increase the release of ^{45}Ca from prelabeled bone into the culture medium. They also showed that 1α,25(OH)₂D₃ is

about 80 times more potent than 25(OH)D₃ in increasing the ^{45}Ca release from prelabeled bone (Fig. 2b). From these results, they concluded that the metabolite of vitamin D₃ which stimulates bone mineral mobilization is indeed 1α,25(OH)₂D₃.

In 1981, Abe *et al.* discovered the cell differentiation-inducing activity of 1α,25(OH)₂D₃ using mouse and human myeloid leukemic cells. HL-60 is a human promyelocytic leukemia cell line established from a leukemia patient, and the cells can be induced to differentiate into granulocytes by retinoic acid and monocyte–macrophages by 1α,25(OH)₂D₃. 1α,25(OH)₂D₃ was a potent and selective inducer of differentiation of HL-60 cells into macrophages. Furthermore, 1α,25(OH)₂D₃ directly induced the fusion of alveolar macrophages at a very high rate. Approximately 80% of the macrophages fused to form multinucleated giant cells by stimulating the differentiation and fusion of macrophages. However, the multinucleated giant cells formed from alveolar macrophages in response to 1α,25(OH)₂D₃ did not satisfy the criteria of osteoclasts.

III. ESTABLISHMENT OF A MOUSE CO-CULTURE SYSTEM TO EXAMINE OSTEOCLASTOGENESIS

It is well recognized that osteoclasts are derived from hematopoietic cells of the monocyte–macrophage lineage. Hematopoietic monocytic cells are present in almost all tissues, whereas osteoclasts, the cells responsible for bone resorption, are present only in

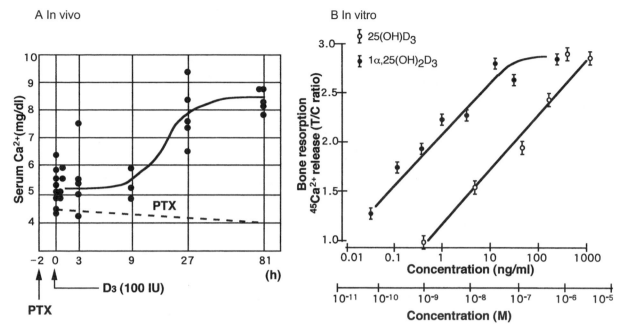

FIGURE 2 (A) Discovery of bone mineral mobilization activity of vitamin D *in vivo*. PTX, parathyroidectomy. Reprinted from Carlsson (1952), with permission from Blackwell Publishing Ltd. (B) The comparison of the *in vitro* activity to increase the release of ^{45}Ca from prelabeled bone between 25(OH)D₃ and 1α,25(OH)₂D₃. Reprinted from Raisz *et al.* (1972), *Science* 175, 768–769. Copyright 1972 American Association for the Advancement of Science.

bone. This led to the speculation that some local factors or local mechanisms are involved in this tissue-specific localization of osteoclasts in bone. Special attention was given to the role of osteoblasts in osteoclast development, since osteoblasts are present only in bone. The process of osteoclast development consists of several steps, including proliferation, differentiation, fusion, and activation.

In 1988, Takahashi *et al.* established an efficient mouse co-culture system to recruit osteoclasts. Osteoblastic cells were isolated from mouse calvaria, and spleen cells were used as hematopoietic osteoclast progenitors. They were either separately cultured or co-cultured together with or without 10^{-8} M 1α,25(OH)₂D₃. When osteoblastic cells alone or spleen cells alone were cultured, no osteoclasts were formed even in the presence of 1α,25(OH)₂D₃. In contrast, numerous multinucleated osteoclasts were formed when spleen cells and osteoblastic cells were co-cultured in the presence of 1α,25(OH)₂D₃. Cell-to-cell contact between spleen cells and osteoblastic cells appeared to be important for osteoclast formation, since no osteoclasts were formed when spleen cells and osteoblastic cells were co-cultured but separated by a membrane filter even in the presence of 1α,25(OH)₂D₃. From these results, it was hypothesized that the direct contact of spleen cells and

osteoblastic cells is essential for osteoclast differentiation, suggesting the requirement of a membrane-associated factor for osteoclast formation. Spleen cells represented osteoclast progenitors, in other words, "the seeds," and osteoblastic cells represented supporting cells that provide a suitable microenvironment for osteoclast formation in bone, in other words, "the farm."

After extensive studies, it was found that not only 1α,25(OH)₂D₃ but also PTH, IL-1, PGE2, IL-6, and IL-11 similarly stimulated osteoclast formation in mouse co-cultures (Fig. 3). The target cells of these bone-resorbing factors were osteoblastic cells but not hematopoietic osteoclast precursors. These bone-resorbing factors were classified into three diverse signaling pathways mediated by the VDR, cAMP, and gp130 (Fig. 3). These three signals appeared to stimulate osteoclast differentiation independently, since osteoclasts were formed both in VDR null mutant mice and in gp130 knockout mice. In other words, there is a redundancy in bone-resorbing factors to recruit osteoclasts. It was proposed that the "osteoclast differentiation factor" (ODF) is commonly induced on the plasma membrane of osteoblastic cells in response to these bone-resorbing factors (Fig. 3). Osteoclast precursors having ODF receptors recognize ODF by cell-to-cell contact and

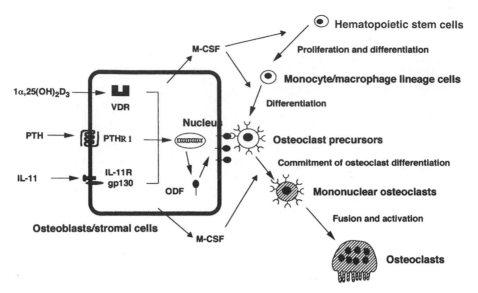

FIGURE 3   A hypothetical concept of osteoclast differentiation, proposing the requirement of a membrane-associated factor, osteoclast differentiation factor (ODF), in osteoblasts/stromal cells for osteoclastogenesis.

differentiate into osteoclasts. Macrophage-colony stimulating factor (MCSF, also called colony stimulating factor-1, CSF-1) appeared to play an important role in the proliferation and differentiation of osteoclast progenitors, since M-CSF-deficient op/op mutant mice showed severe osteopetrosis with the complete absence of osteoclasts.

IV. MOLECULAR MECHANISM OF OSTEOCLASTOGENESIS

In 1997, the research groups of Amgen and Snow Brand Milk Products independently succeeded in the molecular cloning of a factor that strongly inhibits osteoclastogenesis. Amgen named it "osteoprotegerin" (OPG) and Snow Brand named it "osteoclastogenesis inhibitory factor" (OCIF). OPG and OCIF were the same molecule, which belongs to the TNF receptor family. OPG/OCIF lacked the membrane-bound domain, indicating that OPG/OCIF is a soluble receptor. It was speculated that OPG/OCIF could compete with the ODF receptor for the binding of ODF.

Using radioactive OCIF, the molecular cloning of a membrane-associated factor responsible for osteoclastogenesis was finally accomplished. The Amgen group also succeeded in the molecular cloning of such a factor. Amgen named it OPG ligand (OPGL), which was identical to ODF. Figure 4 schematically shows the molecular mechanism of osteoclast formation. All bone-resorbing factors such as 1α,25(OH)$_2$D$_3$, PGE2, PTH, and IL-11 act on osteoblastic cells to

induce ODF. ODF recognizes osteoclast progenitors having an ODF receptor by a mechanism involving cell-to-cell contact. M-CSF is also an essential factor for osteoclast differentiation and is produced by osteoblastic cells in bone. Osteoclast progenitors differentiate into osteoclasts by binding to ODF. When OPG/OCIF covers ODF, osteoclast progenitors having the ODF receptor are unable to bind ODF; thus, osteoclast formation is inhibited.

The molecular cloning of ODF revealed that this molecule was identical to "receptor activator of NF-κB ligand" (RANKL), "TNF-related activation-induced cytokine" (TRANCE), and OPGL, all of which were independently identified by different research groups as a novel member of the TNF ligand family. ODF, OPGL, TRANCE, and RANKL are the same molecule, and it is important in the

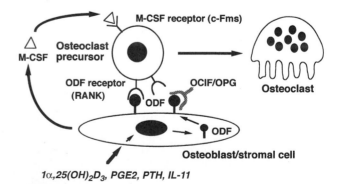

FIGURE 4   The molecular mechanism of osteoclast formation from its precursors supported by osteoblasts/stromal cells.

development of T cells and dendritic cells as well as the development of osteoclasts. "Receptor activator of NF-κB" (RANK), which has been cloned as a receptor of RANKL, is the transmembrane signaling receptor for ODF as well. OPG/OCIF is a soluble receptor for ODF and it appears to function as a decoy receptor.

ODF is involved not only in osteoclast differentiation but also in osteoclast activation. The lifetime of osteoclasts can be divided into three steps: the first step is proliferation and differentiation, the second step involves survival and fusion, and the third step is the activation of osteoclasts. Proliferation and differentiation of osteoclasts essentially require ODF together with M-CSF. The survival and fusion of osteoclasts are induced by either ODF or M-CSF. Activation of osteoclasts is induced by ODF but not by M-CSF. Thus, ODF appears to be involved throughout the lifetime of osteoclasts.

V. ROLE OF 1α,25(OH)$_2$D$_3$ IN MAINTAINING SERUM CALCIUM HOMEOSTASIS

It should, however, be recognized that physiological plasma levels of 1α,25(OH)$_2$D$_3$ do not stimulate osteoclastic bone resorption *in vivo*; only pharmacological or toxic doses of 1α,25(OH)$_2$D$_3$ are capable of stimulating it. Figure 5 shows the difference in dose levels of 1α,25(OH)$_2$D$_3$ required to stimulate intestinal calcium transport activity and bone mineral mobilization activity. In this particular experiment, the intestinal calcium transport activity was measured by the everted gut sac method (serosal/mucosal ^{45}Ca ratio) in vitamin D-deficient rats after administration of graded doses of 1α,25(OH)$_2$D$_3$. The bone mineral mobilization activity was monitored by determining serum calcium levels in rats fed a vitamin D-deficient, low-calcium diet after administration of graded doses of 1α,25(OH)$_2$D$_3$. Physiological dose levels (0.1–0.25 μg/rat) of 1α,25(OH)$_2$D$_3$ greatly increased intestinal calcium transport activity but did not increase serum levels of calcium appreciably. Approximately 10 to 50 times higher dose levels of 1α,25(OH)$_2$D$_3$ were required to induce bone mineral mobilization activity. In our co-culture system, 10^{-8} M 1α,25(OH)$_2$D$_3$ was required to generate osteoclasts *in vitro*, a level that was 50 to 100 times higher than the serum concentration of 1α,25(OH)$_2$D$_3$ in healthy subjects. Thus, it may be concluded that physiological concentrations of 1α,25(OH)$_2$D$_3$ are not capable of inducing bone mineral mobilization and that pharmacological or toxic levels of 1α,25(OH)$_2$D$_3$ are required for inducing bone resorption.

VI. SUMMARY

Physiological doses of vitamin D preferentially stimulate intestinal calcium absorption, which in

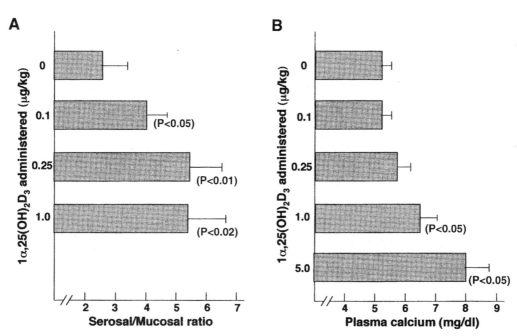

FIGURE 5 Differences in the dose levels of 1α,25(OH)$_2$D$_3$ required to stimulate intestinal calcium transport activity (A) and bone mineral mobilization activity (B).

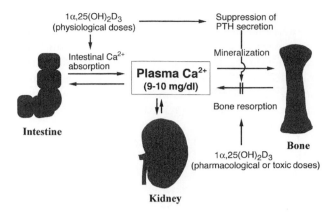

FIGURE 6 The role of 1α,25(OH)₂D₃ in maintaining plasma calcium homeostasis.

turn stimulates bone mineralization (Fig. 6). The recent findings of VDR knockout mice and of those mice fed a rescue diet containing high levels of calcium indicate that the stimulating effect of vitamin D on bone formation and mineralization is indirect, occurring through the stimulation of intestinal absorption of calcium by this vitamin. In contrast, osteoclastic bone resorption can be induced by vitamin D directly but only by pharmacological or toxic doses (Fig. 6). Physiological doses of vitamin D never stimulate bone resorption.

It is interesting that osteoclast formation requires cell-to-cell contact with osteoblastic cells, which generates ODF/RANKL as a membrane-associated factor in response to several bone-resorbing factors including vitamin D. In normal bone remodeling, bone formation by osteoblasts always occurs in a programmed manner accurately and quantitatively just after bone resorption by osteoclasts. Thus, it is possible that cell-to-cell contact between osteoclast progenitors and osteoblastic cells may leave some template for bone formation in osteoblasts/stromal cells. This possibility must be proved by future experiments.

Glossary

osteoblasts The cells responsible for bone formation, which derive from mesenchymal progenitors and synthesize bone matrix proteins containing type III collagen and other noncollagenous proteins such as osteocalcin, osteopontin, osteonectin, and bone sialoproteins.

osteoclast differentiation factor (ODF) The factor responsible for osteoclast formation and activation, which belongs to the tumor necrosis factor (TNF) ligand family. ODF consists of 316 amino acid residues and is also called receptor activator of NF-κB ligand (RANKL).

osteoclasts The cells responsible for bone resorption, which originate from hematopoietic cells of the monocyte–macrophage lineage and which are present only in bone.

osteoprotegerin (OPG) The decoy receptor of ODF/RANKL, which belongs to the TNF receptor family. OPG is also called osteoclastogenesis inhibitory factor (OCIF). OPG/OCIF is a soluble receptor having no membrane-associated domain.

receptor activator of NF-κB (RANK) The receptor of ODF/RANKL, which belongs to the TNF receptor family.

VDR The specific receptor for the hormonal form of vitamin D₃, 1α,25(OH)₂D₃, in target tissues.

See Also the Following Articles

Bone Morphogenetic Proteins ● Osteoporosis: Hormonal Treatment ● Osteoporosis: Pathophysiology ● Vitamin D ● Vitamin D and Cartilage ● Vitamin D and Human Nutrition ● Vitamin D: Biological Effects of 1,25(OH)₂D₃ in the Intestine and the Kidney ● Vitamin D Deficiency, Rickets and Osteomalacia

Further Reading

Abe, E., Miyaura, C., Sakagami, H., Takeda, M., Konno, K., Yamazaki, Y., Yoshiki, S., and Suda, T. (1981). Differentiation of mouse myeloid leukemia cells induced by 1α,25-dihydroxy-vitamin D₃. *Proc. Natl. Acad. Sci. USA* **78**, 4990–4994.

Carlsson, A. (1952). Tracer experiments on the effects of vitamin D on the skeletal metabolism of calcium and phosphorus. *Acta Physiol. Scand.* **26**, 212–220.

Lacey, D. L., Timms, E., Tan, H. L., Kelley, M. J., Dunstan, C. R., Burgess, T., Elliott, R., Colombero, A., Elliott, G., and Scully, S. (1998). Osteoprotegerin ligand is a cytokine that regulates osteoclast differentiation and activation. *Cell* **93**, 165–176.

Matsuzaki, K., Katayama, K., Takahashi, Y., Nakamura, I., Udagawa, N., Tsurukai, T., Nishinakamura, R., Toyama, Y., Yabe, Y., Hori, M., Takahashi, N., and Suda, T. (1999). Human osteoclast-like cells are formed from peripheral blood mononuclear cells in a co-culture with SaOS-2 cells transfected with the parathyroid hormone (PTH)/PTH-related protein receptor gene. *Endocrinology* **140**, 925–932.

Raisz, L. G., Trummel, C. L., and DeLuca, H. F. (1972). 1,25-Dihydroxycholecalciferol: A potent stimulator of bone resorption in tissue culture. *Science* **175**, 768–769.

Simonet, W. S., Lacey, D. L., Dunstan, C. R., Kelley, M., Chang, M. S., Luthy, R., Nguyen, H. Q., Wooden, S., Bennett, L., Boone, T., Simamoto, G., DeRose, M., Elliott, R., Colombero, A., Tan, H. L., Trail, G., Sullivan, J., Davy, E., Bucay, N., Renshaw-Gegg, L., Hughes, T. M., Hill, D., Pattison, W., and Campbell, P. (1997). Osteoprotegerin: A novel secreted protein involved in the regulation of bone density. *Cell* **89**, 309–319.

Suda, T., Takahashi, N., and Martin, T. J. (1992). Modulation of osteoclast differentiation. *Endocr. Rev.* **13**, 66–80.

Suda, T., Takahashi, N., and Martin, T. J. (1995). Modulation of osteoclast differentiation: Update 1995. *Endocr. Rev. Monograph* **4**, 266–270.

Suda, T., Takahashi, N., Udagawa, N., Jimi, E., Gillespie, M. T., and Martin, T. J. (1999). Modulation of osteoclast differentiation and function by the new members of the tumor necrosis factor receptor and ligand families. *Endocr. Rev.* 20, 345–357.

Takahashi, N., Akatsu, T., Udagawa, N., Sasaki, T., Yamaguchi, A., Moseley, J. M., Martin, T. J., and Suda, T. (1988). Osteoblastic cells are involved in osteoclast formation. *Endocrinology* 123, 2600–2602.

Takeda, S., Yoshizawa, T., Nagai, Y., Yamato, H., Fukumoto, S., Sekine, K., Kato, S., Matsumoto, T., and Fujita, T. (1999). Stimulation of osteoclast formation by 1,25-dihydroxyvitamin D$_3$ requires its binding to vitamin D receptor (VDR) in osteoblastic cells: Studies using VDR knockout mice. *Endocrinology* 140, 1005–1008.

Tsuda, E., Goto, M., Mochizuki, S., Yano, K., Kobayashi, F., Morinaga, T., and Higashio, K. (1997). Isolation of a novel cytokine from human fibroblasts that specifically inhibits osteoclastogenesis. *Biochem. Biophys. Res. Commun.* 234, 137–142.

Yasuda, H., Shima, N., Nakagawa, N., Mochizuki, S., Yano, K., Fujise, N., Sato, Y., Goto, M., Yamaguchi, K., Kuriyama, M., Kanno, T., Murakami, A., Tsuda, E., Morinaga, T., and Higashio, K. (1998). Identity of osteoclastogenesis inhibitory factor (OCIF) and osteoprotegerin in vitro. *Endocrinology* 139, 1329–1337.

Yasuda, H., Shima, N., Nakagawa, N., Yamaguchi, K., Kinosaki, M., Mochizuki, S., Tomoyasu, A., Yano, K., Goto, M., Murakami, A., Tsuda, E., Morinaga, T., Higashio, K., Udagawa, N., Takahashi, N., and Suda, T. (1998). Osteoclast differentiation factor is a ligand for osteoprotegerin/osteoclastogenesis-inhibitory factor and identical to TRANCE/RANKL. *Proc. Natl. Acad. Sci. USA* 95, 3597–3602.

Yoshizawa, T., Handa, Y., Uematsu, Y., Takeda, S., Sekine, K., Yoshihara, Y., Kawakami, T., Arioka, K., Sato, H., Uchiyama, Y., Masushige, S., Fukamizu, A., Matsumoto, T., and Kato, S. (1997). Mice lacking the vitamin D receptor exhibit impaired bone formation, uterine hypoplasia and growth retardation after weaning. *Nat. Genet.* 16, 391–396.

Vitamin D: Biological Effects of 1,25(OH)$_2$D$_3$ in the Intestine and the Kidney

JOOST G. J. HOENDEROP, CAREL H. VAN OS, AND RENÉ J. M. BINDELS

University of Nijmegen, The Netherlands

I. INTRODUCTION
II. BIOLOGICAL EFFECTS IN THE INTESTINE
III. BIOLOGICAL EFFECTS IN THE KIDNEY
IV. SUMMARY

Calcitriol or 1,25-dihydroxyvitamin D$_3$ [1,25-(OH)$_2$D$_3$] is essential for the development and maintenance of bone. This hormone plays a crucial role in Ca^{2+} and P$_i$ homeostasis and exerts its biological actions on the intestine and kidney; the absorbing activity of these target organs ultimately determines the mineral balance for the entire body. 1,25(OH)$_2$D$_3$ has strong stimulatory effects on Ca^{2+} transport proteins; thus, transepithelial Ca^{2+} transport in the small intestine and kidney is dependent on vitamin D. Less is known regarding the transport of P$_i$ in the kidney and intestine. However, it is well established that vitamin D stimulates Na$^+$-dependent P$_i$ transport in the small intestine, although the molecular mechanism responsible has not yet been elucidated.

I. INTRODUCTION

Calcitriol or 1,25-dihydroxyvitamin D$_3$ [1,25(OH)$_2$D$_3$] plays a critical role in Ca^{2+} and phosphate (P$_i$) homeostasis and is essential for the development and maintenance of bone. The intestine and kidney are main target organs for the action of this hormone. The absorbing activity of intestine and kidney determines the net intake and excretion of minerals for the entire body and, therefore, the mineral balance. In normal adults, the renal excretion of Ca^{2+} and P$_i$ is critically balanced by gastrointestinal absorption. On the other hand, the distribution of Ca^{2+} within the body is determined by exchanges of Ca^{2+} between interstitium and bone. These pathways are primarily regulated by vitamin D metabolites and parathyroid hormone (PTH). Alterations in these regulatory processes are present in many physiological and pathophysiological states.

The biological actions of calcitriol on the target organs are mediated by both genomic and rapid posttranscriptional mechanisms. The genomic response is linked to the nuclear vitamin D receptor (VDR). Upon binding 1,25(OH)$_2$D$_3$, the VDR undergoes a conformational change and forms a complex with a retinoid X receptor (RXR). The VDR/RXR complex binds to DNA elements in the promoter regions of target genes described as vitamin D-response elements (VDREs). Binding to the VDREs may control the rate of gene transcription. The rapid response is believed to utilize another signal transduction pathway that is likely linked to a putative cell membrane receptor for 1,25(OH)$_2$D$_3$, but its physiological role is still not well understood.

II. BIOLOGICAL EFFECTS IN THE INTESTINE

The most critical role of 1,25(OH)$_2$D$_3$ in the gut is to regulate the absorption of Ca^{2+} and P$_i$ during variations in dietary intake and body demand. The most obvious stimulatory effect of 1,25(OH)$_2$D$_3$ in this tissue takes place in the proximal small intestine and is mediated by VDR-controlled genomic actions.

A. Calcium Absorption

There is ample evidence that vitamin D is an important determinant of intestinal Ca^{2+} absorption. For instance, in vitamin D deficiency, intestinal Ca^{2+} absorption is low, resulting in an increased risk of developing negative Ca^{2+} balance and bone loss. Conversely, plasma levels of 1,25(OH)$_2$D$_3$ are increased as a primary response to low dietary Ca^{2+} intake and increased Ca^{2+} requirements during growth, pregnancy, and lactation, affecting primarily the rate of active Ca^{2+} absorption in duodenum. During transcellular Ca^{2+} transport, Ca^{2+} ions pass across the lumenal brush-border membrane, then transverse through the cytosol, and exit against an electrochemical gradient across the basolateral membrane. The epithelial Ca^{2+} channel, ECaC (or Ca^{2+} transporter, CaT), the vitamin D-dependent Ca^{2+}-binding protein, calbindin-D$_{9K}$, and the plasma membrane Ca^{2+}-ATPase, PMCA, represent the major Ca^{2+} transporters that mediate this three-step process in the small intestine. 1,25(OH)$_2$D$_3$ stimulates this vectorial Ca^{2+} transport primarily via a genomic action and the contribution of each individual transporter to the overall stimulatory action of 1,25(OH)$_2$D$_3$ has been elucidated in several studies.

The molecular identity of the Ca^{2+} entry mechanism across the lumenal brush-border membrane has recently been established. By an expression cloning strategy, the epithelial calcium channels ECaC1 and ECaC2 (also known as CaT1) were identified. These highly homologous channels represent a new class of Ca^{2+}-selective channels, which are predominantly expressed in 1,25(OH)$_2$D$_3$-responsive epithelia such as small intestine, kidney, and placenta. Analysis of the 5' upstream region of the human ECaC1 gene revealed putative VDREs at a distance of approximately 1.5–0.5 kb from the transcription initiation site, which supports the previous findings that ECaC1 is a target gene for 1,25(OH)$_2$D$_3$. The role of the VDREs in 1,25(OH)$_2$D$_3$-mediated ECaC1 gene transcription remains to be established. However, it is likely that 1,25(OH)$_2$D$_3$ regulates the transcription of these Ca^{2+}

channels. Surprisingly, in two initial studies no significant effect of 1,25(OH)$_2$D$_3$ on the expression of these channels could be found, thus far for unexplained reasons. Northern blot analysis did not reveal vitamin D-dependent regulation of ECaC2 expression in the duodenum of rats and no significant relationship was shown between human ECaC2 expression in duodenal samples and serum 1,25(OH)$_2$D$_3$ levels of healthy volunteers. The first indication that ECaC in the intestine is regulated by vitamin D was recently shown in animal studies. A single pharmacological dose of 1,25(OH)$_2$D$_3$ in wild-type mice stimulated the duodenal level of ECaC1 mRNA by a factor of 1.6 and that of ECaC2 mRNA by more than sixfold. In a study from two independent groups, using mice strains in which the VDR was inactivated, it was further investigated whether these channels are indeed prime targets for hormonal regulation by 1,25(OH)$_2$D$_3$. These mice display a phenotype similar to that observed in hereditary hypocalcemic vitamin D-resistant rickets, namely, rickets, hypocalcemia, and hypophosphatemia. This phenotype could be rescued by high dietary Ca^{2+} intake, confirming that the intestinal absorption of Ca^{2+} is critical in 1,25(OH)$_2$D$_3$ action on Ca^{2+} homeostasis. ECaC1 and ECaC2 mRNA levels were considerably and consistently down-regulated in the duodenum of these VDR-knockout mice on a normal Ca^{2+} diet. Similar studies were performed in mice homozygous for the disrupted Na$^+$–P$_i$ co-transporter (Npt2) gene. These hypophosphatemic mice exhibit hypercalcemia and hypercalciuria resulting from duodenal Ca^{2+} hyperabsorption, secondary to elevated serum 1,25(OH)$_2$D$_3$ levels. In these mutants, the duodenal expression of ECaC1 and ECaC2 mRNAs is higher than in wild-type littermates, suggesting that the corresponding proteins are involved in mediating the increase in duodenal Ca^{2+} absorption. Finally, the expression of ECaC2 is rapidly up-regulated by 1,25(OH)$_2$D$_3$ and precedes vitamin D-stimulated Ca^{2+} transport in Caco-2 cells, a human intestinal cell line. Taken together, these results suggest that the expression of these novel duodenal epithelial Ca^{2+} channels is strongly vitamin D-dependent.

There is ample evidence that calbindin-D$_{9K}$ is highly responsive to 1,25(OH)$_2$D$_3$. In animal models and cell lines, it has been documented that 1,25(OH)$_2$D$_3$ stimulates the expression of calbindin-D$_{9K}$ on both mRNA and protein levels, involving a genomic pathway. This results in an increase in the capacity of diffusional flow of Ca^{2+} ions through the cytosol. The linear correlation between the intestinal content of calbindin-D$_{9K}$ and the rate of active Ca^{2+}

transport in the intestine underscores the important role of calbindin-D$_{9K}$ in active Ca^{2+} absorption. The molecular basis for regulating the calbindin-D$_{9K}$ gene by 1,25(OH)$_2$D$_3$ is not completely understood since the previously identified VDREs in the promoter region seem not to be responsible for the stimulatory effect.

PMCA is ubiquitously expressed in Ca^{2+} transporting epithelia and is encoded by four distinct genes (PMCA1–4) that can be further posttranscriptionally modified. PMCA1b is the only isoform predominantly expressed in small intestine and kidney. It has been shown experimentally that in variable circumstances the extrusion capacity of PMCA is more than adequate, suggesting that the Ca^{2+} exit step is not necessarily a prime target for regulation by 1,25(OH)$_2$D$_3$. This could perhaps explain the difficulty in observing a consistent stimulatory effect of 1,25(OH)$_2$D$_3$ on PMCA. In VDR knockout mice strains, the expression of PMCA1b is not altered in duodenal samples, whereas in 1,25(OH)$_2$D$_3$ repletion studies performed in chicken, rat, and mice, an increase in intestinal PMCA1b expression was observed.

The overall conclusion is that the stimulatory effect of 1,25(OH)$_2$D$_3$ on intestinal Ca^{2+} absorption results primarily from an increased expression of ECaC and calbindin-D$_{9K}$. Thus, during periods of high Ca^{2+} demand, the activity of ECaC is increased in the brush-border membrane of the enterocyte via a 1,25(OH)$_2$D$_3$-dependent genomic mechanism. The concomitant increase in the cytosolic content of calbindin-D$_{9K}$ serves two important physiological functions. It guarantees sufficient buffering and inactivation of Ca^{2+} ions in the close vicinity of the channel to prevent a Ca^{2+}-induced inactivation of channel activity and accelerates the transfer of Ca^{2+} to the basolateral extrusion pumps. In this way, 1,25(OH)$_2$D$_3$ can efficiently promote high rates of transcellular Ca^{2+} absorption in the small intestine.

B. Phosphate Absorption

The intestinal P$_i$ absorption process occurs both by a Na$^+$-independent, nonsaturable pathway and by an active, Na$^+$-dependent mechanism present mainly in duodenum and jejunum. This latter process is subject to chronic regulation by 1,25(OH)$_2$D$_3$. Ample studies have demonstrated that the stimulatory effect of 1,25(OH)$_2$D$_3$ occurs through an increased rate of Na$^+$–P$_i$ co-transport present in the brush-border membrane, but the molecular details have not been elucidated. To date, three different families of Na$^+$–P$_i$

co-transporters have been identified, but the physiological role of these transporters in intestinal P$_i$ absorption remains to be firmly established. The so-called NaP$_i$ type IIb co-transporter is expressed in the small intestine and is located in the apical membrane. The abundance of this transporter is up-regulated by 1,25(OH)$_2$D$_3$, but a concomitant increase in mRNA levels was not observed in adult animals. This suggests that posttranscriptional mechanisms are involved in Na$^+$-dependent P$_i$ co-transporter activity, contributing to the observed 1,25(OH)$_2$D$_3$-induced stimulation of P$_i$ absorption. Little is known about the molecular mechanisms responsible for the extrusion of P$_i$ across the intestinal basolateral membrane into the circulation. Future work, in which all apical and basolateral P$_i$ transporters will be identified, must be completed before a comprehensive molecular description of 1,25(OH)$_2$D$_3$ action on intestinal P$_i$ absorption can be provided.

III. BIOLOGICAL EFFECTS IN THE KIDNEY

Renal tubular reabsorption of Ca^{2+} and P$_i$ is a key element in overall mineral homeostasis and also involves hormone-regulated active transport mechanisms. The molecular identification of the responsible Ca^{2+} and P$_i$ transporters provided tools to study the regulation of tubular transport function at the cellular and organ levels and will ultimately disclose the full-delineated mechanisms involved in vitamin D-controlled mineral excretion.

A. Calcium Reabsorption

The distal part of the nephron is the main site of hormone-regulated transcellular Ca^{2+} transport, which is at the cellular level realized by a three-step process similar to that described for the intestine. However, there are distinctive differences between intestinal and renal active Ca^{2+} transport. For instance, renal Ca^{2+} reabsorption is tightly controlled by PTH, but this calciotropic hormone has no direct effect on intestinal Ca^{2+} absorption. The kidney contains a 28 kDa calbindin to facilitate the cellular Ca^{2+} flow, but thus far only mouse, bovine, and rat also contain calbindin-D$_{9K}$. In addition, the kidney utilizes primarily the Na$^+$–Ca^{2+} exchanger to extrude Ca^{2+}.

Although there has been some controversy concerning the role of 1,25(OH)$_2$D$_3$ in renal Ca^{2+} transport and the mechanisms behind 1,25(OH)$_2$D$_3$ responsiveness, there is now accumulating evidence that this seco-steroid stimulates transcellular Ca^{2+}

transport in the distal part of the nephron. In a primary culture of rabbit distal tubular cells, 1,25(OH)$_2$D$_3$ increases transcellular Ca^{2+} transport in a dose-dependent manner. In addition, extensive immuno-histochemical and *in situ* hybridization studies revealed that the VDR is expressed in both proximal and distal segments but is highly enriched in the distal part of the nephron, a site known to be primarily involved in active transcellular Ca^{2+} transport.

Comparable to the intestine, ECaC1 is the postulated gatekeeper of transepithelial Ca^{2+} transport in the kidney and is, therefore, a candidate target for the action of 1,25(OH)$_2$D$_3$. The first indication that ECaC1 is indeed controlled by 1,25(OH)$_2$D$_3$ came from a vitamin D-deficient rat model. In kidneys of these depleted animals, ECaC1 mRNA and protein levels were significantly reduced. Repletion with 1,25(OH)$_2$D$_3$ completely restored the abundance of ECaC1, which was accompanied by a normalization of the plasma Ca^{2+} concentration. This suggests a crucial function of this Ca^{2+} influx channel in renal Ca^{2+} handling.

The vitamin D-induced stimulation of ECaC in this rat model was accompanied by a comparable enhancement of calbindin-D$_{28K}$, confirming the established vitamin D dependence of this calcium-binding protein. In kidneys obtained from VDR knockout mice, the expression of calbindin-D$_{9K}$ was virtually abolished at both the mRNA and protein levels, whereas calbindin-D$_{28K}$ was only modestly decreased. Another mouse model for the study of vitamin D-dependent processes was established by ablation of the 25-hydroxyvitamin D 1α-hydroxylase gene [1α(OH)ase]. The synthesis of 1,25(OH)$_2$D$_3$ from its precursor 25-hydroxyvitamin D is catalyzed by the mitochondrial cytochrome P450 enzyme 25-hydroxyvitamin D 1α-hydroxylase D, which is primarily expressed in the kidney. The 1,25(OH)$_2$D$_3$ dependency was confirmed by the marked reduction in mRNA levels encoding renal calbindin-D$_{9K}$ and calbindin-D$_{28K}$ in the 1α(OH)ase null mice relative to wild-type littermates. These data clearly demonstrate that in mouse kidney, calbindin-D$_{9K}$ and calbindin-D$_{28K}$ are regulated by the VDR-mediated action of 1,25(OH)$_2$D$_3$.

The physiological implication of the concomitant increase in ECaC1 and calbindin-D levels is similar to the findings for the intestine, where the expression of ECaC2 and calbindin-D$_{9K}$ is closely coupled to vitamin D dependency of Ca^{2+} absorption. Together with the fact that both calcium transport proteins are co-expressed in the same tissues, these findings suggest an obligatory functional coupling between ECaC and calbindin-D in order to mediate vitamin D-dependent Ca^{2+} transport.

The effect of 1,25(OH)$_2$D$_3$ on the basolateral extrusion systems, NCX (Na$^+$–Ca^{2+} exchanger) and PMCA, is less clear and remains controversial. Although NCX plays a dominant role in the extrusion process, many studies failed to establish a direct regulation by vitamin D. Exposure of 1,25(OH)$_2$D$_3$ to primary cultures of rabbit connecting tubules did not noticeably alter NCX expression. Surprisingly, a single pharmacological dose of 1,25(OH)$_2$D$_3$ significantly reduced the expression of NCX in mouse kidney. As in small intestine, 1,25(OH)$_2$D$_3$ up-regulates PMCA1b protein expression and activity in kidney distal tubules and derived cell lines. Furthermore, 1,25(OH)$_2$D$_3$ enhanced PMCA1b mRNA stability. However, other reports in which primary cultures of renal cells or mice exposed to 1,25(OH)$_2$D$_3$ were used as model systems failed to show significant regulation of PMCA1b expression levels. Conversely, runoff reporter gene assays using 1.7 kb of the human PMCA1 promoter expressed in distal tubular cell lines demonstrated mRNA down-regulation by 1,25(OH)$_2$D$_3$. Taken together, a consistent stimulatory effect of 1,25(OH)$_2$D$_3$ on the Ca^{2+} extrusion mechanisms in the kidney remains to be established.

B. Phosphate Reabsorption

The reabsorption of P$_i$ in the proximal tubule plays a primary role in overall P$_i$ homeostasis and involves an active P$_i$ transport mechanism. Vitamin D has been suggested to enhance the proximal tubular P$_i$ reabsorption in rats. It is, however, difficult to distinguish between direct and indirect effects since the vitamin D status is closely associated with plasma Ca^{2+} and PTH concentrations. In contrast to the small intestine where 1,25(OH)$_2$D$_3$ has a direct effect on lumenal Na$^+$-dependent P$_i$ uptake, it remains, therefore, unclear whether 1,25(OH)$_2$D$_3$ directly regulates proximal tubular P$_i$ reabsorption.

The cellular scheme for the P$_i$ reabsorption process includes three different Na$^+$–P$_i$ co-transporters, namely, type I, type IIa, and type III; the type I and type IIa transporters are localized along the apical membrane, whereas type III is expressed in the basolateral membrane. A single study demonstrated that NaP$_i$-type IIa mRNA and protein were markedly decreased in the juxtamedullary cortex of vitamin D-deficient rats, but not in the superficial cortex. Luciferase reporter studies in COS7 cells, expressing the human VDR, confirmed the existence of a

TABLE I The Expression Level of Ca^{2+} and P$_i$ Transporters during 1,25(OH)$_2$D$_3$-Stimulated Transport in Small Intestine and Kidney

Ca^{2+} (re)absorption	P$_i$ (re)absorption
Intestine	
ECaC1 ↑	NaP$_i$-IIb ↑
ECaC2 ↑	
Calbindin-D$_{9K}$ ↑	
PMCA1b ↓ ↑	
Kidney	
ECaC1 ↑	NaP$_i$-IIa ↑ ?
Calbindin-D$_{9K}$ ↑	
Calbindin-D$_{28K}$ ↑	
PMCA1b ↓ ↑	
NCX ↓ ↑	
1α(OH)ase ↓	

functional VDRE approximately 2 kb upstream from the transcription initiation site of the NaP$_i$-type IIa gene. At present, sufficient data are not available to postulate a direct role of 1,25(OH)$_2$D$_3$ on proximal P$_i$ reabsorption in general and on the individual P$_i$ transporters in particular.

IV. SUMMARY

Recently, detailed insights in the vitamin D action on Ca^{2+} and P$_i$ homeostasis were obtained from several animal models including vitamin D-depleted rats and knockout mice in which the VDR and 1α(OH)ase genes were inactivated. The delineated effects on the individual Ca^{2+} and P$_i$ transporters are summarized in Table 1. In general, 1,25(OH)$_2$D$_3$ has profound stimulatory effects on the Ca^{2+} transport proteins, explaining the vitamin D dependency of transepithelial Ca^{2+} transport in small intestine and kidney. The situation is less clear for renal and intestinal P$_i$ handling. Only in the small intestine it is well established that vitamin D stimulates Na$^+$-dependent P$_i$ transport, but the elucidation of the molecular mechanism awaits future investigations.

Glossary

calbindin-D Vitamin D-dependent Ca^{2+}-binding proteins consisting of a 28 kDa protein (calbindin-D$_{28K}$) and a 9 kDa protein (calbindin-D$_{9K}$) that bind Ca^{2+} with high affinity and facilitate diffusion of cytosolic Ca^{2+}.

ECaC Epithelial calcium channels that were identified in kidney and small intestine as ECaC1 and ECaC2 (also known as CaT1), respectively, and are the gatekeepers in active Ca^{2+} (re)absorption.

NaPi Sodium–phosphate co-transporters that mediate the movement of extracellular phosphate into cells driven by the existing Na$^+$ gradient. To date, three different families, named types I, II, and III, have been identified.

NCX Na$^+$–Ca^{2+} exchanger present in the plasma membrane and the kidney; it is primarily responsible for the basolateral extrusion of Ca^{2+} in the distal tubular cells.

1α(OH)ase knockout mice A mouse strain in which the key enzyme 25(OH)D-1α-hydroxylase has been inactivated, mimicking the genetic disorder vitamin D-dependent rickets type I, also known as pseudo-vitamin D-deficiency rickets.

PMCA Plasma membrane Ca^{2+} ATPase that mediates the extrusion of Ca^{2+} across the basolateral membrane. To date, four different genes have been identified; PMCA1b is the predominant isoform expressed in the small intestine and the distal part of the nephron.

VDR knockout mice A mouse strain in which the vitamin D receptor has been inactivated, mimicking the autosomal recessive disorder hypocalcemic vitamin D-resistant rickets.

See Also the Following Articles

Vitamin D • Vitamin D and Human Nutrition • Vitamin D-Binding Protein • Vitamin D: Biological Effects of 1,25(OH)$_2$D$_3$ in Bone • Vitamin D Deficiency, Rickets and Osteomalacia • Vitamin D-Dependent Calbindins (CaBP) • Vitamin D Metabolism

Further Reading

Beck, L., Karaplis, A. C., Amizuka, N., Hewson, A. S., Ozawa, H., and Tenenhouse, H. S. (1998). Targeted inactivation of Npt2 in mice leads to severe renal phosphate wasting, hypercalciuria, and skeletal abnormalities. *Proc. Natl. Acad. Sci. USA* **95**, 5372–5377.

Brown, A. J., Dusso, A., and Slatopolsky, E. (1999). Vitamin D. *Am. J. Physiol.* **277**, F157–F175.

Colnot, S., Ovejero, C., Romagnolo, B., Porteu, A., Lacourte, P., Thomasset, M., and Perret, C. (2000). Transgenic analysis of the response of the rat calbindin-D$_{9k}$ gene to vitamin D. *Endocrinology* **141**, 2301–2308.

Dardenne, O., Prud'homme, J., Arabian, A., Glorieux, F. H., and St-Arnaud, R. (2001). Targeted inactivation of the 25-hydroxyvitamin D$_3$-1(alpha)-hydroxylase gene (CYP27B1) creates an animal model of pseudovitamin D-deficiency rickets. *Endocrinology* **142**, 3135–3141.

Hattenhauer, O., Traebert, M., Murer, H., and Biber, J. (1999). Regulation of small intestinal Na-P(i) type IIb cotransporter by dietary phosphate intake. *Am. J. Physiol.* **277**, G756–G762.

Hoenderop, J. G., Dardenne, O., van Abel, M., van Der Kemp, A. W., van Os, C. H., St. Arnaud, R., and Bindels, R. J. (2002). Modulation of renal Ca^{2+} transport protein genes by dietary Ca^{2+} and 1,25-dihydroxyvitamin D$_3$ in 25-hydroxyvitamin D$_3$-1α hydroxylase knockout mice. *FASEB J.* **16**, 1398–1406.

Hoenderop, J. G. J., van der Kemp, A. W., Hartog, A., van de Graaf, S. F., van Os, C. H., Willems, P. H. G. M., and Bindels, R. J. M. (1999). Molecular identification of the apical Ca^{2+}

channel in 1,25-dihydroxyvitamin D$_3$-responsive epithelia. *J. Biol. Chem.* **274**, 8375–8378.

Hoenderop, J. G. J., Nilius, B., and Bindels, R. J. M. (2002). Molecular mechanisms of active Ca^{2+} reabsorption in the distal nephron. *Annu. Rev. Physiol.* **64**, 529–549.

Katai, K., Miyamoto, K., Kishida, S., Segawa, H., Nii, T., Tanaka, H., Tani, Y., Arai, H., Tatsumi, S., Morita, K., Taketani, Y., and Takeda, E. (1999). Regulation of intestinal Na$^+$-dependent phosphate co-transporters by a low-phosphate diet and 1, 25-dihydroxyvitamin D$_3$. *Biochem. J.* **343**, 705–712.

Murer, H., Hernando, N., Forster, I., and Biber, J. (2000). Proximal tubular phosphate reabsorption: Molecular mechanisms. *Physiol. Rev.* **80**, 1373–1409.

Murer, H., Hernando, N., Forster, L., and Biber, J. (2001). Molecular mechanisms in proximal tubular and small intestinal phosphate reabsorption (plenary lecture). *Mol. Membr. Biol.* **18**, 3–11.

Norman, A. W., Song, X., Zanello, L., Bula, C., and Okamura, W. H. (1999). Rapid and genomic biological responses are mediated by different shapes of the agonist steroid hormone, 1alpha,25(OH)$_2$vitamin D$_3$. *Steroids* **64**, 120–128.

Panda, D. K., Miao, D., Tremblay, M. L., Sirois, J., Farookhi, R., Hendy, G. N., and Goltzman, D. (2001). Targeted ablation of the 25-hydroxyvitamin D 1alpha-hydroxylase enzyme: Evidence for skeletal, reproductive, and immune dysfunction. *Proc. Natl. Acad. Sci. USA* **98**, 7498–7503.

Peng, J. B., Chen, X. Z., Berger, U. V., Vassilev, P. M., Tsukaguchi, H., Brown, E. M., and Hediger, M. A. (1999). Molecular cloning and characterization of a channel-like transporter mediating intestinal calcium absorption. *J. Biol. Chem.* **274**, 22739–22746.

Slatopolsky, E., Dusso, A., and Brown, A. (1999). New analogs of vitamin D$_3$. *Kidney Int. Suppl.* **73**, S46–S51.

Tenenhouse, H. S., Gauthier, C., Martel, J., Hoenderop, J. G., Hartog, A., Meyer, M. H., Meyer, R. A., Jr., and Bindels, R. J. (2002). Na/P$_i$ cotransporter (Npt2) gene disruption increases duodenal calcium absorption and expression of epithelial calcium. *Pflugers Arch.* **444**, 670–676.

Van Cromphaut, S. J., Dewerchin, M., Hoenderop, J. G. J., Stockmans, I., Van Herck, E., Kato, S., Bindels, R. J. M., Collen, D., Carmeliet, P., Bouillon, R., and Carmeliet, G. (2001). Duodenal calcium absorption in vitamin D receptor-knockout mice: Functional and molecular aspects. *Proc. Natl. Acad. Sci. USA* **98**, 13324–13329.

Vitamin D Deficiency, Rickets and Osteomalacia

DAVID FELDMAN AND PETER J. MALLOY
Stanford University

The complex interplay of 1,25-dihydroxyvitamin D$_3$ (calcitriol) and parathyroid hormone regulates mineral metabolism and proper delivery of minerals to the skeleton. Supply of adequate calcium and phosphate to bone-forming sites is critical for synthesizing normal bone and for preventing rickets or osteomalacia. A defect in any step in the pathway of synthesis or action of 1,25-dihydroxyvitamin D$_3$ can cause these diseases.

I. INTRODUCTION

Bone is a complex, living tissue composed of a mineralized protein matrix that forms a hard and rigid skeletal framework. Osteoblasts are the bone-forming cells that secrete the malleable collagen matrix that is eventually mineralized with hydroxyapatite, a calcium phosphate crystal. Bone is constantly turning over; osteoclast-mediated resorption in specific areas of bone is coupled to bone formation carried out by osteoblasts. In order to maintain normal mineralization of newly formed bone, adequate calcium and phosphate must be delivered to the osteoblasts at bone-forming sites. To meet this mineral requirement for normal bone formation and turnover requires the ingestion of adequate calcium and phosphate in the diet and the presence of adequate amounts of vitamin D, the hormone responsible for regulating mineral absorption from the gastrointestinal tract. If calcium or phosphate delivery to the bone-forming site is inadequate, undermineralized bone is formed. This process is called osteomalacia. If osteomalacia develops during childhood, while active bone growth is underway, the undermineralization of both bone and cartilage leads to rickets. This involves failure or delay of mineralization in the growth plates and joints as well as in other skeletal sites.

Undermineralized bone is characterized by excess osteoid, the collagenous bone matrix, relative to mineral. Normally, most osteoid is rapidly mineralized and only a small rim of unmineralized matrix can be found on bone trabeculae. However, in rickets or osteomalacia, the level of unmineralized osteoid is increased. Initially, osteoid surface and volume are increased, but osteoid thickness and lag times (delay in mineralizing osteoid) are normal. In more severe cases, osteoid thickness exceeds 15 μm and mineralization lag time exceeds 100 days. In the most florid cases, no mineralization is detected. The strength of unmineralized osteoid is greatly diminished compared to normally mineralized bone, leading to metabolic bone disease and increased susceptibility to fracture. In the case of rickets, a number of additional skeletal abnormalities are found, including bowing of the long bones, joint pain and swelling, bone pain, and abnormalities of the teeth. In severe vitamin D insufficiency, infants with rickets may show delayed development and even respiratory failure if thoracic cage development is impaired sufficiently to restrict breathing.

II. NORMAL VITAMIN D PHYSIOLOGY

A. Synthesis

Calcium is absorbed in the upper small intestine under the control of the active vitamin D hormone, 1,25-dihydroxyvitamin D_3 [1,25(OH)$_2$D$_3$], also known as calcitriol (in this article these terms are used interchangeably). There are two forms of vitamin D: vitamin D_2 (ergocalciferol), of plant origin, and vitamin D_3 (cholecalciferol), of animal origin. Vitamin D_3 can be synthesized in the skin with the aid of sunlight or it is ingested in the diet. The distribution of vitamin D_3 in food is quite restricted, being substantial mainly in oily fish. Because dietary vitamin D is so limited, in some countries various foods (milk, cereals, etc.) have been fortified with either vitamin D_2 or vitamin D_3 in order to avoid widespread vitamin D deficiency. Even in countries with standard vitamin D fortification programs, however, nutritional sources of vitamin D may be limited and exposure to sunlight is critical for adequate endogenous production of vitamin D_3.

As outlined in Fig. 1, vitamin D is ingested in the diet or is endogenously manufactured following exposure to ultraviolet rays of sunlight, which causes conversion of the precursor 7-dehydrocholesterol to vitamin D_3 in the skin. Vitamin D_3 is subsequently converted to the active hormone by a two-step process, first by 25-hydroxylation in the liver to 25-hydroxyvitamin D_3 and then by 1-hydroxylation in the kidney to 1,25-dihydroxyvitamin D_3. 1,25-Dihydroxyvitamin D_3 then acts via the intranuclear vitamin D receptor (VDR) to regulate target genes, in a pathway similar to those of other steroid hormones. The target genes are involved in regulation of calcium and phosphate delivery to the bone-forming sites to mineralize osteoid.

Any step in the pathway of calcitriol synthesis or action that is defective can result in rickets/osteomalacia. The usual causes of rickets/osteomalacia are shown in Fig. 1 and are detailed in Table 1. The most common cause of rickets/osteomalacia worldwide is nutritional vitamin D deficiency, combined

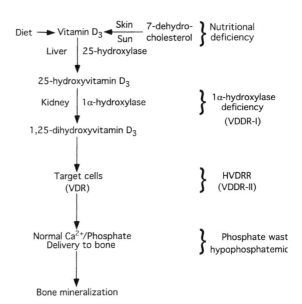

FIGURE 1 Calcitriol synthesis and action. Defects at various points in the synthetic pathway of calcitriol (1,25-dihydroxyvitamin D_3) cause osteomalacia or rickets due to interference with normal mineralization of bone. VDR, Vitamin D receptor; VDDR-I/II, vitamin D-dependent rickets types I and II; HVDRR, hereditary 1,25-dihydroxyvitamin D_3-resistant rickets.

with insufficient synthesis in the skin. This can be caused by inadequate dietary consumption of vitamin D and/or by malabsorption of vitamin D in the gastrointestinal tract, coupled with inadequate sunlight exposure. Because vitamin D supplementation

TABLE 1   Etiology of Rickets or Osteomalacia

Nutritional: vitamin D deficiency
  Deficient synthesis due to inadequate sunlight exposure
  Dietary deficiency
Gastrointestinal disorders
  Malabsorption syndrome
  Hepato-biliary disease
  Pancreatic disease
Renal insufficiency
Tumor-induced osteomalacia (TIO)
Hereditary causes
  X-Linked hypophosphatemic rickets (XLH)
  1α-Hydroxylase deficiency (vitamin D-dependent rickets, type I)
  Hereditary vitamin D-resistant rickets (HVDRR, vitamin D-dependent rickets, type II)
  Autosomal dominant hypophosphatemic rickets (ADHR)
Miscellaneous causes
  Acidosis
  Phosphate depletion
  Renal tubular disorders

of milk or other dietary products reduces nutritional causes of rickets/osteomalacia in the United States and in other developed countries, other etiologies are becoming more important. Other causes of rickets/osteomalacia include the inability to synthesize calcitriol due to renal failure or due to a genetic defect in 1α-hydroxylase, the key enzyme involved in calcitriol synthesis. Abnormalities that cause excess loss of phosphate include genetic defects or tumors that produce phosphaturia. Finally, mutations in the vitamin D receptor, the protein that mediates calcitriol actions in the intestine and other target tissues, can cause rickets in children.

B. Regulation of Calcium and Phosphate Homeostasis

Control of calcium levels in the serum is tightly regulated by the interplay of calcitriol and parathyroid hormone (PTH). As depicted in Fig. 2, serum calcium concentration is monitored by the calcium-sensing

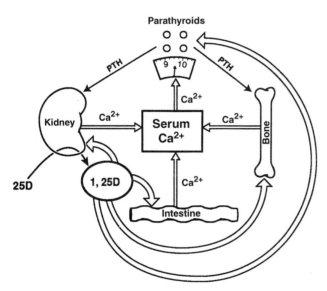

FIGURE 2 Regulation of serum Ca^{2+} levels. The control of calcium levels in the blood is tightly regulated by vitamin D and parathyroid hormone (PTH). Gastrointestinal absorption of calcium from the diet is controlled by the activity of 1,25-dihydroxyvitamin D_3 (1,25D). The active form of vitamin D is synthesized in the kidney by 1α-hydroxylation of circulating 25-hydroxyvitamin D_3 (25D). 1,25-Dihydroxyvitamin D_3 also acts on bone to resorb calcium and on the parathyroid glands to suppress PTH. The calcium-sensing receptor in the parathyroids detects the concentration of serum calcium. When calcium levels begin to fall, PTH secretion is increased, which acts on the kidney to stimulate 1α-hydroxylase activity and increase 1,25-dihydroxyvitamin D_3 synthesis. PTH also acts on bone and kidney to elevate serum calcium levels. Reproduced from Feldman *et al.* (2001), with permission from Elsevier Science.

receptor present in the parathyroid glands and possibly also in the kidney and other sites. PTH synthesis is negatively regulated by calcium and by calcitriol. When the calcium concentration falls, the PTH level rises in an attempt to restore serum calcium to normal. The actions of PTH on the skeleton increase bone resorption whereas the actions of PTH on the kidney reduce the level of calcium excretion. Both processes help to maintain serum calcium within the normal range. Importantly, the actions of PTH on the kidney also result in increased activation of the 1α-hydroxylase enzyme, which augments conversion of circulating 25-hydroxyvitamin D_3 to the active hormone calcitriol. The increased concentration of calcitriol activates intestinal cells to increase calcium absorption along the length of the intestine. These combined actions restore the circulating calcium concentration to normal. Elevated levels of PTH return to normal in response both to normalization of serum calcium and to feedback inhibition of PTH production by a direct action of calcitriol on the parathyroid glands.

Control of phosphate levels is in part controlled by vitamin D but, importantly, is also regulated by other systems that are incompletely understood. Calcitriol increases both calcium and phosphate absorption from the intestine. PTH, although it increases calcium reabsorption in the kidney, inhibits phosphate reabsorption, causing phosphaturia. Renal phosphate transport is controlled by sodium phosphate cotransporter type IIa (NPT2), which is responsible for the bulk of phosphate reabsorption in the proximal tubule of the kidney. It is postulated that there is a phosphate-regulating hormone, phosphatonin, that regulates NPT2. Recent data suggest that fibroblast growth factor 23 (FGF 23) may be the phosphate-regulating molecule. Abnormalities of phosphatonin balance contribute to several causes of rickets/osteomalacia (see Section IV,A).

C. The Vitamin D Receptor

Although called a vitamin, 1,25-dihydroxyvitamin D_3 is actually a member of the steroid hormone family. 1,25-Dihydroxyvitamin D_3 regulates calcium metabolism and promotes other physiologic actions through the vitamin D receptor, a member of the steroid/thyroid/retinoid receptor gene superfamily. These receptors regulate gene transcription by acting as ligand-activated transcription factors (see Fig. 3). Members of this receptor family share a modular structure comprising an N-terminal transactivation domain of variable length, a DNA-binding domain

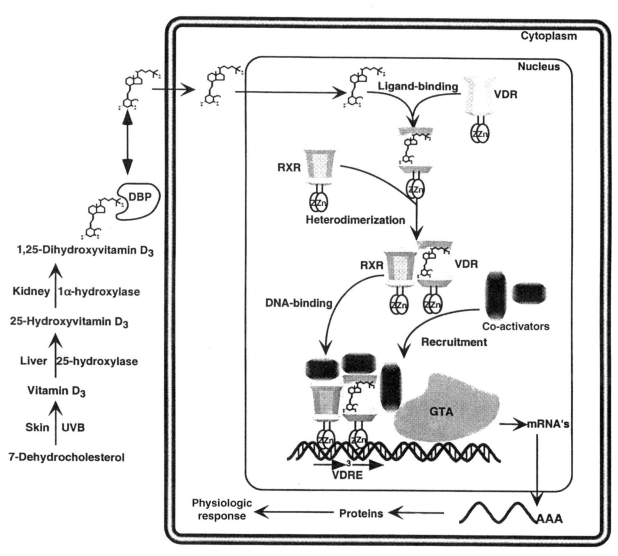

FIGURE 3 Mechanism of 1,25-dihydroxyvitamin D_3 action on target cells. After conversion of 7-dehydrocholesterol in the skin by ultraviolet B (UVB) light, the active form of vitamin D, 1,25-dihydroxyvitamin D_3, is synthesized by sequential hydroxylation steps in the liver and kidney. Once in the circulation, some of 1,25-dihydroxyvitamin D_3 is bound by the vitamin D-binding protein (DBP), and a small amount remains free. The free 1,25-dihydroxyvitamin D_3 enters the cell and binds to the vitamin D receptor (VDR). The occupied VDR heterodimerizes with the retinoid X receptor (RXR) and binds to vitamin D response elements (VDREs) on target genes. Binding to DNA is carried out by the two zinc (Zn) finger DNA-binding domains of the VDR. Co-activators are recruited to the VDR-RXR complex, allowing the general transcription apparatus (GTA) to initiate gene transcription. Reproduced from Malloy, P. J., Pike, J. W., and Feldman, D. (1999). The vitamin D receptor and the syndrome of hereditary 1, 25-dihydroxyvitamin D-resistant rickets. *Endocr. Rev.* 20, 156–188. Copyright The Endocrine Society.

(DBD) that enables interaction of the receptor proteins with hormone response elements in promoter regions of target genes, and a C-terminal ligand-binding domain (LBD). In addition, a highly conserved region at the C-terminus of the LBD, defined as the activation function-2 domain (AF-2), regulates transcription. Like other steroid receptors, the VDR LBD binds specifically to its cognate ligand,

calcitriol, triggering a series of molecular events leading to the activation of vitamin D-responsive genes. Regulation of specific gene transcription by the VDR requires its binding as a heterodimer with the retinoid X receptor (RXR). RXR heterodimerizes with a number of other receptors in the steroid/thyroid/retinoid gene superfamily, including thyroid receptor, retinoic acid receptor, and the peroxisome proliferator-activating receptor. Initiation of gene transcription also involves the recruitment of co-activator proteins that act as bridging factors linking the VDR to the preinitiation complexes and RNA polymerase II. Co-activators include a family of closely related p160 proteins such as SRC-1/NcoA1, TIF2/GRIP1/NcoA2/SRC-2, and pCIP/Rac3/ACTR/AIB1/SRC-3. Other co-activators include a group of proteins collectively called vitamin D receptor-inter-acting proteins (DRIPs). These co-activator proteins associate with nuclear receptors in a ligand-dependent manner to enhance transactivation of target genes.

D. Mechanism of Action

How do cells respond to calcitriol? A simplified model of calcitriol action is shown in Fig. 3. After the hormone is produced and secreted by the kidney, it is transported in the blood either bound to vitamin D-binding protein (DBP) or in the free state. The free hormone is lipid-soluble and readily gains entry into cells by permeating the lipid bilayer of the cell membrane. Cells that respond to calcitriol have VDRs located in the cell nuclear compartment, where they are loosely associated with the RXR. Once inside the cell, calcitriol encounters the VDR and binds in the ligand-binding pocket in the LBD. Calcitriol binding causes the VDR to bind more tightly to the RXR and to interact with vitamin D response elements (VDREs) on target genes. When calcitriol occupies the ligand-binding pocket, helix H12 in the VDR LBD swings into position, locking the hormone inside the binding domain and at the same time forming a new surface interface for interaction with co-activators. The co-activators that are recruited by the VDR, such as steroid receptor co-activator-1 (SRC-1), are then able to remodel the chromatin so that assembly of the transcriptional apparatus can take place. The VDR can then recruit the DRIP complex and begin activating gene transcription.

III. VITAMIN D DEFICIENCY, RICKETS AND OSTEOMALACIA

A. Nutritional Deficiency

Vitamin D deficiency causes a constellation of metabolic abnormalities that combine to cause osteo-malacia or rickets. The insufficiency of vitamin D, if severe, can result in diminished intestinal calcium absorption and hypocalcemia. The calcium-sensing receptor present in the parathyroid gland detects the low serum calcium level. This leads to an increase in PTH synthesis and results in secondary hyperpara-thyroidism. The elevated levels of PTH allow correction of the hypocalcemia by three actions on bone and kidney. One action is aimed at stimulating renal 1α-hydroxylase activity to cause increased renal production of calcitriol. However, for increased production of calcitriol, this step requires adequate vitamin D_3 and 25-hydroxyvitamin D_3 substrate, which is inadequate in vitamin D deficiency. A second PTH action on bone is to increase bone resorption, thus increasing calcium and phosphate flux from bone to serum. A third PTH action is to increase renal calcium reabsorption and decrease calciuria. How-ever, PTH, while decreasing calciuria, increases phosphaturia, thus reducing the availability of this mineral component for bone mineralization. The overall result of vitamin D deficiency is hypocalcemia, secondary hyperparathyroidism, and defective miner-alization of osteoid, leading to the development of osteomalacia.

It is clear that adequate calcium and vitamin D_3 are required for bone health. The vitamin D_3 requirement is estimated to be 400 international units (IU) per day, although elderly subjects may require 600 IU or more. Most infants and children in the United States have adequate vitamin D intake because of vitamin D supplementation of milk. During adolescence, when consumption of milk and dairy products diminishes, decreased dietary vitamin D may adversely affect calcium absorption and thereby lead to impaired skeletal health. Vitamin D insufficiency in the elderly population greatly increases their risk for both osteoporosis and osteo-malacia. This problem is more severe in countries that do not supplement milk or other foods with vitamin D and where sunlight exposure may be inadequate.

Except for oily fish, most dietary components lack substantial levels of vitamin D_3. In the United States, milk is ostensibly fortified with 400 IU of vitamin D_3 per quart, although amounts vary. For the many individuals who do not include in their diet adequate amounts of milk or dairy products, exposure to ultraviolet radiation from sunlight is necessary to achieve normal vitamin D status. Endogenous vitamin D production occurs in the skin, which contains a vitamin D_3 precursor, 7-dehydrocholesterol; this compound undergoes photolysis on exposure to solar irradiation and is converted to vitamin D. Thus, inadequate dietary intake and inadequate sun exposure lead to vitamin D insufficiency. This problem is exacerbated by several modern trends, including avoidance of dairy products to control weight or high cholesterol and avoidance of sunlight to reduce the risk of skin cancer. Also, many elderly individuals have limited mobility and do not have the opportunity for adequate sunlight exposure. These circumstances have led to a substantial increase in the frequency of osteomalacic bone disease and fractures in the elderly, especially among the nursing home population. In wintertime, the problem of reduced sunlight further diminishes vitamin D_3 synthesis and worsens the tendency toward vitamin D_3 insufficiency. Races of people with dark skin have further difficulty with adequate vitamin D_3 synthesis, because the melanin in the skin is a natural sunscreen that reduces the penetration of ultraviolet rays into the layers of the dermis where vitamin D_3 is formed.

Deficient dietary calcium intake may also cause osteomalacia or exacerbate the problem of vitamin D insufficiency. There exists a spectrum of etiologies ranging from pure vitamin D deficiency with normal calcium to adequate vitamin D sufficiency with inadequate calcium. Worldwide, many cases of osteomalacia are due to vitamin D insufficiency combined with relative calcium insufficiency. Certain dietary habits common in selected populations may exacerbate vitamin D insufficiency by inhibiting vitamin D absorption or by increasing the metabolic clearance of 25-hydroxyvitamin D_3. The consumption of chapattis, an East Asian bread made from wheat flour with high phytate levels, impairs both calcium and vitamin D absorption. Thus, inadequate sunlight exposure and dietary habits combine in a variety of situations—e.g., because of customs, life-style choices (vegetarianism, high-fiber diets), or economic, age-related, and geographic circumstance (living at high altitude, calcium-deficient diets)—to exacerbate vitamin D insufficiency, thus determining the risk and severity of osteomalacic bone disease.

B. Gastrointestinal Problems and Malabsorption of Vitamin D

In parts of the world where there are no programs to fortify foodstuffs with vitamin D, the diet of much of the population is estimated to contribute only one-quarter to one-third of the daily requirement of vitamin D. In such populations, therefore, gastrointestinal malabsorption may worsen the vitamin D insufficiency, but is not often the sole cause of osteomalacia. Some gastrointestinal problems are associated with increased metabolic clearance of vitamin D metabolites, compounding the malabsorption problem. Gastrointestinal diseases associated with osteomalacia include celiac disease (gluten

enteropathy), cirrhosis, biliary obstruction, pancreatic insufficiency, inflammatory bowel disease, and post-gastrectomy or jejuno-ileal bypass surgery. Patients receiving total parenteral nutrition (TPN), usually because of chronic bowel disease, develop osteomalacia due to inadequate mineral or vitamin D supplementation. Anticonvulsant therapy increases the metabolic clearance of vitamin D metabolites, requiring vitamin D supplementation.

C. Renal Osteodystrophy

Renal failure is associated with complex abnormalities of vitamin D and calcium metabolism. Phosphate retention due to inadequate kidney function causes hypocalcemia by complexing calcium and inhibiting renal 1α-hydroxylase activity, and therefore diminishing calcitriol synthesis. Also, as kidneys shrink and renal functional tissue declines, 1α-hydroxylase activity is further diminished, leading to deficiency of calcitriol production. These changes also lead to secondary hyperparathyroidism, compounding the bone abnormality. The constellation of hypocalcemia, secondary hyperparathyroidism, and calcitriol deficiency causes osteomalacia and renal osteodystrophy. Recognition of this sequence of events has led to important changes in the medical management of renal failure in an attempt to prevent the development of renal osteodystrophy. Two major therapeutic measures include the use of phosphate binders to minimize and/or prevent the development of elevated phosphate concentration and its consequent hypocalcemia, and supplementation with calcitriol to avoid deficiency of active vitamin D.

D. Tumor-Induced Osteomalacia

Some small mesenchymal tumors (hemangiopericytomas, fibromas, angiosarcomas, etc.) can cause phosphaturia and hypophosphatemia, leading to osteomalacia. The syndrome is known as tumor-induced osteomalacia (TIO), or oncogenic osteomalacia. The mechanism involves the synthesis and secretion of excessive amounts of a phosphaturic factor. Currently, the major candidate for this role is FGF 23. How FGF 23 causes phosphaturia is still not completely understood. However, recent findings from the study of X-linked hypophosphatemia and autosomal dominant hypophosphatemic rickets have shed light on TIO and on the mechanisms for all three phosphaturic entities. The tumors causing TIO originally were thought to be benign and of mesenchymal origin, but malignant tumors have also been reported to cause the syndrome. Often the tumors are small and difficult to locate. The levels of calcitriol are inappropriately low (hypophosphatemia should stimulate calcitriol production) and so the tumor product is also thought to interfere with renal 1α-hydroxylation. The osteomalacia responds to treatment with large phosphate supplements, which restore phosphate levels to normal. The syndrome can be cured by successfully removing the tumor.

IV. HEREDITARY RICKETS

A comparison of hereditary causes of rickets is shown in Table 2.

A. Hypophosphatemic Rickets

1. X-Linked Hypophosphatemic Rickets

X-Linked hypophosphatemia (XLH), an X-linked dominant disorder caused by renal phosphate wasting, results in severe skeletal abnormalities and growth retardation. The primary mechanism, defective phosphate reabsorption in the renal proximal tubule, impairs phosphate reabsorption. The clinical presentation is usually not apparent until 6–12 months of age and ranges from mild abnormalities of the bones to severe rickets and osteomalacia. Children exhibit rachitic bone deformities, including enlargement of the wrists and knees and bowing of the lower extremities. Defects in tooth development and premature cranial synostoses may also be present. Low or inappropriately normal circulating levels of calcitriol are found despite the hypophosphatemia. The low serum phosphate normally causes an increase in 1α-hydroxylase activity and enhanced calcitriol production, suggesting that XLH may also result in abnormal regulation of 1α-hydroxylase.

The gene causing XLH has been cloned; it is a phosphate-regulating gene with homologies to endopeptidases and is located on the X-chromosome, thus it has been named *PHEX*. The *PHEX* gene is homologous to a family of endopeptidases that includes endothelin-converting enzyme-1 and neutral endopeptidase. The *PHEX* gene encodes a 749-amino-acid membrane-bound protein that is expressed in bone, adult ovary, lung, and fetal liver. A number of genetic defects in the *PHEX* gene have been found in patients with XLH. Because many of the mutations are inactivating mutations, the X-linked dominant expression of the disorder is likely the result of the loss of a single functioning allele (haploinsufficiency) coded by the X-chromosome rather than the result of a dominant negative effect.

2. Autosomal Dominant Hypophosphatemic Rickets

Autosomal dominant hypophosphatemic rickets (ADHR), an autosomal dominant disorder caused by phosphate wasting, has findings commonly seen in other phosphate wasting disorders. Patients have short stature, bone pain, rickets, and osteomalacia. The patients also have inappropriately normal serum calcitriol concentrations.

The gene causing ADHR has been cloned; recent data have suggested that fibroblast growth factor 23 is the phosphate-regulating molecule, thus the ADHR gene has been named *FGF23*. The *FGF23* gene encodes a member of the fibroblast growth factor family, a 251-amino-acid protein that is expressed in heart, lymph node, thymus, and liver. Three unique mutations have been found in the *FGF23* gene in patients with ADHR. These mutations affect two arginine residues located in a consensus proteolytic cleavage site. The mutations prevent degradation of *FGF-23* and thus result in enhanced or prolonged action leading to phosphate wasting and the syndrome of ADHR.

TABLE 2 Comparison of Genetic Causes of Rickets[a]

Component	1α-Hydroxylase deficiency	HVDRR	XLH	ADHR
Gene	*CYP27B1*	*VDR*	*PHEX*	*FGF23*
$1,25(OH)_2D_3$	Low	High	(Normal)	(Normal)
PTH	High	High	Normal	Normal
Calcium	Low	Low	Normal	Normal
Phosphate	Low	Low	Low	Low
Alopecia	No	Yes	No	No

[a]1α-Hydroxylase deficiency, causes vitamin D-dependent rickets, type I; HVDRR, hereditary vitamin D-resistant rickets; XLH, X-linked hypophosphatemic rickets; ADHR, autosomal dominant hypophosphatemic rickets; (normal) indicates inappropriately normal relative to decreased serum phosphate concentration.

3. Mechanism of Phosphate Loss in XLH, ADHR, and TIO

How are *PHEX* and *FGF23* involved in the pathophysiology of XLH, ADHR, and TIO? One current hypothesis is that under conditions of normal phosphate regulation the *PHEX*-encoded enzyme regulates the bioavailability of the *FGF23*-encoded protein, the putative phosphatonin molecule. As *FGF23* product is secreted from cells, some of it is degraded to inactive metabolites by the membrane-bound *PHEX* endopeptidase. The remaining active *FGF23* product enters the circulation and interacts with a receptor protein on the renal tubule cells. Binding transmits a signal to down-regulate the activity of the sodium-dependent phosphate cotransporter (NPT2) in the kidney and to decrease phosphate reabsorption. In XLH patients, the mutant *PHEX* protein or lack thereof is unable to degrade the *FGF23* protein. This leads to excess amounts of *FGF23* protein in the circulation. As a result, the signal to down-regulate NPT2 activity is magnified, leading to renal phosphate wasting. In ADHR, on the other hand, mutations in *FGF23* prevent the proteolytic processing step by the *PHEX* product and therefore there is an overabundance of active *FGF23* protein, which then leads to down-regulation of NPT2 activity, which causes phosphate wasting. In TIO, tumors overexpress *FGF23* protein, and elevated secretion by the tumors also leads to phosphate wasting and osteomalacia in this condition.

B. 1α-Hydroxylase Deficiency

This disease was originally known as vitamin D-dependent rickets type I (VDDR-I). Other names include pseudo-vitamin D deficiency type I and pseudo-vitamin D deficiency rickets (PDDR). We prefer to refer to the entity as 1α-hydroxylase deficiency because it has been shown to be caused by mutations in the cytochrome P450 enzyme, 25-hydroxyvitamin D 1α-hydroxylase (1α-hydroxylase). The human 1α-hydroxylase gene (*CYP27B1*) is located on chromosome 12. A number of mutations that disrupt 1α-hydroxylase activity are found scattered throughout the entire region of the *CYP27B1* gene. 1α-Hydroxylase deficiency is a rare autosomal recessive disease that is manifested at an early age. Patients exhibit hypocalcemia, elevated levels of PTH and alkaline phosphatase, and low levels of urine calcium. Affected children present with hypotonia, muscle weakness, growth failure, and rickets. Tetany and convulsions may occur with severe hypocalcemia. Patients have normal serum concentrations of 25-hydroxyvitamin D_3 but low levels of $1,25(OH)_2D_3$ due to the defective synthesis of $1,25(OH)_2D_3$. PTH infusion does not increase circulating $1,25(OH)_2D_3$ levels, consistent with a defect in 1α-hydroxylase activity. Very large doses of vitamin D_3 or 25-hydroxyvitamin D_3 are required for adequate treatment of 1α-hydroxylase deficiency; often, daily vitamin D doses of 20,000 to over 100,000 IU are needed. On the other hand, modest doses of $1,25(OH)_2D_3$ (0.25–2 μg/day) tend to be sufficient to restore calcium to normal and to heal the rickets. Because mutations in 1α-hydroxylase block $1,25(OH)_2D_3$ synthesis, this latter treatment bypasses the defect and reverses the abnormalities caused by the disease.

C. Hereditary 1,25-Dihydroxyvitamin D₃-Resistant Rickets

Hereditary 1,25-dihydroxyvitamin D_3-resistant rickets (HVDRR) is known as vitamin D-dependent rickets type II (VDDR-II), or pseudo-vitamin D deficiency type II. This rare genetic disease arises as a result of mutations in the VDR; HVDRR is an autosomal recessive disease characterized by early-onset rickets, hypocalcemia, secondary hyperparathyroidism, and normal or elevated serum $1,25(OH)_2D$ levels. Parents of children with HVDRR usually have a history of consanguinity and have no evidence of bone disease. In many cases, the affected child exhibits total body alopecia, lacking all body hair, including eyelids and eyelashes. The alopecia, which usually occurs within the first year after birth, provides evidence for the HVDRR syndrome.

Several missense mutations have been identified in the VDR DBD. These usually occur in highly conserved amino acids. In a few families, nonsense mutations that result in premature termination of the VDR have also been found. Some premature termination signals result from mutations that cause exon skipping or affect RNA splicing. A number of missense mutations in the VDR LBD have also been identified. In one case, an arginine at codon 274 was mutated to leucine, which affected $1,25(OH)_2D_3$ binding. Arginine 274 is the contact point for the 1-hydroxyl group of $1,25(OH)_2D_3$ in the ligand-binding pocket of the VDR. In a second case, histidine was mutated to glutamine at codon 305, which caused a 5- to 10-fold reduction in $1,25(OH)_2D_3$ binding and a similar reduction in gene transactivation. Histidine 305 is the residue that makes contact with the 25-hydroxyl group of $1,25(OH)_2D_3$. Some mutations also disrupt RXR heterodimeriztion with the VDR. An arginine to cysteine mutation at codon 391 interfered with RXR binding but did not affect $1,25(OH)_2D_3$ binding, whereas another mutation, phenylalanine to cysteine at codon 251, affected both $1,25(OH)_2D_3$ binding and RXR heterodimeriztion. Interestingly, there has been one case of HVDRR in which no mutations were found in the VDR. The patient exhibited all the signs of HVDRR, including alopecia. This case highlights the fact that proteins other than VDR are involved in $1,25(OH)_2D_3$ signaling and that defects in these proteins may also cause the HVDRR syndrome. Genetic defects in co-activators may also be the molecular basis for other steroid hormone-resistant syndromes.

Some children with HVDRR respond to large doses of calcitriol, which can overcome the VDR ligand-binding defects, whereas others respond to large doses of calcium and calcitriol. However, in cases in which the VDR is completely inactivated, the patients are unresponsive to large doses of vitamin D derivatives or oral calcium supplements. Successful treatment of these children has been achieved by chronic intravenous administration of calcium infusions, given nightly over a period of many months. This treatment bypasses the intestinal defect in calcium absorption and over time is able to correct the hypocalcemia. The treatment eventually results in normalization of serum calcium levels, correction of secondary hyperparathyroidism, and normal mineralization of bone and healing of rickets, as evidenced on X-rays. Clinical improvement can be sustained if adequate serum calcium and phosphorus concentrations are maintained. Although intravenous calcium may have been required to render the child normocalcemic, the benefits can sometimes be maintained thereafter by oral calcium. However, alopecia, if present, does not improve as a consequence of the treatment.

V. SUMMARY

Many forms of rickets/osteomalacia are due to genetic defects in the synthesis or action of calcitriol or to conditions that cause phosphate loss. Recent improvements in our understanding of the molecular mechanisms by which these defects cause rickets or osteomalacia have led to improved diagnostic and treatment strategies. However, the commonest cause of rickets/osteomalacia worldwide is deficiency of vitamin D. Fortification of dietary foodstuffs or provision of vitamin D_3 supplements to individuals at risk would greatly reduce the impact of this devastating disease of the skeleton.

Glossary

1α-hydroxylase Cytochrome P450 enzyme that converts 25-hydroxyvitamin D_3 to 1,25-dihydroxyvitamin D_3 by catalyzing the addition of a hydroxyl group at the C-1 position.

osteomalacia Bone disease in which mineralization of the collagen matrix of bone is defective, causing softening of the bones and susceptibility to fracture.

osteoporosis Bone disease causing increased susceptibility to fracture; although the bones have a normal content of mineral and matrix, bone loss causes porosity and fragility.

PHEX Gene on the X chromosome that encodes a membrane-bound protein with endopeptidase activity; mutations have been found in the disease X-linked hypophosphatemia.

rickets Osteomalacic disease in a growing child; caused by inadequate mineralization of bone and cartilage, resulting in bowing of the weight-bearing bones of the extremities, joint swelling, pain in bones and joints, and other skeletal problems due to softening of the bones.

vitamin D receptor Member of the steroid/retinoid/thyroid superfamily of nuclear receptors; mediates 1,25-dihydroxyvitamin D_3 actions to regulate gene expression in target cells.

See Also the Following Articles

Osteoporosis: Hormonal Treatment • Osteoporosis: Pathophysiology • Vitamin D • Vitamin D and Human Nutrition • Vitamin D-Binding Protein • Vitamin D: Biological Effects of $1,25(OH)_2D_3$ in Bone • Vitamin D: Biological Effects of $1,25(OH)_2D_3$ in the Intestine and Kidney • Vitamin D: 24,25-Dihydroxyvitamin D • Vitamin D Metabolism • Vitamin D: Nuclear Receptor for $1,25(OH)_2D_3$

Further Reading

Bishop, N. (1999). Rickets today—Children still need milk and sunshine. *N. Engl. J. Med.* **341**, 602–604.

Brown, A. J., Dusso, A., and Slatopolsky, E. (1999). Vitamin D. *Am. J. Physiol.* **277**, F157–F175.

Feldman, D., Glorieux, F. H., and Pike, J. W. (1997). "Vitamin D" Chaps. 31–56, Academic Press, San Diego.

Feldman, D., Malloy, P. J., and Gross, C. (2001). Vitamin, D: Biology, action and clinical implications. *In* "Osteoporosis" (R. Marcus, D. Feldman, and J. Kelsey, eds.), pp. 257–304. Academic Press, San Diego.

Grieff, M., Mumm, S., Waeltz, P., Mazzarella, R., Whyte, M. P., Thakker, R. V., and Schlessinger, D. (1997). Expression and cloning of the human X-linked hypophosphatemia gene cDNA. *Biochem. Biophys. Res. Commun.* **231**, 635–639.

Haussler, M. R., Whitfield, G. K., Haussler, C. A., Hsieh, J. C., Thompson, P. D., Selznick, S. H., Dominguez, C. E., and Jurutka, P. W. (1998). The nuclear vitamin D receptor:

Biological and molecular regulatory properties revealed. *J. Bone Miner. Res.* **13**, 325–349.

Heaney, R. P., Barger-Lux, M. J., Dowell, M. S., Chen, T. C., and Holick, M. F. (1997). Calcium absorptive effects of vitamin D and its major metabolites. *J. Clin. Endocrinol. Metab.* **82**, 4111–4116.

Holick, M. F. (1994). McCollum Award Lecture, 1994: Vitamin D—New horizons for the 21st century. *Am. J. Clin. Nutr.* **60**, 619–630.

Holm, I. A., Nelson, A. E., Robinson, B. G., Mason, R. S., Marsh, D. J., Cowell, C. T., and Carpenter, T. O. (2001). Mutational analysis and genotype-phenotype correlation of the *PHEX* gene in X-linked hypophosphatemic rickets. *J. Clin. Endocrinol. Metab.* **86**, 3889–3899.

Jones, G., Strugnell, S. A., and DeLuca, H. F. (1998). Current understanding of the molecular actions of vitamin D. *Physiol. Rev.* **78**, 1193–1231.

Malloy, P. J., Pike, J. W., and Feldman, D. (1999). The vitamin D receptor and the syndrome of hereditary 1,25-dihydroxyvitamin D-resistant rickets. *Endocr. Rev.* **20**, 156–188.

Miller, W. L., and Portale, A. A. (1999). Genetic causes of rickets. *Curr. Opin. Pediatr.* **11**, 333–339.

Shimada, T., Mizutani, S., Muto, T., Yoneya, T., Hino, R., Takeda, S., Takeuchi, Y., Fujita, T., Fukumoto, S., and Yamashita, T. (2001). Cloning and characterization of FGF23 as a causative factor of tumor-induced osteomalacia. *Proc. Natl. Acad. Sci. U.S.A.* **98**, 6500–6505.

Strewler, G. J. (2001). FGF23, hypophosphatemia, and rickets: Has phosphatonin been found? *Proc. Natl. Acad. Sci. U.S.A.* **98**, 5945–5946.

Takeyama, K., Kitanaka, S., Sato, T., Kobori, M., Yanagisawa, J., and Kato, S. (1997). 25-Hydroxyvitamin D_3 1alpha-hydroxylase and vitamin D synthesis. *Science* **277**, 1827–1830.

White, K. E., Jonsson, K. B., Carn, G., Hampson, G., Spector, T. D., Mannstadt, M., Lorenz-Depiereux, B., Miyauchi, A., Yang, I. M., Ljunggren, O., Meitinger, T., Strom, T. M., Juppner, H., and Econs, M. J. (2001). The autosomal dominant hypophosphatemic rickets (ADHR) gene is a secreted polypeptide overexpressed by tumors that cause phosphate wasting. *J. Clin. Endocrinol. Metab.* **86**, 497–500.

Vitamin D-Dependent Calbindins (CaBP)

Angela Porta, Puneet Dhawan,
Kristen Gengaro, Yan Liu, Xiaorong Peng, and
Sylvia Christakos

University of Medicine and Dentistry of New Jersey

I. INTRODUCTION
II. LOCALIZATION AND FUNCTIONAL SIGNIFICANCE
III. REGULATION OF CALBINDIN GENE EXPRESSION
IV. SUMMARY

Calbindin-D_{9k} and calbindin-D_{28k} are intracellular calcium-binding proteins that are present in many different tissues whose production is stimulated by the steroid hormone $1\alpha,25(OH)_2D_3$. The calbindins serve different functions and are regulated by several steroids as well as by factors that affect signal transduction pathways. Understanding their functions and activities may lead to therapeutic intervention in disorders of calcium metabolism and bone development.

I. INTRODUCTION

Increased synthesis in the intestine and kidney of the calcium-binding protein, calbindin, the first identified molecular target of vitamin D action, is one of the most pronounced effects of vitamin D known. There are two major subclasses of calbindin: calbindin-D_{9k} (a 9000-Da protein that is present in highest concentrations in mammalian intestine and in mouse and neonatal rat kidney, placenta, and uterus) and calbindin-D_{28k} (a 28,000-Da protein that is highly conserved in evolution and is present in highest concentrations in avian intestine and mammalian and avian kidney, brain, and pancreas). There is no amino acid sequence homology between calbindin-D_{9k} and calbindin-D_{28k}. The calbindins belong to a family of intracellular proteins that bind calcium with high affinity. Other members of this family include calmodulin, parvalbumin, troponin C, calretinin, calcineurin, the myosin light chains, and S100α and S100β. A characteristic of all of these proteins is the EF-hand structural motif. The EF-hand domain is an octahedral calcium-binding structure formed by a helix–loop–helix conformation of the polypeptide chain. The loop contains the side chain oxygens necessary for binding the calcium cation, and within one protein, amino acid linker sequences connect multiple EF hands. Calbindin-D_{28k} contains six EF hands but only four are functional and bind calcium. Calbindin-D_{9k} contains two EF hands and both bind calcium. Studies related to the distribution of calbindin and its cellular colocalization with the vitamin D receptor have resulted in key advances in our understanding of the diversity of the vitamin D endocrine system (Table 1). The focus here is on the localization, proposed functional significance, and regulation of these calcium-binding proteins. Insights obtained by studying these proteins allow an understanding of the multiple actions of the vitamin D endocrine system.

TABLE 1   Distribution of Calbindin

Calbindin-D$_{9k}$	Calbindin-D$_{28k}$
Mammalian intestine	Avian intestine
Mouse and neonatal rat kidney	Avian, reptilian, amphibian, and mammalian kidney (mouse, rat, bovine, and human kidney)
Rat and mouse yolk sac	Hen eggshell gland (uterus)
Rat uterus	Mouse reproductive tissues (uterus, oviduct, and ovary)
Rat and mouse placenta	Avian and mammalian beta cells of the pancreas Alpha cells of the rat pancreas
Rat growth cartilage	Rat growth cartilage
Ameloblasts and osteoblasts of rodent teeth	Ameloblasts and osteoblasts of rodent teeth; mouse osteoblasts
Rat lung	Brain (avian, reptilian, amphibian, molluskan, fish, and mammalian brain)

II. LOCALIZATION AND FUNCTIONAL SIGNIFICANCE

A. Intestine

One of the most important findings in the vitamin D field was the discovery by Robert Wasserman and Alan Taylor in 1966 of the 28,000-Da vitamin D-dependent calcium-binding protein in avian intestine. The intestinal calbindins (both avian and mammalian) are present in high concentrations in the intestine (0.15 mM or more) and are found in the highest concentration in the duodenum (specifically, in the cytosol of the columnar epithelial cells). Early studies in chicks established a strong correlation between the level of calbindin and an increase in intestinal calcium transport. The active form of vitamin D, 1,25-dihydroxyvitamin D$_3$ [1,25(OH)$_2$D$_3$] affects overall intestinal calcium absorption in three phases: (1) the transfer of calcium across the lumenal brush-border membrane, (2) the transfer of calcium across the cell interior, and (3) the energy-requiring extrusion of calcium from the basolateral membrane. A vitamin D-dependent apical calcium channel has recently been identified in 1,25(OH)$_2$D$_3$-responsive epithelia (proximal duodenum and distal tubule of the kidney), suggesting a mechanism of calcium entry in the first phase of the transcellular process. It is thought that 1,25(OH)$_2$D$_3$ functions in the second phase of the calcium absorptive process by interacting with the intestinal vitamin D receptor (VDR) to induce the genomic production of calbindin. Intestinal calbindin is thought to facilitate the diffusion of calcium in the absorptive cells toward the basolateral membrane. Indeed, in VDR knockout mice (VDR-ablated mice that have been generated by gene targeting), the major defect is in intestinal calcium absorption, which is accompanied by a 50% reduction in intestinal calbindin-D$_{9k}$. It has also been suggested that calbindin can act in the second phase as a cytosolic calcium buffer to prevent toxic levels of calcium from accumulating in the intestinal cell. In the third phase, calbindin is thought to stimulate calcium extrusion indirectly by increasing the local concentration of calcium adjacent to the basolateral plasma membrane calcium ATPase (PMCA).

B. Kidney

In the kidney, relatively high levels of calbindin (2–7 µg/mg protein) are present, specifically in the distal nephron (distal convoluted tubule, connecting tubule, and cortical collecting duct). The vitamin D receptor is localized predominantly in the distal nephron, the site of localization of both calbindin-D$_{9k}$ and calbindin-D$_{28k}$, which are induced by vitamin D. Similar to intestinal calcium absorption, regulation by 1,25(OH)$_2$D$_3$ of calcium transport in the distal nephron is thought to involve a transcellular process. Calcium enters through the apical plasma membrane, diffuses through the cytosol, and is actively extruded across the opposing basolateral membrane. A model of distal tubule renal calcium transport, involving calbindin, has been proposed. Calbindin-D$_{28k}$ has been reported to increase the influx of calcium at the apical membrane. Whether calbindin-D$_{28k}$ affects the activity of the recently identified apical calcium channel in the distal tubule, which has been reported to be up-regulated by vitamin D, is not yet known. Calbindin-D$_{28k}$ may then act as a diffusional carrier of calcium through the cytosol to the basolateral membrane. In addition, renal calbindin-D$_{28k}$ may also act to lower cytosolic calcium levels, preventing the accumulation of toxic levels of calcium. In the vicinity of the basolateral membrane, the calbindin-D_{9k} protein binds the calcium and stimulates the extrusion of calcium via the PMCA (a calbindin-D_{9k} binding domain has been identified in the PMCA). Thus, in the mouse distal nephron and the perinatal rat distal nephron, which contain both calbindin-D_{9k} and calbindin-D_{28k}, these proteins have different functions. The different functions of these proteins suggest mechanisms by which $1,25(OH)_2D_3$ (which induces the calbindins) may function to enhance calcium reabsorption in the distal nephron. Future studies utilizing calbindin-D_{9k} knockout mice as well as calbindin-D_{9k} and calbindin-D_{28k} double-knockout mice should provide additional insights about both intestinal and renal calcium transport. In addition, studies exploring the relationship of $1,25(OH)_2D_3$ and calbindin to the apical calcium channels will further define their respective roles in calcium transport.

C. Bone

Previous studies using immunocytochemical analyses have indicated that calbindin-D_{9k} and calbindin-D_{28k} are found in chondrocytes of growth plate cartilage in rats and in ameloblasts and osteoblasts of rodent teeth. It has been suggested that the calbindins may be involved in the movement of intracellular calcium in the chondrocyte. It has also been suggested that elevated expression of the calbindins may characterize cells involved in the elaboration of mineralized tissues and bone. In a recent study, calbindin-D_{28k} was found to be expressed at low levels in several osteoblastic cell lines and at much higher levels in primary cultures of murine osteoblastic cells. Transient transfection of calbindin-D_{28k} in MC3T3-E1 osteoblastic cells protected against tumor necrosis factor α (TNFα)-induced apoptotic cell death. Extracts from the TNFα-treated cells expressing high levels of calbindin-D_{28k} as well as purified calbindin-D_{28k} inhibited the activity of caspase 3, a protease known to be an important mediator of apoptosis. These findings are novel because they demonstrate that calbindin-D_{28k} is unique among the family of calcium-binding proteins in its ability to interact with and consequently inhibit caspase, thereby preventing apoptotic cell death in osteoblasts, independent of its calcium-binding capabilities. Thus far, calbindin-D_{28k} is the only other known natural inhibitor of caspase besides the inhibitor of apoptosis proteins (IAPs). A further understanding of the mechanisms whereby calbindin-D_{28k} attenuates apoptosis, including which regions of calbindin-D_{28k} are involved in caspase 3 inhibition, will have

important implications for the prevention of degeneration in bone cells (as well as in other cells) and therefore could prove important for the therapeutic intervention of many diseases, including osteoporosis.

D. Pancreas

The pancreas was the first nonclassical target tissue reported to contain vitamin D receptors. Immunocytochemical and autoradiographic studies have indicated that receptors for $1,25(OH)_2D_3$ and calbindin-D_{28k} are both present in the pancreatic beta cell. In chicks and rats, pancreatic calbindin-D_{28k} has been reported to be responsive to $1,25(OH)_2D_3$. In the rat, calbindin-D_{28k} is localized in alpha as well as beta cells of the pancreatic islet. Because $1,25(OH)_2D_3$ receptors are not present in a cells, it has been suggest that beta cell calbindin-D_{28k}, but not alpha cell calbindin, may be regulated by $1,25(OH)_2D_3$. Recent studies using calbindin-D_{28k} null mutant (knockout) mice and beta cell lines have shown that calbindin-D_{28k} can modulate depolarization-stimulated insulin release. These findings suggest that calbindin-D_{28k} can control the rate of insulin release by regulation of intracellular calcium. In addition to modulation of insulin release, more recent studies have indicated that cytokine-mediated destruction of pancreatic beta cells, a cause of insulin-dependent diabetes, can be inhibited by calbindin-D_{28k}. In beta cells transfected with the calbindin-D_{28k} gene, cytokine-mediated stimulation of free radical formation is inhibited. It has been suggested that calbindin-D_{28k}, by stabilizing cellular calcium, could prevent calcium-mediated mitochondrial damage and consequent generation of free radicals. These findings have important therapeutic implications for the prevention of autoimmune destruction of beta cells in type 1 diabetes.

E. Nervous Tissue

In brain tissue, calbindin-D_{28k} is present in most neuronal cell groups and fiber tracts but it is not regulated by $1,25(OH)_2D_3$; i.e., calbindin-D_{28k} is expressed constitutively. Neurons containing calbindin-D_{28k} are found in the cerebral cortex, hippocampus, amygdala, pyriform region, thalamus, and hypothalamus. The highest concentration of calbindin-D_{28k} is in the cerebellum (1–2% of the total soluble protein), where it is specifically localized in the Purkinje cells. The phenotype of the calbindin-D_{28k} knockout mouse (the calbindin-D_{28k} gene is specifically ablated by gene targeting) is impaired motor coordination. This phenotype may be the result of abnormal cerebellar activity because of altered depolarization-induced calcium transients in the Purkinje cells in the absence of calbindin. It has been suggested that calbindin-D_{28k}, by regulating depolarization-induced potentials, may also be involved in the control of hormone secretion from hypothalamic neuroendocrine neurons. In addition, specific neuronal sensory cells (cochlear and vestibular hair cells in the inner ear, cone but not rod photoreceptor cells of the avian and mammalian retina, and photoreceptor cells of pineal transducers) contain calbindin-D_{28k}. Thus, calbindin-D_{28k} in these cells is involved in mechanisms of signal transduction.

In the nervous system, besides affecting induced calcium transients and signal transduction mechanisms, calbindin-D_{28k} protects neurons against calcium-mediated neurotoxicity. Studies using hippocampal cells in culture showed a direct relationship between calbindin-positive neurons and protection against damage induced by glutamate or calcium ionophore. Correlative evidence between decreases in neuronal calbindin and neurodegeneration have been reported in studies of chronic neurological diseases (Parkinson's, Alzheimer's, and Huntington's diseases), epilepsy, aging, and ischemic injury. Direct evidence of a protective role of neuronal calbindin-D_{28k} against a variety of insults, including exposure to glucocorticoid, cyclic adenosine monophosphate (cAMP), immunoglobulin G (IgG) from amyotrophic lateral sclerosis patients, and hypoglycemia, has been shown in primary neuronal cells in culture or in neuronal cell lines in which the calbindin-D_{28k} gene has been transfected, resulting in overexpression of calbindin.

Overexpression of calbindin in neural cells is also found to suppress the proapoptotic actions of mutant presenilin 1 (PS-1). Mutant PS-1 is causally linked to approximately 50% of the cases of early-onset familial Alzheimer's disease. Mutant PS-1 sensitizes cells to apoptosis induced by amyloid β-peptide (Aβ), the cleavage product of the amyloid precursor protein and the major component of plaques in Alzheimer's disease. It has been suggested that Aβ damages neurons by a mechanism involving oxidative stress and disruption of calcium homeostasis. Calbindin-D_{28k} protected against the proapoptotic action of mutant PS-1 by attenuating the increase in intracellular calcium and preventing the impairment of mitochondrial function. Thus, calbindin-D_{28k} in the nervous system (as well as in osteoblasts and pancreatic beta cells) has an important role in protecting against cell death. A further understanding of the mechanisms whereby calbindin-D_{28k} protects

against apoptotic cell death may have important therapeutic implications for the prevention of cellular degeneration.

F. Placenta, Yolk Sac, and Uterus

Immunocytochemical and/or biochemical studies have indicated the presence of calbindin-D_{9k} in bovine placenta, in the placenta and yolk sac of rats and mice, and in the endometrium and myometrium of pregnant and nonpregnant rat uterus and in the uterine epithelium of pregnant rats. In placenta and yolk sac, calbindin-D_{9k} increases in late gestation (when fetal mineralization occurs), suggesting a role for calbindin-D_{9k} in the transport of calcium to the fetus. Calbindin-D_{28k} is not present in rat reproductive tissues. However the 28,000 M_r calbindin is present in the uterus of the laying hen and in mouse reproductive tissues (endometrium and glandular epithelium of mouse uterus, mouse oviduct epithelium, and primary follicles of mouse ovary). Calbindin-D_{28k} in these tissues is not affected by $1,25(OH)_2D_3$. However, calbindin-D_{9k} and calbindin-D_{28k} in rat and chick uterus, respectively, are up-regulated by estradiol. The presence of calbindin in epithelial cells of the uterus and oviduct suggests a role for calbindin in transepithelial calcium transport. The presence of calbindin in the myometrium suggests the involvement of calbindin in intracellular calcium regulation that may affect the frequency and strength of uterine contractions.

III. REGULATION OF CALBINDIN GENE EXPRESSION

A. Calbindin-D_{28k}

1. Genomic Organization
The structure of the chicken calbindin-D_{28k} gene has been elucidated. The size of the gene is 18.5 kb; it consists of 11 exons and 10 introns. The coding regions in the mouse and chicken calbindin-D_{28k} gene share 77% sequence homology.

2. Regulation by $1,25(OH)_2D_3$
Regulation of the calbindin-D_{28k} gene is a complex phenomenon. Its induction by $1,25(OH)_2D_3$ in avian intestine and in avian and mammalian kidney is well known. In response to $1,25(OH)_2D_3$ treatment, the expression of the calbindin-D_{28k} gene is induced by a small early increase in calbindin-D_{28k} transcription followed by a sustained accumulation of mRNA long after $1,25(OH)_2D_3$ treatment, suggesting stabilization of calbindin-D_{28k} mRNA by

$1,25(OH)_2D_3$. Similar observations have been made for chicken intestinal and rat renal calbindin-D_{28k}. A putative vitamin D response element (VDRE) has been found in the promoter of the chicken calbindin-D_{28k} gene and a VDRE that responds to $1,25(OH)_2D_3$ has been identified in the promoter of the mouse calbindin-D_{28k} gene. The putative VDRE in the chicken promoter is relatively inactive and the response of the mouse calbindin-D_{28k} promoter to $1,25(OH)_2D_3$ is modest (maximal fivefold response). The modest response reflects the *in vivo* findings of a small transcriptional response. There is increasing evidence that the large induction of calbindin-D_{28k} mRNA in both chick intestine and mouse kidney is due primarily to posttranscriptional mechanisms. In addition, in VDR-ablated mice, only a minor reduction in basal levels of renal calbindin-D_{28k} is observed. However, the response of renal calbindin-D_{28k} to injection of $1,25(OH)_2D_3$ is compromised. Thus, the regulation of calbindin-D_{28k} mRNA by $1,25(OH)_2D_3$ appears to be more complex than the conventional genomic mechanism of steroid hormone action, which involves steroid receptor binding to specific DNA sequences and transcriptional activation. Regulation of calbindin-D_{28k} by $1,25(OH)_2D_3$ may involve other factors and is mostly posttranscriptional.

3. Regulation of Calbindin-D_{28k} by Factors Other Than $1,25(OH)_2D_3$

In the intestine of vitamin D-treated chicks, glucocorticoids inhibit the levels of calbindin-D_{28k} protein and mRNA, resulting in a decrease in intestinal calcium absorption. Although a putative glucocorticoid-responsive element has been identified by sequence homology in the chicken calbindin-D_{28k} promoter, it is not yet known whether the effect of glucocorticoids is an indirect or a direct effect on the calbindin gene. The complexity of calbindin-D_{28k} gene regulation is also indicated in studies showing a modulation by calcium of calbindin-D_{28k} gene expression in avian intestine as well as in avian and mammalian kidney.

In the central nervous system, calbindin-D_{28k} is not regulated by $1,25(OH)_2D_3$. Various other factors that affect signal transduction pathways, including neurotropin-3, brain-derived neurotropic factor, insulin-like growth factor-I, fibroblast growth factor, and tumor necrosis factors, have all been reported to induce neuronal calbindin-D_{28k}. Because neurotropic factors can protect against cytotoxicity, the induction of calbindin-D_{28k} by these factors may be one mechanism involved in calbindin's neuroprotective

role. In addition to factors that affect signal transduction pathways, neuronal calbindin is also regulated by corticosterone and retinoic acid. Corticosterone has been shown to up-regulate calbindin-D_{28k} in the hippocampus. Because corticosterone causes cell death in non-calbindin-D_{28k}-containing areas of the hippocampus, the induction of calbindin may be a compensatory mechanism to promote neuronal survival. Retinoic acid has also been reported to induce calbindin-D_{28k} in medulloblastoma cells that are derived from the cerebellum and express a neuronal phenotype. Because retinoic acid has profound effects on embryogenesis, it is possible that retinoic acid may have a role in the induction of calbindin in the developing nervous system. Thus, although neuronal calbindin-D_{28k} is unresponsive to $1,25(OH)_2D_3$, it can be regulated by neurotropic factors as well as by other steroids.

As previously discussed, calbindin-D_{28k} is present in the avian eggshell gland as well as in mouse ovary, uterus, and oviduct. In these tissues, calbindin is not regulated by $1,25(OH)_2D_3$ but rather by estradiol. Analysis of the mouse calbindin-D_{28k} promoter indicates that multiple imperfect half-palindromic estrogen-responsive elements (between -1075 and -702 and between -175 and -78) contribute to the induction by estradiol.

B. Calbindin-D_{9k}

1. Genomic Organization

The size of the calbindin-D_{9k} gene is 2.5 kb. The calbindin-D_{9k} gene contains three exons interrupted by two introns. The first exon contains almost the entire $5'$ noncoding region. The second exon codes for the first calcium-binding site. The third exon codes for the second calcium-binding site and the $3'$ untranslated region.

2. Regulation of Calbindin-D_{9k} by $1,25(OH)_2D_3$

Similar to the regulation of calbindin-D_{28k}, calbindin-D_{9k} is regulated by $1,25(OH)_2D_3$ by a small, rapid transcriptional stimulation followed by a posttranscriptional effect, accounting for the sustained increase of calbindin-D_{9k} mRNA. Unlike renal calbindin-D_{28k}, in VDR-ablated mice there is a marked inhibition of both basal and $1,25(OH)_2D_3$-induced calbindin-D_{9k} mRNA levels. These findings suggest that basal levels of intestinal calbindin-D_{9k} mRNA are more sensitive to control by VDR-mediated mechanisms than are basal levels of renal calbindin-D_{28k} mRNA. In addition, recent studies using transgenic mice indicate that 4580 base pairs of the $5'$ regulatory sequence of the calbindin-D_{9k} gene are needed for intestine-specific expression as well as for the responsiveness to $1,25(OH)_2D_3$. The proximal promoter of the calbindin-D_{9k} gene, from -117 to $+400$, and a distal element located at -3500, together, but not separately, confer the $1,25(OH)_2D_3$-induced transcriptional response. In addition, an intestine-specific transcription factor, caudal homeobox-2 (Cdx-2), binds to a Cdx-2-binding site in the distal element of the calbindin-D_{9k} promoter and plays a crucial role in the transcription of the calbindin-D_{9k} gene in the intestine.

3. Regulation of Calbindin-D_{9k} by Other Steroids

In the intestine, calbindin-D_{9k} expression is inhibited by glucocorticoids. This decrease may be involved in the reported decrease by glucocorticoids in intestinal calcium absorption. It is not yet known whether the mechanism of the effect of glucocorticoids on calbindin-D_{9k} expression is direct or indirect.

In the uterus, calbindin-D_{9k} expression is unaffected by $1,25(OH)_2D_3$ but rather is under strong estrogen control. An imperfect estrogen response element (ERE) that binds the estrogen receptor (ER) has been identified in the first $5'$ splice site of the rat calbindin-D_{9k} gene. Because the ERE has been found to contribute only weak estrogen induction, it has been suggested that the ER may cooperate with other transcription factors or co-activators to result in efficient transcriptional activation of the calbindin-D_{9k} gene.

IV. SUMMARY

Calbindin-D_{9k} and calbindin-D_{28k} were previously thought to be exclusively vitamin D-dependent proteins. It is now evident that these proteins are present in many different tissues, that they serve different functions, and that they are regulated by several steroids as well as by factors that affect signal transduction pathways. In future studies the generation of calbindin-D_{9k} null mutant mice as well as increasingly refined cellular and molecular approaches will provide new insights into the mechanism of action of the calbindins, including the role of calbindin in intestinal calcium absorption, in calcium reabsorption in the distal nephron, and in protection against cell death.

Glossary

apoptosis Biological process of programmed cell death that occurs in normal physiology as well as in response to adverse conditions.

calbindin-D_{9k} A 9000-Da calcium-binding protein that is present in highest concentrations in mammalian intestine, in mouse and neonatal rat kidney, and in placenta and uterus.

calbindin-D_{28k} A 28,000-Da calcium-binding protein present in highest concentrations in avian intestine and mammalian and avian kidney, brain, and pancreas.

1,25-dihydroxyvitamin D_3 Active steroid hormone form of vitamin D, which is synthesized in the kidney.

vitamin D receptor Member of the steroid/nuclear receptor superfamily; binds 1,25-dihydroxyvitamin D_3 and to specific DNA sequences and activates or represses the transcription of specific target genes.

See Also the Following Articles

Apoptosis • Vitamin D • Vitamin D: Biological Effects of $1,25(OH)_2D_3$ in Bone • Vitamin D: Biological Effects of $1,25(OH)_2D_3$ in the Intestine and Kidney • Vitamin D Effects on Cell Differentiation and Proliferation • Vitamin D: Nuclear Receptor for $1,25(OH)_2D_3$ • Vitamin D Metabolism

Further Reading

Bellido, T., Huening, M., Raval-Pandya, M., Manolagas, S. C., and Christakos, S. (2000). Calbindin-D_{28k} is expressed in osteoblasts and suppresses their apoptosis by inhibiting caspase-3 activity. *J. Biol. Chem.* **275**, 26328–26332.

Bronner, F., and Pansu, D. (1999). Nutritional aspects of calcium absorption. *J. Nutr.* **129**, 9–12.

Christakos, S., Barletta, F., Huening, M., Kohut, J., and Raval-Pandya, M. (2000). Activation of programmed cell death by calcium: protection against cell death by the calcium binding protein, calbindin-D_{28k}, in calcium. *In* "The Molecular Basis of Calcium Action in Biology and Medicine" (R. Pochet, R. Bonato, J. Haiech, C. Heizmann and V. Gerke, eds.), pp. 259–275. Kluwer Academic Publishers, The Netherlands.

Christakos, S., Beck, J. D., and Hyllner, S. J. (1997). Calbindin-D_{28k}. *In* "Vitamin D" (D. Feldman, F. Glorieux and J. W. Pike, eds.), pp. 209–221. Academic Press, San Diego, CA.

Christakos, S., Gabrielides, C., and Rhoten, W. B. (1989). Vitamin D dependent calcium binding proteins: Chemistry, distribution, functional considerations and molecular biology. *Endocr. Rev.* **10**, 3–26.

Colnot, S., Romagnolo, B., Porteu, A., Lacourte, P., Thomasset, M., and Perret, C. (1998). Intestinal expression of calbindin-D_{9k} gene in transgenic mice. *J. Biol. Chem.* **273**, 31939–31946.

Hoenderop, J. G., Muller, D., Van Der Kemp, A. W., Hartog, A., Suzuki, M., Ishibashi, K., Imai, M., Sweep, F., Willems, P. H., Van Os, C. H., and Bindels, R. J. (2001). Calcitriol controls the epithelial calcium channel in kidney. *J. Am. Soc. Nephrol.* **12**, 1342–1349.

Li, Y. C., Pirro, A. E., and Demay, M. B. (1998). Analysis of vitamin D-dependent calcium binding protein messenger ribonucleic acid expression in mice lacking the vitamin D receptor. *Endocrinology* **139**, 847–851.

Rabinovitch, A., Suarez-Pinzon, W. L., Sooy, K., Strynadka, K., and Christakos, S. (2001). Expression of calbindin-D_{28k} in a pancreatic islet beta cell line protects against cytokine induced apoptosis and necrosis. *Endocrinology* **142**, 3649–3655.

Sooy, K., Kohut, J., and Christakos, S. (2000). The role of calbindin and 1,25-dihydroxyvitamin D_3 in the kidney. *Curr. Opin. Nephrol. Hypertens.* **9**, 341–347.

Sooy, K., Schermerhorn, T., Noda, M., Surana, M., Meyer, M., Fleischer, N., Sharp, G. W. G., Rhoten, W. B., and Christakos, S. (1999). Calbindin-D_{28k} controls $[Ca^{2+}]_i$ and insulin release: Evidence obtained from β cell lines and calbindin-D_{28k} knockout mice. *J. Biol. Chem.* **27**, 34343–34349.

Van Cromphaut, S. J., Dewerchin, M., Hoenderop, J. G., Stockmans, I., Van Herck, E., Kato, S., Bindels, R. J., Collen, D., Carmeliet, P., Bouillon, R., and Carmeliet, G. (2001). Duodenal calcium absorption in vitamin D receptor-knockout mice: functional and molecular aspects. *Proc. Natl. Acad. Sci. U.S.A.* **98**, 13324–13329.

Vitamin D: 24,25-Dihydroxyvitamin D

ANTHONY W. NORMAN AND HELEN L. HENRY

University of California, Riverside

I. INTRODUCTION
II. PRODUCTION OF $24R,25(OH)_2D_3$
III. BIOLOGICAL EFFECTS OF $24R,25(OH)_2D_3$
IV. RECEPTORS FOR $24R,25(OH)_2D_3$
V. SUMMARY

24,25-Dihydroxyvitamin D_3 [$24R,25(OH)_2D_3$] and 1α,25-dihydroxyvitamin D_3 are the two major dihydroxylated vitamin D metabolites circulating in the blood. Although both forms are produced from the parent vitamin D_3, it appears that the less well-studied $24R,25(OH)_2D_3$ form plays distinct biological roles.

I. INTRODUCTION

In comparison to $1α,25(OH)_2D_3$, the biological actions of $24R,25(OH)_2D_3$ have been relatively less studied. Although it is clear that $24R,25(OH)_2D_3$ is produced by the same enzyme system that inactivates $1α,25(OH)_2D_3$ in its target cells, there is substantial evidence that the important biological activities of $24R,25(OH)_2D_3$ and $1α,25(OH)_2D_3$ are distinctly different. One key question that has attracted atten-

tion is whether $1α,25(OH)_2D_3$ acting alone can generate all of the biological responses that are attributed to the parent vitamin D_3, or whether, for some responses, a second vitamin D_3 metabolite is required. There is evidence to support the view that the presence of both $1α,25(OH)_2D_3$ and $24R,25-(OH)_2D_3$ is required to generate the complete spectrum of biological responses attributable to the parent vitamin D_3. The purpose of this article is to summarize results from biological systems in which $24R,25(OH)_2D_3$ has been shown to produce biological effects.

II. PRODUCTION OF $24R,25(OH)_2D_3$

The $25(OH)D_3/1α,25(OH)_2D_3$-$24R$-hydroxylase ($24R$-hydroxylase) is induced by and responsible for the inactivation and catabolism of $1α,25(OH)_2D_3$ in its target cells. In addition, $24R$-hydroxylase in the kidney utilizes $25(OH)D_3$ as substrate to produce significant amounts (2–5 ng/ml) of circulating $24R,25(OH)_2D_3$.

A mouse knockout (KO) of $25(OH)D_3$-$24R$-hydroxylase has been generated. The newborn mice are viable but develop significant bone abnormalities. Although these deficiencies have been attributed to elevated levels of plasma $1α,25(OH)_2D_3$ rather than to a deficiency of $24R,25(OH)_2D_3$, there is experimental evidence that $24R,25(OH)_2D_3$ has biological activity in its own right.

III. BIOLOGICAL EFFECTS OF $24R,25(OH)_2D_3$

A. Parathyroid Gland Regression

In vitamin D-deficient hypocalcemic animals, the parathyroid glands undergo marked hypertrophy and hyperplasia. The first suggestion that $24R,25-(OH)_2D_3$ could generate biological responses when $1α,25(OH)_2D_3$ given alone did not elicit responses was obtained by measuring regression of hypertrophied parathyroid glands typically present in vitamin D-deficient, hypocalcemic chicks. Coadministration of physiological concentrations of $24R,25(OH)_2D_3$ and $1α,25(OH)_2D_3$ resulted in significant reduction in parathyroid gland size, whereas $1α,25(OH)_2D_3$ alone was ineffective in reducing parathyroid gland size. Concomitantly with these observations, several studies reported on the effects of $24R,25(OH)_2D_3$ on parathyroid (PTH) secretion in animal systems and in patients with renal osteodystrophy.

B. Chick Egg Hatchability

Long-term studies of White Leghorn hens that received only exogenous vitamin D metabolites from the day of hatching have shown that $24R,25(OH)_2D_3$ is required in combination with $1\alpha,25(OH)_2D_3$ for the normal hatchability of the fertilized eggs. In a follow-up study of Japanese quail, only the naturally occurring $24R,25(OH)_2D_3$ [i.e. not the artificial $24S,25(OH)D_3$] in combination with $1\alpha,25(OH)_2D_3$ supported normal egg hatchability.

C. Fracture Healing

In an *in vivo* model of fracture healing in the chick, the renal 24R-hydroxylase activity increases three-fold approximately 1 week following imposition of a tibial fracture; this is accompanied by a similar increase in the levels of circulating $24R,25(OH)_2D_3$. When the degree of fracture healing as reflected in bone strength is measured, $24R,25(OH)_2D_3$, but not $24S,25(OH)D_3$, when given in combination with $1\alpha,25(OH)_2D_3$ (a dose that is ineffective by itself), results in bone strength equivalent to that seen in control animals receiving $25(OH)D_3$.

Based on these observations, it is possible to envision the existence of an endocrine system linking a bone fracture to the kidney $25(OH)D_3$-24R-hydroxylase, resulting in the subsequent elevation of

the serum $24R,25(OH)_2D_3$ levels. The increased availability of this steroid hormone allows occupancy of the proposed vitamin D receptor ($VDR_{mem\ 24,25}$), which then initiates, in collaboration with $1\alpha,25(OH)_2D_3$, appropriate transduction signals that orchestrate the competent healing of the fracture (see Fig. 1).

D. Cartilage Cells

$24R,25(OH)_2D_3$ has biological effects distinct from those of $1\alpha,25(OH)_2D_3$ on a subset of cells in growth plate cartilage. One hallmark of a steroid hormone is that it is preferentially accumulated by its target cells *in vivo* on a high-affinity receptor that tightly binds the hormone and effectively removes it from the blood compartment. This standard has been achieved for $24R,25(OH)_2D_3$ in relation to growth plate cartilage cells of the rat. These cells selectively accumulate tritiated $24R,25(OH)_2D_3$ that is been administered *in vivo* to rats.

IV. RECEPTORS FOR $24R,25(OH)_2D_3$

Unlike $1\alpha,25(OH)_2D_3$, which has a widely distributed nuclear receptor that mediates an array of biological responses, the seco steroid $24R, 25(OH)_2D_3$ likely produces biological responses in a more limited

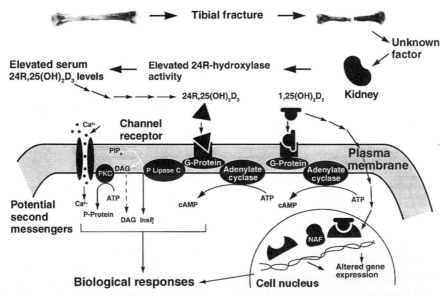

FIGURE 1 Proposed mode of action of $24R,25(OH)_2D_3$ for the process of fracture healing. After imposition of a bone fracture, an unknown factor is produced and delivered systemically to the kidney proximal tubule, leading to a significant increase in the activity of the $25(OH)D_3$-24R-hydroxylase. The resultant elevation of the plasma level of $24R,25(OH)_2D_3$ leads to occupation of membrane vitamin D receptors believed to be present in the fracture-healing callus, and thereby initiating signal transduction processes and contributing to the process of fracture healing. PKC, Protein kinase C; DAG, diacylglycerol; InsP3, inositol 1,4,5-trisphosphate; NAF, nuclear activation factor.

TABLE I   Biological Responses Attributed to 24R,25(OH)$_2$ Vitamin D$_3$

Organ cell system	Response studied
Parathyroid gland	Regression of hypertrophied glands; inhibition of PTH secretion
Egg hatchability	Required in combination with 1α,25(OH)$_2$D$_3$ for normal egg hatchability
Bone	Healing of rachitic lesions with increased bone strength; healing of fractures with increased bone strength
Chondrocytes (resting zone)	Activation of protein kinase C; inhibition of prostaglandin E2 production; increased activity of phospholipase C

sphere, consisting of cartilage and bone cells and possibly parathyroid hormone-secreting cells. Table 1 summarizes the biological responses that have been reported to be mediated by 24R,25(OH)$_2$D$_3$.

The stereospecificity at the C-24R position of 24R,25(OH)$_2$D$_3$ vs 24S,25(OH)D$_3$, for the effects described for parathyroid glands, egg hatchability, and bone fracture healing, suggests the existence of a receptor that can distinguish between the two compounds. The search for 24R,25(OH)$_2$D$_3$-specific receptors is an active area of current investigation. Thus far, there has been no evidence for the existence of a nuclear receptor, but preliminary evidence suggests that there is a membrane-associated receptor-binding protein ($K_d \approx 18 \pm 1.9$ nM) for 24R,25- (OH)$_2$D$_3$ in the chick fracture-healing callus. The binding of [^{3}H]1α,25(OH)$_2$D$_3$ to the callus membrane receptor-binding protein is specific in that it is competed for only by nonradioactive 24R,25- (OII)$_2$D$_3$, and not by 24S,25(OH)D$_3$, 1α,25(OH)$_2$- D$_3$, or 25(OH)D$_3$. Evidence has also been obtained that growth zones cartilage cells of bone and osteoblasts have a membrane receptor for 24R,25(OH)$_2$D$_3$.

The first mechanistic insight into the signal transduction pathways activated by 24R,25-(OH)$_2$D$_3$ in cartilage resting zone cartilage cells includes activation of protein kinase C (PKC) via effects on phospholipase A$_2$, as well as possible effects on increasing the activity of phospholipase C.

V. SUMMARY

Results from a number of studies support a role for 24R,25(OH)$_2$D$_3$ in the parathyroid gland and in hatching of the avian embryo. Current evidence also supports the concept that 24R,25(OH)$_2$D$_3$, acting through its receptor, plays an important role in bone fracture healing and in the maturation of growth plate cartilage cells. Biochemical details of these proposed receptors and further details on the signal

transduction pathways that they activate might emerge in future studies.

Glossary

endocrine system Network of endocrine glands (sources of a hormones) and target cells (locations of the hormones receptors) involved in integrated interactions that generate regulated, selective biological responses necessary to maintain the system viability.

hormone Any of several chemical classes of compounds produced in regulated quantities by an endocrine gland; acts as a chemical messenger, usually delivered through the circulatory system to a target cell, which, by definition, possesses a receptor for that hormone so that a specific biological response is generated.

receptor Protein molecule that binds very specifically to its cognate hormone; binding generates a receptor–hormone complex that initiates a cellular signal transduction process, resulting in one or more biological responses.

steroid Member of the lipid class of compounds; composed of the cyclopentano-perhydro-phenanthrene nucleus, a four-ring structure that is the basic structural component of steroid hormone families such as estrogens, progestogens, androgens, mineralocorticoids, and glucocorticoids.

vitamins Essential organic substances present in trace amounts in food; effect the normal cellular metabolic processes.

See Also the Following Articles

Steroid Nomenclature • Vitamin D • Vitamin D and Cartilage • Vitamin D and Human Nutrition • Vitamin D-Binding Protein • Vitamin D Deficiency, Rickets and Osteomalacia • Vitamin D Metabolism

Further Reading

Bouillon, R., Okamura, W. H., and Norman, A. W. (1995). Structure–function relationships in the vitamin D endocrine system. *Endocr. Rev.* 16, 200–257.

Boyan, B. D., Bonewald, L. F., Sylvia, V. L., Nemere, I., Larsson, D., Norman, A. W., Rosser, J., Dean, D. D., and Schwartz, Z.

(2002). Evidence for distinct membrane receptors for 1α, 25-(OH)$_2$D$_3$ and 24R,25-(OH)$_2$D$_3$ in osteoblasts. *Steroids* 67, 235–246.

Henry, H. L. (2001). The 25(OH)D$_3$/1α,25(OH)$_2$D$_3$-24R-hydroxylase: A catabolic or biosynthetic enzyme? *Steroids* 66, 391–398.

Henry, H. L., and Norman, A. W. (1978). Vitamin D: Two dihydroxylated metabolites are required for normal chicken egg hatchability. *Science* 201, 835–837.

Henry, H. L., Taylor, A. N., and Norman, A. W. (1977). Response of chick parathyroid glands to the vitamin D metabolites, 1,25-dihydroxycholecalciferol and 24,25-dihydroxycholecalciferol. *J. Nutr.* 107, 1918–1926.

Kato, A., Seo, E.-G., Einhorn, T. A., Bishop, J. E., and Norman, A. W. (1998). Studies on 24R,25-dihydroxyvitamin D$_3$: Evidence for a non-nuclear membrane receptor in the chick tibial fracture-healing callus. *Bone* 23, 141–146.

Malluche, H. H., Henry, H. L., Meyer-Sabellek, W., Sherman, D., Massry, S. G., and Norman, A. W. (1980). Effects and interactions of 24R,25(OH)$_2$D$_3$ and 1α,25(OH)$_2$D$_3$ on bone. *Am. J. Physiol.* 238, 384–388.

Norman, A. W., Leathers, V. L., and Bishop, J. E. (1983). Studies on the mode of action of calciferol. XLVIII. Normal egg hatchability requires the simultaneous administration to the hen of 1-α,25-dihydroxyvitamin D$_3$ and 24R,25-dihydroxyvitamin D$_3$. *J. Nutr.* 113, 2505–2515.

Pedrozo, H. A., Schwartz, Z., Rimes, S., Sylvia, V. L., Nemere, I., Posner, G. H., Dean, D. D., and Boyan, B. D. (1999). Physiological importance of the 1,25(OH)$_2$D$_3$ membrane receptor and evidence for a membrane receptor specific for 24,25(OH)$_2$D$_3$. *J. Bone Miner. Res.* 14, 856–867.

Schwartz, Z., Sylvia, V. L., Del Toro, F., Hardin, R. R., Dean, D. D., and Boyan, B. D. (2000). 24R,25-(OH)$_2$D$_3$ mediates its membrane receptor-dependent effects on protein kinase C and alkaline phosphatase via phospholipase A(2) and cyclooxygenase-1 but not cyclooxygenase-2 in growth plate chondrocytes. *J. Cell Physiol.* 182, 390–401.

Seo, E.-G., Einhorn, T. A., and Norman, A. W. (1997). 24R,25-dihydroxyvitamin D$_3$: An essential vitamin D$_3$ metabolite for both normal bone integrity and healing of tibial fracture in chicks. *Endocrinology* 138, 3864–3872.

Seo, E.-G., and Norman, A. W. (1997). Three-fold induction of renal 25-hydroxyvitamin D$_3$-24-hydroxylase activity and increased serum 24,25-dihydroxyvitamin D$_3$ levels are correlated with the healing process after chick tibial fracture. *J. Bone Miner. Res.* 12, 598–606.

Seo, E.-G., Schwartz, Z., Dean, D. D., Norman, A. W., and Boyan, B. D. (1996). Preferential accumulation *in vivo* of 24R,25-dihydroxyvitamin D$_3$ in growth plate cartilage of rats. *Endocrine* 5, 147–155.

St.-Arnaud, R., Arabian, A., Travers, R., Barletta, F., Ravel-Pandya, M., Chapin, K., Mathieu, C., Christakos, S., Demay, M. B., and Glorieux, F. H. (2000). Abnormal intramembranous ossification in mice deficient for the vitamin D 24-hydroxylase. *Endocrinology* 141, 2658–2666.

Varghese, Z., Moorhead, J. F., and Farrington, K. (1992). Effect of 24,25-dihydroxycholecalciferol on intestinal absorption of calcium and phosphate and on parathyroid hormone secretion in chronic renal failure. *Nephron* 60, 286–291.

Vitamin D Effects on Cell Differentiation and Proliferation

CHANTAL MATHIEU, ANNEMIEKE VERSTUYF, SIEGFRIED SEGAERT, AND ROGER BOUILLON
Katholieke Universiteit Leuven, Belgium

1α,25-dihydroxyvitamin D$_3$ [1α,25(OH)$_2$D$_3$] exerts its effects via the vitamin D receptor (VDR), which belongs to the steroid/thyroid hormone receptor superfamily, leading to gene regulation mediating various biological responses. Within the past two decades, the receptor has been shown to be present not only in classical target tissues such as bone, kidney, and intestine but also in many other nonclassical tissues, e.g., in the immune system (T and B cells, macrophages, and monocytes), in the reproductive system (uterus, testis, ovary, prostate, placenta, and mammary glands), in the endocrine system (pancreas, pituitary, thyroid, and adrenal cortex), in muscles (skeletal muscle, smooth muscle, and heart muscle), in brain, in skin, and in liver.

I. INTRODUCTION

In addition to the almost universal presence of vitamin D receptors (VDRs), some cell types (e.g., keratinocytes, monocytes, bone, and placenta) are capable of metabolizing 25-hydroxyvitamin D$_3$ to 1,25(OH)$_2$D$_3$ by the enzyme 1α-hydroxylase. The combined presence of 25(OH)D$_3$-1α-hydroxylase and the specific receptor in several tissues introduced the idea of a paracrine role for 1,25(OH)$_2$D$_3$. Moreover, it has been demonstrated that 1,25(OH)$_2$D$_3$ can induce differentiation and inhibit proliferation of normal and malignant cells. In addition to the treatment of bone disorders with 1,25(OH)$_2$D$_3$, these newly discovered functions of 1,25(OH)$_2$D$_3$ open new therapeutic applications as an immune modulator (e.g., for the treatment of autoimmune diseases or prevention of graft rejection), inhibitor of cell proliferation (e.g., psoriasis), and inducer of cell differentiation (e.g., cancer).

This article discusses the effect of 1,25(OH)$_2$D$_3$ in three important tissues wherein differentiation is essential, namely, in cancer tissues, skin, and tissues of the immune system.

II. CANCER

A wide variety of malignant cells and tissues possess nuclear receptors for 1,25(OH)$_2$D$_3$. Several laboratories have demonstrated that immature mouse myeloid cells, upon treatment with 1,25(OH)$_2$D$_3$, differentiate toward more mature macrophage-like cells that are characterized by a decreased growth rate. The same effect was later observed in human leukemia cell lines such as HL-60 and U937. These cells acquire the morphology of monocytes, are able to perform phagocytosis, and possess differentiation-specific characteristics [such as expression of nonspecific esterases, production of superoxides, and expression of surface markers (e.g., CD14, CD11b)]. The antiproliferative and prodifferentiating effects of 1,25(OH)$_2$D$_3$ are not limited to leukemia cells but are also seen in a wide variety of other cancer cells possessing the vitamin D$_3$ receptor such as melanoma, breast cancer, colon cancer, and prostate cancer.

The molecular mechanisms responsible for cell growth arrest and terminal differentiation are still unclear. It has been demonstrated that 1,25(OH)$_2$D$_3$-treated cancer cells accumulate in the G1 phase of the cell cycle. The regulation of cell cycle genes could be a possible explanation for the anti-proliferative effects of 1,25(OH)$_2$D$_3$. Table 1 gives an overview of genes regulated by 1,25(OH)$_2$D$_3$ at the transcriptional level

in cancer cells. 1,25(OH)$_2$D$_3$ increases the expression level of the cell cycle inhibitory proteins p21 and p27 in a wide variety of cancer cell lines such as leukemia, prostate cancer, and breast cancer cells. The promoter region of p21 even contains a vitamin D-response element (VDRE), suggesting that p21 is a direct target of 1,25(OH)$_2$D$_3$. However, treatment of MCF-7 breast cancer cells with 1,25(OH)$_2$D$_3$ and antibodies neutralizing transforming growth factor-β (TGF-β) completely abrogates 1,25(OH)$_2$D$_3$-induced up-regulation, whereas the growth inhibitory effect was only partially reversed. Moreover, a recent report questions the inhibitory function of p21 in 1,25(OH)$_2$D$_3$-induced growth reduction as an *in vitro* and *in vivo* down-regulation of p21 was observed in squamous cell carcinoma after treatment with 1,25(OH)$_2$D. The cyclin-dependent kinase (cdk) inhibitors p15 and p18 are up-regulated in myeloid U937 cells following treatment with 1,25(OH)$_2$D$_3$. Cell cycle arrest and differentiation in these cells are preceded by a proliferative burst and a transient increase in cyclin D1, A, and E protein levels. The activity of cdk2 and cdk6, involved in the transition from G1 to S, is reduced following treatment with 1,25(OH)$_2$D$_3$ and may contribute to the observed growth inhibitory effect.

Incubation of HL-60 cells with 1,25(OH)$_2$D$_3$ increases cdk5 activity, which is thought to facilitate the G1 to S phase transition in cells approaching replicative quiescence and to enhance concomitant monocytic differentiation. In addition to cell cycle genes, other genes such as proto-oncogenes and tumor suppressor genes are also regulated by 1,25(OH)$_2$D$_3$ (Table 1). It is not always clear whether this modulation represents a direct effect of 1,25(OH)$_2$D$_3$ or is

TABLE 1 Genes Regulated by 1,25(OH)$_2$D$_3$ at the Transcriptional Level in Cancer Cells

Angiogenesis	*Apoptosis regulatory genes*	*Receptors*
VEGF ↓	p53 ↑	VDR ↑
	Clusterin ↑	AR ↑
		ER ↓
Growth factors	*Proto-oncogenes and tumor suppressor genes*	*Cell cycle regulatory genes*
TGF-β ↑	c-myc ↓	Cyclin A ↓
IGF-II ↓	c-fos ↑	Cyclin E ↓
IGF-BP3 ↑	c-fms ↑	Cyclin D1 ↓
IGF-BP5 ↑	c-jun ↑	p21 ↑
PTHrP ↓	E-cadherin ↑	P27 ↑
IL-1β ↓	BRCA1 ↑	
IL-6 ↑		

Note: AR, androgen receptor; BP, binding protein; BRCA1, breast cancer susceptibility gene; ER, estrogen receptor; IGF, insulin-like growth factor; IL, interleukin; PTHrP, parathyroid hormone-related peptide; TGF-β, transforming growth factor-β; VDR, vitamin D receptor; VEGF, vascular endothelial growth factor.

TABLE 2   Anti-Tumor Effects of 1,25(OH)$_2$D$_3$ in Different Animal Models of Cancer

Administration	Tumor model	Anti-tumor effect
Oral	Colon cancer	Reduction of tumor incidence
Intraperitoneal	Head and neck squamous cell carcinoma	Suppression of tumor growth
Intraperitoneal	Lymphoma	Increase in survival time
Intraperitoneal	Liver cancer	Suppression of tumor growth
Intravesical	Bladder cancer	Reduction of tumor incidence
Hepatic arterial infusion	Liver cancer	Suppression of tumor growth

Note: Data are from studies published in 2000–2001.

rather a consequence of its overall effect on proliferation and differentiation. Suppression of c-*myc* transcription in HL-60 cells following treatment with 1,25(OH)$_2$D$_3$ is thought to be mediated by binding of the nuclear phosphoprotein HOXB4 to the promoter region of the gene. A rapid up-regulation of the proto-oncogene c-*fos* has been reported in several cell lines treated with 1,25(OH)$_2$D$_3$. This up-regulation is thought to be a direct effect of 1,25(OH)$_2$D$_3$ mediated by a VDRE in the promoter region of the gene. Exposure of HL-60 cells to 1,25(OH)$_2$D$_3$ induces the expression of c-*fms*, which is the receptor for macrophage colony-stimulating factor, concomitantly with the induction of the monocytic phenotype.

Enhanced expression of some tumor suppressor genes was reported in breast cancer cells after incubation with 1,25(OH)$_2$D$_3$. The cell surface adhesion molecule E-cadherin and the breast cancer susceptibility gene BRCA1 are up-regulated following treatment with 1,25(OH)$_2$D$_3$. Recently, it was demonstrated that 1,25(OH)$_2$D$_3$ promotes the differentiation of colon carcinoma cells by the induction of E-cadherin and the inhibition of β-catenin signaling.

Another mechanism by which 1,25(OH)$_2$D$_3$ and its analogues inhibit cell growth is the induction of programmed cell death (apoptosis) in various cancer cells including breast, colon, and prostate cancer cells. A whole set of genes involved in the cascade of apoptosis are influenced by 1,25(OH)$_2$D$_3$. However, some contradictory reports have been published on the role of apoptotic cell death in the growth inhibition caused by this compound.

The *in vitro* studies showing the anti-proliferative and prodifferentiating effects of 1,25(OH)$_2$D$_3$ on cancer cells have been confirmed *in vivo* in different animal models (Table 2). Indeed, the tumor incidence or tumor growth was reduced in different cancers such as colon, liver, or bladder cancer. To overcome the calcemic side effects of 1,25(OH)$_2$D$_3$ (hypercalciuria, hypercalcemia, and increased bone resorption), attempts were made to generate chemically modified 1,25(OH)$_2$D$_3$ molecules (analogues) that retain the beneficial anti-proliferative and prodifferentiating effects but not the unwanted calcemic side effects. Some of these potent analogues with beneficial effects on tumor growth in animals are now being further investigated in clinical trials (Table 3). These drugs can be used not only as monotherapy but also as adjuvant therapy in combination with chemotherapeutics or hormone therapy. The combined agents may act in concert and produce additional or synergistic effects on cell proliferation and differentiation but also allow dose reduction, thereby decreasing adverse side effects.

III. SKIN

The skin occupies a central position in the vitamin D endocrine system: it is not only the site of synthesis of vitamin D$_3$, as cutaneous cells are also capable of converting vitamin D$_3$ to its active form, 1,25-(OH)$_2$D$_3$. Moreover, they contain the VDR, rendering them responsive to the actions of 1,25(OH)$_2$D$_3$. The exact physiological function of vitamin D in the skin is still elusive. However, humans or mice with a dysfunctional VDR display a postnatal alopecia, which cannot be cured by normalization of calcium levels by dietary means. These findings firmly indicate that the VDR is directly implicated in hair follicle biology. In this context, recent mechanistic studies refer to a ligand-independent role for VDR–retinoic acid X receptor dimers in anagen initiation in the epithelial (keratinocyte) component of the hair follicle apparatus.

Whereas almost every cutaneous cell type contains the VDR (Table 4), the epidermal keratinocyte is generally considered the main vitamin D target cell in the skin. 1,25(OH)$_2$D$_3$ at pharmacological concentrations is a potent inducer of keratinocyte growth arrest and differentiation. These properties were the basis for the successful application of 1,25(OH)$_2$D$_3$ analogues in the treatment of hyperproliferative skin

TABLE 3   Clinical Trials with $1,25(OH)_2D_3$ and Analogues

Compound	Administration	Tumor	Effects
$1,25(OH)_2D_3$	Oral	Hormone refractory metastatic prostate cancer	No toxicity; no reduction of tumor mass
$1,25(OH)_2D_3$	Oral	Myelodysplastic syndrome	Clinical response in 70% of patients; no toxicity
$1,25(OH)_2D_3$	Oral	Myelodysplastic syndrome	No clinical effect
Calcipotriol	Topical	Breast cancer	Reduction of tumor diameter in 20% of patients
EB 1089	Oral	Advanced breast and colon cancer	Stabilization of the disease in 17% of patients
$1,25(OH)_2D_3$ + docetaxel	Oral	Androgen-independent prostate cancer	Reduction in PSA; limited or no toxicity
$1\alpha(OH)D_3$ + surgery + chemotherapy + radiotherapy	Oral	Glioblastomas and anaplastic astrocytomas	Progressive and durable tumor regression in 20% of patients; no toxicity

Note: EB 1089, 22,24-diene-24,26,27-trihomo-$1\alpha,25(OH)_2D_3$.

diseases such as psoriasis and certain forms of ichthyosis. The $1,25(OH)_2D_3$-dependent growth arrest and differentiation in keratinocytes are likely to be based on a similar mechanism of action as described for cancer cells: $1,25(OH)_2D_3$-treated keratinocytes fail to progress from the G_1 to the S phase of the cell cycle due to induction of the negative cell cycle regulators p21 and p27 and suppression of the proto-oncogene c-myc. Induction of autocrine or paracrine growth regulators such as transforming growth factor-β, tumor necrosis factor α (TNFα), and parathyroid hormone-related peptide may also contribute to the anti-mitotic $1,25(OH)_2D_3$ effect in epidermal cells. $1,25(OH)_2D_3$-dependent keratinocyte differentiation is accompanied by induction of cornified envelope precursors such as involucrin and its cross-linking enzyme transglutaminase type I. There is also a stimulatory effect on stratification by translocation of E-cadherin to assembling adherens junctions, which will further enhance the prodifferentiative actions of $1,25(OH)_2D_3$.

Low concentrations of $1,25(OH)_2D_3$ exert mitogenic activity rather than a growth-inhibiting effect on keratinocytes, especially in cells that are committed to differentiate. Increased proliferation is also observed following application of $1,25(OH)_2D_3$ compounds to normal mouse or human skin. In contrast, hyperproliferative epidermis (in psoriasis or induced by application of mitogens) responds to $1,25(OH)_2D_3$ derivatives with growth arrest. These data indicate that $1,25(OH)_2D_3$ exerts a normalizing rather than an unidirectional anti-proliferative effect on epidermal growth.

Skin fibroblasts also respond to $1,25(OH)_2D_3$ treatment with normalization of their growth rate and collagen production. Therefore, $1,25(OH)_2D_3$ compounds can be therapeutically used for diseases with excessive fibroblast activity (scleroderma) or insufficient fibroblast activity (skin atrophy). $1,25(OH)_2D_3$ stimulates the production of melanin in melanocytes, a feature that can be applied in the treatment of vitiligo. Despite the obvious role for the VDR in hair biology, no application of $1,25(OH)_2D_3$ analogues in hair disorders is yet available; however, animal models open promising perspectives for the prevention of chemotherapy-induced alopecia.

TABLE 4   Vitamin D Target Cells in the Skin with Effects of $1,25(OH)_2D_3$ and Clinical Application of $1,25(OH)_2D_3$ Analogues

Target cell	Effect of $1,25(OH)_2D_3$	Clinical use
Keratinocyte	Regulation of growth and differentiation	Psoriasis; hyperproliferative ichthyosis
Fibroblast	Regulation of growth and collagen production	Scleroderma; skin atrophy
Hair follicle cell	Hair cycle regulation	Alopecia (chemotheraphy)?
Melanocyte	Stimulation of melanogenesis	Vitiligo

IV. IMMUNE SYSTEM

The detection of VDRs in almost all cells of the immune system, especially antigen-presenting cells (macrophages and dendritic cells) and activated T lymphocytes, led to the investigation of a potential for $1,25(OH)_2D_3$ as an immunomodulator. Application of the molecule *in vitro* and *in vivo* has led to interesting observations, confirming a role for $1,25(OH)_2D_3$ and its analogues in the immune system. Not only is the VDR present in all cells of the immune system, activated macrophages are able to synthesize and secrete $1,25(OH)_2D_3$. These cells indeed express the enzyme $25(OH)D_3$-1α-hydroxylase, as could recently be demonstrated at the molecular level by reverse transcription-polymerase chain reaction (RT-PCR) in activated macrophages. Although cloning and sequencing of the mRNA clearly demonstrated this enzyme to be identical to the known renal form, its regulation seems to be under completely different control. The macrophage enzyme mainly runs through immune signals, with interferon-γ (IFN-γ) being a powerful stimulator. In macrophages, no clear down-regulation of the enzyme by $1,25(OH)_2D_3$ could be observed, explaining the hypercalcemia occurring in situations of macrophage overactivation such as tuberculosis or sarcoidosis. The secretion of classical macrophage products such as cytokines [interleukin-1 (IL-1), TNFα, and IL-12] precedes the transcription of the enzyme and as a consequence the secretion of $1,25(OH)_2D_3$. Therefore, its timing is compatible with that of a suppressive signal, allowing first an activation and further recruitment of the other members of the immune system, followed by inhibiting signals, such as prostaglandin E2 (PGE2), to limit the extent of the reaction (Fig. 1).

As a true immunomodulator, $1,25(OH)_2D_3$ not only interacts with T cells but also targets the central cell in the immune cascade, the antigen-presenting cell.

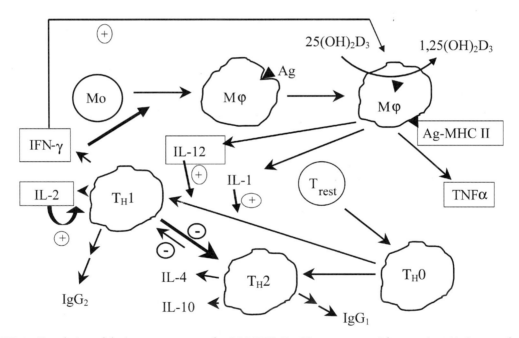

FIGURE 1 Regulation of the immune response by $1,25(OH)_2D_3$. Upon contact with an antigen (Ag), e.g., a bacterial component, blood monocytes (Mo) or dendritic cells will become activated (Mφ) and present this antigen in the context of MHC class II molecules to the rest of the immune system. Moreover, by secretion of chemokines and activating cytokines [e.g., interleukin-12 (IL-12), tumor necrosis factor α (TNFα)], these activated cells will recruit T lymphocytes (CD4 cells) and activate them, depending on the cytokine environment, into T helper 1 (T_H1) or T_H2 cells. T_H1 cells, which produce mainly interferon-γ (IFN-γ) and IL-2, will further activate the macrophage and close a positive feedback loop, leading to amplification of the immune response. $1,25(OH)_2D_3$ and its analogues can modulate the immune response via several mechanisms. $1,25(OH)_2D_3$ inhibits IL-12 production and down-regulates co-stimulatory molecule expression by dendritic cells, thus inhibiting the development of T_H1 cells along the T_H1 pathway and favoring the induction of $CD4^+CD25^+$ regulatory T cells. $1,25(OH)_2D_3$ also exerts direct effects on T cells by inhibiting IL-2 and IFN-γ production and by inducing, in particular, T_H2 cells in target tissues. In addition, $1,25(OH)_2D_3$ inhibits the recruitment of T_H1 cells to sites of inflammation. Macrophages (Mφ) can synthesize $1,25(OH)_2D_3$ and this may also contribute to the regulation of the immune response.

Here, $1,25(OH)_2D_3$ stimulates the differentiation of monocytes toward "good" phagocytosis and killing of bacteria. Differentiation of monocytes into dendritic cells and further differentiation of these cells from immature to mature dendritic cells is almost completely inhibited by $1,25(OH)_2D_3$. Incubation of monocytes with $1,25(OH)_2D_3$ *in vitro* results in a cell type totally different from classical dendritic cells, but also different from monocytes. CD14 is highly expressed on the surface, but human leukocyte antigen class II proteins and B7.2 proteins are down-regulated. Antigen-presenting cells are not able to promote an immune response, since they are not able to properly stimulate T cells to proliferation or cytokine secretion. On the other hand, these cells have also not differentiated into macrophages, since they are unable to perform chemotaxis or phagocytosis of bacteria. Also, the crucial signals secreted by antigen-presenting cells for the recruitment and activation of T cells are directly influenced by $1,25(OH)_2D_3$. A key cytokine in the immune system, IL-12 is clearly inhibited by $1,25(OH)_2D_3$ and its analogues. This monocyte-produced substance is the major determinant of the direction in which the immune system will be activated. IL-12 stimulates the development of CD4 T helper 1 (T_H1) cells and inhibits the development of CD4 T_H2 lymphocytes. T_H1 lymphocytes secrete mainly IL-2 and IFN-γ and are considered to be the most important cells in graft rejection and autoimmunity. T_H2 cells secrete IL-4, IL-5, and IL-10 and are considered to be regulator cells. The observation of clear inhibition of IL-12 by $1,25(OH)_2D_3$ and its analogues (*in vitro* by enzyme-linked immunosorbent assay or by intracellular fluorescence-activated cell sorting (FACS) analysis or *in vivo* by RT-PCR) is essential in understanding the observed effects of these substances *in vitro* on T-cell proliferation and cytokine production and *in vivo* on graft survival and autoimmunity prevention (Table 5). By inhibiting IL-12 secretion, $1,25(OH)_2D_3$ directly interferes with the heart of the immune cascade and shifts the reaction toward a T_H2 profile. $1,25(OH)_2D_3$ also influences the secretion of other cytokines secreted by monocyte-derived cells: the suppressive PGE2 is stimulated and the monocyte recruiter granulocyte/macrophage colony-stimulating factor is suppressed. Several T-cell cytokines, especially the T_H1 type, are also direct targets for $1,25(OH)_2D_3$ and its analogues. $1,25(OH)_2D_3$-mediated inhibition of IL-2 secretion occurs through impairment of nuclear factor of activated T cells (NFAT) complex formation, since the receptor complex itself binds to the distal NFAT-binding site in the human IL-2 promoter. Another key

TABLE 5 Beneficial Effects of $1,25(OH)_2D_3$ and its Analogues in Animal Models of Autoimmunity and Transplantation

Autoimmunity
Autoimmune diabetes
Chemically induced diabetes mellitus
Collagen-induced arthritis
Experimental allergic encephalomyelitis
Experimental autoimmune thyroiditis
Heyman nephritis
Lupus nephritis
Mercuric chloride-induced glomerulonephritis

Transplantation
Aorta
Bone marrow
Heart
Kidney
Liver
Pancreatic islets
Skin
Small bowel

T-cell cytokine that by itself further stimulates antigen presentation, IFN-γ, is directly (via a VDRE) down-regulated by $1,25(OH)_2D_3$. Moreover, progressive deletion analysis of the IFN-γ promoter revealed that negative regulation by $1,25(OH)_2D_3$ is also present at the level of an upstream region containing an enhancer element. Finally, it was recently demonstrated that $1,25(OH)_2D_3$ also directly stimulates IL-4 production by T_H2 cells. The combination of these effects on dendritic cell phenotype and cytokine secretion, with the direct effects on T-cell cytokine profile, results in the differentiation of T cells toward a T_H2 profile. This profile is beneficial in achieving prolonged organ graft survival and in prevention of organ-specific autoimmune diseases such as multiple sclerosis or type 1 diabetes.

The fact that $1,25(OH)_2D_3$ and its analogues influence the immune system, not by pure immunosuppression, but by immunomodulation through induction of immune shifts and regulator cells, makes these products very appealing for clinical use, especially in the treatment and prevention of autoimmune diseases (Table 5). In autoimmune diabetes in the non-obese diabetic (NOD) mouse, up-regulation of regulator cells and a shift from T_H1 toward T_H2 locally in the pancreas and islet grafts of treated mice could be observed, and other effects on the immune system have also been described, the most important being a restoration of defective apoptosis sensitivity in lymphocytes, leading to better elimination of potentially dangerous autoimmune effector cells.

This increase in immunocyte apoptosis in NOD mice by 1,25(OH)$_2$D$_3$ and its analogues has been reported to occur following different apoptosis-inducing signals and could explain why an early short-term treatment with these products, before the onset of autoimmunity, can lead to long-term protection and a restoration of tolerance.

Finally, clear additive and even synergistic effects were observed between 1,25(OH)$_2$D$_3$ or its analogues and other more classical immunomodulators such as cyclosporin A and sirolimus (rapamycin). These effects were observed *in vitro* and could be confirmed *in vivo* in models of autoimmunity (diabetes and experimental allergic encephalomyelitis) and in graft destruction (Table 5).

In conclusion, these data suggest a physiological role for 1,25(OH)$_2$D$_3$ in the immune system as an inhibiting signal secreted by activated macrophages and received by activated T cells, thus limiting the immune reaction (Fig. 1). Analysis of the VDR knockout mouse model, however, confirms that all immune effects of 1,25(OH)$_2$D$_3$ are mediated through the VDR but demonstrate that 1,25(OH)$_2$D$_3$ is possibly a redundant signal in the immune system.

V. SUMMARY

The combined presence of 25(OH)D$_3$-1α-hydroxylase and the VDR in several nonclassical tissues introduced the concept of a paracrine role for 1,25(OH)$_2$D$_3$ outside that of calcium and bone metabolism. Moreover, the fact that 1,25(OH)$_2$D$_3$ was found to be capable of regulating cell differentiation and proliferation of normal (keratinocytes and immune cells) and malignant cells (leukemia, breast, prostate, and colon cancer cells) gave new perspectives on this molecule. The efforts made by companies and laboratories worldwide to develop analogues of 1,25(OH)$_2$D$_3$ with reduced calcemic effects opened therapeutic applications for these compounds as inhibitors of cell proliferation (e.g., treatment of psoriasis or cancer), as inducers of cell differentiation (e.g., treatment of cancer), and as immune modulators (e.g., treatment of autoimmune diseases or prevention of graft rejection). Moreover, the synergistic effects of 1,25(OH)$_2$D$_3$ analogues with retinoids, anti-estrogens, conventional chemotherapeutics, and classical immunomodulators may result in better response rates for the treatment of cancer and immune disorders. However, more research and clinical trials are needed to select the best 1,25(OH)$_2$D$_3$ analogue for each application.

Glossary

alopecia Hair loss that can occur in patches (alopecia areata) or globally. Causes range from hormones to autoimmunity.

anagen The growth phase of the growth cycle of mature hair follicles; anagen is followed by regression (catagen), rest (telogen), and shedding (exogen).

apoptosis Programmed cell death; cells undergoing apoptosis are cleared from the system silently without the initiation of inflammation.

autoimmune diseases Disorders initiated by the activation of autoreactive T cells that result in the destruction of tissues and cells by the body's own immune system.

cornified envelope Proteinaceous reinforced structure beneath the plasma membrane in differentiated keratinocytes consisting of cross-linked precursor proteins.

epidermis Outer epithelial layer of the skin consisting mainly of cells called keratinocytes.

ichthyosis Skin disease in which the skin is very dry and exhibits fish-like scales.

1,25(OH)$_2$D$_3$ The dihydroxylated, biologically active form of vitamin D. It is a central hormone in calcium homeostasis and bone metabolism, but has also a number of other functions and notably powerful immunomodulatory properties.

vitamin D receptor (VDR) A member of the superfamily of nuclear receptors for steroid hormones, thyroid hormone, and retinoic acid. The VDR functions as a 1,25(OH)$_2$D$_3$-activated transcription factor that ultimately influences the rate of RNA polymerase II-mediated transcription. VDRs are present not only in cells typically involved in calcium and bone metabolism, but also in other cell types, such as cells of the immune system.

vitamin D A vitamin/hormone with a central role in calcium and bone metabolism; it can be absorbed from the diet or can be synthesized by the skin via stimulation by ultraviolet light. Deficiency of vitamin D leads to a disorder known as rickets or osteomalacia.

vitamin D analogues Chemically modified molecules derived from 1,25(OH)$_2$D$_3$. Modifications have been made throughout the molecule, to obtain analogues with the desired properties. More than 1000 different vitamin D analogues have been synthesized worldwide.

See Also the Following Articles

Adrenocorticosteroids and Cancer ● Apoptosis ● Cancer Cells and Progrowth/Prosurvival Signaling ● Glucocorticoids and Autoimmune Diseases ● Sex Hormones and the Immune System ● Vitamin D ● Vitamin D Metabolism ● Vitamin D: Nuclear Receptor for 1,25(OH)$_2$D$_3$ ● Vitamin D Receptors and Actions in Nonclassical Target Tissues

Further Reading

Abe, E., Miyaura, C., Sakagami, H., Takeda, M., Konno, K., Yamazaki, T., Yoshiki, S., and Suda, T. (1981). Differentiation of mouse myeloid cells by 1α,25-dihydroxyvitamin D₃. *Proc. Natl. Acad. Sci. USA* **78**, 4990–4994.

Bikle, D. D., and Pillai, S. (1993). Vitamin D, calcium and epidermal differentiation. *Endocr. Rev.* **14**, 3–19.

Bouillon, R. (2001). Vitamin D: From photosynthesis, metabolism, and action to clinical applications. *In* "Endocrinology" (L. J. DeGroot and J. L. Jameson, eds.), 4th ed., Vol. 2, pp. 1010–1028. Saunders, Philadelphia.

Bouillon, R., Okamura, W. H., and Norman, A. W. (1995). Structure–function relationships in the vitamin D endocrine system. *Endocr. Rev.* **16**, 200–257.

Casteels, K., Bouillon, R., Waer, M., and Mathieu, C. (1995). Immunomodulatory effects of 1,25-dihydroxyvitamin D₃. *Curr. Opin. Nephrol. Hyperten.* **4**, 313–318.

Fogh, K., and Kragballe, K. (1997). Vitamin D₃ analogues. *Clin. Dermatol.* **15**, 705–713.

Lehmann, B., Knuschke, P., and Meurer, M. (2000). UVB-induced conversion of 7-dehydrocholesterol to 1α,25-dihydroxyvitamin D₃ (calcitriol) in the human keratinocyte line HaCaT. *Photochem. Photobiol.* **72**, 203–209.

Mathieu, C., Van Etten, E., Gysemans, C., Decallone, B., Kato, S., Laureys, J., Depovere, J., Valckx, D., Verstuyf, A., and Bouillon, R. (2001). *In vitro* and *in vivo* analysis of the immune system of vitamin D receptor-knockout mice. *J. Bone Miner. Res.* **16**, 2057–2065.

Overbergh, L., Decallonne, B., Valckx, D., Verstuyf, A., Depovere, J., Laureys, L., Rutgeerts, O., Saint-Arnaud, R., Bouillon, R., and Mathieu, C. (2000). Identification and immune regulation of 25-hydroxyvitamin D-1-α-hydroxylase in murine macrophages. *Clin. Exp. Immunol.* **120**, 139–146.

Penna, G., and Adorini, L. (2000). 1α,25-dihydroxyvitamin D3 inhibits differentiation, maturation, activation, and survival of dendritic cells leading to impaired alloreactive T cell activation. *J. Immunol.* **164**, 2405–2411.

Sakai, Y., Kishimoto, J., and Demay, M. (2001). Metabolic and cellular analysis of alopecia in vitamin D receptor knockout mice. *J. Clin. Invest.* **107**, 961–966.

Van Leeuwen, J. P. T. M., and Pols, H. A. P. (1997). Vitamin D: Anticancer and differentiation. *In* "Vitamin D" (D. Feldman, F. H. Glorieux, and J. W. Pike, eds.), pp. 1089–1105. Academic Press, San Diego.

Vitamin D Metabolism

HELEN L. HENRY

University of California, Riverside

Vitamin D₃ is produced in the skin through the action of ultraviolet light and is subsequently hydroxylated in the liver and then in the kidney to form 1α,25-dihydroxyvitamin D₃, the biologically active form of vitamin D. The biochemical reactions that occur in vitamin D metabolism, the enzymes that catalyze these reactions, and the genes that encode these enzymes are discussed in this article. In addition, the factors that regulate the pathways of vitamin D metabolism are examined.

I. INTRODUCTION

Ultraviolet light and heat bring about the conversion of 7-dehydrocholesterol to vitamin D₃ in the skin of vertebrates on exposure to sunlight (Fig. 1). In the liver, vitamin D₃ is hydroxylated at carbon 25 on the side chain to form 25-hydroxyvitamin D₃ [25(OH)D₃], the major circulating vitamin D₃ metabolite. 25(OH)D₃ serves as the substrate for the production in the kidney of the biologically active steroid hormone, 1α,25-dihydroxyvitamin D₃ [1α,25-(OH)₂D₃] and of 24R,25-dihydroxyvitamin D₃ [24R,25(OH)₂D₃]. The cytochrome P450-dependent enzymes that catalyze these three reactions are

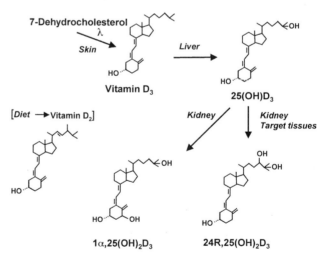

FIGURE 1 Metabolism of vitamin D. Following its production in the skin through the action of ultraviolet light, vitamin D₃ is hydroxylated in the liver by 25-hydroxylase (CYP27A) and then in the kidney by 25(OH)D₃-1α-hydroxylase (CYP27B) to form 1α,25(OH)₂D₃, the steroid hormonally active form of vitamin D. 25(OH)D₃ is also hydroxylated in the kidney and in 1α,25(OH)₂D₃ target tissues at carbon 24 by the 24R-hydroxylase (CYP24). Vitamin D₂, which is derived from and differs only in the side chain from vitamin D₃, which is derived from ergosterol, can undergo the same activation steps to 1α,25(OH)₂D₂.

the vitamin D3-25-hydroxylase (CYP27A1), 25(OH)-D₃-1α-hydroxylase (CYP27B1), and 25(OH)D₃-24R-hydroxylase (CYP24), each of which is discussed in more detail below.

The side chain of both 25(OH)D₃ and 1α,25(OH)₂D₃ is subject to further metabolism, as shown in Fig. 2. Following 24R-hydroxylation, the same cytochrome P450 catalyzes further hydroxylation, oxidation, and cleavage of four carbons from the side chain; another pathway leads to the formation of 26,23-lactone derivative.

Vitamin D₂ (Fig. 1) is derived from the plant sterol ergosterol and is used as a dietary supplement for humans and domesticated animals. In humans, it is considered to be metabolized to 1α,25(OH)₂D₂ in a manner that is qualitatively and quantitatively similar to that of vitamin D₃. However, the presence of the double bond between carbons 22 and 23 and the methyl group attached to carbon 24 impedes the side chain metabolism of the vitamin D metabolites derived from ergosterol.

The enzymes that catalyze the transformations of vitamin D and its metabolites are cytochrome P450-dependent mixed-function oxidases or steroid hydroxylases. In general, these enzymes depend on a source of electrons to reduce molecular oxygen and either one (for microsomal enzymes) or two (for mitochondrial enzymes) accessory proteins to transport the electrons to the specific cytochrome P450 responsible for the stereospecific hydroxylation of the substrate.

II. VITAMIN D₃-25-HYDROXYLASE

The most abundant circulating form (15–60 ng/ml) of vitamin D₃ is the 25-hydroxylated derivative, 25(OH)D₃, which is formed in the liver by the mixed-function oxidase, vitamin D₃-25-hydroxylase. Although other tissues, such as the kidney and intestine, are capable of catalyzing this reaction, the liver makes by far the largest and physiologically most significant contribution to the circulating levels of the prohormone, 25(OH)D₃.

The experimental evidence for the subcellular localization of 25-hydroxylase activity depends on the species under investigation. For example, in rats and rabbits, activity has been reported in both microsomes and mitochondria and both subcellular forms have been purified to homogeneity. In humans, only a mitochondrial form of 25-hydroxylase activity has been demonstrated; on this basis, as well as the fact that in rats microsomes contain fivefold less activity than do mitochondria, some authors have questioned the physiological significance of the microsomal 25-hydroxylase activity and most recent investigations have focused on the mitochondrial enzyme.

The mammalian mitochondrial vitamin D₃-25-hydroxylase that has been cloned is CYP27A1, which also catalyzes the hydroxylation of carbons 26 and 27 of cholesterol, during steps in the formation of bile acids. CYP27A1 cDNA expressed in *Escherichia coli* hydroxylates vitamin D₃ at several positions on the side chain in addition to carbon 25 and carbon

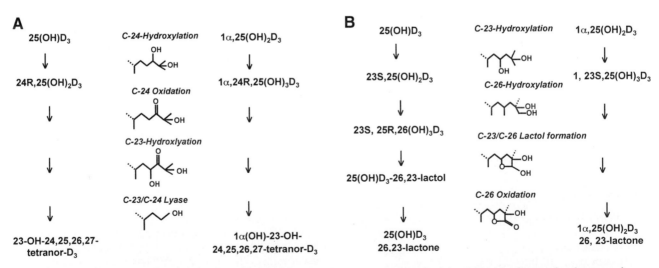

FIGURE 2 Metabolism of the vitamin D side chain. (A) The reactions carried out by CYP24 leading to the cleavage of four carbons. In the kidney, a significant amount of 24R,25(OH)₂D₃ is released prior to the subsequent oxidation steps. The complete C-24 oxidation pathway occurs in most target tissues of 1α,25(OH)₂D₃. (B) The C-23 oxidation pathway leading to the formation of the C-23/C-26 lactone derivatives. As indicated, both pathways can operate on substrates with or without the hydroxylation at carbon 1 in the A ring.

1. Whether CYP27A is the only enzyme responsible for the formation of 25-hydroxylated vitamin D derivatives, however, is brought into question by lack of evidence that it forms 25(OH)D$_2$, the predominant circulating derivative of vitamin D$_2$, as efficiently as it forms 25(OH)D$_3$.

III. 25(OH)D$_3$-1α-HYDROXYLASE

It has been appreciated for three decades that the kidney is the major site of production of circulating 1α,25(OH)$_2$D (20–60 pg/ml), although, as discussed below, other tissues and cell types, notably skin, placenta, and cells of hematopoietic lineage, have been shown to produce 1α,25(OH)$_2$D$_3$ from 25(OH)D$_3$. In the kidney and in other tissues in which subcellular localization has been investigated, 1α-hydroxylase activity is exclusively mitochondrial.

cDNA sequences for the rat, mouse, pig, and human enzymes show that the primary structure of the 1α-hydroxylase is most similar to that of CYP27A1; therefore, it has been designated CYP27B1. The CYP27B1 gene, which is located on mouse chromosome 10 and human chromosome 12, is composed of nine exons and appears to be present in a single copy.

Although studies in vitamin D-deficient animals suggest that 1α-hydroxylase enzymatic activity is localized in the proximal tubule of the renal nephron, recent *in situ* hybridization and immunohistochemical studies of normal human kidney indicate that the enzyme and its message are more highly expressed in the distal portions of the nephron. It is likely that differential localization of the enzyme along the nephron under different conditions of vitamin D status reflects the dual autocrine/paracrine and endocrine roles of the kidney in calcium homeostasis.

Although the belief that the kidney is the principal site of 1α,25(OH)$_2$D$_3$ production is supported by studies in uremic animals as well as by clinical experience with patients with chronic renal failure, there is also evidence for the extrarenal production of 1α,25(OH)$_2$D$_3$. The most studied of these include keratinocytes and skin *in vivo*, various placental preparations, and the cells of the hematopoietic system. 1α-Hydroxylase activity in these cell latter types is not regulated by those components of the calcium homeostatic system described below for the renal 1α-hydroxylase but rather by immune cell regulators such as interferon-γ and lipopolysaccharide. It is thought that these occurrences of extrarenal 1α-hydroxylase activity serve autocrine/paracrine functions.

IV. 25(OH)D$_3$/1α,25(OH)$_2$D$_3$-24R-HYDROXYLASE

Whereas the 1α-hydroxylase has but one naturally occurring substrate, the 24R-hydroxylase has two. The same enzyme catalyzes the 24-hydroxylation and subsequent side chain modification of both 25(OH)D$_3$ and 1α,25(OH)$_2$D$_3$ (Fig. 2). Depending on the enzyme preparation and assay conditions used, the affinity of the enzyme for 25(OH)D$_3$ is either much greater than or much less than that for 1α,25(OH)$_2$D$_3$. Given the fact that circulating levels of 25(OH)D$_3$ are approximately three orders of magnitude greater than those of 1α,25(OH)$_2$D$_3$ and that the turnover number is greater for 25(OH)D$_3$ than for 1α,25(OH)$_2$D$_3$, there is, in the whole animal, considerable capacity to produce 24R, 25(OH)$_2$D$_3$.

The cDNA encoding CYP24 has been cloned from rat, mouse, pig, and human kidneys. Expression studies in *E. coli* have shown that all of the reactions depicted in Fig. 2, C-24-hydroxylation, C-24 oxidation, C-23-hydroxylation, and C-23/C-24 cleavage, are catalyzed by a single cytochrome P450.

The 24R-hydroxylase gene, which contains 12 exons, has been localized to human chromosome 20 and mouse chromosome 2. The promoter region of the rat gene contains two vitamin D-response elements that are likely involved in the induction of the 24-hydroxylase by 1α,25(OH)$_2$D$_3$ (see below).

Although first identified and characterized in the kidney, where it is notable for its regulation that is reciprocal to that of the 1α-hydroxylase, the 24R-hydroxylase is actually very widespread, occurring in all target tissues that contain the receptor for 1α,25(OH)$_2$D$_3$, VDR. In fact, the inducibility of the 24R-hydroxylase by 1α,25(OH)$_2$D$_3$ is often taken as *prima facie* evidence of a cell being a target of 1α,25(OH)$_2$D$_3$ action. Like the 1α-hydroxylase, the 24R-hydroxylase is exclusively mitochondrial.

Although there is no controversy regarding the fundamental importance of the 1α-hydroxylase in the production of a biologically important steroid hormone, 1α,25(OH)$_2$D$_3$, the biological significance of the 24R-hydroxylase is less clear-cut. It is undoubtedly important to the inactivation and catabolism of 1α,25(OH)$_2$D$_3$ in the target cells in which is it induced by this steroid through the nuclear actions of the VDR. A 24R-hydroxylase knockout mouse has been produced in which observed deficiencies in bone metabolism were attributed not to the absence of 24R,25(OH)$_2$D$_3$ but to excess 1α,25(OH)$_2$D$_3$ resulting from its impaired catabolism.

On the other hand, the fact that substantial amounts of 24R,25(OH)$_2$D$_3$ are produced by the kidney along with evidence that 24R,25(OH)$_2$D$_3$ may have biological actions distinct from those attributable to 1α,25(OH)$_2$D$_3$ leaves open the possibility of an endocrine role for the kidney in the production of 24R,25(OH)$_2$D$_3$ as well as 1α,25(OH)$_2$D$_3$.

V. REGULATION OF VITAMIN D METABOLISM

The overall pathway leading to the production of the hormonally active 1α,25(OH)$_2$D$_3$ begins with the availability of vitamin D either from production in the skin or from the diet. If the supply of the parent vitamin is limited, deficiency of 1α,25(OH)$_2$D$_3$ will result in bone abnormalities. There is no documented physiologically significant regulation of the 25-hydroxylation of vitamin D by the liver, and in fact, circulating levels of 25(OH)D$_3$ are widely used to assess vitamin D status.

A. Kidney

The production of 1α,25(OH)$_2$D$_3$ by the kidney is tightly regulated by factors that generally have the opposite effects on the production of 24R,25(OH)$_2$D$_3$. The most thoroughly studied of these factors, and probably the most important in normal physiological circumstances, are the prevailing levels of 1α,25-(OH)$_2$D$_3$ itself and of parathyroid hormone (PTH). As depicted in Fig. 3, 1α,25(OH)$_2$D$_3$ inhibits its own synthesis and increases that of 24R,25(OH)$_2$D$_3$. The effect of 1α,25(OH)$_2$D$_3$ on 24R-hydroxylase is primarily if not exclusively mediated through increased mRNA levels, but the mechanism by which 1α,25(OH)$_2$D$_3$ reduces the 1α-hydroxylase is not as clear.

The second important physiological regulator of the renal hydroxylation of 25(OH)D$_3$ is PTH, which increases the synthesis of 1α,25(OH)$_2$D$_3$ and decreases that of 24R,25(OH)$_2$D$_3$. Low dietary calcium has the same effects on the two hydroxylase activities, which are probably mediated through increased PTH secretion. Intracellular signaling systems involved in mediating the effects of PTH on the two hydroxylases include cyclic AMP-dependent protein kinase as well as protein kinase C. The steady-state level of mRNA encoding CYP27B (1α-hydroxylase) is increased and that for CYP24 is decreased by PTH, but whether the entire effect of the peptide hormone on the activity of the two hydroxylases can be accounted for by alterations in mRNA levels has not been established.

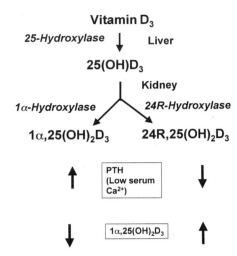

FIGURE 3 Regulation of vitamin D metabolism. The hydroxylation of vitamin D in the liver is not regulated in physiological circumstances so that the circulating levels of 25(OH)D$_3$ are a reflection of vitamin D status. In the kidney, 1α-hydroxylation and 24R-hydroxylation of 25(OH)D$_3$ are regulated in a reciprocal fashion by 1α,25(OH)$_2$D$_3$ and by PTH.

Changes in the levels of other hormones have been reported to influence the amounts of 1α,25(OH)$_2$D$_3$ and/or 24R,25(OH)$_2$D$_3$ produced by the kidney. These include calcitonin, glucocorticoids, growth hormone, and sex steroids. The direction and magnitude of the effects of these hormones on 1α-hydroxylase and 24R-hydroxylase activities are variable, depending on the animal model under investigation. It is likely that although the effects of these hormones on vitamin D metabolism may be important in certain special endocrine circumstances, they are of less significance than 1α,25(OH)$_2$D$_3$ and PTH in the normal homeostatic control of the renal hydroxylation of 25(OH)D$_3$.

B. Bone and Intestine

Studies of the regulation of the mRNA for 24R-hydroxylase in bone and intestine have shown that, as in the kidney, these are increased by 1α,25(OH)$_2$D$_3$. However, as shown in Fig. 4, the effects of PTH and activation of protein kinase C on 24R-hydroxylase mRNA are tissue specific.

VI. OTHER PATHWAYS OF VITAMIN D METABOLISM

A. C-23 Oxidation

As shown in Fig. 2, the side chain of either 25(OH)D$_3$ or 1α,25(OH)$_2$D$_3$ can undergo hydroxylation at

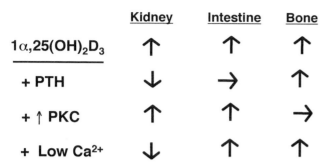

	Kidney	Intestine	Bone
1α,25(OH)₂D₃	↑	↑	↑
+ PTH	↓	→	↑
+ ↑ PKC	↑	↑	→
+ Low Ca²⁺	↓	↑	↑

FIGURE 4 Tissue-specific regulation of 24R-hydroxylase mRNA. In all three tissues, $1\alpha,25(OH)_2D_3$ is required to induce the 24-hydroxylase from basal levels. Once induced, the 24R-hydroxylase is modulated differentially by PTH, activation of protein kinase C, and low dietary calcium in the three tissues.

carbon 23, leading to the formation of the 23(S), 25(R)-26,23-lactone derivatives. Human CYP24, expressed in *E. coli*, is capable of catalyzing all of these reactions with both substrates, but other enzymes may be involved *in vivo*. In terms of their contribution to the catabolism of $1\alpha,25(OH)_2D_3$ and $25(OH)D_3$, there is considerable species variation in the utilization of the C-23 and C-24 oxidation pathways. For example, rats and mice use the C-24 pathway almost exclusively, whereas C-23 derivatives predominate in the guinea pig.

B. 3-Epimerization

The formation of 3-epi-$1\alpha,25(OH)_2D_3$ has been reported in human keratinocytes, bone cells, and parathyroid cells. Although metabolites of this compound have been reported to possess biological activity, the physiological importance of this pathway has not been established.

Glossary

cytochrome P450 In eukaryotes, a family of microsomal and mitochondrial heme-containing proteins (named for their characteristic absorption of light of 450 nm when carbon monoxide is bound) that reduce molecular oxygen, one atom of which is incorporated stereospecifically into the substrate as a hydroxyl group; those that use endogenous steroids for substrates are sometimes called steroid hydroxylases and many catalyze steps subsequent to the initial hydroxylation.

prohormone A precursor (either peptide or steroid) to an active hormone that is produced in significant amounts as an intermediate in the pathway of production of the active hormone.

protein kinase C A family of serine/threonine protein kinases that are activated by Ca^{2+} and/or phospholipids in response to extracellular signals.

VDR The specific target tissue receptor for $1\alpha,25$dihydroxyvitamin D_3, the steroid hormone form of vitamin D.

vitamin D-response element The specific vitamin D receptor-binding DNA sequence in the promoter regions of genes whose transcription is altered by $1\alpha,25$-dihydroxyvitamin D_3.

See Also the Following Articles

Steroid Nomenclature • Vitamin D • Vitamin D and Cartilage • Vitamin D and Human Nutrition • Vitamin D-Binding Protein • Vitamin D: 24,25-Dihydroxyvitamin D • Vitamin D Receptors and Actions in Nonclassical Target Tissues

Further Reading

Adams, J. S., Sharma, O. P., Gacad, M. A., and Singer, F. R. (1983). Metabolism of 25-hydroxyvitamin D_3 by cultured pulmonary alveolar macrophages in sarcoidosis. *J. Clin. Invest.* **72**, 1856–1860.

Astecker, N., Reddy, G. S., Herzig, G., Voriesk, G., and Schuster, I. (2000). 1α25-Dihydroxy-3-epi-vitamin D_3 a physiological metabolite of 1α25-dihydroxyvitamin D_3: Its production and metabolism in primary human keratinocytes. *Mol. Cell. Endocrinol.* **170**, 91–101.

Feldman, D., Glorieux, F. H., and Pike, J. W. (eds.) (1997). "Vitamin D," pp. 1–1285. Academic Press, San Diego, CA.

Gascon-Barre, M., Demers, C., Ghrab, O., Theodoropoulos, C., Lapointe, R., Jones, G., Valiquette, L., and Menard, D. (2001). Expression of CYP27A, a gene encoding a vitamin D-25-hydroxylase in human liver and kidney. *Clin. Endocrinol.* **54**, 107–115.

Mawer, E. B., Taylor, C. M., Backhouse, J., Lumb, G. A., and Stanbury, S. W. (1973). Failure of formation of 1,25-dihydroxycholecalciferol in chronic renal insufficiency. *Lancet* **1**, 626–628.

Murayama, A., Takeyama, K., Kitanaka, S., Kodera, Y., Kawaguchi, Y., Hosoya, T., and Kato, S. (1999). Positive and negative regulations of the renal 25-hydroxyvitamin D_3 1αhydroxylase gene by parathyroid hormone, calcitonin, and $1\alpha,25(OH)_2D_3$ in intact animals. *Endocrinology* **140**, 2224–2231.

Panda, D. K., Kawas, S. A., Seldin, M. F., Hendy, G. N., and Goltzman, D. (2001). 25-Hydroxyvitamin D 1α-hydroxylase: Structure of the mouse gene, chromosomal assignment, and developmental expression. *J. Bone Miner. Res.* **16**, 46–56.

Reichel, H., Koeffler, H. P., and Norman, A. W. (1987). Synthesis in vitro of 1,25-dihydroxyvitamin D_3 and 24,25-dihydroxyvitamin D_3 by interferon-γ-stimulated normal human bone marrow and alveolar macrophages. *J. Biol. Chem.* **262**, 10931–10937.

Sakaki, T., Sawada, N., Koami, K., Shiozawa, S., Yamada, S., Yamamoto, K., Ohyama, Y., and Inouye, K. (2000). Dual metabolic pathway of 25-hydroxyvitamin D3 catalyzed by human CYP24. *Eur. J. Biochem.* **267**, 6158–6165.

Sawada, N., Sakaki, T., Ohta, M., and Inouye, K. (2000). Metabolism of vitamin D_3 by human CYP27A1. *Biochem. Biophys. Res. Commun.* **273**, 977–984.

Zehnder, D., Bland, R., Walker, E. A., Bradwell, A. R., Howie, A. J., Hewison, M., and Stewart, P. M. (1999). Expression of 25-hydroxyvitamin D_3-1α-hydroxylase in the human kidney. *J. Am. Soc. Nephrol.* **10**, 2465–2473.

Zehnder, D., Bland, R., Williams, M. C., McNinch, R. W., Howie, A. J., Stewart, P. M., and Hewison, M. (2001). Extrarenal expression of 25-hydroxyvitamin D_3-1α-hydroxylase. *J. Clin. Endocrinol. Metab.* **86**, 888–894.

Zierold, C., Reinholz, G. G., Mings, J. A., Prahl, J. M., and DeLuca, H. F. (2000). Regulation of the porcine 1,25-dihydroxyvitamin D_3-24-hydroxylase (CYP24) by 1,25-dihydroxyvitamin D_3 and parathyroid hormone in AOK-B50 cells. *Arch. Biochem. Biophys.* **381**, 323–327.

Vitamin D: Nuclear Receptor for $1,25(OH)_2D_3$

J. Wesley Pike and Nirupama K. Shevde
University of Wisconsin

The biological actions of 1,25-dihydroxyvitamin D_3 [$1,25(OH)_2D_3$] in tissues and cells are orchestrated within the nucleus through complex changes in gene expression. These changes lead to cell-specific alterations in the level of proteins that regulate the cell cycle, modulate differentiated cell function, or regulate subsequent levels of gene expression through their additional actions on genes or cells. Most, if not all, of the molecular actions of $1,25(OH)_2D_3$ in the nucleus are mediated by a receptor protein termed the vitamin D receptor (VDR). This receptor is a specific member of a large gene family of transcription factors that function to mediate the actions of all the known steroid hormones, among them the estrogens and androgens, progesterone, the glucocorticoids, and thyroid hormone. As discussed in this article, the structural features of the VDR are well adapted to this functional role in regulating gene expression.

I. INTRODUCTION

Vitamin D_3, derived from 7-dehydrocholesterol through the actions of heat and ultraviolet light, undergoes further enzymatic activation first to 25-hydroxyvitamin D_3 in the liver and then to 1,25-dihydroxyvitamin D_3 [$1,25(OH)_2D_3$] in the kidney. This final metabolic conversion, which is highly regulated by parathyroid hormone as well as a variety of additional hormones and circulating factors, leads to what is now considered to be the active form of vitamin D_3. By virtue of its small size, lipophilic nature, and mechanism of action, $1,25(OH)_2D_3$ is not considered to be a vitamin but rather a steroid hormone.

The classical role of $1,25(OH)_2D_3$ is to regulate mineral homeostasis, achieved in part through regulatory actions on the parathyroid gland and through coordinate actions on intestine, kidney, and bone. Accordingly, the discovery of the vitamin D receptor (VDR) was initially made through investigations in those tissues. Currently, however, the VDR is found in a wide variety of cells and tissues, including those of skin, liver, pancreas, muscle, breast, prostate, adrenal, and thyroid and in cells of mesenchymal and hematopoietic origin. Although the VDR in these tissues is derived from the same chromosomal gene, its role in cellular function is pleiotropic and not necessarily involved in the control of mineral balance. Indeed, one of its most basic functions appears to be that of regulating cellular proliferation and differentiation, an activity that may be found associated with most steroid and adrenal hormones. This regulatory feature is likely a fundamental component of all biological responses to $1,25(OH)_2D_3$, including those that involve mineral homeostasis.

II. STRUCTURAL ORGANIZATION OF THE VDR

Evidence for the existence of a receptor for $1,25(OH)_2D_3$ predated the discovery of the hormone itself and supported the idea that the mechanism of action of vitamin D might be similar to that of other steroids. Over the ensuing years, research revealed numerous biochemical features of the VDR. These characteristics included the ability of the receptor to bind its ligand, $1,25(OH)_2D_3$, with very high affinity and selectivity and, perhaps just as importantly, to bind to DNA. Both were features consistent with those of a protein capable of mediating vitamin D-dependent gene expression. It was the molecular cloning of the VDR, however, that led to new insights into receptor structure and function and which enabled the tremendous progress that has been made recently in understanding how hormones such as 1,25(OH)$_2$D$_3$ function to regulate gene expression.

A. General Organization of Steroid Receptors

The general structural organization of the VDR and other members of the steroid receptor family is illustrated in Fig. 1a. As can be seen, the typical hormone receptor is composed of an amino-terminal domain, a more centrally located DNA-binding domain (DBD), which is the hallmark of the nuclear receptor family, a linker region, and a large carboxy-terminal ligand-binding domain (LBD) that is capable of binding not only hormonal ligands but also additional transcriptional co-regulators that are directly responsible for the activation (or repression) of gene expression. Receptors that contain large amino-terminal extensions can also modulate gene expression through this region. As seen in Fig. 1b, the overall structure of the VDR is generally similar with the exception that its amino-terminal domain is somewhat abbreviated relative to that of other receptor family members. As a consequence, the VDR relies heavily on the activation region found within the carboxy-terminal LBD. The key structural elements of the VDR (as well as other family members) are, therefore, the DNA-binding domain, which specifies the genes that are to be regulated, and

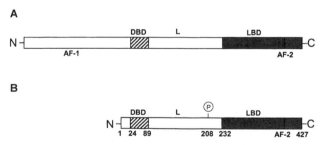

A

B

FIGURE 1 General structural organization of members of the nuclear receptor gene family. (A) Organization of a prototypical steroid receptor. N, amino-terminus; C, carboxy-terminus; DBD, DNA-binding domain; L, hinge or linker region; LBD, ligand-binding domain; AF, activation function. (B) Organization of the human vitamin D receptor. Designations are as in (A). Numbers indicate amino acid residues. P, phosphorylated serine 208.

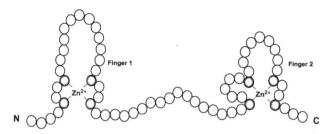

FIGURE 2 Organization of the two zinc-finger structures found in the DNA-binding domain of the VDR as well as all members of the steroid receptor gene family. C, cysteine residue; Zn, zinc atom.

the carboxy-terminal domain, which mediates the transcriptional regulatory process following binding and activation by 1,25(OH)$_2$D$_3$ or other steroidal ligands.

B. The DNA-Binding Domain of the VDR

The DBD of the VDR and the nuclear receptor family consists of two similar modules, each composed of a zinc-coordinated finger structure (Fig. 2). Each zinc atom is coordinated in a tetrahedral fashion through four highly conserved cysteine residues that serve to stabilize the finger structure itself. Although the two zinc modules of the VDR appear to be highly related structurally, topologically they are not equivalent as a result of differing chirality of the residues in each module that coordinate the zinc atom. More importantly, the function of each of these modules in DNA binding is known to be substantially different. Whereas the amino-terminal module functions to direct specific DNA binding in the major groove of the DNA-binding site, the carboxy-terminal module serves as a dimerization interface for interaction with DNA-binding protein partners. Recent studies have led to the elucidation of the three-dimensional structure of the DNA-binding domain of several nuclear receptors while bound to DNA.

C. The Ligand-Binding Domain of the VDR

The LBD of the VDR is responsible for the receptor's functional activity. This region contains both a dimerization domain that permits essential interaction with the retinoid X receptor (RXR), a key DNA-binding protein partner, and an activation domain that directs the recruitment of co-regulatory proteins such as steroid receptor co-activator-1 (SRC-1), glucocorticoid receptor-interacting protein (GRIP), and D receptor-interacting protein 205 (DRIP$_{205}$). These factors as well as others mediate linkage to large

TABLE I   Target Gene, Promoter Location, and Nucleotide Sequence of Natural Vitamin D-Response Elements

Target gene	Location	Nucleotide sequence		
Rat osteocalcin	−460/−446	GGGTGA	atg	AGGACA
Human osteocalcin	−499/−485	GGGTGA	acg	GGGGCA
Mouse osteopontin	−757/−743	GGTTCA	cga	GGTTCA
Rat calbindin D-9K	−489/−475	GGGTGT	cgg	AAGCCC
Rat 24-hydroxylase	−150/−136(Prox)	AGGTGA	gtg	AGGGCG
	−258/−244(Dist)	GGTTCA	gcg	GGTGCG
Human 24-hydroxylase	−169/−155(Prox)	AGGTGA	gcg	AGGGCG
	−291/−277(Dis)	AGTTCA	ccg	GGTGTG
Human p21	−779/−765	AGGGAG	att	GGTTCA

protein machines responsible for altering chromatin structure and facilitating recruitment of RNA polymerase II, both of which are integral to the modulation of gene expression. Most importantly, however, the structural integrity and functional activity of both of these protein-interacting domains within the VDR are under the control of 1,25(OH)$_2$D$_3$. This tight regulatory capacity of the hormone is achieved by its ability to occupy a small pocket within the receptor and to induce significant conformational changes necessary for activity. Thus, the limited functional capabilities of a very small molecule such as 1,25(OH)$_2$D$_3$ are expanded through its interaction with a much larger macromolecule to confer multifunctional cellular capabilities. Recent efforts have resulted in determination of the three-dimensional structure of the LBD of the VDR. The crystal structure both confirms previous biochemical and molecular studies of VDR and provides new avenues of research aimed at understanding the structure and function of this important molecule.

III. REGULATION OF GENE EXPRESSION THROUGH DNA BINDING

The vitamin D hormone is known to regulate a host of genes, a few of which are indicated in Table 1. Perhaps the first to be identified was the chicken vitamin D-dependent calbindin gene, whose product is involved in facilitating intestinal calcium absorption. More recently, gene targets include the 25-hydroxyvitamin D$_3$-24-hydroxylase, osteocalcin, osteopontin, and p21. An initial understanding of how 1,25(OH)$_2$D$_3$ and its receptor might regulate gene expression was derived initially from studies of the human osteocalcin gene. Accordingly, a hexanucleotide repeat DNA sequence separated by 3 bp that represented a specific binding and transcriptional activation site (vitamin D-response element or

VDRE) for the VDR was discovered upstream of the start site of transcription within the human osteocalcin gene promoter. This element as well a similar sequence found in the rat osteocalcin gene provided a first glimpse at a binding site for the VDR within a 1,25(OH)$_2$D$_3$-regulated gene. The sequences of these VDREs as well as several additional ones that were discovered in the mouse osteopontin gene, mouse calbindin -D-28K, rat calbindin D-9K, the rat and human 25-hydroxyvitamin D$_3$-24-hydroxylase genes (two apparent VDREs), and the human p21 gene are documented in Table 1.

IV. THE VDR FUNCTIONS AS A HETERODIMER

The duplicated nature of the VDRE in the osteocalcin gene and other gene promoters suggested that VDR might bind as a homodimer to DNA identical to that for other steroid receptors. Despite this precedent, the VDR was surprisingly found to bind to VDREs as a heterodimer with a previously identified protein, termed the RXR (Fig. 3). This interaction requires a protein dimerization surface within the DBD of both VDR and RXR as well as one located within the carboxy-terminus of both proteins. Additional studies indicate that the VDR/RXR interaction with DNA exhibits polarity. As seen in Fig. 3, RXR binds to the 5′ or upstream promoter half-site of the VDRE and the VDR occupies the downstream site. There are three RXR isotypes that can interact with the VDR, thereby increasing the potential complexity of gene regulation. Interestingly, each of these forms also interacts with other nuclear receptors, including the thyroid hormone receptor and the retinoic acid receptor. Thus, all receptors that utilize RXR as a common partner in a single cell likely compete for this protein during transcriptional activation.

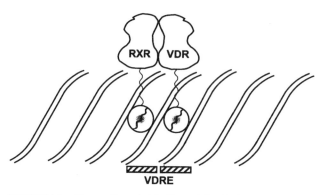

FIGURE 3 Heterodimeric binding of the VDR to a VDRE in a hormone-sensitive gene promoter. RXR, retinoid X receptor; VDR, vitamin D receptor.

V. ROLE OF 1,25(OH)$_2$D$_3$ IN VDR ACTIVATION

1,25(OH)$_2$D$_3$ induces conformational changes in the VDR that lead to significant rearrangements within the receptor, particularly those that form important protein-interacting surfaces. Although these changes have not been visualized directly within the VDR using X-ray crystallography, as has been accomplished for certain steroid receptors, three-dimensional modeling studies based upon similarity in receptor structure strongly support such hormone-induced rearrangements. A variety of biochemical and cellular assays also support in an indirect fashion these conformational changes. For example, ligand binding significantly enhances VDR stability and induces strong resistance to proteolytic degradation *in vitro*. It is now known that the molecular changes that are induced by 1,25(OH)$_2$D$_3$ within the VDR have a functional consequence, namely, to promote the dimerization of VDR with its RXR partner. Indeed, initial studies suggested that the affinity of the VDR for RXR increased almost 10-fold for its protein partner when 1,25(OH)$_2$D$_3$ was present. Since these interactions occurred in the absence of VDRE DNA, it suggests that the initial event in vitamin D-dependent gene activation is the formation of a functional receptor module composed of ligand-occupied VDR and RXR. Formation of this complex is followed by VDRE binding. It is now clear that the conformational changes induced by 1,25(OH)$_2$D$_3$ also lead to the formation of a new surface or surfaces capable of binding directly to members of at least several different classes of co-modulatory proteins. These proteins are essential to the complex transcriptional regulatory process. Thus, a host of latent activities within receptors such as VDR are uncovered

when hormonal ligand is present converting the VDR into a transcriptionally active protein.

VI. VDR RECRUITMENT OF TRANSCRIPTIONAL CO-REGULATORS

Early working models of steroid receptor action placed the receptor in contact with the general transcriptional apparatus, thus directly modulating transcription. Transcriptional regulation is considerably more complicated than originally envisioned, however. Complex sets of molecular machinery capable of modifying chromatin structure and recruiting RNA polymerase II are involved in facilitating transcription and different sets promote transrepression. Thus, 1,25(OH)$_2$D$_3$ functions to target this machinery to the promoters of vitamin D-sensitive genes. These targeting events are mediated by the VDR, first through its interaction with selective sequences of DNA and then through its ability to sequentially recruit additional regulatory complexes.

A. p160 Co-activators and Acetylation

Activation of gene expression requires numerous alterations in chromatin architecture. Thus, protein machines that are initially recruited by steroid receptors to hormonally responsive promoters contain histone acetyltransferases (HATs) capable of modifying lysine residues on histones and increasing transcription factor accessibility to DNA (Fig. 4). HATs exhibit different specificities for lysine residues on histones, providing a likely explanation why multiple proteins within the complex contain residual acetylating capabilities. Direct linkage between the receptor and these large protein complexes is provided in part by several proteins termed p160 co-activators, which contain HAT activity as well. SRC-1 represents the prototypic member. The primary interaction surface or docking site on the VDR that mediates receptor/SRC-1 interaction is designated activation function-2 (AF-2). The formation of this binding site is highly dependent upon the presence of hormone, which alters the placement of several of the approximately 12 α-helices in the receptor LBD and completely rearranges the position of α-helix 12. The p160 co-activators (as well as other proteins that bind to AF-2) interact with the receptor in turn through a specific leucine-charged helix termed the nuclear receptor box that contains central core residues of the pattern LXXLL. The VDR together with the RXR also interacts in a ligand-dependent manner with SRC-1 and other members of

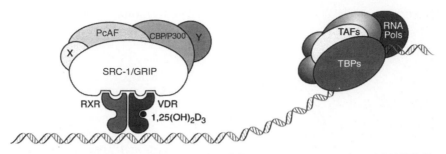

FIGURE 4   Arrangement of the SRC-1/GRIP complex following recruitment to a 1,25(OH)$_2$D$_3$-sensitive gene promoter. SRC-1 or GRIP binding to hormone-activated VDR and its silent partner RXR leads to the subsequent recruitment of additional transcription factors including CBP/p300 (CREB-binding protein/p300, where CREB denotes Ca^{2+}/cyclic AMP-response element-binding protein), P/CAF (p300/CBP-associated factor), and perhaps other unknown proteins (X and Y). This complex mediates transactivation though modification of chromatin-associated histone residues and through direct contacts with specific TAFs (transcription activating factor). RNA pols, RNA polymerase II; TBP, TATA box-binding protein.

the p160 co-activators, thus initiating the recruitment of machinery essential for the initial phase of the transcriptional activation process. Since the co-activator family of genes exhibits little specificity for individual receptors, it is likely that selectivity for the different co-activators that are found within a cell may be promoter context dependent. Despite this, it is clear that the recruitment of these HAT-containing complexes and additional proteins capable of chromatin modification are essential to the process of transactivation.

B. Co-repressor Complexes and Deacetylation

Steroid receptors also function to suppress transcriptional activity. Not surprisingly, repression requires the recruitment of complexes that remove acetyl residues from histones, thereby producing a transcriptionally resistant form of chromatin. These proteins are histone deacetylases (HDACs). Nuclear receptors recruit such HDACs to specific chromatin templates indirectly via proteins such as nuclear receptor co-repressor (N-CoR) and silencing mediator for retinoic acid and thyroid hormone (SMRT). Although the interaction site within the nuclear receptor for these repressors is also located at AF-2, the leucine-charged LXXLL motif within the nuclear co-repression is somewhat altered to a slightly different configuration. Both N-CoR and SMRT also interact with the VDR following activation by 1,25(OH)$_2$D$_3$, presumably to decrease the ability of the receptor to activate transcription. Interestingly, several receptors including the thyroid hormone and retinoic acid receptors suppress gene expression in the absence of hormone. In these cases,

N-CoR and SMRT are recruited to the promoter via receptors that are not bound to their respective hormonal ligands.

C. The DRIP Complex

The DRIP complex, a fundamentally different molecular machine, also interacts with the VDR. The DRIP complex is composed of 10 or more proteins, none of which appear to contain either HAT or HDAC activity. The DRIP complex interacts not only with other members of the nuclear receptor family such as estrogen receptor, but with certain basal transcription factors as well. Recruitment of DRIP is achieved by the VDR through DRIP$_{205}$, a protein that contains several LXXLL motifs that interact with 1,25(OH)$_2$D$_3$-activated VDR at AF-2. Although the function of the DRIP complex is not precisely understood at present, it may be involved in mediating the recruitment of RNA polymerase II to the DNA template.

The discovery that transcriptional regulation by nuclear receptors is mediated by downstream co-regulatory factors highlights the complexity of gene regulation. The diversity of these co-regulators is enormous. In addition to those mentioned, additional factors that provide synergistic regulation, that link nuclear receptors to unrelated transcription factors, and that enable mechanisms whereby receptors are degraded have been identified. Imposing these additional sets of factors into the steroid receptor functional pathway provides important ways in which a cell can modulate receptor action and integrate its actions with other incoming signals important for survival and function.

VII. HEREDITARY RESISTANCE TO 1,25(OH)$_2$D$_3$

The central importance of the VDR to 1,25(OH)$_2$D$_3$ action is emphasized through studies of the human syndrome of hereditary 1,25(OH)$_2$D$_3$-resistant rickets. Early studies suggested that this genetic disease was due to defects in vitamin D signal transduction and experiments in cells from patients with the disease eventually implicated the VDR in this resistance pathway. However, it was cloning and structural and sequence analyses of the chromosomal gene for the VDR that enabled direct analysis of the VDR gene from patients with hereditary resistance. These efforts led to the discovery of a series of different mutations within the VDR that compromised its ability to function. Accordingly, mutations were found in the DBD as well as in the LBD. The former led to an inability of the receptor to bind to DNA, whereas the latter resulted in a receptor unable to bind 1,25(OH)$_2$D$_3$ or to interact with its RXR dimerization partner. Additional mutations continue to be found. Each of these alterations in VDR structure results in the loss of transcriptional activity and leads to significant defects in the skeleton as a result of altered calcium and phosphorus homeostasis. Genetic ablation of the VDR gene in mice has revealed many of the skeletal features found in the human and now provides an excellent animal model with which to study 1,25(OH)$_2$D$_3$ and VDR function.

VIII. SUMMARY

1,25(OH)$_2$D$_3$ is a steroid-like hormone that functions to regulate mineral homeostasis and other biological events in higher organisms. This regulation is achieved in target tissues through selective control of gene expression, a process that is mediated by the VDR. The VDR is an intracellular receptor protein that belongs to the steroid receptor family of transcription factors and whose functional activities are activated by 1,25(OH)$_2$D$_3$. Functional activities include selective VDR/RXR binding to DNA sequences or VDREs followed by VDR-mediated recruitment of additional protein complexes essential to the transcriptional regulatory process. Significant details associated with this highly intricate regulatory step are now beginning to emerge. The importance of the VDR in the biological actions of vitamin D is seen in humans with genetic abnormalities in the VDR as well as in animals in which the VDR has been genetically ablated. It is likely that a fuller understanding of the mechanism of action of the vitamin D hormone and its receptor will be forthcoming during the next few years.

Glossary

activation function A domain located within the ligand-binding region of steroid receptors that interacts with co-regulators, thus modulating transcription.

co-regulators Transcription factors that are recruited to active gene promoters via DNA-binding proteins such as the vitamin D receptor.

hereditary A human syndrome of generalized resistance to 1,25-dihydroxyvitamin D$_3$ due to inherited mutations in the vitamin D receptor.

histone modification Acetylation or deacetylation of lysine residues within DNA-bound histones that alter chromatin structure and transcription factor accessibility.

retinoid X receptor A member of the steroid receptor gene family that functions as a heterodimeric DNA-binding partner for the vitamin D receptor.

steroid or nuclear receptor gene family A large family of eukaryotic genes whose protein products both function as receptors for steroid and thyroid hormones, retinoic acid, and 1,25-dihydroxyvitamin D$_3$ and modulate transcription.

target genes Genes that can be regulated by a specific hormone because their promoters contain regulatory elements that can interact with the hormone's receptor.

vitamin D receptor A specific protein that binds 1,25-dihydroxyvitamin D$_3$ and mediates the actions of this hormone in target tissues.

vitamin D-response element A specific DNA-binding site for the vitamin D receptor that is located within the promoter region of a gene that is regulated by 1,25-dihydroxyvitamin D$_3$.

See Also the Following Articles

Vitamin D • Vitamin D and Cartilage • Vitamin D and Human Nutrition • Vitamin D: Biological Effects of 1,25(OH)$_2$D$_3$ in Bone • Vitamin D: Biological Effects of 1,25(OH)$_2$D$_3$ in the Intestine and Kidney • Vitamin D: 24,25-Dihydroxyvitamin D • Vitamin D Effects on Cell Differentiation and Proliferation • Vitamin D Metabolism • Vitamin D Receptors and Actions in Nonclassical Target Tissues

Further Reading

Baker, A. R., McDonnell, D. P., Hughes, M., Crisp, M., Mangelsdorf, D. J., Haussler, M. R., Shine, J., Pike, J. W., and O'Malley, B. W. (1988). Molecular cloning and expression of human vitamin D$_3$ receptor complementary DNA: Structural homology with thyroid hormone receptor. *Proc. Natl. Acad. Sci. USA* 85, 3294–3298.

Feldman, D., Glorieux, F. H., and Pike, J. W. (1997). "Vitamin D." Academic Press, San Diego.

Freedman, P. L., and Lemon, B. D. (1997). Structural and functional determinants of DNA binding and dimerization by the vitamin D receptor. *In* "Vitamin D" (D. Feldman,

F. H. Glorieux, and J. W. Pike, eds.), pp. 127–148. Academic Press, San Diego.

Gamble, M. J., and Freedman, L. P. (2002). A coactivator code for transcription. *Trends Biochem. Sci.* **27**, 165–167.

Haussler, M. R., Whitfield, G. K., Haussler, C. A., Hsieh, J.-C., Thompson, P. D., Selznick, S. H., Encinas Dominguez, C., and Jurutka, P. W. (1998). The nuclear vitamin D receptor: Biological and molecular regulatory properties revealed. *J. Bone Miner. Res.* **13**, 325–349.

Malloy, P. J., Pike, J. W., and Feldman, D. (1999). The vitamin D receptor and the syndrome of hereditary 1,25-dihydroxyvitamin D-resistant rickets. *Endocr. Rev.* **20**, 156–188.

Mangelsdorf, D. J., Thummel, C., Beato, M., Herrlich, P., Schutz, G., Umersono, K., Blumberg, B., Kastner, P., Mark, M., Chambon, P., and Evans, R. M. (1995). The nuclear receptor superfamily: The second decade. *Cell* **83**, 835–839.

McInerney, E. M., Rose, D. W., Flynn, S. E., Westin, S., Mullen, T. M., Krones, A., Inostroza, J., Torchia, J., Nolte, R. T., Assa-Munt, N., Milburn, M. V., Glass, C. K., and Rosenfeld, M. G. (1998). Determinants of coactivator LXXLL motif specificity in nuclear receptor transcriptional activation. *Genes Dev.* **12**, 3357–3368.

McKenna, N. J., Xu, J., Nawaz, Z., Tsai, S. Y., Tsai, M. J., and O'Malley, B. W. (1999). Nuclear receptor coactivators: Multiple enzymes, multiple complexes, multiple functions. *J. Steroid Biochem. Mol. Biol.* **69**, 3–12.

Perissi, V., Staszewski, L. M., McInerney, E. M., Kurokawa, R., Krones, A., Rose, D. W., Lambert, M. H., Milburn, M. V., Glass, C. K., and Rosenfeld, M. G. (1999). Molecular determinants of nuclear receptor-corepressor interaction. *Genes Dev.* **13**, 3198–3208.

Rochel, N., Wurtz, J. M., Mitschler, A., Klaholz, B., and Moras, D. (2000). The crystal structure of the nuclear receptor for vitamin D bound to its natural ligand. *Mol. Cell* **5**, 173–179.

Sone, T., Kerner, S. A., and Pike, J. W. (1991). Vitamin D receptor interaction with specific DNA: Association as a 1,25-dihydroxyvitamin D3-modulated heterodimer. *J. Biol. Chem.* **266**, 23296–23305.

Vitamin D Receptors and Actions in Nonclassical Target Tissues

MARIAN R. WALTERS

Tulane Medical School, New Orleans

I. INTRODUCTION
II. RANGE OF 1,25(OH)$_2$D$_3$ TARGETS AND ACTIONS
III. 1,25(OH)$_2$D$_3$ FUNCTIONS IN NONCLASSICAL TARGETS: COMMONALITIES AND GENERALITIES
IV. 1,25(OH)$_2$D$_3$ FUNCTIONS IN NONCLASSICAL TARGETS: TISSUE-SPECIFIC EFFECTS
V. 1,25(OH)$_2$D$_3$/VDR INHIBITS BREAST AND PROSTATE CANCER GROWTH
VI. SUMMARY

Intestine, kidney, and bone tissues have long been known to have receptors for vitamin D. Vitamin D receptors are now known to exist in many other tissues, including those of skeletal and vascular smooth muscles, central nervous system components, the heart, endocrine and reproductive organs, the lungs, and the liver. 1,25-Dihdroxyvitamin D$_3$ interacts specifically with receptors in these tissues; the effects of these interactions are mediated by many intracellular signaling pathways. Genetic characterizations of the receptors and activation pathways hold promise in further understanding the roles of vitamin D in health and disease.

I. INTRODUCTION

Traditional studies of vitamin D receptors (VDRs) and their actions have focused on plasma calcium-regulating vitamin D targets such as intestine, kidney, and bone. However, in 1979, putative VDR sites were first described in "nonclassical" tissues—for example, in tissues as diverse as the pancreas, pituitary gland, and uterus. Thus began a new era in which the concept of the actions of the hormonal form of vitamin D, 1,25-dihydroxyvitamin D$_3$ [1,25(OH)$_2$D$_3$], changed from its being considered solely a hormone that regulates plasma calcium homeostasis to understanding that it plays roles in numerous cellular processes, including proliferation/differentiation, hormonal secretion, and neuroprotection.

II. RANGE OF 1,25(OH)$_2$D$_3$ TARGETS AND ACTIONS

As detailed in Table 1, vitamin D receptors have now been described in numerous targets, including many cells of the immune system, cardiovascular tissues, skeletal muscle, reproductive and other endocrine sites, central nervous system, and a host of other tissues. Evidence for the presence of VDR sites in these tissues has come from a variety of experimental approaches (Table 2). Moreover, through the years, increasingly sophisticated approaches have been used to probe for the presence of VDRs in putative new target tissues. For example, a recent immunoblotting study has demonstrated the presence of VDRs in tissue extracts from the hippocampus, with more specific localization demonstrated by immunocytochemistry in the neuronal and glial cells in pyramidal and granule cell layers, including CA1, CA2, CA3, and the dentate gyrus. More functional studies have indicated that hippocampal extracts contain a VDR-like species capable of binding to the specific osteopontin VDR

TABLE 1 Overview of Nonclassical 1,25(OH)$_2$D$_3$ Target Tissues

Cardiovascular tissue and muscle	Other endocrine organs
Cardiac myocytes	Adrenals
Skeletal muscle	Pancreatic beta cells
Vascular smooth muscle	Parathyroid gland[a]
	Pituitary
	Salivary glands[b]
	Thyroid
Reproductive tissues	**Other targets**
Chicken egg shell gland[b]	Adipose tissue
Epididymis	Central nervous system
Mammary gland[b]	Choroid plexus
Ovary	Colon[b]
Oviduct	Hematolymphopoietic cells
Prostate	Liver
Placenta[b]	Lung
Testis	Retina
Uterus	Skin
	Stomach
	Thymus
	Variety of cancers

[a]Site of a key hormonal role for 1,25(OH)$_2$D$_3$/VDR in regulating the Ca^{2+} homeostatic endocrine system.

[b]Although these tissues are not "classical" sites of plasma calcium regulation, regulation of Ca^{2+} translocation is likely to be a principal function of 1,25(OH)$_2$D$_3$/VDR therein.

DNA response element sequence in gel-shift studies. Collectively, studies using all of these approaches provide a large body of complementary data about the receptors and their putative sites of action.

III. 1,25(OH)$_2$D$_3$ FUNCTIONS IN NONCLASSICAL TARGETS: COMMONALITIES AND GENERALITIES

Many effects have been described for 1,25(OH)$_2$D$_3$ actions in nonclassical targets (Table 3). Although

TABLE 2 Types of Analyses Used to Define New VDR Targets

Approach	Example
Biochemical	[^{3}H]-1,25(OH)$_2$D$_3$ binding studies and Scatchard analysis
	Sucrose density-gradient analysis
	DNA cellulose chromatography
	Immunoblotting
Histological	Autoradiography
	Immunohisto/cytochemistry
Molecular	Northern analysis
	Gel shift

some of these effects (e.g., effects on signal transduction pathways, Ca^{2+} buffering, and growth regulation) parallel events known to occur in classical targets in the regulation of plasma Ca^{2+} homeostasis, tissue-specific effects also occur, and knowledge of their existence will likely continue to grow. Moreover, in contrast to many other effects, 1,25(OH)$_2$D$_3$ induction of the vitamin D-related calbindins—which is typical of the traditional Ca^{2+}-translocating tissues—does not occur in many of the nonclassical targets.

The hormonal effects of 1,25(OH)$_2$D$_3$ in its targets involve two separate, but likely interdependent, mechanisms, termed "genomic" and "nongenomic" processes. Genomic actions are those in which the nuclear VDR regulates gene transcription at the DNA level. Interestingly, although this is the classical mechanism of action of the vitamin D endocrine system, specific details (e.g., the identity of the regulated genes) are not well delineated in most nontraditional targets. Nongenomic actions of 1,25(OH)$_2$D$_3$ are those mediated principally through actions at/on the cellular membrane. Although several laboratories have exerted considerable effort to identify the putative membrane receptors for 1,25(OH)$_2$D$_3$, details of the molecular structures are not yet available. In other steroid receptor systems, there may be multiple membrane receptor forms—some with identity to the nuclear receptor forms and some with totally different molecular origins. It is hoped that it will soon be known whether this interesting pattern of diversity of membrane receptor forms also holds for the vitamin D hormone. Despite both the lack of definition of the precise membrane effectors and the relatively recent focus on membrane-related events, a plethora of data exist defining apparent nongenomic signal transduction mechanisms of 1,25(OH)$_2$D$_3$ in these systems. It is important to note that many signal transduction pathways have been implicated in the nongenomic actions of 1,25(OH)$_2$D$_3$, sometimes occurring in different tissues but sometimes all within one tissue (e.g., skeletal muscle). Moreover, it is increasingly clear that these pathways are all intimately intertwined, and thus often affect one another in the response process.

1,25(OH)$_2$D$_3$ exerts important tissue- and development-specific effects on growth and differentiation. Its hormonal effects are important both in regulating normal growth processes and in clinically relevant conditions such as cancer (e.g., breast or prostate) and in tissue regeneration processes. In many tissues (e.g., cells of the hematolymphopoietic lineage),

TABLE 3   Examples of 1,25(OH)$_2$D$_3$ Effects in Nonclassical Targets

Mechanism	Tissue
Regulation of intracellular signaling pathways	Many
Proliferation/differentiation	Many
Protection against cellular damage (including Ca^{2+} buffering)	A growing list that includes the CNS, heart, and pancreas
Hormone secretion	Pancreas, ovary?
Regulation of 1,25(OH)$_2$D$_3$ responsiveness	
24-Hydroxylase	Universal
VDR levels	Pancreas and skin (not heart, testis, or lung)
Calbindin levels	Rare

growth inhibition correlates with specific effects to induce differentiation.

A. Cytoprotective Effects of 1,25(OH)$_2$D$_3$

1,25(OH)$_2$D$_3$ exerts important cytoprotective effects in a number of targets, especially by increasing antioxidant activity or by attenuating increases in free intracellular Ca^{2+} ([Ca^{2+}]$_i$). Thus, the hormone protects against damage from a long list of toxins and carcinogens known to act principally via release of free radicals. Buffering of [Ca^{2+}]$_i$ may occur through several mechanisms, including, for example, increased Ca^{2+} channel activity or increases in Ca^{2+}-binding proteins such as calbindin-D$_{28k}$.

B. Regulation of Vitamin D-Related Responses

In many tissues, 1,25(OH)$_2$D$_3$ alters processes that contribute to the ability of the molecule to regulate its own responsiveness within the tissue. 1,25(OH)$_2$D$_3$ treatment almost universally up-regulates 24-hydroxylase activity, which is an early step in 1,25(OH)$_2$D$_3$ clearance pathways. In more tissue-specific patterns, such treatment also regulates VDR levels and 1α-hydroxylase activity. In the latter case, up-regulation of tissue 1α-hydroxylase activity is thought to provide a local enhancement of the hormonal action with minimal effects on plasma calcium levels. Uncontrolled elevation of this paracrine system may be responsible for the hypercalcemia associated with some diseases such as sarcoidosis. There are also emerging reports of other cellular proteins (e.g., a heat-shock 70-related protein and the Ca^{2+}-binding protein calreticulin) that interfere with genomic actions of the VDR, and their regulation by 1,25(OH)$_2$D$_3$ may be a feedback mechanism to turn off 1,25(OH)$_2$D$_3$ responsiveness.

IV. 1,25(OH)$_2$D$_3$ FUNCTIONS IN NONCLASSICAL TARGETS: TISSUE-SPECIFIC EFFECTS

A. Skeletal Muscle: a Tissue with Well-Delineated Nongenomic Effects of 1,25(OH)$_2$D$_3$

Vitamin D deficiency has long been known to be associated with a generalized muscle weakness, which can lead to muscle atrophy and which is reversed by vitamin D treatment. It now appears that there are both nongenomic and genomic mechanisms through which 1,25(OH)$_2$D$_3$ regulates skeletal muscle function. In a long and elegant series of studies, the research team of Boland and de Boland has delineated the nongenomic mechanisms induced by 1,25(OH)$_2$D$_3$, principally using models from chick skeletal muscle. Their studies define a system in which there is an intricate interplay between numerous intracellular signaling pathways, which likely also interact with the nuclear VDR mechanisms. In this system, 1,25(OH)$_2$D$_3$ treatment results in rapid activation of phospholipase C, producing inositol 1,4,5-trisphosphate (InsP$_3$) and diacylglycerol (DAG). These effectors result in an increase in [Ca^{2+}]$_i$ levels, with an initial release (1 min) from internal stores and then a sustained phase (up to 5 min) of uptake through both L-type and store-operated Ca^{2+} channels. These effects parallel, but are not dependent on, increases in adenylyl cyclase and protein kinase A activities. However, the increases in [Ca^{2+}]$_i$ are dependent on activation of calmodulin, protein kinase C, and tyrosine kinase pathways. In fact, the relationship between 1,25(OH)$_2$D$_3$ stimulation and activation of tyrosine kinases is complex in this system. 1,25(OH)$_2$D$_3$ induces tyrosine kinase cascades, which result in increased phosphorylation of tyrosine residues in several proteins, including, in particular, phospholipase C-γ (which increases [Ca^{2+}]$_i$ from internal stores and by uptake through Ca^{2+} channels), the mitogen-activated protein kinases (MAPKs) ERK1 and ERK2, and c-myc. The $1,25(OH)_2D_3$ effect on MAPK activation is dependent on $[Ca^{2+}]_i$ and protein kinase C (PKC). In addition, $1,25(OH)_2D_3$ treatment increases Src kinase activity and decreases its tyrosine phosphorylation, and also causes increases in the levels of a VDR–Src kinase complex that is associated with elevated tyrosine phosphorylation of the VDR. The function of this tyrosine-phosphorylated VDR–Src kinase complex and its relationship to nuclear actions of the VDR have not yet been established. In rat skeletal muscle, $1,25(OH)_2D_3$ also activates phospholipase D, which results in a second phase of DAG release from phosphatidylcholine. This activation step is dependent on elevated $[Ca^{2+}]_i$ and G-protein activity, but its contributions to the $1,25(OH)_2D_3$ effects in this system have not been fully delineated.

The rapid $1,25(OH)_2D_3$ effects, via tyrosine kinase cascades, on the growth-related MAPK activity and the mitogenic effects of c-myc highlight the concept of cross-talk between the nongenomic pathways activated by $1,25(OH)_2D_3$ and nuclear actions of the VDR. The effects of $1,25(OH)_2D_3$ on growth and differentiation in this system are complex and depend on the developmental state. For example, in undifferentiated chick embryo myoblasts, there is stimulation of DNA synthesis and inhibition of myogenesis. As cultures form more differentiated myotubes, the $1,25(OH)_2D_3$ effects result in inhibition of DNA synthesis and an increase in differentiation as defined by increased synthesis of biochemical markers typical of differentiated muscle. Moreover, PKC α activation was associated with the proliferation phase, whereas its activity was decreased during the differentiation stage.

B. CNS: Neuroprotective Roles of $1,25(OH)_2D_3$

Numerous sites throughout the central nervous system contain VDRs, but the effects of VDRs are not well understood in each of these sites. The cerebellum contains high levels of the vitamin D-related calbindin-D_{28k}, where its expression is not altered by $1,25(OH)_2D_3$/vitamin D status. Nevertheless, there is evidence for roles of $1,25(OH)_2D_3$ in the brain under a variety of conditions. For example, changes in VDR distribution patterns in the central nervous system (CNS) during development suggest possible roles in this process. In cerebral cortex, $1,25(OH)_2D_3$ treatment alters the levels of some enzyme activities (e.g., acetylcholinesterase, citrate

synthase, and acyl phosphatase), but not others (e.g., cytochrome c oxidase and acid phosphatase).

Chronic treatment with $1,25(OH)_2D_3$ has been reported to provide neuroprotective roles in models of both aging and stroke. The rationale for the aging studies comes in part from putative links between altered calcium homeostasis and the development of Alzheimer's disease. Consistent with this hypothesis, when rats are treated chronically with $1,25(OH)_2D_3$, there is an increase in neuronal density in the hippocampus, wherein a loss of neurons is considered a reliable biomarker for aging. In the cerebral artery ligation model of stroke, $1,25(OH)_2D_3$ pretreatment decreases ischemic brain injury concomitant with elevated levels of plasma calcium. In this model, $1,25(OH)_2D_3$ treatment also increases levels of glial cell-derived neurotropic factor in the cortex, which has been associated with reduced cerebral infarction in this model. $1,25(OH)_2D_3$ pretreatment in culture models also protects dopaminergic neurons against cytotoxic effects of numerous insults, including reactive oxygen species, glutamate, specific dopaminergic toxins, or elevated Ca^{2+} entry induced by Ca^{2+} ionophores. Mechanistic studies have indicated that these $1,25(OH)_2D_3$ protective effects may be via direct actions on neurons, in that physiological doses of $1,25(OH)_2D_3$ can reduce the damage to hippocampal neurons *in vitro* that results from excess/inappropriate neurotransmitter release and the resulting sustained excitation. Similar doses of $1,25(OH)_2D_3$ also reduce L-type Ca^{2+} channel levels by effects at the mRNA level, suggesting that the resulting decrease in Ca^{2+} entry into the cell may play a role in the neuroprotective effect. Another clue to the neuroprotective role of $1,25(OH)_2D_3$ comes from a study in which $1,25(OH)_2D_3$ treatment increased the activity of γ-glutamyl transferase, an enzyme that has been implicated in scavenging reactive oxygen species, particularly in pericytes and peripheral astrocytes in rat brain.

CNS inflammatory disease can be associated with excess production of inducible nitric oxide synthase (iNOS). In mice with clinical signs of experimental allergic encephalitis, $1,25(OH)_2D_3$ treatment reduces CNS iNOS levels in a region- and cell-specific pattern and results in improvement of the clinical signs of the disease. Subsequent studies have documented loss of paralysis, decreased white matter and meningeal inflammation, and decreased CNS macrophage accumulation after $1,25(OH)_2D_3$ treatment. These results suggest that $1,25(OH)_2D_3$ provides a protective role in iNOS-associated CNS diseases. Although these $1,25(OH)_2D_3$ effects may relate more to immunomodulatory effects rather than direct neuronal actions, the beneficial effects of $1,25(OH)_2D_3$ treatment in this experimental model of multiple sclerosis are particularly interesting in light of prior suggestions that multiple sclerosis in humans may correlate with diminished activity of the vitamin D endocrine system.

C. Pancreas: Nongenomic and Cytoprotective Effects of $1,25(OH)_2D_3$

There is evidence indicating that insulin secretion and synthesis are impaired in vitamin D deficiency and are restored with $1,25(OH)_2D_3$ treatment. The defects have been shown to relate to the loss of $1,25(OH)_2D_3$ effects on several signal transduction pathways important in effecting glucose-signaled insulin secretion in pancreatic beta cells, including those involved in regulating $[Ca^{2+}]_i$, phospholipase C, PKC, and adenylyl cyclase. These insulinotropic effects of $1,25(OH)_2D_3$ are likely mediated through nongenomic mechanisms, as evidenced in part by their inhibition by a membrane-specific $1,25(OH)_2D_3$ antagonist $[1\beta,25(OH)_2D_3]$. In addition, $1,25(OH)_2D_3$ stimulates the production of a number of specific, but as yet unidentified, proteins in islet cells by a mechanism that seems to involve genomic pathways. These observations may also be important in clinical situations associated with transient defects in glucose signaling. For example, in patients with gestational diabetes, $1,25(OH)_2D_3$ treatment reduces plasma glucose levels, possibly by increasing insulin sensitivity.

Unlike most of the other nonclassical $1,25(OH)_2D_3$ targets, in addition to nuclear VDRs, pancreatic beta cells (and alpha cells in some species) contain the vitamin D-related calbindin-D_{28k}, and it is regulated by $1,25(OH)_2D_3$ in the beta cells. However, studies designed to identify a role for calbindin-D_{28k} in $1,25(OH)_2D_3$ effects on insulin secretion have thus far produced negative results. Pancreatic tissue damage, induced experimentally, for example, by oxidative stress, can result in islet cell destruction by cytokine-induced pathways. In this model of beta cell destruction and diabetes onset or islet allograft rejection, $1,25(OH)_2D_3$ exposure reduces several markers of oxidative stress and decreases immune/cytokine activation, suggesting that the hormone can exert a protective effect against immune destruction in these systems. In another model of diabetes in the nonobese diabetic (NOD) mouse, $1,25(OH)_2D_3$ prevents the development of diabetes by a mechanism that results in reduced resistance to apoptotic

signals in NOD thymocytes and thus disrupts the autoimmune response.

D. Cardiac Myocytes, Including the Atrial Endocrine Myocytes

There are complex effects of vitamin D deficiency, $1,25(OH)_2D_3$ supplementation, and vitamin D or $1,25(OH)_2D_3$ excess in the heart. The complexity derives in part from the attendant changes in parathyroid hormone (PTH) and plasma or tissue calcium. For example, low $1,25(OH)_2D_3$ levels may play a role in the cardiac disease associated with chronic renal failure (Table 4), and vitamin D

TABLE 4 Possible Vitamin D Effects on the Cardiovascular System

Effect[a]	Vitamin D/ $1,25(OH)_2D_3$ levels[b]	
	High	Low
Decreased blood pressure		
Opposes PTH excess?	✔	
Increased blood pressure		
↑Vascular smooth muscle force generation	✔	
↑Vascular smooth muscle cell $[Ca_i^{2+}]$	✔✔✔	
↑PTH production		✔
Cardiac contractility		
↓Contractility		✔
↑Contractility		✔✔✔
Left ventricular mass		
↑Hypertrophy		✔
↑Myocardial collagen content		✔
↓Endothelin-induced myocardial hypertrophy	✔	
Vascular smooth muscle cells		
↑Cell growth	✔	
↓Cell growth/↑cell maturation		✔
Atherosclerosis		
Tissue calcification		
↑Calcium phosphate deposits in vessel wall		✔
↑Heart valve calcification		✔✔✔

[a]PTH, Parathyroid hormone.
[b]A check mark indicates the condition in which the change in cardiovascular function occurs; ✔✔✔ indicates that protracted or severe conditions are required. Adapted from Rostand and Drüeke (1999).

supplementation in these patients results in improved cardiac function. However, the therapeutic improvement may also be due to indirect effects of $1,25(OH)_2D_3$ replacement on other physiological parameters, because impaired vitamin D status may also alter cardiovascular-related systems, including vascular smooth muscle and blood pressure, or other components of calcium homeostasis, in particular PTH and calcium levels (Table 4).

VDR sites have been described in cardiac muscle, with some concentration in atrial natriuretic peptide (ANP)-producing cells of the atria. $1,25(OH)_2D_3$ effects in cardiac tissues, as in many nontraditional targets, are independent of traditional $1,25(OH)_2D_3$ effects such as induction of calcium-binding proteins or changes in VDR levels. $1,25(OH)_2D_3$ stimulation in these systems does include nongenomic, and perhaps genomic as well, effects on Ca^{2+} uptake pathways, as well as developmental roles and genomic effects on ANP production. In nongenomic pathways in cardiac muscle, adenylyl cyclase and G-proteins are involved in $1,25(OH)_2D_3$-induced Ca^{2+} uptake through L-type Ca^{2+} channels and this effect is accompanied by cyclic adenosine monophosphate (cAMP)/protein kinase A (PKA)-dependent increases in microsomal protein phosphorylation.

Vitamin D deficiency results in reduced cardiac contractility, an effect reversed by $1,25(OH)_2D_3$. These effects on contractility are probably mediated at many levels: specific effects of $1,25(OH)_2D_3$ treatment include altered myocyte numbers, altered myosin isoenzyme patterns, and altered activity of many metabolic enzymes in the heart. In neonatal ventricular myocytes, $1,25(OH)_2D_3$ has complex effects on maturation and growth. It inhibits differentiation by a mechanism that may involve PKC. $1,25(OH)_2D_3$ inhibits proliferation by blocking entry into the cell cycle S phase, though there are conflicting reports on whether it also induces hypertrophy. These growth effects are paralleled by events *in vivo*, whereby vitamin D deficiency induces morphological changes in the heart that reflect cardiac myocyte hyperplasia and are accompanied by elevated c-myc levels. Also, in hearts of rat pups from mothers fed diets with low levels of vitamin D, there is evidence of slowed cardiac development. In contrast, excess vitamin D can result in protease-induced cardionecrosis, accompanied by damage to the cardiac contractile apparatus. In the ANP-producing endocrine myocytes of the atria, $1,25(OH)_2D_3$ inhibits ANP synthesis (decreased mRNA) and release, and these genomic effects are Ca^{2+} independent.

E. Vascular Smooth Muscle

$1,25(OH)_2D_3$ also seems to play a role in maintaining normal function of vascular smooth muscle by effects on a number of important processes. For example, the cardiovascular defects due to impaired vitamin D status in renal failure also include effects on smooth muscle elements (Table 4). Most $1,25(OH)_2D_3$ effects described to date in vascular smooth muscle seem to be mediated by genomic pathways, in contrast to the presence therein of well-described membrane-linked (nongenomic) effects of estrogen in these systems.

Recent studies of $1,25(OH)_2D_3$ effects in vascular smooth muscle have indicated that the responses differ in different areas of the vascular tree. In rat mesenteric resistance vessels, $1,25(OH)_2D_3$ treatment *in vivo* prior to vessel isolation increases contractile force and the force response to stress hormones. These long-term effects in more distal vessels seem to reflect a genomic effect of the hormone, but do not involve effects on myosin expression. Conversely, in the aorta, $1,25(OH)_2D_3$ treatment increases the expression of myosin light and heavy chains. When the mesenteric vessels are cultured, they lose the force response to stress (e.g., norepinephrine exposure) and this loss parallels altered patterns of myosin heavy chain expression. These detrimental effects are prevented by $1,25(OH)_2D_3$ treatment. Consistent with $1,25(OH)_2D_3$ effects on vascular contractility, $1,25(OH)_2D_3$ treatment increases blood pressure in *in vivo* models, likely via a genomic mechanism.

Soft tissue calcification, particularly in kidney and heart, is a serious consequence of the hypercalcemia caused by $1,25(OH)_2D_3$/vitamin D excess. Studies of vascular calcification have shown that $1,25(OH)_2D_3$ treatment increases *in vitro* calcification of cultured vascular smooth muscle cells, apparently by inhibiting expression of PTH-related peptide (PTHrP) (which inhibits calcification) and by stimulating expression and activity of procalcification proteins such as alkaline phosphatase and osteopontin.

F. Endocrine and Reproductive Tissues

$1,25(OH)_2D_3$ alters the function of a number of endocrine tissues. It increases thyrotropin-releasing hormone (TRH)-stimulated thyroid-stimulating hormone (TSH) and prolactin secretion in the pituitary. It has a wide range of effects in thyroid C cells, including inhibiting calcitonin gene expression and altering cell structure. It affects the synthetic pathways for adrenal catecholamines by regulating a number of the key enzymatic steps. Moreover, it is required for normal gonad function and estrogen synthesis in both males and females.

In many tissues, $1,25(OH)_2D_3$ exerts its activities through alterations in cAMP pathways. For example, in rat FRTL-5 thyroid cells, $1,25(OH)_2D_3$ regulates (reduces) TSH/cAMP signaling and affects basal cAMP levels. Inhibition of TSH-induced cAMP production is associated with a reduction in TSH-induced growth and iodide uptake in these thyroid-derived cells. TSH receptor levels and the levels of the G-protein $G_{\alpha s}$, which transduces the TSH receptor response to cAMP, are not affected. Conversely, $1,25(OH)_2D_3$ treatment specifically increases the levels of the inhibitory G-protein $G_{\alpha i2}$, but not $G_{\alpha i1}$ or $G_{\alpha i3}$. Because there is evidence of $1,25(OH)_2D_3$ effects beyond the cAMP effects, its effect on PKA subunits has also been also assessed, with a rather complex result. $1,25(OH)_2D_3$ treatment increases levels of the PKA regulatory subunit RIIβ. Additional studies have confirmed that the post-cAMP $1,25(OH)_2D_3$ inhibition in this system is due to the resultant increase in the relative levels of the PKA subunit tetrameric complex RIIβ_2C_2, which thus decreases the relative levels of the alternate tetrameric form RIα_2C_2, because PKA I is the predominant effector in this system. These effects of attenuating the cAMP response pathway at several steps are long term and thus are likely to be genomic effects of $1,25(OH)_2D_3$.

Many reproductive tissues, including testis, epididymis, and uterus, contain modest VDR levels. However, the levels of these VDR sites and of the vitamin D-related calbindins are not regulated by $1,25(OH)_2D_3$ in these tissues. In the uterus, for example, they are estrogen regulated. Moreover, although there are least modest effects (the degree seems to vary among animal models) of vitamin D deficiency on reproduction in males and females, it is possible that the attendant hypocalcemia is responsible for at least some of these effects.

When male and female rats are treated neonatally with $1,25(OH)_2D_3$, there are important changes in their sexual behavior as adults, suggesting that $1,25(OH)_2D_3$ may interfere in sexual imprinting and normal sex steroid receptor actions. Similarly, male pups from mothers exposed to $1,25(OH)_2D_3$ during pregnancy exhibit enlarged prostates but no change in seminal vesicle size. Moreover, there is a high rate of sudden death in these uncastrated male pups at puberty. Thus, there seem to be tissue-specific effects of $1,25(OH)_2D_3$ on development and genetic imprinting in the prostate.

When parameters of the calcium homeostatic endocrine system were assessed in women with fertility problems (especially arrest of follicular development) due to polycystic ovarian disease, despite normocalcemia in all of the patients, a subset exhibited relatively low $25(OH)D_3$ levels and some had elevated PTH levels. Vitamin D and calcium repletion resulted in two pregnancies and the return to normal menstrual cycles for several women. These observations were interpreted as indicating that abnormal calcium homeostasis may contribute to polycystic ovarian disease and/or the problems in follicular development associated with the disease.

In mammary glands, VDR levels vary from puberty to maturation and during pregnancy and lactation. The calcium-supplemented VDR knockout mouse has been used as a model to assess possible effects of $1,25(OH)_2D_3$/VDR on mammary gland development. In this system, the initial stage of development, ductal branching after puberty, is seen to be normal. However, later stages of branching and ductal development show some degree of undifferentiation, suggesting roles for $1,25(OH)_2D_3$/VDR in normal differentiation in this system. Moreover, these observations may explain part of the correlation of reduced activity of the vitamin D endocrine system and mammary tumor development, in that undifferentiated structures are a target of agents that cause cancer transformation in this system.

G. Lung

In the adult rat lung, there are low levels of VDRs and the calbindin-D$_{9k}$, but regulation of both proteins is $1,25(OH)_2D_3$ independent. In the near-term fetal (but not neonatal) rat lung, type II alveolar cells express VDRs and respond to $1,25(OH)_2D_3$ treatment with increased phospholipase activity, including synthesis and release of disaturated phosphatidylcholine and improved surfactant release and advancement of other maturation processes. In contrast, fetal lung fibroblasts do not express VDRs, but do exhibit 1α-hydroxylase activity, which can produce $1,25(OH)_2D_3$. These observations suggest that there is a paracrine $1,25(OH)_2D_3$ response system in the fetal lung for communication between epithelial and mesangial cells; this system may be involved in achieving the degree of lung maturation that is necessary to reduce the respiratory distress syndrome of premature birth.

H. Liver

Chronic liver disease is often associated with vitamin D depletion. Alternatively, $1,25(OH)_2D_3$ treatment induces the activity of a number of metabolic enzymes in the liver and reduces the hepatic damage from some toxins. Moreover, the liver has long served as a system for studies of nongenomic $1,25(OH)_2D_3$ effects.

Impaired calcium metabolism has been shown to interfere in hepatic regeneration processes—for example, after partial hepatectomy. Studies of $1,25(OH)_2D_3$ and calcium effects on specific markers of hepatic regeneration [e.g., mRNAs for hepatocyte growth factor and transforming growth factor-α (TGF-α)] and cell cycle regulators (e.g., cyclin D1 and cyclin A) indicate that both factors are important in optimal liver regeneration and that impaired regrowth occurs through molecular changes that reduce G1 transit efficiency in the cell cycle. In fetal rat hepatocytes, $1,25(OH)_2D_3$ treatment potently inhibits synthesis of α-fetoprotein and corticosteroid-binding globulin (CBG). $1,25(OH)_2D_3$ inhibition of CBG synthesis is much more potent than are the effects of activators of the retinoic acid receptor (RAR) or retinoic acid X receptor (RXR) and is not affected by the stimulation of CBG synthesis by the thyroid hormone triiodothyronine (T_3).

Studies of the antioxidant role of $1,25(OH)_2D_3$ in the liver show that vitamin D supplementation in the rat is more potent than vitamin E supplementation with respect to changes in a number of antioxidant activities, underscoring the notion that many of the cytoprotective effects of $1,25(OH)_2D_3$ may be mediated through antioxidant effects. More recent studies indicate that chronic $1,25(OH)_2D_3$ treatment inhibits hepatocyte damage following injection of the carcinogen diethylnitrosamine, likely by inhibiting lipid peroxidation, which in turn protects cell membranes from damage induced by free radicals.

V. $1,25(OH)_2D_3$/VDR INHIBITS BREAST AND PROSTATE CANCER GROWTH

VDR sites have been described in both breast and prostate epithelial cells. Reports of growth inhibitory $1,25(OH)_2D_3$ effects (particularly in cell models) in cancers from a number of tissues soon followed. These antiproliferative effects led to the hypothesis that $1,25(OH)_2D_3$ might be useful in treatment of a variety of cancers. To date, there is an active interest in these treatments and their mechanisms, but the issue is, of course, complicated by the hypercalcemic effect of $1,25(OH)_2D_3$ treatment. Thus, a number of pharmaceutical companies are actively seeking to develop noncalcemic analogues of the hormone.

In breast cancer, VDR is expressed in most breast cancer cell lines and in about 80% of human tumors. VDR levels in breast cancer do not correlate to sex steroid receptor levels nor to the stage of tumor development, and there is not always a good correlation between VDR levels in breast cancer models and the ability of $1,25(OH)_2D_3$ to inhibit tumor/cell growth. $1,25(OH)_2D_3$ inhibition of breast cancer cell growth includes both antiproliferative (altered cell cycle proteins) and pro-apoptotic effects.

In prostate cancers, the presence of VDR is required for the $1,25(OH)_2D_3$ effects, but there is not a good correlation of VDR levels and $1,25(OH)_2D_3$ responsiveness across cell models. Thus, other factors must contribute to $1,25(OH)_2D_3$ responsiveness in these systems. Recent studies have indicated that inhibition of 24-hydroxylase activity in VDR-containing but relatively $1,25(OH)_2D_3$-insensitive cells restores $1,25(OH)_2D_3$ sensitivity, suggesting that enhanced $1,25(OH)_2D_3$ clearance can contribute to the differences in apparent VDR responsiveness. Nevertheless, studies to date implicate only genomic mechanisms in the growth inhibitory effects of $1,25(OH)_2D_3$ in prostate cancer cells. Specific effects of $1,25(OH)_2D_3$ in these systems include alterations in the cell cycle (although the details differ among cell types), increases in the prostate cell differentiation marker prostate-specific antigen (PSA), and reduced activity of several growth factors. However, in most cases, the details of the $1,25(OH)_2D_3$ effects are not yet well understood. The ability of $1,25(OH)_2D_3$ to induce androgen receptor levels in these systems has led to the suggestion that it may also be useful to restore sensitivity to therapy in patients who have developed anti-androgen resistance. Finally, a small clinical trial of the effectiveness of $1,25(OH)_2D_3$ treatment in patients with prostate cancer has demonstrated that $1,25(OH)_2D_3$ treatment does slow prostate cancer growth *in vivo*, although hypercalcemia is a problem, as expected.

VI. SUMMARY

There are numerous effects of $1,25(OH)_2D_3$ in nonclassical target tissues, including both somewhat general effects on cell/tissue function and tissue-specific effects. The initial impetus for studying $1,25(OH)_2D_3$ effects in many of these tissues was

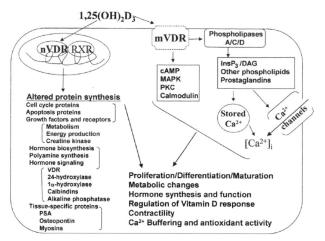

FIGURE 1 A schematic diagram showing the range of $1,25(OH)_2D_3$ effects in nonclassical target tissues. Left: A summary of many of the proteins/processes regulated at the transcriptional level by the nuclear vitamin D receptor (nVDR). Right: A summary of some of the intracellular signaling processes affected through the putative membrane VDR (mVDR) and systems they may affect. Abbreviations: RXR, retinoic acid X receptor; cAMP, cyclic adenosine monophosphate; MAPK, mitogen-activated protein kinase; InsP3, inositol 1,4,5-trisphosphate; DAG, diacylglycerol; PSA, prostate-specific antigen.

the finding of significant (albeit perhaps low) levels of VDR sites in the tissues. The initially described VDR sites in these tissues were likely the traditional nuclear VDRs, which regulate cell function at the level of gene transcription (Fig. 1). However, in many of these tissues, many effects of $1,25(OH)_2D_3$ may be mediated by the as yet uncharacterized membrane VDR sites via a plethora of intracellular signal transduction pathways (Fig. 1). Defining the gene targets of the traditional nuclear VDR sites in these tissues, as well as characterizing the membrane VDR sites and their targets, are exciting directions for future studies.

Glossary

calbindin Vitamin D-regulated calcium-binding protein (two forms, with molecular masses of 9 and 28 kDa) strongly induced by $1,25(OH)_2D_3$ in classical target tissues.

classical $1,25(OH)_2D_3$ target tissues The earliest identified $1,25(OH)_2D_3$/vitamin D targets, such as kidney, bone, and intestine, in which the predominant hormonal effect is Ca^{2+} translocation.

1α-hydroxylase The final enzyme in the biosynthetic pathway that produces the active hormone $1,25(OH)_2D_3$.

24-hydroxylase The initial enzyme in the clearance pathway for $1,25(OH)_2D_3$.

membrane vitamin D receptor Newly hypothesized membrane receptor of as-yet unknown structure that seems to mediate some actions of $1,25(OH)_2D_3$ through well-known membrane receptor-induced signal transduction pathways.

nonclassical $1,25(OH)_2D_3$ target tissues A number of tissues other than those in the earliest studies describing vitamin D receptor and $1,25(OH)_2D_3$ effects.

nuclear vitamin D receptor The traditional $1,25(OH)_2D_3$/vitamin D receptor that exerts its actions as a $1,25(OH)_2D_3$-activated nuclear transcription factor.

See Also the Following Articles

Vitamin D ● Vitamin D-Dependent Calbindins (CaBP) ● Vitamin D Effects on Cell Differentiation and Proliferation ● Vitamin D Metabolism ● Vitamin D: Nuclear Receptor for $1,25(OH)_2D_3$

Further Reading

Basak, R., Bhattacharya, R., and Chatterjee, M. (2001). 1α,25-Dihydroxyvitamin D₃ inhibits rat liver ultrastructural changes in diethylnitrosamine-initiated and phenobarbital promoted rat hepatocarcinogenesis. *J. Cell Biochem.* **81**, 357–367.

Berg, J. P., and Haug, E. (1999). Vitamin D: A hormonal regulator of the cAMP signaling pathway. *Crit. Rev. Biochem. Mol. Biol.* **34**, 315–323.

Blutt, S. E., and Weigel, N. L. (1999). Vitamin D and prostate cancer. *Proc. Soc. Exp. Biol. Med.* **221**, 89–98.

Brown, A. J., Dusso, A., and Slatopolsky, E. (1999). Vitamin D. *Am. J. Physiol.* **277**, F157–F175.

Feldman, D., Glorieux, F. H., and Pike, J. W. (1997). "Vitamin D." Academic Press, San Diego.

Feldman, D., Zhao, X.-Y., and Krishnan, A. V. (2000). Vitamin D and prostate cancer. *Endocrinology* **141**, 5–9.

Gross, C., Stamey, T., Hancock, S., and Feldman, D. (1998). Treatment of early recurrent prostate cancer with 1,25-dihydroxyvitamin D₃ (calcitriol). *J. Urol.* **159**, 2035–2040.

Jones, G., Strugnell, S. A., and DeLuca, H. F. (1988). Current understanding of the molecular actions of vitamin D. *Biol. Rev.* **4**, 1193–1231.

Jono, S., Peinado, C., and Giachelli, C. M. (2019). Phosphorylation of osteopontin is required for inhibition of vascular smooth muscle cell calcification. *J. Biol. Chem.* **275**, 20197–20203.

Kinuta, K., Tanaka, H., Moriwake, T., Aya, K., Kato, S., and Seino, Y. (2000). Vitamin D is an important factor in estrogen biosynthesis of both female and male gonads. *Endocrinology* **141**, 1317–1324.

Langub, M. C., Herman, J. P., Malluche, H. H., and Koszewski, N. J. (2001). Evidence of functional vitamin D receptors in rat hippocampus. *Neuroscience* **101**, 49–56.

Morelli, S., Buitrago, C., Vazquez, G., DeBoland, A. R., and Boland, R. (2000). Involvement of tyrosine kinase activity in 1α,25(OH)₂-vitamin D₃ signal transduction in skeletal muscle cells. *J. Biol. Chem.* **275**, 36021–36028.

Narvaez, C. J., Zinser, G., and Welsh, J. (2001). Functions of 1α,25-dihydroxyvitamin D₃ in mammary gland: From normal development to breast cancer. *Steroids* **66**, 301–308.

Rostand, S. G., and Drüeke, T. B. (1999). Parathyroid hormone, vitamin D, and cardiovascular disease in chronic renal failure. *Kid. Int.* **56**, 383–392.

Walters, M. R. (1995). Newly identified effects of the vitamin D endocrine system: Update 1995. *Endocr. Rev.* **4**, 47–56.

Walters, M. R. (1997). Other vitamin D target tissues: Vitamin D actions in cardiovascular tissue and muscle, endocrine and reproductive tissues, and liver and lung. *In* "Vitamin D" (D. Feldman, F. Glorieux and J. W. Pike, eds.), pp. 463–482. Academic Press, San Diego.

Wheeler, D. G., Horsford, J., Michalak, M., White, J. H., and Hendy, G. N. (1995). Calreticulin inhibits vitamin D₃ signal transduction. *Nucleic Acids Res.* **23**, 3268–3274.

Wnt Protein Family

BENJAMIN N. R. CHEYETTE* AND
RANDALL T. MOON†

*University of California, San Francisco • †University of Washington

I. HISTORY AND BIOLOGICAL SIGNIFICANCE
II. THE Wnt PROTEIN FAMILY: STRUCTURE AND BIOCHEMISTRY
III. RECEPTOR STRUCTURE AND BIOCHEMISTRY
IV. CYTOPLASMIC SIGNAL TRANSDUCTION PROTEINS
V. THE CANONICAL Wnt/β-CATENIN PATHWAY
VI. NONCANONICAL PATHWAYS: PLANAR CELL POLARITY AND Wnt/CALCIUM SIGNALING
VII. SUMMARY: BEYOND DEVELOPMENT AND CANCER

Wnts are a family of secreted signaling proteins. Wnt signaling is critical during animal development, contributing to the regulation of cell fate specification, cell morphology, cell proliferation, cell migration, cell polarity, and tissue patterning. Misregulation of Wnt signaling is a likely etiologic factor in human disease and has been strongly implicated in oncogenesis.

I. HISTORY AND BIOLOGICAL SIGNIFICANCE

The manner in which Wnt signaling was discovered reflects its biological importance across animal species. Mutations in the *wingless* (*wg*) gene of the fruit fly *Drosophila melanogaster* lead to a spectrum of developmental phenotypes. Null mutations cause severe segmental patterning defects that are lethal during embryogenesis. Some hypomorphic mutations are viable—the first mutation identified produces adult flies without wings, which gave the *Drosophila* gene its name. The *int-1* proto-oncogene was separately discovered as a target of the mouse mammary tumor virus (MMTV), a retrovirus that does not carry its own oncogene, but induces carcinomas in the mammary glands of susceptible mice by activating a host gene at its DNA integration site (int). The discovery that *Drosophila wg* and mouse *int-1* are orthologues and are part of a large evolutionarily conserved group of genes in multicellular animals led to the contracted family name "*Wnt.*"

A. Cancer

The initial identification of *Wnt1/int-1* as a proto-oncogene has been extended by further investigation. Alteration in the Wnt/β-catenin signaling pathway is now a well-established etiologic agent in tumorigenesis. The evidence is most striking for two downstream intracellular signaling components: the gene product of the *adenomatous polyposis coli* (*APC*) locus and the β-catenin protein. APC is a negative regulator of the canonical Wnt/β-catenin pathway that is mutated in the majority (>80%) of sporadically occurring colorectal adenomas and carcinomas. In addition, mutations in this gene are responsible for the genetic disease familial adenomatous polyposis, characterized by the proliferation of initially benign colonic polyps that predispose afflicted individuals to intestinal cancer. Similarly, mutations in β-catenin, the transcription cofactor that is activated by canonical Wnt signaling, have been described in a wide array of different cancer types. Mutations in other Wnt pathway components have likewise been associated with cell transformation *in vitro* and with the pathogenesis of an array of cancer types *in vivo* (Table 1).

B. Other Diseases

Given the prevalence and biological significance of Wnt signaling, it should not be surprising that it has

TABLE I   Wnt Signaling Molecules[a] in Human Cancer

Wnts	sFRPs	CK2	Axin	APC	β-Catenin
Breast cancer (WNT1, WNT5a)	Breast cancer	Breast cancer	Liver cancer	Colorectal cancer (spontaneous)	Colorectal cancer; liver cancer; ovarian cancer
Leukemia (WNT16)				Familial ademomatous polyposis (genetic precancerous condition)	pancreatic cancer; prostatic cancer; skin cancer (melanoma); stomach cancer; uterine cancer

[a]See text (Sections V and VI) for full molecule names and roles in Wnt signal transduction.

been linked to many other diseases besides cancer. A rare childhood disorder of bone formation, osteoporosis–pseudoglioma syndrome, is caused by a genetic disruption in canonical Wnt signaling. Disruptions in Wnt signaling have been proposed to underlie an assortment of other diseases as well. This is an area of understandably intense scientific and biomedical interest (Table 2).

C. Vertebrate Development

The first clue to a role for Wnt/β-catenin signaling in vertebrate development came from overexpression studies in the classical embryonic system, the frog *Xenopus laevis*. When Wnt1 is ectopically expressed in cells that would normally contribute to the ventral embryo (i.e., the future belly), they instead adopt a dorsal and anterior fate (i.e., they become the future head). This induction of a "secondary dorsal axis" produces a striking phenotype: two-headed tadpoles. The ability of ectopic Wnt1 to induce a secondary

dorsal axis derives from the participation of the canonical Wnt/β-catenin signaling pathway in the natural process of dorsal cell fate specification early in vertebrate embryogenesis. However, it remains unclear whether an endogenous intercellular Wnt signal, or only the downstream intracellular signaling cascade, is normally responsible for dorsal fate determination. Further developmental analyses in vertebrates have included both overexpression and loss-of-function studies in *Xenopus*, zebrafish, and mice and have established the importance of Wnt signaling in an array of processes in early development (Table 3).

D. Invertebrate Development

In *Drosophila*, the contribution of wg signaling to developmental tissue patterning has been intensely investigated in several processes, especially the segmentation of the embryonic cuticle and the compartmentalization of the wing epithelial primordium

TABLE 2   Wnt Signaling Molecules[a] Implicated in Human Disease

Wnt signaling (general)	Wnt4	sFRP	Fz	LRP5	Dvl	GSK3	β-Catenin
Polycystic kidney disease (Polycystin-1 activates canonical Wnt signaling pathway)	Injury-induced renal fibrosis; wound healing	Heart failure	Ulcerative colitis	Osteoporosis-pseudoglioma syndrome (genetic syndrome of defective bone formation)	Ulcerative colitis; schizophrenia (mouse knockout model)	Familial Alzheimer's disease (through interaction with presenilin-1); schizophrenia (reduced levels in prefrontal cortex); bipolar disorder (enzymatic activity reduced by therapeutic agents)	Familial Alzheimer's disease (through interaction with presenilin-1)

[a]See text (Sections V and VI) for full molecule names and roles in Wnt signal transduction.

TABLE 3   Some Wnt Signaling Developmental Activities across Species

	Caenorhabditis elegans (nematode)	*Drosophila melanogaster* (fruit fly)	*Xenopus laevis* (frog)	*Danio rerio* (zebrafish)	*Mus musculus* (mouse)
Canonical	Embryonic polarity; mesoderms vs endodermal specification through asymmetric cell divisions (note: this pathway may be noncanonical)	Embryonic segmentation & wing disc compartment-alization	Embryonic axis specification & specification of axial vs somitic mesoderm	Patterning of neural ectoderm, mesoderm at gastrulation; specification of neural crest derivatives; specification & patterning of rostral midbrain/ hindbrain; specification & patterning of head cartilage & tail	Embryonic axis specification, specification of caudal structures, specification of neural crest derivatives, specification & patterning of rostral midbrain/hindbrain, specification & proliferation; specification & patterning of urogenital system, differentiation of hair shaft precursors, placental development, osteogenesis, angiogenesis, adipogenesis
Noncanonical	Cell migration?	Wing hair orientation; compound eye facet orientation	Cell movements (convergent extension) during gastrulation	Cell movements (convergent extension) during gastrulation	Limb outgrowth?

(wing disc). In the embryonic cuticle, a band of cells positioned at the posterior border of a future parasegmental boundary first expresses wg. Secreted wg activates expression of the engrailed (en) transcription factor in adjacent cells on the other (anterior) side of the parasegmental boundary. The en transcription factor activates the expression of a second secreted signaling molecule, hedgehog (hh), in the anterior cells. Hedgehog secreted by the anterior cells signals back across the future parasegmental boundary to the original wg-secreting cells, stabilizing their wg expression. The result is an intercellular positive-feedback loop that establishes each parasegmental boundary with cells expressing wg on the anterior border and cells expressing en/hh on the posterior border. In the wing disc, wg secreted by cells at the future dorsal–ventral boundary similarly helps pattern the surrounding tissue by inducing the expression of different genes in neighboring cells on both sides.

E. NONCANONICAL SIGNALING

Genetic studies in *Drosophila* unexpectedly uncovered a completely different class of tissue patterning events that shares some (but not all) of the same genes implicated in the patterning of the embryonic segments and the wing disc. This "planar cell polarity" (PCP) pathway establishes the transverse orientation of cells making up an epithelial sheet. Examples of planar cell polarity in *Drosophila* include the orientation of facets making up the compound eye or the direction in which bristles point on the animal's back. During development, a subclass of wg receptors activate a distinct group of intracellular signaling molecules to regulate planar cell polarity. Because PCP signaling uses wg receptors but a different downstream signal transduction cascade than canonical wg signaling, it represents a separate "noncanonical" wg signaling pathway in *Drosophila* (see Section VI). A noncanonical signaling pathway has also been identified in vertebrates, where it is involved in coordinating major cell movements such as those of gastrulation. However, the correspondence between PCP signaling in *Drosophila* and noncanonical signaling in vertebrates remains ambiguous (see Section VI). Some of the more important and well-studied developmental events regulated by Wnt signaling in vertebrates and invertebrates are summarized in Table 3.

II. THE Wnt PROTEIN FAMILY: STRUCTURE AND BIOCHEMISTRY

There are a total of 7 related *Wnt* genes in the *Drosophila* genome and 19 in the human genome (some with multiple isoforms) that generally have close orthologues in mice (Fig. 1). Orthologous Wnt gene products (proteins with the same function in different species) are often very highly conserved. For example, the mouse and human Wnt1 proteins are 99% identical, differing at only 4 amino acid residues within a cleavable secretory signal sequence at the amino-terminus. More distantly related Wnt family members can share less than 30% identity. The length of vertebrate Wnt protein precursors varies from approximately 100 amino acids to over 400 amino acids. All Wnt proteins contain a cleavable amino-terminal signal peptide that targets them for secretion, a conserved cysteine-rich composition, and multiple N-linked glycosylation sites. Wnt proteins synthesized *in vivo* are glycosylated. Once outside the cell, mature Wnt glycoproteins associate with extracellular matrix and bind to heparin sulfate proteoglycans (HSPGs). Genetic studies in *Drosophila* have demonstrated the importance of HSPGs in stabilizing extracellular wg protein and in regulating its distribution. The importance of proteoglycans for intact Wnt signaling *in vivo* has been confirmed independently in vertebrates. In *Drosophila*, non-wg-producing cells endocytose wg that has been secreted by neighboring cells. Genetic studies have demonstrated that this endocytic activity is important both for facilitating wg signaling and for regulating its distribution.

In *Drosophila* and in vertebrates, it is clear that Wnt proteins often act over a relatively short range: on cells located within a few cell diameters of the secretory source. More controversial is whether Wnt proteins may also act over longer distances. The morphogen hypothesis, which predicts that some signaling molecules specify distinct cellular identities along a concentration gradient, remains contested in the field of developmental biology. Nonetheless, some of the strongest experimental evidence in favor of a morphogen concerns the action of wg in the *Drosophila* wing disc.

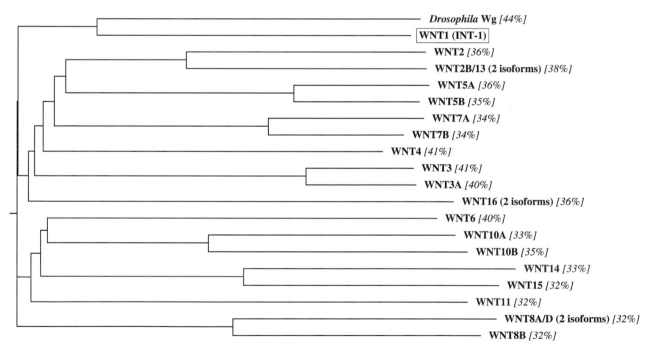

FIGURE 1 A sequence relatedness tree among the 19 human WNT gene products. *Drosophila* wg is included for comparison. The percentage of amino acid residues in each protein that are identical to WNT1 (boxed) is indicated. WNT1/INT-1 was chosen as the index sequence for comparison purposes purely for historical reasons (it is not evolutionarily ancestral to the other WNTs). This tree is based on overall identity among predicted Wnt gene products and is *not* meant to convey absolute evolutionary relationships. Horizontal distance from a node correlates with the degree of sequence divergence; vertical distance is arbitrary. Sequences were obtained from the protein database of the National Center for Biotechnology Information and compared using the default matrix settings of MacVector 6.5.3 (Oxford Molecular Group).

In addition to intercellular signaling, autocrine signaling by Wnt proteins (self-activation by a Wnt-secreting cell) may be important, both as a feedback mechanism during normal biological processes and in disease pathogenesis. Tumors induced by MMTV are clonal—suggesting that once the virus activates the *Wnt1* gene in a single mouse mammary gland cell, Wnt secretion stimulates uncontrolled proliferation by that cell and possibly other oncogenic changes as well. Similarly, some tissue culture cell lines transfected either with a *Wnt* gene or with DNA from MMTV-induced tumors become transformed and clonally tumorigenic. In *Drosophila*, there is evidence that autocrine signaling through wg occurs and activates a downstream signaling cascade that is genetically partly distinct from paracrine wg signaling.

It has been proposed that the vertebrate *Wnt* genes can be subdivided into functional classes based on whether they activate the canonical or noncanonical signaling pathways. However, recent studies have shown that in *Xenopus*, the developmental response to a Wnt of one proposed class can be switched to that of the other class by co-expressing a specific Wnt receptor. In the developing *Drosophila* eye and wing, the response to wg is influenced by the relative abundance and ligand affinity of the wg receptor proteins expressed in the target tissue. Synthesis of the available data from vertebrates and *Drosophila* suggests that the response to a specific Wnt signal *in vivo* is likely to be influenced both by the particular Wnt protein secreted and by the different receptor types (and downstream intracellular signaling molecules) present in the target tissue.

III. RECEPTOR STRUCTURE AND BIOCHEMISTRY

There are two types of cell-surface molecules that are known to be necessary for Wnt/β-catenin signal transduction in responsive cells: the Frizzled (Fz) receptor family and a subclass of the low-density-lipoprotein-related protein (LRP) receptor family.

A. Fz

Fz proteins constitute a family of seven-transmembrane domain receptors with a cysteine-rich extracellular domain. As a class, Fzs are structurally related to the superfamily of trimeric G-protein-coupled receptors (GPCRs). There are 4 *Fz* genes in *Drosophila* and 10 in humans, with close orthologues in mice. As a class, Fz proteins participate in both canonical and noncanonical signaling, but individual Fz receptors may differ in their basal (minus ligand) ability to activate signaling of each type, suggesting that structural differences among the Fz proteins contribute to functional specificity. There is contradictory evidence regarding the importance of the Fz extracellular domain for this specificity, but it is clear that the carboxyl-terminal tail and intracellular loops contribute. In other fields, there is mounting evidence that many seven-transmembrane domain proteins exist and act as multimers on the cell surface. In the case of the Fz receptors, there is no direct functional evidence for this, but crystallization studies have revealed a conserved dimerization interface in the extracellular cysteine-rich domain.

B. LRP

LRP5 and *LRP6* are closely related genes in humans and mice that are structurally distinct from other *LRP* family members. A single *Drosophila* orthologue exists and is called *arrow*. The proteins are single-transmembrane domain receptors with an extracellular domain composed of four amino-terminal epidermal growth factor-like repeats and three low-density-lipoprotein (LDL) receptor type A repeats. They have a relatively short proline-rich intracellular domain. Genetic evidence in *Drosophila* and loss-of-function and overexpression evidence in vertebrates support the conclusion that arrow and LRP5/6 are essential Wnt co-receptors with the Fz proteins. Based on initial genetic and mutational analyses in humans and mice, LRP5 is likely to be partly functionally redundant with LRP6. Unlike the Fz proteins, evidence from both vertebrates and *Drosophila* supports a role for these proteins only in the canonical Wnt signaling pathway, not in noncanonical signaling.

In *Drosophila*, arrow is essential for all aspects of canonical wg signaling, as demonstrated by the observation that the phenotype of an *arrow* null mutation closely resembles that of a *wg* null mutation. Similarly, an *LRP6* mutation in mice causes defects that are a combination of those seen with mutations in canonical mouse *Wnt* genes, whereas overexpression of LRP6 in vertebrates causes ectopic canonical pathway activation. The extracellular domain of LRP6 binds Wnt and interacts with the extracellular domain of Fz in a Wnt-dependent manner, whereas LRP5 activates canonical Wnt signaling when ectopically expressed in mammalian fibroblasts and interacts with canonical pathway cytoplasmic signaling components (see Section V).

IV. CYTOPLASMIC SIGNAL TRANSDUCTION PROTEINS

It remains unclear how signals from the Wnt receptors at the cell surface are coupled to distinct downstream cytoplasmic signal transduction cascades. However, at least two types of proteins have been proposed to functionally link the receptors to downstream effectors in both canonical and PCP signaling: heterotrimeric G-proteins and the Dishevelled (Dvl) family of cytoplasmic proteins.

A. G-Proteins

The topological resemblance of the Fz proteins to other seven-transmembrane receptors that couple to heterotrimeric G-proteins begs the question of whether Fz proteins signal through G-proteins as well. Positive evidence that G-proteins might be involved in Fz-mediated signal transduction has only recently begun to accumulate and at this time is restricted to overexpression studies in vertebrate systems and some antisense (loss-of-function) evidence in tissue culture cells. For example, stimulation of mammalian tissue culture cells by expressing one of the Wnt/Fz combinations implicated in canonical signaling can be blocked by pertussis toxin and other G-protein inhibitors. In *Xenopus* embryos, ectopic expression of a regulator of G-protein signaling (RGS) protein antagonizes canonical signaling and causes defects resembling those caused by ectopic expression of other Wnt pathway inhibitors.

Similarly, overexpression of Wnt5a in mammalian tissue culture cells, zebrafish, and *Xenopus* embryos activates a noncanonical signaling pathway that is selectively blocked by several G-protein inhibitors, including pertussis toxin. Work with chimeric Fz receptors containing the extracellular and transmembrane domains of the β_2-adrenergic receptor suggests that G-proteins may couple to the intracellular domain of Fz proteins. These experiments implicate $G_{\alpha o}$ and $G_{\alpha q}$ for Fz receptors activating canonical signaling and $G_{\alpha o}$ and $G_{\alpha t2}$ for Fz receptors activating noncanonical signaling. It should be noted here that the noncanonical pathway measured in these experiments is the Wnt/calcium pathway, which may or may not be distinct from PCP signaling in *Drosophila* (see Section VI). To date, neither a Wnt/calcium pathway nor a genetic requirement for heterotrimeric G-proteins has been described for wg signaling in *Drosophila*. Accordingly, it remains unclear whether G-proteins couple to Fz receptors to transduce all Wnt signals.

B. Dvl

A well-established component of both canonical and PCP signaling is the cytoplasmic molecule Dvl. There are three Dvl paralogues each in mice and humans and a single gene (*dsh*) in *Drosophila*. All Dvl family members share three well-conserved domains (DIX, PDZ, and DEP, in order from amino-terminus to carboxyl-terminus). The domains have been shown through mutational analyses in both vertebrates and in *Drosophila* to mediate different aspects of Wnt signaling: the DIX and PDZ domains are most critical for canonical Wnt signaling, whereas the PDZ and DEP domains are most important for PCP signaling. These domains have no known intrinsic enzymatic activity, but instead act as protein–protein interaction interfaces. Consequently, Dvl is considered to be a regulative adapter or scaffold protein that brings together cytoplasmic signaling components in response to events at the cell membrane. In most cell types, Dvl proteins display a predominantly cytoplasmic, punctate distribution, though a more diffuse nuclear component has also been described. In *Xenopus* embryos, overexpression of Fz protein can cause a redistribution of Dvl to the inner cell membrane. Whether translocation of Dvl to the membrane is an important component of physiological Wnt signaling is somewhat unclear, and there are no reliable data that Dvl actually interacts with Fz. There is evidence from both *Drosophila* and vertebrates that activation of Wnt signaling is accompanied by phosphorylation of Dvl. Exactly how signals are transduced from the transmembrane Wnt receptors to Dvl, whether through heterotrimeric G-proteins or some other mechanism, remains an area of intense experimental investigation.

V. THE CANONICAL Wnt/β-CATENIN PATHWAY

The canonical Wnt/β-catenin pathway is typified in vertebrates by responses to a subclass of the vertebrate Wnt proteins and Fz receptors and to LRP5 or LRP6; in *Drosophila* it is typified by wg, DFz2, and arrow. The central feature of this pathway is a multiprotein complex (degradation complex) that controls cytoplasmic concentration levels of the multifunctional protein β-catenin. β-Catenin plays a structural role at the inner cell membrane of adherens junctions, but also acts as a transcriptional coactivator in the nucleus. The concentration of soluble β-catenin in the cytoplasm, and therefore in the nucleus, is primarily determined by its rate of degradation through ubiquitination-dependent targeting to the proteosomal pathway. Glycogen synthase kinase-3 (GSK3 in vertebrates, zeste-white/shaggy in *Drosophila*) regulates this process by phosphorylating β-catenin, targeting it for degradation. In addition to GSK3 itself, other components of the degradation complex include Dvl, Axin, and APC. Whereas Dvl is a Wnt pathway activator, GSK3, Axin, and APC are all inhibitors. Axin and APC help to stabilize the activity of GSK3, thereby keeping β-catenin levels low and Wnt target gene transcription turned off in the absence of a Wnt signal (Fig. 2A).

During Wnt signaling, several molecular events that change the composition of the degradation complex occur. It remains unclear whether any of these events are directly mediated by the transmembrane receptor or associated proteins. As mentioned

in Section V, in response to canonical Wnt signaling, Dvl becomes phosphorylated. Several different kinases, including casein kinase I (CK1), casein kinase 2 (CK2), and the Par1 kinase from *Drosophila*, have been implicated in this process and in Wnt-pathway activation, but which of these is most important *in vivo* remains unclear. Another protein called GSK3-binding protein (GBP or FRAT) binds both GSK3 and Dvl in response to canonical signaling, possibly preventing the continued association of GSK3 with other members of the degradation complex. There is also evidence that binding of a Wnt protein to LRP5 causes the translocation of Axin from the degradation complex to the inner cell membrane, followed by Axin degradation. Regardless of which of these molecular events is the key to cytoplasmic transduction of the Wnt signal, the net effect is to destabilize and/or inhibit the degradation

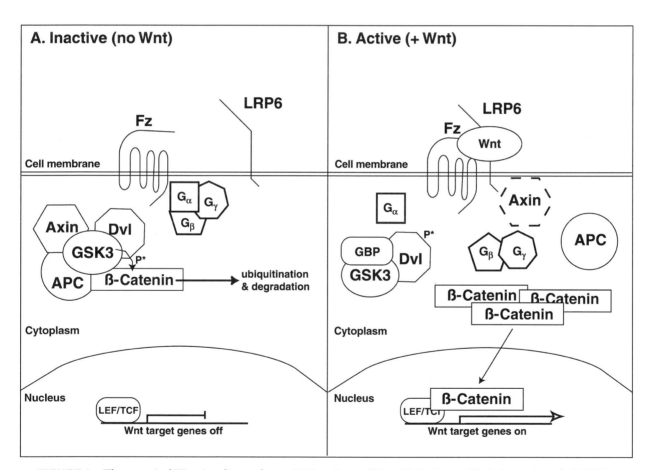

FIGURE 2 The canonical Wnt signaling pathway. (A) Inactive (no Wnt). (B) Active (+ Wnt). Activation of a Fz/LRP6 receptor by a Wnt causes the phosphorylation of Dvl, translocation of Axin to the membrane, and association of GSK3 with GBP. The net effect of these changes is to down-regulate the phosphorylation-dependent degradation of β-catenin in the cytoplasm. β-Catenin accumulates and translocates into the nucleus where it acts as a transcriptional co-activator with members of the LEF/TCF gene family. There is evidence that heterotrimeric G-proteins may couple to the Fz receptor upstream of Dvl in this pathway, but this remains controversial (see text).

complex and thereby to prevent phosphorylation of β-catenin by GSK3. As a result, soluble β-catenin—no longer phosphorylated, ubiquitinated, and degraded—accumulates and translocates to the nucleus. In the nucleus, β-catenin acts with members of the LEF/TCF family of transcription factors to regulate the expression of Wnt target genes (Fig. 2B).

In addition to the well-established canonical pathway members mentioned above and depicted in Figs. 2A and 2B, several other cytoplasmic inhibitors of canonical Wnt/β-catenin signaling that generally share the ability to bind Dvl have been identified in recent years. These include the *Drosophila* gene *naked cuticle* (*nkd*) and the vertebrate proteins Idax and Dapper (Dpr). Both nkd and Dpr have been demonstrated to play crucial roles in the development of *Drosophila* and *Xenopus*, respectively. There are also several secreted extracellular inhibitors of canonical Wnt/β-catenin signaling that are biologically important for development and disease. These include cerberus (cer) and secreted Frizzled-related proteins (sFRPs), which bind Wnt and therefore act as general Wnt inhibitors; Dickkopf (dkk), which binds to LRP6 and is therefore specific for canonical signaling; and Wnt inhibitory factor-1 (WIF-1), which resembles the LRP extracellular domain but whose exact mechanism of action is unknown.

VI. NONCANONICAL PATHWAYS: PLANAR CELL POLARITY AND Wnt/CALCIUM SIGNALING

Noncanonical Wnt signaling in *Drosophila* is defined by the planar cell polarity pathway mediated by the Fz receptor (which has redundant activity with DFz2 in the canonical pathway). Despite the fact that wg has been shown to bind to Fz and is often assumed to be the PCP effector, there is as yet no absolutely conclusive *in vivo* evidence that the endogenous ligand for Fz during PCP signaling is wg. The PCP pathway downstream of Fz has been defined on the basis of a combination of genetic and molecular data. As with the canonical Wnt pathway, the *Drosophila* Dvl homologue, dsh, is one of the most upstream cytoplasmic components of PCP signaling, although the requirement for the domains of dsh differ in the two pathways (see Section IV). As with canonical Wnt signaling, several dsh-interacting proteins that participate in PCP signaling have been identified, including the putative calcium-sensitive protein nkd and the Formin homology protein Daam1, which also

binds the small GTPase RhoA. PCP signaling through dsh activates RhoA, which in turn activates a cascade of signaling proteins through the Jun-N-terminal kinase (JNK). The JNK cascade can alter gene expression through activation of the AP-1 transcription factor in the nucleus; the significance of this for PCP signaling is unknown. RhoA also activates the *Drosophila* Rho-associated kinase (Drok), which causes cytoskeletal changes by phosphorylating the nonmuscle myosin regulatory light chain and possibly other proteins (Fig. 3A).

Aside from the *Drosophila* PCP pathway molecules that fit into the signaling pathway described above, several other genetically identified components play roles that are not yet understood at a biochemical level. Although arrow/LRP6 is not required for PCP signaling through Fz, at least three other transmembrane proteins that could act as co-receptors or independently of Fz proteins have been implicated in PCP signaling: flamingo (fmi), a seven-transmembrane domain protein; strabismus (stbm or vang), a three-transmembrane domain protein; and fuzzy (fy), a four-transmembrane domain protein. Also implicated is the membrane-associated daschous (ds) protein, a member of the cadherin superfamily. Cytoplasmic proteins that play a role include the gene products of *prickle* (*pk*), *inturned* (*in*), and *multiple wing-hair* (*mwh*). How these proteins connect to other components of the *Drosophila* PCP pathway is not yet understood, but the noncanonical signaling function of at least some of them is conserved in vertebrate cells. For example, vertebrate Stbm and the DEP domain of Dvl have been demonstrated to participate in JNK cascade activation in mammalian cells.

In vertebrates, noncanonical Wnt/calcium signaling antagonizes canonical Wnt/β-catenin signaling and is typified by embryonic responses to Wnt5a and Wnt11. Based on studies primarily in zebrafish and *Xenopus*, these responses include an IP$_3$-mediated rapid increase of intracellular calcium, followed by activation of protein kinase C (PKC) and calcium/calmodulin-regulated kinase II (CamKII) (Fig. 3B). As mentioned in Section IV, there is considerable evidence that initial signaling downstream of Fz in the Wnt/calcium signaling pathway occurs through heterotrimeric G-proteins. Studies in mammalian cultured cells and in *Xenopus* embryos have demonstrated that Wnt5a activates the JNK cascade, providing a possible link between the vertebrate Wnt/calcium signaling pathway and the *Drosophila* PCP pathway. Furthermore, activators of the Wnt/calcium pathway (e.g., Wnt5a) and activators of PCP

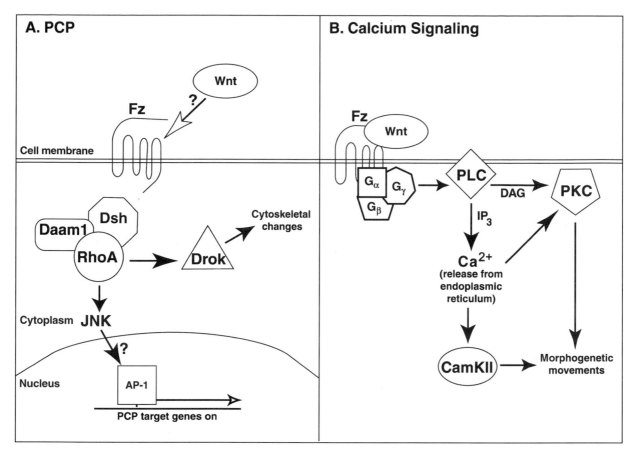

FIGURE 3 The noncanonical Wnt signaling pathways. (A) PCP signaling in *Drosophila*. Signaling through a Fz receptor activates dsh (the *Drosophila* Dvl homologue) through an unknown mechanism. dsh, with the dsh/RhoA-binding protein Daam1, activates RhoA. RhoA has multiple signaling outputs, which include the JNK cascade, which can regulate gene expression, and Drok, which is a component of cytoskeletal regulation. Multiple molecules not shown here, including several membrane-associated proteins, have been implicated genetically (see text). (B) Wnt/calcium signaling pathway in vertebrates. Signaling through some Wnt proteins such as Wnt5a activate heterotrimeric G-proteins and cause a transient increase in intracellular calcium, probably by acting through the second messengers inositol 1,4,5-triphosphate (IP$_3$) and diacylglycerol (DAG), released through membrane phospholipid hydrolysis by phospholipase C (PLC). Calcium (and DAG) activate protein kinase C (PKC) and calcium/calmodulin-regulated kinase II (CamKII). It is possible that the noncanonical pathways presented in A and B are alternate facets of a single conserved noncanonical Wnt pathway (see text).

signaling (e.g., Stbm and Nkd) similarly affect convergent extension movements during gastrulation in zebrafish and in *Xenopus*. One attractive hypothesis is that the Wnt/calcium signaling pathway and the PCP pathway are two aspects of the same molecular cascade. The reason that this is unclear is that the Wnt/calcium signaling pathway represents cellularly defined signaling events in frog and fish embryos, whereas the PCP pathway represents genetically defined signaling molecules in *Drosophila*. It is plausible but unproven that both are part of a single evolutionarily conserved noncanonical pathway. Resolution of this issue awaits the results of ongoing experimental studies in *Drosophila*,

Xenopus, and zebrafish and the investigation of whether Wnt/calcium signaling occurs in mammalian cultured cells.

VII. SUMMARY: BEYOND DEVELOPMENT AND CANCER

The *Wnt* genes, first identified as a single developmental mutation in fruit flies and as a proto-oncogene in a mouse model of cancer, are now established as critically important, evolutionarily conserved intercellular signaling molecules. Although general mechanisms of Wnt signal transduction have been determined, many details remain to be experimentally elucidated. Current studies of cross talk between canonical and noncanonical signaling pathways, as well as of the concordance between these pathways in different biological contexts, are expected to yield exciting new conceptual advances.

In addition to its fundamental importance in developmental patterning events, cell fate determination, cell movements, cell morphology, cell polarity, cell proliferation, and neoplasia, there is emerging evidence that Wnt signaling contributes significantly to disease processes ranging from scar formation to heart failure to neuropsychiatric disorders. Further research into the role of Wnt signaling in these processes offers both the promise of fascinating scientific insights into basic biological processes and the hope of revolutionary therapeutic innovations that may one day alleviate human suffering.

Acknowledgments

Thanks are extended to members of the Moon laboratory for helpful comments. B.N. R.C. was supported by National Institutes of Health Grant MH01750 K08 and a NARSAD/Browning Foundation Young Investigator Award; R.T.M. is an Investigator of the Howard Hughes Medical Institute.

Glossary

canonical Wnt/β-catenin pathway The Wnt signaling pathway as first elucidated in *Drosophila* wing development, *Drosophila* embryonic segmentation, vertebrate axis specification, and mammalian tumorigenesis, which modulates gene activity through the regulated degradation of β-catenin.
noncanonical pathway Signaling by a Wnt or a Wnt receptor that occurs in a β-catenin-independent manner.
planar cell polarity pathway The noncanonical pathway in *Drosophila melanogaster* composed of genes affecting the transverse orientation of cells in an epithelial sheet.
Wnt/calcium pathway A proposed noncanonical pathway, best described in frog and fish embryos.

See Also the Following Article

Cancer Cells and Progrowth/Prosurvival Signaling

Further Reading

Cadigan, K. M., and Nusse, R. (1997). Wnt signaling: A common theme in animal development. *Genes Dev.* **11**, 3286–3305.
Cheyette, B. N. R., Waxman, J. S., Miller, J. R., Takemaru, K., Sheldahl, L. C., Khlebtsova, N., Fox, E. P., Earnest, T., and Moon, R. T. (2002). Dapper, a dishevelled-associated antagonist of β-catenin and JNK signaling, is required for notochord formation. *Dev. Cell* **2**, 449–461.
Jönsson, M., Dejmek, J., Bendahl, P., and Andersson, T. (2002). Loss of Wnt-5a protein is associated with early relapse of invasive ductal breast carcinomas. *Cancer Res.* **62**, 409–416.
Koslovsky, N., Belmaker, R. H., and Agam, G. (2001). Low GSK-3 activity in the frontal cortex of schizophrenic patients. *Schizophr. Res.* **52**, 101–105.
Kuehl, M., Sheldahl, L. C., Park, M., Miller, J. R., and Moon, R. T. (2000). The Wnt/calcium pathway. *Trends Genet.* **16**, 279–283.
Malbon, C. C., Wang, H., and Moon, R. T. (2001). Wnt signaling and heterotrimeric G-proteins: Strange bedfellows or a classic romance? *Biochem. Biophys. Res. Commun.* **287**, 589–593.
McMahon, A. P., and Moon, R. T. (1989). Ectopic expression of the proto-oncogene int-1 in *Xenopus* embryos leads to duplication of the embryonic axis. *Cell* **58**, 1075–1084.
Miller, J. R. (2001). The Wnts. *Genome Biol.* **3**, 3001.1–3001.15.
Morata, G., and Lawrence, P. A. (1977). The development of *wingless*, a homeotic mutation of *Drosophila*. *Dev. Biol.* **56**, 227–240.
Nusse, R., and Varmus, H. E. (1982). Many tumors induced by the mouse mammary tumor virus contain a provirus integrated in the same region of the host genome. *Cell* **31**, 99–109.
Pinson, K. I., Brennan, J., Monkley, S., Avery, B. J., and Skarnes, W. C. (2000). An LDL-receptor-related protein mediates Wnt signalling in mice. *Nature* **407**, 535–538.
Polakis, P. (2000). Wnt signaling and cancer. *Genes Dev.* **14**, 1837–1848.
Rijsewijk, F., Schuermann, M., Wagenaar, E., Parren, P., Weigel, D., and Nusse, R. (1987). The *Drosophila* homolog of the mouse mammary oncogene int-1 is identical to the segment polarity gene *wingless*. *Cell* **50**, 649–657.
Yamanaka, H., Moriguchi, T., Masuyama, N., Kusakabe, M., Hanafusa, H., Takada, R., Takada, S., and Nishida, E. (2002). JNK functions in the non-canonical Wnt pathway to regulate convergent extension movements in vertebrates. *EMBO Rep.* **3**, 69–75.
Zecca, M., Basler, M., and Struhl, G. (1996). Direct and long-range action of a wingless morphogen gradient. *Cell* **87**, 833–844.

GLOSSARY

A

abscission The rejection of plant organs at a site where hydrolytic enzymes reduce cell adhesion.

acne vulgaris A disorder of the sebaceous gland; characteristic lesions include open (blackhead) and closed (whitehead) comedones, papules, pustules, and nodules.

acromegaly A clinical syndrome characterized by overgrowth of extremities and organs and by metabolic disturbances secondary to growth hormone excess, usually due to a growth hormone-secreting pituitary adenoma.

ACTH see ADRENOCORTICOTROPIC HORMONE.

activating enhancer binding protein 2α A transcription factor that is important in embryogenesis and is expressed in the developing respiratory epithelium.

activating (gain-of-function) mutation A structural alteration of the receptor that makes it constitutively activated, i.e., in the absence of ligand hormone. Activating mutation can also increase the receptor's affinity for the ligand hormone, alter its binding specificity, or permit new functions.

activational effect A postpubertal process by which sex steroids exert an effect that transiently activates preexisting hormone-sensitive neural circuits.

activation function regions Segments in a steroid receptor that mediate transcriptional activation through their interaction with co-activators or proteins of the basic transcriptional machinery of the cell.

activin receptor type I A component of the activin receptor complex. It is a serine/threonine kinase that phosphorylates intracellular mediators after being phosphorylated by a type II activin receptor.

activin receptor type II A component of the activin receptor complex. It binds to activins and in turn phosphorylates type I receptors via its intracellular serine/threonine kinase domain.

activins Protein hormones belonging to the transforming growth factor-β superfamily that regulate many developmental and physiological processes, particularly reproduction. They are either homo- or heterodimers of two related inhibin β-subunits, βA and βB.

activity-based anorexia (ABA) A condition in animals in which they run excessively and lose control over body weight if very little food is provided and they enter a state of ABA, which is conspicuously similar to self-starvation in humans.

adapter protein A protein that contains multiple docking sites for other proteins but lacks enzymatic activity; it functions as an "adapter" by allowing the assembly of complexes of signaling proteins that generate signal transduction.

adaptive immune system A limb of the immune system that responds slowly and that depends on interactions between components of pathogens and antigen-specific T-cell or B-cell receptors. Adaptive immunity improves qualitatively and quantitatively with continued or repeated exposure to pathogen antigens. B and T cells are the primary cells of the adaptive limb.

adaptors Proteins composed of protein-protein and/or protein-phospholipid interaction domains, but without an enzymatic activity.

Addison's disease An autoimmune condition leading to adrenal hypofunction; it may be isolated or associated with polyglandular autoimmune syndrome, including diabetes, hypoparathyroidism, hypothyroidism, and mucocutaneous candidiasis.

adenohypophysis Endocrine subdivision of the pituitary; composed of the pars distalis (i.e., the anterior lobe of the pituitary gland), the pars intermedia (i.e., the intermediate lobe of the pituitary gland), and the pars tuberalis.

adenomyosis The infiltration or invagination of the myometrium with endometrial glands.

adenylyl cyclase An enzyme that catalyzes conversion of adenosine triphosphate (ATP) to cyclic adenosine monophosphate (cAMP). There are 10 known isoforms of the enzyme; 9 are membrane bound and 1 is soluble. The various forms of adenylyl cyclase (AC) are differentially regulated; however, all membrane-bound forms are stimulated by the stimulatory GTP-binding protein of AC, $G_{\alpha s}$. All but one membrane-bound AC isoform are stimulated by forskolin.

adipocytes Specialized triglyceride-storing cells found throughout the body, commonly known as fat cells. In addition to being an important site for the storage and release of metabolic energy, adipocytes are the primary source of circulating leptin.

adipokinetic hormone A peptide hormone in insects involved in the mobilization of substrates (predominantly lipids and carbohydrates) for energy generation needed by contracting flight muscles.

adrenocorticotropic hormone (ACTH) A hormone released by the anterior pituitary that stimulates the production of glucocorticoids and catecholamines by the adrenal gland.

adult T-cell leukemia An aggressive malignancy of mature CD3-, CD4-, and CD25- (IL-2Rα) expressing lymphocytes, found predominantly in Japan, the Caribbean Islands, and sub-Saharan Africa; caused by the retrovirus human T-cell lymphotropic virus I.

advanced sleep phase syndrome A disturbance in which sleep occurs intractably early.

AF-1 and AF-2 Amino-terminal and carboxyl-terminal activation function regions of a nuclear receptor.

afferent neuron A neuron that conveys incoming nerve impulses to another neuron or nerve center with which it synapses.

affinity The degree of attraction between a ligand and a specific receptor. It is based on a high degree of structural complementarity between the ligand and the binding site of the receptor.

agonist A chemical that specifically interacts with and activates a receptor by stabilizing the active conformation. The effects of agonists can be prevented by chemicals called antagonists or inverse agonists, which are usually synthetic compounds that interact with the receptor but oppose its activation.

Agrobacterium tumefaciens A plant pathogen causing crown gall tumors on susceptible plants. Tumor induction results from the transfer of a small piece of DNA, called transfer DNA, from the bacterium to the plant cell during infection. The transfer DNA becomes integrated into plant cell nuclear DNA and expression of genes on this segment causes the plant cell to differentiate into a tumor cell.

airway hyperresponsiveness Exaggerated bronchoconstrictor response to a wide variety of endogenous and exogenous stimuli. Airway hyperreactivity is generally assessed by inhalation challenge with metacholine or histamine.

Akt (PKB) An insulin-regulated downstream serine/threonine kinase important in thyroid-stimulating hormone receptor-regulated signaling of growth and function.

alarm reaction The first stage of Selye's General Adaptation Syndrome (see) in which gastric ulcerations, adrenal hypertrophy, and shrinkage of the thymus and lymphatic tissues are consistently seen within 48 h following exposure to noxious stimuli.

aldosterone The main salt-retaining (mineralocorticoid) hormone; a steroid synthesized from cholesterol in the zona glomerulosa of the adrenal cortex under the control of three principal physiological activators: angiotensin II, extracellular potassium, and adrenocorticotropic hormone.

aleurone Layers of cells surrounding the starchy endosperm in cereal grains; on stimulation by gibberellins during germination, the cells synthesize hydrolytic enzymes to break down starch and other storage materials in the starchy endosperm.

allatectomy The removal of the corpora allata, the source of insect juvenile hormone.

allatostatin A neuropeptide that inhibits the biosynthesis of juvenile hormone by the corpora allata.

allatotropin A neuropeptide that activates the biosynthesis of juvenile hormone by the corpora allata.

allele One of two or more alternative forms of a gene, each of which possesses a unique nucleotide sequence.

alopecia Hair loss that can occur in patches (**alopecia areata**) or globally. Causes range from hormones to autoimmunity.

alpha-helix A basic structural element of proteins consisting of a continuous coil that contains 3.6 amino acids per turn.

alternative oxidase The terminal oxidase of the alternative respiratory pathway; unlike the cytochrome respiratory pathway, which conserves energy from electron flow as chemical energy (ATP), the alternative respiratory pathway releases this energy as heat.

alternative splicing A pre-mRNA processing pathway in which a single gene gives rise to different versions of the mRNA and, ultimately, to different proteins.

alveolar proteinosis A rare human respiratory disorder characterized by the accumulation of periodic acid-Schiff-positive lipoproteinaceous material (derived from pulmonary surfactant) in the distal airspaces.

amenorrhea A loss of ovarian cyclicity; the absence of menstruation.

γ-aminobutyric acid see GABA.

amnion The sac in which the embryo and fetus develop; a tough fibrous membrane that surrounds the fetus; has a simple (usually low-cuboidal with microvilli) epithelium facing inward.

anabolic androgenic steroids Synthetic derivatives of testosterone having pronounced anabolic properties and relatively weak androgenic properties.

anabolic steroid Any substance related to the male sex hormone testosterone that promotes the growth of skeletal muscle (anabolic effects) and the development of male sexual characteristics (androgenic effects).

anagen The growth phase of the growth cycle of mature hair follicles; anagen is followed by regression (catagen), rest (telogen), and shedding (exogen).

analogue A molecule that is chemically similar to another.

androgen A steroid hormone, such as testosterone or dihydrotestosterone, that promotes the development and maintenance of male secondary sex characteristics and structures.

androgen-binding protein A protein identical in sequence to the plasma sex hormone-binding globulin that is produced in the Sertoli cells of the testis. In rats, this protein displays a preference for biologically active androgens.

androgenic gland Strands of cells associated with the male gametic duct. These cells produce androgenic gland hormone, which induces primary and secondary male sexual characteristics.

androgen insensitivity syndrome 46,XY genetic males with an androgen receptor gene mutation that results in infertility or partial or complete lack of masculinization of the genitalia. The androgen insensitivity syndrome has also been referred to as testicular feminization.

androgen receptor A member of the steroid receptor superfamily of genes that mediates the action of androgens on the target cell; a ligand-activated transcription factor.

androgen resistance Unresponsiveness or insensitivity of tissues toward the action of androgens or estrogens, caused by a functional defective androgen or estrogen receptor.

andropause A controversial term used to describe the clinical syndrome associated with the age-related decline in serum testosterone concentrations in older men. There is debate over whether the age-related decline in serum testosterone concentrations is clinically important and whether this should be corrected by testosterone replacement.

anemia A significant reduction in red cell mass and a corresponding decrease in the oxygen-carrying capacity of the blood.

ANF (atrial natriuretic factor) A peptide produced by the heart that causes the kidney to excrete sodium.

angiogenesis The formation of new blood vessels from existing capillaries.

angiotensin One of a family of peptide hormones derived from the protein angiotensinogen.

angiotensin II A potent vasoconstrictor peptide that stimulates aldosterone synthesis and secretion from the adrenal zona glomerulosa and participates in the regulation of local and systemic hemodynamic regulation.

anorexia nervosa An eating disorder with severe, self-imposed starvation; commonly associated with a high level of physical activity and hypothermia.

anorexigenic Describing a compound that inhibits or decreases food intake.

antagonist A naturally occurring or synthetic compound that binds to a receptor and opposes the actions of an agonist.

anterior pituitary Major lobe of the adenohypophysis; composed of a heterogeneous mixture of cell types, such as corticotrophs, somatotrophs, lactotrophs, thyrotrophs, and gonadotrophs, each of which secretes specific hormones that act on particular end organs to exert biological effects.

anti-estrogens Drugs such as tamoxifen and raloxifene that bind to the estrogen receptor and inhibit transcriptional activation of estrogen-regulated genes; they are commonly used for the treatment and prevention of breast cancer.

antigen Literally, any molecule that binds to an antibody. Frequently used to refer to any foreign molecules that stimulate an adaptive immune response.

antigen-presenting cells Cells such as macrophages and dendritic cells that can bind and engulf antigens (foreign substances), break them down into smaller units, and insert them into their cell surface membranes where they are "presented" for interaction with T lymphocytes.

antral follicles Follicles that are either tertiary or ovulatory, also called Graafian follicles; characterized by the presence of a fluid-filled antrum in the granulosa layer.

antrum An extracellular matrix-containing cavity that divides the oocyte from granulosa cells in the antral follicle.

apical hook In plants, a structure that forms at the uppermost portion of the hypocotyl that serves to reorient the cotyledons and apical meristem to prevent damage from soil-borne obstructions.

apolipophorin III (apoLp-III) An exchangeable apolipoprotein in the hemolymph of insects engaging in long-distance flights for which lipids are used as an energy source.

apoptosis A genetically programmed process of physiological cell death characterized at the light and electron microscopic levels by separation of the cell from its neighboring cells and/or its extracellular matrix, a loss of cell volume, chromatin condensation and margination along the nuclear envelope (pyknosis), and the final budding and fragmentation of the cell into plasma membrane-bound vesicles that are cleared by phagocytosis.

Arabidopsis thaliana A small member of the mustard family (Brassicaceae), commonly used as a model system for plant genetics, physiology, and molecular biology.

arachidonic acid A polyunsaturated fatty acid that has 20 carbons and four double bonds.

aromatase A cytochrome P450 enzyme that converts androgens to estrogens; an important signaling pathway by which testosterone affects neural development and function.

arrestins Proteins that arrest receptor function by uncoupling the receptor from its cognate G-proteins to target the receptor to the intracellular compartment of the cell by means of endocytosis. The arrestin family consists of visual arrestins (rod and cone arrestins), which have limited tissue distribution, and β-arrestin 1 and β-arrestin 2, which have a more widespread distribution.

arteritis A condition in which the walls of arteries are infiltrated with inflammatory cells, causing damage to the arterial walls and often leading to compromised blood flow and local clotting.

arthropods Animals possessing a hard, jointed exoskeleton and constituting the largest group (phylum) in the animal kingdom in terms of numbers of species, e.g., insects, crabs, spiders, and centipedes.

aryl hydrocarbon receptor An intracellular protein expressed in several tissues of most mammals, including humans, whose three-dimensional structure and endogenous ligand are unknown. It is assumed that this receptor mediates the toxic effects of 2,3,7,

8-tetrachlorodibenzo-*p*-dioxin and structurally related halogenated aromatic hydrocarbons, including polychlorinated biphenyls.

asthma A chronic inflammatory disorder of the airways characterized by recurrent episodes of wheezing, breathlessness, chest tightness, and coughing in response to physical, chemical, or immunological stimuli. The inflammation also causes an associated increase in the existing bronchial hyperresponsiveness. Asthma is frequently associated with atopy.

astrocytes Nonneuronal glial cells that are required for the integration of cell–cell communication within the nervous system, regulation of synaptic transmission, facilitation of neuronal activity, generation of neurons, and production of growth factors needed for the integrity of neuronal function.

asymmetric carbon A carbon atom in a complex molecule that is chemically bonded to four different substituents.

atherosclerosis A condition caused by progressive thickening and hardening of the walls of medium-sized and large arteries as a result of extensive fat and cellular deposits on their inner lining, ultimately leading to arterial occlusion.

atopic disorder A condition resulting from the immediate hypersensitivity based on the abnormal production of immunoglobulin E (IgE) against environmental antigens. Atopic disorders have different clinical manifestations, such as hay fever, asthma, urticaria, or chronic eczema. Antigen, usually called allergen, cross-links allergen-specific IgE bound to FcεRI on mast cells and activates them to release various chemical mediators and cytokines, leading to development of pathological alterations.

atresia The process whereby oocytes are lost from the ovary other than by ovulation.

autocrine Describing the action of a factor produced by a cell that has an action on that cell itself; self-regulation.

autoimmune diseases Diseases that are caused by defects of self-tolerance and are divided into two groups based on their effector mechanisms. Abnormal production of autoantibodies against autoantigen results in immune complex-induced systemic or autoantigen-specific disorders, depending on the properties of autoantibodies. Self-reactive T cells also cause tissue-specific disorders.

autonomic nervous system Collectively, the sympathetic and parasympathetic nervous systems. The sympathetic nervous system readies the body for action, mobilizing energy stores; actions of the parasympathetic nervous system predominate in energy uptake and storage. The sympathetic nervous system acts on some targets via direct contact of nerves with these tissues, but also mediates systemic effects by promoting release of adrenaline from the adrenal medulla. Elevation of sympathetic nervous system activity increases heart rate, blood pressure, etc.

autophosphorylation A process whereby a kinase phosphorylates itself or kinase-associated receptors in a dimeric complex phosphorylate one another.

autosomes A term for any chromosome other than the X or Y sex chromosome.

avidity The functional combining strength of the contact between a protein and an interaction partner (or protein complex, e.g., antibody or receptor, containing multiple binding sites for the interaction partner, e.g., antigen or ligand). Avidity is governed by the affinity of the individual reaction, the number of binding epitopes (valency), and sterical hindrance of the interacting components.

axon projection Long extensions of neurons that conduct nerve impulses to terminals distant from the nerve cell body. The axon projection is the defined path and destination point of the axon.

axons Thin processes of neurons contacting a target; they rapidly conduct action potentials (waves of depolarization) from the cell body to the terminals and slowly transport peptide to be secreted from the terminals.

azoospermia The absence of sperm in the ejaculate.

B

B7 family molecules Cell surface molecules involved in both stimulation and inhibition of immune cells.

basal repression Target gene transcription repression by unliganded thyroid hormone receptor and its recruitment of corepressors.

base pair Two nucleotides located on complementary strands of DNA and paired by hydrogen bonds.

basic helix–loop–helix proteins A family of transcription factors; they bind to DNA as dimers. DNA binding depends on a stretch of basic amino acids adjacent to the dimerization domain formed by a helix–loop–helix structure.

B cells see T CELLS/B CELLS.

Bcl-2 family A group of structurally and/or functionally related proteins that can either promote or prevent cell death and are considered to be the primary regulators of apoptosis, via their actions at the level of intracellular organelles, particularly mitochondria.

BERKO A term for mice with inactivated, knocked-out versions of estrogen receptor-β.

beta cell Pancreatic cells that form 70–80% of the endocrine cell mass. They contain insulin, which is formed by proteolytic cleavage from a precursor molecule, proinsulin. The resulting by-product, C-peptide (connecting peptide), is secreted together with insulin at a 1:1 molar ratio.

beta-cell mass The total mass of all beta cells in the endocrine pancreas. The beta-cell mass is a functional unit and expands in insulin-resistant states. In humans with type 2 diabetes, the beta-cell mass is reduced.

betaglycan The TGF-β type III receptor that increases the affinity of inhibin A for the activin type II receptor.

binding protein Soluble binding proteins that bind circulating ligands and prolong their half-life. They are devoid of intrinsic signaling properties, but may interfere with membrane-receptor signaling by forming inactive heterodimers (one soluble receptor and one membrane-bound receptor). In many species, prolactin- and growth hormone-binding proteins are generated and result either from alternative splicing of transcripts encoding full-length receptors or from limited proteolysis of membrane-bound receptors.

biomagnification A phenomenon in which the tissue concentrations of some pollutants are increased as they transfer from one organism to another through the food chain, due to their lipophilic nature.

blastocyst The stage of embryo development at which implantation occurs.

body mass index An indicator used to define nutritional status and derived from the formula: weight divided by the square of height (kg/m^2). The acceptable range is 19–24 in women.

bombesin-related peptides Members of the bombesin-like peptide subfamily; phylogenetically related to amphibian bombesin and to date have been found only in frogs.

bone marrow transplantation The transplantation of a patient's own bone marrow (autologous) or bone marrow from a different donor (allogeneic) into a patient to provide a source of hematopoietic stem cells from which the entire hematopoietic system can be reconstituted after high-dose chemotherapy or radiotherapy.

bone mineralization The process by which calcium and phosphate are deposited onto the extracellular matrix of bone, resulting in the formation of hydroxyapatite.

bone morphogenetic protein (BMP) A member of the transforming growth factor-β superfamily.

bone morphogenetic protein receptors Serine/threonine kinase receptor complexes of type II and type I components, responsible primarily for ligand binding and signal transduction, respectively.

brain-derived neurotrophic factor A protein purified from pig brain in the 1980s by monitoring its ability to prevent the death of peripheral sensory neurons.

bronchopulmonary dysplasia A chronic lung disease that can occur in premature infants; characterized by abnormal lung structure, tachypnea, and continuing need for supplemental oxygen.

bulimia nervosa An eating disorder with episodes of excessive food intake, followed by compensatory methods to maintain a normal body weight.

C

cachexia A state of malnutrition associated with disease and consisting of a combination of anorexia, increased metabolic rate, and wasting of lean body mass.

calbindin-D Vitamin D-dependent Ca^{2+}-binding proteins consisting of a 28 kDa protein (calbindin-D_{28K}) and a 9 kDa protein (calbindin-D_{9K}) that bind Ca^{2+} with high affinity and facilitate diffusion of cytosolic Ca^{2+}.

calbindin-D_{9k} A 9000-Da calcium-binding protein that is present in highest concentrations in mammalian intestine, in mouse and neonatal rat kidney, and in placenta and uterus.

calbindin-D_{28k} A 28,000-Da calcium-binding protein present in highest concentrations in avian intestine and mammalian and avian kidney, brain, and pancreas.

calcineurin (protein phosphatase 2B) A calmodulin target protein that dephosphorylates proteins including enzymes and transcription factors in a Ca^{2+}-dependent manner.

calciosome A theoretical organelle, or subcellular fraction, that is specifically involved in storing and releasing Ca^{2+} during Ca^{2+} signaling.

calcitonin A 32-amino-acid peptide hormone produced by the C cells of the thyroid. Immunologically similar molecules have also been identified in other tissues, suggesting additional local autocrine or paracrine actions of calcitonin.

calcium influx factor A hypothetical factor released from the endoplasmic reticulum following Ca^{2+} depletion, which diffuses to the plasma membrane and activates Ca^{2+} channels.

calcium oscillations Cycles of regenerative, all-or-none rises in cytoplasmic Ca^{2+} superimposed on a stable baseline. Also called **calcium spikes**. Calcium feedback properties of the $(1,4,5)IP_3$ receptor may underlie these oscillations, at least in some cell types.

calmodulin An intracellular Ca^{2+}-binding protein that acts as a sensor and mediator of the Ca^{2+} signal by binding and regulating specific target proteins.

calmodulin-regulated kinases Enzymes that are activated by Ca^{2+}–calmodulin during the Ca^{2+} signal.

calmodulin target proteins Enzymes, ion pumps, and channels that bind calmodulin and change their activity in a Ca^{2+}-dependent manner.

cAMP (cyclic adenosine monophosphate) A major intracellular signaling molecule that is regulated by a number of extracellular effectors. It is synthesized from adenosine triphosphate via adenylyl cyclase and is metabolized to adenosine monophosphate by cyclic nucleotide phosphodiesterase.

cAMP response element Consensus nucleotide sequence 5′-TGACGTCA-3′; found in the promoter of many hormone-regulated genes, including somatostatin; a specific binding site for the transcriptional activator cAMP response element binding protein (CREB).

cAMP response element binding protein Nuclear transcription factor that mediates effects of cAMP to alter gene expression.

capacitative calcium entry A process by which the depletion of intracellular endoplasmic reticulum Ca^{2+} stores, either artificially or by the signal $(1,4,5)IP_3$, initiates a signaling process to open channels in the plasma membrane.

capillary The smallest-diameter vessel in the body; the site of origin of new vessels.

carboxyamidation The biosynthetic modification of the most C-terminal amino acid residue in the peptide so that the free acid group ($-COOH$) is α-amidated ($-CONH_2$). Many biologically active peptides are carboxyamidated.

carpopedal spasm A spasm of the wrist and foot produced by hypocalcemia and tetany.

casein kinase II (CKII) A ubiquitous protein kinase that phosphorylates over 160 known substrates. Among its many actions, CKII changes the activity of transcription factors, proteins involved in DNA replication and DNA repair (topoisomerase II, DNA ligase), and growth factors (p53, p21).

caspases A cohort of cysteine aspartic acid-specific proteases that function either as initiators (e.g., caspase-8 and -9) or as executioners (e.g., caspase-2, -3, -6, and -7) of the apoptotic cell death program in vertebrates. More than 10 members have been identified. Caspase-1, originally termed interleukin-1β (IL-1β)-converting enzyme, has the capacity to cleave biologically inactive precursors IL-1β and IL-18 into the corresponding biologically active forms.

catalytic domain Amino acid sequence that contains a specific enzymatic activity associated with a protein.

catecholamines A class of neurotransmitters, including epinephrine and norepinephrine, involved in autonomic nervous system actions.

caveolae Sub-domains of the cell's plasma membrane that have a typical flask-like membrane structure where signal transduction molecules may congregate.

caveolin The principal protein component of caveolar membranes.

cdc2 protein kinase A protein kinase that associates with cyclin A or B to form a complex resembling the invertebrate mitosis-promoting factor (MPF).

cDNA (complementary DNA) DNA strand created *in vitro* by reverse transcription of a messenger RNA molecule.

cDNA microarray A method for high-throughput simultaneous analysis of multiple gene expression changes.

cell-mediated immunity Host defenses mediated by antigen-specific T cells, which protect against intracellular bacteria, viruses, and cancer.

cell membrane receptor A hormone-binding transmembrane protein. Binding of the ligand hormone triggers a cascade of responses: conformational change of the receptor → activation of the intracellular second-messenger response(s) → secondary intracellular response(s) → functional target cell response(s) to hormone stimulation.

cGMP (3′,5′-guanosine monophosphate) A cyclic nucleotide that promotes the intracellular reactions that generate a visual signal in the brain.

chaperone A protein that assists in the correct folding (and assembly) of another protein.

chemical library A term for a group of chemical compounds generally related by structure and method of preparation.

chemokines Small proteins characterized by the presence of a four-cysteine motif in their primary structure and by their ability to promote chemotactic responses in leukocytes. Chemokines are divided into subclasses (CCL, CXCL, and CX3CL) on the basis of the spacing between their two conserved N-terminal cysteine residues (adjacent cysteines; cysteines separated by a single amino acid; and cysteines separated by three amino acids, respectively). Chemokines exert their functions by binding G-protein-coupled seven-transmembrane receptors.

chemotaxis The migration of a biological entity toward the source of a chemical stimulus. e.g., a growth factor.

chemotherapy The use of toxic chemicals to attempt to kill (usually) cancer cells in patients. Side effects usually include the killing of normal hematopoietic cells (myelotoxicity), leading to infections, and the killing of intestinal and hair precursor cells, leading to vomiting and hair loss, respectively. Myeloablative chemotherapy is high-dose chemotherapy that permanently destroys the hematopoietic system and would prove fatal without bone marrow transplantation.

chirality Chemical nomenclature for an organic molecule, describing the right- or left-handedness of an asymmetric carbon; any carbon with four different groups attached to it is a chiral center.

cholecystokinin (CCK) A peptide hormone that is secreted by mucosa endocrine cells (I cells) of the upper small intestine and that stimulates pancreatic exocrine secretion, stimulates gallbladder contraction, and inhibits gastric emptying.

cholera toxin An A-B-type bacterial toxin produced by the bacterium *Vibrio cholerae*; catalyzes transfer of the ADP-ribose moiety of nicotinamide dinucleotide to the α-subunit of G-proteins of the G_s subfamily, resulting in their constitutive activation.

cholesterol side chain cleavage enzyme A P450 enzyme (P450scc) located on the matrix side of the inner mitochondrial membrane in all steroidogenic cells studied to date. It is the rate-limiting enzymatic step in steroidogenesis and utilizes the substrate cholesterol to form pregnenolone, the first steroid synthesized in the steroidogenesis pathway.

cholesterol transfer The transfer of cholesterol to the inner mitochondrial membrane and to the P450scc enzyme; this constitutes the true regulated and rate-limiting step in the process of steroid hormone biosynthesis. Therefore, the mechanism of transferring cholesterol to P450scc is of critical importance.

chondrocyte A cartilage cell.

chromaffin Tissue of neuroectodermic origin with the specialized function of synthesizing and secreting catecholamines.

chromatin DNA packaged into nucleosomes or histone octamers.

chromogranin A A glycoprotein that is abundant in the secretory granules of chromaffin and other neuroendocrine cells. This protein may function as a prohormone precursor of biologically active peptides.

Chvostek's sign A spasm of the facial muscles in response to tapping of the facial nerve; caused by hypocalcemia and tetany.

chyme A semifluid mixture consisting of partly digested food and gastric juices; passes from the stomach into the small intestine.

circadian rhythm Endogenous adaptations of physiology and behavior made by organisms in response to day and night cycles; i.e., about 24 hours.

circannual rhythm Endogenous adaptations having a period of about 365 days.

circhoral rhythm Endogenous adaptations having a period of about 1 hour.

climacteric A substantial increase in aerobic respiration coupled with high levels of ethylene production; associated with the ripening of fruits such as tomatoes, avocados, and apples (which are therefore termed climacteric fruits).

clone A purified, specific DNA sequence, such as the sequence that provides the template for synthesis of a particular receptor.

clustering A term for the occurrence of crowded groups of receptors or ligands on the cell membrane.

co-activators Proteins that interact with activated transcription factors at target gene promoters and facilitate their contact with the general transcription apparatus in cells. In addition, co-activators nucleate the assembly of a large complex of proteins at target gene promoters that enhance transcriptional activation by enzymatically modifying histones and effecting a local decondensation of chromatin.

codon A sequence of three nucleotides that encodes a particular amino acid or signals the initiation or termination of protein synthesis.

coleoptile The outermost sheathing leaf of a grass seedling, which serves as a protective sheath for the leaf plumule and shoot apical meristem.

colloid A gelatinous substance within the lumen of thyroid follicles that contains thyroglobulin with attached iodine and thyroid hormone.

colony-stimulating factor (CSF) A term for a group of four growth factors defined by their ability to stimulate hematopoietic progenitor cells to form colonies of mature progeny cells in semisolid culture media. CSF-1 supports the formation of macrophage colonies, granulocyte CSF supports formation of granulocyte colonies, granulocyte/macrophage CSF supports formation of colonies of granulocytes and macrophages, and interleukin-3, also known as multilineage CSF, supports formation of colonies containing cells derived from multiple lineages.

common cytokine receptor γ-chain (γc) A transmembrane protein that was first identified for its contribution to interleukin-2 (IL-2) binding and signaling. It has subsequently been shown to be involved in binding and signaling from a number of other cytokines, which are collectively known as the γc-utilizing cytokines. These include IL-2, IL-4, IL-7, IL-9, IL-15, and IL-21.

co-modulator A substance that interacts with a nuclear receptor and modifies transcriptional activity.

complementary DNA see cDNA.

conformation A particular structure or three-dimensional state that can be assumed by a chemical, such as a receptor protein. Receptor proteins can exist in several conformations and a given receptor molecule can transition between these conformations.

conformational coupling A theory for signaling capacitive calcium entry whereby depletion of intracellular Ca^{2+} stores causes a conformational change in $(1,4,5)IP_3$ receptors, which in turn interact with plasma membrane Ca^{2+} channels, resulting in their activation.

congenital lipoid adrenal hyperplasia A inherited metabolic disease characterized by markedly impaired adrenal and gonadal steroid hormone synthesis due to mutations in the *StAR* gene.

constitutive activity Describing the ability of a receptor protein to adopt an active conformation and to signal in the absence of ligand.

constitutive signaling Receptor signaling that occurs in the absence of agonist binding; also termed basal or agonist-independent signaling.

co-regulators Transcription factors that are recruited to active gene promoters via DNA-binding proteins such as the vitamin D receptor.

co-repressors Proteins that interact with inactive transcription factors and help to inhibit the activity of these proteins by nucleating a large complex of proteins, which functions to condense chromatin structure and repress transcription.

cornified envelope A proteinaceous reinforced structure beneath the plasma membrane in differentiated keratinocytes consisting of cross-linked precursor proteins.

corpus allatum *plural,* **corpora allata** In insects, a typically paired, retrocerebral endocrine gland of a single cell type, which synthesizes and secretes juvenile hormones. The corpus allatum is innervated by nerves from the brain and the subesophageal ganglion.

corpus cardiacum *plural,* **corpora cardiaca** In insects, a typically paired, retrocerebral neurohemal organ for the neurosecretory cells of the brain. The corpus cardiacum contains intrinsic neurosecretory cells, which release a variety of neurohormones, as well as the axons of cerebral neuron and neurosecretory cells, which traverse this organ to reach the corpus allatum.

corpus luteum The progesterone-producing tissue in the ovary that is formed from dominant follicles under the influence of luteinizing hormone.

cortical bone The dense surface layer of mature compact bone.

corticosteroids Steroid hormones secreted by the adrenal cortex that play crucial roles in nutrition, stress, and tissue responses to injury. In humans, cortisone and its synthetic analogues, such as prednisone and dexamethasone, are used therapeutically to control rheumatism and other inflammatory ailments.

corticotropin see ADRENOCORTICOTROPIC HORMONE.

corticotropin-releasing hormone (CRH) The hypothalamic neuropeptide that stimulates pituitary production and secretion of adrenocorticotropin, a hormone that regulates adrenal function. CRH is characterized as the major factor that orchestrates the endocrine stress response in mammals. Urocortin (Ucn) is a mammalian CRH-related peptide; two new members of the CRH peptide family, stresscopin-related peptide/urocortin II (Ucn II) and stresscopin/urocortin III (Ucn III), have recently been identified in humans, mice, and fish.

cortisol A physiological glucocorticoid hormones, produced in the zona fasciculata of the adrenal cortex. In most species, cortisol is the predominant glucocorticoid, but in rats and mice, **corticosterone** is the sole glucocorticoid.

coumestans A potent subgroup of phytoestrogens found in fodder crops.

CRAC channels Calcium release-activated calcium channels located in the cell membrane; CRAC channels are activated on release of calcium from intracellular stores, thus contributing to the replenishment of these stores.

craniotabes A condition caused by softening of the cranium and associated with parietal flattening of the sides of the skull, frontal bossing or exaggeration of the curvature of the forehead, and widened sutures or sites of attachment of bones to one another.

cretinism A developmental condition due to congenital or early-onset hypothyroidism characterized by arrested physical and mental development, dystrophy of bones and soft tissues, and depressed basal metabolism.

CRH see CORTICOTROPIN-RELEASING HORMONE.

cripto A novel growth factor that is normally expressed during embryonic development in a select group of fetal tissues. Cripto is also expressed at high levels in several types of human cancers.

critical period The time during development when sex steroids exert their organizational effects.

Crohn's disease A form of inflammatory bowel disease in which TNF (tumor necrosis factor) is inappropriately produced and contributes to disease.

crosstalk The ability of various signal transduction pathways to influence the signaling processes of one another. Crosstalk often occurs via phosphorylation/dephosphorylation events or through a physical interaction, e.g., tethering.

cryptorchidism A disorder in which one testis or both testes do not descend into the scrotum, as detected at birth. This condition can originate from impairment at an early step or at later steps in testis descent. When cryptorchidism is not reversed spontaneously, surgical placement of the undescended testis into the scrotum is required to obtain normal spermatogenesis and fertility with the onset of adulthood.

crypts of Lieberkühn The base of tubular invaginations in the intestinal mucosa containing rapidly dividing undifferentiated stem cells that continuously produce new epithelial cells.

cumulus cells The layer of granulosa cells surrounding the oocyte that make up the cumulus oophorus.

Cushing syndrome A metabolic disorder relating to chronic oversecretion of adrenal glucocorticoids (mainly cortisol); may result from increased secretion of adrenocorticotropic hormone due to pituitary or nonpituitary tumors or to a benign or malignant adrenal tumor. First described by Harvey Cushing in 1912.

cyclic adenosine monophosphate see cAMP.

cyclic olefin A member of a class of cyclic carbon structures that contain at least one carbon–carbon double bond that may competitively block ethylene binding.

cyclo-oxygenase A enzyme that catalyzes the formation of prostanoids from arachidonic acid.

cystine knot proteins A superfamily of proteins, including four growth factor families, all of which contain a distinctive motif made up of a circle of two disulfides (and the intervening peptide chains) through which passes a third disulfide bond.

cytochrome P450 In eukaryotes, a family of microsomal and mitochondrial heme-containing proteins (named for their characteristic absorption of light of 450 nm when carbon monoxide is bound) that reduce molecular oxygen, one atom of which is incorporated stereospecifically into the substrate as a hydroxyl group; those that use endogenous steroids for substrates are sometimes called steroid hydroxylases and many catalyze steps subsequent to the initial hydroxylation.

cytokine A member of a large family of secreted proteins, hormone-like messenger molecules that mediate cell-to-cell communication through binding to specific receptors on target cells and triggering postreceptor signaling pathways that alter cellular behavior. Cytokines are involved in reproduction, growth and development, injury repair, and the immunoendocrine system. Usually classified as interleukins, interferons, colony-stimulating factors, tumor necrosis factors, or growth factors, their classification is evolving.

cytokine receptor A family of single-pass transmembrane receptors identified in the late 1980s based on sequence comparison of receptors for prolactin, growth hormone, erythropoietin, interleukin-2 (IL-2), and IL-6. Additional members of the class I hematopoietic cytokine receptor superfamily include receptors for leptin, thrombopoietin, and many cytokines regulating the immune system, such as most interleukins. Cytokine receptors are devoid of intrinsic enzymatic activity and signal through associated kinases, the most classical of which are Janus tyrosine kinases.

Receptors for prolactin and growth hormone are very similar with respect to overall structure and signaling properties.

cytotoxic T cell (T lymphocyte) A white blood cell (lymphocyte) defined by expression of CD8 ($CD8^+$) on the cell surface; it expresses a specific T-cell receptor and has the ability to specifically recognize and kill target cells.

cytotoxic T-lymphocyte-associated antigen-4 A surface molecule on T cells that binds to the B7 molecule on antigen-presenting cells, resulting in delivery of a negative signal to the T cell and consequent down-regulation of the immune response.

D

death domain Signature motif of the type I TNF (tumor necrosis factor) receptor, responsible for inducing programmed cell death. Also found in other members of the TNF receptor superfamily.

decidua The endometrial lining shed at the end of pregnancy.

decidualization The collective morphological and functional changes that the endometrium undergoes, in mammalian species with invasive implantation. The endometrial stromal cells proliferate and differentiate into decidual cells that ultimately form the maternal component of the placenta.

decoy receptor A receptor that interacts with the ligand with high affinity and specificity but that is unable to signal or to be part of signaling receptor complexes. Decoy receptors act as a sink for the ligand and, in some cases, as dominant negatives for signaling receptors.

dehiscence In plants, the release of mature pollen grains via degradation of the callose cell wall that surrounds a tetrad of microspores.

dehydroepiandrostenedione A neurosteroid that is synthesized in the central nervous system. The most abundant human steroid hormone, it and its sulfated derivative are produced by the adrenal gland (approximately 30 mg/day), and are universal precursors for androgenic and estrogenic steroids. Conversion and metabolism occur in the peripheral tissues.

deiodinase One of three different enzymes (D1, D2, and D3) responsible for removal of iodine from tyrosine residues to activate or inactivate thyroid hormone.

delayed sleep phase syndrome A disturbance in which sleep occurs intractably late.

deletion Mutation that results in the removal of a sequence of DNA from a chromosome.

dendrikines Factors made by dendritic cells and acting on themselves (autocrine activity), on other cells locally in the lymph node or tissues where they reside (paracrine activity), or on immune cells at other distant sites or tissues (endocrine activity).

dendrites Thick nerve cell processes that receive synapses (contacts) from other nerve cells; also capable of secreting.

dendritic cells Specialized bone marrow-derived cells with dendritic processes and the most potent capacity to take up, process, and present antigens to T lymphocytes.

desensitization Loss of functional response; can be short-term (seconds or minutes) or long-term (hours).

desoxycorticosterone acetate An adrenal cortical steroid with predominant effects on electrolytes such as sodium and potassium.

diabetes Specifically, **diabetes mellitus.** The metabolic syndrome characterized by elevated blood glucose levels, resulting from lack of insulin action, either due to absolute lack of insulin (type 1 diabetes) or the inability to produce enough insulin to overcome insulin insensitivity (type 2 diabetes).

diabetic ketoacidosis Disease state characterized by hyperglycemia and acidosis, in which plasma ketones (β-hydroxybutyrate and acetoacetate) accumulate due to insulin deficiency and elevated glucagon levels.

1,2-diacylglycerol The active lipid product of phospholipase C-mediated hydrolysis of phospholipids; a neutral lipid with fatty acyl chains at positions 1 and 2; activates protein kinase C.

diazepam-binding inhibitor One of the putative releasing factors for cholecystokinin.

dietary steroidal supplements Compounds such as dehydroepiandrosterone (DHEA) and androstenedione that can be purchased in the United States without a prescription through many health food stores. They are often taken because the user believes they have anabolic effects. Steroidal supplements such as DHEA and androstenedione can be converted into testosterone and other sex steroids in the body.

differential immunoprecipitation A technique for the isolation and visualization of interacting proteins using distinct antisera to individual proteins.

differentiation The process of morphological and functional maturation that occurs in cells as they progress from a blast cell stage to the mature cell (e.g., granulocyte).

dihydrotestosterone Testosterone is metabolized via 5α-reductase to the potent androgen dihydrotestosterone, which binds directly to the androgen receptor and cannot be aromatized to estrogen.

1,25-dihydroxyvitamin D_3 The active steroid hormone form of vitamin D; a principal regulator of calcium homeostasis. It is synthesized in the kidney.

dimeric protein (dimer) A protein formed by the joining of two similar or identical proteins (or subunits).

dimerization The generation of a multiprotein functional unit comprising proteins of the same class. A monomer is a single unit, and a dimer is two units. In homodimers, the receptors are the same, whereas in heterodimers the receptors are different. This represents a central concept in the function of nuclear hormone receptors, as the majority work as heterodimers or homodimers.

dim light melatonin onset The time when melatonin levels rise under dim light conditions; a useful marker for the endogenous circadian pacemaker phase.

directed exocytosis The mechanism by which cells can communicate via soluble mediators across an immunologic synapse when they are in close proximity to other cells; cytokines are delivered from a region of one cell adjacent to another, usually after a series of triggering events between the two cells.

diseases of adaptation Maladies observed during the course of the General Adaptation Syndrome (see) in experimental animals; Hans Selye believed the maladies were the counterpart of diseases in humans with similar pathologic changes.

DNA-binding domain Region of steroid receptors that makes specific contact with DNA; has a conserved structural motif among members of the nuclear receptor family and can function autonomously.

DNA response element The DNA nucleotide sequence of a gene promoter that confers specific interaction with a signal-activated DNA-bound transcription factor.

domain Portion of a protein that has a tertiary structure of its own. In large proteins, each domain is connected to other domains by flexible regions of polypeptide.

dominance The status of the follicle (**dominant follicle**) destined to ovulate, given its presumed key role in regulating the size of the ovulatory quota; emerges during the menstrual cycle as a result of stimulation by follicle-stimulating hormone.

dominant negative mutation A mutation in a receptor that must be dimerized to evoke the functional response. When the mutated receptor dimerizes with wild-type receptor, the heterodimer remains functionally inactive.

dominant negative protein A defective protein that interferes with the function of the normal protein in the same cell.

dopamine β-hydroxylase The only enzyme in the catecholamine biosynthetic pathway located within the catecholamine-containing granules of the chromaffin cell, where it catalyzes the conversion of dopamine to noradrenaline.

dormancy A resting condition with reduced metabolic rate.

dose–response interface function A function (e.g., a logistic function) whose response output is an instantaneous rate of hormone synthesis, mass accumulation, or release.

down-regulation Transient loss of cell surface receptors following exposure to tropic hormone.

Drosophila The fruit fly, a commonly used model organism.

E

ecdysis A specific behavior that represents the final step in the molt of an insect—the shedding of the old cuticle—that differs among different insects and that may include distinct subbehaviors.

ecdysone A generic term denoting the biologically active ecdysteroids that initiate and coordinate an insect molt. A precursor form of the steroid hormone 20-hydroxyecdysone.

ecdysone receptor An insect-specific nuclear receptor that mediates the action of the steroid hormone 20-hydroxyecdysone.

ecdysone-response element A specific DNA regulatory sequence found near the transcription start site of ecdysone-regulated genes that is bound by the ecdysone receptor heterodimer.

ecdysteroids A member of a family of steroids characteristic of arthropods, possessing the full cholesterol side chain (unlike most vertebrate steroids) and several hydroxyl groups. They act as hormones (regulators) controlling molting and aspects of reproduction.

eclosion The specific ecdyses of embryonic and adult stage insects.

EcR A nuclear receptor that is the protein product of the ecdysone receptor gene.

effector Any of a number of enzymes or regulatory molecules within a cell that is stimulated or inhibited following receptor activation; responsible for transducing a cellular response to external stimuli.

efferent ductules Series of ductules connecting the testis to the head of the epididymis; their primary function is to resorb fluid leaving the testis in order to concentrate sperm on entry to the epididymis.

EGF see EPIDERMAL GROWTH FACTOR.

eicosanoids Polyunsaturated fatty acids with 20 carbons.

elicitors Compounds present in minute quantities in the saliva of herbivores, in the exudates of pathogens, or as degradation products of cell walls that are recognized by receptor proteins. Elicitors induce defensive responses in the affected plant.

embryogenesis The development of an individual from a fertilized ovum; the process of embryo formation.

enantiomers Different compounds that have the same molecular formula (isomers) but that are mirror reflections of each other; enantiomers are designated as cis or trans, R or S, or E or Z and occur only when the isomers contain chiral molecules.

endemic cretinism Mental retardation, associated with various neurological phenotypes, due to the deleterious effect of iodine deficiency on fetal brain development. This pathology occurs in areas where normal diets are iodine deficient, in the absence of an efficient program of iodination.

endochondral bone formation Bone development that occurs at growth plates by mineralization of a cartilaginous framework.

endochondral ossification Bone formation by replacement of a preformed cartilage scaffold that occurs during skeletal development and fracture repair.

endocrine Describing the action of a factor that is produced by one tissue and circulates through the bloodstream to reach another target organ on which it has an effect. This is the classical definition of all hormones.

endocrine disrupter (disruptor) An exogenous agent that interferes with the production, release, transport, metabolism, binding, action, or elimination of the natural hormones that are responsible for maintenance of homeostasis and regulation of developmental processes. Disrupters can directly affect an exposed individual and can affect fetuses through *in utero* exposure.

endocrine rhythm An oscillation of hormone secretion that is generated endogenously.

endocrine system The network of endocrine glands (sources of a hormones) and target cells (locations of the hormones receptors) involved in integrated interactions that generate regulated, selective biological responses necessary to maintain the system viability.

endocytosis The process by which molecules on the surface of cells are brought into the cell and then degraded or recycled back to the cell surface.

endometriosis The presence of endometrial glands and stroma outside their normal location within the endometrial cavity.

endometrium The inner lining of the uterine cavity; comprises the mucosal and glandular-containing submucosal lining of the uterus.

endonuclease The enzyme that cleaves a nucleotide chain.

endopeptidases The enzymes responsible for the limited proteolysis of proproteins, usually on the carboxylic side of dibasic amino acid sequences, to yield the active mature protein.

endoplasmic reticulum Cellular organelle consisting of sheets of membranes; it functions in the synthesis of lipids and membrane proteins.

β-endorphin A peptide possessing analgesic properties mediated through the opioid receptors.

endothelium The monolayer of cells lining the inner wall of the vascular system.

endotoxic shock A severe, acute disorder caused by gram-negative infection; excess TNF is produced in response to bacterial lipopolysaccharide as a result of signaling via Toll-like receptor 4. Marked by fever, hypotension, and inadequate tissue perfusion.

endowment A term for the first step of follicle formation in which the oocyte is associated with surrounding somatic cells to form a primordial follicle.

enhancers DNA sequences that increase the rate of gene transcription from a distance, irrespective of their orientation relative to the transcription start site in the gene.

enhansons Subunits of enhancers; some enhancers are composed of separate 15- to 20-bp elements that cooperate with one another to enhance transcription. These elements are made up of enhansons, which can be duplicated or interchanged to create new enhancer elements. Unlike enhancers, enhansons are sensitive to changes in spacing.

enteric nervous system Network of neuronal cells and fibers embedded within the gut wall that serve as a relay for signals to and from the brain or spinal cord. This network can respond to stimuli from various sensory receptors and generate changes in neuronal activity independent of the central nervous system.

enterochromaffin-like cells (ECL cells) Endocrine cells dispersed in the fundic part of the gastric mucosa. These cells are important relay stations for the effect of carboxyamidated gastrin. They are well equipped with gastrin receptors and on stimulation they release histamine, which in turn stimulates gastric acid secretion from fundic parietal cells.

enterodiol A lignan metabolite derived by gastrointestinal bacteria.

enteroendocrine cells Specialized, phenotypically distinct endocrine cells; found within the mucosa of the gastrointestinal tract, they produce one or more peptide hormones.

enterogastrone An intestinal hormone that is secreted in response to fat or its digestion products and that inhibits gastric acid secretion.

enteroglucagons Hormones produced in the intestinal glucagon cells (L-cells) through processing of the proglucagon molecule.

enteroinsular axis Nutrient, neural, and hormonal signals arising from the gut that regulate hormone secretion from the endocrine pancreas; triggered by ingested sugars and amino acids.

enterolactone A lignan metabolite derived by gastrointestinal bacteria.

entrainment Regulation of rhythm period and phase by time cues in the external environment.

environmental stress Biotic (insects, pathogens, etc.) and abiotic (drought, hail, temperature extremes, etc.) factors in the environment that can damage plants due to herbivory, disease, wounding, and physiological maladies (such as water stress).

enzyme A protein that catalyzes the transformation of a substrate into a product.

eosinophilia The presence of highly elevated numbers of eosinophils.

eosinophils White blood cells thought to be important in asthma and in defense against parasitic infections.

epidermal growth factor (EGF) A small mitogenic protein involved in regulating normal cell growth, oncogenesis, and wound healing.

epidermal growth factor homology region A domain common to all receptors of the low-density lipoprotein family; adjacent to the ligand-binding site.

epidermal growth factor receptor (EGFR) A cell surface transmembrane protein that specifically binds cognate ligands and transduces a biologic response, usually related to the control of cell proliferation.

epidermis The outer epithelial layer of the skin consisting mainly of cells called keratinocytes.

epinephrine A catecholamine hormone released from the adrenal medulla in response to hypoglycemia.

epiphyseal growth plate A specialized strip of cartilage located at the ends of long bones, in which programmed proliferation and maturation of chondrocytes result in the production of cartilage to form a template for new bone formation during linear growth.

epitope Site on an antigen that is recognized by a particular antibody or T-cell receptor.

erythrocyte A mature red blood cell that circulates within the body to deliver oxygen to tissues and, in exchange, remove carbon dioxide and hydrogen ion from tissues.

erythrocytosis An abnormal increase in red blood cells in the circulating blood.

estradiol A steroid hormone that belongs to the family of estrogens. 17β-estradiol is the "traditional" estrogen, although numerous substances have estrogenic activity.

estrogen A naturally occurring or synthetic steroid that binds to the estrogen receptor and stimulates the development of female secondary sex characteristics and promotes growth and maintenance of the female reproductive system. One of the two major ovarian steroid hormones upon which implantation depends.

estrogen receptor Protein target for the steroid hormone estrogen. Two distinct forms of this nuclear receptor have been identified, ER-α and ER-β (see following).

estrogen receptor α The first identified receptor for estrogen.

estrogen receptor β A second receptor for estrogen that was identified more recently; encoded by a separate gene.

estrogen receptor knockouts Mouse lines developed using gene targeting strategies to disrupt expression of endogenous genes encoding ER-α (αERKO) or ER-β (αERKO).

estrogen response element Specific binding sequence for the estrogen receptor; located in the promoter of estrogen target genes. The consensus estrogen response element is a 13-base-pair inverted palindrome containing a 3-base-pair spacer (GGTCAnnnTGACC).

eustress Hans Selye's term for "good" stress that promotes health.

exon The portion of the DNA sequence in a gene that contains the codons that specify the sequence of amino acids in a polypeptide chain, as well as the beginning and end of the coding sequence.

exopeptidase An enzyme involved in the mechanism of proprotein processing. It selectively removes the carboxylic basic amino acids exposed after the endopeptidase cleavage.

expression gradient Graded expression of a molecule (protein, RNA) in a defined compartment of the organism.

extracellular matrix The complex, collagenous matrices to which cells are attached within a tissue; it includes both interstitial matrix and basal lamina.

F

F-actin (filamentous actin) A protein that results from the self-assembly of G-actin into head-to-tail polymers. This assembly is regulated by a large class of actin-binding proteins.

fat body An organ whose functional role in insects is analogous to the combined functions of liver and adipose tissue in mammals. Fat body is the chief site of intermediary metabolism, detoxification, storage of nutrient reserves, and, in some species, deposition of nitrogenous waste products.

fatty acid Long-chain aliphatic carboxylic acid found in fats, oils, membrane phospholipids, and glycolipids.

fecundity Offspring produced per female. Combines fertility (ability to produce offspring) and prolificacy (number of offspring).

5′,3′ flanking region Noncoding region upstream (5′ flanking) or downstream (3′ flanking) of a gene. A cis-regulatory element for gene expression is often found in the 5′ flanking region.

Flt3 The fms-like tyrosine kinase 3 receptor that acts as the cell surface mediator of biological effects induced by its ligand upon specific receptor binding.

Flt3 ligand (FL) A type 1 transmembrane protein that in soluble or transmembrane form binds to Flt3 and elicits the intracellular signaling cascade that guides hematopoietic stem and progenitor cells to proliferate, survive, and develop. For most activities, FL has modest effects by itself, but it is a potent co-stimulating molecule and actively synergizes with other cytokines for optimal biological effects.

follicle A small, narrow cavity or sac in an organ or tissue, such as those in the ovaries that contain developing eggs.

follicle-stimulating hormone (FSH) A pituitary polypeptide hormone that acts on granulosa cells to promote follicle survival and estrogen production.

follicular phase The approximately 2-week-long stage of the human menstrual cycle, prior to the luteinizing hormone surge, during which ovarian follicles develop prior to subsequent ovulation.

folliculogenesis The process by which oocytes and ovarian somatic cells develop to ovulate a fertilizable egg. The first steps in follicle development are directed by intraovarian factors and result in proliferation of granulosa cells surrounding the oocyte and the recruitment of a layer of theca cells.

follistatin A molecule that binds and inactivates β/β transforming growth factor-β family members, thereby indirectly inhibiting follicle-stimulating hormone transcription.

forward/reverse signaling Traditionally, the signal transduction mechanism originating from activated receptors is referred to as forward signaling. Reverse signaling, a signaling cascade within the ligand-expressing cell, is triggered on receptor binding to membrane-bound ligands.

frameshift mutation A change in the DNA sequence that occurs by insertion or deletion of some number of nucleotides that is not a multiple of 3, thus altering the reading frame for protein translation.

free hormone hypothesis Plasma-specific binding proteins sequester circulating hormones and therefore only the non-protein-bound fraction (= free) of hormones is available for movement out of capillaries and for cell biodisposal, where it may either initiate a biological response or be metabolized and cleared from the circulation.

free radical A molecule, usually short-lived and highly reactive, that contains an unpaired electron. All molecules containing an odd number of electrons are free radicals.

FSH see FOLLICLE-STIMULATING HORMONE.

functional complementation A technique in which co-expression of two receptors that are nonfunctional or partially functional leads to improved functional activity.

functional hypothalamic amenorrhea A clinical state of subfertility in women resulting from stress exposure.

G

GABA(γ-aminobutyric acid) The principal inhibitory neurotransmitter in the mammalian central nervous system (CNS), inhibiting virtually every neuron in the adult CNS at physiological concentrations.

G-actin (globular actin) The major protein of the microfilament system in eukaryotic cells.

gain-of-function mutations Gene alterations that render a receptor constitutively active, in the absence of hormone. In the thyroid-stimulating hormone receptor, such mutations usually result in hyperthyroidism.

galactorrhea Production and secretion of milk from breast tissue.

gastrin A gastrointestinal polypeptide hormone produced by G cells of the gastric antrum; stimulates gastric acid secretion.

gastrin cells (G cells) Endocrine cells dispersed in the antral part of the gastric mucosa and in the proximal part of the duodenal mucosa. G cells produce by far most of the gastrin in the adult organism. The synthesis of gastrin is regulated by negative feedback from gastric acid via antral somatostatin cells.

gelsolin A calcium- and polyphosphoinositide-regulated F-actin severing and capping protein found in both cytosol and serum.

gene A specific sequence of DNA at a particular chromosomal location; it codes for a specific protein.

gene knock-in A technique in which the coding sequences of one gene are replaced with those of another.

gene knockout A technique for selectively inactivating a gene in the germ-line of an animal by replacing the gene with a mutant allele; a method of evaluating the functional significance of that gene product in cell, tissue, or organ function.

General Adaptation Syndrome Hans Selye's term for the manifestations of stress in the whole body following prolonged stress exposure; the syndrome develops over time in three phases: the alarm reaction, the stage of resistance, and the stage of exhaustion.

generalized inherited (familial) glucocorticoid resistance A rare inherited syndrome characterized by elevated plasma cortisol levels but lacking the symptoms characteristic of Cushing's syndrome because of general target tissue resistance to glucocorticoids.

genetic polymorphism A heritable genetic difference between two individuals at a specific location in the genome that is present in the general population.

genomic Relating to gene transcription and its regulation.

genotype The entire array of genes carried by an individual, or the particular allele at a specified locus in an individual.

germ cell A cell that can grow to form the reproductive cells (sperm or eggs). In the testis, these are the gonocytes, spermatocytes, spermatids, and spermatozoa.

germ-line mutation A heritable genetic alteration not present in the general population.

ghrelin Polypeptide growth hormone secretagogue predominantly produced by the stomach; exerts a direct or indirect stimulatory effect on growth hormone secretion by somatotrophs.

glial cells Nonneuronal support cells of the nervous system. Schwann cells are found in the peripheral nervous system and astrocytes and oligodendrocytes are found in the central nervous system.

glicentin Intermediary 69-amino-acid peptide processed from proglucagon and cleaved to form glicentin-related polypeptide and oxyntomodulin.

glucagon A hormone secreted by the pancreatic alpha cell in response to hypoglycemia.

glucagon-like peptides Two small peptides, glucagon-like peptide-1 and glucagon-like peptide-2, derived from posttranslational processing of proglucagon; found in endocrine cells of the gastrointestinal tract and in the brain. They exhibit sequence similarity to glucagon.

glucagonoma syndrome A disorder caused by elevated glucagon levels from a pancreatic alpha-cell tumor, leading to necrolytic migratory erythema, cheilosis, diabetes mellitus, impaired glucose tolerance, anemia, venous thrombosis, and psychiatric symptoms.

glucocorticoid Any of a group of cholesterol-derived steroid hormones (e.g., corticosterone) that are the primary product of the adrenal cortex. Some glucocorticoids are produced in adipose and other tissues, as well. Glucocorticoids bind to nuclear glucocorticoid receptors to modulate transcription of target genes. Glucocorticoids are often referred to as catabolic steroids, promoting the breakdown of cellular proteins and potentiating the effects of counterregulatory hormones. They are essential for life and are key regulators in the stress response. The term also encompasses synthetic hormones with a similar structure and function.

glucocorticoid receptor An intracellular protein that specifically binds glucocorticoids and functions as a transcription factor by activating or repressing the transcription of target genes. This receptor is a member of the nuclear hormone receptor family of ligand-inducible transcription factors.

glucocorticoid-response element A specific glucocorticoid receptor-binding DNA element that is located in the promoter regions of glucocorticoid target genes.

gluconeogenesis Production in the liver of glucose from noncarbohydrate precursors.

glucose $C_6H_{12}O_6$, a 6-carbon aldose that is the major sugar in the blood and a key intermediate in metabolism. Used as a fluid and nutrient replenisher, usually given intravenously. The major energy source for the brain.

glucose toxicity Adverse biochemical effects in many tissues within the body resulting from prolonged elevations of glucose.

glutamate The principal excitatory neurotransmitter in the mammalian central nervous system, stimulating virtually every neuron in the adult CNS at physiological concentrations.

glycogenolysis The glucagon-stimulated breakdown of glycogen stores in the liver.

glycogen phosphorylase An enzyme that catalyzes the sequential removal of glycosyl residues from the nonreducing end (i.e., with a free 4'-OH group) of the glycogen molecule, using orthophosphate as a co-substrate and releasing glucose-1-phosphate.

glycogen synthase The main rate-limiting enzyme in glycogen synthesis; inhibited by glucagon.

glycoprotein hormones Family of heterodimeric (two dissimilar subunits) glycosylated proteins in vertebrates that includes thyrotropin, follitropin, lutropin, and choriogonadotropin.

glycosylation The conjugation of carbohydrate residues, which for proteins can occur through the side-chain oxygen atom of serine or threonine residues by O-glycosidic linkages or to the side-chain nitrogen of asparagine residues by N-glycosidic linkages.

GnRH see GONATROPIN-RELEASING HORMONE.

GnRH pulse generator The cellular and molecular mechanisms that produce and sustain pulsatile gonadotropin-releasing hormone neurosecretion; these mechanisms are incompletely understood.

goiter Enlargement of the thyroid gland; occurs in hypothyroid states, when thyroid cells are under TSH stimulation to produce more hormone, or in hyperthyroid states, when stimulating substances, usually antibodies, bind to the TSH receptor and stimulate thyroid function.

Golgi apparatus A complex cytoplasmic organelle consisting of a series of layered cisternae and associated small vesicles; it is involved in terminal glycosylation, membrane flow, secretion, and delivery of cellular products either to the cell surface or to the appropriate intracellular destination.

gonadal dysgenesis A disorder of gonadal development affecting all gonadal compartments.

gonadotropes Pituitary cells that make and secrete gonadotropins (follicle-stimulating hormone and luteinizing hormone).

gonadotropin A collective term for two related, but functionally distinct, peptide hormones (luteinizing hormone and follicle-stimulating hormone) synthesized and secreted from the gonadotrope cells in the mammalian pituitary. Gonadotropins bind to receptors on the gonads, the ovaries, and testes, and individually influence either sex steroid production (primarily luteinizing hormone) or the development of eggs and sperm.

gonadotropin-releasing hormone (GnRH) A decapeptide that is synthesized in neurons of the basal forebrain, released into the hypophyseal portal vasculature, and conveyed to the anterior pituitary gland, where it stimulates the synthesis and secretion of the gonadotropins luteinizing hormone and follicle-stimulating hormone; it is also referred to as luteinizing hormone-releasing hormone.

gonads A collective term for the testes and ovaries; these develop from the urogenital ridge through a bipotential gonad. This process is mediated through differentiated genetic control.

G-protein Any of a class of guanine nucleotide-binding proteins associated with the cytoplasmic face of the plasma membrane of mammalian cells; proteins involved in transmitting signals from certain types of hormone and neurotransmitter receptors to intracellular pathways. These proteins are composed of three subunits; the α-subunit binds GTP (guanine triphosphate) and has GTPase activity, the β- and γ-subunits form stable heterodimers, and both G_α and $G_{\beta\gamma}$ can independently activate effector proteins in response to hormone stimulation.

G-protein-coupled receptor A family of cell surface receptor proteins consisting of seven transmembrane regions. The intracellular region interacts with GTP-binding proteins, which, on ligand binding, transduce signals within the cell, leading to a cellular response (e.g., secretion, motility, and growth).

granulocyte A white blood cell containing granules in the cytoplasm that is involved in attacking bacterial infections. There are three types, depending on the type of granules, called neutrophils, eosinophils, and basophils. The term granulocyte is sometimes used to mean only neutrophils, e.g., in the case of granulocyte colony-stimulating factor.

granulocyte colony-stimulating factor A hematopoietic cytokine responsible for the regulation of neutrophil production.

granulocyte colony-stimulating factor (G-CSF) receptor The protein displayed on the surface of cells that specifically recognizes, interacts with, and responds to G-CSF.

granulosa cells Hormone-producing somatic cells that surround the oocyte and become differentiated into cumulus cells, which are closest to the oocyte, and antral and mural cells.

Graves' disease A disorder caused by overexpression of thyroid-stimulating hormone receptor (TSHR) signaling, which is induced by TSHR autoantibodies.

growth factor A small peptide hormone that regulates cell production and differentiation in the tissue in which it is produced; often is produced in excess by tumor cells.

growth factor receptor A transmembrane protein that consists of an extracellular ligand-binding domain and an intracellular effector domain; often is associated with a kinase activity that is activated on ligand binding.

growth hormone (GH) A polypeptide hormone (191 amino acids in humans) that adopts the α-helix-bundle fold typical of hematopoietic cytokines. GH is secreted mainly by the pituitary gland, although it is also produced by other cell types, such as lymphoid cells. Its actions are related mainly to growth (soft tissues, long bones, etc.) and metabolism. It belongs to a family of hormones that includes prolactin and placental lactogens, as well as other placental factors.

growth hormone-binding protein A soluble, circulating form of the growth hormone receptor that is composed of the receptor's extracellular ligand-binding domain and can be formed in different species by proteolytic cleavage of the membrane-bound form or by alternative splicing of the growth hormone receptor primary transcript.

growth hormone-releasing hormone The hypothalamic peptide, found in several molecular forms, that stimulates the pituitary to secrete growth hormone.

growth hormone secretagogue A synthetic or naturally occurring peptide that interacts with the growth hormone secretagogue receptor to stimulate secretion of pituitary growth hormone.

growth hormone secretagogue receptor The unique receptor for a growth hormone-releasing peptide.

GTPase accelerating proteins (GAPs) Proteins that accelerate the hydrolysis of GTP (guanosine triphosphate) on distinct types of G-protein α-subunits. GAPs occur in four of the five families of RGS-like proteins and the effector protein phospholipase C-β.

guanine nucleotide-binding protein see G-PROTEIN.

guanosine triphosphate A nucleoside triphosphate used in RNA synthesis and in some energy-transfer reactions. It also plays a special role in protein synthesis, cell signaling, and microtubule assembly.

gubernaculum A paired ligamentous cord present in both sexes that attaches to the gonad at the superior end and attaches to the bottom of the abdomen at the expanded inferior end (gubernacular bulb). Development and relative shortening of the gubernaculum, which occur only in the male, are essential for the first abdominal phase of testis descent. Later changes in the configuration of the gubernaculum are involved in passage of the testes through the inguinal canal into the scrotum.

gynecomastia Abnormal enlargement of the breast; usually used in reference to the male breast.

H

HDLp High-density lipophorin (density approximately 1.12 g/ml), the abundant and generally single lipoprotein particle in insect hemolymph, transporting several classes of lipids between organs and tissues in the resting situation.

heat shock proteins Proteins that are synthesized by cells in response to increased temperature and function mainly as molecular chaperones protecting cellular proteins by aiding in protein folding.

helminths Parasitic worms such as *Nippostrongylus brasiliensis*, which pass through the intestine and provoke a strong T_H2-mediated immune response that normally results in clearance of the worms from the system.

hematopoiesis The development of multiple lineages of blood cells from a pluripotential stem cell. These include red blood cells, platelets, lymphocytes (T and B), natural killer cells, monocytes, and granulocytes (neutrophils, eosinophils, and mast cells). This process is regulated by soluble and membrane-bound growth factors, cell contact, and interaction with the extracellular matrix.

Hemimetabola An insect subclass in which insects go through several nymphal stages, then molt directly to the adult stage.

hemolymph The blood of insects, which circulates in the body cavity between the various organs, bathing them directly. It consists of a fluid plasma in which the blood cells or hemocytes are suspended.

heparin binding The ability of a protein to bind tightly to heparin or heparan sulfate proteoglycan.

hepoxilins Eicosanoids that are the products of the 12-lipoxygenase pathway.

heptahelical receptors Another term for G-protein-coupled receptors.

hermaphroditism A developmental condition in which an individual displays both male and female sexual phenotypes.

heterodimerization Physical association between nonidentical proteins (heteromers).

heterozygote An organism with two different alleles at a particular locus.

heterozygous Having different alleles at one locus.

hippocampus A curved, elongated ridge in the medial temporal lobe of the brain; thought to be responsible for consolidation of short-term memories and their conversion to long-term memories; also involved in spatial learning. Hippocampal morphology is markedly altered in epilepsy (in which certain hippocampal neurons die and others sprout aberrant connections) and Alzheimer's disease (in which there is degeneration of hippocampal neurons).

hirsutism Excess facial and body hair in women in a pattern similar to that found in men.

histone acetylase A protein with enzymatic activity that results in covalent acetylation of histones and other proteins.

histone deacetylase A protein with enzymatic activity that results in removal of acetyl groups from histones and other proteins.

histone modification Acetylation or deacetylation of lysine residues within DNA-bound histones that alter chromatin structure and transcription factor accessibility.

Holometabola An insect subclass in which insects have a pupal stage in their life cycle. There usually are several larval stages followed by a pupal stage, then the adult stage.

homeodomain proteins A family of transcription factors; contain a DNA-binding domain with a helix–turn–helix motif originally described in homeotic genes in *Drosophila*.

homeostasis A term for the body's tendency to maintain physiological stability in response to influences that threaten to disturb the steady state.

homodimerization Physical association between identical proteins (homomers).

homologous recombination A natural chromosomal recombination mechanism that has been harnessed to "knock out" genes in mice in order to test for their functional importance.

homologues Compounds that have a similar core structure but have carbon skeletons that vary by one or more atoms.

homozygote An organism with the same alleles at a particular locus.

homozygous Having identical alleles at one locus.

hormone Any of several chemical classes of compounds produced in regulated quantities by an endocrine gland; a hormone acts as a chemical messenger, usually delivered through the circulatory system to a target cell, which, by definition, possesses a receptor for that hormone so that a specific biological response is generated. Most hormones act on distant sites, but they may also act on the cell that secreted them (autocrine action) or on nearby cells (paracrine action).

hormone antagonist A drug that counteracts the action of a hormone by binding to a nuclear receptor.

hormone receptor A protein in or on the surface of target cells; functions as a sensor for the hormone by binding the hormone and initiating a cellular response.

hormone receptor signaling cascade The chain of intracellular events beginning from the activation of a hormone receptor that ends in the final response to the hormone. Also known as a signal transduction pathway.

hormone resistance A disease condition in which a specific hormone is unable to exert its biological actions; it is usually caused by an inactivating receptor mutation.

hormone response element A regulatory DNA sequence in the promoter region of a gene; interacts with factors that bind hormone receptors, altering transcription of specific genes.

human chorionic gonadotropin A glycoprotein hormone similar to luteinizing hormone that is produced by the trophoblast cells of the early embryo and placenta.

human leukocyte antigen A member of a family of cell surface heterodimers expressed on antigen-presenting cells that are responsible for presenting foreign antigens to T cells, via the T-cell receptor.

human T-cell lymphotropic virus I (HTLV-I) A retrovirus that is found predominantly in Japan, the Caribbean Islands, and sub-Saharan Africa that induces the expression of IL-2 and IL-15 and their receptors and that is the etiological agent of a number of human diseases, including adult T-cell leukemia and autoimmune disorders such as tropical spastic paraparesis/HTLV-I-associated myelopathy.

humoral hypercalcemia of malignancy A syndrome characterized by elevated calcium levels in cancer patients without metastases.

humoral immunity Host defenses, mediated by antibodies, which protect against extracellular bacteria and other foreign macromolecules.

hydroperoxyeicosatetraenoic acids Eicosanoids that are the products of the lipoxygenase pathway.

20-hydroxyecdysone A biologically active ecdysteroid that induces molting and metamorphosis.

hydroxyeicosatetraenoic acids Eicosanoids that are the products of the P450 and lipoxygenase pathways.

1α-hydroxylase Cytochrome P450 enzyme that converts 25-hydroxyvitamin D_3 to 1,25-dihydroxyvitamin D_3 by catalyzing the addition of a hydroxyl group at the C-1 position.

11β-hydroxysteroid dehydrogenase An enzyme that catalyzes the oxidation of hydroxy groups in the 11β position of steroids. 11β-HSD2, the second isoform of this enzyme, has high affinity for endogenous glucocorticoids and is expressed specifically in aldosterone target cells.

5-hydroxytryptamine A neurotransmitter long known to inhibit food intake; it is the focus of many treatment interventions aimed at normalizing disordered eating behavior. Also known as 5-HT or serotonin.

hyperglycemia Elevated blood glucose level.

hyperparathyroidism A condition defined by excess parathyroid hormone secretion; leads to accelerated bone turnover.

hyperplasia Increase in the size of an organ due to excessive proliferation of the constituent cells.

hypersensitive response A reaction manifested by the formation of necrotic lesions at the site of pathogen entry; thought to play a role in reducing pathogen growth and spread.

hyperthyroidism A condition of thyroid hormone excess; commonly associated with weight loss, tachycardia, excessive sweating, heat intolerance, moist skin, and fatigue; usually due to excessive thyroid gland production of thyroid hormone.

hypertrehalosemia A condition characterized by an increase in the level of trehalose in the hemolymph (insect blood) to values that significantly exceed the normal resting level.

hypertrehalosemic hormone In insects, a peptide hormone from the corpus cardiacum involved in the mobilization of fat body glycogen to fuel flight activity. For transport to the flight muscles, glycogen is converted into the disaccharide trehalose, the carbohydrate transport form in insects, whose level in hemolymph is raised during flight.

hypocotyl The stem-like axis between the seed leaf or leaves and the root in an embryo or seedling.

hypoglycemia A decrease in blood glucose concentration to below the normal level, which can generally be considered 65 mg/dl (3.6 mM).

hypoglycemia unawareness syndrome A condition that occurs in some insulin-treated patients with diabetes who experience frequent bouts of hypoglycemia. Such patients are unable to mount a counterregulatory response to hypoglycemia or develop symptoms of hypoglycemia until blood glucose falls below the level at which neuroglycopenia occurs (generally below 40 mg/dl or 2.2 mM).

hypophysectomy Surgical removal of the pituitary gland.

hypophyseotropic hormones Neurotransmitters, including neuropeptides, dopamine, and γ-aminobutyric acid; secreted from tuberoinfundibular neurons and conveyed as hormones through the long portal vessels, acting at a distance on pituitary cells and regulating their function.

hypophysial portal vasculature The circulatory system that connects the median eminence (perfused by the dense capillary network stemming from the superior hypophysial artery) to the anterior pituitary via portal vessels, through which releasing and inhibiting factors are transported.

hypophysiotropic Relating to regulation of anterior pituitary secretion.

hypophysiotropic hormone-secreting neurons Hypothalamic neurons that secrete into the hypophysial portal circulation various releasing or inhibiting hormones, which in turn control secretion of the six anterior pituitary tropic hormones.

hypothalamic–hypophyseal portal vessels The specialized vasculature that forms a plexus in the median eminence of the hypothalamus and collects into larger vessels that extend into the hypophysis (pituitary gland); a major function of this vascular network is to convey substances that undergo neurosecretion from neurovascular junctions in the median eminence to the anterior pituitary gland, where these factors, such as gonadotropin-releasing hormone, can regulate hormone secretions.

hypothalamic-pituitary-adrenal axis (HPA axis) Cells and pathways that form the communications between the hypothalamus, the pituitary, and the adrenal gland. The major hypothalamic factors are corticotropin-releasing hormone and vasopressin, both of which stimulate the release of pituitary adrenocorticoticopic hormone, which in turn stimulates the release of glucocorticosteroids from the adrenal cortex (principally corticosterone and cortisol).

hypothalamus The part of the diencephalon in the subconscious brain that integrates various environmental stimuli to regulate motivation, physiology, and endocrine function. The hypothalamus contains nerve centers (nuclei) that regulate the autonomic nervous system and that regulate the production of pituitary releasing factors. It lies at the base of the brain, overlying the pituitary gland, and is connected to the pituitary gland by a stalk and a specialized portal circulation that carries releasing factors to the anterior pituitary.

hypothyroidism A condition of thyroid hormone deficit; commonly associated with weight gain, slow mentation, decreased energy, cold intolerance, edema, and dry skin; usually due to failure of the thyroid gland to synthesize and release thyroid hormone.

hypoxia A deficiency of oxygen reaching the body tissues.

I

IA-2 (ICA-512) A protein tyrosine phosphatase-like molecule that is one of the major autoimmune targets in type 1 diabetes.

ichthyosis Skin disease in which the skin is very dry and exhibits fish-like scales.

IgE An immunoglobulin class that mediates many allergic-type responses; functions by binding to high-affinity FcεRI receptors on mast cells and basophils. When IgE molecules are cross-linked, by binding their cognate antigen, they signal the release of preformed mediators and the synthesis and secretion of cytokines.

IGF see INSULIN-LIKE GROWTH FACTOR.

IL-10R Interleukin-10 receptor complex, composed of the ligand-binding IL-10R1 and the signal-transducing IL-10R2 chains.

ileal brake A term for inhibitory effects on upper gastrointestinal motor activity; triggered by a distal intestinal hormone that is released in response to intralumenal fat.

ileoanal anastomosis Surgical end-to-end connection between the terminal ileum and distal rectum after total colonic resection.

ileostomy A procedure in which the terminal ileum is exteriorized through the abdominal wall; allows intestinal waste to be collected in a bag.

immune response The series of events that occurs after T and B cells are exposed to antigens for which they have a specific receptor. T cells that are thus activated produce cytokines that foster the proliferation of activated cells (clonal expansion) plus the recruitment and activation of other cells of the immune system. B cells also proliferate as a result of the actions of cytokines and secrete the antibody specific for the antigen.

immune system The physiologic system consisting mainly of white blood cells that specializes in protecting the organism from infection and clearing debris after tissue injury.

immunocytochemistry A microscopy technique that identifies cells containing peptides or proteins recognized by specific antibodies, which are labeled.

immunoglobulin-like domain Domain of about 100 amino acids; predicted to adopt a seven-stranded immunoglobulin-like fold that in cytokine receptors has been shown to participate in ligand binding.

immunoglobulins Also known as antibodies; a secreted form of B lymphocyte antigen receptors that bind to pathogens.

impaired glucose tolerance An early aspect of diabetes mellitus when the subject is unable to secrete sufficient insulin for a given carbohydrate load, leading to higher than normal plasma glucagon levels.

impaired insulin secretion Inability of the pancreatic beta cells to secrete sufficient amounts of insulin to maintain normal glucose tolerance.

implantation Establishment of a stable tissue interface between the maternal endometrium and the embryo.

implantation window A restricted period of time during which the endometrium permits implantation of a competent blastocyst.

inactivating (loss-of-function) mutation A mutation that inactivates the function of a receptor by one of the following mechanisms: decreased synthesis, aberrant intracellular processing, impaired or missing ligand binding, impaired or missing signal transduction, inability to anchor to plasma membrane (cell membrane receptors), inability to dimerize (if needed for action), or increased degradation.

incretin A hormone that is released from the intestine in response to the ingestion of glucose; stimulates insulin secretion from pancreatic β-cells.

induced systemic resistance A self-defense mechanism induced by nonpathogenic rhizobacteria that initiates the systemic production of pathogenesis-related proteins, leading to broad resistance against pathogens.

infertility The inability to produce offspring; typically defined in a clinicla context as a failure to achieve pregnancy within a year of unprotected intercourse.

inflammation In higher organisms, a defense mechanism that protects the organism from infection and injury by localizing and limiting tissue damage, so that healing can begin. An inflammatory response lasting only a few days is called acute inflammation, whereas a response of longer duration is referred to as chronic inflammation.

inflammatory mediators The endogenous compounds that mediate inflammation (autocoids) and related exogenous compounds including the synthetic prostaglandins.

innate immune system The primitive defensive system, including barriers between the inner and the outer environments, defensive proteins in the circulation, and immune competent cells except for T cells and B cells. Recently, it was shown that innate immunity can strictly discriminate microbe products from self-molecules by the corresponding receptors.

inositol phosphates A series of phosphorylated derivatives of the hexitol, D-*myo*-inositol. In mammalian cells, inositol phosphates are derived from inositol 1,4,5-trisphosphate, formed by cleavage of phosphatidylinositol 4,5-bisphosphate by phospholipase C.

***in situ* hybridization** A microscopy technique that identifies cells containing messenger RNA for specific peptides or proteins by hybridization to labeled complementary nucleotide probes.

insulin A hormone synthesized in the beta cells of the islets of Langerhans, which form the endocrine pancreas. The main function of insulin is the regulation of carbohydrate metabolism. It is used as a therapy for diabetes and can cause hypoglycemia.

insulin-like factor 3 A protein hormone that may be involved in the control of testis descent. During fetal development, insulin-like factor 3 (Insl3) is produced by the testis, in the interstitial Leydig cells, but not by the ovary. Inactivation of the gene encoding Insl3 in the mouse (*Insl3* knockout) results in complete blockade of testis descent.

insulin-like growth factor A member of a class of hormones structurally related to insulin, but exhibiting proliferative and differentiative, rather than metabolic, effects.

insulin resistance A pathophysiological condition in which the action of insulin is impaired, so that a higher insulin concentration is needed to result in the same effect.

insulin secretory granule The intracellular compartment of the pancreatic islet beta cells where insulin is stored, ready to be released when an appropriate stimulus triggers the beta cell. The insulin secretory granule is formed in the *trans*-Golgi, where proinsulin, the precursor of insulin, is sorted into the clathrin-coated immature insulin secretory granule. Secretory granule maturation comprises clathrin uncoating, granule acidification, and conversion of proinsulin to insulin.

insulin signal transduction The intracellular events [tyrosine phosphorylation of the insulin receptor and insulin receptor substrate-1 (IRS-1), association of the p85 regulatory subunit of phosphatidylinositol 3-kinase (PI3-kinase) with IRS-1, and activation of PI3-kinase] whereby insulin binding to its receptor stimulates, glucose transport.

integrins Heterodimeric molecules on the surface of leukocytes that mediate strong adhesion between cells, including adhesion between leukocytes and endothelial cells, which is necessary for proper trafficking. Integrins that are activated have increased affinity for their ligands, which are members of the immunoglobulin superfamily.

interferon A member of a family of species-specific vertebrate proteins, some of which are glycoproteins, that confer nonspecific resistance to a broad range of viral infections, affect cell proliferation, and modulate immune responses.

interferon-α A family of highly homologous species-specific interferons, the natural forms of which are derived primarily from either leukocytes or lymphoblastoid cells upon exposure to live or inactivated virus.

interferon-β An interferon produced primarily by fibroblasts in response to stimulation by live or inactivated viruses or by certain synthetic polynucleotides.

interferon γ A cytokine that is a member of the interferon/interleukin-10 family; it mediates a wide variety of cellular functions, particularly the enhancement of the microbicidal activity of macrophages.

interferon-τ A relatively new class of type I interferon that is not virus inducible but is constitutively produced by the trophectoderm of the ruminant conceptus during a very short period in early pregnancy. This interferon displays high antiviral and antiproliferative activities with a prominent lack of cytotoxicity *in vitro* and possibly *in vivo*.

interferon-ω An interferon first described in 1985 and now recognized as sufficiently distinct from IFN-α to deserve the separate ω-subtype status. It appears to possess comparable biologic activity to many Hu-IFN-αs but its particular function is not understood.

interleukin The generic description for a group of protein factors that affect primary cells; derived from macrophages and T cells that have been activated. A term meaning "between leukocytes"; originally coined to describe the first cytokines known to be involved in the regulation of the immune and inflammatory systems. (see the text for entries on specific interleukins.)

internalization Also termed sequestration; the loss of surface receptor number determined by a combination of the effects of endocytosis and recycling. A commonly used route for G-protein-coupled receptor internalization is via clathrin-coated pits.

intracellular receptors A family of related transcription factors, some of which have affinity for specific hormones. These proteins mediate a wide range of physiological processes and are directly responsible for the effect of retinoids, estrogens, glucocorticoids, progestins, androgens, and thiazolidinediones, among others.

intracellular signaling pathway The series of chemical and physical reactions within a cell following external stimuli that lead to the overall response of the cell.

intracrine Describing a mechanism of signaling in which a hormone produced by a cell is rapidly transported to the nucleus of that same cell where it exerts its effects.

intracytoplasmic sperm injection Fertilization of an oocyte by direct injection of a sperm into its cytoplasm.

intramembranous ossification Bone formation by direct transformation and ossification of condensed mesenchyme that occurs during development of flat bones, including the skull, mandible, scapula, and ileum.

intrinsic activity A term for the maximal response caused by a drug in a tissue preparation relative to the endogenous ligand or another reference compound, if the endogenous ligand is not known. A full agonist causes a maximal response and a partial agonist causes less than a maximal response. The terms "intrinsic activity" and "efficacy" are often used interchangeably, although efficacy requires both intrinsic activity and potency.

intrinsic efficacy The property of a molecule that changes the conformation of a receptor, leading to a functional response.

intrinsic osteoinductive activity Induction of bone formation by specific geometric configurations of biomimetic matrices in the absence of exogenously applied bone morphogenetic proteins/osteogenic proteins.

introns Intervening segments of DNA separating sequences that code for proteins; introns carry no protein-coding information.

invasive cytotrophoblasts Mononuclear trophoblasts that migrate into the uterine interstitium and vasculature.

inverse agonist A ligand with negative intrinsic efficacy; induces a functional response that is opposite to that of an agonist and decreases basal or constitutive receptor activity.

in vitro transcription The study of RNA synthesis from a DNA template in cell extracts.

ion channels Macromolecular pores in cell membranes; they play a central role in cell excitability, calcium signaling, and transport of small molecules. At rest, the channels remain closed, blocking ion entry into the cell. A group of voltage-gated channels can rapidly activate in response to a change in membrane potential, allowing ions to flow through the aqueous pore of the channel. The direction of ion flow is determined by an electrochemical gradient. After only a few milliseconds, or even as long as several hundred milliseconds, the channels inactivate and the flow of ions is again blocked.

ionotropic receptor A membrane receptor with an intrinsic ion channel.

islets of Langerhans Small clusters of neuroendocrine cells scattered throughout the pancreas, consisting of alpha, beta, delta, and gamma cells that produce the hormones glucagon, insulin, somatostatin, and pancreatic polypeptide, respectively.

isoflavones A subgroup of phytoestrogens derived from legumes, e.g., soybeans.

isomers Different compounds with the same molecular formula, but differing in the order in which their atoms are joined (structural isomers) or in the arrangement of their atoms in space (stereoisomers, diastereoisomers).

isostere A chemical equivalence in which an undesired chemical moiety is replaced by an atom or groups of atoms that retain the desired properties of the moiety being replaced.

isotype switching A process by which a B cell switches from production of an immunoglobulin isotype, such as IgM, to production of another isotype, such as IgA; accomplished by switching to the transcription of an alternative antibody heavy chain C region.

J

JAK see JANUS FAMILY KINASES.

Janus family kinases (JAKs) A family of protein tyrosine kinases that are activated by cytokines binding to their receptors. They function as second messengers, acting intracellularly to signal molecules in the cytoplasm and nucleus by catalyzing the phosphorylation of tyrosine residues on target molecules. Their best-characterized substrates are members of the signal transducers and activators of transcription family.

Janus kinase 2 A nonreceptor tyrosine kinase that associates with the growth hormone receptor and is activated by growth hormone, leading to the initiation of multiple pathways of intracellular signal transduction.

Janus kinase/signal transducers and activators of transcription pathway(JAK/STAT pathway) The most typical signaling pathway activated by cytokine receptors. This involves a family of four tyrosine kinases designated "Janus" or "JAK" kinases (members are JAK1, JAK2, JAK3, and Tyk2). JAK2 is the main JAK involved in growth hormone and prolactin receptor signaling. Substrates of JAK tyrosine kinases include cytokine receptors and STAT factors. The eight members of the STAT protein family must interact with tyrosine-phosphorylated cytokine receptor complexes to be activated by tyrosine phosphorylation (by JAKs); they then migrate into the nucleus and transactivate cytokine target genes.

Janus tyrosine kinases see JANUS FAMILY KINASES.

juvenile hormone (JH) A major insect hormone family, a group of similar sesquiterpenoid molecules that facilitate retention of juvenile characteristics in larval and nymphal insects and thus prevent metamorphosis. The identical molecules function as gonadotropic hormones in the majority of adult insects by promoting the production of the yolk protein precursor, vitellogenin.

juxtacrine Describing a mode of cell-to-cell signaling mediated by interaction of a transmembrane growth factor on one cell with its receptor on another cell.

K

K$^+$ channels Multisubunit structures located in the plasma membrane that gate the flux of potassium into the cell. These include the so-called delayed inward rectifier channels that open to repolarize the cell after a contraction. Some of the genes for individual subunits are regulated by thyroid hormone.

Kallmann's syndrome A genetic disorder associated with an X chromosome deletion at Xp22.3, resulting in anosmia and hypogonadism due to failure of olfactory nerve ingrowth and GnRH neuronal migration during embryonic development.

Kennedy's disease (spinal bulbar muscular atrophy) A progressive degenerative neuromuscular disease of genetic origin resulting from expansion of a polyglutamine repeat in the androgen receptor gene.

keratinocytes A specialized type of epithelial cell that covers the body surfaces of mammals.

ketone bodies Any of three compounds that arise from acetyl coenzyme A and that may accumulate in excess amounts as a result of starvation, diabetes mellitus, or other defects in carbohydrate metabolism.

kinase Any protein that catalyzes phosphorylation (the transfer of a phosphate group from a donor to a substrate molecule).

kinins Small diuretic peptides that were first isolated as myotropins on the basis of their ability to stimulate muscle contractions and act synergistically with the corticotropin-releasing factor-like diuretic peptides.

knockout Describing a mouse or other animal with a gene that has been specifically inactivated (or "knocked out") so that the protein is no longer made.

kyphosis Enhanced curvature of the spine as seen from the side, or hunchback.

L

labyrinthine zone A murine placental complex of trophoblast, mesoderm, and vascular derivatives; functionally analogous to the floating chorionic villi in humans.

lactotrophs A class of anterior pituitary cells that produce prolactin. They constitute over one-third of all pituitary hormone-secreting cells. Lactotrophs are heterogeneous in structure and function and are normally subjected to inhibition by dopamine.

L cells Endocrine cells localized in the intestine; they produce and secrete GLP-1 and GLP-2 and are categorized as "open" cells because the apical microvilli are in contact with the intestinal lumen.

LDLp Low-density lipophorin (density approximately 1.04 g/ml), the adipokinetic hormone-induced form of lipoprotein in the hemolymph of insects.

leptin A cytokine-like peptide composed of 146 amino acids, mainly secreted by adipocytes.

leucine-rich repeats Tandem repeats of a versatile protein–protein interaction domain that often consists of 24 residues with a consensus sequence, LxxLxxLxxLxLxxNxxxGxIPxx, where x represents any amino acid.

leukemia inhibitory factor A pleiotropic cytokine that was originally identified as a factor that inhibits leukemic cells and exhibits many biological activities, e.g., induction of monocytic differentiation of the murine leukemic cell line M1, suppression of differentiation of pluripotent embryonic stem cells, and inhibition of adipogenesis.

leukemia inhibitory factor receptor A signal-transducing receptor component; closely related to gp130 and binds leukemia inhibitory factor with nanomolar affinity.

leukocyte Any kind of white blood cell, divided into two main subgroups: phagocytes and lymphocytes. Phagocytes, which include neutrophils, monocytes, eosinophils, and dendritic cells, directly engulf microbes and other particulate matter. Lymphocytes, which include T cells and B cells, attack targets either directly, in the case of cytotoxic T cells, or indirectly, in the case of plasma cells, a terminally differentiated B cell specialized to produce antibodies.

leukotrienes Eicosanoids that are the products of the lipoxygenase pathway.

Leydig cells Somatic cells of the testes secreting testosterone after stimulation by luteinizing hormone or chorionic gonadotropin.

LH see LUTEINIZING HORMONE.

LH surge A midcycle surge of pituitary luteinization hormone initiating the ovulatory cascade.

ligand A molecule that binds specifically to another molecule, i.e., a target molecule or a receptor. The binding between the ligand and its target molecule is usually not covalent and does not usually result in a chemical alteration of the ligand. However, the interaction triggers changes in the target molecule that lead to changes in function in the target cells.

ligand agonist A small molecule that upon binding to the receptor induces a conformation in the ligand-binding domain that results in activation of transcription, leading to an increase in gene expression.

ligand antagonist A small molecule that upon binding to the receptor induces a conformation in the ligand-binding domain that results in an inhibition of transcription activation by agonists, leading to a decrease in gene expression.

ligand-binding domains Large C-terminal domains that are well conserved among members of the nuclear hormone receptor superfamily. Composed of several α-helices, these domains are involved in hormone binding, dimerization, and activation of hormone-dependent transcription.

ligand inverse agonist A small molecule that upon binding to the receptor induces a conformation in the ligand-binding domain that results in an inhibition of the basal ligand-independent activity of the receptor, leading to a decrease in gene expression.

lignans A subgroup of phytoestrogens found in vegetables, fruits, nuts, and seeds.

linkage The association between two genes that are located near each other on the same chromosome and that as a result tend to be inherited together.

lipophorin The abundant and generally single lipoprotein particle in insect hemolymph. The density of lipophorin (lipid-bearing protein) is similar to that of human high-density lipoprotein (HDL); for the insect lipophorin, HDLp is used to distinguish it from HDL.

lipopolysaccharide One of a group of related compounds released when the cell walls of gram-negative bacteria are degraded. Also known as endotoxin, lipopolysaccharide is a potent stimulator of the immune system and the vasculature, acting on the specific receptors (toll-like receptor 4) on B cells, macrophages, and endothelial cells.

lipoxins Eicosanoids that are the products of the 5- and 15-lipoxygenase pathways.

lipoxygenase An enzyme that catalyzes the formation of leukotrienes, hepoxilins, and lipoxilins from arachidonic acid.

local regulation Autocrine, paracrine, or juxtacrine regulation of cells by growth factors or cytokines made locally within a tissue.

locus The position in a chromosome of a particular gene or allele.

long-term potentiation A cellular model of learning and memory that uses stereotyped *in vitro* or *in vivo* stimulation of defined neural pathways to elicit long-term increases in synaptic strength; thought to be a general model for how brain synapses are altered by experience and learning.

losartan A nonpeptidic, selective antagonist of the AT_1 receptor subtype; widely used to block cardiovascular effects of angiotensin II.

loss-of-function mutations Gene alterations that reduce or abolish receptor activity; result in impaired ligand–receptor interaction. Such mutations in thyroid-stimulating hormone receptor produce resistance to TSH, which, when severe, causes hypothyroidism. Such mutations in thyroid hormone receptor produce resistance to thyroid hormone.

low-density lipoprotein (LDL) A molecule that is a mixture of lipid and protein, characterized as having a density of $1.019–1.063$ g/cm^3 and a particle size of $180–250$ Å.

low-density lipoprotein receptor A specific receptor for low-density lipoproteins; the first identified member of a large receptor family.

low-density lipoprotein receptor-related protein A receptor that binds many different ligands, including low-density lipoproteins; a member of the low-density lipoprotein receptor family.

lumenal Facing the interior of a cell or the interior cavity (lumen) of an organ; e.g., a releasing factor may be secreted directly into the intestinal lumen where it acts on the lumenal side of gut hormone cells localized in the intestinal epithelium.

luteal peptide/protein production The synthesis and secretion of nonsteroid hormones, notably inhibin A and relaxin, by the primate corpus luteum.

luteal phase The approximately 2-week-long stage of the human menstrual cycle, after ovulation has occurred, during which the corpus luteum produces progesterone and inhibin A.

luteal–placental shift The transfer of critical hormonal functions from the corpus luteum to the placenta during gestation; thereafter, the corpus luteum is not essential for maintaining intrauterine pregnancy.

luteal steroidogenesis The synthesis and secretion of steroid hormones, notably progesterone and estrogens, by the primate corpus luteum.

luteinization The ovulatory-related process of formation of the corpus luteum from the ovulatory follicle. The corpus luteum comprises luteal and nonluteal cell types. The luteal cells differentiate from the theca and granulosa cells and have the capacity to produce steroids and peptide hormones.

luteinizing hormone (LH) A pituitary polypeptide hormone that promotes ovarian steroidogenesis and triggers ovulation.

luteolysis The processes whereby the corpus luteum regresses near the end of the nonfertile menstrual cycle or, presumably, after the luteal–placental shift in early pregnancy.

luteolytic factors Putative local substances, such as prostaglandin $F_{2\alpha}$, that cause regression of the corpus luteum.

luteotropic hormones Blood-borne factors, particularly luteinizing hormone from the pituitary gland and chorionic gonadotropin from the placenta, that promote the structure and function of the primate corpus luteum.

luteotropin Any substance that stimulates the function of the corpus luteum.

lymphangiogenesis Growth of lymphatic vessels.

lymphatic system An open-ended network of vessels that collect fluid from tissue spaces and ultimately drain it into the venous system.

lymphedema Swelling of tissue due to accumulation of lymphatic fluid.

lymphocytes White blood cells that bear variable cell surface antigen receptors. The two main classes of lymphocytes, B lymphocytes (B cells) and T lymphocytes (T cells), mediate humoral and cell-mediated immunity, respectively.

lymphokines Soluble proteins (generally 12–30 kDa) produced by various lymphocyte populations following their stimulation by an antigen or another mode of cell activation.

lymphotoxin The closest paralogue of TNFα, but produced by different cells; also referred to as LTα and as TNFβ; important for normal immune development and function.

M

macrophage A term for leukocytes that reside in tissues and have innate and immune host defense functions.

macrophage colony-stimulating factor A hematopoietic cytokine responsible for regulation of monocyte/macrophage production and osteoclast function.

MafA A transcription factor of the Maf family originally described in chick eye development; contains a basic leucine-zipper-type DNA-binding domain and binds to and activates through the insulin promoter C1 element.

major histocompatability complex (MHC) A set of genetic regions and encoded antigenic proteins that present intracellular peptides to T-cells. MHC molecules are also involved in antigen processing and host defense.

major proglucagon-derived fragment The C-terminal half of the proglucagon molecule containing the glucagon-like hormones glucagon-like polypeptide-1 and glucagon-like polypeptide-2.

male pseudo-hermaphroditism A condition in which the gonads are testes but the genital ducts and/or external genitalia are incompletely masculinized, caused by defective masculinization of the male embryo. Can result from defects of testicular androgen synthesis or defects in androgen action.

Malpighian tubules Blind-ended hollow tubules that function as the insect "kidneys," forming an isosmotic primary urine by cation secretion.

MAP kinase A family of mitogen-activated protein kinases that phosphorylate proteins on serine or threonine residues.

mast cells Large cells containing granules that store a variety of mediator molecules, including histamine. They have high-affinity IgE receptors, which can trigger degranulation and play a crucial role in allergies.

matrix vesicles Extracellular organelles produced by chondrocytes that are sites for initiation of calcification and also contain matrix-processing enzymes.

median eminence The neural tissue at the base of the medial hypothalamus that contains neurovascular junctions, from which releasing factors, such as gonadotropin-releasing hormone, are secreted into the hypothalamic–hypophyseal portal vessels.

median neurosecretory cells (MNC) Insect cells functionally analogous to the vertebrate hypothalamus, the MNC have axon endings in the corpora cardiaca.

megalin A multifunctional, transmembrane clearance receptor of the low-density lipoprotein family that mediates the uptake and lysosomal degradation of numerous ligands, particularly in renal proximal tubular cells.

meiosis A specialized cell division program completed during the formation of haploid gametes.

melanocortins Peptide hormones (e.g., α- and γ-melanocyte-stimulating hormones and adrenocorticotropic hormone) derived from the precursor protein proopiomelanocortin. Following their release, melanocortins mediate intercellular signaling by binding and regulating one or more of the four known melanocortin receptors on the surface of target cells.

membrane vitamin D receptor A newly hypothesized membrane receptor of as-yet unknown structure that seems to mediate some actions of $1,25(OH)_2D_3$ through well-known membrane receptor-induced signal transduction pathways.

memory B/T cells B or T cells (or their descendants) that have been activated by their cognate antigen and undergone phenotypic changes resulting in a lower activation threshold and the capability to migrate into peripheral tissues in addition to (or rather than) secondary lymphoid organs.

menarche The time of first menstrual bleeding.

Mendelian ratio The ratio of progeny with particular phenotypes or genotypes that is expected in accordance with Mendelian law.

menstruation The process whereby the functional layer of the endometrium is shed, accompanied by bleeding at the end of each nonpregnant cycle.

meristem A group of undifferentiated and proliferating cells that continuously give rise to all plant organs and tissues throughout the plant life cycle.

mesangial cell A contractile cell of the glomerular mesangium, which is a thin membrane that helps support the capillary loops in a renal glomerulus. Vasopressin stimulates contraction of these cells and stimulates their growth in cell culture.

mesenchyme Embryonic tissue from which are formed the connective tissues, blood, and lymphatic vessels.

metabolic syndrome A term for a condition defined by insulin resistance, hyperinsulinemia, and dyslipidemia (generally elevated serum triglycerides and decreased high-density lipoprotein cholesterol).

metamorphosis Changes in form from the immature to the sexually mature stage in the life cycle of an organism. The change varies in degree with evolutionary lineage of the orders from primitive to more highly evolved: very little change (ametabolous); some change (incomplete or hemimetabolous); extreme change (complete or holometabolous).

methyl farnesoate (MF) A sesquiterpenoid compound that is a member of the insect family of juvenile hormones (JH). MF has been detected in crustaceans and may function as their JH.

methyltransferases Enzymes that promote methylation of substrates.

mevalonic acid pathway A biosynthetic pathway present in all organisms. It involves a group of enzymes responsible for the production of mevalonate, which is the universal intermediate in terpene metabolism.

microsomes Closed vesicles formed during fragmentation of the endoplasmic reticulum membrane system in eukaryotic cells, i.e., cells having the nucleus separated from the cytoplasm by a nuclear membrane and the genetic material borne on a number of chromosomes.

microvilli Finger-like extensions along the apical surface of intestinal mucosal cells. On enterocytes, microvilli increase the absorptive surface of the cell; on endocrine cells, microvilli allow potential stimuli greater exposure to their targets (e.g., receptors).

midgut The organ for digestion and absorption of food in insects that also has important roles in water balance, nutrient metabolism, and detoxification.

migrating motor complex A repetitive pattern of contractile activity that begins in the stomach and moves caudally throughout the small intestine during the interdigestive period. This pattern of activity is also known as the migrating myoelectric complex and the interdigestive housekeeper.

milieu intérieur Claude Bernard's term for the internal environment of the body, or the "soil" in which all biologic reactions occur.

mineralocorticoid One of the main steroid hormones synthesized by the adrenal cortex. Its function is focused on the regulation of electrolyte balance through stimulation of renal sodium retention. Aldosterone is the principal circulating mineralocorticoid.

mineralocorticoid receptor A protein with a ligand-binding site for specific ligands, in this case, those related to aldosterone, which is the primary ligand in the human. The receptor is not ubiquitously distributed throughout the body, like the glucocorticoid receptor, but is found mainly in epithelial cells that line lumens (tubes).

miniglucagon A product of proteolytic cleavage of glucagon by endopeptidase; of uncertain physiological significance, despite its greater biological potency.

missense mutation A change in the DNA sequence that alters a codon so that it codes for a different amino acid.

mitochondria Oval-shaped subcellular organelles in eukaryotic organisms that are responsible for producing ATP, the immediately available energy store.

mitogen A substance that induces an increase in cell proliferation, usually by stimulating DNA, RNA, and protein synthesis.

mitogen-activated protein kinase (MAPK) pathway (cascade) One of the major pathways activated by membrane receptors. It involves a cascade of serine/threonine and dual-specificity (Tyr/Ser/Thr) kinases, leading to the activation of several target genes. The MAPK pathway has been historically linked to cell proliferation, but recent data have shown that it is involved in many cell responses and crosstalk with other pathways, including the Janus kinase/signal transducers and activators of transcription pathway. Activation of the MAPK cascade by prolactin and growth hormone receptors involves Box 1 but not the phosphotyrosines of the receptor.

mitosis Cell division that produces daughter cells with the same DNA content as the parental cell. The process begins after DNA replication and involves four phases as follows: (1) prophase, which is subdivided into stages describing chromosome morphology; (2) metaphase, when condensed chromosomes are aligned; (3) anaphase, when chromatids separate to opposite poles; and (4) telophase, which is followed by nuclear and cytoplasmic division.

modulators Small-molecule drugs that mimic endogenous steroids by binding to intracellular steroid hormone receptors, but on binding allow only a subset of the molecular, cellular, and physiological responses that would be induced by the native steroid hormone to occur, thus effecting a desired pharmaceutical outcome.

molting In insects, the process of shedding the exoskeleton between developmental stages. This process is also called ecdysis or eclosion.

mononuclear phagocytic lineage A term used to describe the lineage of the colony-stimulating factor-1-responsive hematopoietic precursor of macrophage → monoblast → promonocyte → monocyte → macrophage. Mononuclear phagocytes generally include tissue macrophages, microglia, Kupffer cells, Langerhans cells, synovial type A cells, and osteoclasts. These cells are derived from common hematopoietic precursors and their differentiation is regulated by CSF-1.

monooxygenases A class of enzymes (catalysts) also called "mixed-function oxygenases" because one atom of oxygen appears in the reaction product and the other in water. The majority of hydroxylases, including the steroid hydroxylases, belong to this class of enzymes.

motilide A macrolide antibiotic that acts as a motilin receptor agonist at subantibiotic doses and mimics the physiological and pharmacological effects of motilin.

α-MSH, β-MSH, γ-MSH α-, β-, and γ-Melanocyte-stimulating hormones, collectively called the melanocortins. These peptides are thought to stimulate pigmentation and may be involved in appetite and feeding behavior.

Müllerian ducts Paired ducts, formed of epithelial cells surrounded by mesenchymal cells, present in male and female embryos before sexual differentiation. Also known as paramesonephric ducts. In the male fetus, they degenerate under AMH action; in the female fetus, they give rise to the Fallopian tubes, the uterus, and the upper third of the vagina.

Müllerian inhibitory substance (MIS) A member of the transforming growth factor-β superfamily.

mucosa The innermost layer of the gastrointestinal tract that is in intimate contact with lumenal contents. This layer is composed of epithelial cells with interspersed enteric endocrine cells.

multiple hormone resistance syndrome A rare syndrome characterized by partial resistance to several steroid hormones, including glucocorticoids, mineralocorticoids, and androgens; may be caused by a defect in a co-activator molecule that is shared by multiple steroid receptor pathways.

mutation A change in the DNA sequence of a gene.

myenteric plexus Also known as Auerbach's plexus; a system of nerves and ganglia lying within the longitudinal and circular muscle layers of the intestine. Nerves of the myenteric plexus innervate numerous targets, including the myenteric externa, mucosa, and sympathetic prevertebral ganglia.

myoepithelial cells Contractile cells surrounding the milk-secreting glands in the lactating mammary gland.

myometrium Contractile, muscular tissue of the uterus.

myosins Proteins that are part of the contractile fibers found in myocytes. The genes for myosin heavy chain α (MHCα) and myosin heavy chain β (MHCβ) are regulated by thyroid hormone in some species. In rodents, MHCα is predominant in the adult heart and MHCβ can be strongly induced by hypothyroidism.

myositis Inflammation of muscle.

N

naive B/T cells Mature B or T cells that have never been activated by their cognate antigen. Naive cells can migrate only into secondary lymphoid organs and have a higher threshold for activation than memory cells.

NaPi Sodium–phosphate co-transporters that mediate the movement of extracellular phosphate into cells driven by the existing Na^+ gradient. To date, three different families, named types I, II, and III, have been identified.

nasal (olfactory) placode Thickening of nasal ectoderm bilaterally; the precursor of the olfactory and vomeronasal epithelia.

natriuresis Stimulated sodium excretion by the kidney.

natural killer cells (NKcells) White blood cells (leukocytes) that can nonspecifically kill virally and bacterially infected cells and tumor cells.

N cells Enteroendocrine cells localized to the intestine; they produce and secrete neurotensin and neurotensin-related peptides; categorized as "open" cells, in which the apical microvilli are in contact with the intestinal lumen.

N/C interaction Interaction between the NH_2-terminal and carboxyl-terminal (N/C) regions of the androgen receptor that is selectively induced by the binding of a biologically active androgen, testosterone or dihydrotestosterone. This interaction is mediated by FXXLF- and WXXLF-binding motifs in the NH_2-terminal region and activation function 2 in the ligand-binding domain.

NCX Na^+–Ca^{2+} exchanger present in the plasma membrane and the kidney; it is primarily responsible for the basolateral extrusion of Ca^{2+} in the distal tubular cells.

necrolytic migratory erythema The characteristic rash seen in glucogonoma syndrome, consisting of macules and papules in the lower extremities, perineum, and perioral areas, which blister, leaving central erosions and necrosis. They are often pruritic and painful.

negative feedback The inhibition of the action or function of a factor, cell, or organ by another factor or hormone. This type of system is often described as a feedback loop because of its autoregulatory nature.

nerve growth factor (NGF) The first neurotrophin to have been identified in the 1950s. It was purified on the basis of its ability to elicit neurite outgrowth from ganglionic explants. The extraordinary and unexplained abundance of NGF in the adult male mouse submandibular gland was a prerequisite for its early characterization.

nestin An intermediate neurofilament found in proliferating neural precursor cells. Nestin mRNA and protein are temporarily expressed in developing GnRH neurons.

neural cell adhesion molecule A large cell surface glycoprotein along which neurons may migrate.

neural network A group of interconnected neurons and associated glial cells that perform a specific brain function.

neuroD1 A bHLH protein present in neurons and islet cells; heterodimerizes with ubiquitous bHLH proteins, binds to the E elements in the insulin promoter, and stimulates insulin gene transcription.

neuroendocrine Describing the regulation by neural factors reaching the anterior pituitary gland via the portal vessels.

neurohemal organs Sites of neuronal terminals specialized for release of neurohormones into the hemolymph (circulating body fluid in insects).

neurohormones Hormones produced by neurons and released into the hypophyseal portal system in the median eminence of the hypothalamus for transport to the pituitary gland to stimulate or inhibit the release of hormones; for example, gonadotropin-releasing hormone stimulates gonadotropin secretion from pituitary gonadotrophs.

neurohypophyseal Describing neuronal projections from the supraoptic and paraventricular hypothalamic nuclei to the posterior pituitary gland.

neurohypophysis The posterior (neural) and intermediate lobes of the mammalian pituitary gland.

neuromedin N A hexapeptide that is encoded on the same gene as neurotensin and has a similar distribution pattern.

neuropeptide Y A hormone thought to increase food intake; a 36-residue neuropeptide hormone with considerable homology to pancreatic polypeptide.

neurophilic neuronal migration Movement of neurons that occurs via the preferential adherence of the neurons to the surface of apposing axons.

neurosecretion A process in which peptides, produced by cells of the nervous system, regulate numerous functions. Some act locally, diffusing to target organs through local extracellular space (paracrine), and others circulate in the body fluid to act at distant target organs (neuroendocrine or humoral).

neurotensin A tridecapeptide that is found in the brain and gastrointestinal tract.

neurotransmitter A chemical messenger found in and released from particular nerve cells that possess the protein machinery necessary for its biosynthesis, reuptake and degradation; interacts with a distinct set of plasma membrane-bound proteins called receptors to produce an electrochemical signal associated with cell-to-cell communication. Synonym neuromodulator.

neurotrophic factor Any one of several hormonal substances that provide tropic support for neurons by interacting with cell surface receptors and stimulating the metabolic and transcriptional responses required for

maintenance of viability, differentiation, and other activities.

neurotrophin One of a family of growth factors that includes nerve growth factor, brain-derived neurotrophic factor, neurotrophin-3, neurotrophin-4/5 (NT-4/5), neurotrophin-6, and neurotrophin-7. All have been shown to have growth- or survival-promoting actions on subpopulations of peripheral or central nervous system neurons.

neutral antagonist A ligand with no intrinsic efficacy; binds to the receptor without inducing a functional response on its own and blocks functional responses mediated by agonists.

neutropenia A reduction in the normal circulating numbers of neutrophilic granulocytes from $4000-10,000/\mu l$ to $1000/\mu l$ or less. The reduction can be due to genetic diseases (congenital neutropenias) or to the myelotoxic effects of chemotherapeutic drugs.

NGF (nerve growth factor) A neurotrophic factor that promotes a wide range of responses in its target cells. These include neuronal differentiation, maintenance of survival, and regulation of metabolic activity.

nitric oxide A molecule composed of one atom of oxygen and one atom of nitrogen, with the chemical formula NO, which chemically is a free radical. NO is one of the body's many hormones; it is unique in that it is the only animal hormone that is a gas.

nongenomic Describing a process independent of RNA transcription.

nonsense-mediated decay The process whereby cells degrade mRNAs containing premature stop codons to prevent the synthesis of truncated proteins.

nonsense mutation Change in the DNA sequence that results in a codon that specifies an amino acid being replaced by a stop codon (codon that terminates protein synthesis).

nonsteroidal anti-inflammatory drugs (NSAIDs) A class of drugs that inhibit the formation of prostanoids. NSAIDs are used in clinic mainly for the treatment of fever and pain.

nuclear co-factor A protein that enables a transcription factor to modify nucleosomal structure and/or gene transcription.

nuclear factor κB A pro-inflammatory transcription factor that is responsible for the activation of many inflammatory genes.

nuclear localization sequence A consensus sequence that is short, is single or bipartite, and contains clusters of basic amino acids. It functions as a nuclear-targeting motif.

nuclear receptors A class of transcription factors that regulate gene expression in response to binding of small molecules called ligands. The ligand-bound receptor can activate or repress gene expression by binding to specific DNA-response elements. In the absence of ligand, these receptors generally repress gene transcription.

nuclear receptor superfamily An evolutionarily conserved family of ligand-dependent transcription factors that includes the steroid, vitamin D, retinoic acid, and thyroid hormone receptors.

nucleotide The hydrolysis product of a nucleic acid, consisting of a purine or pyrimidine base combined with a ribose or deoxyribose sugar and a phosphate group; a phosphate ester of a nucleoside.

O

ob mouse A leptin-defective mouse model of obesity.

octadecanoid pathway A signaling pathway in many plants; it regulates a variety of cell-specific responses and is initiated by release of linolenic acid from membranes, in response to specific signals. Free linolenic acid is converted to jasmonic acid, a second messenger that activates genes, via several enzymes that cumulatively comprise this pathway.

octreotide A commonly used eight-residue peptidyl analogue of SS14 with a long biological half-life and efficacy as an agonist at SSTR2 and SSTR5.

Olf-1 A transcription factor that is expressed in cells, including developing GnRH cells, in the olfactory epithelium.

oligomenorrhea A menstrual cycle pattern consisting of fewer menstrual periods within a given time, typically fewer than nine menstrual periods in 12 months.

oligozoospermia A count of 3 million sperm/ml in the ejaculate.

oncogene A gene that can cause or contribute to cancerous growth or other unregulated cell proliferation.

oocyte A developing egg cell.

oocyte retrieval A procedure for recovering oocytes by follicular aspiration using a needle guided by transvaginal ultrasound.

oral hyperglycemic agents Drugs that can be taken by mouth to treat hyperglycemia.

orexigen A compound that stimulates or increases food intake.

organelle An intracellular, membrane-bounded compartment (e.g., mitochondrion, Golgi, lysosome, endoplasmic reticulum with membrane-bound ribosomes, nucleus) with specialized functions, reflecting division of labor within cells.

organification The oxidation of iodide and attachment to organic molecules such as thyroglobulin in the thyroid gland by thyroid peroxidase for iodine retention, storage, and hormone production.

organizational effect Early developmental process by which sex steroids exert an effect that causes permanent, hard-wired differences in the structure and function of the central nervous system.

organotypic culture An *in vitro* experimental tissue preparation in which the organization of the (brain) cells resembles their *in vivo* organization.

orthologues Peptides from a pair of genes in related species, derived from a single gene in the last common ancestor, which arose as a result of a speciation event; genes of different species that have a common origin. Orthologue assignments do not involve function.

osteoblast One of the cells responsible for bone formation, which derive from mesenchymal progenitors and synthesize bone matrix proteins containing type III collagen and other noncollagenous proteins such as osteocalcin, osteopontin, osteonectin, and bone sialoproteins.

osteoclast One of the large, multinucleated cells that are responsible for the resorption of bone in the cycle of bone turnover that comprises bone removal and bone formation. Osteoclasts are sensitive to CT, which rapidly and potently inhibits their bone-resorbing activity.

osteoclast differentiation factor (ODF) The factor responsible for osteoclast formation and activation, which belongs to the tumor necrosis factor (TNF) ligand family. ODF consists of 316 amino acid residues and is also called receptor activator of NF-κB ligand (RANKL).

osteomalacia A bone disease that occurs in adults as a result of vitamin D deficiency and that is caused by abnormal mineralization of the skeleton and weak bone that is prone to bend and fracture.

osteonecrosis A condition in which there is decreased blood supply to bones—usually weight-bearing bones near joints. It is also known as avascular necrosis.

osteoporosis A progressive systemic skeletal disease characterized by low bone mass and deterioration of bone tissue, causing increased bone fragility and susceptibility to fracture. It commonly occurs after menopause, after long periods of inactivity, and as a result of drug treatment, particularly with glucocorticoids.

osteoprotegerin (OPG) The decoy receptor of ODF/RANKL, which belongs to the TNF receptor family. OPG is also called osteoclastogenesis inhibitory factor (OCIF). OPG/OCIF is a soluble receptor having no membrane-associated domain.

ovarian hyperstimulation syndrome A potentially life-threatening condition that is triggered by superovulation treatment of women with polycystic ovaries.

ovulation The release of a fertilizable ovum from the graafian follicle. In its broader sense, the ovulatory response defines the cascade of events following the LH surge and including the resumption of meiosis and oocyte maturation, luteinization, and the rupture of the follicular wall.

ovulation rate The number of mature eggs released from the ovaries during one reproductive cycle.

ovulatory cascade A highly synchronized and exquisitely timed cascade of specific gene(s) expression to ensure the correct process of ovulation.

oxylipins Octadecanoid pathway products, including volatile six-carbon aldehydes (hexenal and hexenol), traumatin, cutin monomers, 12-oxo-dodecenoic acid, 9S,13S-12-oxo-phytodienoic acid, jasmonates, and methyl ester or amino acid conjugates of many of these. Oxylipins can function as signal molecules in plants and/or in attracting parasitic wasps.

oxyntic mucosa The acid-secreting portion of the stomach.

oxyntomodulin A 37-amino-acid peptide that is processed from proglucagon in the intestinal L-cells and in the brain, but not in the pancreatic A-cells.

oxytocin A polypeptide hormone closely related to vasopressin. Composed of 9 amino acids, oxytocin is synthesized in and released from neurosecretory cells in the hypothalamus of mammals; it promotes uterine contractions, salt excretion, and milk ejection.

P

P450 see CYTOCHROME P450.

pancreastatin A chromogranin A-derived peptide that inhibits secretion and impairs insulin action.

pancreatic islet see ISLETS OF LANGERHANS.

pancreatic polypeptide A 36-residue peptide hormone found predominantly in the pancreas.

pancreatitis Acute or chronic inflammation of the pancreas.

Paneth cells A specialized type of secretory cell located at the bottom of small intestine crypts of Lieberkühn.

paracrine Describing the relationship between a hormone-releasing cell and its target cell. Hormones that act in a paracrine manner are released from a cell into the extracellular space and act on adjacent target cells without reaching the general circulation.

paralogue Describing the duplication of a peptide gene, giving rise to two copies in the genome; this involves a duplication and not a speciation event.

paraneoplastic syndromes Clinical syndromes experienced by some cancer patients due to the production of hormones or other substances by a tumor. The symptoms of the syndrome depend upon the exact substance(s) produced.

parathyroid hormone (1–34) The N-terminal biologically active portion of parathyroid hormone, which is produced by the parathyroid glands and increases bone resorption and tubular reabsorption of calcium by the kidney.

paraventricular nucleus A collection of small (parvocellular) and large (magnocellular) neurons in the hypothalamus that contain the neurons of origin of the thyrotropin-releasing hormone tuberoinfundibular system.

parietal cells Acid-producing cells located in the gastric glands of the stomach.

partial agonist A ligand with intrinsic efficacy lower than that of the agonist. Partial agonists either activate the receptor, inducing a response, or block the response induced by an agonist.

pathogenesis-related proteins Several families of proteins that are expressed first in the inoculated and subsequently in the uninoculated leaves of plants resisting pathogen attack; due to the correlation between *PR* gene expression and development of hypersensitive response and systemic acquired resistance, increased *PR* expression is frequently used as a marker for these phenomena.

pattern alopecia The androgen-dependent thinning of hair that occurs progressively with advancing age in genetically susceptible men and women; the process is mainly the result of miniaturization of terminal to vellus hair follicles.

Pax6 Paired-homeodomain transcription factor; contains both paired domain and homeodomain DNA-binding motifs; present in all islet cells and binds to the C2 site in the insulin promoter and stimulates insulin gene transcription.

P-box A segment of the DNA-binding domain of nuclear receptors that is responsible for the specificity of DNA binding by the receptor protein.

PCR (polymerase chain reaction) A laboratory technique for exponentially amplifying the number of copies of a short segment of DNA.

PDGF (platelet-derived growth factor) A dimeric protein that acts as a mitogen for almost all mesenchymally derived cells.

PDX1 A para-hox class homeodomain transcription factor; present in duodenum and pancreas, with high-level expression in mature beta cells; binds to the A elements in the insulin promoter and stimulates insulin gene transcription.

PDZ domain An approximately 90-amino-acid segment with a distinctive three-dimensional shape that contains a binding cleft for protein interaction. The PDZ domain typically allows homologous and heterologous recruitment and assembly into larger protein complexes.

P-element A widely used transposable genetic element in *Drosophila* that is used to create transgenic animals and/or to mutate specific genes.

Pendrin (PDS gene product) An apical membrane iodide porter controlling iodide export from the thyrocyte into the follicular lumen.

peptide A compound formed by two or more amino acids, in which a carboxyl group of one is united with the amino group of another. Many hormones are peptides.

peptideYY A 36-residue peptide hormone found predominantly in the gut; it shows homology to both neuropeptide Y and pancreatic polypeptide.

peptidomimetic A nonpeptide structure designed to be recognized by a receptor and modeled by comparison to peptide structures.

peptidylglycine α-amidating monooxygenase An enzyme that synthesizes the amino-terminal amide group on neuropeptides through use of the nitrogen from the adjacent glycine residue.

peripheral tissues Extraglandular tissues, i.e., extratesticular and extra-adrenal tissues.

peroxisome A subcellular organelle in the cytoplasm of eukaryotic cells; involved in the β-oxidation of long-chain fatty acids.

pertussis toxin An A-B-type bacterial toxin produced by the bacterium *Bordetella pertussis;* catalyzes transfer of the ADP-ribose moiety of nicotinamide dinucleotide to the α-subunit of G-proteins of the $G_{i/o}$ subfamily, resulting in their inactivation.

pharmacokinetics The study of the kinetics of drugs in humans, animals, and *in vitro* test systems, including the processes of absorption, distribution, metabolism, and excretion.

pharmacophore A conceptualization of features, both steric and electronic, minimally required in a molecule in order to elicit some desired biological response.

phenotype The appearance or other characteristics of an organism, resulting from the interaction of its genetic constitution with the environment, as opposed to its underlying hereditary determinants, or genotype.

phenylbutyrate A butyrate derivative used in differentiation therapy.

phenylethanolamine N-methyltransferase An enzyme that catalyzes the final step in the catecholamine biosynthetic pathway, i.e., the N-methylation of noradrenaline to result in the synthesis of adrenaline.

pheromone A chemical (or blend of chemicals) that is released by an organism and that causes specific behavioral or physiological reaction(s) a in one or more individuals of the same species.

pheromone biosynthesis-activating neuropeptide A 33- or 34-amino-acid peptide produced in the brain that triggers pheromone production in many species of Lepidoptera.

PHEX A gene on the X chromosome that encodes a membrane-bound protein with endopeptidase activity; mutations have been found in the disease X-linked hypophosphatemia.

phosphatidylinositol 3-kinase (PI3-kinase) A kinase that directly binds to tyrosine kinase receptors (or to insulin substrate-1) via a SH2 domain in its p85 subunit. PI3-kinase converts phosphatidylinositol 4,5-biphosphate to phosphatidylinositol 3,4,5-triphosphate. The PI3-kinase signal transduction pathway mediates cell survival and proliferative responses to a variety of growth factors and insulin.

phosphodiesterases Cyclic nucleotidases that hydrolyze cAMP and cGMP.

phosphoinositide-dependent protein kinase-1 A protein kinase that is activated by phosphatidylinositol 3-kinase and in turn directly phosphorylates and enzymatically activates serum- and glucocorticoid-inducible protein kinase.

phosphoinositides A family of lipid molecules important in intracellular signaling. The minor membrane component, phosphatidylinositol 4,5-bisphosphate, is hydrolyzed by phospholipase C to yield inositol 1,4,5-trisphosphate and 1,2-diacylglycerol. The former compound is responsible for release of intracellular calcium stores, and the latter component functions with phosphatidylserine and often calcium to activate protein kinase C.

phospholamban A small 6 kDa protein that associates with SERCa2a and regulates the calcium pump activity dependent on the phospholamban phosphorylation status.

phospholipase C A member of the family of phospholipases responsible for the hydrolysis of phosphatidylinositol 4,5-bisphosphate to inositol 1,4,5-trisphosphate and diacylglycerol. Enzymatic activity of the phospholipase C-β isoform is regulated by subunits of the G-proteins.

phosphorylase kinase A regulatory enzyme that modifies the action of glycogen phosphorylase by phosphorylation.

phosphorylation The binding of a phosphate group onto a molecule.

phosphotransferase An enzyme that catalyzes the transfer of a phosphate group from one molecule to another.

phosphotyrosine phosphatase An enzyme that catalyzes the dephosphorylation of tyrosine residues from signaling molecules and thereby opposes the action of protein tyrosine kinases, which are key mediators of cellular responses such as proliferation and differentiation.

photochemical reaction A chemical reaction mediated or enhanced by some wavelength of light.

photoperiod Annual variation of daily changes in a physiological response that results from exposure of an organism to a natural light/dark cycle. Long photoperiodic responses are associated with longer days and shorter duration of the melatonin peak, because light inhibits melatonin synthesis.

phytoalexins Low molecular-weight compounds that exhibit antimicrobial activity.

phytoestrogen A plant compound with binding affinity for the estrogen receptor.

pilosebaceous unit A skin appendage consisting of a hair follicle, a hair shaft, and a sebaceous gland.

pineal gland An epndocrine gland (also called the pineal body) located in the center of the brain; main site of production of the hormone melatonin.

pituitary gland An endocrine organ located ventral to the hypothalamus and connected to it neurally and by a specialized vasculature called the hypophyseal portal system.

pituitary gonadotrope cells The cells in the anterior pituitary gland responsible for producing follicle-stimulating hormone and luteinizing hormone, which regulate the function of the gonad. The gonadotropes are one of the primary sites of action for inhibin.

plasticity Ability of a cell, cell body, or organelle (i.e., generally a system) to adapt to a changed environment.

pleiotropic Having more than one effect; through pleiotropism a single stimulus can often evoke several different cellular responses, often mediated by distinct intracellular messengers or pathways.

PMCA Plasma membrane Ca^{2+} ATPase that mediates the extrusion of Ca^{2+} across the basolateral membrane. To date, four different genes have been identified; PMCA1b is the predominant isoform expressed in the small intestine and the distal part of the nephron.

point mutation A change in one nucleotide in a DNA molecule.

polyadenylation A process by which a sequence of adenylic acid residues is added to the 3′-end of many eukaryotic mRNA molecules immediately after transcription.

polycystic ovary An ovary containing numerous antral follicles, which is associated with a clinical profile varying from regular ovulatory cycles to anovulation with virilization (polycystic ovary syndrome).

polycystic ovary syndrome A disease characterized by obesity, insulin resistance, ovarian dysfunction, and cutaneous symptoms.

polyhalogenated hydrocarbons Synthetic chemicals, chlorinated or brominated, such as polychlorinated biphenyls, dioxin, or polybrominated biphenyls.

polypeptide Describing hormones found ubiquitously in animals as two major classes: those synthesized in the endoplasmic reticulum, processed through the secretory pathway, stored in vesicles, and released in response to an appropriate signal, and those synthesized in the secretory pathway, anchored to membranes with the hormone domain in the extracellular space, and released by proteolysis in response to an appropriate signal. Polypeptide hormones have been identified only recently in plants, and their mode of synthesis, storage, and release is poorly understood.

polyphenism The occurrence of several distinct phenotypes or forms in a given species, each of which develops facultatively in response to some cue from the internal or external environment; sequential polyphenism occurs in the metamorphosis of insects (larval, pupal, and adult forms).

polyprotein prohormone A hormone precursor that is posttranslationally processed into multiple active peptide hormones.

portal vessels A venous system connecting the capillary loops formed by the superior hypophyseal artery in the median eminence of the hypothalamus with the sinusoids of the anterior pituitary gland.

posterior pituitary lobe (gland) A region of the pituitary that houses vasopressin- and oxytocin-containing axon terminals, fenestrated capillaries, and a large population of astrocyte-like cells, the pituicytes. Developmentally, a downgrowth from the hypothalamus of the brain.

posttranslational modifications Changes in the structure of a protein hormone that include glycosylation, phosphorylation, and cleavage. These modifications affect hormone binding to the receptor or clearance from the circulation and thus alter its biological properties.

potency The dose or concentration of a drug required to produce an effect. The relative potencies of two or more ligands are determined from the ratio of concentrations or doses required to produce the same effect. By convention, EC_{50}/ED_{50}, or the concentrations/doses producing a 50% of maximum effect, are usually compared.

POU-homeodomain-1 Transcription factor-1, previously known as pituitary transcription factor-1; responsible for development of pituitary cell lines (somatotroph, lactotrophs, and thyrotrophs).

PP cell One of four endocrine cell types in pancreatic islets where pancreatic polypeptide is located. Also known as the F cell.

PP-fold The U-shaped structural fold assumed by members of the pancreatic polypeptide (PP) family (PP, peptide YY, and neuropeptide Y).

preantral follicle An oocyte surrounded by several layers of granulosa and theca cells. Includes all growing follicle stages after the primary follicle stage up to the formation of the antrum.

precursor processing The specific proteolytic cleavage of larger precursor proteins to release biologically active peptides or proteins, e.g., insulin from proinsulin.

pregnenolone sulfate A neurosteroid that modulates glutamate channel activity.

preprohormone The entire polypeptide encoded by an mRNA for a peptide hormone or hormones before processing by prohormone convertase enzymes to remove signal sequences and other nonfunctional regions.

prepro structures (zymogens) Precursor forms of proteins that are exported from the cell by removal of the pre sequence (to initiate transfer into the endoplasmic reticulum) and then the pro peptide, to yield the active mature protein. Such structures are common for hormones and hydrolases, for example.

primary follicle An opocyte surrounded by one clearly visible cuboidal-shaped layer of granulosa cells and a thin layer of theca cells.

primary lymphoid organs Sites of lymphocyte development and maturation. In humans, these are the bone marrow (B cells, NK cells) and thymus (T cells).

primary oocyte An oocyte in the process of undergoing the first meiotic division, arrested in meiotic prophase.

primary spongiosum A region of trabecular bone forming the interface between the growth plate and bone marrow and the site for neovascularization and osteoblast invasion during endochondral ossification.

primordial follicle The first stage of follicle development, consisting of the oocyte surrounded by a thin layer of granulosa cells.

proconvertase enzymes Proteolytic enzymes of the subtilisin/kexin-like family that participate in the conversion of peptide precursors to their final biologically active forms by cleaving at the C-terminal basic amino acids.

progesterone One of the two major ovarian steroid hormones upon which implantation depends.

progesterone receptor A nuclear transcription factor that binds the steroid hormone progesterone and modulates progesterone-mediated transcription of hormone-regulated genes such as STAT5A.

proglucagon A 160-amino-acid peptide processed in a tissue-specific manner. In the pancreatic alpha cells, proglucagon is processed to glucagon, whereas in intestinal endocrine L cells, proglucagon is processed to several biologically active peptides, including glucagon-like peptide-1 and glucagon-like peptide-2.

prohormone A precursor (either peptide or steroid) to an active hormone that is produced in significant amounts as an intermediate in the pathway of production of the active hormone.

prohormone convertase A class of proteolytic enzymes responsible for cleaving proopioimelanocortin into biologically active peptides.

proinsulin The precursor of insulin; it has less than 5% of the biological activity of insulin. Proinsulin is processed to mature, active insulin by limited proteolysis.

prolactin (PRL) A polypeptide hormone (199 amino acids in humans) that adopts a four-α-helix-bundle fold typical of hematopoietic cytokines. PRL is secreted mainly by the pituitary gland, although it is also produced by other cell types and tissues, such as mammary gland, endometrium, lymphoid cells, and prostate. Its actions are essentially related to reproduction and lactation, but its involvement in an extremely wide spectrum of biological responses has been reported.

prolactinomas Nonmalignant tumors of the anterior pituitary that are composed of lactotrophs and result in hyperprolactinemia or abnormally high serum prolactin levels. They usually develop from a single cell (monoclonal) but their etiology is unclear.

prolactin promoter A DNA sequence that is used to regulate the transcription of the prolactin gene. The pituitary proximal promoter is located immediately 5′ upstream of the transcription initiation site, whereas the extrapituitary superdistal promoter is located 5.8 kb further upstream.

promoter The region of a gene that directs regulation of transcription of its specific mRNA.

proopioimelanocortin A prohormone expressed in the neuroendocrine system.

prostaglandins Cyclic, unsaturated fatty acids derived from arachidonic acid, a phospholipid that is an integral component of the cell membrane. Inflammatory stimuli induce the rapid release of arachidonic acid, which is converted to prostaglandins, prostacyclin, and thromboxanes by cyclooxygenase (COX) enzyme activity.

prostate-specific antigen (PSA) A protein that serves as a tumor marker for prostate cancer; elevated concentrations in the bloodstream may indicate the presence of prostate cancer.

prosystemin The precursor of a systemin.

proteasome A large protein complex responsible for degrading proteins that have typically been modified by ubiquitination.

protein kinase An enzyme that adds a phosphate group to a target, usually as a means to control the activity of the target.

protein kinase A A serine/threonine protein kinase, also denoted as cyclic adenosine monophosphate (cAMP)-dependent protein kinase, containing two regulatory (R) and two catalytic (C) subunits.

protein kinase C A family of serine/threonine protein kinases that are activated by Ca^{2+} and/or phospholipids in response to extracellular signals. Kinases phosphorylate their substrates, generally promoting activation.

protein phosphatase An enzyme that removes a phosphate group from a protein by hydrolysis.

proteinuria Elevated urinary protein as a result of renal dysfunction.

prothoracic glands Paired organs in the prothorax (region between the head and thorax) of insects, which are the major site of ecdysteroid synthesis in insect larvae.

prothoracicostatic peptide A peptide hormone that acts on the prothoracic glands and inhibits ecdysone secretion.

prothoracicotropic hormone A neuropeptide hormone that is secreted in the insect brain and stimulates the prothoracic glands to secrete ecdysone.

pseudo-fracture A thickening of periosteum or bone surface and formation of new bone over what appears to be a fracture on X ray. It is usually found at the site of a pulsating artery and may result from softening of bone and arterial pulsation.

pseudo-hermaphroditism A condition in which an individual has sexual organs of only one sex but has either genital openings or external tissue exhibiting one or more traits of the opposite sex.

psoriasis Hyperproliferative skin disorder with infiltrating lymphocytes and neutrophils in the epidermis and dermis.

pulmonary neuroendocrine cells Airway epithelial cells that secrete a variety of neuropeptides, growth factors, and amines; may also be involved in oxygen sensing.

pulsatile neurosecretion Rhythmic releases of neurohormone pulses from neurovascular junctions in the median eminence into the hypothalamic–hypophyseal portal vessels.

pulse generator A process, possibly modulated by feedback, that governs the resulting, variable-pulse time-release pattern for a pulsatile secreting gland.

R

racemic Denoting a mixture of optically active compounds (enantiomers), with the mixture itself being optically inactive because it is composed of equal amounts of all the enantiomers; a single enantiomer is optically active because it rotates the plane of a beam of plane-polarized light passing through it.

radioimmunoassay A solution-based assay for the competition and separation of unlabeled and radioactive isotope-labeled molecules bound to specific antibodies that allows for the identification and quantification of the molecules in tissue extracts and chromatography fractions.

raloxifene A selective estrogen receptor modulator that is an agonist for bone and, unlike estrogen, is an antagonist for uterine and breast tissue.

receptor A protein molecule that binds very specifically to its cognate hormone; binding generates a receptor–hormone complex that initiates a cellular signal transduction process, resulting in one or more biological responses.

receptor isoforms Variants of a receptor.

receptor-mediated endocytosis Cellular entry of an agonist via a specialized region of the cell where receptor molecules, capable of specifically binding hormones, are localized.

receptor-mediated system A physiological system (e.g., a hormonal axis) whose linkages are interconnected via receptor mechanisms (interface functions).

receptor recycling Movement of a receptor from an internal compartment to the cell surface.

receptor serine/threonine kinase A cell surface protein that can catalyze the phosphorylation of serine or threonine residues in target proteins.

receptor tyrosine kinases A superfamily of plasma-membrane-bound glycoproteins that specifically bind hormones and growth factors, leading to activation of their intracellular tyrosine kinase domains and thus inducing any of several signaling cascades, usually by sequential activation of other kinases.

recessive allele An allele that is not expressed in the phenotype of a heterozygote, due to the presence of the dominant allele.

Recommended Dietary Allowance (RDA) Recommendations for the amounts of various dietary nutrients (e.g., vitamins and minerals) required to maintain human health.

recruitment The process wherein a follicle departs from the resting pool to begin a well-characterized pattern of growth and development. Recruitment, although obligatory, does not guarantee ovulation. Stated differently, recruitment is necessary but not sufficient for ovulation to occur.

redox state Ratio of total reducing equivalents (NADH, GSH, etc.) to their oxidized form (NAD, GSSG, etc.).

red pigment concentrating hormone Peptide hormone from the eyestalk of crustaceans, a member of the adipokinetic hormone/red pigment-concentrating hormone family that comprises structurally related but functionally diverse peptides.

5α-reductase Enzyme responsible for the conversion of testosterone to 5α-dihydrotestosterone.

5β-reductase A cytosolic enzyme that reduces a 4,5 double bond with the formation of a *cis*-bond between cycles A and B.

regulatory element A stretch of DNA sequence in the promoter region of genes that when bound by a specific transcription factor results in the regulation of gene transcription.

regulatory peptide A peptide that is released in response to a stimulus and that exerts specific biological actions. It may function as an autocrine, paracrine, or endocrine agonist or antagonist.

releasing and inhibiting hormones Polypeptides or small molecule neurotransmitters that are released from the terminals of hypothalamic neurosecretory cells; these hormones are transported from the median eminence via the hypophysial portal vasculature to the anterior pituitary, where they act to stimulate or inhibit the release of specific adenohypophysial hormones.

releasing factor A small peptide/protein produced in the gastrointestinal tract and/or pancreas that stimulates the secretion of gut hormones; levels of these releasing factors in the gut lumen may be regulated, in part, by degradation from pancreatic enzymes.

renin A proteolytic enzyme that is released by the kidney in response to a drop in blood pressure, sympathetic nerve activity, or decreased sodium excretion; generates angiotensin I in the circulation by cleaving the 10 N-terminal amino acids of a large a_2-globulin produced by the liver, angiotensinogen.

renin–angiotensin–aldosterone system The primary mechanism by which blood pressure and volume are maintained; prolonged activation of this system is associated with deleterious outcomes in patients with congestive heart failure and hypertension.

response element A short region of DNA that is bound by a transcription factor and the deletion or addition of which affects the transcription of genes containing such elements. For nuclear hormone receptors, most response elements consist of two 6 bp half-sites that have variable spacing and orientation with respect to each other.

retinoid Any of a number of small molecules that can bind to and regulate the activity of the nuclear hormone retinoic acid receptor.

retinoid X receptor A member of the steroid receptor gene family that functions as a heterodimeric DNA-binding partner for the vitamin D receptor.

retrograde menstruation The flow of menstrual effluent via the fallopian tubes into the peritoneal cavity.

reverse transcriptase-polymerase chain reaction A method through which RNA is transcribed into complementary DNA and then the amounts of a specific cDNA are amplified in an exponential manner to enable detection. This approach can be used to determine the mRNAs expressed by single neurons.

rexinoids Any of a number of small molecules that can bind to and regulate the activity of the nuclear hormone retinoid X receptor.

RGS proteins A newly discovered family of proteins that are regulators of G-protein signaling.

rheumatoid arthritis An atoimmune inflammatory disorder, affecting joints and other tissues, in which TNF is inappropriately produced and contributes to disease.

rickets A bone disease in infants and children characterized by a reduction of bone calcium content that results from a dietary deficiency of vitamin D or lack of adequate exposure to sunlight.

ring gland An endocrine gland in the higher Diptera (flies) that encircles the foregut and that is composed of fused corpora allata, corpora cardiaca (which release neuropeptides), and prothoracic glands (which secrete ecdysteroids).

RNA editing The process of making posttranscriptional changes in the RNA sequence by enzymatic mechanisms; in a classic example, this process is involved in the formation of different forms of the glutamate receptor.

S

salicylate hydroxylase An enzyme encoded by the bacterial *nahG* gene; converts salicylic acid into catechol, a compound that does not induce defense responses.

salmon calcitonin A hormone produced by the parafollicular C cells of the thyroid gland; it inhibits osteoclastic bone resorption and tubular reabsorption of calcium by the kidney. Salmon calcitonin has a different structure than human calcitonin and is more potent.

sarcoplasmic-endoplasmic reticulum calcium ATPase pump (SERCA pump) The predominant active Ca^{2+} transport molecule responsible for concentrating Ca^{2+} in the sarcoplasmic and endoplasmic reticulum.

sarcoplasmic reticulum A membranous organelle system of muscle cells, composed of vesicular and tubular components, that stores calcium ions involved in muscle contraction.

scaffold protein A protein capable of binding to multiple signaling components, thereby providing a platform to relay signals and achieve specificity of communication among components.

scoliosis A lateral curvature of the spine.

seasonal rhythm Endogenous rhythm synchronized to the time of the year by the natural change in the length of the daily light phase.

sebaceous gland A small sacculated organ within the dermis; composed of acini, which are attached to a common excretory duct that is continuous with the wall of the piliary canal and, indirectly, with the surface of the epidermis.

secondary complications Adverse effects on many structures and organs in the body resulting from chronic diabetes.

secondary lymphoid organs Sites of primary stimulation of B and T cells by specific antigen. These include, among others, lymph nodes, spleen, and Peyer's patches.

second messenger A small molecule that is formed in or released into the cytosol in response to an extracellular signal; helps to relay the signal to the interior of the cell; e.g., cyclic AMP, inositol 1,4,5-triphosphate, diacylglycerol, or Ca^{2+} and other stimuli.

secretory granules Granules that contain insulin crystals made up of zinc–insulin hexamers. Beta cells contain ~ 9000 secretory granules. Upon stimulation, their contents are released by exocytosis.

seedling triple response An ethylene-dependent phenotype found in dark-grown seedlings characterized by exaggerated apical hook formation, shortening and thickening of the hypocotyl and root, and proliferation of root hairs.

selection The final winnowing of the maturing follicular cohort by atresia down to a size equal to the species-specific ovulatory quota.

selective estrogen receptor modulators (SERMs) Natural or synthetic ligands that exhibit either estrogen agonist or antagonist activity among different cells and tissues. Most likely, this is due to the differential expression of cell- and tissue-specific factors, such as co-activator and co-repressor proteins.

selective serotonin reuptake inhibitors (SSRIs) Widely used anti-depressants that enhance serotonin availability at synaptic sites thought to be altered in patients with eating disorders.

serine protease inhibitors (SERPINs) A superfamily of proteins that undergo a relaxed/stressed transition state on binding with serine protease to form an inactive complex. The subgroup including corticosteroid-binding globulin, α1-anti-trypsin, and α1-antichymotrypsin derives from a common ancestral gene by gene duplication.

Sertoli cells Somatic cells of the testes that form the seminiferous tubules where the germ cells giving rise to the gametes are embedded. The tissue surrounding the seminiferous tubules is called interstitial tissue and contains Leydig cells.

serum- and glucocorticoid-inducible protein kinase Protein kinase that is regulated by hormones and other extracellular signals at three distinct levels of cellular control and is a unique point of cross talk in hormone signaling cascades.

sesquiterpene A class of hydrocarbon compounds having a 15-carbon skeleton, built from five-carbon (isoprene) units that are linked head to tail or in rings; many contain oxygen.

severe oligozoospermia A count of ≤ 1 million sperm/ml in the ejaculate.

sex hormone-binding globulin (SHBG) A protein made in the liver that binds certain steroids with high affinity, making them less available for uptake by tissues compared to albumin-bound or free (bioavailable) steroids. The binding affinity of SHBG is highest for dihydrotestosterone and testosterone but less for estradiol.

sexual determination Gonadal development via genetically determined pathways.

sexual differentiation The developmental process by which the two sexes become different.

sexual dimorphism Sex difference in brain structure or function.

SH2 domain Src homology domain; a protein domain common to many cytoplasmic signal transduction molecules; interacts specifically with a linear epitope containing a phosphorylated tyrosine residue as part of defined consensus sequences.

SH3-binding motif A consensus motif, PXXP, where P denotes proline and X denotes an unspecified amino acid. The motif is recognized by Src homology (SH) domains of *Src* and other nonreceptor tyrosine kinases, permitting the SH domain to bind to SH-binding motifs.

SH3 domain Src tyrosine kinase homology domain 3; a conserved regulatory region of many signaling molecules that interacts with other proteins.

signal peptide An additional peptide sequence of 12–30 amino acids, having a hydrophobic central stretch of 8–12 strongly hydrophobic amino acids, usually located at or near the N-terminus of a nascent secreted protein, that serves as a signal for its segregative transfer into the secretory pathway. The signal peptide is then removed by the signal peptidase when this function has been completed.

signal transducers and activators of transcription (STATs) A family of latent cytoplasmic transcription factors whose members contain an SH2 domain, are activated by phosphorylation at a single carboxy-terminal region tyrosine residue in response to cytokine or growth factor receptor stimulation, and when activated, dimerize and translocate to the nucleus where they induce transcription of specific target genes.

signal transduction A set of events taking place in a cell in response to extracellular stimuli, including input reception, intracellular transmission of the information from the membrane to the nucleus, and integration of concomitant signals, resulting in production of a suitable biological response.

signal transduction pathway A series of molecules activating one another through physical contacts and/or enzymatic modifications, leading to a specific effect, such as cell growth, survival, or migration.

signaling crosstalk see CROSSTALK.

signaling molecule An extracellular or intracellular molecule that cues the response of a cell to the stimulus of other cells.

single-nucleotide polymorphism Single-nucleotide differences in the DNA sequence identified when sequences from multiple individuals are compared.

sinus gland/X-organ complex A neurosecretory complex in the eyestalk of decapod crustaceans. Several important peptide hormones are produced and released by this complex.

Smads A group of intracellular proteins that mediate signaling by members of the TGF-β superfamily. They are vertebrate homologues of *Drosophila* Mad (mother against *dpp*) and *Caenorhabditis elegans* Sma. They include receptor-mediated Smads that are phosphorylated and activated by type I receptors, common Smads that form complexes with receptor-mediated Smads, and inhibitory Smads that antagonize signaling by members of the TGF-β superfamily.

SOCS Suppressor of cytokine synthesis; inhibitory molecules that bind to receptor docking sites, preventing Stat activation and inhibiting signal transduction.

sodium/potassium ATPase A physiological membrane-associated protein that pumps two potassium ions into the cell and three sodium ions out of the cell for every adenosine triphosphate that is split to form adenosine diphosphate and inorganic phosphate.

somatic cells A collective term for all cells of the body except the germ cells. In the testis, the somatic cells include the Sertoli cells, peritubular myoid cells, Leydig cells, and macrophages.

somatic mutation An induced or spontaneous genetic alteration in a differentiated cell that is not transmitted to the next generation.

somatostatin A 14- or 28-amino-acid peptide, found in the hypothalamus and elsewhere, that inhibits pituitary secretion of growth hormone and, to a lesser degree, other pituitary hormones, such as thyroid-stimulating hormone. The prototype is SS14, or somatotropin release-inhibiting factor, so named for one of its biological activities, inhibition of the secretion of pituitary growth hormone.

somatotrope (somatotroph) A secretory cell type in the anterior pituitary that is the major site for synthesis and secretion of growth hormone.

somatotropin release-inhibiting factor see SOMATOSTATIN.

spermatids Haploid germ cells that undergo differentiation from an early, rounded form to a mature, elongated form.

spermatocytes Tetraploid germ cells that undergo two meiotic divisions, yielding haploid spermatids.

spermatogenesis The process by which undifferentiated male germ cells form into mature spermatozoa.

spermatogonia Diploid germ cells that divide and differentiate; the most immature germ cell type.

sphincter of Oddi A muscular region surrounding the distal ends of the common bile duct and pancreatic duct as they enter the duodenum. When constricted, this sphincter prevents flow of bile and pancreatic juice into the duodenum and restricts reflux of duodenal contents back into the bile and pancreatic ducts.

splanchnic glucose uptake The amount of glucose taken up by the splanchnic tissues (liver plus gastrointestinal tissues) during the postabsorptive state and/or following glucose ingestion. The great majority (~ 80–90%) of splanchnic glucose uptake occurs in the liver.

spongiotrophoblast Anm intermediate layer in the murine placenta that, like the trophoblast giant cells, arises from the ectoplacental cone; with the giant cell layer, separates the labyrinthine zone from the maternal decidua.

Src homology 2 (SH2) domains Protein segments able to recognize and bind to phosphorylated tyrosines. They are present in several intracellular proteins acting as signal transducers.

stage of exhaustion The third and final stage of the General Adaptation Syndrome (see), during which the ability to adapt to stress is exhausted and death often ensues.

stage of resistance The second stage of the General Adaptation Syndrome (see), during which the body's resistance to stress is maximized.

Stat Kinase signaling molecules downstream of Jak; involved in IL-10R signal transduction and activation of transcription.

stem cell A primitive cell that has an unlimited capacity to divide and that can differentiate into different functional cell types.

stem cell transplantation The transfer of stem cells, classically hematopoietic stem cells, from either another organism or the same organism to a recipient animal to reconstitute an entire multilineage cellular system.

stereological Describing methodology that allows structural information (for instance, estimation of cell number) to be derived from sections of a structure.

steroid (hormone) One of a family of lipid structures related to the parent substance, cholesterol, which is modified by enzymes in certain tissues that synthesize highly active products with hormonal functions, such as estrogen and progesterone in ovary, testosterone in testis, and cortisol in the adrenal cortex.

steroid 5α-reductase An enzyme complex that converts testosterone to 5α-dihydrotestosterone. It has two isoforms that have different biochemical properties and tissue distribution.

steroid biosynthesis Synthetic pathways that start with cholesterol; defined enzymatic steps produce the final products, glucocorticoids, mineralocorticoids, and sex steroids. Intermediate products may induce distinct hormonal actions, as is seen in enzymatic pathway defects that lead to abnormal hormonal profiles and defined disorders in humanz.

steroid hormone receptor family Subfamily of nuclear receptors consisting of the receptors for androgens, glucocorticoids, estrogens, mineralocorticoids, and progesterone.

steroidogenesis The production and secretion of steroids from cholesterol precursors, occurring in tissues such as the ovaries and testes. The process can occur only in cells that contain the steroidogenic acute regulatory protein, a transport protein that brings the cholesterol ester to the inner mitochondrial membrane for modification, and specific cytochrome P450 enzymes, which are located in the mitochondria and endoplasmic reticulum. The enzymes contain heme and reduce molecular oxygen, incorporating one atom specifically into the substrate as a hydroxyl group.

steroidogenic acute regulatory protein (StAR protein) see STEROIDOGENESIS.

steroidogenic enzymes A family of enzymes, many of which belong to the P450 gene family, that catalyze the synthesis and metabolism of the sex steroid hormones, estrogens, androgens, and progestogens.

steroidogenic factor 1 An orphan nuclear receptor that plays a key role in controlling the transcription of the *StAR* gene.

steroid or nuclear receptor gene family A large family of eukaryotic genes whose protein products both function as receptors for steroid and thyroid hormones, retinoic acid, and 1,25-dihydroxyvitamin D_3 and modulate transcription.

steroid receptor co-activators A family of proteins of 160,000 molecular weight (p160); interact with transcriptional activation domains of nuclear hormone receptors and act as bridging factors between the DNA-bound receptor and the general transcriptional machinery.

sterols Compounds having three 6-sided carbon rings, one 5-sided carbon ring, and a side chain, e.g., cholesterol.

stomata Small openings located in the epidermal layers of plants allowing uptake of CO_2 and loss of water. Stomata are surrounded by two guard cells that control the pore size.

stress An internal or external condition that presents a physiological challenge to the body's state of homeostasis (equilibrium).

stressor Hans Selye's term for any stimulus that produces a state of stress.

stress response The ability of cells to survive or to undergo apoptosis in response to environmental stress conditions, such as changes in osmolarity, nutrient deprivation, or extreme temperatures. Generally considered to be initiated by receptor-mediated events.

subesophageal ganglion A large nerve center consisting of the fused ganglia of the original mandibular, maxillary, and labial segments, situated in the head, beneath the esophagus.

submucosal plexus A network of nerves and small ganglia found in the submucosa of the intestine. It is composed of outer and inner layers and transmits secretomotor and vasodilator stimuli to the mucosa. Primary sensory nerves are contained in this plexus, which also communicates with the myenteric plexus.

substrate A molecule that will be altered by the actions of an enzyme.

subtilisin-like proprotein convertases The seven-member family (in mammals) of precursor-processing endoproteolytic enzymes that are all derived in evolution from the bacterial serine protease subtilisin; function in the secretory pathway of most of the body's cells to process a wide variety of protein precursors.

sulfhydryl group A chemical group (thiol, -SH) containing sulfur and hydrogen found in cysteine, glutathione, and other molecules.

suppressor of cytokine signaling (SOCS) A recently identified family of proteins that play an important role in regulating the Janus kinase/signal transducers and activators of transcription (JAK/STAT) pathway. They are currently viewed as negative regulators of this pathway, either by interfering with Janus kinase activity or by competing with STATs for binding to phosphorylated tyrosines of the receptor complex.

suprachiasmatic nucleus (SCN) Hypothalamic nuclei; the major endogenous pacemaker of circadian rhythms in mammals, i.e., the endogenous circadian clock.

supraoptic and paraventricular nuclei Clusters of neurons in the mammalian hypothalamus with axons that project to the neurohypophysis; they synthesize vasopressin and oxytocin.

sympathetic nervous system A division of the autonomic nervous system (see) that mediates responses to stress, e.g., increased heart rate, blood pressure, and energy mobilization.

synaptic plasticity A general term for a variety of alterations in synapses, both strengthening and weakening; may involve alterations in neurotransmitter receptors, neurotransmitter release, or propensity for activation of intracellular second messengers.

syncytiotrophoblasts Multinucleate trophoblasts that line the surface of floating villi.

synergism The action of two or more hormones to achieve a response that each hormone is incapable of achieving individually.

systemic acquired resistance A self-defense mechanism induced by pathogen infection that initiates the systemic production of pathogenesis-related proteins, leading to broad resistance against pathogens.

systemins Polypeptide plant hormones that are released following attack (wounding) by insects and pathogens; they regulate activation of defense-related genes.

T

target cell A type of cell in which a specific hormone exerts its actions (e.g., the prostate is a classic androgen target tissue).

target genes Genes that can be regulated by a specific hormone because their promoters contain regulatory elements that can interact with the hormone's receptor.

TATA-, CAAT-, GC-boxes Sequences present in the promoter region of eukaryotic genes that recognize and bind ubiquitous transcription factors and allow transcription by RNA polymerase II.

T cells/B cells Lymphocytes in general are divided into T and B cells. Subgroups of T cells exhibit diverse activities including production of cytokines, mediation of delayed-type hypersensitivity, regulation of on-going immune responses, cytotoxic functions, and "help" for the activation of B cells. T cells interact with APCs via an antigen-binding molecule, the T-cell receptor (TCR). The general T-cell population has TCRs for all the antigens that they would encounter in an individual's lifetime. B cells produce antibodies. The B-cell surface receptor molecule is an antibody and when it binds to its specific antigen, activated B cells secrete antibodies of the same specificity.

T-cell selection The process that T-cells undergo during cell proliferation that eliminates potentially self-reactive cells and favors the survival of those cells that can recognize foreign antigens.

T-cell-stimulating factor Originally identified by Hermann and Rude as a factor promoting T-cell function, survival, and cluster formation; subsequently identified as being identical to interleukin-12.

T-DNA activation tagging A novel mutagenesis method utilizing transferred DNA (T-DNA). T-DNA is derived from *Agrobacterium tumefaciens* and is used to introduce multiple copies of a viral transcriptional enhancer element randomly into a plant genome, resulting in transcriptional activation of a plant gene that is near the introduced T-DNA.

terminal nerve A ganglionated cranial nerve that is in part embedded within the olfactory nerves in the nasal area, enters the brain caudal to the olfactory bulbs, and has projections to the septal and preoptic areas of the brain.

testosterone Male sex hormone (androgen) secreted by interstitial Leydig cells of the testis; responsible for triggering development of sperm and secondary sexual characteristics.

testosterone esters The compounds that result from esterfication of testosterone at the 17β-hydroxy position. Two common, clinically used testosterone esters include testosterone enanthate and testosterone cypionate.

tethering Physical interaction between two different transcription factors, forming a heteromeric complex independent of DNA binding. Tethering may also occur on the DNA at the point where one of the transcription factors is attached. This interaction often leads to a mutual repression of the transcriptional ability of either of the factors.

3α,5α-tetrahydrocorticosterone A neurosteroid that modulates GABA$_A$ channel activity.

3α,5α-tetrahydroprogesterone (allopregnanolone) A neurosteroid that modulates GABA$_A$ channel activity.

tetramer A polymer that is assembled from four identical monomers.

TGF see TRANSFORMING GROWTH FACTOR.

TGF-β superfamily A group of more than 30 structurally related dimeric proteins involved in diverse processes, including cell growth, differentiation, homeostasis, and hormone secretion.

Th1/Th2 see T HELPER CELL.

thalamus A deep brain structure involved in processing and transmitting peripheral sensory information to the cerebral cortex. The lateral geniculate nucleus of thalamus receives visual input from the retina and transmits it to the visual cortex in the occipital lobe.

theca cells Hormone-producing somatic cells differentiated into a vascularized interna and externa layer, recruited from the stroma to lie around the basal lamina outside the granulosa layer.

T helper cell A white blood cell (lymphocyte) defined by expression of CD4 (CD4$^+$) on the cell surface and that is capable of expressing a specific T-cell receptor. T helper 1 cells are defined by their ability to express IFN-γ, whereas T helper 2 cells are defined by their lack of expression of IFN-γ and expression of interleukin-4.

thermogenesis The physiological generation of heat.

Thiry–Vella fistula Loop of intestine with ends exteriorized through the abdominal wall; allows easy access to intestinal contents. The loop retains its blood and neural supply through intact mesentery.

thromboembolic events Blood clots in the venous system leading to pulmonary embolism and possibly death.

thyrocytes The cells from the thyroid gland that produce thyroid hormones.

thyroglobulin The primary protein synthesized by thyrocytes; it is both the precursor of thyroid hormone formation and a feedback regulator controlling thyroid-stimulating hormone receptor signaling.

thyroid follicle Structural component of the thyroid, composed of thyrocytes that surround a central lumen and whose function and growth are controlled by thyroid-stimulating hormone receptor signaling.

thyroid hormone Triiodothyronine (T3) or thyroxine (T4); secreted by the thyroid gland and converted by peripheral deiodination.

thyroid hormone receptor Nuclear receptor for triiodothyronine (T3, the active form of thyroid hormone). The two thyroid hormone receptor genes, α and β, are located on human chromosomes 17 (q21–q22) and 3 (p22–p24.1), respectively. Various splicing arrangements of these genes result in several isoforms of both α and β.

thyroid hormone response elements Discrete enhancer sequences in the promoters of target genes to which thyroid hormones bind and regulate transcription.

thyroid peroxidase The enzyme catalyzing the iodination of thyroglobulin and catalyzing the coupling of iodotyrosine residues to form thyroid hormones, whose activity is controlled by thyroid-stimulating hormone receptor signaling.

thyroid-stimulating hormone (TSH) see THYROTROPIN.

thyroid transcription factor-1 Thyroid-restricted transcription factor controlling thyroid-specific gene expression, whose levels and activity are controlled by thyroid-stimulating hormone receptor signaling.

thyroid transcription factor-2 Thyroid-restricted transcription factor controlling thyroid-specific gene expression, whose levels and activity are controlled by insulin signaling but which influences thyroid-stimulating hormone receptor signaling.

thyrotoxicosis Clinical condition due to overactivity of the thyroid gland and excess thyroid hormone production characterized by rapid heart rate, elevated basal metabolism, goiter, exophthalmia, nervous symptoms, and weight loss.

thyrotrophs Cells from the anterior pituitary that secrete thyrotropin.

thyrotropin (thyroid-stimulating hormone) The pituitary hormone that stimulates the thyroid gland to produce thyroxine and triiodothyronine.

thyrotropin-releasing hormone (TRH) A tripeptide amide originally isolated from the hypothalamus and expressed in many extrahypothalamic brain nuclei, especially the medulla. Hypothalamic TRH regulates thyroid function by releasing pituitary thyrotropin hormone, whereas medullary TRH regulates autonomic function by acting as an excitatory neurotransmitter on autonomic regulatory neurons.

Toll-like receptors Primary sensors of the innate immune system; named after the *Toll* gene found in *Drosophila*, they provide essential signals for TNF production under conditions of infection.

trabecular bone Interior network of organized calcified spongy bone, the space between which contains bone marrow and communicates with the marrow cavity.

trans-acting factors Transcription factors (specific proteins) that bind to relatively short DNA sequence motifs, or cis-acting elements, to regulate gene transcription. The cis-acting elements can occur in various locations and at different distances and directions relative to the transcriptional start and stop sites within the gene.

transactivation The ability of a factor, e.g., the glucocorticoid receptor, to induce gene expression.

transcription The formation of a nucleic acid molecule using another molecule as a template, particularly the synthesis of an RNA using a DNA template.

transcriptional activation domain A region of steroid receptors that binds co-activators and mediates transcriptional enhancement activity.

transcriptional crosstalk The crosstalk of two signaling pathways converging on a gene promoter.

transcription factor A protein that regulates the transcription of a gene by interacting with DNA regulatory elements, directly or indirectly.

transfection The introduction of new genetic material into a cell.

transforming growth factor-α (TGF-α) A growth factor closely related to EGF (epidermal growth factor). TGF-α is often expressed in neoplastic tissue together with gastrin, and TGF-α (or EGF) stimulates gastrin gene transcription.

transforming growth factor-β (TGF-β) A cytokine capable of regulating cell growth, extracellular matrix protein synthesis, and immune cell functions. The first isolated member of a family of factors controlling the growth, differentiation, and death of most tissues in invertebrates and vertebrates.

transforming growth factor-β superfamily A group of more than 30 structurally related dimeric proteins involved in diverse processes, including cell growth, differentiation, homeostasis, and hormone secretion.

transgenic Describing animals that are generated by insertion of new DNA into the germ line via DNA microinjection into the one-cell-stage embryo.

transgenic adenocarcinoma of the prostate (TRAMP) mouse A transgenic mouse model of prostate cancer.

transgenic mice Mice with heritable, engineered manipulations of the genome. These mice can have genes introduced for ectopic expression or can have endogenous genes or sequences altered. When the expression of an endogenous gene is completely abrogated, mice homozygous for the null allele are called knockout mice.

translation The processing of information coded in messenger RNA to form amino acid sequences; results in cytoplasmic peptide and protein synthesis.

translocation The process of movement within a cell; usually the movement of a subcellular molecule or organelle from one site to another.

transmembrane domain The segment of a membrane protein that passes through the membrane. The transmembrane domain is often composed of an abundance of lipid-preferring (hydrophobic) amino acids that form an α-helix.

transrepression The ability of a factor, e.g., the glucocorticoid receptor, to suppress gene expression.

transsynaptic The mode of communication between neurons, which convey information to one another via chemical signals released into specialized points of contact known as synapses.

tritrophic interactions Relationships involving species at three different trophic levels within an ecosystem. In the case of jasmonates, these interactions involve wounded plants, herbivorous insect larvae, and parasitic wasps.

trophoblast cells Progenitor cells, important in the formation of the placenta and responsible for various functions, including nutrition of the differentiating embryo and the growing fetus and secretion of hormones indispensable for the maintenance of pregnancy.

trophoblast giant cells Polyploid mouse trophoblast cells that surround the conceptus and lie in direct contact with the maternal decidua.

tropical spastic paraparesis/human T-cell lymphotropic virus I (HTLV-I)-associated myelopathy A demyelinating neurological disease that is caused by the retrovirus HTLV-I and that is associated with progressive weakness and bowel and bladder dysfunction.

tropism A growth response that is directionally oriented with respect to the stimulus.

tropomyosin receptor kinases (Trks) A small group of closely related tyrosine kinase membrane receptors that are activated by neurotrophin binding. Trk was first recognized as an oncogene made up of the kinase domain of Trk fused with a portion of *tropomyosin*. The proto-oncogene was later found to be a nerve growth factor receptor.

tuberoinfundibular system The collection of neurons in the brain and their axon trajectory that terminate in the neural–hemal contact zone of the hypothalamic median eminence.

tumor necrosis factor (TNF) Proinflammatory cytokine mediator essential for normal immune development and function; the factor first discovered to be produced primarily by macrophages, also referred to as TNFα and as TNF.

two-component regulator (system) A protein–sensor system commonly found in bacteria, yeast, and plants that serves to detect changes in specific environmental stimuli.

type1, type 2 diabetes see DIABETES.

tyrosine hydroxylase The enzyme that catalyzes the oxidation of tyrosine to dihydroxyphenylalanine; it is the rate-limiting enzyme in the catecholamine synthetic pathway in the adrenal medulla.

tyrosine kinases A group of transmembrane proteins with tyrosine-specific phosphorylating activity. The extracellular domain of receptor tyrosine kinases serves as a receptor for agonists, such as growth factors and hormones. The binding of a specific ligand to the extracellular domain of the receptors turns on the kinase activity of their catalytic domain, which is located on the cytoplasmic side of the membrane. Nonreceptor tyrosine kinases lack an extracellular binding domain, and they are activated by phosphorylation of their tyrosine residues.

U

ubiquitin A small protein that becomes covalently linked to lysine residues in other intracellular proteins. This reaction is catalyzed by ubiquitin ligases. Ubiquitinylated proteins are usually degraded in the proteasome.

ultraspiracle The insect homologue of vertebrate retinoid X receptor, an obligatory partner of the ecdysone receptor.

upstream Describing events that control and/or initiate subsequent events in a regulatory pathway.

USP A nuclear receptor that is the protein product of the *ultraspiracle* gene.

V

vagovagal reflex Signal transmitted through afferent vagal fibers to the dorsal vagal complex and then back to an abdominal target through efferent vagal fibers.

vagus nerve The 10th cranial nerve that emerges from the brainstem and passes through the neck and thorax to the abdomen, innervating visceral organs including the heart, lungs, and digestive organs; it plays a major role in the parasympathetic regulation of gut functions.

vascular endothelial growth factor A protein acting on endothelial cells to induce vascular leakage; it is of critical importance for vasculogenesis and angiogenesis.

vascular permeability factor Another name for vascular endothelial growth factor.

vasculogenesis Establishment of the vascular system during embryonic development.

vasopressin A polypeptide hormone composed of 9 amino acids. Synthesized and released from neurosecretory cells in the hypothalamus of mammals, vasopressin increases blood pressure and promotes water reabsorption from the kidneys.

VDR see VITAMIN D RECEPTOR.

VDR knockout mice A mouse strain in which the vitamin D receptor has been inactivated, mimicking the autosomal recessive disorder hypocalcemic vitamin D-resistant rickets.

vellus hair Thin, short, usually nonpigmented hair.

vitamin Any of a group of essential organic substances provided in trace amounts in food components to effect the normal function of a cellular metabolic process.

vitamin D A vitamin/hormone with a central role in calcium and bone metabolism; it can be absorbed from the diet or can be synthesized by the skin via stimulation by ultraviolet light. Deficiency of vitamin D leads to a disorder known as rickets or osteomalacia.

vitamin D analogues Chemically modified molecules derived from $1,25(OH)_2D_3$. Modifications have been made throughout the molecule, to obtain analogues with the desired properties. More than 1000 different vitamin D analogues have been synthesized worldwide.

vitamin D-binding protein An abundant serum protein of the albumin family that functions to bind and solubilize vitamin D sterols for transport to target tissues and for storage; it is also an extracellular G-actin-binding and sequestration protein.

vitamin D receptor (VDR) A member of the superfamily of nuclear receptors for steroid hormones, thyroid hormone, and retinoic acid. The VDR functions as a $1,25(OH)_2D_3$-activated transcription factor that ultimately influences the rate of RNA polymerase II-mediated transcription. VDRs are present not only in cells typically involved in calcium and bone metabolism, but also in other cell types, such as cells of the immune system.

vitamin D-response element A specific DNA-binding site for the vitamin D receptor that is located within the promoter region of a gene that is regulated by 1,25-dihydroxyvitamin D_3.

vitellin A storage form of the major yolk protein.

vitellogenesis A major stage during egg maturation in egg-laying animals during which yolk protein precursors are synthesized and accumulate in developing oocytes.

vitellogenin A precursor form of the major yolk protein vitellin.

vivipary The ability of a plant embryo to bypass dormancy and proceed directly from embryogenesis to germination if rescued from the normal dehydration that occurs during seed maturation.

vomeronasal organ A chemosensory organ that sends projections to the accessory olfactory bulbs and transmits pheromone-related stimuli to the brain.

W

Wnt/calcium pathway A proposed noncanonical pathway, best described in frog and fish embryos.

X

xenograft A tumor maintained in host animals.

xyloglugan endotransglycosylase A cell-wall-modifying enzyme that cleaves xyloglucan polymers internally and then religates the newly generated ends to other xyloglucan ends.

Y

yolk protein Major yolk protein in flies.

Y-organ Paired glands of ectodermally derived cells that produce ecdysteroids.

Z

zinc-finger A motif of amino acids with a characteristic spacing of cysteines that may be involved in binding zinc and that is also characteristic of some proteins that bind DNA.

zona pellucida A layer of highly glycosylated proteins regulated by the oocyte Fig α gene; it forms the unique surface coat of the oocyte and is traversed by extensions of cumulus cells that form gap junctions with the oocyte.

INDEX

Volume numbers are boldfaced, separated from the first page reference with a colon. Subsequent references to the same material are separated by commas.

A

AA, *see* Arachidonic acid
AADC, *see* Aromatic L-amino acid decarboxylase
AASs, *see* Androgenic anabolic steroids
ABA, *see* Abscisic acid
ABP, *see* Androgen-binding protein
Abscisic acid (ABA)
  degradation, **1:** 3
  discovery, **1:** 1
  functions
    germination and seedling growth inhibition, **1:** 4–5
    root and shoot growth control, **1:** 5
    seed maturation and dormancy, **1:** 4
    stomata closure during water stress, **1:** 2–4
    wound response, **1:** 6
  gene regulation targets
    cis-acting elements, **1:** 9
    inducible genes, **1:** 9
    trans-acting factors, **1:** 9
  mutant studies of biosynthetic and signaling genes, **1:** 5, 9
  occurrence, **1:** 1
  prospects for study, **1:** 10
  receptors, **1:** 6
  signal transduction
    calcium channels, **1:** 6
    cyclic nucleotides, **1:** 7
    farnesylation, **1:** 8
    G-proteins, **1:** 8
    inositol phosphates, **1:** 7
    phosphatidic acid, **1:** 7
    potassium channels, **1:** 6
    protein phosphorylation, **1:** 7–8
    proton channels, **1:** 6–7
    RNA cap-binding proteins, **1:** 8
    sphingosine-1-phosphate, **1:** 7
  structure, **1:** 1
  synthesis, **1:** 1–3
  synthetic analogs and applications, **1:** 9
  transport, **1:** 3
AC, *see* Adenylyl cyclase
ACE, *see* Angiotensin-converting enzyme

Acetylcholine
  hormone secretion regulation
    corticotropin-releasing hormone, **2:** 708
    gonadotropin-releasing hormone, **2:** 710
    growth hormone-releasing hormone, **2:** 708
    prolactin, **2:** 708
    thyroid-stimulating hormone, **2:** 710
  neurons, **2:** 706
  receptor mutations and disease, **2:** 655–656
  synthesis, **2:** 704
Acid sphingomyelinase, oocyte apoptosis role, **1:** 163
Acne vulgaris
  androgen roles, **3:** 205
  definition, **3:** 205
  treatment, **3:** 205
Acromegaly, growth hormone secretion defects, **2:** 212, 233
ACTH, *see* Adrenocorticotropic hormone
Actin
  F-actin, **3:** 608
  G-actin, **3:** 608
  vitamin D-binding protein scavenger activity, **3:** 606–607
Activating receptor mutation
  cell membrane receptors, **1:** 13
  classification, **1:** 11
  definition, **1:** 16
  nuclear receptors, **1:** 11–12
  types, **1:** 12
Activation tag mutant, production, **1:** 378
Activators of G-protein signaling (AGS)
  discovery, **2:** 270–271
  GoLoco domains, **2:** 271
  types, **2:** 271–272
Activin receptor
  definition, **1:** 22
  signal transduction
    FYVE domain proteins, **1:** 20–22
    inhibitors
      follistatin, **1:** 20, 24
      inhibin, **1:** 20, 24–25; **2:** 300–302
      Smads, **1:** 20–22, 24; **2:** 300
    termination, **1:** 20

    type I receptors
      domains, **1:** 19
      ligands, **1:** 20
      type II receptor dependence, **1:** 19–20, 24
    type II receptors
      domains, **1:** 18–19
      gene cloning and structure, **1:** 18–19
      knockout mouse, **1:** 19
      ligand specificity, **1:** 19
      types, **2:** 300
Activins
  assays, **1:** 26, 28
  biological activity, **1:** 24–25
  biosynthesis, **1:** 23
  definition, **1:** 22
  follicle-stimulating hormone regulation, **1:** 650–651
  inhibitors, *see* Follistatin; Inhibins
  knockout and transgenic mouse studies, **1:** 25–26
  male functions, **2:** 308–309
  paracrine effects within pituitary gland, **2:** 308
  roles
    bone resorption and formation, **1:** 28
    cancer, **1:** 28
    inflammation, **1:** 27
    pregnancy, **1:** 27
    renal regeneration after ischemic injury, **1:** 27, 28
    wound repair, **1:** 28
  subunits, **1:** 23–24; **2:** 298–300, 307
  transforming growth factor-β superfamily, **1:** 18, 23, 26–27
    overlapping functions, **1:** 26–27
Acute-phase reaction
  interleukin-1 role, **1:** 363; **2:** 411
  interleukin-6 modulation, **2:** 437
AD, *see* Alzheimer's disease
Adaptive immunity
  definition, **3:** 348
  overview, **1:** 326
Adaptor
  definition, **1:** 555
  epidermal growth factor receptor signaling, **1:** 551
Adenylyl cyclase (AC)
  activation, **1:** 476–477, 479